NANDA DIAGNOSES, 1995–1996

Activity intolerance
Activity intolerance, risk for
Adaptive capacity, decreased: intracranial
Adjustment, impaired
Airway clearance, ineffective
Anxiety
Aspiration, risk for
body image disturbance
Body temperature, altered, risk for
Bowel incontinence
Breastfeeding, effective
Breastfeeding, ineffective
Breastfeeding, Interrupted
Breathing pattern, ineffective
Cardiac output, decreased
Caregiver role strain
Caregiver role strain, risk for
Communication, impaired verbal
Community coping, ineffective
Community coping, potential for enhanced
Confusion, acute
Confusion, chronic
Constipation
Constipation, colonic
Constipation, perceived
Coping, defensive
Coping, family: potential for growth
Coping, ineffective family: compromised
Coping, ineffective family: disabling
Coping, ineffective individual
Decisional conflict (specify)
Denial, ineffective
Diarrhea
Disuse Syndrome, risk for
Diversional activity deficit
Dysreflexia
Energy field disturbance
Environmental interpretation syndrome, impaired
Family processes, altered: alcoholism
Family processes, altered
Fatigue
Fear
Fluid volume deficit
Fluid volume deficit, risk for

Fluid volume, excess
Gas exchange, impaired
Grieving, anticipatory
Grieving, dysfunctional
Growth and development, altered
Health maintenance, altered
Health-seeking behaviors (specify)
Home maintenance management, impaired
Hopelessness
Hyperhemia
Hypothermia
Incontinence, functional
Incontinence, reflex
Incontinence, stress
Incontinence, total
Incontinence, urge
Infant behavior, disorganized
Infant behavior, disorganized: risk for
Infant behavior, organized: potential for enhanced
Infant feeding pattern, ineffective
Infection, risk for
Injury, perioperative positioning: risk for
Injury, risk for
Knowledge deficit (specify)
Loneliness, risk for
Management of therapeutic regimen, community: ineffective
Management of therapeutic regimen, families: ineffective
Management of therapeutic regimen, individuals: effective
Management of therapeutic regimen, individuals: ineffective
Memory, impaired
Mobility, impaired physical
Noncompliance (specify)
Nutrition, altered: less than body requirements
Nutrition, altered: more than body requirements
Nutrition, altered: potential for more than body requirements
Oral mucous membrane, altered
Pain
Pain, chronic
Parent/infant/child attachment, risk for altered
Parental role conflict
Parenting, altered
Parenting, risk for altered

Peripheral neurovascular dysfunction, risk for
Personal identity disturbance
Poisoning, risk for
Post-trauma response
Powerlessness
Protection, altered
Rape-trauma syndrome
Rape-trauma syndrome: compound reaction
Rape-trauma syndrome: silent reaction
Relocation stress syndrome
Role performance, altered
Self-care deficit, bathing/hygiene
Self-care deficit, dressing/grooming
Self-care deficit, feeding
Self-care deficit, toileting
Self-esteem disturbance
Self-esteem, chronic low
Self-esteem, situational low
Self-mutilation, risk for
Sensory/perceptual alterations (specify) (visual, auditory, kinesthetic, gustatory, tactile, olfactory)
Sexual dysfunction
Sexuality patterns, altered
Skin integrity, impaired
Skin integrity, impaired, risk for
Sleep pattern disturbance
Social interaction, impaired
Social isolation
Spiritual distress (distress of the human spirit)
Spiritual well-being, potential for enhanced
Suffocation, risk for
Swallowing, impaired
Thermoregulation, ineffective
Thought processes, altered
Tissue integrity, impaired
Tissue perfusion, altered (specify type) (renal, cerebral, cardiopulmonary, gastrointestinal, peripheral)
Trauma, risk for
Unilateral neglect
Urinary elimination, altered
Urinary retention
Ventilation, inability to sustain spontaneous
Ventilatory weaning process, dysfunctional
Violence, risk for: self-directed or directed at others

From NANDA Nursing Diagnosis Definitions and Classification 1995-1996; North Americn Nursing Diagnosis Association, Philadelphia, 1994.

PSYCHIATRIC MENTAL HEALTH NURSING

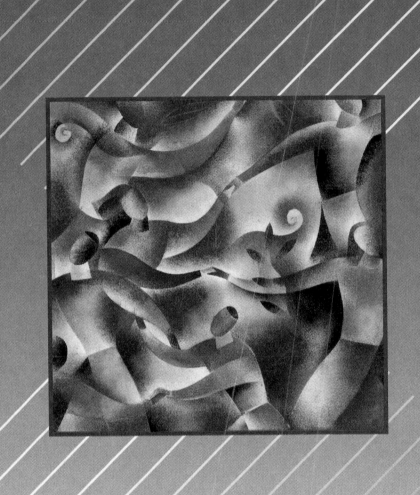

PSYCHIATRIC-MENTAL HEALTH NURSING

Katherine M. Fortinash, MSN, RNCS

Certified Clinical Specialist, Adult Psychiatric-Mental Health Nursing
Clinical Nurse Specialist and Clinical Educator
Sharp Behavioral Health Services
Sharp HealthCare
San Diego, California

Patricia A. Holoday-Worret, MSN, RN, CS

Certified Clinical Specialist, Adult Psychiatric-Mental Health Nursing
Associate Professor, Psychiatric-Mental Health Nursing
Department of Nursing
Palomar College
San Marcos, California
Instructor, Statewide Nursing Program
California State University-Dominguez Hills
Carson, California

with 120 full-color illustrations

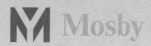 Mosby

St. Louis   Baltimore   Boston   Carlsbad   Chicago   Naples   New York   Philadelphia   Portland
London   Madrid   Mexico City   Singapore   Sydney   Tokyo   Toronto   Wiesbaden

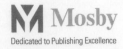

Dedicated to Publishing Excellence

A Times Mirror
Company

Publisher: Nancy L. Coon
Editor: Jeff Burnham
Associate Developmental Editor: Linda Caldwell
Project Manager: Mark Spann
Senior Production Editor: Jerry Schwartz
Designer: Dave Zielinski
Manufacturing Supervisor: Betty Richmond
Cover Art: Linda Frichtel
Editorial Assistant: Rae Robertson
Editorial Intern: Natalie Gehl

A Note to the Reader:

The author and publisher have made every attempt to check dosages and nursing content for accuracy. Because the science of pharmacology is continually advancing, our knowledge base continues to expand. Therefore we recommend that the reader always check product information for changes in dosage or administration before administering any medication. This is particularly important with new or rarely used drugs.

Printed in the United States of America
Project management, composition and prepress by GTS Graphics, Inc.
Printing/binding by Von Hoffman

Mosby–Year Book, Inc.
11830 Westline Industrial Drive
St. Louis, Missouri 63146

Library of Congress Cataloging-in-Publication Data
Psychiatric-mental health nursing / [edited by] Katherine M.
    Fortinash, Patricia A. Holoday-Worret.—1st ed.
            p.   cm.
        Includes bibliographical references and index.
        ISBN 0-8151-3348-0
        1. Psychiatric nursing.   I. Fortinash, Katherine M.   II. Holoday
    -Worret, Patricia A.
        [DNLM: 1. Psychiatric Nursing.   2. Mental Disorders—nursing.   WY
    160 P972035   1996]
    RC440.P7338   1996
    610.73′68—dc20
    DNLM/DLC
    for Library of Congress   95-39307
                                                                          CIP

96 97 98 99 00 / 9 8 7 6 5 4 3 2 1

CONTRIBUTORS

Donna C. Aguilera, PhD, FAAN, MFC, FIAEP

Consultant in Private Practice
Beverly Hills and Sherman Oaks, California
Chapter 21, Crisis Intervention

Merry A. Armstrong, DNSc, RN, CNS

Assistant Professor of Nursing
Intercollegiate Center for Nursing Education
Washington State University, Eastern Washington
    University, and Whitworth College
Spokane, Washington
Chapter 20, Adjustment Disorders

Mary Ann Barbee, RN, MS

Executive Director of Clinical Services
Cedar Springs Psychiatric Hospital
Colorado Springs, Colorado
Chapter 26, Suicide

Margaret T. Barker, RN, MSW, LCSW

Psychiatric Social Worker
Grossmont Hospital Behavioral Health Services
Sharp HealthCare
Private Practice
La Mesa, California
Chapter 9, The Adult

Marjorie F. Bendik, RN, DNSc

Associate Coordinator, San Diego Area
Statewide Nursing Program
California State University-Dominguez Hills
Carson, California
Chapter 13, The Schizophrenias

Pamela Bricker, MSN

Private Practice
Colorado Springs, Colorado
Chapter 26, Suicide

Gloria B. Callwood, PhD, RN

Associate Professor of Nursing
University of the Virgin Islands
St. Thomas, U.S. Virgin Islands
Chapter 5, Theoretical Perspectives

Anne Clarkin-Watts, MSW, LCSW

Private Practice
San Diego, California
Chapter 18, Eating Disorders

Katherine M. Fortinash, MSN, RNCS

Clinical Nurse Specialist and Clinical Educator
Sharp Hospital Behavioral Health Services
Sharp HealthCare
San Diego, California
Instructor, Statewide Nursing Program
California State University-Dominguez Hills
Carson, California
Chapter 6, The Nursing Process

†George G. Glenner, MD, FCAP

Rescarch Pathologist
School of Medicine
University of California at San Diego
Medical Director
The George G. Glenner Alzheimer's Family Centers, Inc.
San Diego, California
*Chapter 16, Delirium, Dementia, and Amnestic and
    Other Cognitive Disorders*

Ruth N. Grendell, DNSc, RN

Professor of Nursing and Assistant Chair
Department of Nursing
Point Loma Nazarene College
San Diego, California
Chapter 29, Psychologic Aspects of Physiologic Illness

†Deceased

Bonnie Hagerty, RN, PhD, CS

University of Michigan
Ann Arbor, Michigan
Chapter 12, Mood Disorders: Depression and Mania

Linda M. Hollinger-Smith, PhD, RN

Associate Chairperson and Associate Professor
Rush-Presbyterian-St. Luke's Medical Center
College of Nursing
Rush University
Chicago, Illinois
Chapter 10, The Elderly

Patricia A. Holoday-Worret, MSN, RN, CS

Associate Professor, Psychiatric-Mental Health Nursing
Department of Nursing
Palomar College
San Marcos, California
Instructor, Statewide Nursing Program
California State University-Dominguez Hills
Carson, California
Chapter 1, Foundations of Psychiatric Nursing
Chapter 2, Student Issues Regarding Client and
*   Environment*

Charles Kemp, RN, MS

Lecturer
School of Nursing
Baylor University
Dallas, Texas
Chapter 27, Grief and Loss

Joyce K. Laben, RN, MSN, JD, FAAN

School of Nursing
Vanderbilt University
Nashville, Tennesssee
Chapter 3, Legal-Ethical Issues

Richard C. Lucas, MD, JD

Supervising Psychiatrist
San Diego County Mental Health Services, Child, Youth,
   and Family Services
Assistant Clinical Professor of Psychiatry
University of California at San Diego
San Diego, California
Chapter 17, Disorders of Childhood and Adolescence

Shelly F. Lurie, MS, RN, CS

Associate Director of Nursing
Clifton T. Perkins Hospital Center
Jessup, Maryland
Faculty Associate, School of Nursing
Johns Hopkins University
Nurse Psychotherapist, Private Practice
Baltimore, Maryland
Chapter 19, Sexual Disorders

Gay Mallon-Frank, MA, CBT

Certified Bioenergetic Therapist
Dallas, Texas
Chapter 27, Grief and Loss

Pamela E. Marcus, RN, MSCS-P

Nurse Psychotherapist, Private Practice
Upper Marlboro, Maryland
Chapter 14, Personality Disorders

Margaret McDonald, RN, MS

Doctoral Student
School of Nursing
University of Maryland
Baltimore, Maryland
Chapter 31, Community Mental Health and Home
*   Care*

Susan Fertig McDonald, MSN, RN, CS

Operations Coordinator
Behavioral Health Services, Sharp Cabrillo Hospital
Sharp HealthCare
San Diego, California
Chapter 7, Principles of Communication

Monica Ann Molloy, MSN, RN, CS

Clinical Nurse Specialist for Research
Division of Psychiatric Nursing
Department of Psychiatry and Behavioral Sciences
Medical University of South Carolina
Charleston, South Carolina
Chapter 11, Anxiety and Related Disorders

Diane Podsedly Oran, MN, RN, CS

Clinical Manager, Behavioral Medicine
Midcoast Hospital
Brunswick, Maine
Chapter 8, Children and Adolescents

Vincent R. Pieranunzi, MSN, PhD, RN

Associate Professor
Department of Nursing
Point Loma Nazarene College
San Diego, California
Chapter 4, Cultural Issues
Chapter 17, Disorders of Childhood and Adolescence

Barbara Redding, RN, EdD

Associate Professor
College of Nursing
University of South Florida
Tampa, Florida
Chapter 15, Substance-Related Disorders

Nan Rich, RN, CS, PMHNP, PhD(c)

Psychiatric Mental Health Nurse Practitioner
Josephine County Mental Health Department
Grants Pass, Oregon
Instructor, Psychiatric-Mental Health Nursing
Oregon Health Sciences University
Portland, Oregon
Nursing Care in the Community

Ona Z. Riggin, EdD, RN

Professor and Chair
Psychiatric-Mental Health Nursing Graduate Program
College of Nursing
University of South Florida
Tampa, Florida
Chapter 15, Substance-Related Disorders

Patricia F. Schmidt, RN, EdD

Associate Professor and Interim Dean
Nursing Education Department
Palomar College
San Marcos, California
Psychobiology Research

Alwilda Scholler-Jaquish, RN, MN, MS, CS-P

Instructor
Department of Psychiatric and Community Health Nursing
University of Maryland
Baltimore, Maryland
Chapter 30, Persons with Chronic Mental Illness

Jay D. Sherr, PharmD

Clinical Assistant Professor
School of Pharmacy
Research Assistant Professor
Maryland Psychiatric Research Center
School of Medicine
University of Maryland at Baltimore
Chapter 23, Psychopharmacology and Other Biologic Therapies
Drug Cards

Bonnie Neil Spangler, RN, MS

Clinical Supervisor, Psychiatric Program
Sharp Home Health and Hospice
San Diego, California
Chapter 31, Community Mental Health and Home Care

Rachel E. Spector, PhD, RN, CTN, FAAN

Associate Professor
School of Nursing
Boston College
Chestnut Hill, Massachusetts
Chapter 4, Cultural Issues

Geraldine I. Strachan, RN, MSNEd

Nursing Education Supervisor
School of Dementia Care
The George G. Glenner Alzheimer's Family Centers, Inc.
San Diego, California
Chapter 16, Delirium, Dementia, and Amnestic and Other Cognitive Disorders

Judith A. Strasser, RN, DNSc

Associate Professor of Community Health Nursing
University of Maryland
Baltimore, Maryland
Chapter 31, Community Mental Health and Home Care

Kathryn Thomas, PhD, RN, CS-P

Assistant Professor
Union Memorial Hospital
Associate Director
The Hancial Institute for the Study, Prevention and Treatment of Sexual Trauma
Baltimore, Maryland
Chapter 19, Sexual Disorders

Joan C. Urbancic, PhD, RN, CS

Associate Professor of Nursing
University of Detroit, Mercy
Detroit, Michigan
Chapter 25, Survivors of Violence

Gwen van Servellen, RN, PhD, FAAN

Professor
School of Nursing
University of California, Los Angeles
Los Angeles, California
Chapter 28, Persons with AIDS

Mary Magenheimer Webster, MS, CS

Psychiatric Nurse Liaison
Grossmont Hospital Behavioral Health Services
Sharp HealthCare
La Mesa, California
Chapter 5, Theoretical Perspectives
*Chapter 22, Interactive Therapies and Methods of
    Implementation*

William R. Whetstone, PhD

Associate Professor
Assistant Chair/Undergraduate Coordinator
Statewide Nursing Program
California State University-Dominguez Hills
Carson, California
Nursing Care in the Community

Theresa Williams, MA, MFCC, ATR

Art Therapist and Marriage/Family/Child Counselor
Private Practice
San Diego, California
Chapter 24, Adjunct Therapies

REVIEWERS

Deanah Alexander, MSN, RN, CS
Instructor
West Texas A&M University
Canyon, Texas

Charla Mae Andrews, RNC, MS
Instructor
Spokane Community College
Staff Nurse
Sacred Heart Medical Center
Spokane, Washington

Claudette A. Bachand, MSN
Professor
Bristol Community College
Fall River, Massachusetts

Marjorie Baier, RN, PhDc
Associate Professor
Jewish Hospital College of Nursing
St. Louis, Missouri

Loretta M. Birckhead, EdD, RN
Professor
Department of Nursing
California State University
Los Angeles, California

Linda K. Blazer, MEd, MS, RN
Instructor of Psychiatric/Mental Health Nursing
Lancaster General Hospital School of Nursing
Lancaster, Pennsylvania

Sheila Bollinger, RN, MSN, EdD, CNS
Instructor of Nursing
Houston Community College
Houston, Texas

Gina Bufe, RN, CS, PhD(c)
Psychiatric Clinical Nurse Specialist
Psychiatric Services
Barnes Hospital
St. Louis, Missouri

Teresa Burckhalter, MSN, RN, C
Nursing Faculty, ADN Program
Technical College of the Lowcountry
Beaufort, South Carolina

Patricia A. Chin, RN, DNSc
Assistant Professor
Department of Nursing
California State University
Los Angeles, California

Lou Ann Cook, RN, EdD
Professor
Department of Nursing Education
San Antonio College
San Antonio, Texas

Regina Cundall
Instructor
School of Nursing
Lutheran Medical Center
St. Louis, Missouri

Patricia R. Dean, RN, MSN, CCDN
Associate Professor
School of Nursing
Florida State University
Tallahassee, Florida

Mary Alice Dedinsky, MSN, PhD, RN, NCC
Nurse Educator
Milwaukee Area Technical College
Milwaukee, Wisconsin

Susan Dewey-Hammer, RN, MN
Associate Professor
Suffolk County Community College
Selden, New York

Ellarene Duis-Nittsche, MSN, RN, CNNA
College Station, Texas

Tim Engelhardt, B.Sc.Pharm
Manager-Operations
Pharmacy Department
Rockyview General Hospital
Calgary, Alberta

Thomas Forsell, Pharm.D.
Associate Professor of Clinical Pharmacy
College of Pharmacy
Xavier University of Louisiana
New Orleans, Louisiana

Elaine Gallien, RN, MSN, CS

Assistant Professor
Capstone College of Nursing
University of Alabama
Tuscaloosa, Alabama

Rauda Gelazis, PhD, RN

Associate Professor
Ursuline College
Pepper Pike, Ohio

Karen S. Gingrow, PhD, RN

Professor
College of Nursing
Valdosta State University
Valdosta, Georgia

Nancy Green, RN, MSN

Professor of Nursing
Victor Valley College
Victorville, California

Nancy J. Grover, MSN, CS

Associate Professor and Undergraduate Nursing Chair
Husson College/Eastern Maine Medical Center
Bangor, Maine

Rebecca Crews Gruener, MSN, RN

Associate Professor of Nursing
Louisiana State University at Alexandria
Alexandria, Louisiana

Sandra Halsey, MSN, RN

Associate Professor of Nursing
Sinclair Community College
Dayton, Ohio

Renee Harrison, RN, BSN, MS

Assistant Professor of Nursing
Tulsa Junior College
Tulsa, Oklahoma

Rhonda K. Hollis, PhD, RN, CS

Assistant Professor
Columbus College
Columbus, Georgia

Nelda Jeane, RNC, MSN

Associate Professor of Nursing
Louisiana State University
Alexandria, Louisiana

Barbara Ann Johnston, PhD, RN

Assistant Dean for Continuing Education
Intercollegiate Center for Nursing Education
Spokane, Washington

Doris Jones

Assistant Professor
Creighton University
Omaha, Nebraska

Alice Kempe, RN, BSN, MEd, MSN, PHc

Associate Professor
Ursuline College
Pepper Pike, Ohio

Mary Kunes-Connell, PhD, RN

Assistant Professor
Coordinator, Psychiatric Nursing
Creighton University
Omaha, Nebraska

Joanne Lavin, RN, EdD

Associate Professor
Kingsborough Community College of CUNY
Brooklyn, New York

Barbara J. Limandri, DNSc, RN, CS

Associate Professor
Oregon Health Sciences University
Portland, Oregan

Linda Nance Marks, RN, EdD

Associate Professor
Director of Learning Resources Center
University of Texas at Arlington
Arlington, Texas

Floreine Garvin Marshall

Instructor
Jewish Hospital of Nursing
St. Louis, Missouri

Eleanor Morad, EdD

Associate Professor
Bristol Community College
Fall River, Massachusetts

Rosemarie Nedeau-Cayo, RN, MSN

Director and Instructor
School of Nursing
Bronson Methodist Hospital
Kalamazoo, Michigan

Modesta Soberano Orque, RN, MPH, EdD, JD

Attorney at Law
Nurse Consultant
San Francisco, California

Michael J. Rice, RN, BSN, MSN, PhD

Assistant Professor
Intercollegiate Center for Nursing Education
Spokane, Washington

Mary W. Riley, MSN

Instructor, Psychiatric Nursing
St. Louis Community College at Meramec
St. Louis, Missouri

Mary J. Roehrig, RN, MSN, MA, LPC

Associate Professor of Nursing
Ferris State University
Big Rapids, Michigan

William Shannon Rubush, RN, BSN

Nursing Instructor
Forsyth Technical Community College
Winston-Salem, North Carolina

Cynthia A. Russell, DNSc, RN

Associate Professor
Valparaiso University
Valparaiso, Indiana

Mary Alice Saunders, MEd, MSN

Assistant Professor of Nursing
Ursuline College
Pepper Pike, Ohio

Linda S. Smith, RN, MSN

Nurse Educator
Gateway Technical College
Kenosha, Wisconsin

Marcy J.T. Smith, RN, MSN

Professor
Department of Nursing
Cape Cod Community College
West Barnstable, Massachusetts

Stephanie Stockard Spelic, RN, MSN, CS, CPC

Assistant Professor
Creighton University
Omaha, Nebraska

Susan Speraw, RN, PhD

Director, Division of Pediatric Psychology
T.C. Thompson Children's Hospital
Chattanooga, Tennessee

Barbara Stafford, RN, MSN

Assistant Professor
New Mexico State University
Carlsbad, New Mexico

Mary Steinhoff, MSN

Nurse Program Specialist
Adolescent Psychiatry
Barnes Hospital
St. Louis, Missouri

Joanne S. Stevenson, PhD, RN, FAAN

Professor
The Ohio State University
Department of Adult Health and Illness Nursing
Columbus, Ohio

Sue G. Thacker, RN, AS, BSN, MS

Associate Professor in Nursing
Wytheville Community College
Wytheville, Virginia

Anita L. Throwe, MS, BSN, CS

Associate Professor
Medical University of South Carolina
Satellite Program at Francis Marion University
Florence, South Carolina

Anna M. Tichy, BS, MS, PhD, RN

Professor
Department of Administrative Studies
College of Nursing
University of Illinois at Chicago
Chicago, Illinois

Linda G. Trabucco, BSN, JD

Partner
Kelly, McLaughlin & Foster, PC
Philadelphia, Pennsylvania

Stephanie Valdes, RN, MS

Associate Professor
Black Hawk College
Moline, Illinois

Marianne E. Weiss, RN, BSN, MEd, MS

Instructor
Hocking College
Nelsonville, Ohio

Barbara Wejman, RN, BSN, MN

Instructor in Nursing
St. Francis Hospital School of Nursing
Evanston, Illinois

Mona L. White, RN, MSN, CNS

Assistant Professor
Delta College
University Center, Michigan

Donna Marie Wing, RN, CDNS, EdD

Associate Professor
University of Tulsa
Tulsa, Oklahoma

Jean H. Woods, RNCS, PhD

Professor
Department of Nursing
Temple University College of Allied Health Professions
Philadelphia, Pennsylvania

Lee Anne Xippolitos, RN, MS, CARN, NPP, CS

Clinical Assistant Professor
SUNY at Stony Brook
Stony Brook, New York

PREFACE

Psychiatric-mental health nursing is experiencing extraordinary changes that provide challenge, excitement, and wonder for new nurses as well as seasoned practitioners. Expanding research and discovery in the area of psychobiology, the continuing shift of care to community settings, health care reform, managed care, the evolution of the information superhighway, and increasing societal demands and psychosocial stressors are the most significant of these changes. The scope of psychiatric-mental health nursing has expanded dramatically over the past forty years, and change will continue to be its constant companion. These challenges need to be analyzed and addressed in a proactive manner, as they influence nurses and clients in innumerable ways.

The past decade, which produced this explosion of information in the psychobiological sciences, presented psychiatric nurses with the responsibility of integrating biological bases of knowledge into education, practice, and research. Congress has declared the 1990s the "Decade of the Brain," indicating that research, diagnostic technology, and treatment modalities have greatly expanded in the direction of psychobiology. The implication for psychiatric nursing is that these findings must be incorporated into all areas of the specialty. This is particularly true for psychopharmacology, "to ensure safe and effective care of people with mental illness and the advancement of the specialty" (ANA, 1994).

Revolutionary changes in the entire health care industry over the past few years have strongly affected the care of individuals who require treatment through the mental health care delivery system. In the past, people who required intervention for acute psychiatric problems were admitted to an inpatient, acute care psychiatric facility for observation, assessment, and treatment. If the problems were resolved within expectations, the person was discharged to an appropriate level of care and perhaps continued with outpatient treatment, medication therapy, and sometimes rehabilitative or educational services. Now, inpatient hospitalization is often replaced with alternative care options in community settings. Inpatient psychiatric care continues to be available for people whose illness demands it, although the typical lengths of stay in acute care have been dramatically reduced.

APPROACH AND INTENDED USE

Although this first edition of *Psychiatric-Mental Health Nursing* strongly addresses the biological revolution as well as new concepts in health care delivery, the clients' psychosocial needs and the behavior of nurses and associated professionals to attain, maintain, and promote the clients' integrity related to those needs, remain the principal focus of this text.

The text provides a balanced nursing and medical approach with strong coverage of DSM-IV and related treatments. It is not tied to any specific nursing framework, although psychiatric nursing is thoroughly discussed in relation to various well-respected theorists.

This revolutionary, state-of-the-art text is primarily intended to help students and practicing psychiatric nurses deliver professional nursing care for clients and their families, regardless of time, place, or circumstances.

The nursing process, a time-proven, six-step problem-solving method is featured as a distinct section in relevant chapters. Interesting case studies depicting "real-life" situations followed by a series of questions are interspersed throughout the various stages of the nursing process section to stimulate student learning and critical thinking skills. This section also includes comprehensive nursing care plans that begin with a case study, followed by relevant DSM-IV and NANDA diagnoses. Client outcomes are identified, interventions with rationales are presented, and an evaluative statement is provided.

The major organizing structures for the disorders chapters include both the diagnoses of the North American Nursing Diagnosis Association (NANDA, 1994) and the American Psychiatric Association *Diagnostic and Statistical Manual of Mental Disorders,* Fourth Edition (DSM-IV, 1994). We strongly believe in the practicality and effectiveness of the collaborative efforts of nursing and medicine whenever possible. We contend that the use of current NANDA terminology most accurately describes the therapeutic services and contributions of nurses, and also reflects contemporary nursing actions and responses. Application and use of refined diagnostic labels are essential to the evolution of the language and discipline of nursing.

STRUCTURE AND ORGANIZATION

Part One, Introduction to Psychiatric-Mental Health Nursing, presents concepts and issues fundamental to psychiatric-mental health nursing. The reader is introduced to concepts that not only define nursing as an art and a science, but also reveal the substantive changes and trends that currently shape and challenge traditional professional nursing roles in the area of mental health. Typical student issues, dilemmas, and concerns, specific to the role of psychiatric nursing, are uniquely presented in the form of clinical *challenges* and *solutions*. This information will be very helpful for students as they enter and interact in the psychiatric setting. Legal and ethical issues specific to clients with mental disorders are described. Patients' rights related to mental illness are carefully defined, while citing relevant case law. Cultural issues are discussed, offering a cross-section of the various cultures. Explanation of how cultural beliefs affect clients' attitudes toward health care and care giving practices is provided, with emphasis on mental health and mental disorders. Theoretical perspectives, including psychotherapeutic and biological components, that provide the framework for mental and emotional disorders are discussed. Clear, concise examples of each therapeutic modality are presented as well as vivid and precise **full-color** illustrations of biological effects on brain chemistry.

Part Two, Dynamics of Nursing Practice, discusses the two essential components of the nursing role. The chapter on the nursing process presents the foundations of critical thinking, intuitive skills, and problem-solving approaches used by nurses as they practice their discipline in a variety of clinical and community settings. Several helpful assessment and interview tools are featured, including a treatment plan, a standardized care plan, and a clinical pathway. Each phase of the nursing process is carefully explained, with examples provided. The second chapter of this unit discusses the most valuable tool of the psychiatric nurse—that of communication—with emphasis on the essential components of the therapeutic nurse-client relationship.

Part Three, Developmental Aspects Across the Life Span, analyzes the stages of growth and development in separate chapters about childhood and adolescence, adulthood, and the elderly. Critical tasks that need to be met or mastered in order for clients to move forward developmentally are discussed from a variety of theoretical perspectives.

Part Four, Mental/Emotional Disorders, focuses on ten major disorders generated by DSM-IV criteria. Each disorder is presented in terms of a brief description, history, etiology, epidemiology, and prognosis. The nursing process is presented as a separate section at the end of each chapter, with discussion of each nursing process step. A detailed nursing care plan is presented in this section, beginning with a case study, followed by DSM-IV multiaxial diagnoses and relevant nursing diagnoses. Client outcomes are identified based on the nursing diagnosis statement, interventions and their rationales are presented, and an evaluation is noted. Collaboration between nursing and medicine is evident throughout the nursing process section, most notably in columns depicting a side-by-side listing of DSM-IV and NANDA diagnoses and in the multiaxial diagnostic segments preceding the nursing care plans.

Part Five, Therapeutic Modalities, emphasizes the four major therapeutic modalities used to treat clients in the psychiatric setting. Crisis intervention is discussed, tracing the historical development of this modality and describing its major components. The chapter on interactive therapies presents discussion of the different theoretical concepts in the form of practical examples and scenarios typically found in a mental health facility. The discussion of psychopharmacology offers a thorough description of medications typically used to treat mental illness, as well as their therapeutic and nontherapeutic effects, usual dosages, nursing implications, and other valuable information. Thirty-nine perforated, detachable drug cards in the back of the book accompany this chapter for the learner's convenience. A unique separate chapter is devoted to adjunct therapies, such as occupational, recreational, art, music, and dance therapies, emphasizing the text's interdisciplinary focus. Special consideration is given to the nurse's role in each therapeutic task, function, or activity.

Part Six, Nursing Implications for Contemporary Issues, describes a variety of timely issues and concerns experienced by clients in different settings and treated by psychiatric nurses. Such important topics as surviving violence, grief and loss, AIDS, psychological aspects of physiological illness, and chronic mental illness are discussed in this unit. The text concludes with an in-depth discussion of the shift of care to the community and home settings.

DESIGN AND KEY FEATURES

Bright and vivid **full-color** design is used throughout this text to promote visual appeal, emphasize and distinguish key pedagogical features, and graphically portray illustrations of important psychiatric nursing concepts for today's students. Numerous **full-color** brain scans and drawings of psychobiological concepts are presented in relevant chapters. Many boxes, tables, and other figures summarize and highlight important information.

Each chapter has several standard features that make important information more accessible:

- *Learning Objectives,* placed at the beginning of the chapter, emphasize the most important concepts.
- The *Chapter Outline* presents the major topical headings.
- *Key Terms* with definitions are presented at the beginning of the chapter and are highlighted throughout the chapter in bold.
- A *Summary of Key Concepts* concludes each chapter, summarizing the most significant ideas to be remembered.

Other important key features are highlighted by a unique design. The location of these features is detailed in a handy feature locator on the inside back cover of the book.

A detailed *Nursing Care Plan* is presented as part of the nursing process section. It begins with a case study, followed by DSM-IV multiaxial diagnoses and relevant nursing diagnoses. Client outcomes based on the nursing diagnosis statements are identified, interventions with rationales are presented, and an evaluative statement concludes the care plan.

Case Study with Critical Thinking Questions integrates critical thinking questions following realistic case studies to foster students' problem solving skills and application of the concepts presented.

Nursing Care in the Community boxes discuss community perspectives on particular disorders and issues.

Clinical Alerts interspersed throughout the text highlight critical information relevant to clinical practice.

DSM-IV Criteria boxes present the DSM-IV criteria for particular disorders.

Collaborative Diagnoses boxes present DSM-IV and NANDA diagnoses relevant for a certain disorder.

Client and Family Teaching Guidelines provide education for both the client and the family on various concerns for a particular disorder.

Clinical Symptoms boxes summarize the symptoms that indicate a certain disorder.

Additional Treatment Modalities boxes summarize various modalities and interventions that are used in conjunction with nursing interventions in the treatment of a particular disorder.

Understanding and Applying Research boxes summarize a research study related to a disorder and its application to nursing interventions.

Nursing Assessment Questions boxes present questions that should be included in the assessment of a particular disorder.

Thirty-nine perforated *Drug Cards* containing essential information about the most common and important psychiatric medications are in the back of the book. These cards can be torn out and easily used for reference in clinical settings.

Five *Clinical Pathways,* for various disorders and from different institutions, are presented in both Chapter 6 and Appendix D to demonstrate the importance and usefulness of this interdisciplinary tool in the treatment of mental disorders.

A *Glossary* in the back provides concise definitions of the key terms found in the book.

Complete listings of *NANDA diagnoses* (1995–1996) and *DSM-IV diagnoses* are in Appendixes A and B.

A *listing of mental health organizations* is provided in Appendix C, as a resource for further information about mental disorders and other mental health issues.

TEACHING-LEARNING PACKAGE

A complete ancillary package to enhance teaching and learning is provided for this text.

Instructor's Resource Manual and Test Bank

The Instructor's Resource Manual and Test Bank to accompany *Psychiatric-Mental Health Nursing* includes many features that will supplement and enhance teaching and learning from the textbook. Critical thinking questions, enrichment activities, and multimedia resources are provided for each text chapter. Strategies for teaching psychiatric nursing and suggested course outlines for courses of varying lengths are presented. Student worksheets for each chapter are included. The test bank has 700 questions in NCLEX format and provides the applicable nursing process step, cognitive level of each question, and answer rationale.

Mosby's Psychiatric Nursing Transparency Acetates, second edition

The second edition of Mosby's *Psychiatric Nursing Transparency Acetates* contains 48 two-color and **full-color** transparencies covering many topics in psychiatric nursing. These transparencies provide a visual learning experience to reinforce knowledge and understanding.

Computerized Test Bank

The computerized version of the Test Bank is available in IBM and Macintosh versions. It comes with an instruction manual and allows users to edit, add, delete, or select questions on the computer.

TERMINOLOGY AND LANGUAGE

We have made every effort to remove evidence of sexism from this text. Whenever possible, we have attempted to use plural nouns and pronouns in place of the singular *his* or *her.* We recognize the contribution of both men and women to the nursing profession. However, clarity sometimes has dictated the use of *she* for nurse and *he* for client.

We have chosen to use the term *client* instead of *patient* because we view individuals receiving treatment as significant participants in the reciprocal process of treatment. We also recognize that *family* can refer not only to blood relatives, but friends and significant others. However, the term *family* is generally used for simplicity.

ACKNOWLEDGMENTS

We would like to thank the following individuals who provided valuable assistance to us in so many ways.

- Elizabeth Campbell Trottier, OTR, Clinical Supervisor, Therapies, Sharp Behavioral Health Services, San Diego, California, for writing the behavioral theory section of Chapter 5, Theoretical Perspectives.

- Cindy Peternelj-Taylor, RN, BScN, MSc, College of Nursing, University of Saskatchewan, Saskatoon, Saskatchewan, Canada, for writing Nursing Care in the Community in Chapter 31, Community Mental Health and Home Care.

- Marie DeBenedictis, MOT, OTR, Lead Therapies, Grossmont Hospital Behavioral Health Services, Sharp HealthCare, La Mesa, California for her assistance with Chapter 24, Adjunct Therapies.

- Joy Glenner, CEO/President, Jean Stehman, MA, ACC, and Margrit Goodrich, RN, PhD, of the George G. Glenner Alzheimer's Family Centers, San Diego, California, and Jim Strachan, for their assistance with Chapter 16, Delirium, Dementia, and Amnestic and Other Cognitive Disorders.

- Kathy Sweet, LPT, for her library research for several chapters.

- Donna Berger, RN, MN, Director of Operations, Sharp Behavioral Health Services; David Fleming, LCSW, Operations Coordinator, Therapies Inpatient Services; Roseann Giordano, RN, BSN, Operations Coordinator, Grossmont Behavioral Health Services; Richard Jiminez, MD, Medical Director, Older Adult Program, Sharp Cabrillo Hospital; and Susan McDonald, RN, MSN, Operations Coordinator, Sharp Cabrillo Hospi-

tal, all of Sharp HealthCare, San Diego and La Mesa, California, for their assistance with the development of the clinical pathway presented in Chapter 6, The Nursing Process.

We want to thank Jeff Burnham, Editor; Linda Caldwell, Associate Developmental Editor; Jerry Schwartz, Senior Production Editor; Mark Spann, Project Manager; and all those at Mosby who helped with this challenging project.

We would like to pay special tribute to Dr. George G. Glenner, co-contributor for Chapter 16, Delirium, Dementia, and Amnestic and Other Cognitive Disorders. Dr. Glenner passed away on July 14, 1995. His landmark research and findings on Alzheimer's disease have provided the basis for much of the research currently being done on this disorder. Dr. Glenner's work provides a legacy for the research to continue, and hopefully will culminate in, as was Dr. Glenner's fervent wish, "a real cure for Alzheimer's disease."

We are proud of this state-of-the-art textbook and invite psychiatric nursing students and nurses at all levels to meet the challenges presented and to apply the concepts in clinical practice. In the midst of the changes and dynamic forces influencing health care and health care delivery, the time-honored role of psychiatric nursing holds steady in the eye of the storm. It is our hope that the content presented in this textbook will serve as an anchor amid the sea of change. We wish you well in your professional journey and feel confident that you will successfully meet these challenges while experiencing the joy and excitement of psychiatric nursing.

Kathi Fortinash
Pat Holoday-Worret

SYMBOLS

A note about the artwork in symbolic form.

Symbols have always been, and continue to be, an integral part of our lives. Primitive humans began to record their history, fears, hopes, dreams, and basic rules by marking symbols on cave walls, rock formations, and trees. The symbols were meant to convey intended messages, but the events, and the markings that represented them, were sometimes interpreted as mystical when not completely understood by other people. The symbols often became powerful tools for uniting, organizing, governing, and teaching groups of people, and contributed to the development of cultures.

Symbols remain powerful objects in contemporary societies, in such widely varying areas as communication, religion, medicine, weather, international travel, music, engineering, mathematics, chemistry, Braille, and computer science. For example, there is no denying the impact on those who have been influenced by such symbols as the country flag, a cross, a six-point star, a coat of arms, or a swastika! A single symbol can convey many meanings and greatly affect thoughts, emotions, and behaviors. Our alphabet, a set of twenty-six symbols originating in the Near East, was transmitted by the Greeks and evolved into the system we use today. When these individual symbols, with their diverse backgrounds, are purposefully and thoughtfully joined together, they influence us and our history in innumerable ways.

We have selected only a few of the world's countless symbols to represent meanings that may be associated with the six parts of the text. Some are ancient, and some modern. Several complex meanings are often conveyed by a singular symbol. We hope that readers will be positively influenced by the symbolic images, and by the purposeful and thoughtful joining of the alphabet throughout these chapters.

BRIEF CONTENTS

CONTENTS

Introduction to Psychiatric-Mental Health Nursing

Ntesie

ASHANTI, WEST AFRICA

This symbol, signifying wisdom, knowledge, and prudence, is derived from the Ashanti people of Ghana, West Africa. A literal translation of the symbol is, "What I hear, I keep . . . I consider and keep what I learn." The Ashanti often stamp cloth with many symbols in graphic patterns that represent and convey their ideals, proverbs, history, and beliefs.

This symbol is a fitting representation for the chapters in Part One of this text, which impart fundamental concepts of psychiatric nursing for the readers to "learn and keep" throughout their endeavors in this field.

CHAPTER 1

Foundations of Psychiatric-Mental Health Nursing

Patricia A. Holoday-Worret

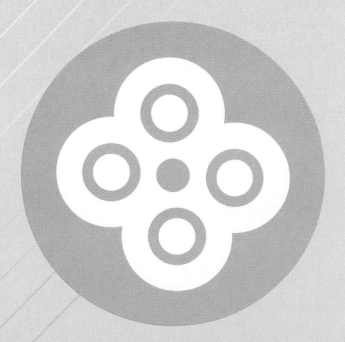

Autodiagnosis Examination of one's own thoughts, feelings, perceptions, and attitudes about a particular client.

Ego defenses Automatic psychological processes that keep the threat of internal and external stressors and dangers out of awareness and protect the person. Also known as defense mechanisms or mental mechanisms.

Epigenesis Developmental concept developed by Erikson that genetics and environmental experiences, which begin with conception and continue throughout life, determine the person's personality and the mentally healthy or destructive responses to the world.

Euthymia A state of mental tranquility; joyful feelings.

Incidence The frequency of occurrences of a specific disorder within a designated period (number of new cases).

Objectivity Remaining free from bias, prejudice, and personal identification in an interaction with another person and being able to process information based on facts.

Prevalence The number of existing cases of a specific disorder in a normal population at a given time.

Primary prevention Prevention efforts that focus on reduction of the incidence of mental disorders within the community. It is directed toward occurrence of mental health problems, with emphasis on health promotion and prevention of disorders.

Secondary prevention Prevention efforts directed toward reducing the prevalence of mental disorders through early identification of problems and early treatment of those problems. This stage occurs after the problem arises and aims to shorten the course or duration of the episode.

Subjectivity Emphasizing one's own words, attitudes, and opinions in an interaction with another person.

Tertiary prevention Prevention efforts that have the dual focus of reducing residual effects of the disorder and rehabilitating the individual who experienced the mental disorder.

- Define and describe psychiatric-mental health nursing.
- Distinguish between a therapeutic and a social relationship.
- Explain the four stages of the nurse-client relationship.
- Identify the American Nurses Association Standards of Care.
- Describe specific ego defense mechanisms.
- Compare and contrast mental health and mental disorder.
- Discuss the roles of several members of the mental health team.
- Identify significant trends in health care and their effects on psychiatric nursing.

P sychiatric-mental health nursing is a specialty within the discipline of nursing that is recognized as one of the four core mental health practice areas, which also include psychiatry, psychology, and social work (NIMH, 1992). The National Mental Health Act of 1946 designated these four disciplines in the interest of increasing the supply of mental health professionals in the United States during the post–World War II time of need.

PSYCHIATRIC-MENTAL HEALTH NURSING

Definition and Description

Psychiatric-mental health nursing (PMHN) is defined by the American Nurses Association as a "specialty area of nursing practice employing theories of human behavior as its science and the purposeful use of self as its art" in the "diagnosis and treatment of human responses to actual or potential mental health problems" (ANA, 1994b). The discipline of nursing is relatively young and continues to define itself. With this growth come many changes that keep nursing in a constant state of flux. Psychiatric nursing has made dramatic strides in its art and science, and most of those changes have occurred in the past few decades.

Traditional Roles

Traditionally, psychiatric nurses have focused on psychosocial aspects of the client (individual, group, family, or community) as the client conducted life and managed or failed to manage the challenges, tasks, demands, and problems of life. In this endeavor, psychiatric nurses have been concerned primarily with the client's perceptual, mental, emotional, and behavioral responses to internal and external stressors and crises. In addition, they assessed factors that enhanced or inhibited the client's ability and capacity to cope with these challenges and with real or perceived threats to stability. At the heart of psychiatric nurses' interactions was the interpersonal relationship, which still remains the emphasis of treatment. Even though many other biologic and scientific factors have major influence, the nurse-client interaction is the catalyst for client participation and progression toward wellness.

Psychiatric nursing has changed considerably over time. Actual formalization of this specialty did not begin until the mid-1950s. Nursing texts prior to this were often vague and ambiguous when describing interpersonal nurse-client interactions. They offered little information about specific nursing interventions or rationale for those interventions. Although most authors agreed that the nurse-client relationship was a key to client wellness, examples of successful interactions with clients were not clearly defined to help nurses learn how to be effective therapeutic communicators.

Following passage of the National Mental Health Act in 1946, the nursing profession responded to a mandate calling for an increase of activity in mental health nursing. Several graduate programs in psychiatric nursing were begun, and produced the nursing leaders who "set the stage in the 1950s for the importance of the one-to-one nurse-patient relationship" (Lego, 1995). The significance of that alliance has never diminished. Following is a description of the art and science of the nurse-client relationship.

THE NURSE-CLIENT RELATIONSHIP
The Art of the Nurse-Client Relationship

The art of caring is embodied in the therapeutic nurse-client relationship, which is the basis for psychiatric-mental health nursing. The relationship is used as a therapeutic vehicle to effect change, promote growth, and heal mental and emotional wounds. It has been identified as one of the most crucial components of the entire health care delivery process (Lego, 1995; Peplau, 1952; Ruben, 1990; Thompson, 1990) and has a primary purpose of optimal well-being of the client (Bernstein and Bernstein, 1985).

Hildegard Peplau, a pioneer in psychiatric nursing, first described the nurse's relationship with the client in her text, *Interpersonal Relations in Nursing* (1952).

Thereafter, Peplau and other psychiatric nurse practitioners and authors continued to develop and refine nursing theory that described and interpreted the relationship. Even though significant changes occurred between 1974 and 1994 in the care of people with actual and potential mental disorders, "the one-to-one relationship remained a core modality in psychiatric mental health nursing practice" (Beeber, 1995).

The art of a therapeutic relationship includes essential characteristics of the nurse that facilitate client participation in his or her own care toward the ultimate purpose of wellness. These essential characteristics of a successful therapist were first identified nearly 30 years ago by Carkhoff (Carkhoff, 1969; Carkhoff and Traux, 1967) and have become classic, core conditions for facilitative interpersonal relationships. The characteristics are empathy, warmth, genuineness, respect, concreteness, immediacy, confrontation, and self-disclosure. They are described in Box 1-1.

CONCEPT OF HELPING

A major objective for nurses is client participation in his or her own care within the client's capacity. The ultimate goal is eventual client self-sufficiency, achieved through self-searching and self-help. Nurses facilitate this growth process by understanding that concept before undertaking the role of care provider in the psychiatric setting.

The helping process is complex. It is not unique to health care providers but is practiced by all caring and concerned individuals. Many motives exist for the act of helping. It is imperative that psychiatric nurses, who work with an exceptionally vulnerable population, assess their own interests in helping and become aware of their personal needs and reasons for serving others. Some reasons cited by Brammer (1993) and Sussman (1992) are the following:

- *Desire to contribute to society.* A feeling of wanting to give back to the world describes this altruistic urge to make things better than they are. By contributing to society, the person feels more worthwhile. Beginning to help in tangible, concrete ways versus grandiose ways is recommended.

- *Need to protect others.* Helping may take the form of protecting the individual. Sometimes, rescuing others from consequences of their own decisions and behaviors is counterproductive. (For example, a family member's codependent protective behaviors toward a person with alcoholism). Objective assessment of the client's condition and situation is necessary in knowing when protection for health and safety's sake is legitimate and when it fosters dependence or encourages, rather than eliminates, maladaptive behavior.

- *Need for love.* If when helping others the focus is on the helper's own need for love and attention, the result becomes counterproductive. Awareness of the need to be needed is important, because a conse-

Box 1-1   Essential Characteristics of a Successful Therapist

Empathy   Considered by many to be the most important element of a therapeutic relationship and necessary for client to feel understood. It encompasses placing self in client's internal perception without losing objectivity or identity.

Warmth   The nurse is wholly and intently attentive to the interaction, resulting in client feeling accepted and significant. Conveyance of warmth also means nonpossessive caring and avoiding emotional entanglements while maintaining boundaries.

Genuineness   Nurse's verbal and nonverbal messages are entirely congruent with way he or she feels. Honest, sincere, open; "real" responses; does not imply "tell all." Requires discriminating responses.

Respect   Unconditional positive regard for client's uniqueness regardless of his or her present life situation. Valuing the client and conveying recognition of client's human worth. Does not mean allowing or condoning inappropriate behaviors.

Concreteness   Involves use of specific, realistic terminology rather than vague, abstract jargon or concepts. Assists client to speak concretely, clearly fosters self-understanding, and helps in problem solving and formulation of plans and alternatives.

Immediacy   Interactions and communication focus on interpersonal relationship as it exists at the moment. Client relationship with the nurse is a "snapshot" of problems experienced in other relationships and needs to be addressed.

Confrontation   Constructive confrontation is necessary for client behavioral changes. If the client remains unaware of problems or if problems go unaddressed, he or she will continue to conduct life in the same self-defeating patterns and will avoid getting well. The nurse discusses discrepancies and incongruities. Timing is important. The nurse avoids outbursts that may occur for the sake of relief of the nurse's frustration.

Self-Disclosure   Here, the nurse volunteers personal information (ideas, feelings, experiences) only when relevant to the client's concerns and interests. The client is the focus in the nurse-client relationship, so the nurse should redirect conversation back to client problems, situations, or events. The purpose of self-disclosure is to assist clients in recognizing that problems being experienced are not unique—that the client is not alone, and others will support the client through difficult times. The nurse models success in problem solving.

---

quence of serving others to the exclusion of getting one's own needs met leads inevitably to disappointment and burnout, resulting in decreased capacity and ability to help others. Clients must not be the source of this love.

- *Need for control or power.* Clients often see helpers as more powerful because of their presumed knowledge, coupled with the client's sense of vulnerability during both acute and chronic dysfunction or disorder. When helpers are aware of this need to influence others or to gain prestige and praise, they can act to correct their motive for helping and focus on the client's needs. Gratitude and praise are then received appropriately.

- *Need for personal satisfaction.* Balanced, healthy individuals who work in helping professions often describe personal satisfaction from working with and watching individuals overcome adversity, achieve goals, and experience growth. To know that the helper facilitated these changes is rewarding and often brings great satisfaction to the helper.

- *Need for personal insight.* While working with clients who have personal problems, a helper may use the relationship to solve his or her own problems. Awareness of this vicarious learning is important, with a constant reminder to focus on clients and their issues. Many helpers who have worked through their own similar problems become effective therapists, able to offer empathy and insight to their clients who move toward change and growth.

Above are some reasons why helpers enter the psychotherapeutic arena. Many motives are unconscious and can be brought to awareness through a process of **autodiagnosis,** examination of one's own thought, feelings, perceptions, and attitudes about a particular client. Motives can also be discovered through continual education and supervision by effective instructors, mentors, or professional peers who will assist the helper in confronting areas that may be problematic.

Helping is a process that aims to assist another person:

- help himself or herself
- choose a direction in life

- find purpose for existing
- solve problems
- survive crises
- share life with others in work, play, and love

Helping is not about doing "to" or "for" another when the person can function autonomously or with guidance and assistance. Only when the client takes responsibility for life through independence, within his or her own ability and age, stage of development, and life situation, can that person experience the freedom to grow. The helper's task is awareness of self, awareness of client needs, and utilization of skills to set the client free with tools to forge his or her own life.

The Science of the Nurse-Client Relationship

The term *science* is used here broadly, to describe the systematic operationalization of the nurse-client relationship. The essential characteristics mentioned earlier and the desire to help people in the psychiatric setting are only beginnings. The nurse also needs to know how to help. This requires learning tangible skills that are used in conjunction with the helping characteristics previously described—skills that are put into action in the form of specific interventions directed at identified client needs and problems.

Only four decades ago, nurses' interventions with clients in psychiatric settings were focused primarily on keeping them safe, carrying out medical orders, and helping them (by whatever nursing means were available) to be comfortable. Care was largely custodial. Nursing textbooks lacked specific instructions for effective, meaningful interactions to benefit clients and were vague, ambiguous, abstract, and general regarding nursing interventions. Today, instructions are clear and specific regarding nursing activities with psychiatric clients (Fortinash and Holoday-Worret, 1995).

The nurse-client interpersonal relationship involves the integration of many components to be successful. In addition to previously defined characteristics and the willingness or desire to help people solve their problems, the nurse also must have knowledge of content that includes, but is not limited to:

- principles of the nurse-client relationship
- nursing scope of practice
- mental health versus mental disorder
- psychiatric diagnoses
  - DSM (Diagnostic and Statistical Manual of Mental Disorders)
  - NANDA (North American Nursing Diagnoses Association)
- nursing process
- protective defenses
- therapeutic treatment modalities

- epidemiology and research
- prevention of disorders
- roles of the mental health team
- trends and the future

Principles of the Nurse-Client Relationship

The therapeutic interpersonal relationship that develops between nurse and client is a vehicle for effecting client change and growth. There are principles and guidelines for developing and maintaining the relationship:

- The relationship is therapeutic rather than social.
- The focus remains on the client's issues rather than on the nurse's or other issues.
- The relationship is purposeful and goal-directed.
- It is objective versus subjective in quality.
- It is time-limited versus open-ended.

THERAPEUTIC VERSUS SOCIAL

A therapeutic relationship is formed to help clients solve problems, make decisions, achieve growth, learn coping strategies, let go of unwanted behaviors, reinforce self-worth, and examine relationships. The meetings between nurse and client are not for mutual satisfaction. Although the nurse can be friendly with the client, the nurse is not there to be the client's friend. Because boundaries define us and our roles and are important in any relationship, especially in a therapeutic relationship, trying to be a client's friend blurs boundaries and confuses roles. The nurse helps the client increase awareness of boundaries and practice boundary-setting (Box 1-2).

Some social conversation is usual at the beginning of meetings and may help to establish or maintain rapport. Occasionally during meetings, superficial or social conversation may briefly reappear, but the majority of conversation is focused and therapeutic. Table 1-1 compares therapeutic and social interactions.

CLIENT FOCUS

Frequently during a session a client redirects the focus away from self by changing the subject, talking about the weather, or focusing on the nurse (nurse's appearance, personal problems, problems in the milieu) or other issues. The nurse recognizes this as a divergent tactic that is probably a form of resistance. The nurse then confronts the behavior in a matter-of-fact way and refocuses the client. Clients do this for one or more of several reasons: resistance to discussing anxiety-producing material, boredom, repetition of material previously discussed with other therapists, or inability to stay cognitively focused because of a mental disorder.

GOAL DIRECTION

The primary purpose of a therapeutic relationship is helping clients to meet adaptive goals. Together the

---

Box 1-2   Signs of Unhealthy Boundaries

- Going against personal values or rights to please another
- Not noticing when someone displays inappropriate boundaries
- Not noticing when someone invades your boundaries
- Talking at an intimate level on the first meeting
- Falling in love with a new acquaintance
- Falling in love with anyone who reaches out
- Being overwhelmed by (preoccupied with) a person
- Acting on first sexual impulse
- Being sexual for partner, not self
- Accepting food, gifts, touch, sex that you do not want
- Touching a person without asking
- Taking as much as you can for the sake of getting
- Giving as much as you can for the sake of giving
- Allowing someone to take as much as they can from you
- Letting others direct your life
- Letting others describe your reality
- Letting others define you
- Believing others can anticipate your needs
- Expecting others to fill your needs automatically
- Falling apart so someone will take care of you
- Self-abuse
- Sexual and physical abuse
- Food abuse
- Loaning money you do not have
- Flirting; sending mixed messages
- Telling all

TABLE 1-1   Therapeutic versus social interactions

Therapeutic	Social
• Offer client therapeutic assistance	• Give and receive friendship equally
• Focus on client's needs	• Meet both person's needs
• Discuss client's perception, thoughts, feelings, behaviors	• Share mutual ideas, experiences
• Actively listen and use therapeutic communication, skills, and techniques	• Socially give opinions and advice
• Encourage client to choose subject for discussion	• Randomly discuss topics at will or whim
• Encourage client to problem-solve toward independence	• Insist on helping as a friend; tolerate dependence
• Keep no secrets that may harm client	• Promise to keep secrets at any cost
• Set goals with client	• Goals of relationship not important
• Remain objective	• Become subjectively involved
• Maintain healthy boundaries	• Accept blurred boundaries
• Evaluate interactions with client	• Avoid relational evaluations

---

client and nurse determine problematic issues and collaboratively decide what the client needs and is able to achieve. Once goals are established, the nurse and client agree to work toward those goals, putting intentions into action and modifying strategies when necessary until the identified goals are achieved. The activities involved are usually many and varied, but each activity is purposefully planned with the client's goals in mind.

OBJECTIVE VERSUS SUBJECTIVE

Nurses can be therapeutic only if they remain objective. **Objectivity** refers to remaining free from bias, prejudice, and personal identification in interaction with the client and being able to process information based on facts. **Subjectivity,** on the other hand, refers to emphasis on one's own feelings, attitudes, and opinions in in-

teraction with the client. When nurses act subjectively in relation to clients' problems or situations, they lose effectiveness in the relationship. By stepping back, the nurse can see things realistically rather than become overly and personally involved with clients' issues.

This, of course, does not imply that the nurse withdraws from feeling, or constructs barriers to protect himself or herself by intellectualizing or avoiding responses. With knowledge, awareness, and practice, the nurse can be both objective and fully attentive to clients' situations and needs.

An example of objectivity versus subjectivity is the nurse's ability to remain empathic instead of becoming sympathetic when interacting with a client, even though the nurse may have experienced a similar, painful situation. For instance, consider a nurse who had lost a child in an accident and then encounters a client who is depressed and grieving the recent death of her own child. The nurse demonstrates objectivity by allowing and facilitating the client's full expression of thoughts and feelings and then responding in a warm, empathic way that remains client-centered. This approach helps the client relieve pent-up feelings in a normal grieving process, allows her to feel understood, and helps the client to process and organize thoughts directed toward solving her own problems.

An example of nontherapeutic subjectivity is a nurse in the same situation who hears the client's expression of feelings and responds with excessive self-disclosure about his or her own similar experience. This approach represents a loss of therapeutic boundaries by identifying with the client's problem—becoming enmeshed in the situation by personalizing it. The client's response will most likely be negative. The client will probably stop sharing information because she feels unimportant and negated, or because he or she worries that the nurse is fragile or inept and cannot even manage his or her own problems.

TIME-LIMITED INTERACTIONS

Before the relationship is established, the nurse sets necessary parameters of the relationship by agreeing with the client on days and times when they will meet, and the numbers of times meetings will take place. Such structure helps the client realize that this relationship has limits and is not open-ended (in other words, the client cannot see the nurse whenever he or she wants, for as long as he or she wants).

The principle of time-limited interaction is important for several reasons. Sometimes clients have not learned during formative relationships that limits are important for all relationships and, without limits, problems are inevitable. When participants define the amount of time they are willing and able to give, then anxiety-provoking guesswork is eliminated and individuals can decide how to make appropriate use of the time they have together. Also, all relationships have inevitable endings. Much grief is avoided if both the nurse and client are certain of the parameters of their relationship and enforce them together. The relationship is a microcosm of the client's relationships outside of their meetings and serves as a model for the client to successfully begin and appropriately let go of subsequent relationships.

Stages of the Nurse-Client Relationship

Every relationship between nurse and client is unique because of the qualities each participant brings to the interaction process and the human chemistry that develops between them. There are, however, definitive phases that relationships undergo. The astute nurse identifies these phases as they occur, to more effectively facilitate the client's progress.

PREORIENTATION PHASE

During this initial phase before nurse and client ever meet, the nurse must accomplish several tasks. The first is to gather data about the client, his or her condition, and present situation. Information is taken from all available sources (client's chart, staff report, and physician's report, and input from family or other reliable sources, such as police and ambulance attendants).

From the information gathered, the nurse engages in a period of autodiagnosis regarding his or her thoughts, feelings, perceptions, and attitudes about this particular client. Judgmentalism, biases, or stereotyping may arise that can influence the pending contact in a nontherapeutic way. For example, if the nurse learns information that reminds him or her of a loved one or of a despised or feared person, the nurse's response to the client could be subjective and ineffective if the facts are not closely examined.

Consider Nurse A, whose father was an alcoholic who verbally abused her mother when he drank. What are some possible responses Nurse A may demonstrate in the following situations if she does not engage in autodiagnosis?

- A male client is admitted to the unit because of inebriation and wife abuse.
- A matronly female is admitted to the unit with major depression. Her husband drinks and abuses her.

Nurse A's conscious efforts to examine each situation and put it in an objective perspective are important if judgmentalism and stereotyping are to be avoided.

ORIENTATION PHASE

Following nurse-client introduction, the relationship begins to grow. During this stage, participants become acquainted, build trust and rapport, and demonstrate acceptance of the process that will take place when the client begins to work on important issues.

THE CONTRACT

A contract is established in the orientation phase of the relationship. The contract may be formal or informal, written or verbal. Nurses most frequently use verbal, informal contracts with clients in acute care settings in which the client and nurse are more continually together. It may be necessary for the nurse to write a more specific, formalized contract for clients who are seen outside of an acute care setting.

The contract may be succinct and still be effective and efficient. For example, the nurse on an inpatient unit may say to the client: "I will be your contact person while you are in the (facility). I work Monday through Friday from 8 A.M. to 4 P.M. Because of your schedule on this unit, it seems that the best time for us to meet is 9 A.M. Is that a good time for you?" If the client agrees, the contract is established.

In a community setting (home care, partial-day treatment program, halfway house) the nurse would probably write a contract for the client, specifying dates, days, and times of meetings, and phone numbers where the nurse can be reached if client has questions between appointments. Some contracts clearly define client behaviors expected to occur between meetings and goals to be reached.

Regardless of the type of contract, the nurse explains the purpose of the meetings, what may be expected during the meetings, and roles of both nurse and client. Together, they determine long-term goals and short-term objectives for reaching those goals.

Dependability is imperative and nurses must keep all appointments with clients. Even at times when circumstances prevent this, the nurse contacts the client to explain the situation and sets a new meeting time. Client dependability is also expected and conveyed.

During the orientation stage, client strengths, limitations, and problem areas are identified by both client and nurse. Outcome criteria are established, and a plan of care is formulated. Clients' responses to this phase vary widely.

WORKING PHASE

The orientation phase ends and the working phase begins when the client takes responsibility for his or her own behavior change. This means committing to working on issues and concerns that have caused disruptions in the client's life.

Prioritization of clients' needs helps determine those problems that require immediate attention and promotes an organized way to manage the problems. A general principle is that safety and health problems supersede any others. For example, it is always assured first that clients are free from danger to self or others and that physical needs are met before traditional therapy begins. Then, behaviors that are socially unacceptable are modified (for example, hostile remarks, swearing, isolation, and poor hygiene). The nurse assists the client to change problematic behaviors in a safe environment where the client can practice new skills and behaviors.

As nurses gain experience, they are more able to recognize when their clients are in the working phase. Sometimes clients tell their "story" but do not do the work to change. Seasoned nurses are able to separate the provocative content from actual process and growth.

TERMINATION PHASE

In this stage, the relationship comes to a close. Termination begins in the orientation phase when the nurse states meeting times with the client. This lets the client know the relationship is about to begin, but that it also has parameters and will end. It avoids confusion on the part of the client who occasionally is unable or unwilling to recognize boundaries of the relationship and wants to contact the nurse outside the facility or after the client is discharged. The nurse does not continue relationships after clients leave treatment.

Termination generally occurs when the client has improved and is discharged, but it may also occur if the client or nurse is transferred. When termination is anticipated, the nurse employs strategies to prepare for the event. Ending treatment may sometimes be traumatic for clients who have come to value the relationship and the help. Some methods that the nurse may use when preparing for termination are the following:

- Reducing amount of time spent with client in each session, and increasing amount of time between sessions, as condition improves.

- Beginning to work on preparation for client's postdischarge situation (plans for future) rather than focusing on new or past problems.

- Having client identify changes he or she has made toward growth; sharing perceptions of the client's growth.

- Helping client express feelings about ending the relationship; telling client if relationship has been pleasurable for him or her.

When nurses recognize relationship stages and are aware of the strategies and responses during each stage, the course of the therapeutic process is smoother. The nurse is not caught off guard or shocked when responses are other than anticipated. When nurses are unaware of potential client responses, they may take responsibility for what seems like failure or may even abandon the relationship because it is unrewarding or unfulfilling. When aware of responses that may occur, however, the nurse is prepared to use strategies that facilitate client growth.

SCOPE OF PSYCHIATRIC-MENTAL HEALTH NURSING PRACTICE

Purpose of Standards

A profession has the task of developing standards of practice that serve as a model for conduct and a gauge by which it measures performance and competence. Standards also communicate values, priorities, and patterns of excellence.

Standards of nursing practice are also guidelines that direct provision of care for clients during promotion and maintenance of health, prevention of illness and injury, and restoration of health.

Standards of care and practice for psychiatric-mental health nurses were developed by the American Nurses Association (ANA, 1994b) and describe nursing functions. They follow the steps of the nursing process and provide a framework within which psychiatric-mental health nursing is implemented and evaluated.

ANA Standards of Psychiatric-Mental Health Clinical Nursing Practice: Standards of Care*

Standard I
Assessment
The Psychiatric-Mental Health Nurse Collects Client Health Data

During the nurse's interview with the client or other reliable reporters, relevant information is obtained that enables the nurse to make decisions about the client's situation and begin to formulate a plan of care. In the interview process, the nurse utilizes multiple skills of observation, communication, and assessment techniques, and then records the review. When data collection is completed, the nurse prioritizes the information.

Standard II
Diagnosis
The Psychiatric-Mental Health Nurse Analyzes the Assessment Data in Determining Diagnoses

Through synthesis and analysis of the collected data, the nurse determines patterns of client responses that represent needs, problems, or actual/potential psychiatric disorders. Nursing diagnoses are derived using the accepted classification of the North American Nursing Diagnosis Association (NANDA). Nursing diagnoses will also be closely associated with the client's psychiatric diagnosis when applicable.

Standard III
Outcome Identification
The Psychiatric-Mental Health Nurse Identifies Expected Outcomes Individualized to the Client

The nurse and client together determine the ultimate goals (expected outcomes) for the client's health that can be expected from health care. The goals are identified and documented. Expected outcomes are realistic, attainable, measurable, and client-focused. They not only provide a target for the client to reach, but also provide a basis of information to measure health status and progress or lack of progress.

Standard IV
Planning
The Psychiatric-Mental Health Nurse Develops a Plan of Care that Prescribes Interventions to Attain Expected Outcomes

An individualized prioritized plan of care is developed by the nurse in collaboration with the client and signifi-
cant others and is used to guide interventions to ultimately achieve the client's expected outcomes. The care plan is utilized by all health team members and is modified as changes occur in client's health status or progress.

Standard V
Implementation
The Psychiatric-Mental Health Nurse Implements the Interventions Identified in the Plan of Care

Psychiatric-mental health nurses practice according to their level of educational preparation and certification. Nurses select interventions according to client need, their own level of practice, and in keeping with the care plan that has been established for the client.

BASIC PRACTICE LEVEL

At the basic level of practice, nurses may intervene in the following ways.

Counseling
The Psychiatric-Mental Health Nurse Uses Counseling Interventions to Assist Clients in Improving or Regaining Their Previous Coping Abilities, Fostering Mental Health, and Preventing Mental Illness and Disability

Counseling is described by the ANA as including interviewing and communication techniques, problem solving, crisis intervention, stress management, and behavior modifications.

Milieu Therapy
The Psychiatric-Mental Health Nurse Provides, Structures, and Maintains a Therapeutic Environment in Collaboration with the Client and Other Health Care Providers

The environment is used as a therapeutic tool to modify behaviors, teach skills, and encourage communication between the client and others. The nurse in milieu therapy provides structure and support, and promotes growth through role modeling and opportunities for interactions.

Self-Care Activities
The Psychiatric-Mental Health Nurse Structures Interventions Around the Client's Activities of Daily Living to Foster Self-Care and Mental and Physical Well-Being

A primary concept in psychiatric-mental health nursing is to encourage independence within a client's ability and capacity. In keeping with this principle, clients are urged to take responsibility for their care, and in turn experience increased self-esteem along with improved function and health.

---

*Reprinted with permission from American Nurses Association: *A Statement on Psychiatric-Mental Health Clinical Nursing Practice and Standards of Psychiatric-Mental Health Clinical Nursing Practice,* Washington, D.C., 1994, ANA.

Psychobiological Interventions
The Psychiatric-Mental Health Nurse Uses Knowledge of Psychobiological Interventions and Applies Clinical Skills to Restore the Client's Health and Prevent Further Disability

Nursing interventions with clients in a psychiatric setting frequently include the use of medications, so nurses have responsibility for thorough knowledge, preparation, and experience in this area. Other psychological interventions also require nurses' participation, observation, and teaching skills.

Health Teaching
The Psychiatric-Mental Health Nurse, Through Health Teaching, Assists Clients in Achieving Satisfying, Productive, and Healthy Patterns of Living

Nurses teach multiple topics to clients in the psychiatric setting, offering feedback for learning and opportunities for practice of skills.

Case Management
The Psychiatric-Mental Health Nurse Provides Case Management to Coordinate Comprehensive Health Services and Ensure Continuity of Care

Nurses participate in client care and comprehensively oversee the care provided by other members of the health team or agencies when appropriate.

Health Promotion and Health Maintenance
The Psychiatric-Mental Health Nurse Employs Strategies and Interventions to Promote and Maintain Mental Health and Prevent Mental Illness

Aside from secondary psychiatric nursing interventions employed after clients' problems have been identified, the nurse at this level also engages in promotion of mental health and prevention of mental disorder.

ADVANCED PRACTICE LEVEL

The following interventions may be employed only by clinical specialists who are certified in advanced psychiatric- mental health nursing.

Psychotherapy
The Certified Specialist in Psychiatric-Mental Health Nursing Uses Individual, Group, and Family Psychotherapy, Child Psychotherapy, and Other Therapeutic Treatments to Assist Clients in Fostering Mental Health, Preventing Mental Illness and Disability, and Improving or Regaining Previous Health Status and Functional Abilities

The psychiatric-mental health nurse clinical specialist uses a wide range of knowledge to intervene with clients. The nurse and client agree to a contract and work within its parameters. The nurse at this level is autonomous in therapeutic modalities, but collaborates appropriately where warranted.

Prescription of Pharmacological Agents
The Certified Specialist Prescribes Pharmacological Agents in Accordance with the State Nursing Practice Act to Treat Symptoms of Psychiatric Illness and Improve Functional Health Status

The nurse at this level, in accordance with government regulation and state nursing practice acts, and with full knowledge of psychopharmacological agents, prescribes medications and manages the client's regimen.

Consultation
The Certified Specialist Provides Consultation to Health Care Providers and Others to Influence the Plans of Care for Clients and to Enhance the Abilities of Others to Provide Psychiatric and Mental Health Care and Effect Change in Systems

The nurse clinical specialist at this level provides consultation regarding changes in agencies or systems when necessary.

Evaluation
The Psychiatric-Mental Health Nurse Evaluates the Client's Progress in Attaining Expected Outcomes

Evaluation of client health status and progress is done at this level.

The above standards of client care provide a framework for psychiatric-mental health nursing practice and evaluation. These criteria help nurses clearly define role responsibilities and outcomes for which they are accountable during the process of caring for clients in any psychiatric setting.

The scope of practice for psychiatric-mental health nursing is also based on knowledge of and compliance with standards of professional performance. Some of these standards are directly related to client care (quality of care, ethics, performance evaluation, collaboration, and use of appropriate resources); others are directed beyond that performance level, but still address the professional role (research, advanced education, specialty certification, advanced practice, continuing education, and memberships in organizations) (ANA, 1994b).

Practice Levels and Settings

Within the specialty of psychiatric-mental health nursing, nurses practice at two levels: generalist or clinical specialist. The previously listed ANA Standards of Care describe criteria that determine the nurse's responsibility and accountability at these two levels. Other standards also govern the nurse's performance and are the following:

- professional standards of practice
- professional code of nursing
- specialty certification
- state-registered nurses license (RN)
- state nursing practice act
- educational level of the RN
- personal competence
- policies and procedures of individual facility
- position description in work setting (clearly defined)

In addition to these standards, nurses also choose to practice in one of the following subspecialty settings:

- clinical
- educational
- administration
- research

MENTAL HEALTH AND DISORDER

Understanding the concepts of mental health and mental disorders is necessary for the nurse who works with clients in the psychiatric setting. This understanding comes from two main sources: education and experience.

Extensive education for the nurse includes theoretical knowledge derived from natural, physical, and behavioral sciences; the humanities; and the art and science of nursing. Psychiatric nurses also need a foundation in communication theory and courses in psychiatric-mental health nursing content and process.

Practitioners agree that to understand mental health and mental disorders, there is no substitute for experience. A strong theory background is the basis for successful practice, but the nurse hones skills only through exposure to challenging psychiatric settings and the clients.

The terms *mental health* and *mental disorder* are complex and defy simplistic operational definitions. A discussion of these concepts follows.

Mental Health

Mental health consists of multiple and varied components, many of which are unmeasurable by scientific standards. For that reason, a concise, encompassing definition of mental health does not currently exist, although many definitions appear in the literature. This emphasizes the fact that human beings are not simply defined or described, or predictable. Each individual brings his or her own uniqueness to the world and interacts with it in a way that is unlike any other person.

No two people have the same experience. Two children born into the same home, of the same parents, have entirely different life experiences. Two people witnessing the same event may have similar but different perceptions. Individual responses are considered healthy or disordered as measured by psychiatric, psychological, and sociocultural standards.

Physical health is more easily defined because of specific parameters rooted in physical science (anatomy, physiology, chemistry, microbiology). These parameters can be measured by exacting diagnostics (for example, laboratory tests, pathology exams, radiology, and nuclear medicine). More precise definitions of physical health can be derived based on the presence or absence of specific anatomical or physiological components.

This is not always so with mental health. Some of the same traits present in mental disorders may be present in individuals who are considered healthy and normal by existing sociocultural standards. Thus, many health professionals choose to work with the physically impaired rather than those with mental disorders because of their inability to tolerate this ambiguity. The ability to suspend judgment and to be open to various interpretations without requiring closure or cure to proceed are necessary qualities in the mental health care professionals.

Often mental health has been presented through linear paradigms that depict optimal mental wellness to extreme mental disorder. The one-dimensional presentation in Figure 1-1 does not incorporate or consider all the components that comprise mental health or that may malfunction to constitute mental disorder. Figure 1-2 shows a more representative illustration of mental health and mental disorder.

To be mentally healthy one need not demonstrate or exhibit all the characteristics that appear in Box 1-3 on page 14. As stated previously, some symptoms of dysfunction are likely to appear in even the healthiest individuals; conversely, healthy components can be found in even the most disordered persons.

Factors that contribute to and influence mental health or mental disorder are also numerous and varied, and can broadly be categorized as intrapersonal, interpersonal, or environmental in nature. (Box 1-4 on page 15).

Every infant comes into the world with certain inborn responses. The child is not a blank slate, or tabula rasa (Kaplan, 1994). Recent research demonstrates that the newborn is endowed with these responses and interacts with the environment to produce behaviors that uniquely define the child.

The concept of **epigenesis,** described first by Erikson (1963), considers several factors that influence development and ultimately shape the individual. Erikson wrote that genetics and environmental experiences, which begin with conception (pregnancy, intrauterine development, and childbirth) and continue throughout life, determine the person's personality and his or her mentally healthy or destructive responses to the world. In addition, the individual must have the capacity to successfully structure experience at every stage of development and contend with and negotiate the given environment in order to maintain health.

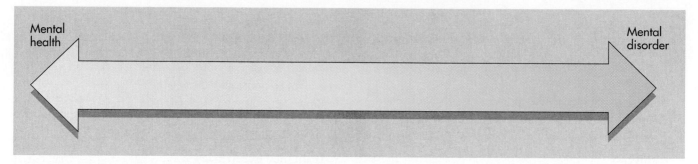

Figure 1-1 One-dimensional presentation of mental health and mental disorder.

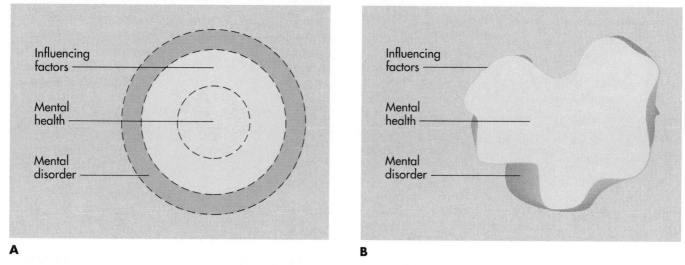

A   **B**

Figure 1-2 A) Mental health is the core; influencing internal and external factors surround the core; mental disorder is the outer layer. Dividing each component are broken lines that represent the dynamic states of each component that change continually across the life span depending on the individual's intrapersonal characteristics, interpersonal relationships, and environmental events and circumstances. **B)** Representation of how this may occur in one instance—in its dynamic state.

The origins of mental health and its influencing factors have been contemplated and shaped by a few influential thinkers and expanded by many of their followers. The question still remains concerning the degree to which the potential toward health or disorder is present at conception, or is modified by effects of the environment (that is, nature versus nurture).

Presently the pendulum has swung back toward biological elements as causal factors of mental health or disorder. Psychiatric nurses need to stay informed of the latest developments, while not losing sight of psychologic, sociologic, behavioral, cultural, and spiritual factors that may also influence their clients' health.

Mental Disorder

It seems logical that deviations in the factors that influence mental health or disorder would define mental disorder. It remains a term, however, that is not easily defined. In its most recent discussions of the term *mental*

disorder, the American Psychiatric Association (APA) states that it "implies a distinction between mental and physical disorders that is a reductionistic anachronism of mind/body dualism" (APA 1994a). In other words, the word *mental* does not adequately include the multiple varied aspects of mental disorders.

Like the concept of mental health, the concept of mental disorder encompasses far too many components and situations to be covered in one operational definition. Mental disorders are well described in the *Diagnostic and Statistical Manual of Mental Disorders,* fourth edition (DSM-IV), but definition remains imperfect. With that qualifier, the APA defines mental disorder as ". . . clinically significant behavioral or psychological syndrome or pattern that occurs in an individual and is associated with present distress (e.g., a painful symptom) or disability (i.e., impairment in one or more important areas of functioning) or with a significantly increased risk of suffering death, pain, disability, or an important loss of freedom" (APA, 1994).

Box 1-3   Components of Mental Health

- Presence of anatomical and physiological components necessary to function in the world
- Absence of signs and symptoms of mental disorder
- Freedom from excessive mental and emotional disability and pain

Ability to

- Perceive self, others, and events correctly
- Recognize own strengths, weaknesses, capabilities and limitations
- Separate fantasy from reality
- Think clearly
    - problem-solve
    - use good judgment
    - reason logically
    - reach insightful conclusions
- Negotiate each developmental stage
- Attain and maintain positive self-system
    - self-concept
    - self-image
    - self-esteem
- Accept self and others as uniquely different, but humanly similar
- Appreciate life
- Find beauty, joy, goodness in self, others, environment
- Be creative
- Be optimistic but realistic
- Use talents to fullest
- Involve self in purposeful, meaningful life work
- Engage in play
- Develop and demonstrate appropriate sense of humor
- Express emotions

- Exhibit congruent behaviors
- Accept responsibility for actions
- Control impulses and behavior
- Be accountable for own behaviors
- Respect societal rules and sanctions
- Learn from experiences
- Maintain wholesome values and belief system
- Cope with internal and external stressors in constructive and adaptive ways
- Return to usual or higher function after crises
- Delay gratification
- Function independently
- Maintain reasonable expectations concerning self and others
- Adapt to social environment
- Relate to others
    - form relationships
    - maintain close, meaningful, loving, adaptive relationships
    - work and play well with others
    - be intimate, appropriately and selectively
    - respond to others in need
    - feel and exhibit compassion and empathy toward others
    - demonstrate culturally and socially acceptable interpersonal interactions
    - manage interpersonal conflict constructively
    - give and receive, gracefully
    - learn from and teach others
    - function interdependently
- Seek self-actualization
- Attain self-defined spirituality

STIGMA OF MENTAL DISORDERS

Mental disorders are presented in the DSM-IV where it openly states that the manual is a classification of disorders and not a classification of people. The meaning of that statement is significant for psychiatric-mental health nurses who act as client advocates in the reduction of judgmentalism, disrespectful labeling, and the stigma that has been associated with mental disorders. Instead of referring to a person by a diagnosis, the nurse refers to the person who has a diagnosis.

Example 1

Correct: "A 19-year-old male is being admitted for suicide threats as a result of several days use of crystal methamphetamine. Put him in the quiet area, on close watch precautions."

Incorrect: "We're going to have to admit a crystal meth addict who is threatening to kill himself. Put him with the alcoholic in Room 25."

Example 2

Correct: "A family has been added to my cases. The father has a diagnosis of Bipolar Disorder, Manic phase. His daughter has out-of-control behavior due to alcoholism."

Incorrect: "They've added a manic to my case load. His daughter is an alcoholic and lives with him. They fight constantly."

Nurses specializing in psychiatric mental health are continually faced with situations where they need to keep reminding themselves, and perhaps each other, that client behaviors and responses are a product of the dis-

Box 1-4   Mental Health or Disorder: Influencing Factors

- Inherited factors
  - predisposition
  - capacities
  - limitations
- The pregnancy environment and experience (from conception to birth)
- Psychoneuroimmunological factors
- Biochemical influences
- Hormonal influences
- Family
  - composition
  - birth position
  - bonding
  - members' mental health
- Developmental events
  - completion of clearly defined stages
  - resolution of developmental crises
- Culture
- Subculture
- Values
- Belief systems
- Perception of self

- Cognitive abilities
  - capacity
  - volition
- Personality traits and states
- Goals, aspirations
- World view
- Internal stressors
- External stressors
- Support systems
  - choice of
  - availability
- Negative influences
  - internal/external
  - mental disorders
  - crime
  - drugs
  - psychosocial stressors
  - poverty
- Demographic factors
- Geographic location
- Health practices and beliefs
- Spirituality/religion

order. *The client is not the disorder.* Respect for the human, regardless of the condition or the situation, remains constant. Limits may have to be set on behavior, but the client needs to maintain dignity, which is facilitated by the nurse.

In addition to immediate practice, nurses have the opportunity to reduce stigma by educating the general public about causes and treatments of mental disorders and the needs of mental health clients. Stigmatizing and stereotyping continue to hover over persons with mental disorder and are fueled by ignorance and fear. Stigma increases the problems faced by mental health clients, and these problems will only increase as the trend of present day funding reroutes essential monies away from their care. Because of economic reallocation, homelessness will increase and the issues surrounding it will become more difficult. Some problems faced by those with mental disorder are the following:

- homelessness
- housing discrimination
- unstable living conditions
- job discrimination
- diminished self-esteem
- inappropriate or inadequate treatment
- inability to seek treatment

- alienation, isolation
- loss of entitlements

With enlightenment and advocacy, these individuals can be provided:

- access to education
- job opportunities
- health insurance coverage
- adequate treatment
- adequate housing
- research
- appropriate personal and human contact

People with mental disorders are feared or perceived as dangerous, violent, and aggressive, and are blamed for their illness. In fact, they are more likely to be passive, withdrawn, and isolated. Nurses can be instrumental in modifying or significantly changing the public's attitude and the client's experience of rejection, to one of acceptance.

PSYCHIATRIC DIAGNOSES

Psychiatric diagnoses are precise descriptions and classifications of mental disorders. They are necessary and important for several reasons, such as communication, treatment, prognosis, and funding.

Communication

Each psychiatric diagnosis represents a specific set of symptoms or a syndrome. The criteria for each disorder enable mental health care providers to communicate with each other without having to explain symptoms when discussing the diagnoses. Staff should bear in mind that each client will present a unique expression of the disorder.

Educating individuals about psychiatric disorders is effective because the psychiatric classification of disorders is clearly defined and therefore can be communicated to learners in an organized way.

Treatment

Staff members are prepared to begin symptom-specific treatment based on a client's diagnosis. They know that the approaches (biological and interpersonal) will vary, depending on the diagnosis. For example, preparation of the staff and the psychiatric setting will be different for a client reported to have a diagnosis of paranoid schizophrenia with acutely psychotic symptoms and aggressive behavior towards others, than will preparation for a client with a diagnosis of major depression and severely withdrawn behavior.

Prognosis

Some psychiatric diagnoses have more favorable prognoses than others. Mental health care providers remain hopeful and convey that hope to clients. However, they are aware that a goal of treatment may be to return a client to a level of function experienced before an acute exacerbation of a chronic disorder without expecting a cure of the disorder. The prognosis for some adjustment disorders, for example, is more favorable than the prognosis for one of the schizophrenias that has a chronic course.

Funding

It is a well-established fact that money is required to pay for services delivered during the care of clients, regardless of the psychiatric setting. Whether the source is private or public, certain criteria must be met to receive payment, and the client's diagnosis is a major factor.

On a larger scale, research monies are targeted for investigation of designated diagnoses. Research may be carried out in the private sector (e.g., drug companies) or public sector (e.g., government mental health agencies).

Nomenclatures

DSM-IV

A nomenclature of psychiatric diagnoses developed by the American Psychiatric Association is widely accepted in the United States as the official diagnostic criteria in clinical, research, and educational settings. The diagnoses are published in the *Diagnostic and Statistical Manual of Mental Disorders,* fourth edition (DSM-IV). See Appendix A for the complete listing of DSM-IV diagnoses.

NANDA

Nursing has formed its own nomenclature of nursing diagnoses. Many of the current diagnoses published by the North American Nursing Diagnosis Association (NANDA) are applicable in the psychiatric setting. The NANDA nursing classification is relatively young, but new diagnoses are evolving for psychiatric clients with each publication.

COLLABORATIVE DIAGNOSES

In the interest of establishing itself as a separate science, nursing has passed through a time when it attempted to use its own classification apart from medical diagnoses. Textbooks for psychiatric nurses were sometimes written with chapter headings directed at client behaviors rather than psychiatric diagnoses. It was more difficult for learners first exposed to psychiatry to associate the psychiatric (admitting) diagnosis of a mental disorder with the nursing diagnosis and subsequent combined treatment. It seems clear that a coexistence of medical and nursing diagnoses is essential for the ultimate collaborative, interdisciplinary care of clients. Only through this synergy will clients' needs be fully met.

The Nursing Process

The nursing process is a scientific, problem-solving method that helps nurses in total client care. This important process consists of six steps: assessment, diagnosis, outcome identification, planning, implementation, and evaluation. An entire chapter in this text, Chapter 6, is devoted to a full description and explanation of the nursing process as it relates to psychiatric nursing.

PROTECTIVE DEFENSES

Most healthy individuals want and strive to feel good about themselves, their accomplishments, and their relationships. They want to be content with their world. They also strive to avoid anxiety, distress, discomfort, and pain, whenever possible.

Mature adults realize that some negative aspects of life, such as disappointments, loss, embarrassment, and nonfulfillment are inevitable and intrinsically woven into the fabric of every life. All people, however, employ mechanisms, techniques, and methods to attain and maintain a state of tranquility and joyful feelings called **euthymia.** They do this either purposefully (consciously) or automatically (unconsciously).

The concept of defenses is widely embraced by clinicians and educators in many disciplines such as nursing, psychiatry, psychology, and social work. Knowledge of the defenses and an awareness of their use are important elements in assessment, diagnosis and treatment. These elements are also necessary in order to understand the value of defenses in a person's development.

The literature presents support for the fact that individuals develop coping styles or defensive styles (APA, 1994; Freud, 1946; Huffman, 1995; Kernberg, 1975). Some styles are adaptive, preserving reality and helping the person to continue to function. Other styles are maladaptive, distorting reality and inhibiting or preventing psychological growth.

Ego Defenses

Ego defenses, also referred to as defense mechanisms or mental mechanisms, are automatic and semi-automatic psychological processes that keep the threat of internal and external stressors and dangers out of awareness and protect the person. The ego mechanisms develop as a means of controlling impulses, desires, and affects (feelings that accompany ideas), thus avoiding conflict and anxiety. But anxiety and conflict cannot be totally avoided.

When anxiety occurs, it is perceived as uncomfortable or even a painful experience. The person takes corrective action to dispel the feelings of anxiety and to continue with the tasks of daily living.

Action may take the form of conscious, purposeful measures, as stated in Box 1-5. Action, on the other hand, may manifest in automatic psychological processes

---

Box 1-5   Conscious Measures as Defenses

- Exercising
- Calling a friend
- Talking to parent, significant others
- Going to a movie
- Crying
- Eating
- Dancing
- Reading
- Volunteering time
- Writing in journal
- Sleeping
- Practicing relaxation techniques
- Going to the theater
- Attending church or community meetings
- Writing letters to friends, family, or others
- Getting involved in purposeful work

---

known as ego defense mechanisms to avoid anxiety and keep the threatening internal and external stressors out of awareness. Ego defense mechanisms and strategies appear in Box 1-6.

Nursing Implication

Nurses are aware that healthy individuals may employ many defenses during stressful situations throughout their life span. Recovery and healthful adaptation following stressful times can be measured by these criteria:

- maintenance of reality orientation
- restoration of equilibrium
- continued involvement in purposeful work
- evidence of continued cognitive and emotional growth
- ability to problem-solve
- continued involvement in nurturing and interdependent interpersonal/social network

Problems may arise in the following situations: when the individual's internal and/or external stressors are greater than the capacity to contend with them; the individual's perception is that the obstacle cannot be overcome; or, when a person uses one or a few defenses exclusively, especially those that distort reality.

When the nurse recognizes the client's use of defenses, it is possible to accept them as part of the individual's attempts to contend with the situation or to intervene if the defenses are inhibiting development or interfering with reality orientation. The nurse's action is dependent on level of education and clinical experience.

An inexperienced psychiatric-mental health nurse will generally not confront or attempt to remove the client's protective defenses. Instead the focus is one of support and assistance in identifying the client's positive characteristics and development of ego strength, through the establishment and maintenance of the nurse-client relationship.

An experienced nurse will move beyond these limits to challenge defenses in the interest of the client's cognitive and emotional growth. Through insight, the client is guided toward subsequent behavioral changes that are practiced in the safety of the relationship, then generalized in the client's life outside of therapy.

THERAPEUTIC TREATMENT MODALITIES

A virtual revolution in mental health care has occurred in the past few years in which traditional inpatient hospitalization has been replaced with an entire range of care options. These optional care modalities may offer cost-effective, creative, client-focused alternatives to traditional treatment. Nurses' awareness of these shifts in treatment methods will ensure optimum client care.

Box 1-6   Defense Mechanisms and Strategies

Repression: The active unconscious process of keeping out or ejecting from the consciousness ideas or impulses that are unacceptable to the person.
Example: An adult male who was sexually abused as a child has no recollection of the events.

Denial: Refusal to perceive or face unpleasant reality as it actually exists.
Example: Non-acceptance of a fatal diagnosis, such as AIDS.

Rationalization: Use of contrived, socially acceptable and logical explanation to justify unpleasant material and to keep it out of consciousness.
Example: A high school graduate who doesn't get accepted to a prestigious military academy says he could never tolerate the regimentation anyway.

Projection: Attributing one's own unacceptable motives or characteristics to another person or group.
Example: A paranoid person uses projection frequently in always seeing "the others" as hostile.

Displacement: The discharge of pent-up feelings (frequently hostility) onto something or someone else in the environment that is less threatening than the original source of the feelings.
Example: After her boss berates her publicly, a woman comes home and starts an argument with her neighbor over parking rights.

Reaction Formation: Prevention of awareness or expression of unacceptable desires by adoption of opposite behaviors in an exaggerated way.
Example: A woman who doesn't want her child before it is born becomes overly protective after the birth, refusing to leave the child's side.

Intellectualization: The overuse of abstract thinking or generalizations to control or minimize painful feelings.
Example: A man who faces a pending divorce engages in lengthy and lofty discourse about divorce statistics and process during a support group but never talks about his own fears and feelings.

Undoing: Atonement for or attempt to dissipate unacceptable acts or wishes.
Examples: 1. A man has an affair with another woman then buys his wife a new car. 2. A professional berates her colleague and causes her to lose her job, then offers to help take care of the colleague's child.

Compensation: Counterbalance for deficiencies in one area by excelling in another area.
Example: A young man who fails at sports studies hard and becomes valedictorian of his graduating class.

Identification: Incorporation of the image of an emulated person, then acting, thinking, and feeling like that person (unconscious mental mimicry).
Example: Gang members dress exactly like their leader and steal from neighbors as the leader does.

Introjection: Treating something outside the self as if it is actually inside the self.
Example: A child who fears dragons "becomes" a dragon in serious play, thus assimilating the fearful experience.

Sublimation: Modification of an instinctual but socially unacceptable impulse into a constructive acceptable behavior.
Examples: 1. An aggressive young man becomes a star hockey player. 2. A woman with strong sexual urges becomes a sculptor.

Regression: Returning to an earlier level of adaptation.
Examples: 1. An adolescent under stress curls up on his bed with a stuffed teddy bear, sucks his thumb, and doesn't speak. 2. An adult client admitted to the psychiatric unit with a diagnosis of psychosis is found smearing feces on the wall.

Suppression: The conscious inhibition of an impulse, idea, or affect. The person has full awareness of the behavior.
Example: A man on his way to give a major speech is told by his wife that she is divorcing him. He decides not to think about it until his speech is over, and puts it out of his mind so he can complete his task.

Humor: Emphasis on ironic or amusing components of a crisis, conflict, or stressor.

Multiple methods may be used during intervention with clients in any psychiatric setting that include, but are not limited to, inpatient hospital or treatment center, outpatient day treatment program, clinic, home, community center, crisis center, place of employment, or school. The choice of methods for intervening with clients' needs and problems is influenced by several factors:

- the client's presenting problems
- the client's knowledge about treatment methods
- client's ability to make treatment choices
- the therapist's theoretic background, training, and philosophy
- type of setting
- available resources

Approaches vary widely among the scores of available therapies, and it is not uncommon practice to incorporate several methods (eclectic approach) during treatment. Generally, clients admitted to an acute care psychiatric setting will receive both interactive and biologic types of therapy. Any range of methods may be employed in community settings.

Interactive therapies include all those in which the client has interpersonal contact with one or more therapists, and includes interaction with other clients. Biologic therapies include use of medications, electroshock

Box 1-6   Defense Mechanisms and Strategies—cont'd

Example: Two people leave a room after being strongly disciplined by their boss and burst into laughter that they had restrained. They jokingly discuss the only thing each focused on—a large piece of the boss's hair stuck straight up in the air and bobbed up and down as he paced around the room and crowed at them.

Splitting: Compartmentalization of opposite affect states and failure to integrate positive and negative aspects of self or others, resulting in polarized images of self and others as "all good" or "all bad."

Example: A client on a psychiatric unit tells Nurse A that she is "the kindest, smartest, most well-prepared nurse on the unit." She tells Nurse B, who sets limits on the client's behavior, that she is "stupid and insensitive, and it's a miracle she ever got an RN license."

Self-Observation: Reflection on one's own behavior, thoughts, and feelings, followed by appropriate response.

Self-Assertion: Expression of thoughts and feelings in direct ways that are not manipulating or intimidating.

Altruism: Devotion of self to serving others as a way to manage conflict and stress. Differs from reaction formation in that it is gratifying but not self-sacrificing.

Example: Some nuns, priests, rabbis, ministers, nurses, physicians, firefighters, and paramedics, to name a few, often serve people for unselfish reasons and gain satisfaction through giving.

Affiliation: Turning to others for support and help when stressed or conflicted, without attempting to make others responsible for taking care of the person.

Example: A woman is widowed and moves across the country to be near her family of origin and friends from her past.

Anticipation: Anticipating consequences of events yet to come and thinking of options, solutions, and alternatives; also can include experiencing the feelings associated with the thoughts (a "mental rehearsal" of future events).

Example: A hard-working attorney, called to interview for partnership in a law firm, spends the rest of the day rehearsing and experiencing the event.

Help-Rejecting Complaining: Repeated requests for help, suggestions, or advice that is then rejected. The request disguises covert feelings of reproach or hostility for others. Complaints may be about problems of life, or physical or psychological symptoms.

Example: A woman constantly calls her grown and married children to complain about her physical pains and loneliness, but constantly refuses to take any helpful steps they suggest to alleviate her situation.

Passive Aggression: Expression of aggression toward others in indirect and nonassertive ways. Covert hostility and resentment are masked by overt compliance.

Example: A girl is jealous because her best friend dated a boy she wanted to date, agrees to meet her friend for lunch, and then arrives an hour late, apologizing profusely and begging forgiveness.

Omnipotence: Feeling or acting as if the individual is superior to others or has special abilities or power.

Example: An inept and underachieving son of a dynamic business tycoon struts around his own plush but token office and treats others condescendingly.

Isolation of Affect: Separation of feelings from thoughts and ideas originally associated with them.

Example: A woman describes in full detail the traumatic event of watching her friend get hit by a truck and killed but displays no emotion.

Fantasy: Gratification of frustrated desires, achievements, and relationships by substituting them with daydreams and imagery.

Example: An unpopular high school senior is left out of social events but spends her spare time imagining herself dressing for and going to the senior prom with the class football hero.

Acting Out: The use of actions versus reflection or true experiencing of feelings in order to deal with stress and conflict.

Example: A student learns he failed a course, then smashes a window in the classroom, leaves, and drinks six beers.

---

therapy, and, more rarely, psychosurgery. Interactive therapies most often used regardless of the theoretic framework, or conceptual model on which they are based, take the form of one-to-one therapy, group therapy, and adjunctive therapies. Box 1-7 lists therapeutic treatment modalities that may be offered in traditional and nontraditional settings. A description of therapies is presented in Chapter 22.

EPIDEMIOLOGY AND RESEARCH RELATED TO MENTAL DISORDERS

Two significant psychiatric epidemiologic studies have revealed startling results about mental disorders. The first landmark survey is the Epidemiologic Catchment Area (ECA) study, and the second is the National Comorbidity Survey (NCS) (Maxman, 1995). Although done at separate times and with different but large sample sizes, the findings are similar and conclude that one-third to one-half of all adult Americans will have a mental disorder in their lifetime.

In the ECA survey, researchers from the National Institute of Mental Health (NIMH) interviewed almost 20,000 adults in multiple sites to establish the one-year and lifetime prevalence of 30 mental disorders (Robins and Regier, 1991). Researchers from the NCS interviewed 8,098 adults regarding 17 of the most commonly occurring disorders (Kessler et al, 1994). The ECA and

Box 1-7   Therapeutic Treatment Modalities

- Psychotherapy
- Crisis intervention
- Milieu therapy
- Support, psychosocial
  - caregiver support
- Therapeutic processes
  - transference (psychology)
  - countertransference (psychology)
- Transactional analysis
- Reality therapy
- Validation therapy
- Symbolism (psychology)
  - metaphor
- Socioenvironmental therapy
  - client passes
  - group psychotherapy
    - psychodrama
- Role playing
- Support groups
- Residential care
- Family therapy
- Marital therapy
- Behavior modification
  - assertiveness training
  - behavior contracting
  - behavior therapy
  - cognitive therapy
  - biofeedback
  - relaxation techniques
    - distraction
    - guided imagery
    - meditation
- Biofeedback
- Hypnosis
- Art therapy
- Play therapy
- Pet therapy
- Music therapy
- Dance therapy
- Bibliotherapy
- Guided imagery
- Substance dependence program
- Rehabilitation, psychosocial

TABLE 1-2   Prevalence rates of mental disorders

Rank	Disorder	Percentage of adult Americans affected
First	Anxiety Disorders	14.4–17.2
Second	Substance Abuse Disorders	8.8–11.3
Third	Mood Disorders	4.3–11.3
Fourth	Cognitive Impairment Disorder	5.9
Fifth	Schizophrenia	0.5–1

Adapted, using one-year figures, from Maxman J and Ward N: *Essential psychopathology and its treatment,* New York, 1995, WW Norton.

NCS concluded that mental disorders affected approximately 20%–30% of adult Americans during the year preceding the interviews and 32%–50% of them throughout their lives (Maxman, 1995). Table 1-2 presents mental disorders in order of their prevalence.

The ECA survey stated that most clients with mental disorders were more likely to be treated by general practitioners, internists, psychologists, nurses, and social workers (nonpsychiatrists). Both studies clarified the need for health care professionals of all fields to be aware of psychopathology (Maxman, 1995).

Psychobiology

Epidemiologic studies have been instrumental in the current paradigm shift that caused the NIMH to name the 1990s the *Decade of the Brain.* Epidemiologic investigation and studies are "based on the assumption that human disease has causal and preventive factors" (Betemps and Ragiel, 1994), identified through systematic assessment of populations that manifest symptoms that can be classified. Epidemiology employs the scientific measures of *prevalence* and *incidence.*

Prevalence refers to the number of cases of a specific disorder in a normal population at a given time. **Incidence** refers to the frequency of occurrences of a specific disorder within a designated time period (number of new cases).

Prior to World War II, the biologic model greatly influenced epidemiology. During World War II, however, it was determined that stress was a major cause of psychiatric disorders. These findings led to an emphasis on social influences, thus changing the study of etiology and epidemiology relating to mental disorders in the United States (Grob, 1992; Klerman, 1990). The development of sociologic and psychologic frameworks of psychiatry during this time dramatically turned the focus of intervention from biology toward social psychologic aspects of mental disorders.

In the 1970s, focus began to turn back toward biologic causes of psychiatric disorders. The greatest momentum for this shift came from the Epidemiologic Catchment Area survey begun by the NIMH (Klerman, 1986). Basic goals of the ECA program were to:

- estimate rates of prevalence and incidence of specific mental disorders
- estimate rates of mental health services use
- study factors influencing the development and continuance of disorders
- study factors influencing use of services (Eaton, 1984)

The ECA surveys created a shift in research that once again focused on biologic causes of mental disorders. From the mid-1980s to the present time, there has been an explosion of research in this area. More has been learned about psychiatric disorders in the last ten years than at any other time in history. Biological research findings appear throughout this textbook.

Evolution of Care

In 1946 the U.S. government awarded state grants through the National Mental Health Act for the purpose of establishing mental health programs in the community away from mental institutional settings. The Community Mental Health Centers Act, passed by Congress in 1963, began the discharge of individuals with mental disorders into the community. Deinstitutionalization had begun.

Between 1955 and 1990, the locus of mental health care in the United States shifted from inpatient to ambulatory services (Redick, 1994), and the trend continues today. (Figure 1-3).

State and county mental hospitals accounted for 63% of inpatient episodes in 1955, compared with only 16% in 1990. On the other hand, private psychiatric hospitals and inpatient services of general hospitals accounted for 30% of inpatient episodes in 1955, but that number rose to 66% in 1990.

Issues for nurses arising from these findings relate to the following:

- future role of state mental hospitals
- balance between state mental hospitals and community-based services
- balance between inpatient and ambulatory services
- contracting by state mental health agencies for the provision of services through the private sector (Redick, 1994)

Across the nation, mental health services staff are experiencing changes in the way health care is delivered; the changes appear to be accelerating continually. Data regarding numbers of psychiatric beds from 1970 to 1990 show a dramatic decrease in state beds and increase in private and general hospital beds. Considerations for the future are influenced by managed care and other cost-saving "mechanisms" that will undoubtedly continue to substitute outpatient partial care for costlier inpatient treatment. Numbers of hospitalizations and lengths of stay will continue to be reduced (Redick, 1994).

The outcome remains to be seen for clients who will inevitably continue to require psychiatric intervention and for the nurses who will care for them. Conjecture is no substitute for data, so interested psychiatric nurses need to stay informed of and involved in the changes that keep rapidly occurring, and the decisions that shape those changes.

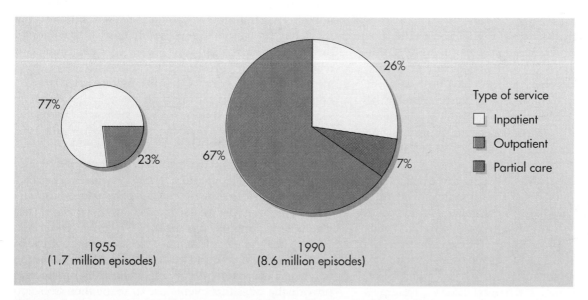

Figure 1-3 Client care episodes in mental health organizations in 1955 and 1990.

(From Center for Mental Health Services, U.S. Department of Health and Human Services, No. 210, May 1994.)

Psychiatric-mental health nurses have the opportunity for involvement through participation in decisions regarding changes in types of care and levels of care. Levels of care refers to *primary, secondary,* or *tertiary prevention,* and is described below.

PREVENTION OF MENTAL DISORDERS

The impetus for deinstitutionalization came from several sources. One was the 1949 government grant awards through the National Mental Health Act for community treatment of clients with mental disorders. A second source was the use of antipsychotic medications that began in the 1950s, and provided more complete relief to clients plagued by life-hampering psychotic symptoms. Because of the medication, clients were able to leave mental institutions and, in many cases, function in society once again. Third was the Mental Health Centers Act of 1963 that called for development of comprehensive community mental health programs across the nation.

In 1964 Gerald Caplan in his textbook *Principles of Preventive Psychiatry* proposed a model for preventive care of persons with mental disorders, in response to the mandate to treat clients in the community setting. Although begun for psychiatry, the model has been widely adopted by many disciplines. Psychiatric nurses use the effective and efficient principles in client care, and the model is a primary focus for nurses who practice community health nursing. It is widely adaptable to biologic, psychologic, or social problems.

The model proposes three levels of prevention of illness and disorder: *primary prevention, secondary prevention,* and *tertiary prevention.* Some subsequent theorists stated that there are actually four levels because the primary level includes two steps: promotion and prevention (Clark, 1992; Leavell, 1965).

Levels of Prevention

Primary prevention focuses on reduction of the incidence of mental disorders within the community. It is directed toward occurrence of mental health problems, with emphasis on health promotion and prevention of disorders. Nursing interventions may concentrate on the client, the environment, or both. For example, the nurse may help the client to learn about and cope with life stressors, or strive to diminish numbers of stressors in the community.

Secondary prevention is directed toward reducing the prevalence of mental disorders through early identification of problems and early treatment of those problems. This stage occurs after the problem arises and aims to shorten the course or duration of the episode.

Tertiary prevention has the dual focus of reducing residual effects of the disorder and rehabilitating the individual who experienced the mental disorder. Examples of primary, secondary and tertiary prevention appear in Box 1-8.

Box 1-8 Examples of Prevention Levels

Primary prevention

- Teach stress reduction and stress management techniques to any population
- Present seminar for school-age children and parents on drug actions and effects
- Teach parenting skills and normal child development expectations to pregnant couples
- Lead a group that cleans cluttered grounds of a troubled tenement lot to begin a garden

Secondary prevention

- Treat individuals in any psychiatric setting (inpatient, home, clinic, day treatment) after diagnosis has been identified, by any approved method of therapy (interactive or biologic medications)
- Refer clients who demonstrate symptoms to other appropriate mental health care providers (psychometric testing; medication consultation; family therapy)

Tertiary prevention

- Provide family support and education to assist in early identification of symptoms that may occur in the future
- Engage couple in therapy to learn new ways to relate to each other in their marriage
- Provide ongoing outpatient therapy group that meets for mutual support of members, education, and assessment of progress

---

Psychiatric nurses who are familiar with this model will benefit as nursing practice continues to move out into the community. As funding becomes more constricted, a primary mission is to increase intervention at the primary prevention level. An even more important reason for primary prevention is to assist clients in avoiding pitfalls whenever possible through increased awareness and education.

ROLES OF THE MENTAL HEALTH TEAM

Clients involved in mental health care are usually treated by an interdisciplinary team of care providers. The roles of mental health team members vary widely, but each role exists primarily to assist the client in achieving and maintaining optimum wellness.

The healthy client-member relationship collaboratively works toward eventual client independence within his or her capacity, whenever possible. Team members provide the tools that clients use to shape their lives and the relationship within which the client practices learned behaviors.

Roles of team members, which are further discussed in Box 1-9, differ with respect to:

- philosophy
- conceptual bases
- theoretical frameworks
- preparatory education
- purpose
- methods of intervention

FUTURE TRENDS IN PSYCHIATRIC-MENTAL HEALTH NURSING

The future of psychiatric-mental health nursing will be affected by many influences. Thus, flexibility will be an essential characteristic of the PMH nurses. One thing is certain: the future will be exciting, dynamic, and chal-

---

Box 1-9   Roles of Mental Health Team

Psychiatric nurse

Nurses have the most widely focused position description of any of the member roles. This depends on their license and certification mandates, the policies of the psychiatric facility or care setting, and experience. They interact with clients in individual and group settings; manage client care; administer and monitor medications; assist with numerous psychiatric and physical treatments; participate in interdisciplinary team meetings; teach clients and families; take responsibility for client records; act as a client advocate; interact with clients' significant others; and assess and intervene with clients' psychiatric, biological, psychosocial, cultural, and spiritual problems.

Licensed vocational nurses provide direct client support. Registered nurses have expanded roles of unit management and decision making in addition to client interaction. Master's- and doctoral-prepared nurses act as clinical specialists in individual group and family therapy, with expanded roles within psychiatric settings; or they act autonomously in private practice.

In some states clinical nurse specialists prescribe medications and manage client case loads. A master's or doctoral degree is required to teach nursing education. Graduate nurses frequently conduct psychiatric research or act as administrators of psychiatric settings.

Psychiatric social worker

This graduate level position allows members to work with clients on an individual basis; conduct group therapy sessions; work with clients' families, and act as liaison with the community to place clients after discharge. They emphasize intervention with the client in the social environment in which he or she will live.

Psychiatric technician

The licensed psychiatric technician has direct client contact in a psychiatric setting and usually reports to the registered nurse. Technicians are trained to observe and record symptoms, and intervene under supervision. In some states they can administer medications under supervision of a registered nurse.

Mental health worker

Some facilities call this position mental health counselor. It is an unlicensed position where the member acts only under supervision of an RN to assist clients in activities of daily living, maintaining the schedule, and providing gen-

eral support. Some have minimal education in psychiatry; others may work in this position while accruing hours toward master's or doctoral degrees. They do not administer medications.

Psychiatrist

A licensed medical physician who specializes in psychiatry. Responsibilities include admitting clients into acute care settings, prescribing and monitoring psychopharmacologic agents, administering electroshock therapy, conducting individual and family therapy, and participating in interdisciplinary team meetings that focus on their clients.

Psychologist

A licensed individual with a doctoral degree in psychology. There are several different psychology tracks. Preparation is for assessment and treatment of psychologic and psychosocial problems of individuals, families, or groups (including industrial, educational, and environmental). Psychologists do not prescribe or administer medications. Many psychologists administer psychometric tests that aid in diagnosis of disorders.

Marriage, family, child counselor

Licensed individuals who frequently work in private practice. They are prepared to work with individuals, couples, families, or groups, and emphasize the interpersonal aspects of achieving and maintaining relationships.

Case managers

This position is being defined and redefined as you read these words. Nurses are qualified for this position because of their diverse education. Case managers facilitate delivery of individualized, coordinated care, in cost-effective ways. *Managed care* and *case management* are not interchangeable concepts. *Managed care* refers to a system of cost containment programs utilized to direct, control, and approve access to services and costs within the health care delivery system. *Case management* is a process in the managed care strategy (Mullahy, 1995). Case managers need to know the various types of hospitalization and outpatient care settings, the coverage offered by different payers (insurance companies, health maintenance organizations, and preferred provider organizations), and the impact of federal and state legislation. Case managers serve as a connection between agencies to provide the most favorable outcomes for the client.

lenging. Persons seeking static, predictable surroundings may not find them in this field.

In addition to the previously discussed changes in the delivery of health care, nurses will also experience changes in other areas:

- emphasis on psychobiology
- expanding technologies
- computer assistance
- new educational demands
  - biologic
  - holistic
- societal demands and stressors
- scientific, geographic, sociopolitical, and economic factors

Nurses do not function in a vacuum, and they will see these and other factors affect the future process and delivery of psychiatric-mental health care. The following discussion of the above criteria does not provide answers or solutions but serves as a source for expanded thinking about the future of psychiatric-mental health nursing.

Emphasis on Psychobiology

The past decade has seen an explosion of psychobiologic information. Research with an emphasis on neurobiology has focused on the structure and function of the brain and nervous system, and how these systems affect health and illness. Research findings support a biological basis for many mental disorders.

This emphasis on the biologic aspect of mental illness greatly affects client care and treatment. Pharmacological interventions are emphasized and new technologies are applied as assessment and treatment measures. Neurobiologic etiologies of major disorders are specifically discussed throughout the book.

Medical Technology

In this text, readers will discover the impact that expanding technology has had on psychiatry. Modern brain imaging techniques, such as MRI, PET, and CAT scans have revolutionized diagnosis of mental disorders. Brain surgery done by stereotactic methods may become even more sophisticated in the future. Research in circadian rhythms and their influence on mental disorders is well documented.

Constant discovery of new psychopharmacologic agents is certain to alter the future treatment of disorders. Clients might be able to automatically monitor their own medication levels and replenish them before minor symptoms become extreme disorders. For example, anxiety levels may be monitored by unobtrusively connected mechanisms that will signal an individual to perform his or her own therapy before a full-blown panic attack occurs.

Computer Technology

Few psychiatric settings currently function without assistance from computers. As a rule, the larger the agency, the more complex the system. There may come a time when clients will be able to turn to computer assisted instruction (CAI) programs or interactive videodiscs (IVD) to input symptoms and effect diagnoses and self-treatment without leaving home.

At the 32nd Biennial Convention of the Sigma Theta Tau National Honor Society, a video was presented to show how nursing is changing (AJN, 1993). The video showed that in a time when more instructors are needed, it may soon be possible to provide safe clinical experiences for student nurses working in multiple community settings by giving each student technologic aids that can communicate to one instructor in a designated setting. With the use of individual computers, students may safely reach community destinations via explicit instructions, send symptoms back to the base, receive laboratory values, answer clients' questions, and teach them about disorder or treatment modalities.

Educational Demands

A nurse's education consists of multiple courses in natural, physical, and behavioral sciences, the humanities, and the art and science of nursing. The task force on the Psychiatric-Mental Health Nursing Psychopharmacology Project of 1994 recommends that nurses include and add additional components in their education where necessary (ANA, 1994a). These components are listed in Box 1-10.

Psychiatric nurses are faced with new educational challenges. They will integrate biologic content for safe and effective care, while still forging the proven basis for optimum client wellness—the art and science of the nurse-client relationship. It must all work together for comprehensive client care.

Psychiatric nurses are also responding to holistic methods of treating clients. These methods (for example, healing touch, nutrition, herbal medicine, massage, acupuncture, and acupressure) are becoming increasingly popular in the United States, and the trend will continue. Increasing numbers of mental health care providers espouse a combination of western and eastern methods for most comprehensive client care. Chapter 29 presents a detailed discussion of holistic health care and alternative therapies.

Societal Demands and Stressors

Genetics and biologic vulnerability have been scientifically implicated in several mental disorders. As previously described, these findings have affected major changes in thinking, and the pendulum of causality has swung far in the biologic direction.

Psychiatric mental health nurses do well to maintain balanced thinking, to avoid minimizing the part that psychosocial stressors play in mental well-being or mental

---

Box 1-10   Components of Psychiatric Nursing Education

- Neuroanatomy
- Physiology
- Biochemistry
- Psychiatry
- Psychology
- Physics
- Genetic/family correlates
- Neurology
- Neurosurgery
- Psychoimmunology
- Psychopharmacology
- Neuroimaging
- Computer sciences
- Psychoendocrinology
- Biologic rhythms
- Psychobiologic dysfunction
- Biologic theories of major mental disorders
- Chronobiology

---

disorder. Biology is influenced by environment and cannot function in a vacuum. For example, a genetically vulnerable individual who may be predisposed to substance dependence will not become dependent if he or she never has access to or chooses not to use mind-altering substances. On the other hand, a person who is faced with intolerable stressors may find drug use a viable alternative. In these instances, stressors and choice are important, as is biologic vulnerability.

As our society becomes more and more complex, it is safe to predict that occurrences of mental disorders may also increase. It seems evident that intolerance of increased societal demands has contributed to psychiatric diagnoses.

Scientific, Geographic, Sociopolitical, and Economic Factors

The United States continually becomes more homogenous. Geographic distances have shortened, and scientific discoveries instantly reach around the world. Present sociopolitical and economic factors remain a constant reminder of the degree to which countries are interdependent. The *International Classification of Mental Disorders* is very similar to the U.S. publication of the *Diagnostic and Statistical Manual of Mental Disorders*. Perhaps one answer to a reduction of symptoms of mental illness and treatment success lies in diverse cultures looking more to each other for common answers and solutions.

Psychiatric nursing and all other nursing disciplines face many changes that depend in large part on the government leaders who will direct and guide health care decisions and the allocation of funds for maintaining health care. In 1994 a major health care reform bill was defeated that included, among others, areas for prevention, maintenance, and restoration concerning mental health issues. Politics greatly affect the outcomes for mental health care. The current administrator has invited psychiatric nurse leaders to give input to this important subject, but the result remains unpredictable and will depend on priorities of future political leaders.

At present the entire country is undergoing countless changes in the operation of businesses and industries in an effort to maintain socioeconomic balance. One of the largest industries in the United States is health care, so we will inevitably continue to see many changes occur in nursing, and in the delivery of care to our clients.

Another factor that will influence mental health delivery systems is the increased influx of immigrants from many and varied countries who will see America as a promised land. The differences in cultures, the expectations of citizens and those wishing to be citizens, and the potential strain on an already compromised system will surely result in changes that are yet unforeseen. When countries cooperate and share information, on the other hand, positive results can occur.

The government is attempting to balance the federal budget which will greatly impact the financial resources available for health care. It remains a simple conclusion that the quantity and quality of future health care, including psychiatric nursing and all other nursing, rests on the decisions of a few, deciding for many.

Neither answers nor solutions have been provided, but the reader should be encouraged to think beyond the obvious. Expanded, creative thinking will need to be a constant for psychiatric-mental health nurses in this coming decade. Proactive rather than reactive involvement by psychiatric nurses in the making and changing of policies affecting our clients and ourselves will be valuable.

Summary of Key Concepts

1. Psychiatric-mental health nursing is a specialty within nursing and is recognized as one of the four core mental health practice areas.
2. The therapeutic nurse-client relationship is the basis of psychiatric-mental health nursing.
3. The client's needs are the focus of a therapeutic relationship.
4. The four stages of the nurse-client relationship are preorientation, orientation, working, and termination.
5. The ANA Standards of Care follow the steps of the nursing process and provide a framework within which psychiatric-mental health nursing is implemented and evaluated.

6. There is no one definition for mental health. Mental health is influenced by numerous and varied factors.

7. Ego defense mechanisms are the psychological processes used to protect the person from internal and external stressors and dangers.

8. Traditional mental health care in an inpatient setting is significantly decreasing as delivery systems in the community and home become more prevalent.

9. The most effective mental health care will be delivered through a team approach, applying the expertise of multiple mental health disciplines.

10. Psychobiologic research supports biologic basis for many mental disorders, with significant implications for psychiatric-mental health nursing.

11. Expanding scientific and computer technology, educational demands, societal stressors, and sociopolitical and economic factors all have important influence on the future of psychiatric-mental health nursing.

REFERENCES

American Journal of Nursing: Health Care Reform (video), 32nd Biennial Convention of Sigma Theta Tau. Alan Trench/Helene Fuld Trust, 1993.

American Nurses Association: *Standards of clinical nursing practice,* Kansas City, Mo., 1991, ANA.

American Nurses Association: *Psychiatric mental health nursing.* Psychopharmacology project. Washington, D.C., 1994a, ANA.

American Nurses Association: *A statement on public mental health clinical nursing practice and standards of public mental health nursing practice,* Washington, D.C., 1994b, ANA.

American Psychiatric Association: *Diagnostic and statistical manual of mental disorders,* ed 4, Washington, D.C., 1994, APA.

Beeber LS: The one-to-one relationship in nursing practice: the next generation. In Anderson CA, editor: *Psychiatric nursing 1974 to 1994: a report on the state of the art,* St. Louis, 1995, Mosby.

Bernstein L and Bernstein R: *Interviewing: a guide for health professions,* Norwalk, Conn., 1985, Appleton Century Crofts.

Betemps E and Ragiel C: Psychiatric epidemiology: facts and myths on mental health and illness, *J Nursing* 32:23, 1994.

Brammer L: *The helping relationship: process and skills,* Boston, 1993, Allyn & Bacon.

Caplan G: *Principles of preventive psychiatry,* New York, 1964, Basic Books.

Carkhoff R: *Helping and human realities,* New York, 1969, Holt, Rinehart, & Winston.

Carkhoff R and Traux C: *Toward effective counseling and psychotherapy,* Chicago, 1967, Aldine Publishing.

Clark MJ: *Nursing in the community,* Norwalk, Conn., 1992, Appleton & Lange.

Eaton W et al: The design of the epidemiologic catchment area surveys, *Arch of Gen Psychiatry* 41: 942, 1984.

Erikson E. Childhood in Society, ed 2, New York, 1963, WW Norton.

Fortinash K, Holoday-Worrett P: *Psychiatric nursing care plans,* ed 2, St. Louis, 1995, Mosby.

Freud A: *Ego and the mechanisms of defense,* New York, 1946, International Universities Press.

Grob GN: Mental health policy in America: *Health Affairs* Fall: 7, 1992.

Huffman K, Vernoy M, Williams B: *Psychology in action,* ed 2, New York, 1995, John Wiley & Sons.

Kaplan H and Sadock B: *Synopsis of psychiatry,* ed 6, Baltimore, 1994, Williams & Wilkins.

Kernberg O: *Borderline conditions,* New York, 1975, Aronson.

Kessler RC et al: Lifetime and 12 month prevalence of DSM-III psychiatric disorders in the United States, *Arch of Gen Psychiatry* 51:8, 1994.

Klerman GL: The National Institute of Mental Health Epidemiology Catchment Area (NIMH-ECA) Program, *Social Psychiatry Psychiatric Epidemiology* 21:159, 1986.

Klerman GL: Paradigm shifts in U.S. epidemiology since World War II, *Social Psychiatry Psychiatric Epidemiology* 25:27, 1990.

Leavell HR et al: *Preventive medicine for the doctor in his community,* ed 3, New York, 1965, McGraw-Hill.

Lego S: The one-to-one nurse-patient relationship. In Anderson CA, editor: *Psychiatric nursing 1974 to 1994: a report on the state of the art* St. Louis, 1995, Mosby.

Maxman J., Ward N: *Essential psychopathology and its treatment,* New York, 1995, WW Norton.

Mullahy C: *The case manager's handbook,* Gaithersburg, Md., 1995, Aspen Publications.

Peplau H: *Interpersonal relations in nursing,* New York, 1952, CP Putnam.

Redick R et al: Expansion and evolution of mental health care in the United States, *Center for Mental Health Services Publications #210,* 1994.

Robins L and Regier D, editors: *Psychiatric disorders in America: the epidemiological catchment area study,* New York, 1991, Free Press.

Ruben BD: The health caregiver-patient relationship: pathology, etiology, treatment. In Ray EB and Donohan L, editors: *Communication and health: systems and applications,* Hillsdale, N.J., 1990, Lawrence Earlbaum.

Sussman M-B *A curious calling,* Northvale, N.J., 1992, Jason Aronson.

Thompson TL: Patient health care: issues in communication. In Ray EB and Donohan L, editors: *Communication and health: systems and applications,* Hillsdale, N.J., 1990, Lawrence Earlbaum.

Witkin M et al: The effect of inflation on expenditures by mental health organizations between 1969 and 1990, *Center for Mental Health Services Publication No. 212,* 1994.

CHAPTER 2

Student Issues Regarding Client and Environment

Patricia A. Holoday-Worret

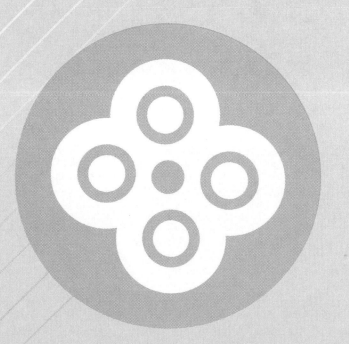

Acting out Behavior displaced from one situation to another in response to inner tension from unconscious impulses; the individual acts out an impulse instead of feeling, thinking, or discussing the tension-causing situation when it happens.

Indifference The manner in which the nurse interacts with the client that manifests as disconnectedness, unconcern, and aloof separation from the client's needs and situation.

Inference Interpreting behavior, finding motive, and forming conclusions.

Neutrality The manner in which the nurse interacts with the client that shows respect and acceptance but not excessive approval or disapproval.

Fear of performance inadequacy Feelings that less experienced nurses have concerning lack of skills for helping clients.

Positive affirmation Self-confirming and self-supporting message that reinforces confidence and enhances performance.

Positive cognitive set A positive outlook toward the world and others, and the belief that success is possible and that one can achieve what one believes.

Stereotype To form an oversimplified, standardized opinion of a person or group of people; often determined without adequate information.

Vicarious learning Learning through imagining the experiences of others as if they are one's own.

- Discuss reasons for nurses' fear of entering the psychiatric setting.

- Explain direction and intention in the psychiatric setting.

- Describe the importance of focusing on client strengths.

- Discuss the clinical priorities of nursing diagnoses and nursing intervention.

- Tell why it is important to think and observe for fluctuating symptoms rather than static behavior patterns and responses (more or less versus all or none).

- Explain the importance of avoiding evaluative responses when communicating with clients.

- Explain why it is better to simply observe client behavior than draw inferences about it.

- Discuss reasons for
  - stating observations versus making inferences
  - presenting alternatives versus solutions.

P sychiatric-mental health nursing is an engaging, challenging, and rewarding specialty. Interviews with experienced psychiatric nurses reveal a loyalty to the discipline, as illustrated in statements such as these:

- "Clients with psychiatric disorders have complex needs—no case is simple."

- "Psychiatric nursing requires and makes use of intuition that results in effective intervention when coupled with expertise."

- "Clients' emotional needs are often profound, and helping them meet those needs is a privilege that is satisfying."

- "The unpredictable environment prevents boredom—no two days are the same."

- "The fulfillment that comes from knowing I have helped a life take new direction is unequaled professionally."

- "I often have to be a detective."

- "Joy can be found in the most simple happenings and at unlikely moments."

Here are some examples of those nursing moments that make a psychiatric nurse's job so rewarding:

- A mute client speaks after weeks of silence.
- A child initiates interaction with the nurse after a lengthy period of being unable to show trust.
- A suicidal teenager states in group that she has several genuine reasons for wanting to live.
- Threatened with a break-up caused by a member's disorder, a family is armed with tools for managing their lives in more loving ways.

Nurses who work in the psychiatric setting are usually genuine, realistic, and able to discuss challenges concerning the practice. For instance, a routine atmosphere is not guaranteed, so the nurse must be ready for the unexpected. For example, clients sometimes say things that can embarrass or shock an inexperienced nurse, or cause hurt feelings. The nurse must remain aware that the client is probably **acting out** as a result of psychiatric disorder. That is, behavior is being displaced from one situation to another in response to inner tension from unconscious impulses; the client is acting out on impulse instead of feeling, thinking, or discussing the tension-

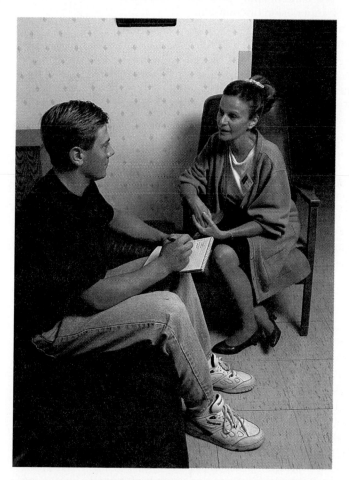

An interaction between a psychiatric nurse and an adolescent client. The nurse and the adolescent are discussing his strengths while he makes a list to keep for personal reference and reflection.

(Copyright Cathy Lander-Goldberg, Lander Photographics)

causing situation as it happens. The nurse is not necessarily a target, and the remarks are not intended as personal. The nurse's patience is frequently tested by the client's behavior or lack of behavior in the psychiatric setting. Nurses can experience excessive sadness or anger over a client's situation if they fail to maintain their personal boundaries.

CHALLENGES, EXPLANATIONS, SOLUTIONS

Student nurses and those just beginning a career in the psychiatric setting may experience situations that can be viewed as problematic. Some of these challenges are presented here. Each challenge is explained and solutions are provided that offer insight about the client, the nurse, and the situation. The challenges and solutions are summarized in Table 2-1 on page 30.

These explanations and solutions are not conclusive, and the readers will undoubtedly be able to discuss additional ones. The interpretations are meant for beginning nurses in an effort to increase insight and decrease discomfort or anxiety through **vicarious learning,** learning through imagining the experiences of others as if they are one's own.

Of course, there is no substitute for experience. Knowing what to do during interactions with clients will improve competence and decrease performance anxiety. Successful communication is more likely if the nurse will tolerate some initial discomfort in this new and dynamic environment, absorb the theory, and practice the skills. There are many rewards in being able to effectively communicate with clients in every psychiatric nursing setting.

Throughout this chapter, both student and graduate nurses are identified as nurse. Whether student or graduate, the challenges can be similar for any nurse, regardless of credentials.

CHALLENGE: FEAR OF ENTERING THE PSYCHIATRIC SETTING

There may be several reasons why the nurse experiences fear and anxiety before beginning a clinical rotation or position in the psychiatric setting. Two major reasons are predetermined stereotyped images of danger and self-doubt.

Stereotyped Images

To **stereotype** means to form an oversimplified, standardized opinion of a person or group of people. A stereotype is often determined without adequate information. Unfortunately, the general public often stereotypes people with mental disorders as insane, out of control, and dangerous. Films and books have reinforced this unrealistic image and have added to the fear. The new nurse, without experience, prepares to feel unsafe in these imagined circumstances.

Solutions to this challenge include:

- Learn and understand the formal psychiatric diagnoses (DSM-IV).
- Select safe units on which to begin interactions.
- Become familiar with unit policies and role expectations.
- Interact with clients.

An understanding of mental disorders, coupled with opportunity to interact with individuals who have the disorders, will quickly dispel stereotypes. Only a small percentage of people with mental disorders are dangerous toward others, and they will usually not be placed directly with other clients on units that are managed effectively. The nurse will soon begin to see clients as humans with problems who are to be helped, not feared.

TABLE 2-1 Suggested solutions to key challenges of working in the psychiatric-mental health nursing setting

Challenges	Solutions
1. Allay fear and anxiety by avoiding stereotyping people with mental disorders.	• Learn and understand formal psychiatric diagnoses (DSM-IV). • Select safe units on which to begin interactions. • Become familiar with unit policies and role expectations. • Interact with clients.
2. Address self-doubt about performance inadequacy and concern about own stability or mental health.	• Learn the principles of psychiatric-mental health nursing. • Learn and use therapeutic communication techniques. • Make yourself available to clients to gain experience. • Practice communication skills. • Review content about personal boundaries. • Seek supervision or counseling. • Maintain a positive cognitive set. • Practice positive affirmations.
3. Become action-oriented through direction and intention.	• Prepare daily objectives that are client-focused. • Validate objectives with client, staff, and the client's treatment plan. • Meet objectives by participating with intent. • Involve client in meeting objectives.
4. Focus on client strengths.	• Identify strengths with the client. • Focus on strengths. • Provide positive feedback to the client regarding strengths. • Encourage activities and behaviors that will increase and reinforce those strengths.
5. Prioritize nursing diagnoses and nursing interventions.	• Attend to safety and health issues first by ensuring client safety and prevention of self-harm or harm to others.
6. Think in terms of more or less versus all or none.	• Keep the client expected outcomes hopeful but realistic. • Avoid predicting client progress. • Be prepared for and accept an unpredictable course toward wellness. • Avoid absolute "black and white" thinking.
7. Avoid evaluative statements and responses when communicating with clients.	• Focus on behaviors; not the person. • Be neutral, but not indifferent. • Avoid evaluative statements. • Use statements of recognition.
8. Make observations instead of inferences.	• Respond through observation instead of inference. • Validate interpretations with the client to reach mutual conclusions. • Explore difficult conclusions with the client.
9. Offer alternatives rather than solutions.	• Help the client express concerns and problems. • Allow expression of feelings. • Help the client problem-solve toward solutions. • Avoid giving advice. • Offer multiple alternatives or options only when the client is unable to do so. • Facilitate choices.

Unit safety, a paramount issue, is the responsibility of the facility and staff. The nurse has a personal obligation to be thoroughly oriented to each unit and familiar with policies, procedures, and role expectations. Nurses with little experience will not be assigned to units where clients are potentially dangerous, unless the units are monitored by teaching staff who assume responsibility for safety. Well-operated units are usually safe.

Of course, the nurse does not provoke a situation that results in disruption. If disruption does occur, the beginning nurse should get experienced assistance immediately and usher uninvolved clients away from the area.

Self-Doubt

Self-doubt comes from several sources. In conjunction with the nurse's role in the psychiatric setting, two main sources of self-doubt are beliefs about performance inadequacy and concern about own stability or mental health.

PERFORMANCE INADEQUACY

Performance inadequacy is a fear experienced by novice nurses who tend to believe that they will not know what to say or do to help clients with their problems. "I don't know what to say to them" is a frequent remark when nurses have had little exposure to or experience with clients in this setting. They hear more experienced staff members who frequently seem to find the perfect words for clients. But they must remember that this seemingly simple process of communication is both an art and a science. The science or skills can be learned, and most communicators become artful with practice!

Solutions to this challenge include:

- Learn principles of psychiatric-mental health nursing.
- Learn and use therapeutic communication techniques.
- Make yourself available to clients to gain experience.
- Practice communication skills.

Nurses just starting in psychiatry have the responsibility of learning correct therapeutic communication techniques and practicing them in order to become skillful communicators. Chapter 7 further discusses these techniques.

Nurses need to be realistic about their performance expectations. They are not expected to be seasoned therapists during early encounters with clients. With opportunity, time, and attention on becoming skillful, they will ultimately succeed. Response selection, correctness, and timing will continue to improve. As a result, both nurses and clients will benefit.

Remember, precise words are not nearly as important as the capacity to convey a sense of caring to the client. Mistakes in communication inevitably will occur. However, they will be overlooked and forgiven if the client senses that the nurse has genuine empathy and a willingness to assist the client on his or her journey to wellness.

CONCERN ABOUT ONE'S OWN MENTAL HEALTH

Some psychiatric-mental health nurses fear that their own stability or mental health is inadequate for, or is compromised by being in the setting. The nurse who has difficulty maintaining personal boundaries may not feel emotionally strong enough to tolerate the depth of human problems in a psychiatric facility. This can be especially true if the nurse has had serious mental or emotional dysfunction in the past, or is currently experiencing overwhelming personal life stressors.

Newcomers sometimes say, "I worry that this could happen to me" or "My problems seem greater than some of theirs—why are they in the hospital and I'm not?" Undoubtedly, the reader has also heard of what is commonly called the "Medical or Nursing Student's Syndrome," meaning that the student believes he or she has symptoms of every disorder studied!

Solutions to this challenge include:

- Review content about personal boundaries.
- Seek supervision or counseling.
- Maintain a positive cognitive set.
- Practice positive affirmations.

Maintaining personal boundaries is essential in a therapeutic relationship. The nurse can then be empathic about the client's situation without becoming so personally involved that he or she loses objectivity and effectiveness. This topic is also covered more thoroughly in Chapters 1 and 7. The nurse with healthy boundaries and ego is prepared to maintain personal mental health.

It is important to discuss concerns about one's own mental health. Relief may come when the topic is addressed during a student or staff conference and the nurse learns that worry is not unique and that solutions are available. Deep concern requires conferring with an instructor or counselor who will objectively assess the problem and advise the nurse whether further counseling will be helpful.

Self-defeating thoughts can become self-fulfilling prophecies if repeated often enough. When the nurse continually focuses on worry, fear, or inadequacy, then successful role performance becomes difficult or impossible. Thinking positive thoughts constitutes possessing a **positive cognitive set.** This is a positive outlook toward the world and others, and the belief that success is possible and that one can achieve what one believes.

In conjunction with conscious effort to maintain a positive cognitive set, the nurse can practice **positive affirmations,** which are self-confirming and self-supporting messages that reinforce confidence and enhance performance. They can be self-fulfilling prophecies toward success. Examples of positive affirmations are the following:

- "I am able to study, learn, and practice this new and challenging content."
- "Every day, I become more proficient in nurse-client interactions."
- "I am as good at interviewing clients as I am supposed to be at this time."
- "I use therapeutic communication techniques."
- "I am relaxed and more capable each day."
- "Instructors and staff are here to assist me."
- "The client heals self, and I facilitate that progress, within my capacity; that capacity grows each day."

Once again—and it can't be said too often—fears will decrease and confidence will increase with greater knowledge, time, experience, and the resulting successful interpersonal interactions.

CHALLENGE: DIRECTION AND INTENTION

Entering any unfamiliar environment that requires performance is a challenge. The nurse who enters the psychiatric setting is there primarily to help clients achieve the following:

- Increase awareness of personal and relational issues that impair mental health and impede growth.
- Discuss difficult issues during therapeutic interactions.
- Engage in the problem-solving process.
- Share thoughts and feelings.
- Identify positive aspects of self and life.
- Accept self and others.
- Learn new skills for building competence and improving relationships.

To assist the client in these areas, the nurse must be action-oriented, rather than merely being an observer. When nurses fail to become active participants in the nurse-client relationship, both the client and the nurse fall short of meeting potential objectives, goals, and needs. Being action-oriented means moving beyond observing and assessing to become an actual facilitator. This does not imply that the nurse takes charge and does things to or for the client. It does imply, however, that client and nurse work together to formulate a personal plan of care and then collaboratively work the plan.

Objectives and goals are met only when there is a purposeful plan that provides direction, and the plan is put into action by intention. Sometimes nurses write exquisite client-focused objectives but fail to refer to or follow the plan in order to meet the objectives. Unless the plan is kept in mind, they revert to merely assessing, observing, and recording, rather than interacting with a purpose.

Solutions to this challenge include:

- Prepare daily objectives that are client-focused.
- Validate objectives with client, staff, and the client's treatment plan.

- Meet objectives by participating with intent.
- Involve client in meeting objectives.

CHALLENGE: FOCUS ON CLIENT STRENGTHS

Some psychiatric-mental health nurses just beginning a nursing rotation or career have a tendency to focus mainly on the client's disorders instead of on their healthy aspects and strengths. Psychiatric disorders often seem dramatic and fascinating, so it is easy to understand why the nurse's attention is directed toward dysfunction instead of health. In addition, there is a great deal to learn about psychiatric disorders, so energy gets channeled into learning and applying this information.

Solutions to this challenge include:

- Identify strengths with the client.
- Focus on strengths.
- Provide positive feedback to the client regarding strengths.
- Encourage activities and behaviors that will increase and reinforce those strengths.

The nurse's contact time with a client will be spent helping him or her overcome problems that stem from the disorders. But, more importantly, the nurse will also help the client build strengths, increase competence, and accentuate and reinforce reasons for living. With the treatment plan in mind, the nurse provides activities and encourages participation that will foster mental and emotional health and growth.

For several reasons, it may not be possible for some clients to identify their strengths directly after admission to the facility. For example, a psychotic state, severe depression, substance intoxication, or low self-esteem could all interfere with this process. However, as soon as these symptoms diminish, the nurse again focuses on the client's strengths. Some techniques for accomplishing this are:

- Ask the client's opinion about personal strengths and attributes.
- Ask the client his or her reasons for getting well.
- Allow time for the client to process thoughts—they may not come easily.
- Suggest that the client write a list of his or her strengths if unable to verbalize them.
- If client is unable to think of strengths, ask what a spouse, child, friend, member of the clergy, or significant other would say about client.
- Have staff members share observations about client strengths.

Staff members can also chart clients' strengths along with other progress to inform other members of the mental health team of important areas of focus. This ensures continuity of care and additional potential for reinforcement.

Clients who are grandiose, or have an exaggerated view of themselves, will probably have little difficulty telling about their real and imagined strengths and attributes. The nurse will be prepared to accept the client's behavior within appropriate limits and use therapeutic techniques to help him or her get more in touch with reality.

CHALLENGE: CLINICAL PRIORITIES

Prioritization of both nursing diagnoses and nursing interventions is essential to meet client's needs in a timely manner.

Nursing Diagnosis

When a client is admitted for psychiatric problems, the admission information may clearly state which problems are more urgent than others. However, often the admitting information is incomplete and the nurse must interview the client and significant others to determine prioritization of nursing diagnoses.

A major principle of psychiatric nursing is that safety and health issues are addressed first, as in the following clinical situation.

A 23-year-old female client was admitted to the unit following a suicide attempt. She had been severely depressed for several weeks, was currently abusing multiple substances, and had been treated at age 16 for anorexia nervosa. She lost 15 pounds over the month prior to admission.

Each problem is of major importance but the primary concern and first priority are to maintain the client's life. This second clinical situation concerns a holistic priority.

A 63-year-old male client was admitted to the acute care psychiatric facility by the police who were called because the client was shouting loudly and incoherently in his apartment and had barricaded his door. He had been grieving his wife's recent death, so the landlord became concerned about his behavior and sought help from the police. Upon admission, the experienced nurse assessed the client during an interview. Amidst his incoherence, he stated that his "wife gave him his insulin because she loved him." The nurse asked the lab to do his blood work, STAT. The client's psychiatric symptoms were actually from an insulin reaction, and the nurse's awareness kept him from becoming more disordered.

In this instance, the experienced psychiatric nurse was aware that medical problems can often affect a client's responses and behaviors. A common problem that can exist in psychiatric settings is the tendency to concentrate solely on psychiatric and communication problems and issues and ignore or forget medical and other aspects. Nursing is a holistic practice and requires assessment of all aspects of the client, regardless of the type of unit to which the client is admitted.

Solutions to such challenges include:

- List all client problems and needs.
- Convert client problems to nursing diagnoses.
- Prioritize nursing diagnoses.
- Practice prioritization.

Following an intake history, the nurse must determine an order of importance for every problem identified during assessment. In the psychiatric setting, it is easy to miss medical problems because psychiatric and communication problems and needs are often so outstanding. Remember safety and health issues. A helpful exercise when beginning psychiatric nursing is to develop hypothetical clinical situations containing multiple client problems, and to practice prioritizing.

Nursing Interventions

Priority of interventions within each nursing diagnosis is also necessary. For instance, consider a care plan that includes the priority nursing diagnosis of *Risk for Violence: Self-Directed*. The nurse is aware that a necessary nursing intervention is establishing a relationship in which the client can express thoughts and feelings about suicide and reasons for living.

But this intervention, even though important and at the heart of psychiatric nursing, is secondary to ensuring client safety and prevention of self-harm.

Solutions to such challenges include:

- Consider the client's unique manifestations of the nursing diagnosis.
- Prioritize nursing interventions under each nursing diagnosis.

CHALLENGE: MORE OR LESS VERSUS ALL OR NONE

Unlike most physical sciences that are predictable and exact, psychiatry can sometimes seem elusive to the beginning nurse. The definition, description, and categorization of psychiatric diagnoses in the *Diagnostic and Statistical Manual of Mental Disorders*, Fourth Edition (DSM-IV) appear exact. However, because of the complex nature of human beings, symptoms of the same name are manifested and expressed in unique ways by each client.

The nurse may initially think in absolutes, seeing symptoms as totally present or totally absent (that is, all or none). In reality, the client's symptoms may change slightly or dramatically over hours or days (that is, more or less). Because psychiatric symptoms can't always be measured by laboratory values, charts, and graphs, they are sometimes overlooked or missed completely by beginning nurses. Subtle changes may be clues that more dramatic changes are coming, so increases or decreases need to be carefully noted. For example, see the clinical situation that follows.

Charlotte was admitted to the psychiatric acute care unit because she was jogging down the center of a busy two-way traffic boulevard and taunting motorists. She was wearing multiple layers of brightly colored clothes, high heels, and excessive jewelry. She was shouting about the indignity of having to be in this facility against her will, which she termed a violation of her "personal, important rights." She was diagnosed with Bipolar Disorder; Manic type.

After several days of quiet surroundings, consistent unit routines, staff interventions, and medication (which she had stopped taking prior to admission), she calmed. Just before discharge, staff reports and charting stated that she seemed ready to return home.

Prior to discharge, her contact staff person noted that she began to change her clothes every few hours and the content of her conversation centered on "very important" things she was planning to accomplish when she got home. The staff member asked her if she had been taking her medication. Charlotte admitted she had been putting it in the toilet because she was getting too "normal" to get her plans accomplished. Discharge was postponed.

Solutions to such challenges include:

- Keep clients' expected outcomes hopeful but realistic.
- Avoid predicting client progress.
- Be prepared for and accept an unpredictable course toward wellness.
- Avoid absolute "black and white" thinking.

Symptoms are dynamic and are more like shades of grey than black and white. So the nurse will observe for fluctuation of symptoms rather than static, set patterns of behaviors and responses.

A client who is paranoid, for instance, may demonstrate mistrust by being loud and accusatory upon admission. He may then quiet down, but remain guarded, suspicious, and controlled on subsequent days. The symptom of paranoia is the same, but the manifestations change, depending on the client's internal stimuli, the unit environment, and present situation or events.

Another point is to write care plans reflecting realistic appraisal of client's symptoms, as seen in the following partial nursing care plan. Note that the correct realistic expectations indicate symptom reduction (more or less) rather than total absence (all or none).

Nursing Diagnosis: Altered thought processes related to impaired ability to process internal and external stimuli; stressful current family and work situation; manifested by guarded and suspicious behavior, statements that other clients are stealing his clothes and staff want to harm him.

Expected Outcomes:

Correct	*Incorrect*
Client will demonstrate decreased delusions of persecution within one week.	Paranoid delusions will be absent in one week.

CHALLENGE: EVALUATIVE RESPONSES

A general principle in psychiatric nursing states that the nurse will avoid using evaluative statements and responses when communicating with clients that indicate approval or disapproval (for example, good or bad, right or wrong) about the client's appearance, progress, or behavior. A more effective response from the nurse is neutral recognition. For example, see the clinical situation that follows.

Mrs. H, a 72-year-old woman, was hospitalized following the death of her spouse of 53 years. Although she suffered from major depression and chronic low self-esteem for several decades, he had remained loyal and loving. After admission, Mrs. H wore dark, drab clothing every day and cared for her hygiene only after constant encouragement from staff. After several days, she showered and came to breakfast wearing a pink printed dress. Jane, a nurse with little experience, was assigned to the unit. She said, "Oh, Mrs. H, you look so pretty in that pink dress. It's so much better than all those dark clothes you've been wearing." Mrs. H lowered her head and returned to her room. She refused breakfast, lunch, and activities, saying she didn't feel well. She came to dinner in her dark, drab clothing.

Withdrawn or depressed people reject praise because it is the opposite of their own present negative self-image. Praise conflicts with the client's mind-set of "I'm ugly," "I'm worthless," "I deserve nothing." The client either fails to hear the praise, or praise is discredited. Disapproval only serves to reinforce pathology, so it too needs to be avoided.

On the other hand, nurses sometimes learn to avoid direct approval or disapproval but mistakenly substitute indifference. Neutrality and indifference are not the same. **Indifference** manifests as disconnected, unconcerned, aloof separation from the client's needs and situation; it is the antithesis of psychiatric nursing. Nurses can still provide a necessary warm human experience and environment by maintaining **neutrality,** interaction with the client that shows respect and acceptance but not excessive approval or disapproval. Showing indifference toward a client who is mentally or emotionally compromised is like having the person take an ice cold shower in the dead of winter. It is certain to snuff out any spark of remaining spirit or soul.

Solutions to showing appropriate evaluative responses include:

- Focus on behaviors; not the person.
- Be neutral, but not indifferent.
- Avoid evaluative statements.
- Use statements of recognition.

Of course, limits may need to be appropriately set on self-defeating behaviors. When doing the latter, the nurse will comment on behaviors while avoiding statements about the person's worth. Compare the nurse's comments to the client in the following two examples.

- *Correct:* "During group yesterday, it was agreed that each client would be ready to go on the field trip by 8 A.M. Because you are refusing to dress, the trip is behind schedule. The bus will leave in 15 minutes." (Comment on behavior.)

- *Incorrect:* "You are so slow and undependable. Everyone is on the bus and thinks you're terrible for holding up the field trip." (Comment on the person's worth.)

Neutral statements recognize the person's behavior. Recall Mrs. H and the pink dress. Appropriate neutral statements to her would be, "I see you showered before breakfast, Mrs. H" and "You're wearing a pink printed dress today." These statements, that imply neither approval nor disapproval, offer recognition and may elicit responses from the client that offer further insight into her problems. Evaluative statements, on the other hand, close communication and the client either withdraws from the interaction or becomes defensive.

Here are two other examples of neutral statements:

- "You decided to join the group today, Tom. Seats are not assigned, so sit anywhere you wish."

- "I notice you received all your points yesterday for attending school and the scheduled activities, Amber."

Evaluative statements are discouraged for other reasons as well. If staff praises the client too soon, he or she may fear support will be withdrawn. Even though rehearsing new behaviors, the client may still feel vulnerable and revert to old behaviors to regain imagined loss of support. Or, a client may believe he or she is acceptable only if he or she looks or behaves in the specified evaluative way. If the client can't comply with the evaluation, he or she may feel even more unworthy.

Some psychiatric nurses may disagree with this practice and freely offer praise for positive behavior. This practice has merit when it is clear that the client is ready to receive praise. Each case is unique, but the nurse has responsibility to understand the client and the situation before choosing responses.

CHALLENGE: INFERENCES VERSUS OBSERVATIONS

It is sometimes difficult for the nurse who is new to the psychiatric setting to avoid inferences about a client's behavior. An **inference** is an interpretation of behavior that is made by finding motive and forming conclusions without having all the information. When inferences are made, the nurse interprets the client's behavior, decides on a reason, assigns a motive, and forms a conclusion. There is great potential for error and unfairness.

Some dangers in drawing inferences are that the nurse is operating from his or her own experience and frame of reference that may have little or no connection to the client's actual behavior. In addition, when the nurse makes an inference and forms a conclusion, the client is robbed of the opportunity to problem-solve and share thoughts and ideas about important issues. A false conclusion may also misdirect treatment objectives.

Interpreting client behaviors and making inferences is not always negative, and seasoned nurses do it frequently. The difference is that experienced nurses take additional steps before final conclusions are reached.

Solutions to this challenge include:

- Respond through observation instead of inference.
- Validate interpretations with the client to reach mutual conclusions.
- Explore conclusions with the client.

To avoid making inferences, the nurse operates from an understanding of the importance of obtaining a client's viewpoint about situations and events that affect his or her own life instead of forming a personal opinion. Also, the nurse draws conclusions by responding to client behaviors without interpreting them. This means that the nurse simply observes behaviors. For example:

- "I saw your wife leave, Jim, and now you're crying."

- "Yesterday you sat alone, Tommy, but today the other children joined you."

- "Marsha, what you just said got a major reaction from the group."

Notice that the nurse does not offer any conclusions to these obviously significant situations. It may be difficult for the nurse to relinquish giving his or her concluding opinion, but it is a necessary, rewarding tactic.

The client will usually respond to the nurse's statement, and then communication, reasoning, and problem solving can begin. The more experienced nurse will continue beyond observation to interpretation. The critical difference is that the nurse immediately validates the interpretation with the client, and a mutual conclusion is formed or at least brought to awareness for future discussion. Here is an example of the entire four step process.

- Step 1. "I saw your wife leave, Jim, and now you're crying." (*Observation*)

- Step 2. "You said earlier that she was coming in today to discuss a divorce." (*Interpretation*)

- Step 3. "Is that the reason you're feeling sad now?" (*Validation*)

- Step 4. "This might be a good time for us to discuss your relationship." (*Offer to engage*)

Notice that the nurse is not guessing but rather is reasoning based on past information. Also, the client now has an opportunity to validate. The last important step is the nurse's willingness to be available to the client for processing this event through therapeutic communication.

CHALLENGE: ALTERNATIVES VERSUS SOLUTIONS

Nurses may feel inadequate before beginning to work in the psychiatric setting because they worry that they don't have answers for the clients' problems. Clients, not nurses, however, are responsible for their lives. This, of course, does not mean that nurses abandon clients who are searching for answers.

Solutions to this challenge include:

- Help the client express concerns and problems.
- Allow expression of feelings.
- Help the client problem-solve toward solutions.
- Avoid giving advice.
- Offer multiple alternatives or options only when the client is unable to do so.
- Facilitate choices.

The nurse engages in therapeutic communication with the client, facilitating expression of thoughts and feelings. When the client is able to hear his or her own words, the problem-solving process has begun and the client starts to reach his or her own solutions.

It is important for the nurse to avoid giving advice. The client probably doesn't want the nurse's opinion as much as he or she wants the nurse to stay engaged while the client talks; there is a relief in expressing problems openly to a willing listener. If the client asks, "What would you do?" or "What do you think I should do?", the nurse can reply, "I think it is more important for you to decide what works best for you. Let's talk about your ideas."

Another reason to avoid offering advice and solutions is that doing so negates the client. He or she feels less worthwhile and maybe even infantilized, as if a parent is dictating how the client should conduct his or her life. Also, the nurse's solutions may not fit the client's lifestyle or self-image.

If the client for any reason (depression, cognitive impairment or deficit, state of crisis) is unable to come up with answers, the nurse can then offer alternatives or options. This means offering assistance and giving some

prompting without providing answers or advising. For example:

- "Some things that have worked for other people in similar situations are . . . (name several options). Do any of these seem reasonable for you?"
- "Have you considered . . . (give several choices)?"
- "What are some of the options you have for placement when you're discharged? Some that come to mind are . . . (give several realistic and appropriate choices)."

The nurse may need to be more definitive in helping the client when the client sees no solutions. For example: "You said you are a workaholic and can't relax since you got your own business. What leisure activities have you enjoyed in the past? Which of those would you enjoy now if you had the time? What did you like most about (golfing, fishing)? Who do you trust to run the business while you take vacations? Since the business is open Monday through Friday, when could you find time to (golf, fish)?"

Most clients possess the solutions they need and only require assistance to bring these solutions to their awareness.

Summary of Key Concepts

1. Students may fear entering the psychiatric setting because of predetermined stereotypes of danger and self-doubt.

2. Students can remain realistic about their performance expectations.

3. Nurses need stable mental health themselves before they attempt to stabilize clients.

4. An action-oriented nurse will meet the client's treatment goals.

5. Focusing on client strengths fosters emotional and mental health and growth.

6. The priority intervention is ensurance of client safety and prevention of harm.

7. Comments to clients should focus on behavior, rather than personal worth.

8. Relating observations rather than inferences leaves the conclusions to the client.

9. Offering alternative problem-solving techniques gives control to the client and builds self-esteem, while providing the solution suggests the client is incapable of handling the situation.

REFERENCES

Fortinash K, Holoday-Worret P: *Psychiatric nursing care plans,* ed 2, St. Louis, 1995, Mosby.

Holoday-Worret P: Accumulated clinical anecdotal notes, (unpublished).

Peplau H: *Interpersonal relations in nursing,* New York, 1982, Putnam.

CHAPTER 3

Legal-Ethical Issues

Joyce Laben

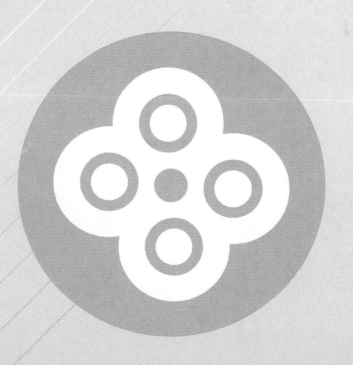

Clear and convincing evidence A burden of proof that requires more than that used in a civil proceeding and less than that used in a criminal proceeding. Civil proceedings call for merely a preponderance of evidence, whereas criminal proceedings require proof beyond a reasonable doubt.

Commitment Court order certifying that an individual is to be confined to a mental health facility for treatment.

Competency to stand trial The ability of the individual to understand the charges and their consequences, to comprehend the nature and object of the legal proceedings, and to advise an attorney and assist in the defense.

Duty to warn Legal obligation of a mental health professional to warn an intended victim of potential harm from a mental health client.

Expert witness Someone with education and experience on a specialized sub-

ject who is qualified as an expert and is allowed to testify, thereby assisting the jury in understanding technical information.

Least restrictive alternative Providing the least restrictive treatment in the least restrictive setting for a mental health client.

Legal duty Something that an individual is required to do by law.

Mandatory outpatient treatment An individual is legally required to undergo mental health treatment in an outpatient setting. The individual usually has been noncompliant and allegedly has a propensity for dangerous acts.

Privileged communication Communication between a professional and a client is confidential and protected from forced disclosure in court unless authorized by the client. The privilege is delegated by statutes in various states.

- Discuss the various historical events that affected the passing of commitment laws.

- Compare and contrast the various forms of admissions to mental health facilities.

- Explain the difference between confidentiality and privileged communication.

- Identify situations in which the duty to warn should be invoked.

- Discuss the rights of mental health clients and identify how these rights apply in practice.

- Distinguish between the concepts of competency to stand trial and insanity defense.

- Apply the elements of malpractice to a current practice situation.

- Describe situations in mental health treatment in which the ethical issues of autonomy and paternalism are prevalent.

HISTORICAL REVIEW

According to Sales and Shuman (1994), law and mental health have been intertwined for many years. Even in ancient Rome the law was concerned about the legal status of the mentally disabled. Should the individual have a guardian? Could the individual enter into a contract? According to Roman law, the person with a mental disability could not form a marriage contract and if made a ward could not have any legal capacity (Brakel et al, 1985).

During the Middle Ages, people with mental illnesses were considered to be possessed by demons. The king could hold custody of property of these people. The profits were applied to the maintenance of the individuals and their households. When a person was thought to be incompetent because of mental illness, a jury of twelve men would decide whether to commit the individual to the care of a friend, who would receive an allowance for maintenance (Brakel et al, 1985).

In the American colonies of the seventeenth century, the lack of facilities meant that families were expected to care for people with mental illnesses. If a person had no family or friends, the individual might wander from town to town—in some instances in the company of transient groups. There was no distinguishing between a vagrant and a person with a mental illness; therefore, all were treated as itinerant poor persons. As early as 1676, a law was passed in the state of Massachusetts to manage people who were considered to have mental illnesses and be dangerous. The individual could be detained, but generally no procedures for commitment of a person with a mental illness were instigated at this time (Brakel et al, 1985).

It was not until 1752 that Pennsylvania Hospital in Philadelphia opened to treat people with mental illnesses (Laben and MacLean, 1989). In Williamsburg, Virginia, in 1773, a facility was opened by the state especially for treatment of people with mental illnesses. The next state institution erected was in Lexington, Kentucky, in 1824 (Brakel et al, 1985).

In 1841 Dorothea Dix began her crusade for placing individuals with mental illnesses in specially built hospitals rather than placing them in almshouses, jails, and hospitals for the mentally ill. During the following years, Dix traveled throughout the United States, pressing for moral and humanistic treatment of people with mental illnesses (Laben and MacLean, 1989).

During the late nineteenth and early twentieth centuries, laws were passed by various states enacting civil commitment procedures for people with mental illnesses. From 1900 to 1955, the population in mental institutions grew from 150,000 to 819,000 inpatients in state and county mental hospitals (LaFond, 1994). Passage of the Community Mental Health Centers Act of 1963 authorized monies to build community treatment centers. Shortly thereafter, civil rights lawyers began to challenge the treatment of people with mental illnesses. During the Vietnam War era, a distrust of government emerged. Judicial activism began with concern about the treatment of people with mental illnesses and maintenance of their rights. More consideration was given to individual rights; especially questioned was the long-standing practice of hospitalizing individuals for many years, in some instances without much treatment (LaFond, 1994).

Commitment to mental hospitals was no longer seen as a medical decision but rather a decision to be entrusted to a neutral decision-maker, such as a judge. Many laws were changed at this time to encompass not only mental illness but also dangerousness. In addition to this criteria, individuals with mental illness who were unable to care for themselves were labeled "gravely disabled" and were committed.

Large numbers of individuals were released into the community, raising concerns that there were not appropriate facilities and services to adequately care for them within the community. Because of the increasing number of people with mental illnesses in the community and the appointment of more conservative judges, who were reluctant to become involved in the administration

of hospitals, recommendations for expanding the mental health commitment laws emerged. A tendency developed in some jurisdictions, such as the state of Washington, where more individuals were committed under the gravely disabled criteria rather than the dangerousness criteria. LaFond emphasizes that once again mental health professionals are being given the responsibility for caring for the people with mental illnesses who are involuntarily committed. "Unfortunately, this broadened mandate is all too seldom accompanied by the resources required for the task" (LaFond, 1994). Efforts to balance the rights of people with mental illnesses vs. the concerns of the community continue as we move toward the twenty-first century.

COMMITMENT

Least Restrictive Alternative

When an individual enters mental health treatment, determining the best location for the individual's treatment is crucial. The concept of **least restrictive alternative** means providing mental health treatment in the least restrictive environment, utilizing the least restrictive treatment. About 30 years ago an elderly woman who was hospitalized at St. Elizabeth's in Washington, D.C., filed a writ of habeas corpus so that she could be released into the community. At that time, there were few alternatives to hospitals for treatment. The court ruled there should be alternatives to inpatient facilities, including halfway houses, nursing homes, and day treatment programs (*Lake v. Cameron,* 1966).

Developing a treatment plan involves consideration of all alternatives, including such options as inpatient treatment, day treatment, and respite, foster, and home health care. An individual residing in a community that has developed many care options is the least likely to be hospitalized. Because health care costs have escalated in the last few years, the most cost-effective, as well as the most appropriate, intervention to assist the client should be selected.

Voluntary Admissions

Legally, **commitment** refers to a court order certifying that an individual is to be confined to a mental health facility for treatment. Generally, there are three types of commitments in each of the states: an emergency commitment, a voluntary commitment, and an involuntary indefinite commitment. The details may vary from state to state as do the mechanisms for admission. Nurses are most familiar with the voluntary admission: individuals come to the hospital and agree to be treated.

Informed Consent

Upon admission, clients should be informed about the treatments involving material risks (that is, risks that a reasonable person would consider significant). For example, the side effect tardive dyskinesia can occur with neurologic drugs and, in some instances, is irreversible and would be considered a material risk. In addition, the client should know alternatives to the treatment and possible side effects of these alternatives. If the individual agrees to a treatment, the consent can be revoked at any time (Laben and MacLean, 1989).

The emphasis should be placed on including the individual in the decision-making process. The problem with admissions into a mental health facility is that, in some instances, the individual's ability to make an informed decision is questionable. Generally, unless the person has been declared incompetent to manage personal matters, the individual is considered able to give consent.

However, in emergency situations, where clients require treatment as the result of behavior that is dangerous to themselves or others, treatment can be provided without the clients' consent. State laws vary, both in emergency and judicial commitment statutes, regarding the limits of such treatment. Under any other conditions, if a person cannot give informed consent, a guardian must be appointed. It is difficult to maintain that a person who is acutely psychotic has the ability to make an informed decision. It is, however, incumbent upon mental health professionals to continually inform clients about treatment and to provide a list of client rights at the time of admission or soon after.

Recently, there was an occurrence that generated national interest. Individuals with schizophrenia were selected to be in a research study. A controversy ensued when some of the clients were withdrawn from antipsychotic medication and suffered severe exacerbations as a result. One individual committed suicide. The purpose of the study was to observe the client's behavior when withdrawn from medication. The question has arisen as to whether the clients were sufficiently informed about the severity of the symptoms that might occur if withdrawn from medication. Some ethicists have stated that it was not ethical to withdraw the medication when, most assuredly, psychotic symptoms would reoccur (Hilts, *New York Times,* March 1994).

Involuntary Admissions

When some individuals become mentally ill, they refuse to seek treatment for a variety of reasons. A person could be suffering from paranoid delusions that someone is going to inflict harm, and therefore help is rejected because of the psychiatric symptomatology. In some instances, the individual can be dangerous because of suicidal ideation or commanding hallucinatory voices that demand that harm be done to another person. This situation poses a likelihood of serious harm to the individual as well as other members of the community. Under these circumstances, an emergency commitment might be appropriate.

Emergency Commitment

Emergency commitment is different from a judicial or indefinite commitment in that it is for a shorter period of time and generally has more restrictive criteria for admission. Usually, a state will require that the individual be seen initially by a mental health official, such as a physician, psychologist, social worker, or advanced practice nurse. Some states require a licensed physician. The examining professional cannot be on the staff of the admitting facility. Once the individual is brought to the inpatient unit, examination by a second mental health professional, usually a physician, must take place. This procedure protects the rights of the individuals. Usually, within a short period (5 days or less, excluding weekends and holidays) a probable cause hearing must take place to continue the person's hospitalization. For emergency admissions, the standard criterion for an involuntary commitment is likelihood of harm to self or others. In some jurisdictions, the term *gravely disabled* recently has come into use (Laben and MacLean, 1989; Appelbaum, 1994).

In Alabama, an individual with paranoid schizophrenia contended his commitment into a psychiatric facility was not proper, because he had not perpetrated any recent dangerous acts. The mental health professional (a psychologist) testified that the client had threatened to harm others on previous occasions, was not compliant with medication, and had threatened a woman who had terminated her relationship with him. The court upheld the commitment by clear and convincing evidence that he needed continued inpatient treatment (*Mink v. Alabama Department of Mental Health and Mental Retardation,* 1993).

The standard of proof that must be offered to uphold a commitment proceeding is **clear and convincing evidence.** A United States Supreme Court decision ruled that the civil standard of preponderance of the evidence as used in civil lawsuits was insufficient to use in a commitment hearing that deprived a person of liberty. The criminal standard of "beyond a reasonable doubt" was not utilized because the purpose of a commitment was not to punish but to treat the individual (*Addington v. Texas,* 1979). Therefore the middle standard of clear and convincing evidence was deemed sufficient.

Civil or Judicial Commitment

An indefinite judicial or civil commitment is for a longer period of time than an emergency commitment. The legal basis for detention of an individual for treatment lies in the *parens patriae* power of the state to protect and care for individuals with disabilities and the police power of the state to protect the community from persons who pose a threat. A judicial commitment allows for involuntary hospitalization not only of persons dangerous to self or others but also for people with other kinds of behavioral problems—such as inability to provide self-care because of mental illness (Laben and MacLean, 1989).

For a judicial commitment, the individual must be given time to prepare a defense to state why hospitalization is not necessary. The client has the right to have his or her attorney cross-examine the mental health professionals regarding the necessity for inpatient treatment. The client may also appeal a decision of a lower court (see Understanding and Applying Research below).

Preventive or Mandatory Outpatient Treatment

In recent years, because of the concept of least restrictive alternative, long-term hospitalization, especially in state hospitals, has decreased. A dilemma has arisen about what to do with individuals who, upon discharge from an inpatient treatment facility, discontinue medication, deteriorate, and exhibit dangerous behavior. Legislation for preventive commitment or involuntary outpatient treatment was subsequently enacted. According to Geller (1991), half of the United States currently support such legislation. In Tennessee, an individual must be judicially committed and **mandatory outpatient treatment** ordered prior to discharge. If the individual does not remain in compliance with the treatment agreement, the treating professional files an affidavit with the court, and the client is ordered to appear in court before a

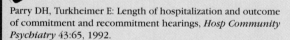
Understanding and Applying
RESEARCH

Parry DH, Turkheimer E: Length of hospitalization and outcome of commitment and recommitment hearings, *Hosp Community Psychiatry* 43:65, 1992.

Researchers describe commitment proceedings at a large state hospital in Virginia over a 3-month period in 1988. More than half of the 190 individuals were at the initial commitment hearing and 184 were at recommitment hearings. As the individuals' time in the hospital increased, attorneys were less likely to consult with the client/respondent to review the information in the charts or to cross-examine the clinical examiner. Judges were less likely to inform the respondents of their right to legal counsel or the right to appeal or to contemplate a voluntary admission. Based on this information, nurses need to take steps to ensure that clients are not confined to mental health facilities for long periods without meaningful treatment and frequent assessments of their ability to be discharged to a less restrictive environment.

judge and to state why compliance has not been maintained. The individual can be returned to the hospital for noncompliance with the treatment plan (*Tenn Ann Code* §33-6-201). Other states do not have a hearing for noncompliance as a criteria for rehospitalization (*Rhode Island Department of Mental Health, Retardation, and Hospitals v. RB*, 1988). The standard for rehospitalization does not have to be dangerousness or likelihood of serious harm, although this is usually a potential result of noncompliance. It is the treating professionals' responsibility to closely follow the individuals mandated to receive treatment. If these people become compliant and no longer need the surveillance demanded by mandatory outpatient treatment, in some instances the treating professionals can remove them from this requirement by writing a letter to the court.

CONFIDENTIALITY

Confidentiality of information is a concept that nurses learn early in their education. Information given to them by clients is considered private and should not be disseminated, either verbally or in writing, without the permission of the client or guardian. Confidentiality of client information is clearly defined in the American Nurses' Association *Code of Ethics*.

A recent court decision was related to a confidentiality issue. A doctor revealed a client's HIV status to the attorney of the client's employer. The individual, a flight attendant, was HIV positive and sought treatment from a physician for an ear and sinus infection. The flight attendant explicitly stated that the HIV status was not to be included on insurance forms because it might endanger his employment. The doctor agreed to this specification. One month later, the client filed a claim with a state workers' compensation board. A subpoena from another state was sent to the physician along with authorization from the client for two earlier workers' compensation claims, but not for this claim. The doctor sent the record with the HIV status to the attorney. A New York appeals court ruled that by revealing the client information to the requesting parties, the doctor had not acted in good faith. The subpoena was voluntary and from another state. This case illustrates that even with a subpoena a health care professional should not release information without consulting with an attorney from the facility where employed (*Doe v. Roe*, 1993).

Questions have been raised also about the confidentiality limits of group therapy. Currently there are no known laws requiring clients to respect the confidentiality of other group members. However, it is important to stress to group members the importance of not revealing information outside of the therapy session. The participants should consider themselves co-therapists who help to ensure the comfort and safety of other group members. In group therapy perhaps each member should sign a contract relative to confidentiality (Appelbaum and Greer, 1993).

Confidentiality must be considered with changing technology. Computer-generated records will become more and more prevalent. They are time-efficient for the provider, and generation of data is useful for utilization review, diagnosing, treatment planning, and communicating through various networks. It is paramount that information be secure; a system of passwords should be included to gain entry to the system. Those who have accessed the network should be monitored (Mordai and Rabinowitz, 1993).

Privileged Communication

Privileged communication is different from confidentiality. It is enacted by statute to designated professionals, such as the clergy, attorneys, psychologists, or physicians. Privilege extends to information elicited in the therapeutic relationship. In many states, nurses are not included. The provisions of these statutes allow certain information given to the professionals by clients to remain secret during any litigation. The privilege belongs to the client and can be asserted or waived only by the client. These statutes exclude reporting child and elder abuse (in some instances), domestic violence, some communicable diseases, and information that could prevent the commission of a felony, such as murder.

Release of Information

States have specific statutes related to release of mental health records. Nurses practicing in this clinical area should be aware of the state and federal statutes and guidelines relative to release of information. When clients are admitted to mental health facilities and have been treated on prior occasions, a request is usually extended to the client to authorize release of prior records. The kind of records requested, and for what period of time, should be clearly spelled out on the authorization form. Contents of records should not be released over the telephone unless the health care professional has a release signed by the client and is familiar with the other professional to whom the information is being given. Courts have generally considered that information contained in health records belongs to the client, and the actual record is the property of the treating professional or health care facility (Laben and MacLean, 1989). Most individuals no longer have problems obtaining records; however, obtaining the information can be expensive.

Duty to Warn

Twenty years ago, a case came to the forefront that changed the manner in which mental health professionals dealt with warning their clients' potential victims. The landmark decision *Tarasoff v. Regents of the University of California* (1976) concerned a young man

from India, Prosenjit Poddar, who was attending the University of California. He had formed a relationship with Tatiana Tarasoff and had misinterpreted a New Year's Eve kiss as a serious romantic gesture. After several months, she conveyed to him that she wished to date other men, and she did not view their relationship as serious. He subsequently became depressed and sought mental health counseling. He communicated to his therapist that he might harm Tarasoff who, at that time, was in South America. One day he ran out of the therapist's office and was detained by the campus police and released. After Tarasoff's return, he went to her home and fatally wounded her with a knife. The family of the victim brought suit against the University of California and, after the case reached the Supreme Court of California, the justices ruled that "protective privilege ends where the public peril begins." This ruling, **duty to warn,** established responsibility of a treating mental health professional to notify an intended, identifiable victim.

Since this time, many states and federal jurisdictions have promulgated decisions and passed statutes that delineate the duty to warn potential identifiable victims. In Vermont, the court imposed the duty to warn when an individual posed a threat of potential harm to property. Mr. Peck was seen by an outpatient counselor to whom he communicated that he was angry with his father and wanted to set fire to his father's barn. The next day, a family session was held with the father present. Five days later, Peck stated that he would set fire to his father's barn. He promised the therapist that he would not burn down the barn; however, despite this agreement, he did later ignite the structure. The court ruled that the therapist had a duty to inform the parents of the threat to their property (*Peck v. the Counseling Service of Addison County, Inc.,* 1985).

Nurses should be aware of any case law related to this matter within their jurisdiction. In addition, several states have passed statutes in relation to this issue defining the responsibility of mental health professionals and the duty to warn potential victims (*Tenn Ann Code* §33-10-103 and *Cal Civ Code* §43.92).

RIGHTS OF CLIENTS

According to Wexler and Winick (1992), mental health law based on the constitutional premise of protecting client rights is a little more than 20 years old. Prior to that time, there was little litigation or attention paid to the rights of individuals in mental health facilities.

Although the number of lawsuits that emerged in the 1970s and 1980s has decreased, certain rights not afforded to people with mental illnesses in institutions prior to that time are now taken for granted. Currently, when individuals enter a mental hospital, it is a rarity (not a probability) that the individuals have had their civil rights removed. Therefore these individuals have retained the right to vote, to manage financial matters, and to assert the constitutional right to seek the advice of an attorney. Other rights usually include the rights to receive mail, to wear one's own clothes, and to receive visitors (although, in forensic units, a limitation on the days and hours could be delineated).

The state of Pennsylvania requires that voluntary clients receive a summary of their rights on admission to an inpatient facility and a more inclusive manual of the rights within 72 hours. A study that was conducted in an urban university-affiliated hospital with 50 subjects concluded that only a minority of the subjects understood their rights after having them read by a nurse, followed up by a written copy. The implications are that, as part of the treatment plan, discussion and reinforcement of client rights should be an ongoing process (Wolpe, Schwartz, and Sanford, 1991). The state of Washington provides for a list of rights to be posted in the facility (*Wash Ann Code* §71.05.370). See Nursing Care in the Community below for a discussion of legal issues and community psychiatric nursing.

Access to Client Records and Confidentiality

The majority of states provide for client access to records. Generally, there is a procedure to be followed. Release forms should be signed if information is provided to a third party (Lyon, Levine, and Susman, 1982).

When a relative or significant other desires information about the client, a release form should be signed by the client prior to release of any data. Especially with people with serious and persistent mental illnesses who have family members involved with their care, it is important to collaborate with the family on treatment to maintain the individual in the community without frequent exacerbations. With the shorter length of stay in a hospital and, in some areas, the lack of wide-based community alternatives, coordination of care with significant others is important. "The issue of confidentiality must be carefully considered but not used as an artificial barrier to collaboration. Formal and informal strategies can resolve the conflict between the patient's confidentiality and the family's compelling need for information fundamental to successful caregiving" (Reinhard, 1994). This stance does not negate the signing of release of information by the client for relatives to receive information but instead stresses the importance of the family in caregiving.

Seclusion and Restraints

Seclusion and restraint were major issues in two well-known cases: the right to treatment suit in Alabama (*Wyatt v. Stickney,* 1972) and the evaluation of seclusion practices at a state hospital in Massachusetts (*Roger v. Okin,* 1980). In the latter case, seclusion had been insti-

Nursing Care in the Community

Legal and Ethical Issues

The expansion of mental health nursing care into the community presents unique legal and ethical concerns for the nurse. The community psychiatric nurse's role is greatly influenced by laws that were initially intended to promote and protect the rights of the individual client but now threaten to engulf the mental health system itself. Often the right of the individual to receive treatment seems to be in conflict with the right of the individual to refuse treatment. The right to refuse treatment usually takes precedence, unless the client is deemed to be a danger to self or others or is in some way gravely disabled. Nurses must often make grim decisions, balancing the expressed desire of the clients against what would be in their best interests mentally, emotionally, and physically.

These decisions can impair the trust implicit in the therapeutic relationship with the client. A broader effect may be felt in the community, because other clients might react defensively in response to the involuntary hospitalization of a friend. Nurses' commitments to advocacy may be called into question, jeopardizing their position in the mental health community. Alternative solutions should be thoroughly explored to ensure that the principle of least restrictive treatment for the client is upheld, while main-

taining the integrity of the environment for the surrounding community. How much deviant behavior is tolerable before the integrity of the community is compromised?

Nurses may also experience internal conflicts among the expectations of meeting legal requirements, containing costs, and satisfying personal ethical values. Mental health nurses practicing in the community have expanded the scope of their independence, which demands greater responsibility and accountability. Documentation must be rigorous, thorough, and accurate, leaving no opportunity for legal challenges. Treatment plans should be clearly stated, with accompanying rationales and anticipated outcomes. Standards of care and client outcome should be measurable in concrete ways and treated as if they were part of a research study. The nurse's ethical ideals will be mollified by painstaking attention to the details of client care in accordance with the requirements of the law. The nurse should have an adequate support system for addressing legal and ethical issues, including a consultant to explore legal ramifications of specific interventions and a working network in which to discuss and explore treatment options.

gated when there was no immediate threat of violence or threatening behavior. *Wyatt* outlines guidelines for instituting seclusion and restraint. Recently, the original 20-year-old guidelines were updated by a federal judge. These standards include the instruction that clients should only be restrained to prevent "physical injury to themselves or others." Only a psychiatrist or licensed physician can order nonemergency seclusion or restraint, and the doctor must be present and evaluate the client before writing the order (News & Notes, 1992). The new guidelines set 8 hours instead of 24 as the maximum of the original order. The client must be observed every 15 minutes instead of every hour as previously outlined. An order for seclusion and restraint can be issued by a nurse for 1 hour, but the nurses must be physically present and document observations in the client's chart. A qualified physician must be notified after the emergency and see the client within 4 hours; however, 1 hour is preferred. Although these guidelines are only binding in Alabama, when originally disseminated, they were used as guidelines in other states and mental health organizations (News & Notes, 1992).

Although research is limited in guiding the nurse about the implementation of seclusion, Outlaw and Lowery (1992) recommend that seclusion be used only when necessary and not for events such as refusing to take medications, participating in activities, or for making loud noises. Research shows that secluding a client is viewed by the staff as upsetting. Some clients also see seclusion as a very negative experience, whereas others view it as a reward.

Norris and Kennedy (1992) recommend that explanations about what is happening be given to the isolated individual and that special attention be given to assessing the individual's physical needs. Every attempt should be made to minimize a struggle, and the person should be placed in seclusion or restraints in the least restrictive manner. Afterward, talking with the client can help decrease the psychological impact.

Nurses should be familiar with the seclusion and restraint rules and regulations of the agency where practicing. Clear documentation delineating the reasons for seclusion and restraint and the less restrictive alternatives initially attempted should be outlined. Recording of the client's behavior, including the nurse's verbal interventions to decrease the behavior that prompted the intervention, is important. If a staff member or other client is injured during an incident related to seclusion or restraint, a postmortem of the incident should take place to assess what happened and to plan for more appropriate interventions in the future.

Right to Treatment

More than 20 years ago, a movement began in Alabama directed at the right to treatment for people with mental illnesses. With financial constraints within the mental health system, employees at Bryce Hospital were laid off because of a budget shortfall. As a result of this situation, a class action suit on behalf of the employees and clients was filed, alleging that with fewer employees the clients could not receive the proper treatment. Eventually, the Fifth Circuit Court of Appeals upheld a right to treatment, and the state of Alabama was placed in receivership to be monitored by the federal system. The case was settled by consent decree in 1986. Although the right to treatment concept applies to this particular federal circuit, the guidelines for treatment promulgated by Judge Johnson of the Federal District Court have been followed in many jurisdictions. Some of the standards specified include the right to privacy and dignity, the right to the least restrictive treatment, and individual treatment plans that include a statement of problems and intermediate and long-range treatment goals (with a timetable for attainment with rationale for the specified treatment) (*Wyatt v. Stickney,* 1972; Laben and MacLean, 1989).

In a United States Supreme Court decision, it was ruled that, if nondangerous and capable of surviving in the community, an individual cannot be kept in a mental hospital without treatment. Mr. Donaldson had been hospitalized in Florida for over 14 years and desired to be released. Because of his religion, he declined to take medication or other treatment. He was denied the privilege of going out on the grounds. He had a friend who was willing to assist him upon discharge from the hospital. The ruling was very limited, but it did set forth the premise that the state cannot detain individuals who are nondangerous without providing some mode of treatment (*O'Connor v. Donaldson,* 1975).

In the later decision *Youngberg v. Romeo* (1982), the U.S. Supreme Court ruled that a young man with profound retardation was entitled to "minimally adequate training" to provide him with safe conditions. The court stated that a qualified professional's judgment about this matter is considered "presumptively valid." There was great concern at the time that the right to treatment movement was over, but that has not proved to be true: courts have upheld the concept of providing adequate treatment (*Woe v. Cuomo* and Appelbaum, 1987). Stefan, however, reports that "conditions and treatment in many state institutions are still so appalling that plaintiffs still can establish a departure from professional judgment in a well-litigated case" (Stefan, 1993, p. 211).

Right to Refuse Treatment

In the late 1970s and early 1980s, two well-known cases were litigated in the states of Massachusetts and New Jersey, based on the right to refuse psychotropic medication. In the New Jersey case, Mr. Rennie was diagnosed with a psychotic disorder (schizophrenia) at one point and manic depression at another time. There was no unanimous conclusion about the appropriate medication to be administered to him. He was given Prolixin and Thorazine at different times. He suffered from such side effects as akathisia and wormlike movements of the tongue. He refused to take his medication. Rennie filed suit in court to prevent the involuntary administration of medications. After the suit was heard on four different occasions, it was decided that voluntary and involuntary clients had the right to refuse medication. During emergency situations, if potential danger is involved, clients can be forcibly medicated. In the case of an involuntary client, as long as due process guidelines are followed as established, and the administration complies with accepted professional judgment, medication can be given (*Rennie v. Klein,* 1979, 1981). The administrative procedure includes the physician communicating with the clients about their mental health condition and outlining the plan of care with the client when possible. If the client refuses, the medical director of the facility reviews the treatment recommendations and is authorized to call in an outside psychiatrist for consultation (Weiner and Wettstein, 1993).

Rogers v. Okin was originally filed in 1975 as a class action suit to enjoin a state hospital from certain seclusion practices and forcibly medicating clients. In this case, the courts reached a different conclusion. Instead of deferring to administrative procedures that rely on professional judgment, the right to refuse treatment is upheld if the client is involuntary and competent. If the person is ruled incompetent, the judge will use the substituted judgment standard to determine administration of medication. The judge will look at whether the client, if competent, would have chosen medication administration. In this decision, the court ruled that only a judicial authority, and not the decision of the physician or the guardian, was paramount (Weiner and Wettstein, 1993).

Recently, the Massachusetts Supreme Court ruled that once a client becomes competent, the substituted judgment should be terminated. The court also ruled that substituted judgment treatment orders should be reviewed periodically to be in compliance with the current treatment plan. All substituted judgment orders should in the future include a termination (*Guardianship of Weedon,* 1991).

Nurses practicing in mental health facilities should be aware of the state and case laws and policies and procedures for that jurisdiction relative to administration of medication to refusing clients. Frequent checks for side effects and listening carefully to clients' complaints about side effects are imperative for adjustment and changing of medication. The reason for the refusal of medication should be carefully analyzed: Is it because of the denial of the illness or symptomatology of the psychosis, or is it because of side effects or anger with the treatment staff? Education of the client and a reassuring therapeutic relationship can assist in diminishing a client's refusal (Laben and MacLean, 1989).

Electroconvulsive Therapy and Psychosurgery

The administration of electroconvulsive therapy (ECT) continues to be controversial; however, in certain instances, it can be a viable treatment. One major issue that arises is providing informed consent for the procedure. The procedure, including the risks and benefits, should be carefully explained to the client. A major side effect continues to be loss of memory, which may not later be recovered.

Another issue is, who can give consent? The American Psychiatric Association advises that if an incompetent client cannot give informed consent, a relative of the client should be sufficient (1978). Parry, however, states that if there is a question of competency, legal consultation or court guidance should take place (1985).

In the state of Washington, a client has the right to refuse such treatment unless there is clear and convincing evidence that it is needed. The state must have a compelling interest: ECT is necessary and would be effective, and other forms of treatment have not been beneficial or are not available (Washington; Antipsychotic Medication; ECT, 1993). Some states, such as Tennessee, have regulations related to administration of ECT to minors (*Tenn Ann Code* §33-3-105). Other states limit the number of treatments that can be given to an individual within a certain time frame (Weiner and Wettstein, 1993).

Research

Guidelines have been established by the federal government that apply to research on human subjects. The major objective is to provide informed consent to the person who has agreed to participate in research projects. Some of the guidelines include a clear statement of the following: the purpose of the research, the risks and possible discomforts to the subject, the possible benefits to the individual or to others, alternative treatment procedures, confidentiality of records, sources for further information, and availability of compensation if injury occurs. Perhaps the most important fact to convey is that the research is voluntary (45 CFR §46.116).

Nurses should be aware of these guidelines, especially when completing research projects to fulfill educational requirements. Many health care facilities are encouraging staff nurses to participate in research, and awareness of these guidelines is imperative.

THE AMERICANS WITH DISABILITIES ACT

The Americans with Disabilities Act is a substantial breakthrough in discrimination against people with mental illnesses; however, there are specific exclusions (42 USC §12101). The definition includes mental impediments that limit the ability of the individual in one or more major activities (42 USC §12102). Enforcement of the statute depends upon the person's limitations. It has been ruled that if a person's mental condition is stabilized, there is no disability (*Mackie v. Runyon,* 1992). Such people are protected, however, if the fact that they once had a mental disability (such as depression) is used against them in the employment situation. Some exclusions include persons who use controlled substances for unlawful purposes and individuals who take prescribed drugs without the supervision of a health care professional (Parry, 1985). In addition, people who pose a direct threat to others are excluded. However, it is important to recognize that this must be based on actual behavior of the individual and not on the mental disability itself.

A person cannot be asked about a prior history of mental health treatment as part of an application process for employment. The individual can be evaluated as to the ability to perform the job functions. Questions about prior use of health care insurance coverage are also not permissible (Weiner and Wettstein, 1993).

Advocacy

As a result of the mental health movement begun in the 1970s, states developed advocacy programs for clients. Internal grievance procedures allowing clients to express views on their treatment have been initiated in many states. Under the Protection and Advocacy for Mentally Ill Individuals Act of 1986, all states were required to designate an agency that is responsible for maintaining the rights of people with mental illnesses. The names vary from state to state. For example, in Tennessee, Effective Advocacy for Citizens with Handicaps, Inc. (EACH) is the organization responsible for implementation of this act. There has been some controversy over this movement; some mental health professionals say that advocacy sets up adversarial relationships. Advocates should have some understanding of the nature of mental illness and how the mental health system works (Laben and MacLean, 1989).

At the least, nurses should have some understanding of each client's rights and should report to administration when those rights are observed to be violated. Nursing has a long history of advocating for the client, and this should be continued, taking into account changing laws and guidelines relative to mental health treatment.

FORENSIC EVALUATIONS

Individuals who have mental health problems and who are charged with or convicted of crimes fall within the category of forensic mental health services. In the 1960s and 1970s exposés of treatment of these individuals were prevalent in the professional journals and newspapers. In many instances, persons were sent to institutions for evaluation and remained for many years in these facilities without resolution of criminal charges. Procedural due process for many was nonexistent. Many forensic units were isolated and provided inadequate treatment. These

conditions began to change in 1972 with the landmark decision *Jackson v. Indiana.* Jackson was mentally challenged and hearing and speech impaired. He was found incompetent to stand trial. Because of his disabilities, he probably would never become competent to stand trial. At that time, Indiana required hospitalization in a mental hospital until return to competency. Jackson was not going to become competent, so hospitalization would literally sentence him to a form of detention for life. His criminal charge was robbery for a total of 9 dollars.

The U.S. Supreme Court ruled that an individual could be hospitalized only for a reasonable length of time (not defined), but that the 3½ years that Jackson had been detained was too long. If the state wanted to hospitalize him longer, he must be civilly committed, meeting commitment standards, or released. Because of this ruling in the state of Tennessee, the population of the forensic unit went from 185 to 50 within 2 years (Laben and Spencer, 1976).

Competency to Stand Trial

Competency to stand trial is a very narrow concept. The criteria include the following: Does the individual charged with the crime understand the criminal charges? Is there an understanding of the legal process and the consequences of the charges? Can the individual advise an attorney and defend the charges? Essentially, it is the person's awareness of the legal process that must be evaluated by the mental health professional.

If the judge or prosecuting or defense attorney believes that competency is an issue, a request by the attorney results in a court order asking for the evaluation of the person's competency to stand trial. Many states recognize not only the psychiatrist as competent evaluator on this issue but also grant psychologists, social workers, and advanced practice psychiatric nurses who have been educated and trained in this evaluation process. Many evaluations are now performed on an outpatient basis, resulting in return to the courts and a speedier resolution of the charges (Laben and MacLean, 1989).

Criminal Responsibility (Insanity Defense)

Competency to stand trial relates to the present mental condition of the defendants and their current ability to make a defense in court. The insanity defense relates to the state of mind at the time of the offense. This concept stems from the legal doctrine of *mens rea.* For a person to be found guilty, the individual must be able to form intent. If, because of mental illness, intent cannot be formed and the person is possibly responding to hallucinatory voices, there is no guilt involved (Shah, 1986).

The first well-known case came from England where the M'Naghten rule was promulgated. The set of circumstances involved Daniel M'Naghten, who shot and mistakenly murdered the secretary to the prime minister instead of his intended victim, Sir Robert Peel. Afterward, he was found not guilty by reason of insanity. This caused great consternation in that country. Subsequently a panel of 15 judges met and defined what has become known as the M'Naghten Rule. An accused will not be held responsible if at the time of the commission of the act, he was "laboring under such a defect of reason, from disease of the mind, as to not know the nature and quality of the act he was doing, or if he did know it, that he did not know he was doing what was wrong" (Shah, 1986, p. 176).

Much criticism of this doctrine emerged in the 1960s and 1970s, and some states subsequently adopted a modern interpretation of the insanity defense, which states that a person is not responsible for criminal conduct if at the time of such conduct, as a result of mental disease or defect, he lacks substantial capacity either to appreciate the criminality (wrongfulness) of his conduct or to conform his conduct to the requirements of the law (*Graham v. State of Tennessee*, 1977). This definition is derived from the Model Penal Code.

Once a person is found not guilty by reason of insanity, he or she is usually hospitalized and sent to a psychiatric unit for evaluation of commitability. Many states have stricter release standards for individuals found not guilty by reason of insanity because, although found not guilty, the person has committed a criminal act (Laben and MacLean, 1989).

Guilty But Mentally Ill

Recently several states have adopted a new plea called Guilty But Mentally Ill (GBMI). The individual is found guilty, but because of the plea that mental illness caused commission of the crime, is sent to prison and treated for the mental illness. It was felt that fewer people would adopt an insanity defense with the GBMI plea. This has not always proved to be the case; in Michigan the numbers of those pleading this form of the insanity defense increased, although in Georgia the numbers have decreased (Callahan et al, 1992).

Nursing Responsibilities in the Criminal Justice System

In at least one state, advanced practice nurses can testify to the issue of competency to stand trial. This should not be undertaken lightly, and special education should be sought out before testifying on this issue. In most states, psychologists with doctoral degrees and psychiatrists testify concerning the insanity defense.

MALPRACTICE

Because of the irreversible side effects of some medications given to individuals with mental health problems and the trend of short-term hospitalizations, nurses working in psychiatric settings must be aware of situations that might later lead to a malpractice lawsuit. Negligence, the primary basis for malpractice lawsuits, is a civil dispute between two or more citizens or a health care facility. A person alleges that a professional omitted or committed an act that a reasonably prudent professional would not do. The action of the professional causes injury resulting in measurable damages.

Elements of a Malpractice Suit Based on Negligence

To bring a suit, the plaintiff must establish that a nurse had a **legal duty** to that person to provide a certain standard of care. The care is measured by the reasonably prudent nurse standard: What would another nurse working in a mental health facility have done in the same situation? Usually **expert witnesses** are brought in to testify to the standard of care. Some jurisdictions look to a reasonably prudent nurse standard; however, with the development of standards by the American Nurses' Association in relationship to psychiatric nursing practice, these guidelines could be adopted in a lawsuit (*Statement on Psychiatric Mental Health Nursing Practice*, 1994). The next element that will be explored is whether or not the injury was foreseeable based upon the nurse's behavior and the set of circumstances that followed. The court will explore whether the nurse was the causal link in the injury that ensued. For example, did the nurse give the wrong medication or did the nurse not know about drug interactions with certain medications that led to the injury? The last element that must be determined is whether or not there is a proven injury from the nurse's behavior (see the clinical example in Box 3-1).

Documentation

The information that must be kept in a mental health record is often regulated by the state or the mental health facility where the nurse is practicing. Many mental health professionals view charting as a burden. However, it is not just a record of the care of the client; it is also a legal document that might be very valuable in any litigation that might take place.

Adequate documentation is the best method to defend against a lawsuit and to validate that the nurse provided a safe standard of care. It is important to be specific and to document symptoms by noting what the client expresses to you, such as, "I am hearing voices that say I am a bad person." Recording the actual words of the client is more definitive than writing, "The client is hallucinating." Charting should be done in a timely manner. Recording at the time something happens is considered more adequate than block charting, which is usually more brief and not as definitive (*Nurse's Handbook of Law & Ethics*, 1992).

In a mental health record, it is especially important to document when the person has achieved the goals outlined in the treatment plan. If the individual has an exacerbation of the illness, the treatment plan should reflect the change. Informed consent concerning the giving of psychiatric medications is an important aspect of the chart, especially medications such as neuroleptics, which can cause irreversible side effects.

Records are an excellent source for communicating with other mental health professionals on the staff of a facility as well as other agencies where the client is being treated. It is also validation for reimbursement that care was given for particular symptoms. Since managed care is becoming prevalent, a clear outline of all the client's symptoms should be carefully recorded to document a necessity for continued hospitalization. For example, if routine hospitalization is for 10 days, but the client continues to verbalize suicidal thoughts daily, recording of this information is critical for extended permission to continue the hospitalization.

Improper abbreviations not authorized by the agency should not be used. Records from other facilities or other treating professionals should be obtained to provide an accurate long-term picture of how the client was treated on prior occasions.

Any client teaching, aftercare plans, or referral to other agencies for care should be written. Accurate recording of blood pressure is essential, especially in relation to the taking of medications such as Clozaril and other antipsychotic medications. Any nursing assessments that are required by the organization should be completed. Words should be spelled correctly and sentences should be grammatically correct.

Sexual Misconduct

In studies that have been conducted with social workers, psychiatrists, and psychologists, estimates range up to 14% that these professionals have had a sexual relationship with a client (Weiner and Wettstein, 1993). There has been no known study of nurses; however, cases for

---

Box 3-1   Clinical Example

Pennie Johnson had been mentally ill for 10 years. She had been an outpatient in a forensic unit, because long-term inpatient treatment was considered nontherapeutic (*Hatley v. Kassen,* 1992). Because of her long-term history, a difficult client file had been established to assist treating physicians. In February of 1988, she was picked up by a state trooper on a tollway road, at which time she threatened suicide. She was taken to a county hospital. In the nursing assessment, Johnson stated that she was feeling increasingly depressed and had ingested medication that exceeded the prescribed dosage. She continued to take this medication in front of the hospital staff, at which time it was removed from her.

She was examined by Dr. Kalra, who decided to discharge her because he felt her condition had not changed. Johnson asked both the nurse who assessed her and the nursing supervisor, Ms. Kassen, RN, to return her medication. She announced that if the medication was not returned, she would throw herself in front of a car. Kassen told her if she would return home in a taxicab paid for by the hospital, Kassen would return the medication. Johnson declined the offer. A security officer was instructed to escort her out of the hospital. There was disputed testimony as to whether the physician knew of her threats. Thirty minutes after leaving the hospital, she stepped in front of a truck and was killed.

An action for damages was brought by Johnson's parents. In the lower court decision, a summary judgment (granted when no genuine issue of material fact is presented) was awarded to the physician and the hospital, and a directed verdict in favor of Kassen (a decision that is directed to the jury by the judge because the opposing party has not sufficiently presented its case) (Weiner and Wettstein, 1993). The Court of Appeals of Texas reversed the decision and remanded the case back to the lower court for further litigation, stating that the doctor and the nurse were not entitled to official immunity because of employment at a government hospital.

The court, in its decision, did note the testimony of three expert witnesses regarding Kassen's nursing care. Two nurse experts testified that Kassen's actions were substandard once she knew that Johnson had communicated suicidal intentions with a specific plan. A psychiatric expert in the field of suicidology testified that Kassen should have sought the advice of the physician or supervisor before releasing Johnson after the suicidal threats.

One judge wrote a dissenting opinion. This justice believed that Johnson had threatened for 10 years to commit suicide and had never done so; therefore, it was not foreseeable that Johnson would follow through with her threat and therefore it was not negligence on Kassen's part. "I would hold that threats of suicide cannot enslave the intended victim to either submission or damages—especially threats that have been 'empty' for years" (*Hatley v. Kassen,* at 382).

This case was remanded for retrial, so the final results are unknown. However, elements of the case can be analyzed. The nurses and doctor had a duty to a client who was brought to the emergency room. Several experts testified that once a client has a suicide plan, some form of hospitalization should be instituted, or—at the least—a supervisor notified or another discussion held with the physician. Based on this testimony, it might be concluded that the nurse fell below the standard of care. Because the nurse permitted the client to leave the hospital, she could be targeted as a causal agent in the resulting death. Damages could be awarded for the incident (*Hatley v. Kassen,* 1992; Weiner and Wettstein, 1993).

removal of a nursing license for such activity are recorded (*Heinecke v. Department of Commerce*, 1991). All mental health professions consider such behavior unethical, and in many states this behavior is considered criminal, especially if it is within a few months of the therapeutic relationship. Some states have mandatory reporting laws for a second therapist who becomes knowledgeable about such behavior (Strasburger, Jorgenson, and Randles, 1991).

Many of the cases are settled out of court (*Hall v. Schulte*, 1992). When information about the relationship is presented to a jury, members tend to be sympathetic to the client, except when a client appears to have encouraged the relationship. Because the client comes to a therapist with a problem, the issue of the transference phenomenon becomes pronounced, resulting in true lack of consent to become involved with the therapist (Weiner and Wettstein, 1993).

Suicide and Homicide

Malpractice suits and wrongful death actions for homicidal clients' injury to a third party and death from suicide have become prevalent. Some states have ruled that individuals working in governmental agencies have sovereign immunity and can be protected from liability in malpractice situations (*Smith v. King*, 1993; *Poss v. Department of Human Resources*, 1992). It should be noted, however, that when an individual threatens suicide and communicates this information to a mental health provider, the appropriate steps, including involuntary commitment, must be taken to escape liability. If there is a question, legal consultation should be sought. However, "clinicians are not liable for errors of clinical judgment; they are liable only for departures from the relevant standard of care, given the clinical situation" (Weiner and Wettstein, 1993).

Because of the previously described *Tarasoff* decision, it is important to communicate with the mental health treatment team when a client threatens to harm someone. Many states require that a potential victim and/or police should be notified of this occurrence. Some states have limited the warning to include only identifiable victims (Rudegair and Appelbaum, 1992; *Leonard v. Iowa*, 1992). Failure to comply with the required notification could lead to liability.

ETHICAL ISSUES

Ethical issues are closely tied to legal implications for nursing care. *Ethics* is that body of knowledge that explores the moral problems that are raised about specific issues. In nursing practice, one should look at the rules, principles, and ethical guidelines that have been developed by the nursing profession to guide conduct (Davis and Aroskar, 1991). Laws reflect the moral fiber of a society and are developed (hopefully) with an ethical basis; therefore ethical principles should be taken into consideration when evaluating a dilemma. Many problems are raised in the area of mental health law when statutes conflict with a nurse's personal beliefs.

Autonomy

Autonomy means having respect for an individual's decision or self-determination about health care issues. This point is especially important with problems such as the right to die and, in mental health, treatment in the least restrictive alternative. When involuntary commitment is necessary, it is very difficult for mental health providers to have to follow the law rather than what the client currently desires. On one hand the caregiver may want to allow the client to make decisions, but, if the individual is threatening suicide with an active plan, proceeding against the wishes of the person may be necessary for safety and compliance with the law. This kind of decision in ethical terms is called a *paternalistic decision,* or *parentalism* (Purtilo, 1993). This can cause a great deal of inner turmoil for the health care professional when first participating in this kind of decision making.

In addition, it is sometimes very difficult for families when the member who is mentally ill and refusing treatment has to be involuntarily hospitalized. Educating the family about the illness, being supportive, and allowing all of the family to ventilate their frustration, anxieties, and (perhaps) anger can be helpful in this time of crisis for the family.

Beneficence

Individuals who work in the health care field have a special duty and responsibility to act in a manner that is going to benefit and not harm clients. *Beneficence* means bringing about good (Purtilo, 1993). The goal in mental health treatment is to assist individuals to return to a mentally healthy way of life.

The moral imperative of *Primum no nocere* ("First do no harm") should be paramount in clinical interventions with people with mental illnesses. Situations in which this issue might arise include giving neuroleptic medications when it is known that certain side effects can be irreversible. Another instance is the consideration of giving ECT to a client who has failed to respond to antidepressive medication and continues to be suicidal. It is known that memory loss can be a side effect. Do the beneficial aspects of the treatment outweigh the possible side effects? This dilemma can cause anxiety for the client, family, and the mental health professional in the decision-making process.

Certainly, when a mental health professional considers a sexual relationship with a client, preventing harm should be the major consideration. According to the literature, the professional who becomes involved with a client uses denial and rationalization that the client desires the relationship, that the therapeutic relationship has been discontinued, or that it took place outside of the therapeutic time (Russell, 1993). Russell writes that it is important for students to become aware of their own sexual feelings and possible attraction to a client, and that this be an important part of the mental health curriculum, especially for students who later hope to specialize in this area.

Distributive Justice

According to Purtilo, distributive justice refers to the "comparative treatment of individuals in the allotment of benefits and burdens" (1993, p. 23). During times of health care cost constraints, who is going to get treatment and for how much are frequently asked questions. In managed care, provisions for mental health care are not always treated equally with provisions for physical health; the mental health needs of clients can be compromised. The nurses working in a mental health setting may find that it is a necessity to become an advocate for the client with the primary care provider to access mental health care. When there is a yearly cap on the amount of money that a managed care organization is allowing for each individual in a health care plan, resistance to treating a person with a serious and persistent mental illness can arise, especially when this person needs a variety of services over a long period of time.

A major question is the treatment site for individuals with medical and mental health problems. It is not uncommon for a mental health unit to not want to admit a person with serious physical health problems, and a medical unit might not want to admit someone with severe mental health problems who also has a physical problem. These issues are going to become more prevalent as the nation moves toward managed care to control health costs. How is the health care dollar going to be divided and where will the people with mental illnesses fit into the picture when it comes to the division of resources (Lazarus, 1994)?

Summary of Key Concepts

1. Balancing the rights of the mentally ill versus the community has been and continues to be a struggle.

2. Alternatives to inpatient mental health treatment should consider the least restrictive environment utilizing the least restrictive treatment.

3. There are three types of commitments for a client with a mental illness: an emergency commitment, a voluntary commitment, and an involuntary indefinite commitment.

4. Clients should be informed about treatment, including risks and alternatives, upon admission.

5. A civil or judicial commitment of a client is legally based in *parens patriae,* power of the state to protect and care for disabled individuals, and the police power of the state to protect the community from persons who pose a threat.

6. Half of the states in the United States have enacted preventive or mandatory outpatient treatment, in which clients can be returned to the hospital if they discontinue treatment medication, deteriorate, and exhibit dangerous behavior after discharge.

7. Clients with mental illnesses retain their civil rights upon entering a mental hospital or other inpatient treatment center. Clients should receive a summary of their rights upon admission.

8. Clients should be restrained only to prevent physical injury to themselves or others, and only a psychiatrist or licensed physician can order nonemergency seclusion or restraint.

9. Clients who are ruled competent and are voluntarily or involuntarily committed have a right to refuse treatment and medication.

10. The U.S. Supreme Court ruled that individuals charged with or convicted of a crime could only be hospitalized for a reasonable length of time. To be committed longer requires a person to be civilly committed or released.

11. Competency to stand trial is based upon a person's current awareness of the legal process as evaluated by a mental health professional.

12. The insanity defense stems from the concept that for a person to be found guilty, the person must be able to form intent and relate to his or her state of mind at the time of the offense.

13. A new plea, guilty but mentally ill (GBMI), has recently been adopted by several states. Because of the plea that states mental illness caused the commission of the crime, the person is sent to prison and treated for mental illness.

14. Nurses working in psychiatric settings must be aware of situations that may lead to potential malpractice lawsuit.

REFERENCES

Addington v. Texas, 441 US 418 (1979).

American Nurses' Association: Code for nurses, Kansas City, Mo, 1982, The Association.

American Psychiatric Association: *Electroconvulsive therapy: task force report 14,* Washington, DC, 1978, The Association.

Americans with Disabilities Act (42 USC §12101).

Appelbaum PS: *Almost a revolution. Mental health law and the limits of change,* New York, 1994, Oxford University Press.

Appelbaum PS, Greer A: Confidentiality in group therapy, *Hosp Community Psychiatry* 44(4):311–312, 1993.

Appelbaum P: Resurrecting the right to treatment, *Hosp Community Psychiatry* 38(7):703–704, 721, 1987.

Black's law dictionary, St. Paul, Minn, 1990, West Publishing Co.

Brakel SJ, Parry J, Weiner BA: *The mentally disabled and the law,* ed 3, Chicago, 1985, American Bar Foundation.

Cal Civ Code §43.92.

Callahan LA et al: Measuring the effects of the guilty but mentally ill (GBMI) verdict, *Law Hum Behav* 16(4):441–462, 1992.

45 CFR §46.116.

Wash Ann Code §71.05.370.

Davis AJ, Aroskar MA: *Ethical dilemmas and nursing practice,* ed 3, Norwalk, Conn, 1991, Appleton & Lange.

Doe v. Roe, 599 NYS2d 350 (NY App Div 1993).

Geller J: Rx: a tincture of coercion in outpatient treatment?, *Hosp Community Psychiatry* 42(10):1068–1070, 1991.

Graham v. State of Tennessee, 541 SW2d 531 (Tenn 1977).

Guardianship of Weedon, 565 NE2d 432 (MA 1992).

Hall v. Schulte, 836 P2d 989 (Ariz Or of App 1992).

Hatley v. Kassen, 859 SW2d 367 (Tex App Dallas 1992).

Hilts, PJ: Agency faults a U.C.L.A. study for suffering of mental patients, *New York Times,* March 10, 1994, pp. A1, B10.

Heinecke v. Department of Commerce, 810 P2d 459 (Utah App 1991).

Jackson v. Indiana, 406 US 715 (1972).

Laben JK, MacLean CP: *Legal issues & guidelines for nurses who care for the mentally ill,* Owings Mills, Md, 1989, National Health Publishing.

Laben JK, Spencer LD: Decentralization of forensic services, *Community Ment Health J* 12(4):405–414, 1976.

LaFond JQ: Law and the delivery of involuntary mental health services, *Am J Orthopsychiatry* 64(2):409–422, 1994.

Lake v. Cameron, 364 F2d 657 (DC Cir 1966 en banc).

Lazarus A: Disputes over payment for hospitalization under mental health "Carve-out" programs, *Hosp Community Psychiatry* 45(2):115–116, 1994.

Leonard v. Iowa, 491 NW2d 508 (Iowa Sup Ct 1992).

Lyon M, Levine ML, Susman J: Patient's bill of rights: a survey of state statutes, *Ment Disab Law Rep* 6(3):178–201, 1982.

Mackie v. Runyon, 804 F Supp 1508 (1992).

Mink v. Alabama Department of Mental Health and Mental Retardation, 620 So2d 22 (1993).

Mordai MD, Rabinowitz IJ: Why and how to establish computerized system for psychiatric case records, *Hosp Community Psychiatry* 44(11):1091–1095, 1993.

News & Notes: *Hosp Community Psychiatry* 43(8):851–852, 1992.

Norris MK, Kennedy CW: How patients perceive the seclusion process, *J Psychosoc Nurs Ment Health Serv* 30(3):7–13, 1992.

Nurse's Handbook of Law & Ethics, Springhouse, Penn, 1992, Springhouse Corp.

O'Connor v. Donaldson, 422 U5 563 (1975).

Outlaw FJ, Lowery BJ: Seclusion: the nursing challenge, *J Psychosoc Nursing Ment Health Serv* 30(4):13–17, 1992.

Parry J: Mental disabilities under the APA: a difficult path to follow, *Ment Physical Disab Law Rep* 17(1):100–112, 1985.

Peck v. The Counseling Service of Addison County, Inc., 449A2d 422 (Vt 1985).

Poss v. Department of Human Resources, 426 SE2d 635 (Go Or App 1992).

Purtilo R: *Ethical dimensions in the health professions,* ed 2, Philadelphia, 1993, W.B. Saunders.

Reinhard SC: Perspectives of the family's caregiving experience in mental illness, *Image* 26(1):70–J4, 1994.

Rennie v. Klein 416 F Supp 1294 (1979); 653 F2d 836 (3rd Cir 1981); 454 US 1978 (1982).

Rhode Island Department of Mental Health, Retardation and Hospitals v. RB, 541 A2d (RI 1988).

Rogers v. Okin 478 F Supp 1342 (D Mass 1979). See also *Rogers v. Okin* 634 F2d 650 (1980).

Rudegair TS, Applebaum PS: On the duty to protect: an evolutionary perspective, *Bull Am Acad Psychiatry Law* 20(4):419–426, 1992.

Russell J: *Out of bounds sexual exploitation in counseling and therapy,* London, 1993, Sage Publications.

Sales BD, Shuman DW: Mental health law and mental health care: introduction, *Am J Orthopsychiatry* 64(2):172–179, 1994.

Shah S: *Criminal responsibility in forensic psychiatry and psychology,* Philadelphia, 1986, F A Davis.

Smith v. King, 615 So2s 69 (Ala Sup Ct 1993).

Stefan S: What constitutes departure from professional judgment? *Ment Physical Disab Law Rep* 17(2):207–211, 1993.

Statement on psychiatric-mental health nursing practice and standards of psychiatric-mental health clinical nursing practice, Washington, DC, 1994, American Nurses Publishing.

Strasburger L, Jorgenson L, Randles R: Criminalization of psychotherapist-patient sex, *Am J Psychiatry* 148:859–863, 1991.

Tarasoff v. Regents of the University of California 529 P2d 553 (Cal 1974) and 551 P2d 334 (Cal 1976).

Tenn Ann Code §33-6-201, 33-10-103, 33-3-105.

Tooke SR, Brown JS: Perceptions of seclusion: comparing patient and staff reactions, *J Psychosocial Nurs Ment Health Serv* 30(8):23–26, 1992.

Washington; Antipsychotic Medication; ECT, Legislative and Regulatory Developments, *Ment Physical Disab Law Rep* 17(2):206, 1993.

Weiner BA, Wettstein RM: *Legal issues in mental health care,* New York, 1993, Plenum Press.

Wexler DB, Winick BJ: Therapeutic jurisprudence and criminal justice mental health issues, *Ment Physical Disab Law Rep* 16(2):225–231, 1992.

Woe v. Cuomo 638 F Supp. 1506 (ED NY 1986).

Wolpe PR, Schwartz SL, Sanford B: Psychiatric inpatients' knowledge of their rights, *Hosp Community Psychiatry* 42(11):1168–1169, 1991.

Wyatt v. Stickney 344 F Supp 373 (1972).

Youngberg v. Romeo 461 US 308 (1982).

CHAPTER 4
Cultural Issues

Rachel E. Spector
Vincent R. Pieranunzi

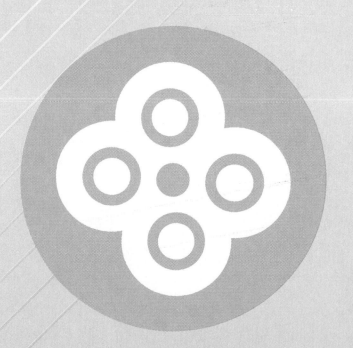

Acculturation The process of adapting to another culture.

Allopathic Health care that refers to the health beliefs and practices derived from contemporary scientific models; involves the use of technology and other modalities of present-day health care, such as immunization, proper nutrition, and resuscitation.

Assimilation To become absorbed into another culture and adopt its characteristics.

Ethnicity A cultural group's sense of identification associated with its common social and cultural heritage.

Ethnocentrism The tendency of members of one cultural group to view the members of other cultural groups in terms of the standards of behavior, attitudes, and values of their own group; belief in the superiority of one's own group.

Heritage consistency The observance of the beliefs and practices of one's traditional cultural belief system.

Homeopathic Health care that refers to health beliefs and practices derived from traditional cultural knowledge to maintain health, prevent changes in health status, and restore health.

Interrelatedness The idea that everything is related to everything; foundation for understanding the cultural issues related generally to health and specifically to mental health.

Socialization The process of being raised within a culture and acquiring the characteristics of the given group.

Xenophobia A morbid fear of strangers and those who are not of one's own ethnic group.

- Analyze the need for a nurse's self-evaluation when providing care to patients from other sociocultural backgrounds.

- Identify demographic issues that are interwoven with cultural aspects of mental health.

- Compare and contrast heritage-consistent and heritage-inconsistent attributes.

- Analyze socialization issues—acculturation, assimilation, ethnocentrism, and xenophobia—as they interrelate with heritage and mental health.

- Compare and contrast traditional cultural issues that define mental health perspectives.

- Differentiate general examples of both health and illness and mental health beliefs and practices of Asian-Americans, African-Americans, Native Americans, and Hispanics.

- Identify selected social issues that interface with mental health beliefs and practices.

- Perform a cultural assessment using the Heritage Assessment Tool.

- Formulate potential nursing diagnoses related to a client's ethnicity.

- Discuss ways in which planning and implementation of nursing interventions can be adapted to a client's ethnicity.

The commitment to provide holistic, culturally sensitive, congruent, and competent psychiatric-mental health nursing care has its foundation in the need to deliver care that is ethical and client-centered. To do this, the nurse must understand the cultural worldview of a given client, family, and community. There are numerous cultural groups represented in our society, each embracing variations in health beliefs and practices. These varied belief systems deeply affect people's daily lives. How clients view illness, their perspectives on what health is, how they heal themselves—all these crucial issues are determined by culture.

In the area of mental health, the definitions of mental illness are largely determined by clients' behaviors and responses to physiological and psychosocial events in their lives. Culture becomes one of the key variables that nurses must understand in order to enter the world of their clients.

All aspects of the nursing process are affected by the cultural perspective of the nurse and the client. In fact, because the key mental health nursing intervention is the therapeutic use of the self, the nurse's ability to relate to and understand the meanings of each client's world, is foundational to effective, ethical, and caring nursing practice.

The nurse needs to know how to interview clients to determine their traditional cultural origins and unique perceptions of health and illness. Knowing where to find relevant information about traditional health and mental health beliefs and practices is also important. The nursing process should incorporate all aspects of an individual's cultural beliefs into his or her care, and be tailored to meet the expectations and needs of the given client, family, and community. The mental health resources within each community must be identified, understood, and respected.

The idea of **interrelatedness**—everything is related to everything—is the foundation for understanding the cultural issues related generally to health and specifically to mental health. The interrelationships between social and cultural trends and mental health issues (Box 4-1) are readily identified when the nurse confronts the complex issues facing the nation.

Many people are trapped in the complex web of spiritual distress, traumatic refugee experiences, suicide, homicide, violence, crises, or other situations. Interpersonal violence in particular is a serious national health problem. The nature of violence between people in intimate relationships is extremely complex. Understanding how culture affects these issues can help the nurse properly interpret and understand them, thereby increasing the efficacy of nursing interventions. Issues related to power and powerlessness are often connected to mental health issues, especially where violence is involved. Many minority groups are disenfranchised and feel powerless. The nurse must seek to understand these complex psychosocial issues within a framework of culture as well as personal history.

A paradox occurs when people seek allopathic treatment in mental health settings for problems that are best handled in their traditional community, or when people delay seeking allopathic treatment because they initially sought "traditional" or homeopathic treatment modalities. **Allopathic** health care refers to health beliefs and practices derived from contemporary scientific models; it involves the use of technology and other modalities of modern health care, such as immunization, proper nutrition, and resuscitation. **Homeopathic** health care refers to health beliefs and practices derived from traditional cultural knowledge to maintain health, prevent changes in health status, and restore health. Family members may often disavow relatives when they seek allopathic care; conversely, many people may accompany a relative when seeking these services. The former may be the result of cultural taboos and shame; the latter the result of cultural resiliency. The needed cultural rituals that generally accompany the crisis or chronic situation may be overlooked by nurses and other caregivers in the intensity of the moment; or, when included, they may be devalued or ignored.

The mental health services providers may not understand the given problem from the person's, family's, and community's point of view and may evaluate the situation in ways that are not culturally appropriate. These situations are frequently observed among the poor, new immigrants, and members of one of the emerging majority communities.

In the twenty-first century, nurses practicing in settings that deliver services to those in need of mental health care will be on the cutting edge of enormous demographic, social, and cultural changes. Many of these changes will play a profound role in both the observed mental health care beliefs and practices and the use of mental health services by individuals, families, and communities. Nurses currently care for people from a wide variety of cultural backgrounds, including recent immigrants. Providing mental health nursing care can be especially challenging when the nurse is from one cultural background and the client is from another. The nurse who is not familiar with the client's cultural background and frame of reference may incorrectly assess and evaluate certain aspects of the client's status. All of this calls for a nurse who can think critically and who understands the multiple meanings inherent in complex health care situations. It demands an ability to respond to clients based on a systematic, critical thought process that allows the nurse to identify personal biases and the barriers that these may present to client interaction.

Box 4-1   The Interrelationship between Social and Cultural Trends and Mental Health Issues

- In 1988–1990 the suicide rate for Native American youth 15–24 years of age (26.8 deaths per 100,000) was nearly twice the rate for Caucasian youth, about 3 times the rate for African-American and Hispanic youth, and 3.6 times the rate for Asian-American youth in the United States (National Center for Health Statistics, 1992).

- In 1988–1990 the homicide rate for African-American youth 15–24 years of age (676 deaths per 100,000) was 2.5–3.6 times the rates for Hispanic and Native American youth and 7.9–9.1 times the rate for Caucasian and Asian-American youth (National Center for Health Statistics, 1992).

- An African-American male in the United States is seven times more likely to be in jail than a black man in South Africa (Hodgkinson, 1992).

This chapter addresses how the cultural aspects of mental health are woven into the scope of mental health nursing practice. Since these issues form a complex web of interrelated factors, this chapter presents a theoretical overview and description of several selected factors:

- demographic change
- concepts of heritage consistency
- socialization issues
- cultural issues related to health and mental health beliefs
- social issues such as poverty and communication

Each factor may serve as facilitator or barrier to the use of mental health services in primary, acute, chronic, and community-based mental health care settings.

Nurses practice in many "worlds" and the following questions may be asked about the nurse's personal and professional worlds as this topic is studied:

- Who am I with respect to my cultural identity?
- What is my personal heritage, and how deeply do I adhere to it?
- What is my nursing heritage, and how deeply do I adhere to it?
- What biases and assumptions do I have, and how do these affect my ability to interact with clients?
- What do I know about mental health and illness from my formative years?
- What have I learned about mental health and illness in nursing?

Nurses should consider aspects of their own culture-bound mental health and illness beliefs and issues that vary from the dominant norms of professional beliefs and practices because the former may impact their delivery of nursing care.

DEMOGRAPHIC ISSUES

It has been said that "demography is destiny" (Hodgkinson, 1986). Evidence of demographic change may be seen in many ways, including a comparison of the 1980 and 1990 census, and a comparison of immigration profiles.

Census Comparison

Figures 4-1 and 4-2 compare the 1980 and the 1990 census, showing how the population of the United States is changing. The data from these two sources may be viewed in two ways. The most commonly presented way is to observe the census that includes Hispanics without breaking out the number of non-Hispanics. When this is the method used, the comparison is as follows: In 1980, the overall population of the United States (226.5 million) broke down as 83.2% Caucasian and 16.8% people of color. It may also be noted that 6.4% of the population claimed Hispanic origin but could be of any race (U.S. Bureau of the Census, 1991).

In 1990, despite an estimated head count shortfall of 5.3 million—many of whom are non-Caucasian and Hispanic city dwellers (Sege and Mashek, 1991)—the overall population of the United States (248.7 million) broke

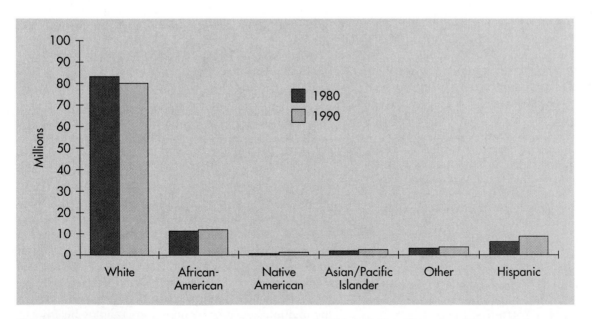

Figure 4-1 United States population comparison, 1980 and 1990, including Hispanic origin population.

From U.S. Bureau of the Census: *Current Population Reports, 1980 General Social and Economic Characteristics Part 1, United States Summary, PC 80-1-C1, United States,* Washington, D.C., 1983, U.S. Government Printing Office, and U.S. Bureau of the Census: *Current Population Reports, 1990 Census of Population and Housing: Summary Populations and Housing Characteristics, United States,* Washington, D.C., 1991, U.S. Government Printing Office.

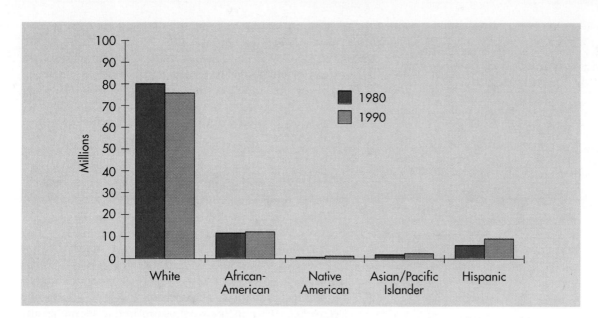

Figure 4-2 United States population comparison, 1980 and 1990, Hispanic origin population not included.

From U.S. Bureau of the Census: *Current Population Reports, 1980 General Social and Economic Characteristics Part 1, United States Summary, PC 80-1-C1, United States,* Washington, D.C., 1983, U.S. Government Printing Office, and U.S. Bureau of the Census: *Current Population Reports, 1990 Census of Population and Housing: Summary Populations and Housing Characteristics, United States,* Washington, D.C., 1991, U.S. Government Printing Office.

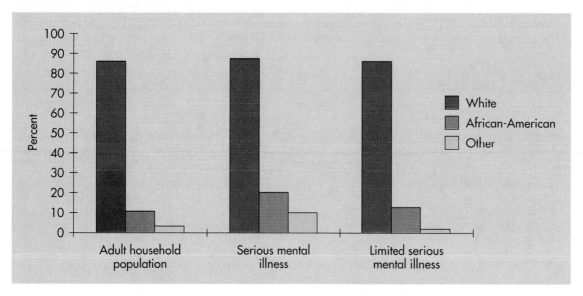

Figure 4-3 Percentage distribution of the adult household population, those with serious mental illness and those limited by serious mental illness, 1989.

From Manderschied RW and Sonnenschein MA, editors: *Mental Health, United States, 1992,* Washington, D.C., 1992, U.S. Government Printing Office.

down as 80.3% Caucasian and 19.7% people of color. It may also be noted that 9.0% of the population claimed Hispanic origin but could be of any race (U.S. Bureau of the Census, 1991). The European majority decreased by about 3%.

When the two sets of data are compared by Hispanic and non-Hispanic origin, the results are as follows: 79.7% Caucasian, 11.5% African-American, 0.6% Native American, and 1.5% Asian/Pacific Islander for 1980, and 75.6%

Caucasian, 11.7% African-American, 0.7% Native American, and 2.8% Asian/Pacific Islander for 1990. The European majority was below 80% for each decade.

Demographic data also serve to illustrate the manner in which mental health issues impact emerging majority populations, compared to the rates of mental illness in the overall population. Figure 4-3 compares the percentage distribution of the adult household population members with serious mental illness to those households

---

Box 4-2   Demographic Trends That Illustrate the Relationship of Demography and Mental Health

- Sixty percent of today's children will live with a single parent at some time.
- There will be fewer women producing fewer children, and there will be a decline in the number of Caucasian children.
- It is predicted that by 2010, 7 states plus the District of Columbia will have an emerging majority youth (ages 0–17) population far greater than 50%.

From Hodgkinson HL: *A demographic look at tomorrow*, Washington, D.C., 1992, Institute for Educational Leadership.

---

with members limited by serious mental illness in 1989. In both instances, the numbers of African-American populations with mental illness are greater than the proportionate percentage of African-American households in the overall population. In 1989, 703,000 adults with serious mental illness received government disabled payment for their mental disorder. Of this particular population, 20.5% were Caucasian and 43.8% were African-American.

These data are not in proportion with the demographic profiles of the United States and raise questions as to why mental health problems are not equally distributed among races. There are many explanations that rationalize these demographic phenomena and other discrepancies related to the differences in the occurrence of mental illness based on race. Certainly the factors of poverty, racism, and significant demographic trends (Box 4-2) play a role in the situation.

Immigration

Another way of illustrating this demographic change is to analyze recent immigration and refugee trends. The countless social and political upheavals in the world, including Cuba, Haiti, the former Yugoslavia, the former Soviet Union, and the famines and civil wars in African nations have created thousands of situations in which people are seeking refuge in the United States.

For example, in 1992, 810,635 immigrants arrived in the United States—the second largest flow of immigrants in 70 years. The majority were from Mexico (91,332), Vietnam (77,728), the Philippines (59,179), the Republics of the former Soviet Union (43,590), and the Dominican Republic (40,840). The Immigration and Naturalization Service expects between 800,000–900,000 immigrants to come to the United States each year under the immigration laws passed in 1990. The Immigration Service uses mental health status to control immigration.

Currently this affects the admission of Haitians and homosexuals (Kraut, 1994).

The relevance of changes in the U.S. population to the study of mental health is readily understood when one realizes that much of the "American norm" of mental health and prevention and treatment of mental illness is based on predominantly allopathic, European-heritage philosophies.

HERITAGE CONSISTENCY

Most of the people who live in the United States are immigrants or have ancestors who were immigrants. The early waves of immigrants were predominantly European, with subsequent waves coming from Asia (in the 1970s and 1980s) and presently from the Americas (especially Mexico and Central America). Every immigrant group has brought its own culture, beliefs, and attitudes (Castillo, 1979), including those related to mental health and illness. It is expected that people, families, and communities learn from their cultural heritage how to maintain health, prevent illness, and treat an episode of illness, including mental illness.

There are many ways to analyze the role that one's cultural background plays in mental health care practices in the context of heritage consistency. **Heritage consistency** is a theory originally developed in 1980 by Estes and Zitzow as a means of assessing and counselling Native American alcoholics within a cultural context. It describes "the degree to which one's lifestyle reflects his/her tribal culture." The theory states that people who tend to identify with their "traditional culture" respond more readily to traditional healing modalities rather than western allopathic models of care (Estes and Zitzow, 1980).

Since 1983 the theory has been further developed and expanded by Spector in an attempt to study to what degree a person's lifestyle reflects his or her traditional culture, whether it is of European, Asian, African, or Hispanic origin. The value characteristics, such as spoken language of preference, food preferences, name, schools attended, family and neighborhood ties, and religious and social activities, that indicate heritage consistency exist on a continuum. People can possess value characteristics of both a heritage-consistent (traditional) and a heritage-inconsistent (accelerated) nature. The theory includes a determination of one's cultural, ethnic, and religious background (Spector, 1996). Thus, heritage consistency theory encompasses three broad concepts: culture, ethnicity, and religion.

Culture

There is no single definition of culture and, all too often, definitions tend to omit prominent aspects or are too general to have real meaning. However, there are countless ideas about the meaning of this term. One way of describing culture is that it is the "sum total of socially inherited characteristics of a human group that comprises everything which one generation can tell, convey, or hand down to the next" (Fejos, 1959). A second description (and the one that is most relevant in areas of mental health) is that culture is a "metacommunication system" wherein not only the spoken words have meaning, but everything else as well (Matsumoto, 1988).

A third way of understanding culture is to view it as a "cultural lens" and understand that all facets of human behavior can be interpreted through it. Culture is the medium of personhood and social relationships, only part of which is conscious, and the way of explaining symbols. Culture is a device for creating and limiting human choices, and can be in two places at once—in a person's mind and in the environment as spoken words or artifacts (Bohannan, 1992).

Culture is a complex phenomenon in which each part is related to every other part. Culture must be learned by each person within the family and social community, and depends on an underlying social matrix that includes knowledge, belief, art, law, morals, and customs (Bohannan, 1992)

Culture is learned to the extent that people learn the ways to see and understand their environment. Culture is the medium of our individuality, the way in which we express ourselves. It is the medium of human social relationships in that it must be shared. The symbols of culture—sounds and acts—form the basis of all languages. Symbols are everywhere: religion, politics, and gender, to name just a few areas. But the meaning of these cultural symbols varies between and within cultural groups (Bohannan, 1992).

Culture is a phenomenon that impacts all groups. For example, nurses form a sub-culture within the larger culture of the American health care system. They share a unique language, employ special technologies, and are socialized with an embedded set of values and perspectives. These meaning systems often clash with those of our clients, especially when the client seeks to retain culture-bound views of health and how to respond to illness.

A person who is heritage-consistent, that is, has a strong sense of the traditional heritage, is also culturally competent. That is, he or she possesses a strong personal cultural identity and has a knowledge of the beliefs and values of a given culture. The attributes of a heritage-consistent person include a sensitivity to the affective process of the culture; the ability to communicate clearly in the language of the given culture; and a willingness to perform socially sanctioned behavior, maintain social relations in the group, and negotiate successfully with the institutional structures of the culture (LaFromboise, 1992). Box 4-3 lists factors that indicate heritage consistency.

Ethnicity

Cultural conditioning is a fundamental component of one's ethnic background. Ethnicity is complex and includes the following characteristics a group may share in some combination:

- common geographic origin
- migratory status
- race
- common language
- religious faith or faiths
- ties that transcend kinship, neighborhood, and community boundaries
- shared traditions, values, symbols, and symbolic meanings
- literature, folklore, music, and food preferences
- settlement and employment patterns
- special political interests

Box 4-3 Factors Indicating Heritage Consistency

- Childhood development occurred in the person's country of origin or in an immigrant neighborhood in the United States of like ethnic group.
- Extended family members encouraged participation in traditional religious or cultural activities.
- Individual engages in frequent visits to country of origin or to the "old neighborhood" in the United States.
- Family homes are within the ethnic community.
- Individual participates in ethnic social events, such as religious festivals or national holidays, sometimes with singing, dancing, and costumes.
- Individual was raised in an extended family setting.

- Individual maintains regular contact with the extended family.
- Individual's name has not been Americanized.
- Individual was educated in a private school with a religious and/or ethnic philosophy similar to the family's background.
- Individual engages in social activities primarily with others of the same ethnic and/or religious background.
- Individual has knowledge of the culture and language of origin.
- Individual possesses elements of personal pride about the heritage of origin.

TABLE 4-1 Nations of family origin of the American population, 1994	
Country of origin	**Family origins (%)**
Germany	20.3
England and Wales	13.4
Ireland	12.2
Africa	9.3
Italy	4.9
Scotland	3.9
American Indian	3.8
Poland	2.4
Mexico	3.1
Norway	1.8

From Smith TW: National Opinion Research Center, Chicago, 1994, University of Chicago (unpublished data).

- an internal sense of distinctiveness
- an external sense of distinctiveness

Ethnicity is the condition of belonging to a particular ethnic group and may often lead to the feelings of **ethnocentrism,** the belief in the superiority of one's own group. **Xenophobia** is a morbid fear of strangers and those who are not of one's own ethnic group. There are at least 106 different ethnic groups in America and more than 170 Native American tribes, or nations (Thernstrom, 1980). Table 4-1 lists the ten leading nations of origin of the American population, according to a 1994 survey by the National Opinion Research Center at the University of Chicago.

The term *ethnic* may arouse strongly negative feelings and is often rejected by the general population. In today's world, ethnic identity is often a reason for scorn and even death. These attitudinal and behavioral responses occur as a result of people's needs, especially when they are foreign born and must find a way to function before they are assimilated into the mainstream. People cluster together against the majority, who in turn discriminate against them (Spector, 1996).

Religion

Religion is the belief in a divine or superhuman power(s) to be obeyed and worshipped as the creator(s) and ruler(s) of the universe, as well as a system of beliefs, practices, and ethical values. Religion provides a frame of reference and a perspective for organizing information. Religious teachings in relation to health and illness help present a meaningful philosophy and a system of practices. These teachings result in a system of beliefs, practices, and social controls that have specific values, norms, and ethics that vary among religious groups (Abramson, 1980). Ethnicity and religion are related because one's religion is quite often the determinant of one's ethnic group.

Religious meanings can impact a client's perspective on illness. For most people, illnesses are "events." They are made up of social, cultural, and psychological meanings that are interwoven with the physiological event. Religion, both the traditional as well as more eclectic approaches to spirituality, is significant in helping the nurse understand the way that a client is interpreting the illness event.

The religious character of American culture may result in some individuals drawing on religious symbols and language within their worldview to articulate and cope with their concerns and problems. There is little doubt that mental health and illness can be manifested in religious expression. However, some mental health care providers have a negative view of religion and there is often a polarization between them and religious believers and leaders (Post, 1993). Nurses, especially psychiatric nurses, must be sensitive to this bias and work to understand the way clients interpret events in their lives. Religious and spiritual practices and beliefs are often deeply connected to client issues, such as grief, depression, and guilt. In addition, delusions and hallucinations can take on a religious character. The nurse must be able to differentiate between legitimate but different religious practices and beliefs and those that have become distorted by mental illness.

Heritage Assessment

The Heritage Assessment Tool (Box 4-4) contains questions that may be used to assess if a person identifies with a "traditional" culture or modern American culture. As the nurse begins to develop skills in this form of assessment, it is suggested to make the initial assessment of an individual a personal one, followed by assessments of parents, family members, and friends. Since most clients (especially people in mental health settings) often do not react well to pencil-and-paper quizzes, it is helpful to memorize the scope and nature of these questions and then piece together the information needed to determine a client's level of heritage consistency.

SOCIALIZATION ISSUES

In the mid-1960s there was a social explosion in the United States that caused a surge of group consciousness. African-Americans, then Hispanics, Asian-Americans, and others began to assert their cultural group identity, and the myth of the "melting pot" eroded. Today, yet another social explosion is occurring, which is caused by the profound forces of demographic change. We are now living in a multicultural society, and it is becoming more and more evident that cultural differences are increasingly isolating and alienating people and com-

---

Box 4-4   Heritage Assessment Tool

1. Where was your mother born?

2. Where was your father born?

3. Where were your grandparents born?

   a. Your mother's mother?

   b. Your mother's father?

   c. Your father's mother?

   d. Your father's father?

4. How many brothers and sisters do you have?

5. What setting did you grow up in?

   a. urban

   b. rural

   c. suburban

6. What country did your parents grow up in?

   a. father

   b. mother

7. How old were you when you came to the United States?

8. How old were your parents when they came to the United States?

   a. mother

   b. father

9. When you were growing up, who lived with you? (ask this way)

   a. nuclear family

   b. extended family

   c. single parent family

   d. other

10. Have you maintained contact with:

    a. aunts, uncles, cousins?   (1) yes   (2) no

    b. brothers and sisters?   (1) yes   (2) no

    c. parents?   (1) yes   (2) no

    d. your own children?   (1) yes   (2) no

11. Did most of your aunts, uncles, and cousins live near to your home when you were growing up?

    a. yes

    b. no

12. Approximately how often did you visit your family members who lived outside of your home when you were young?

    a. daily

    b. weekly

    c. monthly

    d. once a year or less

    e. never

13. Was your original family name changed?

    a. yes

    b. no

14. Do you have a religious preference?

    a. yes (if yes, please specify)

    b. no (1 point for yes, but 0 for no)

15. Is your spouse the same religion as you?

    a. yes

    b. no

16. Is your spouse the same ethnic background as you?

    a. yes

    b. no

17. What kind of school did you go to?

    a. public (0)

    b. private

    c. parochial

Continued

munities. It has been pointed out that merely educating people about the differences that underlie culturally determined beliefs is not enough; one must first confront competing ideals of "truth" (Hunter, 1994). There are several concepts interwoven with the theory of heritage consistency: socialization, acculturation, assimilation, ethnocentrism, and xenophobia.

Socialization

Socialization is the process of being raised within a culture and acquiring the characteristics of the given group.

Education—whether elementary school, high school, college, or nursing school—are forms of socialization. For many people who have been socialized within the boundaries of a "traditional" or nonwestern culture, modern "American" culture becomes a second cultural identity. Those who immigrate here from non-English speaking, nonwestern, or nonmodern countries may find socialization into the American culture, both in schools and in society, an extremely difficult and painful process. They may experience biculturalism, which is a dual pattern of identification that often commands a divided loyalty (LaFromboise, Coleman, and Gerton, 1993).

Box 4-4 Heritage Assessment Tool—cont'd

18. As an adult, do you live in a neighborhood where the neighbors are the same religion and/or ethnic background as yourself?

    a. religion   (1) yes   (2) no
    b. ethnicity   (1) yes   (2) no

19. Do you belong to a religious institution?

    a. yes
    b. no

20. Would you describe yourself as an active member?

    a. yes
    b. no

21. How often do you attend your religious institution?

    a. more than once a week
    b. weekly
    c. monthly (0)
    d. special holidays only (0)
    e. never

22. Do you practice your religion in your home?

    a. yes (please specify, 1 point each example)
    b. praying
    c. bible reading
    d. diet
    e. celebrating religious holidays
    f. no

23. Do you prepare foods of your ethnic background?

    a. yes
    b. no

24. Do you participate in ethnic activities?

    a. yes (if yes, please specify, 1 point for each)
    b. singing

    c. holiday celebrations
    d. dancing
    e. festivals
    f. costumes
    g. other
    h. no

25. Are your friends from the same religious background as you?

    a. yes
    b. no

26. Are your friends from the same ethnic background as you?

    a. yes
    b. no

27. What is your native language (the language your parents may have spoken other than English)?

28. Do you speak this language?

    a. prefer
    b. occasionally (0)
    c. rarely (0)

29. Do you read this language?

    a. yes
    b. no

The greater the number of yes answers, the more likely the client is to strongly identify with a traditional heritage. (The one no answer that indicates heritage identity is "Was your name changed?") This assessment may be scored 1 point for each yes from question 10, except where noted (0), and 2 points for no if the person's family name was not Americanized. Again, a high score, usually greater than 15 points, is indicative of identification with a traditional background.

From Spector RE: *Cultural diversity in health and illness,* ed 4, Norwalk, Conn., 1996, Appleton & Lange.

Acculturation

The process of **acculturation** occurs when a member of a cultural group is forced to adapt to the new dominant culture in order to survive. It is an involuntary process. No matter how competent the person becomes in acquiring the generalities of the new host culture, he or she will always be identified as a member of the nondominant culture. This model of second culture acquisition is what an individual experiences when one lives within or between cultures (LaFromboise, Coleman, and Gerton, 1993).

Assimilation

Assimilation is the process of developing a new cultural identity. Assimilation means becoming, in all ways, like the members of the dominant culture. The process comprises various stages, such as cultural or behavioral assimilation, marital assimilation, identification assimilation, and civic assimilation. The underlying assumption is that the person loses his or her original cultural identity to acquire the new one. However, this is not always possible, and the process of assimilation may cause stress and anxiety (LaFromboise, Coleman, and Gerton, 1993).

Ethnocentrism and Xenophobia

Many prejudices or biases can surface when social situations grow difficult (Box 4-5). Just as Hunter (1994) proclaims that the differences between culturally determined beliefs must be confronted, so must the stereotypes, prejudice, and discrimination. For example, it is impossible to describe traditional beliefs without a tendency to stereotype. When one encounters inexplicable differences in health behaviors, it is most comfortable to view newly learned academic, western theories as "best"—a form of **ethnocentrism.** Also, there is a natural tendency for nurses to fear and distrust the practices of others who are not part of the allopathic system of care—a form of **xenophobia.** But each person is an individual; therefore, levels of heritage consistency will differ within and among ethnic groups as will variations in health beliefs and practices. The nurse who understands the meaning of traditional health practices will be understanding of the client who embraces these practices.

The other issue that surfaces in this arena is prejudice. Prejudice refers to a negative set of beliefs and judgments that become generalized to a whole population of people. The person who has formed the beliefs or made the judgments does not understand the individual or the individual's cultural heritage. Discrimination occurs when a person acts on a prejudice; the result is the denial of the other person's equal rights and opportunity.

Box 4-5   Common Prejudices or Biases

Racism	The belief that members of one race are superior to those of other races
Sexism	The belief that members of one sex are superior to the other sex
Heterosexism	The belief that everyone is or should be heterosexual and that heterosexuality is best, normal, and superior
Ageism	The belief that members of one age group are superior to those of other ages
Ethnocentrism	The belief that one's own cultural, ethnic, or professional group is superior to that of others. One judges others by his or her own "yardstick" and is unable or unwilling to see what the other group is really about.
Xenophobia	The morbid fear of strangers and those who are not of one's own ethnic group

From American Nurses Association: *Multicultural issues in the nursing workforce,* Washington, D.C., 1993, ANA.

TRADITIONAL HEALTH AND ILLNESS BELIEFS

It is within one's heritage that the rules for maintaining health, preventing illness, and restoring health are learned. Although the focus of this chapter and this text is mental health, it is impossible to separate the mind from the physical person in a holistic traditional cultural philosophy. There are culture-specific beliefs and practices related to mental health, but they are interwoven with the entire phenomenon of traditional health beliefs and practices. The dimensions of health in a traditional culture, as shown in Table 4-2, consist of:

- one's body—the physical self—all that is visible from the outside
- one's mind—the invisible self—the culturally determined feelings, attitudes, and behavior that one has, manifests, and experiences (Jalali, 1988)
- one's spirit—the "who am I?"—as expressed through the body, thoughts, etc. (Stoll, 1989)

From a traditional or cultural perspective, health is the balance of these three dimensions. Each dimension—body, mind, and spirit—must be carefully treated because each one's status is inextricably related to the other two. The traditional environment serves to provide the person with the necessary physical, mental, and spiritual support deemed necessary from the person's traditional culture.

Ethnomedicine

The discipline of *ethnomedicine* studies the beliefs and practices relating to disease that are the products of indigenous cultural development and are not based on the tenets of modern medicine. Throughout history, all human communities have developed social institutions and cultural traditions designed to restore and maintain health (Foster, 1983).

Many traditional health beliefs are observed among the cultural groups in the United States. For example, there are culturally based, or folk, beliefs that determine the definitions of health and illness. People of Asian origin may view health as the "balance of yin and yang" and illness as the "imbalance." *Yin* refers to male-positive energy that produces light, warmth, and fullness, and *yang* refers to female-negative energy, the force of darkness, cold, and emptiness. Haitians, Jamaicans, or others of Caribbean origin may view health as "harmony with nature" and illness as "disharmony with nature." Individuals from Hispanic and Latin countries such as Spain, Portugal, Mexico, and Central and South America may view health as the "balance of hot and cold" and illness as the "imbalance." Native Americans may view health as the "ability to live in harmony with nature" and illness as "living in disharmony with nature." Traditional people of European origin may have a philosophy that sees health as

TABLE 4-2   The interrelationship of the body, mind, and spirit in traditional cultures and personal methods used to maintain health, prevent illness, and restore health

	Body	Mind	Spirit
Maintain Health	Proper clothing Proper diet Exercise/Rest	Concentration Social and family support systems Hobbies	Daily religious worship Prayer Meditation

Prevent Illness	Special foods and food
	   combinations
	Symbolic clothing
		Avoid certain people
		   who can cause illness
		Family activities
			Religious customs
			Superstitions
			Wearing amulets and other
			   symbolic objects to prevent
			   the "evil eye" or defray other
			   sources of harm

Restore Health	Homeopathic remedies (liniments)
	Special foods (herb teas)
	Special treatments (massage,
	   acupuncture, moxibustion)
		Relaxation
		Exorcism
		Curanderos and other
		   traditional healers
		Nerve teas
			Religious rituals (special prayers)
			Meditation
			Traditional healings
			Exorcism

Modified from Spector RE: *Cultural diversity in health and illness,* ed 4, Norwalk, Conn., 1996, Appleton & Lange.

"feeling good and able to do one's duty" and illness as "feeling bad" (Spector, 1996).

The traditional, or folk, methods of health maintenance, illness prevention, and the treatment of illness rest in the person's ability to understand the cause of an illness. Ethnomedicine is one way to illustrate these different beliefs because it presents a categorization of causation that includes:

• angry deities who punish those who violate taboos

• ancestors and other ghosts who believe they have been forgotten

• sorcerers and witches who can be hired to cause illness

• the loss of the soul when it is jarred loose from the body by a sorcerer or spirit

• the possession or the intrusion of an object into the body

• loss of the basic body equilibrium because of excessive heat or cold entering the body

• the "evil eye"

Traditional beliefs regarding the causation of illness also differ vastly from the modern model of epidemiology. Yet another model that more fully appreciates the richness of the traditional methods is "Traditional Epidemiology." This model includes three key components: agents, host factors, and environmental factors.

1. Traditional agents refer to concepts such as "hexes," "spells," and the "evil eye." The "evil eye" is a concept that manifests among numerous cultural, religious, and ethnic populations. One of the oldest-held beliefs, it asserts that a power emanates from the eye or mouth that strikes a victim—usually a child—with an injury, illness, or other misfortune. This belief helps to explain misfortune (Budge, 1978). It is also perceived that illness may also be caused by people, or witches, who have the ability to make others—usually children—ill. It is therefore deemed necessary to avoid such individuals. The belief is that the victims can best be cured by removing the evil one's influence from the vulnerable people. This may be accomplished by a variety of rituals, depending on the culture.

2. Traditional host factors include such phenomena as "soul loss"; "spirit possession"; the ability to provoke the envy, hate, and jealousy of a friend, acquaintance, or neighbor; and the religious and social behavior of the person. Health is often viewed as the reward for good behavior, and illness is perceived as the punishment for bad behavior.

3. Traditional environmental factors include air quality, "mal aire" (bad air), and such natural events as a solar eclipse.

Many of these traditional factors are thought to cause not only physical maladies but emotional and spiritual ones as well.

Traditional Practices

Health-promoting behaviors that may be used to maintain the health of the person include maintaining balance of the body by wearing proper clothing. For example, traditional women from Germany may wear shawls to protect themselves from drafts. Another example is eating the proper diet. For example, people from Southeast Asia and China may eat rice daily. The maintenance of mental health may consist of activities that include sports, mental concentration, reading, arts, and crafts. Spiritual health is maintained in the traditional ways by silence, prayer, and meditation.

Traditional practices of prevention developed from the folk beliefs about the causes of illness. To protect the body, it is advocated to wear special clothing, such as the underwear worn by Mormons, the wigs worn by Orthodox Jews, and the scarves worn by Moslem women. People avoided those who were known to cause or transmit hexes and spells, and many elaborate methods were developed to prevent the envy, hate, and jealousy of others. For example, there are those in the Mexican culture who may hide success or choose failure to avoid provoking the envy of friends and neighbors. Countless methods evolved over generations and exist today to protect people from the "evil eye." Every effort is made to avoid situations in which social or religious behaviors are compromised.

The following are additional examples of traditional practices used to maintain health and illness.

USE OF PROTECTIVE/RELIGIOUS OBJECTS

Various protective objects may be worn, carried, or hung somewhere in the home. Amulets are objects with magical powers, such as charms, worn on a string or chain around the neck, wrist, or waist to protect the wearer from the "evil eye" or evil spirits. These spirits are believed to be transmitted from one person to another, or may have supernatural origins. Amulets have been found in societies all over the world and are associated with protecting people from trouble.

In addition to amulets, some people carry or possess talismans (consecrated religious objects). Talismans are believed to possess extraordinary powers.

Finally, some people prevent the "evil eye" by touching a baby when admiring it (Puerto Rico), by drawing a circle around a baby's bed and spitting on the child three times (Eastern Europe), or by placing a red ribbon somewhere on the child's crib or bed (Western Europe).

USE OF SUBSTANCES

One example of substance use is special dietary observances to keep the body in balance or harmony. There are numerous food taboos and combinations that are prescribed in traditional belief systems. For example, people from many ethnic backgrounds eat raw garlic or onion to prevent illness. Garlic or onions may also be worn or hung in the home to protect it from evil spirits.

RELIGIOUS RITUALS

Religion strongly affects the way people choose to prevent illness and plays a strong role in prevention rituals. It dictates social, moral, and dietary practices designed to keep a person healthy and in balance. It also plays a vital role in a person's perception of the prevention of illness.

For example, many people believe that strict adherence to religious codes, morals, and practices prevents illness, and they view illness as a punishment for breaking a religious code.

From a traditional perspective the goal of restoring health is to restore the body's internal and external balance. Thus, in terms of rebalancing the physical self, such homeopathic remedies as liniments, herbal teas, selected foods, massage, acupuncture, and moxibustion may be used. To restore mental health, relaxation, exorcism, or special nerve teas may be the modalities of choice. Spiritual ailments may be treated by prayer, meditation, healers, or exorcism.

Traditional Remedies

Folk medicine is related to other types of medicine that are practiced in our society. It has coexisted with modern medicine and was derived from earlier medical theories. There is ample evidence that the folk practices of ancient times have only in part been abandoned by modern belief systems; many of these beliefs and practices continue to be observed today. There are two types of folk medicine:

- natural folk medicine—the use of elements in the natural environment such as herbs, plants, minerals, and animal substances—to prevent and treat illnesses

- magico-religious folk medicine—the use of charms, holy words, and holy actions to prevent illnesses (Yoder, 1972)

A wide variety of substances may also be ingested for the treatment of maladies. Frequently, the active ingredients of these traditional remedies are unknown. If a nurse believes a client is taking such remedies, he or she must make an effort to determine the active ingredients which can be antagonistic or synergistic to prescribed medications. The medication may have no effect, or a severe overdose may ensue. Plotkin (1993) described his studies of plants that traditional healers have used for thousands of years and the need to understand the nature of these plants, the rain forest, and their connection to health.

Substances may also be used to restore the body's balance, and they may be introduced into the body in other ways. For example, in the Asian practice of coining, a substance, usually Tiger Balm, is rubbed over a certain area of the body with a coin to release "wind" and restore the body's balance.

Illness is also treated through religious beliefs, objects, and other practices. Wearing religious medals and performing sacrifices are not unusual practices. There are currently strong beliefs in religious healing, and people in traditional communities often seek traditional healers.

Traditional Healers

Within a given cultural community, people may consult traditional healers before they seek health care services or during the course of allopathic treatment. Within a community there are specific people who are known to the members of that community to have the power to heal. The healer may be male or female and is most often believed to have received the gift of healing from a divine source.

The relationship between the person and the healer is quite often much closer than that between the person and the health professional. The person views the healer as one who understands the problem within the cultural context, speaks the same language, and shares a similar worldview. The following are examples of traditional healers:

- medicine man: the traditional healer of the Native Americans
- señora: a Puerto Rican woman knowledgeable in the treatment of illness
- esperitista: a Puerto Rican woman who possesses more sophisticated skills than the señora
- curandero: a Mexican man who possesses the God-given ability to heal and uses a religious-psychiatric approach
- partera: a Mexican-American midwife
- root-worker: an African-American man or woman who is able to determine the cause of an illness and the treatment within the cultural context

Traditional healers have been a part of human cultures as long as people have existed. The methods used to heal have been developed over generations by trial and error, with religious beliefs and social circumstances contributing to the methods. The traditional healer is aware of the needs of the person and family and is able to understand them within the cultural context of their contemporary problems. Table 4-3 compares the scope of practice of the traditional healer with that of the modern practitioner. The healer is usually a part of the client's culture and community and is able to help the client interpret and deal with illness events in ways that are congruent with the client's worldview. This decreases anxiety and guilt, issues that often complicate mental illness.

It is not known precisely how many people actually seek treatment from traditional healers. People may tend to seek help first from the traditional healer, they may seek traditional help in conjunction with modern therapy, or they may leave modern therapy entirely (elope) to be treated by the traditional healer.

CROSS-CULTURAL PERSPECTIVES OF MENTAL HEALTH

The following discussion presents an overview of mental health beliefs and practices from different selected cultures. This information is not intended to stereotype any group but merely to describe the known traditional means by which an individual member or family of a given group may cope with a mental health problem.

The nurse's understanding of a client's cultural norms serves as a framework for understanding the client's world. The nurse cannot begin to understand a client with only previously held views of that client's cultural group. Sincere dialogue and genuine interest in the client and his or her culture are necessary elements for beginning the process.

African-Americans

Members of the African-American communities in the United States have their origins in Africa, and a cultural heritage that is a mixture of the Caribbean cultures, Na-

---

TABLE 4-3 Comparison of the practices of the traditional healer and the modern nurse or physician

Traditional healer	Modern nurse or physician
Maintains a friendly, informal relationship with the family	Business-like and formal relationship with client
Care is personalized	Care is depersonalized
Comes to the home day or night	Client must visit the office or clinic, or is receiving inpatient care
Consults with head of family or other family members, creates a mood of awe, and has social rapport	Deals with ill person
Not expensive and may provide in-kind services	Authoritarian manner may create fear
Has ties to the world of the sacred and spirits	Expensive
	Secular, pays little attention to the client and family's religion and the meaning of the illness
Shares the worldview of the client	Does not usually share client's worldview
Speaks the same language	Does not usually speak the same language
Understands client and family's lifestyle	Does not understand client and family's lifestyle

tive American cultures, and northern European cultures (Baker, 1988). In 1990 there were 29,986,000 African-Americans in the United States, or 11.7% of the total population. The following is a brief demographic sketch of this population (Go, 1994):

- the median age is 27.9 years
- 71.9% of the males and 77.9% of the females have a high school education
- 50.2% are married couples
- 70.1% of the men and 57.8% of the women are employed
- the median earning for a family is $20,210
- 30.7% of this group are below the poverty level

The family often has a matriarchal structure, and there are many single-parent households headed by females. There are strong, large extended family networks. There is a continuation of tradition and a strong religious affiliation within the community. Many African-Americans tend to use traditional medicines and healers when the people are knowledgeable and when they have access to this resource.

The traditional people may choose to be treated by a traditional Voodoo priest or the "Old Lady" ("granny" or "Mrs. Markus") or other traditional healers, and herbs are frequently used to treat mental symptoms. Several diagnostic techniques include the use of Biblical phrases and material from old folk medical books, observation, and entering the spirit of the client. The therapeutic measures include various rituals such as the reading of bones, wearing special garments, or some rituals from Voodoo (Spurlock, 1988).

Asian-Americans

Members of the Asian-Pacific Island communities in the United States have their origins in China, Hawaii, the Philippines, Korea, Japan, and Southeast Asia (Cambodia, Laos, and Vietnam). In 1990 there were 7,273,662 Asian-Americans in the United States, or 3% of the total population. The following is a brief demographic sketch of this population (Go, 1994):

- the median age is 30.4 years
- 82% of the members have a high school education
- 80% are married couples
- 72% of the men and 56% of the women are employed
- the median earning for a family is $42,250
- 11% of this group are below the poverty level

The family has a hierarchical structure, and loyalty among members is valued. There is a devotion to tradition; many religions, including Taoism, Buddhism, Islam, and Christianity, are practiced. Many people tend to use traditional medicines and healers such as the "Chinese Doctor" or other traditional healers; herbs are frequently used to treat mental symptoms.

Little knowledge or skill in mental health therapy is seen in the Asian communities. There are two points that must be noted: the importance placed on the family in caring for the mentally ill, and the fact that people may tend to describe mental illness in somatic terms. There is a tremendous amount of stigma attached to mental illness. Asian patients tend to come to the attention of mental health workers late in the course of their illness, and they come with a feeling of hopelessness (Lin, 1982).

One example of cross-cultural therapy is the Japanese practice of Morita therapy. This 70-year-old treatment originated from a treatment for shinkeishitsu, a form of compulsive neurosis with aspects of neurasthenia. The patient is separated from the family for one to two weeks and taught that one's feelings are the same as the Japanese sky and instantly changeable. One cannot be responsible for how one feels, only for what one does. At the end of therapy, the client focuses outside of the self and less on inner feelings, symptoms, concerns, or obsessive thoughts (Yamamoto, 1982).

Hispanics

Members of the Hispanic community have their origins in Spain, Cuba, Central and South America, Mexico, Puerto Rico, and other Spanish-speaking countries. In 1990 there were 22,354,059 in the United States, or 9% of the total population. Hispanics are now the most rapidly growing ethnic group in the American population. The following is a brief demographic sketch of this population (Go, 1994):

- the median age is 26.2 years
- 51% of the members have a high school education
- 56.7% are married couples
- 78% of the men and 51% of the women are employed
- the median earning for a family is $23,400
- 25% of this group are below the poverty level

The family often has a nuclear structure, with strong and large extended family networks and compadrazzo (godparents). There is a continuation of tradition and a strong church affiliation within the community. Many, but not all, Hispanics are Catholic. Many tend to use traditional medicines and healers and are knowledgeable about these resources.

The people may be treated by a traditional healer such as a curandero, santero, or señora, and herbs are frequently used to treat mental symptoms. Diagnostic techniques include the use of divination (foretelling the future), observation, and exorcism.

TABLE 4-4   Cross-cultural examples of selected communication phenomena that affect nursing care

Nations of origin	Language	Space	Time orientation
ASIAN ORIGIN China Hawaii Philippines Korea Japan Southeast Asia Laos Cambodia Vietnam	National language preference Dialects, written characters Use of silence Nonverbal and contextual cuing	Noncontact people	Present
AFRICAN ORIGIN West Coast (as slaves) Many African countries West Indian islands Dominican Republic Haiti Jamaica	National languages Dialect Pidgin Creole Spanish French	Close personal space	Present over future
EUROPEAN ORIGIN Germany England Italy Ireland Other European countries	National languages Many learn English immediately	Noncontact people Aloof Distant Southern countries: closer contact and touch	Future over present
NATIVE AMERICAN 170 Native American tribes Aleuts Eskimos	Tribal languages Many learn English immediately	Space is very important and has no boundaries	Future over present
HISPANIC ORIGIN Spain Cuba Mexico Central and South America	Spanish or Portuguese primary languages	Tactile relationships Touch Handshakes Embracing Values physical presence	Present

From Spector RE: *Cultural diversity in health and illness,* ed 4, Norwalk, Conn., 1996, Appleton & Lange and Giger JN, Davidhizar RE: *Transcultural nursing,* ed 2, St. Louis, 1995, Mosby.

The therapeutic measures related to mental health include various rituals such as reading the palm, eyes, tongue, and head. The practice combines herbalism and magical-religious practices.

Native Americans

The ancestors of Native Americans living in the United States today immigrated to this land long before the Europeans and other immigrants. Today there are approximately 170 Native American nations, or tribes, located mostly in the western states. Many Native Americans have remained on reservations, while others live in urban and rural areas off the reservations on the East Coast. In 1990 there were 1.9 million Native Americans in the

United States, or 0.7% of the total population. They now compose the smallest ethnic group in the American population. The following is a brief demographic sketch of this population (Go, 1994):

- the median age is 23.5 years
- 56% of the members have a high school education
- the median earning for a family is $20,025
- 23.7% of this group are below the poverty level

The family often has a nuclear structure, with strong biological and large extended family networks. Children are taught to respect traditions and community organizations that provide social and cultural services. Many Native Americans tend to use traditional medicines and healers and are knowledgeable of these resources. The people may frequently be treated by a traditional Medicine Man, and herbs are frequently used to treat mental symptoms. Diagnostic techniques include the following:

- divination: the art of foretelling events or revealing secrets

- conjuring: the art of summoning information

- star-gazing: the art of "reading" the stars to find answers to questions

The basis of Native American philosophy is that all of nature, including the holistic person—body, mind, and spirit—is related. If one aspect of this relationship is not in balance, then health does not exist.

SOCIAL ISSUES RELATED TO MENTAL HEALTH CARE

There are many social barriers that prevent clients from using modern mental health services. The major barriers are of communication and poverty because they limit or restrict a person's or family's access to these services. Closely related to but not necessarily occurring only among families who are poor are the selected problems of language, space, time orientation, and transportation. Table 4-4 describes major points of these cross-cultural communication phenomena.

Communication

Communication is a major element of culture because it rests at the root of people's ability to relate to one another. There are two types of communication: verbal and nonverbal. Each has the potential for causing numerous cross-cultural issues between nurses and clients. The impact of verbal versus nonverbal communication is dynamic. People can and do interpret other people's nonverbal behavior. For example, they are able to sense what lies behind a smile or such significant body language as hands on the hips. Nonverbal communication creates problems when the observed behavior does not fit the spoken words. Clients may interpret nonverbal behavior of the caregiver as judgmental or condescending. For example, a smiling nurse may stand with hands on hips, which is viewed as hostile or superior by a client of traditional background. These clients often read nonverbal behavior with greater ease than their nontraditional counterparts.

LANGUAGE

People from traditional cultures experience another problem in verbal communication when the connotation and the denotation of a given word vary. The use of English or medical jargon presents many problems; when the client is unable to understand the conversation there is often a feeling of alienation. The attempt to communicate verbally in English with non-English speaking clients is generally not effective. All too often nurses may shout when a client does not understand English and need to remember that the person is not hearing impaired. Since many "new Americans" tend to retain their native languages, there is a constant demand for qualified interpreters. However, the interpreter must know the client's dialect. For example, a Spanish-speaking interpreter was used in the diagnostic workup of a Puerto Rican, Spanish-speaking child. Being from Spain, the interpreter spoke Castilian Spanish but the child spoke Puerto Rican Spanish. The mental health diagnostic workup was inaccurate, and the child was incorrectly diagnosed. Box 4-6 provides suggestions for communicating with clients who speak other languages.

Box 4-6   Suggestions for Communicating with Clients Who Speak Other Languages

- Respect clients as individuals, regardless of differences in language skills and values. Avoid judging clients' intellectual abilities or emotional states on the basis of how they use language.

- Avoid treating emerging majority group members differently from other clients; such "special" treatment may be interpreted as patronizing.

- Do not assume that clients are angry, aggressive, or hostile if they speak more loudly or emotionally than most European Americans.

- Use titles such as Mr. or Ms. unless you have established a first-name basis for the relationship.

- Never attempt to use ethnic dialects with clients. This may be interpreted as making fun of clients or as condescension.

- Avoid attempting to impress clients by saying you have friends of the same ethnic or racial background.

- Be attentive to clients' nonverbal communication which can help to clarify seemingly confusing verbal communications.

- Make use of ethnic group preferences when giving care. Involve the extended family in communication, for example, or focus on oral rather than written teaching methods.

- Explain medical and nursing terms in simple, everyday terms and be sure that clients truly understand.

- If you do not understand what a client is saying, ask for clarification. Do not let embarrassment at not understanding lead to the risks of misinformation.

SPACE

Space, or proxemics, the personal distance that people prefer to maintain from one another, is a significant cultural issue. The nurse spends a great deal of time in the client's territory and therefore needs to be aware of the person's territorial needs. Touch is another source of communication that varies widely from culture to culture. In some cultures it is expected to shake hands when meeting a stranger, and it is permissible to embrace and caress a person who is only a limited acquaintance. In other cultures this is taboo, and touch may do more harm than good. Eye contact is another variable. It is common among those with a traditional European background to expect eye contact and to think the worst when a person does not make eye contact. Among many people, such as Asian-Americans, eye contact is taboo.

TIME ORIENTATION

Time orientation is manifested in several ways. The orientation to the future versus the present may create conflict in that people from traditional cultures may not be able to adapt to the norms of using the health care system. For example, they may have difficulty with the demand to arrive promptly for an appointment and to wait hours to be seen. In many cultures, such as the Hispanic and Native American cultures, people do not regard the time of day as an essential element. This is exemplified by the common practice of not living by the clock, not being on time, and arriving late or even several days after scheduled appointments.

Poverty

The federal government has defined poverty as living below the poverty threshold. This poverty threshold is based on pre-taxed income only, excluding capital gains, and does not include the value of noncash benefits such as employer-provided health insurance, food stamps, or Medicaid, the state/federal health insurance program available to eligible people and funded 50% by the federal government and 50% by the state. (A form of Medicaid is available in most states.) The average poverty threshold for a family of four was $12,674 in 1989 and $13,359 in 1990. The average poverty thresholds in 1990 varied from $6,652 for a person living alone to $26,848 for a family of nine or more members. The number of persons living below the official government poverty level in 1990 was 33.6 million, 13.5% of the nation's population. This figure represents the first significant rise in poverty since 1982. Nearly 40% of the nation's poor were children under 18 years of age; the poverty rate for children continues, as it has since 1975, to be higher than that for any group. Overall, the poverty rates for Caucasians and Hispanics have increased in 1990; for African-Americans the poverty rate remains at 30.7%.

The poverty rate for children under 18 years of age in 1990 was 15.9% for Caucasian children, 38.4% for Hispanic children, and 44.8% for African-American children.

Cycle of Poverty

Poverty is more than just the absence of money. One way of analyzing the phenomenon is by observing the effects of the "Cycle of Poverty" as illustrated in Figure 4-4. In this cycle, the family lives in a situation that may create poor intellectual and physical development and poor economic production; there is generally a high birth rate. This living situation, in turn, causes poor economic production that creates insufficient family salaries and a subsistence economy that forces the family to most often reside in densely populated areas or remotely located rural areas. There is often a lack of shelter or potable water, and the family members generally suffer from chronically inadequate nutrition. This often leads to high morbidity and accident rates that precipitate high health care costs which, in turn, prevent the family members from seeking health care services. A consequence is frequent increased sickness and decreased production, in a cycle that has yet to be broken.

The effects of poverty on mental health and illness continue to be debated. For example, a recent publication describes the relationship between schizophrenia and poverty. It notes that even though studies of social class and mental illness have become archaic in the current era of neurobiological research, the fact remains that there are important correlations to examine regarding the effects of poverty and social class on the origin and course of mental illnesses such as schizophrenia (Cohen, 1993).

Welfare is a source of available funding for families in poverty. The welfare system is currently under sharp scrutiny by politicians and members of society at large, and significant efforts are underway to reform the welfare system.

Barriers to Care
ACCESS

There are several factors that limit a family's access to the health care delivery system, including availability, location, transportation, and whether or not the family has any type of health insurance. The lack of insurance, whether public (Medicaid) or private, is a rapidly increasing problem. There are more than 30 million people who do not have health insurance. The national discussion that focused on health care reform in the early 1990s was weak when it focused on the type of coverage and benefits that would be available to the mentally ill, and more and more institutions that provide services to the poor and minorities are being closed for the use of community-based care. These issues have yet to be adequately addressed and resolved.

In addition, many chronically mentally ill persons live in board and care facilities or group homes in the com-

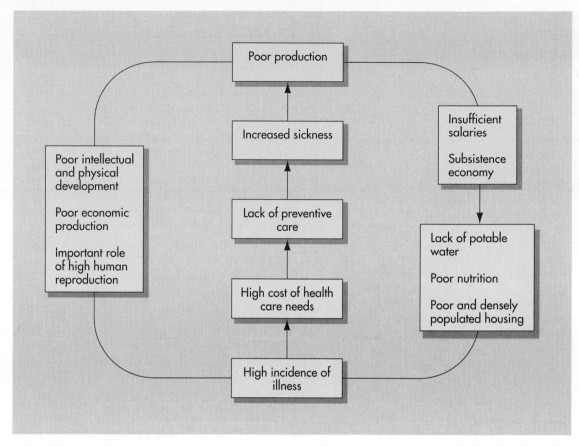

Figure 4-4 The cycle of poverty.

From Spector RE: *Cultural diversity in health and illness,* ed 4, Norwalk Conn., Appleton and Lange.

munity. Often, these facilities are poorly staffed and supervised, and treatment opportunities are limited or nonexistent. Clients must often depend on partial hospitalization or day treatment for care. In the absence of reasonable access to these programs, clients often decompensate and are forced to use inpatient care when a less restrictive alternative might have been as effective and more humane.

TRANSPORTATION

All too frequently families are not able to obtain mental health services because of geographic distance, and they may have to depend on other family members or friends to help them get to the resource. In many settings the hospital that provides free care is not in the same location as the families needing this care. Public transportation may be expensive and unavailable in many locations.

CULTURAL FACTORS AND THE NURSING PROCESS

Understanding the significance of culture and its impact on clients' mental and physical health is of foundational importance for nurses in all settings of health care deliv-

ery. This understanding and awareness are integral to the nursing process; they inform and affect assessment, diagnosis, outcome planning, intervention, and evaluation of clients.

The principal nursing tool in mental health is the therapeutic use of self. It is in the relationship between the nurse and client that the sensitive and usually embedded cultural issues manifest themselves and impact client care.

As the nurse applies the nursing process in the mental health setting, understanding the meanings of the health care problem from both the client's and the nurses's cultural perspective is important. Each step of the nursing process is impacted by an understanding of the complex cultural issues which affect clients and their interpretation of life events.

Assessment

The assessment process is foundational to all other steps of the nursing process. It is during assessment that the nurse formulates a perspective of the client's needs and issues. Far from objective, this process is colored by the nurse's personal biases, assumptions, cultural meanings, and nursing experience.

Understanding and Applying
RESEARCH

Lipson J: Afghan refugees in California: mental health issues, *Issues in Mental Health Nursing* 1:411, 1990

This article describes the mental health problems and their antecedents experienced by Afghan refugees who immigrated to northern California.

Based on an ethnographic study that focused on sequelae related to the invasion, years of war, and the continuing political turmoil in Afghanistan, the article includes and analyzes refugees' stories to determine the antecedents to many of their mental health problems. Their experiences included incidents in Afghanistan, the escape, camp, transit experiences, and continuing trauma in the United States.

Several of the participants told of being imprisoned, of family members imprisoned, and of torture. For example, "My family did not know where I was. Once I was beaten and left for dead, another time they beat me on different parts of my body, they electrocuted me, and so forth." Several other situations of like magnitude are presented in each of these categories of experience.

Mental health care providers should elicit stories from clients about their experiences in their home countries and as immigrants. Nurses play a legitimate role in identifying potential survivors of torture and in helping them to seek appropriate care.

CLINICAL ALERT !

A 3-year-old child enters the emergency room for pneumonia. On assessment, the nurse discovers round bruises covering the child's back, buttocks, and chest. Is this a case of child abuse? Not necessarily! In some southeastern Asian cultures, this could be the result of the practice of "coining." This procedure entails heating a coin and rubbing it across the body to draw out sickness. It is harmless and leaves only superficial bruising. Rather than being abusive, it is an attempt by the family to help the child, and thus is a caring action. The nurse must assess whether or not this practice is used in the client's culture before deciding that abuse has taken place.

Numerous researchers have described cultural factors that impact assessment. Race in particular can alter the assessment of symptoms and level of functioning. Lawson et al (1994) describe how racial differences between client and clinician can lead to a failure to appreciate cultural differences in presentation of symptoms and thus lead to misdiagnosis. In addition, clients from minority groups may delay seeking treatment due to mistrust of the system, which can lead to the application of more serious diagnostic labels.

The nurse must be as informed and sensitive as possible. This enables the client to be truly "heard" and allows for accurate diagnosis. It helps prevent stereotyping and labeling, major problems in mental health care today.

The nurse needs to be aware of his or her own personal and professional cultural heritage, as well as the client's cultural heritage and what mental health means in its context. The use of the Heritage Assessment Tool (see Box 4-4 on pages 61–62) in assessing the client is an entry point for gathering culture-specific data. In addition, the following questions may be asked to gather cultural data.

1. Cultural Background. What is the client's ethnic, religious, spiritual, and racial heritage? If unfamiliar with the client's culture, seek information about the specific cultural group by interviewing the client's family and members of the group. Understanding and Applying Research in the box at left describes a study relating to the assessment of Afghan refugees.

2. Values Orientation. What are the attitudes of the given client, family, or community based on their cultural heritage in regard to this mental health problem?

3. Cultural Sanction and Restrictions. What are the "rules" in this client's cultural background with respect to this mental health problem?

4. Communication. What primary language does this client speak, and are there any interpreters available?

5. Health/Illness Beliefs and Practices. What cultural factors do the client and family associate with the identified problem? What types of traditional healers are available to the family?

6. Nutrition. What are the specific dietary restrictions to consider, if any?

7. Economic Considerations. What economic resources are available to the family?

8. Educational Background. What is the level of education of both client and family? Are they able to read, understand, and follow instructions in English or in their native language? Where have they attended schools and for how long? Have they attended schools in the United States? What role does informal education play in their lives?

9. Spiritual or Religious Affiliation. What role does spirituality or religion play in the life of the client and family? Is a spiritual advisor or a member of the clergy readily available? What are the religious views of this client and family? Do they have special prayers?

Box 4-7 Commonly Misapplied Nursing Diagnoses

Common NANDA nursing diagnoses frequently misapplied due to a lack of understanding of cultural issues:

Impaired social interaction and impaired verbal communication

Misunderstanding occurs when the nurse fails to take into account culture-specific interaction patterns. Silence, infrequent eye contact, shame, fear, and language barriers all impact clients' ability to interact. The gender of the nurse and the gender of the client may also impact communication because many cultures have specific gender-role behavioral codes.

Defensive coping and noncompliance

Clients from minority cultures that have experienced discrimination, bias, and stereotyping may be resistant to appropriate nursing interventions, especially in the area of teaching and discharge planning. Suspicion and mistrust may cause the nurse to misunderstand a client's behaviors, and mislabel them.

Altered role performance and altered parenting

Use of these diagnoses requires an understanding of the client's culture-specific roles and parenting activities. They may be different from those of the nurse and the majority culture.

Altered thought processes

Thought patterns and processes which may appear to be distorted can be related to culture-specific expressions of anxiety and fear. Careful assessment will enable the nurse to accurately diagnose anxiety or fear in many clients, rather than assume that underlying thought processes are altered.

Nursing Diagnosis

The nursing diagnoses are much the same for clients from diverse cultural backgrounds, with a few exceptions. The nurse should be as specific as possible in conducting an assessment to determine that a problem is individualized to the client. Actual culture-related nursing diagnoses include communication barriers, sociocultural dissonance, language barriers, and differences in health and illness beliefs and practices.

The process of assigning a nursing diagnosis is an important one. These diagnostic categories often enable other staff to "frame" a client's health concerns. They must be as accurate as possible and reflect the unique cultural perspective of the client. In other words, they must be culturally congruent.

Often, a nursing diagnosis is chosen based upon an inaccurate assessment. The nurse, viewing client behavior through an ethnocentric "lens," interprets the client's behavior as dysfunctional. Box 4-7 describes common nursing diagnoses that are often misapplied to clients due to culture-related misunderstandings.

Outcome Identification

Client outcomes in the mental health setting are determined based upon the assessment and diagnostic process. An understanding of cultural issues is crucial to assure that the determination of outcomes of nursing care use client input and are congruent with the clients' needs and wishes. Often, clients fail to achieve the desired outcomes because such outcomes are inconsistent with their cultural worldview. Many clients will defer to the nurse whom they see as the "expert." In reality, however, the clients do not plan to follow through with patient educational and discharge planning because it does not make sense to them and is not relevant to their problems from their perspective. This may lead to further misdiagnosis, especially "noncompliance." This happens most often when a client wants to use a traditional healing method or other culture-specific approach and sees the allopathic-oriented nursing intervention as conflicting with the traditional ways of achieving health.

Planning

When establishing goals of care and planning nursing interventions, the nurse considers each client's variables. The family is generally included in the client's treatment plan and, as often as possible, the client's community as well. A client's beliefs will more likely be included in a client's mental health care plans when the nurse is aware of the meaning of the client's behavior and verbalizations in the context of his or her culture and tradition.

Implementation

The implementation of nursing care plans that are holistic and culturally sensitive, congruent, and competent evolves over time and includes the following goals:

1. Maintain the client's cultural mental health practices as much as possible. For example, if the client is using ethno-medications, determine what type and how they react with conventional medications.

2. Maintain effective verbal and nonverbal communication between client and caregivers and obtain an interpreter if necessary.

3. Promote the client's understanding of the allopathic system and the rationale behind the care that is being delivered.

CASE STUDY

Maria, a 20-year-old Hispanic woman, is seen in the psychiatric unit to rule out schizophrenia. She was admitted after she was found screaming in her front yard and acting irrationally. She sat in her room and was well-groomed and quiet. She isolated herself from other clients and appeared suspicious of staff. She had poor eye contact and spoke softly when questioned by the nurse. She remarked that her mother, who has been deceased three years, appears to her and speaks to her. The nature of these "appearances" is comforting; no commands are given.

Critical Thinking Questions

1. What culture-specific issues may be impacting Maria?

2. How might the assessment process be improved with an understanding of Maria's cultural heritage?

3. It is known that Hispanic people often report hearing the voice of deceased relatives in times of stress. How could the nurse differentiate between this cultural phenomenon and a psychotic thought process?

4. What communication barriers may be operating between Maria and the nurse?

The nurse must be aware that trust issues are important in mental health nursing care. Clients who are members of cultural communities may have a deep-seated mistrust of the system in general and the nurse in particular, especially if the nurse comes from a different cultural background. Researchers have noted that race, for example, is a powerful issue in treatment. In particular, it can affect how medication is administered, the level and frequency of interventions, and the outcome of intervention (Adebimpe, 1994).

In a study of the psychiatric treatment of older African-American clients, Baker (1994) noted that the use of social support mechanisms in the intervention process was crucial in effectively caring for these elderly clients. This study is typical of many that suggest that mental health intervention must be done within the framework of culture if it is to be effective (Nelson et al, 1992; Morris and Silove, 1992; Friedman, Paradis, and Hatch, 1994; Hickling and Griffith, 1994). Use of family members and other members of the client's cultural group in the assessment, planning, and intervention process can facilitate nursing care and insure more effective client outcomes.

Evaluation

The nurse evaluates mental health care from a multicultural nursing perspective by determining if the client outcomes have been achieved.

It is important to evaluate whether or not the client has been able to maintain his or her cultural beliefs regarding mental health and illness. The client's needs and beliefs should be respected with open lines of communication. The discharge plan should be realistic and culturally congruent. If the client does not feel invested in the treatment choices, he or she is less likely to be effective after discharge. Thus, evaluation of nursing interventions is based on the attainment of client outcomes that have been determined to be culturally sensitive and realistic.

Summary of Key Concepts

1. Psychiatric-mental health nurses must assess and evaluate clients and implement care plans with a holistic and culturally sensitive perspective toward care.

2. Multicultural nursing in mental health involves an understanding of many issues, including demographic change, heritage consistency, socialization, acculturation, and assimilation.

3. To better assist someone from another culture, nurses should have an awareness of their own cultural heritage.

4. Heritage consistency is the concept that describes the degree to which a person identifies with his cultural background.

5. The Heritage Assessment Tool can assist nurses in assessing a client's heritage consistency.

6. Health can be viewed as three-dimensional, encompassing the body, mind, and spirit.

7. The communication aspects of language, space, and time orientation have various practices among different cultures.

REFERENCES

Adebimpe VR: Race, racism, and epidemiological surveys, *Hosp Community Psychiatry* 45:27, 1994.

Abramson P: Religion. In Thernstrom S, editor, *The Harvard encyclopedia of American ethnic groups,* Cambridge, Mass., 1980, Harvard University Press.

American Psychiatric Association: *Diagnostic and statistical manual of mental disorders,* ed 4, Philadelphia, 1994, The Association.

Baker FM: Afro-Americans. In Comas-Diaz L and Griffith EEH, editors: *Cross-cultural mental health,* New York, 1988, John Wiley & Sons.

Baker FM: Psychiatric treatment of older African-Americans, *Hosp Community Psychiatry* 45:32, 1994.

Bannerman RH, Burton J, and Wen-Chieh C: *Traditional medicine and health care coverage,* Geneva, 1983, World Health Organization.

Barringer F: Census shows profound change in racial makeup of nation, *New York Times,* March 11, 1991, p. 1.

Bohannan P: *We, the alien,* Prospect Heights, Ill., 1992, Waveland Press.

Budge EAW: *Amulets and superstition,* New York, 1978, Dover (originally published London, 1930, Oxford University Press).

Castillo LJ: *Communicating with Mexican Americans—por su bueno salud,* Houston, Tex., 1979, Baylor College of Medicine.

Cohen CI: Poverty and the course of schizophrenia: implications for research and policy, *Hosp Community Psychiatry* 44:951, 1993.

Council on Cultural Diversity in Nursing: *Multicultural issues in the nursing workforce and workplace,* Washington, D.C., 1993, American Nurses Association.

Cross T: Understanding family resiliency from a relational worldview. In *Resiliency in families: racial and ethnic minority families in America,* Madison, Wis., 1994, University of Wisconsin-Madison.

Estes G and Zitzow D: *Heritage consistency as a consideration in counseling Native Americans,* Dallas, Tex., 1980, National Indian Education Association Convention.

Fejos P: Man, magic, and medicine. In Goldstone I, editor: *Medicine and anthropology,* New York, 1959, International University Press.

Fortinash KM and Holoday-Worret PA: *Psychiatric nursing care plans,* ed 2, St. Louis, 1995, Mosby.

Foster GM: An introduction to ethnomedicine. In Bannerman RH, Burton J, and Wen-Chieh C, editors: *Traditional medicine and health care coverage,* Geneva, 1983, World Health Organization.

Friedman S, Paradis C, Hatch M: Characteristics of African-American and white patients with panic disorder and agoraphobia, *Hosp Community Psychiatry* 45:798, 1994.

Gaw A, editor: *Cross-cultural psychiatry,* Boston, 1982, John Wright.

Giger JN and Davidhizar RE: *Transcultural nursing assessment and intervention,* ed 2, St. Louis, 1995, Mosby.

Go GV: Changing populations and health. In Edelman CL and Mandle C, editors: *Health promotion through the life-span,* ed 3, St. Louis, 1994, Mosby.

Goldberg G, et al: *Alternative medicine—the definitive guide,* Puyallup, Wash., 1993, Future Medicine Publishing.

Hand W: *Magical medicine,* Berkeley, 1980, University of California Press.

Hickling FW and Griffith EEH: Clinical perspectives on the Rastafari movement, *Hosp Community Psychiatry* 45:49, 1994.

Hodgkinson HL: *A demographic look at tomorrow,* Washington, D.C., 1992, Institute for Educational Leadership.

Hodgkinson HL: Reform? Higher education? Don't be absurd!, *Higher Education,* 271, December 1986.

Hunter JD: *Before the shooting begins: searching for democracy in America's culture war,* New York, 1994, Free Pres.

Jalali B: Ethnicity, cultural adjustment and behavior: Implications for family therapy. In Comas-Diaz L and Griffith EEH, editors: *Cross-cultural mental health,* New York, 1988, John Wiley & Sons.

Kraut AM: *Silent travelers: germs, genes, and the immigrant menace,* New York, 1994, Basic Books.

LaFromboise T, Coleman HLK, Gerton J: Psychological impact of biculturalism: evidence and theory, *Psychol Bull* 14:395, 1993.

Lawson WB et al: Race as a factor in inpatient and outpatient admissions and diagnosis, *Hosp Community Psychiatry* 45:72, 1994.

Lin KM: Cultural aspects of mental health for Asian Americans. In Gaw A, editor: *Cross-cultural psychiatry,* Boston, 1982, John Wright.

Manderschied RW and Sonnenschein MA, editors: *Mental health, United States, 1992,* Washington, D.C., 1992, Govt. Print. Off., DHHS Pubs. No. (SMA)92-1942.

Marsella AJ and White GM, editors: *Cultural conceptions of mental health therapy,* London, 1982, D. Reidel Publishing.

Matsumoto M: *The unspoken way,* Tokyo, 1988, Kodansha International.

Morris P, Silove D: Cultural influences in psychotherapy with refugee survivors of torture and trauma, *Hosp Community Psychiatry* 43(3):257, 1992.

Nelson SH and others: An overview of mental health services for American Indians and Alaska natives in the 1990s, *Hosp Community Psychiatry* 43(3):257, 1992.

Plotkin MJ: *Tales of a shaman's apprentice,* New York, 1993, Viking.

Post SG: Psychiatry and ethics: the problematics of respect for religious meanings, *Culture, Medicine, and Psychiatry* 17(1):363, 1993.

Sege I and Mashek J: Census total will stand despite undercounting, *Boston Globe,* 1991, V. 240, p. 16.

Spector M: Poverty: The barrier to health care. In Spector R: *Cultural diversity in health and illness,* New York, 1979, Appleton, Century, and Crofts.

Spector RE: Cultural concepts in clinical care, *J Obstetric, Gynecologic, and Neonatal Nursing* 24(3): 243, 1995.

Spector RE: *Cultural diversity in health and illness,* ed 4, Norwalk, Conn., 1996, Appleton & Lange.

Spurlock J: *Black Americans.* In Comas-Diaz L and Griffith EEH, editors: *Cross-Cultural mental health,* New York, 1988, John Wiley & Sons.

Stoll RI: The essence of spirituality. In Carson VB, editor: *Spiritual dimensions of nursing practice,* Philadelphia, 1989, WB Saunders.

Thernstrom S, editor: *The Harvard encyclopedia of American ethnic groups,* Cambridge, Mass., 1980, Harvard University Press.

U.S. Bureau of the Census: *Current population reports, 1980 general social and economic characteristics part 1, United States summary, PC 80-1-cl,* Washington, D.C., 1983, U.S. Government Printing Office.

U.S. Bureau of the Census: *Current population reports, 1990 census of population and housing: summary populations and housing characteristics,* Washington, D.C., 1991, U.S. Government Printing Office.

U.S. Bureau of the Census: *Current population reports, series P-60, no. 175, poverty in the United States: 1990 United States,* U.S. Government Printing Office, Washington, D.C., 1991.

Yamamoto J: Japanese Americans. In Gaw A, editor: *Cross-cultural psychiatry,* Boston, 1982, John Wright.

Yoder D: Folk medicine. In Dorson RH, editor: *Folklore and folklife,* Chicago, 1972, University of Chicago Press.

CHAPTER 5

Theoretical Perspectives

Mary Magenheimer Webster
Gloria B. Callwood

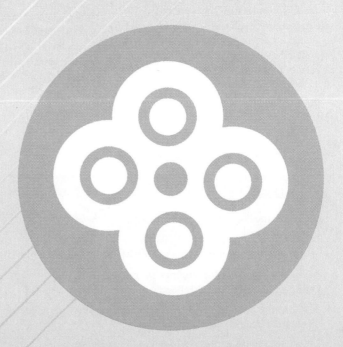

Alter ego A function of the therapist to reflect back the client's attitudes and feelings without including the client's negative connotations.

Autonomic nervous system (ANS) The system contained partly within the peripheral nerves, and partly within the central nervous system, directly connecting with hypothalamus; concerned with emotional states as they are related to specific patterns of autonomic responses.

Brain stem Consisting of the midbrain, pons, and medulla oblongata; it is involved in the transmission of all ascending and descending impulses.

Cognitive triad Pattern of thinking noted in people with depression and characterized by (1) a negative self-assessment, (2) a negative view of the present, and (3) a negative view of the future.

Ego The organizing part of the personality that is in contact with reality and acts as a mediator between the id and reality to find an acceptable satisfaction of needs.

Ego state A coherent set of feelings developed by the child's organization of similar life experiences and accompanied by a related set of coherent and observable behavior patterns. There are three ego states defined in transactional analysis: parent, adult, and child.

Extrapyramidal system (EPS) A system consisting of all the motor nerve tracts and pathways connecting the cerebral cortex, basal ganglia, thalamus, cerebellum, RAS, and spinal cord in complex circuits that are not included in the pyramidal system. It is involved with the regulation of stereotyped reflex movement of muscles, maintenance of muscle tone, and control of body movements.

Faulty information processing Fixed and rigid patterns of thinking that block the contextual aspects of a situation and are characteristic of people with depression.

Figure-background formation The concept that an organism's foremost need or specific interest will define the reality of the moment. Component of Gestalt theory.

Id The part of the personality that holds the instincts, primitive impulses, and all that is inherited, present at birth, and fixed in a person's psychic constitution.

Interactive context of behaviors The concept that behavior is shaped and reinforced by interaction with one's social system while the social system is being shaped and reinforced by the same interaction.

Libido The energy of the instincts held in the id.

Limbic system A set of structures comprising a vertical limbus (border) on each side of the brain surrounding the corpus callosum and a cerebral peduncle, or stemlike connecting part; and a horizontal limbus surrounding the midbrain. It is the principal location for intermediary processes and is primarily concerned with the integration of affective (emotional) aspects of behavior, memory, and basic drives required to preserve the individual.

Neurons Nerve cells made up of a body called the soma and extensions of protoplasm called neutrites.

Neurotransmitters A chemical substance derived from amino acids synthesized within neurons and stored at the nerve terminal in distinct vesicles. Neurotransmitters cause or inhibit responses and are released in response to physiologic situations.

Organismic self-regulation The concept that once the need is satisfied it will recede and allow the emergence of the next need.

Peripheral nervous system (PNS) The system referring to all parts of the nervous systems that lie outside the central nervous system (brain and spinal cord). It includes the twelve pairs of cranial nerves and the thirty-one pairs of spinal nerves and their branches.

Pleasure principle The goal of experiencing pleasure while avoiding pain. This principle represents the id's goal in the personality to satisfy a person's innate needs and instincts.

Reality principle The goal of postponing immediate gratification until a suitable object for this satisfaction is found. The ego is ruled by this principle.

Reframing A technique of changing the viewpoint of a situation and replacing it with another viewpoint that fits the facts equally well but changes the entire meaning.

Superego The part of the personality holding the internalization of the demands, prohibitions, and ideals of significant others (notably the parents). It is organized into two subsystems: the *conscience* (representing the demanding or forbidding aspects of the parents) and the *ego ideal* (representing the values thought to be morally good by the parents).

Synapses Specialized areas of contact between neurons where impulses cross.

Unconditional positive regard The stance of therapist modeling the unconditional acceptance of the client and based on the belief that the client is competent to direct him- or herself in a natural tendency to move forward toward integration.

LEARNING OBJECTIVES

- Discuss the basic concepts and application of each theory presented.
- Compare and contrast the various theoretical approaches.
- Describe the basic concepts of rational emotive therapy (RET) and compare with Beck's newer cognitive therapy.
- Determine the appropriateness of the various therapies to specific client needs.
- Evaluate inpatient and outpatient clients successfully by manipulating one or more theoretical approaches.

- Correlate the appropriateness of the various therapies to specific client needs and symptoms.
- Define and discuss the hemispheres and lobes of the brain, the structure of the brain stem, and their roles.
- Discuss the role of neurotransmitters.
- Describe the structure and purpose of the limbic system.
- Compare and contrast the peripheral nervous system, the autonomic nervous system, and the extrapyramidal system.

- Define and discuss the genetic strategies used to uncover correlates to mental illness.
- Discuss the connection between the endocrine system and psychiatric disorders.

The various theories of human behavior each have the common goal of producing frameworks that promote the understanding of the complexities of human behavior. They represent the theorists' attempts to organize and interpret data derived from human interactions and behaviors into a cohesive format from which one is better able to predict and interpret meanings and thus base effective interventions.

Theories are useful because they provide an organized way to view human behavior and, in so doing, suggest strategies to modify or change behavior. For example, if one views a disturbed behavior as resulting from intrapsychic conflicts, as in psychoanalytic theory, then it would follow that treatment would involve some type of exposure to the conflict, with the purpose of resolving that conflict. However, if one viewed the same behavior as stemming from an irrational thought or belief, as in the cognitive theories, then it would make sense that effective treatment would necessitate changing or altering the faulty belief system. The theory bases provide the framework for cohesive work and consistent treatment.

The difficulty, of course, lies in the multiple ways to view, organize, and interpret human behavior. The variety of theoretical perspectives represents the creativity and worldviews of their founders and reflects the cultural and social influences of their time. There is no dominant theory of human behavior, although all human behavior can be described by each theory. Practitioners either choose a theory that corresponds to their personal worldview and proceed to practice within that theory base or they familiarize themselves with several theories and move fluidly within them, depending on the needs of their clients. For example, a psychoanalyst works consistently with the psychoanalytic model while another practitioner uses the cognitive model to work with a client with depression and a behavioral model for a client with obsessive traits. In either case, it is important that practitioners be well-versed in the theoretical base from which they practice and comfortable with implementing it. Many therapists use an eclectic (varied) approach to treatment.

Therefore, the beginning practitioner is wise to review the various theories and their unique applications. The beginner, as well as seasoned practitioner, needs to consider the perspective of the theory as well as its applicability in various practice settings. Clients in outpatient settings may require a different approach from those in inpatient settings.

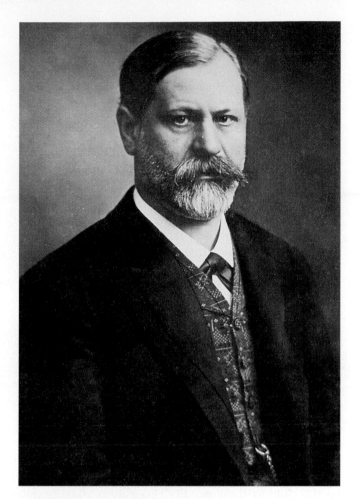

Figure 5-1 Sigmund Freud, 1856–1939.

(From the Bettmann Archive.)

PSYCHOANALYTIC THEORY

Sigmund Freud (1856–1939) developed the first organized theory of personality (Fig. 5-1). Prior to Freud, much of the thinking about personality development was based on vague philosophical approaches. Freud based his theory on clinical observations of the clients in his private practice and on his own subjective interpretations. Because of this subjective approach, the validity of his theory has been challenged. Nevertheless, Freud's theory of personality has formed the basis for psychoanalysis that has been expanded and revised by subsequent theorists.

Theoretical Overview

Freud organized his theory of personality around three major themes: levels of consciousness, sexuality, and functions of the personality. Freud saw individuals as being driven by instinctual impulses and believed that the personality is organized to control these impulses to the individual's best advantage. At times, this control involves repression of certain impulses, thoughts, or experiences. Freud proposed that these repressed impulses continue to affect an individual's behavior throughout his or her lifetime, for good or ill, without the individual's awareness.

Basic Concepts
LEVELS OF CONSCIOUSNESS

Freud's basic assumption was that all behavior is meaningful. The "little daily mistakes" of forgetting something, misplacing something, or misspeaking spring from a purposive desire that may or may not be known to the individual (A. Freud, 1979). If it is unknown, it is said to spring from the unconscious. Freud proposed that people know only a small part of their inner life and nothing of many feelings and thoughts that occur outside their awareness (A. Freud, 1979).

Freud theorized that the unconscious is developed during the early years of life in the following way: a child is born into the world with a variety of physical needs such as hunger, thirst, and physical comfort. When these needs are met, the child experiences pleasure. The child's central purpose in life is the attainment of pleasure (A. Freud, 1979), and the child thoroughly enjoys all the opportunities for attaining this pleasure, such as thumb-sucking, elimination, and/or masturbation. However, around the age of 1 year, the child realizes that the mother, the primary caregiver and satisfier of needs, does not belong only to himself but is shared with other siblings and the father. A jealousy of the others follows and, at about the same time, more demands are placed on the child by these people. The child is asked to give up these pleasures and begin the process of becoming "civilized" via activities such as toilet-training and ending thumb-sucking.* The child eventually gives up these pleasures due to adult interventions that may be perceived as threat of disapproval, withdrawal, or the possibility of physical harm. Initially, the child only pretends to take on the parental attitude but gradually accepts the adult values as truth. For this acceptance to happen, the child must undergo a reversal of feelings associated with the previous physical pleasures. In doing this, the memory rejects the pleasurable experiences and also the whole period of life associated with those memories. That period of life is seen as "unworthy" and "repulsive" compared with the adult standard (A. Freud, 1979). This part of life is relegated to the unconscious, the level of consciousness that holds the "forgotten" or repressed thoughts, feelings, and memories. Freud theorized that this occurs in the first 5 years of life and would explain the absence of memories most people have about their very early childhood. This "forgotten" part of the self remains active, however, and shapes relationships and interactions.

---

*The time frame of rearing a child in nineteenth century Vienna was different from our contemporary world but the process is the same.

FUNCTIONS OF THE PERSONALITY AND LEVELS OF CONSCIOUSNESS

As the child continues to grow, other processes occur in the organization of the personality. Freud saw the personality as consisting of three parts or systems: the id, the ego, and the superego. Each part has its own function within the personality.

Id. The **id** is the part of the personality that holds what is inherited, present at birth and fixed in a person's psychic constitution. The id contains the *instincts,* the primitive forces existing behind the tensions of the id that make somatic (bodily) demands, i.e., hunger, touch, thirst, sexuality. There are multiple instincts. Freud saw these instincts as the "ultimate causes of all activity" (S. Freud, 1960). Freud identified two main and oppositional categories of instincts: the life instinct and the death instinct. The aim of the life instinct is to bind things together into greater and greater unities that it strives to preserve. The death instinct tends to undo connections and destroy things, with the ultimate goal of reducing living things to an inorganic state (S. Freud, 1960). Such is the nature of the id that conflicting instincts can exist together and exert influence on an individual's behavior. The id is characterized by a subjectivity toward experience and a lack of logic, time, or morality. The id's goal in the personality is to satisfy a person's innate needs and instincts. The goal of experiencing pleasure while avoiding pain is called the **pleasure principle.** When acting under the pleasure principle, a person will seek immediate gratification of needs.

Libido. The id holds the individual's instincts and drives for pleasure, and these instincts provide energy for the personality. This energy is called the **libido,** the energy with which sexual instincts function in all phases of life (A. Freud, 1979). The id holds instincts and drives for pleasure, things the child repressed during the early years. Consequently, the id and its energy, the libido, are in the unconscious and exert their influences outside of a person's awareness. Freud considered the id to be the most important influence throughout one's life.

Ego. The **ego** develops from the id to function as an intermediary between the id and external reality. Its function is to mediate between the instincts of the id and the constraints of environment to find an acceptable and efficient satisfaction of needs. The ego is the only part of the personality that is in contact with reality. It is ruled by the **reality principle,** which aims to postpone immediate gratification until a suitable object for this satisfaction is found. Thus the ego is logical, organized, and causal and participates in problem solving. The ego's external, self-preserving function includes perception (storing experiences), adaptation, flight (escape), and activity (an attempt to modify the world to its own advantage). The ego's internal self-preserving functions involve gaining control over the demands of the instincts by deciding whether to satisfy, postpone, or suppress the demands (S. Freud, 1960). The ego functions as the organizer of the personality and strives to achieve harmony between the reality of the external world, the id, and the superego. Often this challenge produces anxiety. The ego is the aspect of the personality that experiences anxiety, as a signal to the self to protect oneself from some perceived danger (S. Freud, 1960). Since the ego has memories that can be recalled, it is associated with a level of consciousness called the preconscious. Preconscious material can move from the unconscious to the conscious but can also be obstructed by resistance (S. Freud, 1960). Consciousness is an awareness of an experience at the moment it occurs. It is the awareness of daily living. When the attention is taken away from one experience and into the next, that experience goes to the preconscious level where it subsequently can be retrieved.

Superego.   The **superego** develops from the ego as an internalization of the demands, prohibitions, and ideals of significant others (notably the parents). In fact, the superego can be viewed as a prolonging of the parental influence (S. Freud, 1960). The superego consists of two subsystems reflective of the parental influence: conscience and the ego ideal. The *conscience* represents the demanding or forbidding aspects of the parents. It represents what the individual thinks the parents considered morally wrong. The *ego ideal* evolves from the individual's perception of what the parents thought was morally good and includes ideals of strength, power, beauty, and success. The individual submits to the standards of conscience and ego ideal and, therefore, continues on in a relationship with the parents. This relationship is acted out in other relationships. The ego must intervene to reach a satisfactory level of interaction with the superego. Conflicts arise when an individual cannot live up to the standards of the superego. Shame and a lowered sense of self-worth occur if a person cannot meet one's ego ideal, and failure to live up to perceived moral standards can cause guilt.

Sexuality.   The second theme woven through Freud's theory of personality is that of sexuality. Prior to Freud, sexuality was thought to exist as an influence only after puberty. One of Freud's greatest contributions was the recognition that sexuality operates from the beginning of a child's development and that it gradually changes form from one phase to the next (A. Freud, 1979). Freud hypothesized that the stages of sexual development are predetermined and that this development is fueled by the energy from the libido. During the child's development, this energy becomes focused on specific body parts called erogenous zones and causes tension in those parts. This tension is relieved by manipulation of the body part, and the tension relief is experienced as pleasure. Freud saw the erogenous zones as progressing from the mouth (the oral phase—birth to 18 months) to the anus (the anal phase—18 months to 3 years) to the penis (the phallic phase—3 years to 5 years) and later to the entire genital area (the genital phase—15 years).*

Freud saw each of these periods as having a task and concomitant development of defense mechanisms to allow for the task accomplishments.

Oral Phase (birth to 18 months)
The oral phase is characterized by the need to suck, and the baby receives pleasure from the satisfaction of that need. The baby will suck its fist, toy, blanket, and so on if the nipple is not available.

Anal Phase (18 months to 3 years)
The anal phase is characterized by increasing awareness of the anal sphincter and the ability or inability to exert control over it. The child receives pleasure from being able to "produce" or expel from this body part during bowel movements.

Phallic Phase (3 years to 5 years)
The phallic phase is arguably the most challenged aspect of Freud's theory. Freud proposed that during this phase the young boy will touch his penis to receive pleasure and imagine sexual activity with the primary female in his life, his mother. However, he fears retaliation from his father in the form of castration. This desire for the mother and the fear of the father's reprisal is called the oedipal conflict (based on the Greek story of Oedipus, who killed his father and married his mother). According to Anna Freud, this conflict is so great that the boy flees to latency, which is marked by an absence of sexual interest (A. Freud, 1979).

According to Freud, girls undergo a different type of trauma at this stage of development. Girls try to be similar to boys but recognize the "inferiority of the clitoris" compared with the penis and in disappointment turn away from sexual life (A. Freud, 1979). This aspect of theory on female sexuality has been challenged by subsequent psychoanalysts as representing a male-dominated view of experience.

Genital Phase (15+years)
The genital phase is marked by sexual maturity and pleasure in heterosexual relations.

Techniques

The techniques of psychoanalysis flow from the premise that the conflicts causing disturbances are held in the unconscious and that it is possible to move this material from the unconscious to the preconscious and finally into consciousness. Once it is in one's conscious awareness, the individual can decide how to deal with it in a more adaptive manner. The two main means to access this unconscious material are through free association in the therapy session and dream analysis.

---

*Freud did not consider the latency period (5–12 years) or the prepubescent period (12–15 years). These were added later by his daughter, Anna Freud, as she continued the theory development.

Clinical Application   Psychoanalytic Theory

The client is a 42-year-old woman who is being treated for a depression of 6 months' duration. She has divorced and has been married to her second husband for 6 years. She has 2 children by her first marriage: a son who is 14 years old and a daughter who is 11 years old. She worked as a bank teller until the symptoms of the depression forced her to stop 4 months ago. Her parents are living in the same city although she rarely sees them.

Peggy has experienced anhedonia (loss of pleasure in life), decreased appetite, anxiety, and insomnia punctuated by nightmares.

The interaction that follows occurs 4 months into the client's treatment with a psychoanalyst. Peggy has previously discussed a recurring dream she has of a young child crying out into the darkness. Instead of stars in the dark sky, there are only eyes. The more the child cries, the smaller the child becomes.

Peggy: (Angry) "You just sit there, like a nothing. I don't even know if you're listening to me."

Therapist: Silence.

Peggy: "Well, are you?"

Therapist: Silence.

Peggy: (With sadness) "This is so typical. I talk and no one listens, even when I pay them to."

Therapist: Silence.

Peggy: "Why is it I'm so unnoticeable? Can't you notice me, you bastard?"

Therapist: Silence.

Peggy: (In small voice) "I feel small."

Therapist: Silence.

Therapist: "This is the experience of your dream: of crying out to eyes that watch but do not take the action that you expect. Because no action or rescue comes, you feel insignificant and angry. It may be helpful for you to consider whom you expected to take action. Your projected anger at me suggests a true anger at your father."

Continuing this work, Peggy eventually uncovers her anger at her father for his absence during her upbringing, a pattern that continued with her husbands.

FREE ASSOCIATION

During the therapy session, the individual is encouraged to relax and to speak whatever comes to mind without judging its appropriateness or relatedness. To facilitate this process, the client reclines on a couch or lounge chair while the therapist sits behind out of view, so as to avoid any eye contact that may impede the client's flow of thoughts. The psychoanalyst listens for themes and recurrent distortions in the material presented and assists in clarifying the material through various means. The analyst may make an *interpretation,* which proposes an underlying cause for a client's expressed feeling. As therapy progresses, the analyst will examine *transference issues,* in which the client's repressed feelings and past relationships are acted out in the current relationship with the therapist. The analyst will examine the *resistance* of the client to the work of therapy. The resistances are exhibited by avoidance (canceling appointments, failure to free-associate, or talking about trivia) or more active means (rejecting an interpretation or acting out of a need). Resistances exist around areas of conflict and are clues to the therapist of repressed material.

DREAM ANALYSIS

Freud viewed dreams as a means of access to the unconscious. Freud believed that every dream demands the satisfaction of some intrinsic need or the solution of a conflict. Furthermore, Freud proposed that dreams make broader use of memory and linguistic symbols, since the id has more liberty in dreams than in waking periods (S. Freud, 1960). Therefore dream analysis involves the client free-associating around a dream so the analyst can determine the deep unconscious meanings and symbols involved.

TRANSACTIONAL ANALYSIS

Transactional analysis (TA) provides an easily understood framework for examining human communication and its problems. It provides a straightforward approach to analyzing and changing communication that can be easily understood by a variety of clients, and it has become a popular mode of therapy since it was introduced by Eric Berne in 1961. Berne originally perceived TA as a powerful adjunct to psychotherapy (Berne, 1964), but since its introduction it has become a major form of psychotherapy in its own right. Basically, TA can be used to identify an individual's dysfunctional life stances through the analysis and correction of communication patterns, both internal (self-talk) and external (communication with others), as well as examining how this dysfunction is communicated over a lifetime.

Theoretical Overview

Berne proposes that young children are constantly organizing their life experiences and that similar thoughts, actions, and feelings become organized into **ego states.** An ego state is defined as a coherent set of feelings accompanied by a related set of coherent behavior patterns that are observable (Berne, 1964). Berne defines three ego states of an individual: *parent, adult, child.* Individuals move fluidly from one ego state to another, depending on which ego state is active at the moment. These ego states are recognizable to observers and are consistent over time.

PARENT EGO STATE

The *parent ego state* reflects the attitudes, beliefs, and behavioral patterns of the parental figures. The parent ego state can be the supportive "good parent" (the *nurturing parent*) or the never-pleased "bad parent" (the *critical parent*). The function of the parent ego state is to set limits, protect, support, and teach. It functions to save time for the individual by making many decisions and responses automatic (Berne, 1964). When a person acts from this ego state, the behaviors, words, and decisions will be automatic and imitative of the parental figures.

ADULT EGO STATE

The *adult ego state* allows the individual to objectively appraise the reality of a situation without self-criticism or conceit. The adult ego state functions as a rational data processing system to assist the individual in problem solving and dealing effectively with the outside world. As the rational ego state, the adult ego state is called upon to mediate conflicts between the automatic parent and the impulsive child. When a person is acting from the adult ego state, the behaviors and decisions represent a rational and informed response to the situation.

CHILD EGO STATE

The *child ego state* holds the spontaneous urges and impulses of an individual. The creative, playful, and intuitive impulses are associated with the *natural child* or *free child* ego state. The shamefulness, fearfulness, anxiety, and inhibitions that result when the natural child is thwarted in some manner by the controlling parental influence is called the *adapted child* ego state. The function of the child ego state is to experience feelings and to act spontaneously and intuitively. When a person acts from this ego state, decisions will be impulsive.

LIFE STANCES

Berne proposes that a person is always acting from one ego state or another but perhaps not consciously. As noted earlier, it is the early life experiences that help organize these ego states. As a cumulative effect of these early life experiences, the individual will develop a *life stance.* The life stance is basically the individual's assessment of personal self-worth compared with others. Berne has identified four life stances: (1) I'm OK, you're OK; (2) I'm OK, you're not OK; (3) I'm not OK, you're OK; and (4) I'm not OK, you're not OK. Berne's position is that the individual's basic stance is enacted in his or her communication with self and others. By analyzing the ineffective communication pattern, the therapist and client can identify both the sources of dysfunction and healthier alternatives. It is the goal of TA to help individuals recognize their various ego states and be able to function within the appropriate one by choice.

Basic Concepts
COMMUNICATION PATTERNS

Since Berne envisions that individuals always speak from one of the three ego states, he uses the ego states to analyze communication. TA represents an individual with three distinct ego states as depicted in the following illustration:

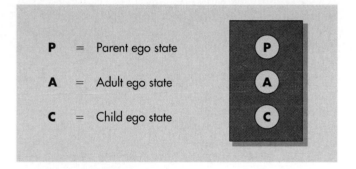

When analyzing communication from one person to another, Berne looks at transactions between the two individuals. A transaction is the smallest unit of interaction between two people and is represented by arrows designating stimulus and response. A transaction between two people is represented in the following illustration:

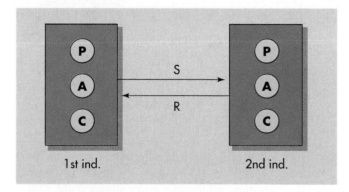

In this example, the first individual spoke from the adult ego state to the second individual's adult ego state, and the second individual responded from the adult ego state as well. This represents a *complementary* transaction or exchange. (A complementary exchange is also called a parallel exchange because the arrows are parallel to each other.) Complementary transactions are between role-appropriate ego states. The example above could be between two coworkers; two adults interacting with each other. The example below shows a complementary transaction between a mother and her child.

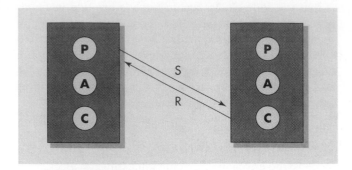

Please note the arrow lines are still parallel. Berne proposes that communication is effective and functions if it is complementary (Berne, 1964) because it is experienced as mutually satisfying and serves to further communication. For example, a child expects a parental response from a parent, and such a transaction is role-congruent (parent-child) and furthers communication.

Differences arise when the transactions are not along complementary (or parallel) lines. This means communication is not between role-appropriate ego states. The figure below represents such a transaction and is known as a crossed transaction:

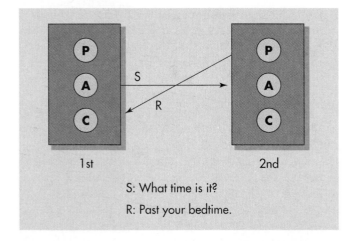

1st   2nd

S: What time is it?

R: Past your bedtime.

In this case, the first person initiated an adult to adult transaction. The second person, however, responded from the parent ego state, as if addressing a child. This is an example of a crossed transaction. Crossed transactions are experienced as dysfunctional and have the effect of stopping or inhibiting further communication. The most common form of a crossed transaction occurs when the stimulus is adult to adult, but the response is either parent to child or child to parent (Berne, 1964).

STROKES

Strokes refer to the TA concepts of validation. All human beings attempt to validate their existence through words and/or touch. Transactions that result in increasing esteem are called positive strokes. Those which produce negative feelings of belittlement are called negative strokes. Conditional strokes are received for accomplishing something while unconditional strokes are given just for being. Complementary communication would tend to increase a person's self-validation because it is effective; crossed transactions are confusing and often discounting.

Techniques

The techniques of TA are actually the steps in the progression of therapy. This is designed to help individuals become aware of their interactive style as a reflection of their life stance and to assist them in choosing the most appropriate ego stances. The approach is educative and challenging. Therapy is divided into four sections: *structural analysis, transactional analysis, game analysis,* and *script analysis.* All are best accomplished in a group situation.

STRUCTURAL ANALYSIS

Structural analysis is the initial part of the therapy. It begins with the client identifying the problem or symptom to be relieved by the therapy. The client is then educated to the functions and purposes of various ego states. Work is done to assist the client in identifying the phenomena associated with his or her own ego state presentations and to clearly separate the various states. This is done through analyzing transactions with the therapist or from examples that the client brings to therapy.

The overall goal of structural analysis is to assist the client to function predominantly from the reality-testing ego state (i.e., the adult ego state) (Berne, 1972). However, to accomplish this the therapist and client must identify the ego state that is carrying the symptoms with which the client presented (Berne, 1972). Consequently, the need exists to activate the adult ego state to rationally mediate between the more reactive and impulsive ego states. The goal of structural analysis is the mastery of internal conflicts through the diagnosis of ego states so the adult ego state can maintain mastery of the personality in stressful situations. At the conclusion of structural analysis, the client may terminate or proceed to the next phase.

TRANSACTIONAL ANALYSIS

Once clients are aware of their various ego states, they begin to examine when and how they are activated. The eventual goal of this phase is to establish the adult ego state in the executive role of the personality and actively choose when to release the child ego state or adult ego state and when to terminate their transactions (Berne, 1972).

Transactional analysis defines the active ego state in a transaction (Berne, 1972). Again, this is done through analyzing various transactions between group members. Clients learn how and when their parent or child ego state overrides their adult ego state, and then learn to formulate adult responses.

One of the specific techniques the TA therapist uses throughout therapy, but especially at this stage, is inviting the client to be responsible for choosing more appropriate responses to situations. This involves changing inappropriate parent or child responses to the realm of the adult. For example, a client complains from her helpless, fearful child state, "I'm scared; I can't do that." The therapist asks the client to take responsibility for that reaction by stating from the adult ego state, "I choose not to do that now," or better yet, "I will do that when I'm ready." This simple change of words serves to reinforce the adult ego state. As much as possible, these invitations are framed in the positive. After analyzing transactions, the client may end therapy or proceed to look at how the various ego states affect larger segments of his or her interactions.

GAME ANALYSIS

Games are defined as a recurring set of transactions that have a concealed or ulterior motivation (Berne, 1972). Berne views games as having their origins in early childhood when they are consciously initiated by the child. Over time, however, they become fixed in patterns, the origins lost, and the ulterior nature obscured (Berne, 1964). According to Berne, games are necessary and desirable because they provide structure for time. Berne views the world as offering little opportunity for intimacy in daily life, and games provide rituals to pursue this. At question is whether the individual's games offer the best outcome for him/her (Berne, 1964).

Indeed, while complementary and crossed transactions follow specific directions, games employ ulterior transactions that are tied to the individual's life stance. An ulterior transaction involves the game player pretending to do one thing but really doing something else. Therefore all games will involve a con of some sort (Berne, 1972). Berne and others have defined many types of games but all games have two characteristics: the ulterior quality and the "payoff" (Berne, 1964). Payoffs are the feelings that the game arouses within the individual.

Rather than examine the many games defined by Berne, one will be used to demonstrate game characteristics. A common game between spouses has been named "If It Weren't For You." As an example of this game, the wife complains that her husband restricts her social activities so that she never learned to dance. When she begins to change certain attitudes during her psychiatric treatment, her husband retreats from his previous

stance and she is able to expand her social activities. She takes dancing lessons only to discover a horrible fear of dance floors! Her domineering husband was actually providing her a real service by preventing her from even becoming aware of her fears.

The transactional analysis of this game is illustrated below. The dotted lines represent the ulterior transaction.

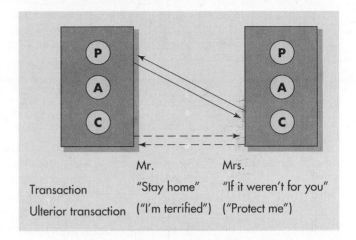

	Mr.	Mrs.
Transaction	"Stay home"	"If it weren't for you"
Ulterior transaction	("I'm terrified")	("Protect me")

Thus on the social level the game was a parent-child one with the husband as parent demanding the wife stay home and care for the house. The wife responded as a child with, "If it weren't for you."

On the ulterior level, the game is played between the child ego states, with the husband using his dominance to hide his child fear of desertion and the wife's child ego state seeking protection from fearful situations (Berne, 1964).

SCRIPT ANALYSIS

Script theory holds that the child makes early decisions about self and begins to make a life plan based on that decision (Goulding and Goulding, 1979). This script is reflected in the predominance of one ego state over another, in the individual's transactions, and in the choice of games. Thus script analysis represents the final stage of therapy and focuses on the analysis of lifelong patterns. The script is seen as the adaptation of early childhood experiences that is played out through life by manipulating others to play the necessary roles (Berne, 1972). Scripts are analyzed by examining the material collected in and out of group until the nature of the script becomes clear (Berne, 1972). Berne has identified many scripts in his book, *What Do You Say After You Say "Hello"?* For example, he identifies the Waif, Cinderella, the Dragon Slayer, and Sigmund.

GESTALT THERAPY

Gestalt therapy was founded by Fred (Fritz) Perls, who began his career as a psychoanalyst. Over time, he became dissatisfied with some of Freud's beliefs. Specifi-

---

Clinical Application   Transactional Analysis

The client, Peggy, has been involved in an outpatient transactional analysis group to deal with the symptoms of her depression. She has so far identified her life stance as "I'm not OK, you're OK," and is currently working with other group members to learn more about the activation of ego states.

The group has been working for about 45 minutes but Peggy has been silent.

Therapist: "Peggy, you've chosen to be quiet tonight."

Peggy: "I don't have much to offer. I learn a lot from listening to you."

Group member: "Do you mean you learn a lot from the therapist or from the group?"

Peggy: "Well, the therapist, I guess. I mean, he is the expert and we are all just trying to learn from him."

Group member: "Sounds like you're coming from your child ego state to me. Big Daddy has all the answers for us poor kids."

Peggy: "Well, I do feel like I need help. I feel ashamed and scared and sad and I want someone to help me."

Therapist: "Perhaps that person is closer than you think. What would your last comment sound like, Peggy, if you were speaking from an adult ego state instead of a child one?"

Peggy: "You mean, about being scared?"

Therapist: "Yes."

Peggy: "Um, I'm having some uncomfortable feelings . . . that will probably pass in time when I choose to let them go . . . I'd like to figure out how to let them go."

In her last statement, Peggy identified the more rational, problem-solving response of the adult ego state.

---

cally, Perls did not see intrapsychic conflicts as originating from conflicts with the id, ego, and superego, but rather from an individual's interactions with society. Gestalt therapy is considered a type of humanistic psychology.

Theoretical Overview

Perls envisioned human beings as "organisms" (beings) with their own nature and also as being a part of nature. Organisms have emotions, impulses, intellect, and a history of experiences which all serve to direct and fulfill the organism in life. Perls theorized that society made demands on organisms (or individuals) to conform to certain standards of behavior. In short, society makes demands on an organism by defining how the individual should function. Perls theorized that as the individual complies with these "should" demands of society, she distances herself from her own emotional experiences and, as a result, dissociates from being a part of nature (Stevens, 1975). The individual can no longer function at full capacity because of this alienation and separation from its nature. In fact, if allowed to continue, the individual may deteriorate in her functioning. In addition, this reliance on society for setting standards of behavior leaves the individual dependent on society for validation and support. In short, the individual organism cannot validate or support herself but instead is dependent on environmental support for approval and direction. To Perls, the result again is one of minimized functioning of

the individual, because she cannot self-regulate but must rely on external factors that may be making inappropriate demands on her.

Basic Concepts
TOP DOG AND UNDERDOG

Perls created the terms *top dog* and *underdog* to represent this struggle. *Top dog* refers to the **superego,** the "shoulds" of life learned in society, and Perls notes that this is so strong a force that it is rarely understood. The *underdog* represents the id, the impulses and desires. The underdog is constantly working at evading the top dog and the two are in constant strife, struggling for control. To a Gestaltist, cure represents the end of this control struggle between top dog and underdog, in that the struggle for supremacy is replaced by their natural acknowledgment and interaction (Stevens, 1975).

FIGURE-BACKGROUND FORMATION

Another tenet of Gestalt therapy is that of **figure-background formation.** Basically, this means that reality is determined by the individual's specific interest and needs and that "whatever is the organism's foremost need, makes reality appear as it does" (Stevens, 1975). For clarification, consider the following situation: three people enter a restaurant. The first person is famished, having worked through the day, skipping both breakfast and lunch. The obvious need is hunger and as the individual enters the restaurant, she notices the dessert tray by the entrance, the smells of cooking coming from the kitchen, and the food being eaten by other diners.

The second person enters the restaurant to use the phone. Her car has broken down just outside and she is late for a dinner meeting with a client. She needs to use the phone to inform the client of her later arrival and to call a cab. She enters the restaurant and scans the lobby for a telephone. She is not particularly aware that this is a restaurant; it just happened to be an open public building close to the spot of her car trouble.

The third person enters the restaurant. A friend arranged for her to meet a blind date here. As she enters she becomes aware of the dim lighting and of the many people in the restaurant and lounge. She begins to worry about whether or not she will be able to find her date.

In each of these cases, reality was experienced differently, demonstrating the Gestaltist point of view that reality is determined by one's needs. While the hungry individual was eating and her hunger pains were disap-

pearing, she was able to look around and notice several business associates dining in the corner. She began to wonder if she should join them or not. Once the second individual made her phone calls, she was able to examine the restaurant and menu while waiting for the cab and decided to return to the restaurant the next time she had an opportunity. When the third individual navigated the room and finally found her date, she was then able to concentrate on getting to know him. These examples demonstrate that once the need is satisfied, it recedes and the next need emerges. Perls saw this as **"organismic self-regulation"** (Stevens, 1975).

However, if the need is not met, conflict ensues because Gestalt theory proposes that an organism cannot tolerate an unfinished situation. Gestalt therapy works to help an individual complete unfinished situations through assisting the individual to differentiate the various aspects affecting any given moment or conflict, and then to integrate them (Stevens, 1975).

Clinical Application   Gestalt Therapy

Peggy is in an outpatient group and is currently the focus of the work. She sits opposite an empty chair in the center of the group's circle. The therapist is standing behind her. She has just told the group that she felt sorry for her father who had to work so hard all his life.

Therapist: "Pretend your father is sitting in that chair. What would you like him to know?"

Peggy: "Hi, Dad. It's been a long time. You're looking good . . . I guess."

Therapist: Silence.

Peggy: "I really don't know what to say to you, Dad . . . except thank you for taking care of me."

Therapist: Silence.

Therapist: "Can you remember a time he took care of you?"

Peggy: "No, I can't."

Therapist: "Tell him."

Peggy: "Dad, I don't know what to say to you, and I think that's a shame. I know you had to work hard to support us, but I work hard, too, and I still have more time for my kids than you did. What was the matter? Was it me?"

Therapist: "Switch chairs and answer your daughter."

Peggy: (As father) "Hello, Peggy. I don't know what to say to you, either . . . I guess I never did. I always counted on your

mother to do that. I tried to show you I loved you, but I guess I'm not good at showing it. Did I hurt you?"

Therapist: "Switch back."

Peggy: "It's not anything big, Dad. It's just all those small little things that make me feel I'm not worth much if . . . if, if even my own father doesn't love me."

Therapist: Silence.

Therapist: "Switch chairs again."

Peggy: (As father) "Well, Peggy, I do love you. I'm just lousy at showing it. You were always such a quiet little girl. I never knew what you were thinking. I don't know how girls think. Hell, I grew up with four brothers! But, Peggy, didn't you know I loved you?"

Therapist: "Switch back."

Peggy: "I guess I did. I remember you carrying me back to my bed after I'd fall asleep watching TV with you. I always liked that."

Therapist: Silence.

Peggy: "I guess I was kind of in awe of you, Dad. I didn't know what to say to you, but I did not think that would be hard for you. You seemed to be able to handle anything. You always knew what to do, so I just guessed you'd know what to do with me, too."

The conversation goes on until both Peggy and the father feel it was completed.

Thus the emphasis in Gestalt therapy is always on the present moment, the "here and now," known as the *foreground.* Past events and experiences are useful in that they influence the present moment. Gestalt therapists illuminate their influence so as to allow the individual to integrate them.

Techniques
CHAIR WORK

Perhaps the most well-known Gestalt therapy technique is *chair work.* In this exercise, the client sits opposite an empty chair, which represents some aspect of the foreground. It may be a person, a physical sensation, or an emotion. The individual has a conversation with the empty chair, stating her concerns and point of view. At the conclusion of her statement, the therapist asks her to switch seats and roles and to make a reply to what has been said. (Thus a man may be speaking to his "empty-chair" father and then be asked to take the father's position, via the chair, and respond to the son.) This switching back and forth is continued until the individual reaches some integration, and the need recedes.

This technique illustrates the Gestalt approach of *differentiation* and *integration.* It allows the client to experience the many aspects of the moment. Indeed, "chairworkers" frequently remember sounds, lights, voice tones, colors, seasons, emotions, and interactions of others, along with their own self-expectations and reactions. This interplay adds to the texture and depth of the experience, which may have been flattened by the conflict of the unmet need. By becoming aware and accepting of the many aspects of the situation and by listening to them, the individual is in a position to integrate them. She does not need to bend only to "top dog," but will find a way to blend all the acknowledged aspects of the situation. Perls has said that "True listening is understanding" (Stevens, 1975).

This aspect of Gestalt work is demonstrated again in the dream work. To Perls, a dream is a message that contains not only the kernels of an individual's life situation but also answers about how to change the nightmare of the situation. In Gestalt dream work, the individual acts out the various aspects of the dream and listens to the message of each aspect. The assumption is that each part of the dream is a projection of some aspect of the individual's life and consequently has a truth message that the individual finds difficult to hear or accept. By actually playing out the various parts of the dream while aware and in therapy, the individual is forced to identify with the various aspects of the dream and, in Gestalt terms, listen to it.

CLIENT-CENTERED THERAPY
Theoretical Overview

Another form of humanistic psychology is called client-centered therapy. It was developed in the 1940s by Carl Rogers, an American psychiatrist (Fig. 5-2), who ac-

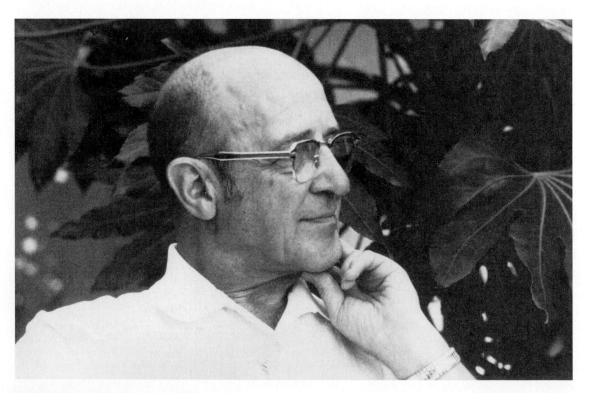

Figure 5-2 Carl Rogers, 1902–1987.

(From the Bettmann Archive.)

knowledges his indebtedness to Gestalt psychology for its recognition of the wholeness and center-relatedness of phenomena (Rogers, 1951). Rogers, too, extols the richness of experiences and the profound potential of human organisms to move forward. Indeed, it is this fundamental belief that the basic tendency of a human being is to move forward toward constructive change and integration that underlies client-centered (or Rogerian) therapy. The central hypothesis is that the individual has "sufficient capacity to deal constructively with all those aspects of his/her life that can potentially come into conscious awareness" (Rogers, 1951). The difficulty is that many aspects of the client's life or experiences are buried in shame, guilt, or denial. The individual's personality then works to continue to suppress thoughts or feelings that are not consistent with the individual's self-image. This suppression can cause difficulties in the individual's definition of self or in interpersonal relations. In addition, Rogers (1951) recognized that as society grew more and more diverse, it was less capable of supporting the individual in his or her definition of self. The goal of client-centered therapy is to bring these buried aspects of one's self to awareness, in full confidence that the individual will be able to accept these various parts, integrate them into an expanded self-concept, and live more fully and freely because energy is not being spent on suppression.

Basic Concepts

Rogers believed that within every human organism is "a whole person, distinctly organized" that can be approached directly in a therapy situation (Kovel, 1976). One of the basic tenets of client-centered therapy is the belief that at the core of the human organism is an organized self whose basic energy is moving forward toward integration of experiences. Another tenet at the core of this therapy is that interpersonal relationships are the basis for both health and neurosis, for it is in these aspects that the self is defined.

It therefore follows that a client-centered therapist would use the therapeutic relationship to support the growth of the client's inner self in its endeavors to comprehend, accept, and integrate those experiences that have been hidden from consciousness and prohibited from acceptance and integration. This is the core of Rogerian therapy.

Techniques

However simplistic the premise of client-centered therapy may sound, the practice of it is demanding on the therapist. It requires therapists to, as much as possible, totally accept the premise that an individual's natural tendency is to move forward toward integration. Therapists must be firmly grounded in this premise because all of their actions and words must flow from this basic premise in a consistent manner. Indeed, the only "technique" of client-centered therapy is to create a therapeutic relationship that is unconditionally accepting of and empathetic to the client. This is called **unconditional positive regard.** That is, the therapist must demonstrate the belief that the client is competent to direct himself (Rogers, 1951).

To demonstrate this belief, the therapist attempts to take on the client's frame of reference and perception of the world and relate it back to the client in an accepting and nonjudgmental way. The therapist does not attempt to change or challenge the client's thoughts or perceptions. In fact, just the opposite occurs. The therapist simply accepts and empathizes with what the client verbalized and relates it back without the negative connotation placed on it by the client. Rogers has described this technique as functioning as an **"alter ego"** for the client's attitudes and feelings, which allows the client to see him/herself "more clearly and to experience him/herself more significantly" (Rogers, 1951). The therapist is just as accepting and empathetic toward the negative or contradictory aspects of an individual's presentation as of the more positive aspects. As the client experiences the safety of acceptance from the therapist, he or she is free to explore these newer or contradictory elements of his or her self with the same acceptance shown by the therapist. In this self-acceptance, the client can accept and assimilate more experiences of the self in a broader way than before and move toward a reorganization of self that is more inclusive and comfortable because it is more consistently acceptable to the self (Box 5-1).

BEHAVIOR THERAPY

Behavior therapy involves attempting to modify an observable behavior. It differs from other therapies in that the focus is on the behavior rather than the cause. The behavior could be an emotional response, verbalization, or action.

Theoretical Overview

One of the early theorists working with the concept of behaviors was Ivan Pavlov (1849–1936). Pavlov described the learned behavior he observed when a stimulus was present and when a response to that stimulus was given. He was well-known for his studies with salivation of dogs. Pavlov first noted that dogs salivate when food is within their sight and that the salivation occurs even before the dog begins to eat. As an experiment, Pavlov would ring a bell and present food to the dog, and the dog would salivate. After repeating this sequence several times, the dog salivated with the ringing of the bell, whether or not the food was present. Pavlov called this *conditioned response* or *classical conditioning.*

Another theorist involved in early behaviorist work was B. F. Skinner (1904–1990). Skinner's belief was that virtually all behavior resulted from learned environmental experiences. He thought not only that human behavior is completely determined by one's history but also that one learns from those experiences that have been repeatedly reinforced. This is known as *operant conditioning.*

Even though both these theorists looked at behavior, Pavlov proved the stimulus occurred before the behavior, and Skinner believed that the reinforcement should come after the behavior occurred. It is obvious then that Pavlov's theories of behavior were more experimentally driven whereas Skinner took a more retrospective approach.

Basic Concepts

All therapies involve learning to some degree, but proponents of behavior therapy view client learning as the primary focus of their work. The behavioral therapist engages the client in an activity that is focused on learning about an unwanted or troubling behavior. By having the client focus on his or her problem behavior, it separates the problem or behavior from the client. The problem is something the client *has* rather than *is.* This process, in essence, allows the client to become a "scientist" and as such, the client is able to study the problem in an intellectual way rather than in an emotional way. Therefore there is some distance placed between the client and the problem behavior.

Once the problem behavior has become separate from the client and the client believes it is something he or she "has," rather than "is," the problem can more clearly be observed, dissected, and attacked. Because the problem is not part of the whole person, aggressive treatment will not interfere with the client/therapist relationship. The aggressive treatment will actually strengthen the therapeutic relationship because the therapist and client work together to diminish the problem.

The first goal of behavior therapy is to narrow the problem down to something tangible, clear-cut, and well-defined. This allows the client to feel the problem can be better controlled and removes the feelings of hopelessness and being overwhelmed. Therefore, defining the problem gives the client some relief from his or her symptoms.

Techniques
SYSTEMATIC DESENSITIZATION

One technique of behavior therapy is known as *systematic desensitization,* created by Joseph Wolpe for treatment of phobias. This treatment begins with a series of graded tasks to be performed by the client. The client is asked to perform an activity that is related to the phobia in some way, but is beneath the client's ability. Because the task is easy for the client to accomplish, successful confidence is established and the client develops the feeling of anticipation and the desire to "get on with the treatment." At this stage the client usually wants to confront the phobia and do even more than what the therapist requires. As treatment progresses, the activities or tasks come closer to approaching the phobia. By the time the client is ready to deal with the phobia, it is generally at the client's insistence since the therapist is still trying to restrain the client somewhat.

When it is time for the "real-life" exposure, the exposure time should be one hour or more. This allows time for any feelings of fear, whether psychologic or physically manifested, to diminish naturally. Prolonged exposure allows the client to develop natural relaxation in spite of the phobic situation.

A common element of the task for the client is to keep a journal or log about the therapeutic experience. This enables the client to be the "scientist" and to record any reactions, feelings, and thoughts as they relate to the tasks of therapy. The process of journalizing also helps keep the problem narrow, clear-cut, and separate from the client. This method also helps keep physical symptoms distinct and accurate and reduces the likelihood that the client will exaggerate his or her reactions to the event at a later date.

RELAXATION TRAINING

Another technique of behavior therapy is relaxation training. There are a variety of relaxation techniques used to decrease anxiety or nervousness and to assist clients who experience sleep disorders.

One technique, known as *abdominal breathing,* can be used on its own or with other relaxation techniques. Abdominal breathing requires that the client breathe deeply by expanding the lower lungs and raising the abdomen and then exhaling. This technique encourages the body to relax and to slow down and thus promotes the feeling of calmness.

Clinical Application Behavior Therapy

Peggy is working with a behavior therapist to deal with various aspects of her depression. Since she lost her job, she has noticed an increased fearfulness in her life, with old fears becoming more predominant. Especially troublesome is her fear of going to the grocery store.

In her first session she discussed experiencing physical sensations when she was in the store. She became dizzy and nauseated and experienced heart palpitations so often she feared she would have a heart attack.

She and the therapist have defined the problem of their focus as "panicky/fearful feelings in grocery store."

The treatment begins with the therapist educating Peggy as to the physiologic basis of her symptoms. Her first assignment is to keep a journal of these feelings, noting their intensity and duration and the precipitating event. This begins the work of segmenting the problem and observing it in a scientific, nonemotional manner.

Progressive relaxation is another relaxation technique in which there is systematic contracting and relaxing of different muscle groups. This allows the client to distinguish between the feeling of tension vs. relaxation, which is the first step toward effective treatment.

Another technique is called *autogenics.* This technique uses self-talk to promote relaxation. For example, telling oneself "I can handle this," "I am calm," or "I am relaxed" can be helpful in ultimately achieving a relaxed state.

RATIONAL EMOTIVE THERAPY
Theoretical Overview

Rational emotive therapy (RET) was developed by Albert Ellis during the 1960s and 1970s as he became disillusioned with the effectiveness of the psychoanalytic approach and yet found the behavioral approach to be limiting as well. Ellis views individuals as being able to actively and consciously choose their orientation toward themselves. His RET is designed to help individuals apply a scientific approach to their own situation to test the validity of their self-assumptions. In this way, Ellis views his approach as "humanistic" in that it encourages individuals to use their most human skill: to think about thinking (Ellis, 1973).

Some theorists have defined RET as a cognitive therapy because of its use of cognitive restructuring, and others regard it as an existential approach because it acknowledges an individual's freedom to choose. Ellis, however, argues that by dealing with the attitudes and beliefs of individuals through activating their human ability to think and by accepting humans as fallible, RET is indeed a humanistic therapy. The goal of RET is to assist individuals in their unconditional self-acceptance, not in terms of performance or accomplishments, but only in terms of "being." Ellis points out that self-acceptance does not involve esteeming the self because esteeming implies rating or valuing oneself. In fact, he considers rating the self in any way to be "ridiculous." According to Ellis, the only aspects of a human being that can be rated are traits and performances, and these are distinctly separate from the self. The self is inherently valued. Yet Ellis sees many people choosing to base their self-worth on irrational philosophic premises about life and self. It is the goal of RET to empower individuals with the skills that scientifically challenge these irrational premises, so that they will behave differently (rationally), and enjoy life (Ellis, 1973). Although Ellis defines himself as a humanist, his groundbreaking work is the precursor to cognitive therapy.

Basic Concepts

Ellis agrees with others that an individual must interpret data from the environment to make sense of it and respond to it. A basic premise of RET is that the way in which an individual interprets the data will affect his

---

Box 5-2 Basic Irrational Ideas According to Albert Ellis (RET)

1. The idea that it is a dire necessity for an adult human to be loved or approved by virtually every significant other person in his/her life.

2. The idea that one should be thoroughly competent, adequate, and achieving in all possible respects, to consider oneself worthwhile.

3. The idea that certain people are bad, wicked, or villainous, and that they should be severely blamed and punished for their villainy.

4. The idea that it is awful and catastrophic when things are not the way one would like them to be.

5. The idea that human unhappiness is externally caused, and that people have little or no ability to control their terrors and disturbances.

6. The idea that it is easier to avoid, than to fail, life's difficulties and self-responsibilities.

7. The idea that one's past history is an all-important determinant of one's present behavior, and that because something once strongly affected one's life, it should indefinitely affect it.

From Ellis A: *Humanistic psychotherapy*, New York, 1973, McGraw-Hill.

---

emotions and actions. For instance, if an individual interprets an argument with a significant other as "terrible" or "destructive," she may feel frightened and vulnerable. If, however, she views the argument as "clearing the air," she may feel validated and assertive. Ellis goes on to propose that much of what individuals base their interpretation and behavior on are faulty assumptions learned so early in their experiences that they are never questioned. These basic irrational ideas are listed in Box 5-2.

A-B-C

Ellis proposes that people upset themselves by holding onto and using these basic misassumptions. He demonstrates this interaction between thoughts and emotions with the ABCs of rational emotive therapy. "A" represents the action, activity, or agent (i.e., person) with whom the individual becomes upset. "B" represents the belief system activated by "A." The belief can be rational or irrational. A rational belief (rB) can be supported by data, while an irrational belief (iB) cannot be supported by any evidence. Irrational beliefs frequently imply a demand for a certain outcome. These demands are frequently couched in phrases containing "should," "ought," or "must." "C" represents the consequence of belief and is either a rational consequence (rC) or an irrational consequence (iC). Irrational consequences present as dysfunctional or self-defeating behaviors.

For an example of this A-B-C schema, consider a student who has received a low grade on an important exam. The grade represents the activating event. The student may evaluate this as a sign of poor performance in the course. This would represent a rational belief because it is reported by the data. As a consequence, the student may ask the teacher for extra instruction, join a study group, or engage a tutor. This would be a rational consequence to the rational belief and promotes a self-enhancing activity. If, however, the student responds with an irrational belief, the scenario would be different. Perhaps the student thinks, "This proves I'm incompetent and that I'll never make anything of myself. I ought to do better." As a consequence of this thinking, the student becomes depressed, avoids interactions around the difficult subject, and eventually drops out of school. This would be the irrational consequence of an irrational belief.

To quickly identify the faulty assumptions and modify the consequent self-defeating behaviors, Ellis proposes that therapy include a combination of cognitive approaches and behavioral techniques, while always working within a therapeutic relationship that encourages the individual to express emotions. The therapist's stance is one of unconditional acceptance of the individual. This models the basic assumption that the self is totally acceptable, while traits or behaviors are to be evaluated. The RET therapist is active and directive, orientating the individual to the scientific method and its application in his or her situation.

Techniques

The therapy begins with an overview of RET. The therapist orients the individual to the premise that thoughts affect emotions, reactions, and behavior, and that many of one's thoughts are inaccurate. The therapist explains that much of the work will be examining the individual's thoughts and evaluating their accuracy, using the scientific method of testing hypotheses for validity.

The therapist then actively questions the individual to uncover the individual's basic stance toward self and the belief system that supports it. The RET therapist is direct, challenging, and often confrontive. The work is done through questioning rather than making interpretations or statements. The attempt is always to assist the individual to become aware of and to challenge self-defeating thinking. RET therapists frequently ask "How do you know that?", "What proof do you have to support that?", or "Are there other possible explanations?"

RET uses behavioral techniques to help undermine the cognitive aspect of self-defeating behavior. Once an individual is oriented to the therapy and has some recognition of that process, the therapist assigns "activity homework." These activities are designed to test some irrational belief held by the individual or to challenge the behavioral consequence of the irrational belief. The work should always focus on the symptom causing the most discomfort to the client. These activities are designed to proceed progressively and are unique to each

Clinical Application   Rational Emotive Therapy

Peggy is in the initial stages of RET and has been educated about the course of therapy, the ABCs, and the irrational ideas of life.

Peggy: "I'm so worthless."

Therapist: "Why do you say that?"

Peggy: "I can't do anything."

Therapist: "What can't you do?"

Peggy: "I can't be a good wife, or mother, or daughter. I even lost my job. I'm a failure in every aspect of my life."

Therapist: "Let's take them one by one. Which do you want to start with?"

Peggy: "Uh, being a mom."

Therapist: "OK. What makes you think you're not a good mom?"

Peggy: "I have no patience with the kids. I snap at them more than I used to . . . I don't do anything for them anymore. I used to make cookies or help them with their schoolwork."

Therapist: "Do you still fix dinner?"

Peggy: "Sure, but the meals are not as good as they used to be."

Therapist: "Do you talk with the kids at all?"

Peggy: "Of course! I keep up with their lives, but I'm not as involved as I should be."

Therapist: "So, you feed them and talk with them. Is that right?"

Peggy: "That's right."

Therapist: "But you don't do all the things you think you should, like helping with schoolwork and making cookies. Is that right?"

Peggy: "Yeah."

Therapist: "So, because you don't do at least two of the things you think you should, you've decided that you're a failure as a mom. Is that what you think?"

Peggy: "Well, yes."

Therapist: "What do you think you're basing that on?"

Peggy: "I guess one of those irrational ideas, that I have to be completely competent all the time and in all ways to be worthwhile."

The therapist continues to point out the irrational beliefs held by Peggy until she recognizes that reality doesn't support those beliefs.

---

individual. For example, Ellis has used role-playing to assist individuals to become desensitized to rejection and has assigned progressive tasks to those who procrastinate. He has also assigned public speaking engagements for shy individuals.

Through all of this, the therapist consistently points out that reality does not support the irrational belief held by the individual. For instance, the individual who is so afraid of rejection does not die or become a worthless person when rejected. The procrastinator does not have to write the world's greatest novel in order to be effective, and the shy person is able to speak publicly although with some anxiety.

COGNITIVE THERAPY

Cognitive therapy was begun by Aaron Beck in the 1970s as an outgrowth of his interest in depression. Beck had accepted the Freudian hypothesis that depression represents hostility and that the client withdraws into self because of a need to suffer. As Beck studied the research, he found that people with depression consistently interpret their experiences in a negative way. As he reviewed this further, he developed a theory of depression and

consequently a therapeutic approach based on identifying and counteracting an individual's negative thoughts (or cognitions). Beck acknowledges the contribution of the behavioral therapies in the development of cognitive therapy (especially evident in some of the techniques) (Beck, 1979). Beck, however, places much more importance on the external (or mental) experiences of his clients than does behaviorism (Beck, 1979).

Theoretical Overview

Beck holds, as do other theorists, that the way in which a person structures the world through thoughts and evaluations largely influences both affect and behaviors. The classic example of the glass filled with water to its midpoint serves to illustrate this point. If one observes the glass to be half empty, one may experience sadness stemming from the loss or fear that there may not be enough water for all. However, if one's reaction is that it is half full, one may be grateful that there is water at all or hopeful that there will be more. How one perceives a situation influences the emotions one has toward that situation. It follows then that actions and behaviors will match the emotions.

Basic Concepts

Beck explored this concept with people who experience depression and found a consistency in the way they structured their experiences. He organized this into a cognitive model of depression with the following components.

COGNITIVE TRIAD

The **cognitive triad** is Beck's term to identify three common characteristics in the thinking of people with depression. *First,* depressed people hold a very negative view of themselves, tending to see themselves as defective in some way (psychologically, morally, or physically). Because of these presumed defects, they tend to view themselves as worthless. *Second,* people with depression tend to evaluate ongoing life events in a negative way (e.g., the glass is *always* half empty). The person with depression tends to misinterpret available data so as to always result in a negative outcome (i.e., defeat, humiliation, rejection, or inadequacy). *Third,* the person with depression assumes that the future holds no promise and that the current difficulties will continue. He or she expects despair, frustration, and failure to persist (Fig. 5-3).

The cognitive triad is basic to Beck's understanding of depression. He views all other symptoms of depression as connecting back to these cognitive patterns of negative self-image, negative interpretation of ongoing experiences, and the negative view of the future.

SCHEMAS

The term *schema* refers to an individual's organization of incoming data into meaningful patterns. Beck points out that while people tend to conceptualize situations in a variety of ways, an individual will be fairly consistent in interpreting similar sets of data. These schemas have been learned over time and represent attitudes or assumptions that have been formed on the basis of one's experiences. Schemas affect how an individual will cognitively structure experiences and consequently respond to them. Beck proposes that in a state of depression, dysfunctional schemas become prevalent and the data from a situation are distorted to fit the dysfunctional schema. The individual is no longer able to match an appropriate schema to a situation because the dysfunctional schema predominates over so much of the thinking. In effect, any stimulus will trigger the negative, dysfunctional schema. This would then explain why people with depression cannot "see" or respond to the many positive aspects of their lives.

FAULTY INFORMATION PROCESSING

This aspect of the cognitive theory of depression refers to the characteristics of a depressed person's thinking. Beck calls depressed thinking "primitive" as opposed to

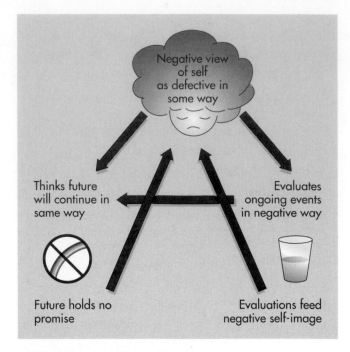

Figure 5-3 The cognitive triad.

more mature thinking. Primitive thinking is more absolute than relative, more judgmental than flexible, and more invariable than variable. It is "black and white" thinking with the emphasis on black. Primitive thinking misses the context and variations of life and tends to be rigid and fixed. It locks the person with depression into a flat and unidimensional way of thinking, an "all-or-none" mentality whereby he or she views self and actions as "all-bad." Faulty patterns of processing information are the following:

- Arbitrary inference: Drawing a conclusion when evidence does not support it, e.g., deciding that one's boss is displeased with one's work because the boss did not greet the person in the morning.

- Selective abstraction: Paying attention to only one detail of a situation, taking that detail out of context, and ascribing the meaning to the situation based on this singular detail. For example, a woman is explaining a plan to save enough money to go on a wonderful vacation to her depressed spouse. In the course of doing this, she mentions, "I've always wanted to go there." The depressed spouse then takes this one side comment out of context and decides he's been a failure as a husband because he hadn't known this and therefore probably had never met her needs in any way.

- Overgeneralization: The practice of drawing a conclusion based on one incident and then applying it in general, e.g., a person nervously spills a glass of water when talking with another person and concludes that he must be totally socially incompetent and unable to carry on even the simplest conversations.

- Magnification and minimization: The inability to evaluate the importance or significance of an event to the point of creating a distortion, e.g., a copy editor misses one minor misprint in a publication and berates herself for months for incompetence.

- Personalization: The tendency to assume that external events are related to one's self when there is no reason to make such a connection. For example, a mother makes cookies for her child's class and the next day a few of the children are ill. The mother assumes it is from her cookies although she does not even know whether the ill children ate the cookies.

- Absolute thinking: The habit of defining experiences in one or two opposite categories, e.g., good or bad, perfect or flawed, healthy or sick, worthwhile or worthless.

In summary, the cognitive triad, the concept of schemas, and faulty information processing are the bases for Beck's cognitive therapy of depression. The techniques of cognitive therapy naturally flow from the theory base.

Techniques

The therapeutic approach in cognitive therapy is a combination of cognitive and behavioral techniques. The cognitive techniques assist clients to notice their own automatic negative thoughts and the connection of those thoughts to moods and actions. The cognitive techniques also help individuals evaluate the presence or absence of evidence supporting the automatic thought, and to replace it with a more reality-based interpretation (similar to Ellis' scientific method approach). The behavioral techniques are used to show individuals that they are capable of interrupting dysfunctional patterns.

USE OF THE THERAPEUTIC RELATIONSHIP

Beck repeatedly advises that the therapist must be well-grounded in the theory before attempting the therapy. He warns that the techniques can seem "gimmicky" or contrived if not based on a solid understanding of the theory. In addition, he stresses the importance of a strong therapeutic relationship and interpersonal skills. It is not enough to simply perform the techniques; the interventions must be based on a sound understanding of the theory and presented within a strong therapeutic relationship of concern, acceptance, and empathy. Beck points out that the effectiveness of a therapeutic relationship depends greatly on the client's ability to experience and express feelings. Very often, people with depression do not think they can honestly say how they feel and perceive a pressure to keep up a facade to hide the depth of their despair. This can lead them to think of themselves as dishonest and describe themselves as deceitful. It is only in an effective therapeutic relationship that they are able to act in an emotionally congruent

manner. This helps to restore a sense of honesty and genuineness (Beck, 1979).

Although Beck proposes that all feelings are acceptable and open to discussion, he advises that the therapy time be structured so that the entire time is not used to express emotions. It is the work of therapy to explore the attitudes that cause the emotions, and this is a collaborative process.

The therapist begins by acknowledging the client's "personal paradigm." In this instance, a paradigm is a person's model or view of the self. The client's paradigm is his or her particular presentation of the cognitive triad, schemas, and faulty information processing. The therapist has the client give examples of past and present events that confirm his or her negative ideas, in an attempt to identify the underlying patterns of thoughts. The therapist makes no attempt to counteract or discount these beliefs. Rather, the cognitive therapist poses questions for the client's consideration. These questions are used to elicit what the client is thinking, as well as to plant the seed of other possibilities the client has ignored. Beck has found skillful questioning to be a useful device for identifying, considering, and correcting cognitions and beliefs (Beck, 1979).

Together, the therapist and client redefine the client's initial chief complaint into a target symptom that can be the focus of their work. A target symptom is defined as "any of the components of depressive disorder that involves suffering or functional disability" (Beck, 1979). Beck identifies five areas: affective symptoms, motivational symptoms (e.g., the desire to escape), cognitive difficulties, behavioral symptoms, and physiologic, or vegetative, symptoms. Selection of the target symptom is made by choosing the one that is most upsetting to the client and also amenable to therapy. The work is then to identify and correct the specific thinking that leads to these symptoms.

REATTRIBUTION TECHNIQUES

Perhaps the best-known specific cognitive techniques are those called reattribution techniques. These techniques are designed to assist the depressed individual who assumes total blame/responsibility for anything that goes wrong based on her automatic negative self-assessment. These techniques are designed to help the person with depression realize that there are many reasons for things to go wrong, not just one's presence in the world. The technique has also been called "de-responsibilitizing" because it assists in relieving the client of the burden of total responsibility for everything in his or her life.

This technique requires that the client keep a record that consists of four columns with the following headings: Situation; Emotions; Automatic Thoughts; Other Interpretations.

The client records situations that trigger negative feelings and records these feelings and the automatic thoughts associated with them. The client is then chal-

Clinical Application   Cognitive Therapy

The following is Peggy's "homework" and is an example of reattribution technique.

Situation	Emotions	Automatic thoughts	Other interpretations
1. Kids were late for school.	Upset/shame. I made a mistake.	I should have helped them more in morning. I did something wrong.	They dawdled (wasted time) on the way. The clocks are off.
2. I forgot name of person I was introducing to friend.	Embarrassed. Humiliated.	I'm losing my mind. I can't do anything right. I'm socially inept.	Everybody forgets sometimes. I'd only met her once a month ago.
3. Burned cookies.	Shamed. Sad.	I'm a failure. I can't even do simple things.	Buzzer didn't go off. Kids didn't call me.

lenged to come up with other possible explanations regarding the situation and, by so doing, begins to evaluate and modify the automatic thoughts.

BEHAVIORAL TECHNIQUES

Behavioral. Beck emphasizes that behavioral techniques are used to supplement the cognitive work. One of the main reasons for using a behavioral technique is to demonstrate to the client that the negative assumptions and conclusions are incorrect and thus pave the way for improvement in performance in those aspects of life that are important to the client.

After the therapist has assisted the client with identification of appropriate data to be studied, he or she designs an experiment to help the client become more specific in his or her observations and thinking and to recognize gradations. For example, the therapist may ask the client to keep an activity schedule to test the hypothesis that inactivity increases negative thinking. If so, then perhaps activity would decrease such thoughts. The client's task is to make a schedule of daily activities and record their effect on cognition, as well as any changes in the level of depressed thinking that accompanies the activity. The point is to get the client to observe (not evaluate) how much is accomplished by the client throughout the day.

Such an "experiment" implies many things, such as: The client can organize activities; there are subtleties to reactions that the client may be missing; and the despair may be influenced by activities. None of this is "told" to the client, but rather left for them to discover through the homework and the skillful questioning of the therapist.

MASTERY AND PLEASURE TECHNIQUE

The next step may be the mastery and pleasure technique. Mastery refers to the sense of accomplishment one feels after a task completion, and pleasure refers to the pleasant feeling associated with it. In this technique,

the client rates a certain activity in terms of his mastery over it, and pleasure in doing the task. This technique begins to counteract the client's unidimensional thinking by having him or her notice even small variations in successes and pleasures (Beck, 1979).

COGNITIVE REHEARSAL

Another technique is known as *cognitive rehearsal* in which the client is asked to imagine all the steps required to complete a task. This is useful in breaking down the repetitive thought patterns that so often prevent a depressed client from accomplishing things.

When the client has demonstrated the ability to observe his or her actions and thoughts, the therapist moves to the higher level of cognitive techniques, to assist the client in discovering his or her own thinking and in testing the validity of his or her automatic thoughts. It is here that the therapist and client act as true collaborators as the client learns to observe and record his thoughts, images, and self-talk, and the therapist continues to assist the client to observe and identify the dysfunctional thinking. After the client has identified an automatic thought, the therapist poses questions that help the client ascertain the connection between the thought and certain behaviors the client has identified, especially those in recent experiences. Homework is assigned to further assist the client in this task.

The therapy continues until the client is able to identify his automatic thoughts and recognize their effects on feelings and behaviors, and develop more balanced cognitions and self-statements more reflective of reality.

STRATEGIC THERAPY

Communication theorists propose that the actual structure of language creates reality for individuals. They suggest that the choice, use, and organization of words influence one's perceptions of one's experiences. In fact, many theorists propose that defining an experience with words limits and confines the experience (Box 5-3). Consequently, communication theorists have extensively investigated how language can influence a person's perceptions and reactions and, in a therapeutic sense, how the use of words can promote health.

Strategic therapy, a form of communication therapy, has become increasingly popular as an effective and time-efficient approach to treatment. There are variations of strategic therapy (i.e., solution-focused therapy, brief therapy), but all types trace their beginnings to the pioneering work of Gregory Bateson, Don Jackson, Paul Watzlawick, John Weakland, and Richard Fisch at the Mental Research Institute (MRI) in Palo Alto, California, in the 1950s and 1960s. This group took a decidedly different approach in its attempt to decrease the time of treatment for individuals and families. They studied the process of change itself. The "Palo Alto Group" examined problem-formulation and maintenance in human systems and how best to promote change in that system (Greene, 1991).

Theoretical Overview

Strategic therapy represents a unique departure from medical model-based approaches. In the medical model, the healer diagnoses a pathology or dysfunction and then treats it. Strategic therapy is based more on the approach of one of its founders, anthropologist Gregory Bateson. While working with psychotic clients at a V.A. hospital, Bateson would ask: "In what human context does this 'crazy' behavior fit?" The anthropologic position is that behavior makes sense in the context in which it occurs. This is one of the underlying assumptions of strategic therapy. The corollary to this is that behavior is continually being shaped and reinforced by the individual's support system (i.e., the family) and vice versa. This is called the **interactive context of behavior** (Fisch et al, 1986). Over time, behavior patterns arise between people, and some patterns may be viewed as problematic. A strategic therapist always examines the problem behavior in the context of the surrounding behaviors.

The MRI group theorizes that the reason behaviors are viewed as problematic has to do with people's perception of reality. Most people assume that there is one real-

ity that is based on objective truths, and that their own thinking aptly reflects this. If this assumption is valid, then it would follow that anyone with a different view of reality than their own must be either "mad" or "bad" (Watzlawick, 1977). The MRI Group proposes that there is no *one* reality. Each person creates his or her own reality through communication with others (Watzlawick, 1977). For example, a child's behavior may be called "stubborn" by one individual and "determined" by another. Each definition creates a different "reality" for the child and other. If the child's behavior is seen as "stubborn," it may also be viewed as problematic and requiring treatment. If it is seen as "determined," it may become the source of pride and esteem. As Shakespeare said, "Nothing is good or bad, but thinking makes it so." The concept of reality as a function of one's communication is essential. Following this, change is approached within the framework of communication and the complainant's* view of reality. To promote change, the strategic therapist must learn the individual's view of the reality of the problem.

The MRI group has done a considerable amount of research on change, and it has defined two types: *first-order change* and *second-order change*. First-order change is defined as a change within the system that remains unchanged. Second-order change is that which changes the system itself. Second-order change is discontinuous and therefore appears illogical from within the system (Watzlawick, 1974). One of MRI's classic examples will help to illustrate first- and second-order changes. *Example of first-order change:* A dreamer is caught in a nightmare. Within her dream, she does many things to end the nightmare: she runs, hides, and tries to change its course. This is first-order change as the dreamer is attempting to change the course of the dream from within the dream. *Example of second-order change:* The only way the dreamer can change the dream is to awaken and be in a different state altogether. This is second-order change because it changes the system itself from without (Watzlawick, 1974).

Strategic therapy creates second-order change in human systems, and these changes seem illogical from within the system. Strategic therapists propose that insight is not a necessary prerequisite for change. Rather, people must learn how to act in a different way if they are to see things in a different way. This is congruent with thinking that reality is created through communication and behaviors are a form of communication.

Basic Concepts

To work within this orientation, it is necessary to understand two concepts: *attempted solutions* and *position*.

---

*Complainant refers to the person who presents with a complaint and is requesting assistance.

ATTEMPTED SOLUTIONS

Basic to this approach is the view of problem development and maintenance. The MRI model defines a problem as a client's concern about some behavior (action, thought, or feeling) in the self, or another behavior that is described as deviant or distressing in some way. Furthermore, *all the client's efforts to stop or change this behavior have failed,* and the client is seeking the therapist's help to change the situation (Fisch et al, 1986). There are two important points here: (1) The client's repeated and best attempts at change have failed. (2) The request for assistance is for a specific problem, not a personality makeover. The strategic therapy approach focuses on change in relation to the identified problem.

In the MRI model, problems are the result of mishandled or wrong attempts at changing an area of difficulty. In other words, it is the attempted solutions that create the problem. An attempted solution is simply the client's best attempt to change a troublesome situation, but the attempt repeatedly fails and further aggravates the situation. Most attempted solutions are first-order changes and are simply repetitions of a theme. For example, a couple presents with complaints of family distress based on their perception of their teenage son's defiant stance toward them, as demonstrated by his consistent disregard of curfew. They scolded and disciplined him to get him to comply with rules, only to see him increase his defiance as the result of their attempts. Their attempted solutions were variations on the theme "You will obey us," and only served to maintain the problem and possibly aggravate it.

There are three ways to mishandle a difficulty: (1) An action is necessary but none is taken (as in the case of denial). (2) An action is taken when it should not be (as in the case when a nonproblem is defined as a problem). (3) An action is taken at the wrong level (i.e., a first-order change is attempted when a second-order change is necessary) (Watzlawick, 1974).

Attempted solutions are called *problem-maintaining behavior:* the attempts to solve the problem actually aggravate it despite the reasonableness of the approach. The MRI group believes that people continue problem-maintaining behavior inadvertently and often with the best of intentions. They do not view the presence of a problem as an indicator of a pathologic condition (Fisch et al, 1986). Because it is the attempted solution that is noted to worsen (or at least maintain) the problem, strategic therapists aim their interventions at the attempted solutions rather than the problem itself (Watzlawick, 1974).

POSITION

To know how to intervene, it is important that the therapist understand the client's *position* on the problem. *Position* refers to values, beliefs, and priorities of the client (Fisch et al, 1986). In brief, position is the client's view of the "reality" of the situation and is demonstrated by the client's language, perception of the problem, and motivations. It is essential that strategic therapists understand the client's position in order to present the intervention in a way that the client will accept and use (Greene, 1991). One of the most basic positions to note is whether the client is "benevolently concerned" about the behavior of feeling victimized. Benevolent concern implies that the problem behavior is not willfully done, i.e., it is caused by a sickness, illness, or weakness. Victimization implies a willful enactment of the behavior and is viewed as bad by the client. In the above example of the teenage boy, the parents' position was that their son was "bad," i.e., willfully stayed out, and that he had control over his behavior. The same case would present differently if their view was that the behavior was out of their son's control due to some infirmity, such as being stressed over exams or being unable to tell time because of a learning disability. The therapist's intervention must always be congruent with the client's position.

Techniques

The techniques of strategic therapy are designed to provide the client with a "chance occurrence" that provides a new frame of reference with which to view the problem. Watzlawick tells the following story to explain chance occurrences.

Suppose a man presents in therapy with a fear of elephants. To keep elephants away, he has begun incessant hand-clapping. There are several ways the therapist can deal with this: the therapist could develop a trusting relationship with the man so that when the therapist says there is no reason to fear elephants, the man would believe the therapist; the therapist could work to uncover the cause of this fear of elephants, with the assumption that understanding the source of fear will stop the fear; or the therapist could introduce elephants into the therapy, and demonstrate that there is no reason to fear them. Or suppose that one day, on the way to therapy, the man is involved in an accident in which both his hands are broken. Despite the fact that he cannot clap, no elephants approach and he learns he no longer needs to apply his solution of hand-clapping. This unplanned occurrence provides a corrective emotional experience. The goal of strategic interventions is to create planned chance occurrences that lead to corrective emotional experiences (lecture, Stanford, Palo Alto, 1991). Planned chance occurrences are accomplished by either interrupting the problem-maintaining behavior or altering the client's view of the problem so it no longer causes distress (Fisch et al, 1986).

SYMPTOM PRESCRIPTION

This involves the therapist prescribing the very symptom from which the client is seeking relief. Symptom prescription is useful when the attempted solution has been to force something that can only occur spontaneously.

This often occurs with bodily functions in which normal fluctuations are defined as problems (e.g., sexual preference, insomnia, memory blocks, GI and urinary functions). The symptom is perceived by the client as spontaneous and out of the client's control (e.g., "I'm frigid," "I'm impotent," "I can't sleep," "I can't remember," "I wet my pants"), and yet clients work very hard to stop these behaviors. However, the attempted solution maintains the symptomatic behavior. Symptom prescription is aimed at having the client stop the attempted solutions by directing the client to perform another behavior. The strategic therapist provides a rationale and directions to fail at "attempted solutions" behaviors. The client is often instructed to bring on the symptom for diagnostic purposes or as a beginning step toward behavioral control (Fisch et al, 1986).

For example, the impotent man is instructed to maintain his impotence so he can study his thoughts during intercourse. He is unable to maintain his impotence and enjoys intercourse. Thus the "attempted solution" ("I have to have an erection") is interrupted with the direction, "Do not, under any circumstances, have an erection," and as a result normal functioning returns.

Another variation of symptom prescription can be employed when the attempted solution revolves around mastering a feared event by avoiding it. This is often the case with fear and anxiety states, such as phobias, performance blocks, public speaking, beginning relationships, etc. In these situations, the client is exposed to the task but instructed not to master it (Fisch et al, 1986). For example, the client with a driving phobia is instructed to sit in the car for 30 minutes a day and consider the hazards of driving. During this time, the driver must never consider the pleasures of driving and does not actually drive at all. This again stops the client's attempted solution of avoiding the task while pushing himself to master it by being presented with an alternate behavior to perform.

REFRAMING

Reframing is a powerful verbal tool used to create a second-order change. It involves changing the conceptual and/or emotional setting or viewpoint in which a situation is seen and placing it "in another frame that fits the facts of the situation equally well or even better, and thereby change its entire meaning" (Watzlawick, 1974). A reframe does not change anything about the client's view of the problem-situation. It works by making the client's old view (or frame) absolute. To work, the reframe must always fit the client's position and be congruent with his or her understanding of the situation. However, the reframe changes the way the situation is viewed.

For example, a 40-year-old woman is hospitalized with suicidal depression. She is despondent because she never seems to be able to please her parents and, indeed, the staff observes her parents frequently criticizing and

---

Clinical Application   Strategic Therapy

Peggy is having her second meeting with a strategic therapist.

Peggy: "I just can't do anything right. I'm a total failure."

Therapist: "What do you fail at?"

Peggy: "Life! You name it, I fail at it. I burn cookies, oversleep, lose my job and my car keys. I don't seem to be able to do anything right. Everybody notices; they're just too nice to say anything."

Therapist: "Well, I have a suggestion, but it may be too much for you to do because you seem to be a perfectionist and perfectionists have a hard time with this."

Peggy: "Tell me, I'll do anything."

Therapist: "This will be difficult for you to do. I want you to plan three perfect mistakes, or failures, as you call them. Now, these failures must be a secret and you must not tell anyone what you've planned. You tell your family you're going to make these mistakes that day and ask them to figure out what they are."

Peggy: "I already make three mistakes a day."

Therapist: "Yes, but I want you to plan these mistakes, not to leave them to chance."

When Peggy returns in two weeks, she delightedly reports that no one even noticed her planned failures.

---

belittling her. She continues to please them, only to be told she'll never be as good as her brothers and sisters who have moved away. In this situation the attempted solution was the client's repeated attempts to please. A reframe of the situation was initiated and proved very successful. The client was congratulated on being such a fine and caring daughter. Obviously her parents feared an end to their parental role, and she provided them an opportunity to continue this role. By allowing them to criticize her, she reassured them that their job was not done and their parental role could continue.

PSYCHOBIOLOGY

This section provides an overview of psychobiology content believed to be essential for psychiatric nurses as stated by the American Nurses Association (ANA) Psychiatric Mental Health Nursing Psychopharmacology Project (1994). Psychobiology as it relates to psychiatry is an extremely complex subject. While effort has been made to present important material, the student is referred to listed references for more in-depth information on topics covered.

Variations in biologic processes and hormonal balances have long been recognized as a cause of some psychiatric disturbances. Behavioral changes that become manifest with some brain lesions give further evidence of possible neurophysiologic determinants of some psychiatric disorders. Introduction of psychotropic agents in the early 1950s, notably reserpine and thorazine, restimulated research on the biochemistry of psychiatric disorders. Over the subsequent 40 years, advances in biotechnology, immunology, genetics, endocrinology, and brain imaging have led to an explosion of investigations into the role of psychobiology in mental illness. Although there are considerable gaps in knowledge as to the specific mechanisms of causation for many psychiatric disorders, it has become generally accepted that there is no real division between the mind and body, the mental and the physical, the brain and thought.

The brain is an organ of the body and is as vulnerable to disease as other body organs. Research on the function of the brain, including the role of neurotransmitters, has led to the reinterpretation of most functional psychiatric disorders (previously considered to have no organic basis) as brain diseases. Despite evidence of brain pathology in these disorders, they still do not fit the traditional view of neurological disorders. The challenge is to find the loci of deficits in brain tissue, chemistry, physiology, and anatomy that cause manifestation of aberrant behaviors labeled mental illness. Then models of comprehensive treatment for these disorders must be developed. This is of particular concern for psychiatric nurses, who may not have been well grounded in the basic sciences in the past. Psychobiology is rapidly becoming the basis for mental health practice. If psychiatric nursing is to remain viable, it cannot afford to be without this body of knowledge (Keltner and Callwood, 1994).

Neuroanatomy

The central nervous system (CNS) consists of the brain, the spinal cord, and associated nerves. **Neurons** are nerve cells made up of a body (*soma*) and extensions of protoplasm called *neutrites* (Fig. 5-4). Neutrites that relay impulses toward the nerve soma are *dendrites,* and those conducting impulses away from the soma are *axons.* **Synapses** are specialized areas of contact between neurons where impulses cross. Billions of neurons in the CNS are connected to one another electrochemically. Most are mediated by chemical substances known as **neurotransmitters.** A more detailed discussion of neurotransmitters will follow.

The brain has two hemispheres: left and right. The *cerebral cortex* is the gray matter at the surface of the two hemispheres of the brain. Fissures (sulci) and con-

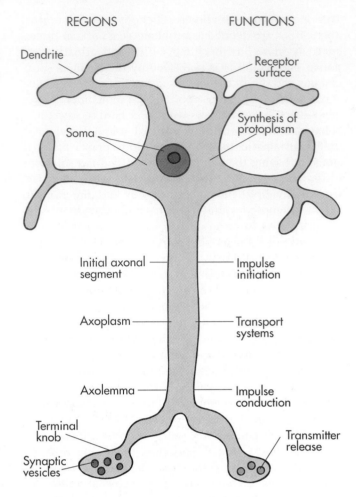

Figure 5-4 Structure/function relationships in neurons.

volutions (gyri) of variable extent make up the cortex. Sulci serve to separate the cortex into areas of distinct function. Gyri are connected by short fibers that link adjacent gyri, and long fibers that link different lobes of the brain. There are four major lobes of the brain on each hemisphere: the frontal, parietal, temporal, and occipital lobes. The *frontal lobes* influence the functions of learned motor activity and the planning and organizing of future expressive behavior; they allow versatile responses of the mind and are concerned with judgment, personality, and intellectual function. *Parietal lobes* affect attention selectivity and span. They integrate somatic stimuli to recall form, texture, and weight. The parietal lobes also integrate these perceptions with other sensations to create self-awareness of both inner and outer worlds. Structures of the *temporal lobes* are critically involved with visual recognition, auditory perception, memory, and emotions. *Occipital lobes* are primarily concerned with vision, including form recognition, color recognition, and integration of visual stimulation from partial objects into perceptions of a coherent whole. The *corpus callosum* interconnects matching areas of the two hemispheres. It contains 300 million fibers and is the largest fiber tract—a superhighway of information exchange between the hemispheres that keeps them working together. Embedded deep within the cerebrum are several large masses of gray matter called the *basal ganglia* (Fitzgerald, 1992). Basal ganglia are extensively connected with association and limbic structures and are involved in complex behavior. Diseases of the basal ganglia, such as Huntington's and Parkinson's diseases, are usually associated with major changes in mental states (Mesulam, 1988). Figure 5-5 depicts the major structures of the brain.

Gathering, processing, integrating, and storing information about internal and external conditions is done through a hierarchy of neural interconnections that form networks distributed throughout the cerebrum. The neurons of the central nervous system are concerned with the three major operations responsible for thoughts, feelings, and behavior. These are: (1) input, receiving and registering sensory stimuli from outside and from within; (2) output, planning and execution of complex motor acts; and (3) intermediary processing interposed between input and output. Manifestations of intermediary processing include functions of thought, language, memory, self-awareness, and many aspects of mood and affect. The limbic system is the principal location for these intermediary processes and is primarily concerned with the integration of affective (emotional) aspects of behavior, memory, and basic drives required to preserve the individual (Mesulam, 1988). A basic principle of psychiatry is that thoughts, feelings, and behaviors are deviant from some norm and therefore induce distress in the individual and those close to him or her (Klerman, 1988). The limbic system is believed to be the point of origin for these psychiatric disorders of mood and thought (Fitzgerald, 1992).

Limbus means a border. The **limbic system** refers to a set of structures comprising a vertical limbus on each side of the brain surrounding the corpus callosum and a cerebral peduncle, or stemlike connecting part; and a horizontal limbus surrounding the midbrain (Fig. 5-6). Among structures included in this system are the hippocampus, thalamus, hypothalamus, and amygdala. The components of the limbic system are interconnected through many neural circuits and may contain common immunological properties (Mesulam, 1988). One can conceptualize the limbic circuits as divided into hippocampal and amygdaloid spheres of influence, with the *hippocampus* and its connections being more closely associated with memory functions while the *amygdala* and its pathways are more closely related to affective

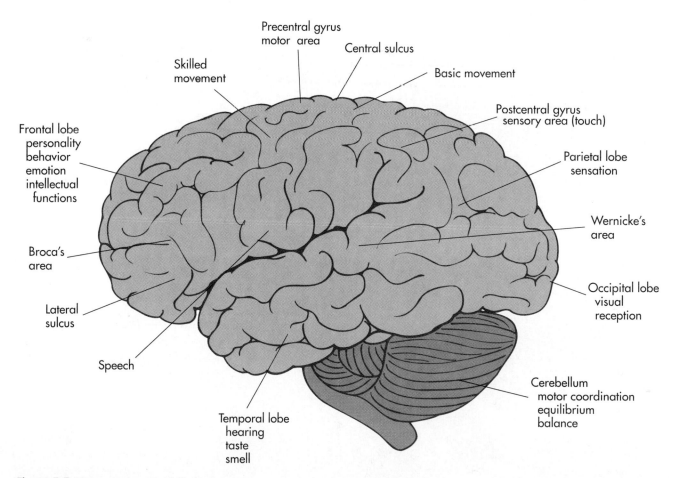

Figure 5-5 Major structures of the brain.

components of events. The *thalamus,* besides being part of the limbic system, is integrated into the motor and sensory systems, regulating activity, sensations, and emotions. It relays impulses up to the hippocampal and to wide areas of the cerebral cortex. The *hypothalamus* is the gray matter below the thalamus. It is the chief coordinator of instincts and drives. Its homeostatic and survival functions act to regulate body temperature, the circulation of blood, food and water intake, the sleep cycle, defensive mechanisms, and sexual drives. Emotion is thought to be generated and coordinated chiefly by the hypothalamus through the integration of endocrine and motor responses, including autonomic responses. The amygdala is thought to be associated with strong emotional experiences but not with the generation of the emotion itself. It acts to direct the emotion to the proper object and to the proper mental content. The largest concentration of opiate receptors in the entire brain is found in the amygdala. Acute stressful situations activate the amygdala, releasing endogenous opiates into the bloodstream. The limbic system and higher brain structures link the hypothalamus to the outside world.

The *cerebellum* is the largest part of the hind brain. It lies below the cerebrum and under the occipital lobes and is the center for motor coordination. It is responsible for the smooth contraction and relaxation of muscle groups and is essential for muscle tone and balance. Smoothing action is also crucial for both automatic and voluntary movement. However, the cerebellum does not initiate movement, nor does it have any role in intelligence and perceptions of conscious sensations. This process takes place on an entirely unconscious level. Staggering gait, clumsiness, and slurred speech observed in acute alcoholic states are symptoms of a generalized malfunction of the cerebellum (Mesulam, 1988).

The **brain stem** is involved in the transmission of all ascending and descending impulses. Structures of the brain stem are, in descending order, the midbrain, pons, and medulla oblongata. They provide the many motor neurons, fibers, and tracts that relay information to and from the forebrain. The *midbrain* merges into the thalamus and hypothalamus, thus interacting with the limbic system that was previously identified as the emotional center of the brain. *Pons* and *medulla structures* are connecting pathways with the spinal cord. Norepinephrine cells in the pons called *locus coeruleus* and other norepinephrine systems are implicated in the production of anxiety. The medulla contains autonomic centers that are vital for the regulation of the heart and blood vessels, respiration, salivation, and swallowing (Fitzgerald, 1992).

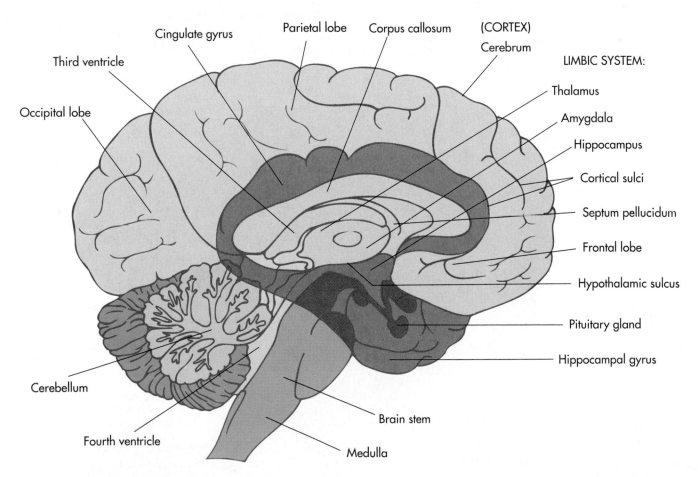

Figure 5-6 The limbic system.

Permeating the core of the brain stem is a network of neurons known as *reticular formation (RF)*. The ascending limb of the RF that extends into the thalamus and hypothalamus is the *reticular activating system (RAS)*, where signals from the internal and external environment meet (Cutting, 1992; Fitzgerald, 1992) and decide the level of arousal of the cerebral cortex (Fig. 5-7). Level of consciousness and sleep-wake cycles are affected by the reticular activating system. The hypothalamus with which the RAS is linked has anatomical connections to the optic nerve that respond to light. Within the hypothalamus are the basic mechanisms of the circadian clock that regulates the rhythm of many body functions, including sleep. Therefore disturbances of the RAS have significance for sleep irregularities and seasonal affective disorders and may exacerbate other psychiatric disorders (Fitzgerald, 1992). Investigators have found that this clock can be reset through planned exposure to a light stimulus (Gallagher, 1993).

The *pyramidal tracts* take their name from the pyramid-like structures of the medulla. These are a collection of nerve fibers that originate in the motor cortex and travel through the pyramids of the medulla en route to the spinal cord. Within the pyramids, at the *pyramidal decussation,* nerve fibers cross from one side of the brain to the opposite side of the spinal cord. The pyramidal tracts mediate voluntary movement, especially those that are coordinated and purposeful and require skill. The **extrapyramidal system (EPS)** consists of all the motor nerve tracts and pathways connecting the cerebral cortex, basal ganglia, thalamus, cerebellum, RAS, and spinal cord in complex circuits that are *not* included in the pyramidal system (Fitzgerald, 1992). It is involved with the regulation of stereotyped reflex movement of muscles, maintenance of muscle tone, and control of body movements as in walking. Disturbances in EPS characteristically produce hypertonicity of muscles. This is evident in dystonic reactions often seen with the use of antipsychotic medications (Baldessarini, 1988).

The **peripheral nervous system (PNS)** refers to all parts of the nervous systems that lie outside the CNS (brain and spinal cord). It includes the twelve pairs of cranial nerves and the thirty-one pairs of spinal nerves and their branches. Cranial nerves enter and exit the brain and primarily supply the head and neck (Fig. 5-8). Spinal nerves enter and exit from the length of the spinal cord and enervate the rest of the body (Fig. 5-9). Peripheral nerves carry messages from organs, glands, and muscles to the CNS and back. *Afferent* nerves relay impulses to the CNS, while *efferent* nerves relay impulses from the CNS to areas of the body. Nerves of the PNS carry fibers that can functionally be divided into *somatic* and *autonomic* fibers. Somatic fibers innervate the skeletal, voluntary muscles. Autonomic fibers innervate the smooth involuntary muscles and regulate bodily functions that are mostly out of conscious control, such as the heart and intestinal movement (Fitzgerald, 1992).

The **autonomic nervous system (ANS)** is of particular interest, as emotional states are related to specific patterns of autonomic responses (Nemiah, 1988). It is partly contained within the peripheral nerves and partly within the CNS, directly connecting with the hypothalamus (Fig. 5-10). This association with the limbic system accounts for the powerful influence the amygdala and hypothalamus have on autonomic function. The ANS further subdivides into the *sympathetic* and the *parasympathetic* systems. The *sympathetic* system prepares the body for the "fight-or-flight" response by increasing the body alertness. It speeds the heart, dilates the pupils of the eye, causes the hair to stand on end, makes skin sweat, and releases *norepinephrine* as a neurotransmitter. The *parasympathetic* system counteracts the responses induced by the sympathetic system and releases the neurotransmitter *acetylcholine.* Interplay of the two systems is important to the maintenance of equilibrium in the face of external and internal challenges to the organism. Sustained arousal of the sympathetic system related to stressors can result in physiologic changes. Physical conditions commonly cited as being affected by "psychologic factors" are hypertension, peptic ulcer, migraine, and colitis (Rogers and Reich, 1988).

Neuroregulation

When a neuron is stimulated, an impulse is generated that causes the release of a neurotransmitter from the portion of the neuron closest to a neighboring neuron

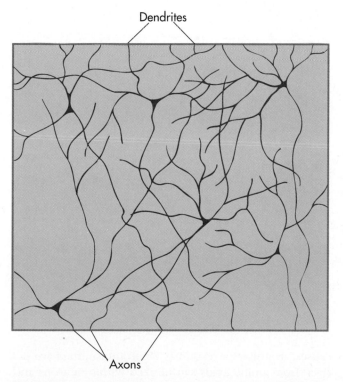

Figure 5-7 Network of neurons in the reticular activating system located in the brainstem.

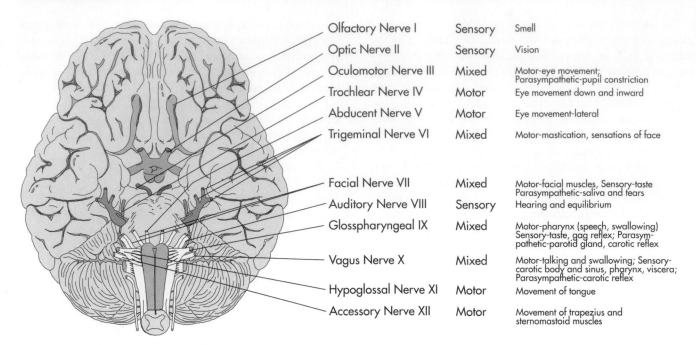

Olfactory Nerve I	Sensory	Smell	
Optic Nerve II	Sensory	Vision	
Oculomotor Nerve III	Mixed	Motor-eye movement; Parasympathetic-pupil constriction	
Trochlear Nerve IV	Motor	Eye movement down and inward	
Abducent Nerve V	Motor	Eye movement-lateral	
Trigeminal Nerve VI	Mixed	Motor-mastication, sensations of face	
Facial Nerve VII	Mixed	Motor-facial muscles, Sensory-taste Parasympathetic-saliva and tears	
Auditory Nerve VIII	Sensory	Hearing and equilibrium	
Glosspharyngeal IX	Mixed	Motor-pharynx (speech, swallowing) Sensory-taste, gag reflex; Parasym-pathetic-parotid gland, carotid reflex	
Vagus Nerve X	Mixed	Motor-talking and swallowing; Sensory-carotic body and sinus, pharynx, viscera; Parasympathetic-carotic reflex	
Hypoglossal Nerve XI	Motor	Movement of tongue	
Accessory Nerve XII	Motor	Movement of trapezius and sternomastoid muscles	

Figure 5-8 The cranial nerves.

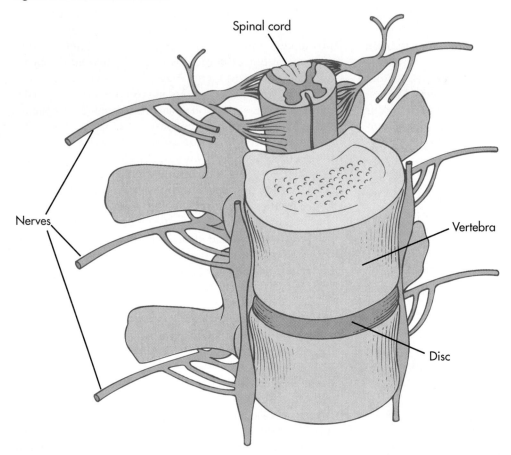

Figure 5-9 The nerve structures of the spine.

(dendrite) into a space between two neurons called the *synaptic cleft* (Fig. 5-11). The neurotransmitter crosses the synapse and binds to a *receptor* on the neighboring neuron, triggering an extracellular electrical signal that causes or inhibits a response. Neurotransmitters are derived from amino acids synthesized within neurons and stored at the nerve terminal in distinct *vesicles*. The ability of a neuron to generate an *action potential* depends

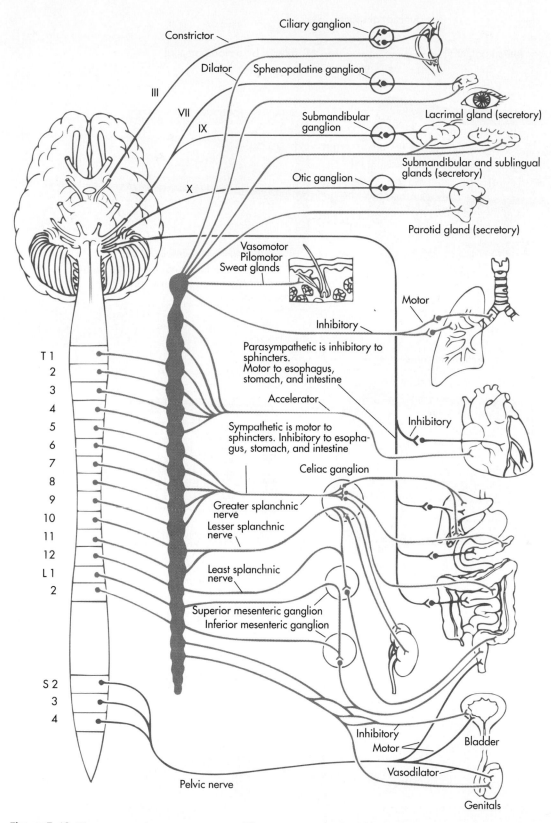

Figure 5-10 The autonomic nervous system. The parasympathetic division is shown in red; the sympathetic division is shown in blue.

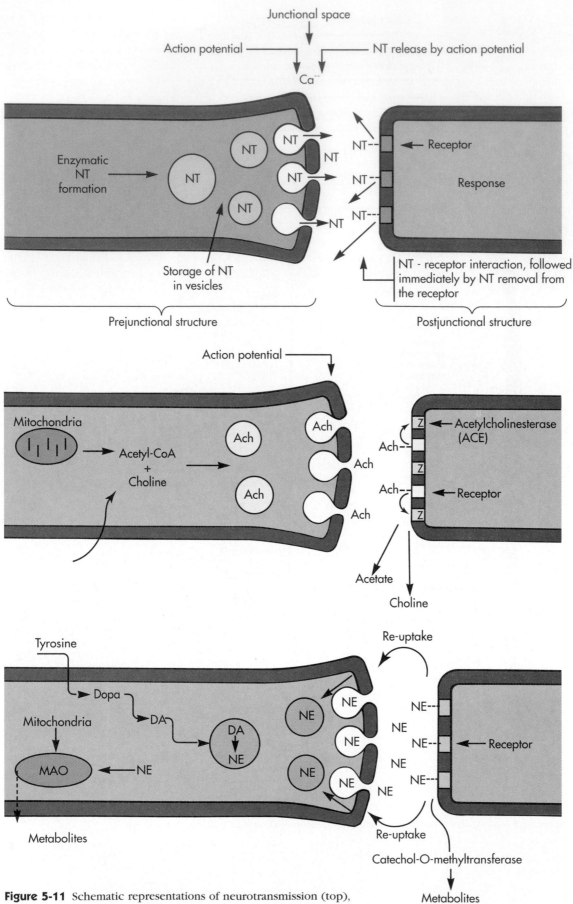

Figure 5-11 Schematic representations of neurotransmission (top), a cholinergic junction (middle), an adrenergic junction (bottom).

on the presence of sodium (Na^+), chloride (Cl^-), potassium (K^+), and calcium (Ca^{++}) ions that affect the permeability of the cell membrane through electrical polarization and depolarization. A rise in concentration of Ca^{++} causes release of neurotransmitter molecules by fusing the wall of the vesicles to the nerve terminal, creating an opening through which the neurotransmitter is expelled into the synaptic cleft. The neuron releasing the neurotransmitter is the *presynaptic neuron,* and the neuron receiving the neurotransmitter is the *postsynaptic neuron* (Snyder, 1988; van Praag, 1978).

Transmission by a neurotransmitter can be increased or decreased in response to a given physiologic situation. Major neurotransmitters of concern with psychiatric disorders are *acetylcholine (Ach), dopamine (DA), norepinephrine (NE), serotonin (5-HT), gamma aminobutyric acid (GAMA),* and *beta endorphin (B-END)* (Fig. 5-12). Ach is synthesized by the enzyme *choline acetyltransferase (CAT)* from choline and acetyl coenzyme A (which comes from the mitochondria structure

of the nerve cell). Release of acetylcholine stimulates cholinergic (parasympathetic) receptors that act on blood vessels, glands, and most of the internal organs. Dopamine, norepinephrine, and serotonin are *catecholamines* that chemically contain a benzene ring with adjacent hydroxyl groups (catechol) and an amino group on a side chain. This is the reason these compounds are also known as *monoamines.* Dopamine and norepinephrine are synthesized from the amino acid *tyrosine.* The sequence is tyrosine to dopa (dihydroxyphenylalanine), which is decarboxylized to dopamine by the enzyme aromatic L-amino acid decarboxylase. The sequence can continue, with the presence of appropriate neuronal enzymes, from dopamine to norepinephrine to *epinephrine* (Green et al, 1988). Catecholamine levels are regulated by changes in activity of the enzymes tyrosine hydroxylase and *monoamine oxidase (MAO)* localized in the nerve terminals. Monoamine oxidase is involved in the metabolism of dopamine and a number of other monoamines, including serotonin, in the presynap-

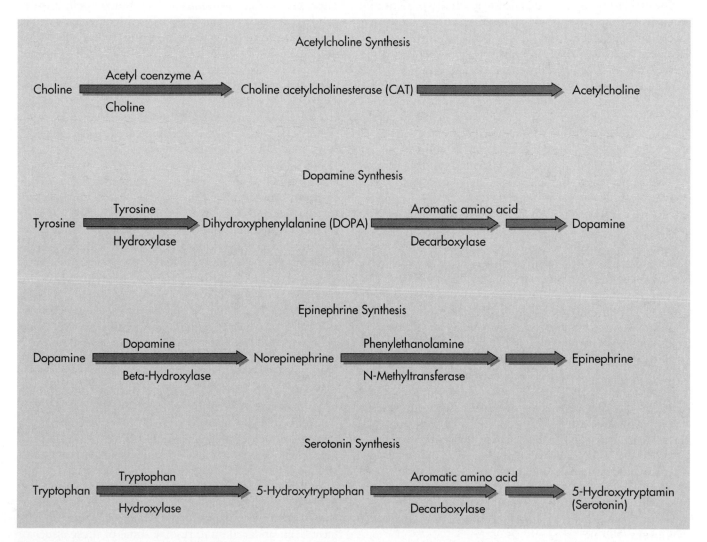

Figure 5-12 Synthesis of neurotransmitters.

tic neuron. Under stressful conditions, including vigorous exercise, release of dopamine is greatly increased. Build up of concentrations of dopamine serves to ready the body for action by increasing the heart beat, raising blood pressure, and constricting key blood vessels. Dopamine plays an important role in controlling emotions, cognition, movement and in the side effects observed with the use of antipsychotic drugs. A number of neurologic and psychiatric disorders are linked to the dysfunction of dopamine. These include Parkinson's disease, schizophrenia, mood disorders and Tourette's syndrome (Daly, 1994; Snyder, 1988; van Praag, 1978).

Serotonergic pathways originate in the lower midbrain and the upper pons. Serotonin synthesis begins with tryptophan and is widely distributed in tissues, particularly that of the CNS and intestinal wall and in blood platelets. As tryptophan is an essential amino acid not synthesized by the body, the synthesis of serotonin depends on dietary intake to make tryptophan available. Serotonin is implicated in depression and sleep disturbances, but the exact mechanism is not well understood. Gamma aminobutyric acid is the major inhibitory neurotransmitter in the brain and is estimated to be present in 30% of all synapses. Gamma aminobutyric acid binds to receptors and decreases neuronal firing. It inhibits activation of neurons containing monoamines that mediate arousal and anxiety-related behaviors (Dubovsky, 1992). When an individual is clinically anxious, it is thought that there is a change in balance between inhibitory neurotransmitters such as gamma aminobutyric acid and excitatory neurotransmitters like acetylcholine. This imbalance results in a lack of inhibitory control over noradrenergic firing in the locus coeruleus and the manifestation of symptoms of anxiety. Beta-endorphin is a polypeptide neurotransmitter that consists of 31 amino acids. B-End is one of the endogenous opiates, low levels of which occur in the CNS, where the hypothalamus extends to the limbic system and the brain stem. There are other endogenous opiates under investigation. Some are concentrated in areas associated with pain, while others are concentrated in limbic structures, causing questions about their role in depression (Snyder, 1988).

A number of neurologic and psychiatric symptoms are caused by problems in the activity of neurotransmitters as they interact at critical sites in the brain. Drugs that affect the nervous system most often adjust the neurotransmission process. They can increase or decrease the synthesis, storage, release, metabolism, or receptor activity of neurotransmitters. Correction of neurotransmitter defects implicated in the disorder is the therapeutic purpose of these drugs. For instance, the antipsychotic drug thorazine affects receptor activity resulting in reduction of dopamine transmission. However, the exact mechanisms by which specific drugs intervene in neurotransmission processes are still under investigation (Dubovsky, 1992).

Genetics and Familial Correlates

Genetic research seeks to determine the contribution of inherited factors to the development of disease. Discovering that a disorder runs in families provides the epidemiological evidence that focuses on genetic research. The basic structures of interest in genetics are the *chromosomes, genes, deoxyribonucleic acid (DNA),* and *ribonucleic acid (RNA).* Every cell in the body carries the individual's own code, unlike any other. Genes decide the message the code carries. Scientists have yet to discover, locate, and map thousands of human genes; however, genes are known to be grouped into various types. *Structural genes* decide the biochemical makeup of proteins; *regulatory genes* govern the rate of protein production; *architectural genes* integrate protein into the structure of cells, and *temporal genes* control the temporal and spatial actions of other genes. They also have a role in the differentiation of body cells and tissues. Genes are arranged linearly along the length of DNA in the cell nucleus. Bundles of long double-filament DNA coiled into a helix with associated proteins form chromosomes. There are 46 chromosomes in each human cell, 23 contributed by each parent. The DNA molecule can copy itself exactly through replication, transferring all genetic information to the daughter cell with cell division. Changes in DNA cause *mutations.* RNA occurs in the nucleus and cytoplasm of cells and is concerned with the synthesis of protein.

There are a growing number of disorders for which scientists have demonstrated biochemical or gene defects that serve as genetic markers. Among these are Down's syndrome, galactosemia, phenylketonuria, and Huntington's disease. Diseases transmitted by major genes or where major genes control important risk factors have a higher probability for discovery of mode of transmission (Buckle et al, 1989). However, it appears that most mental disorders where there is evidence of genetic influence are not transmitted as classical Mendelian traits (Kety and Matthyssc, 1988). These disorders are probably polygenic, representing small effects from many genes. Nevertheless, investigators are using most strategies to uncover genetic and familial correlates to mental illness. The questions listed in Box 5-4 determine which strategy is most appropriate (Malaspina et al, 1992).

Family studies can illustrate the relative risk for an illness in first-degree relatives of an identified patient as compared to the general population. For example, a number of epidemiological studies have confirmed the higher incidence of schizophrenia among parents and siblings of schizophrenics than in the general population. While providing valuable information, this strategy is unable to distinguish whether the risk is genetic or due to shared environmental factors. *Twin* and *adoptive studies* have been undertaken to resolve some of these issues of

Box 5-4 Questions and Related Strategies for Investigating the Genetics of Neuropsychiatric Disorders

Question	Strategy
Is the disorder familial?	Family studies
Is it inherited?	Twin studies, Adoption studies
What is being inherited in the disorder? What "epigenetic" factors influence development of the disorder?	High risk studies
How is the disorder inherited?	Segregation analysis, Pedigree analysis
Where is (are) the abnormal gene(s)?	Linkage analysis
What is the abnormal gene? What is its molecular and pathological effect?	Molecular approaches

Adapted from Malaspina D; Qutkin, AB; Kaufman CA; Yudofsky SC; Hales RE; eds: "Epidemiology and Genetics of Neuropsychiatric Diseases," in *Textbook of Neuropsychiatry*, ed. 2, 187–226. Washington, D.C., 1992; American Psychiatric Press.

genetic contributions. This strategy is based on the fact that monozygotic (MZ) and dizygotic (DZ) twin pairs differ in their genetic inheritance, with the monozygotic sharing 100% of genes and the dizygotic sharing 50%. The heritability of a disorder can be measured by comparing the concordance rates for monozygotic and dizygotic twins. By heritability, we mean that part of difference that can be credited to genetics as opposed to environmental and other factors. In adoption studies, offspring of affected mothers adopted at birth are compared to adopted offspring of control mothers. Biologic relatives of the affected and control adoptees are matched, then the rates of illness of the adoptees are compared.

Segregation analysis and *pedigree analysis* are sophisticated research methods that allow direct comparison of monogenic and polygenic models. Segregation analysis uses a statistical genetic hypothesis to compare the distribution of illness observed in family members to that predicted. It provides estimates of gene frequency and penetration. An important limitation is that each family is treated as a separate observation, although there is the assumption that the same disorder is present in all families. Pedigree analysis looks at affected individuals over several generations, and is therefore less likely to fail to support a particular genetic model because of observed differences.

Linkage analysis, through a complex and statistical process, maps the chromosomal location of genes involved in transmitting a disorder. It depends on finding

within pedigrees coinheritance of the disorder with identifiable genetic markers at a known location on a chromosome. Linkage analysis narrows the field by providing markers of particular regions of the chromosome where the disease gene is located. Molecular biologic techniques can then be applied to examine the genetic material for specific flaws. This strategy has produced the most promising hope of progress in identifying specific genetic defects implicated in mental illness (Malaspina et al, 1992). These scientific techniques help to decide what is genetically transmitted, how it is transmitted, and how it is expressed.

Psychoendocrinology

There is clear evidence of prominent neuropsychiatric symptoms with some endocrine disorders. With endocrine disturbances there is often manifestation of affective and anxiety symptoms with mild cognitive impairment. This evidence has led clinicians and researchers to consider possible connections between the endocrine system and psychiatric disorders. Discovery that the hypothalamus modulates the activity of the pituitary gland has focused attention on the following complex and well-integrated axes: the hypothalamus-pituitary-adrenal axis (HPA), the hypothalamus-pituitary-thyroid axis (HPT), and the hypothalamus-pituitary-gonadal axis (HPG).

The hypothalamus exerts regulatory control of the activities of the anterior and posterior lobes of the pituitary in two ways. Hormones from the hypothalamus reach the anterior lobes of the pituitary indirectly through a specialized vascular system. These neurohormones control the synthesis and secretion of hormones of the anterior pituitary, which in turn regulate the peripheral endocrine glands: the adrenal, thyroid, and gonads. In contrast, the posterior pituitary is directly connected to the hypothalamus through axons originating in neurons located in the hypothalamus. Peptide hormones synthesized in the hypothalamus, which act in the periphery to regulate water balance, milk secretion, and uterine contraction, are stored in these axons. Primary concern in neuropsychiatry is focused on the hypothalamic link with the anterior pituitary.

In the HPA axis a hypothalamic peptide, corticotropin-releasing hormone (CRH), stimulates the release of adrenocorticotropic hormone (ACTH) from the pituitary. ACTH stimulates the adrenal cortex to secrete cortisol, which modulates further release of CRH from the hypothalamus. Similarly, in the HPT axis, the hypothalamus releases the peptide thyrotropin-releasing hormone (TRH) into the anterior pituitary. TRH stimulates the pituitary to release the hormone thyrotropin (TSH), which regulates the production of the thyroid hormones. These thyroid hormones exert a feedback control over the axis. Gonadotropin-releasing hormone (GnRH) is the hypothalamic neurohormone released in the HPG axis. It stimulates the pituitary to release both luteinizing hormone (LH) and follicle-stimulating hormone (FSH) that stimulate both male and female gonads. Gonadal hormones exert feedback control over the axis. Both the HPA and HPT axes are implicated in mood disturbances. Investigations have centered on studies of hormonal levels in body fluids under various circumstances. Persons who are depressed often exhibit increased levels of cortisol in plasma, urine, and cerebral spinal fluid (Goldman, 1992; Green et al, 1988).

Hormones produced by the hypothalamus and pituitary are secreted in a pulsating mode, with periods of activity interspersed with periods of inactivity. These rhythmic circadian cycles vary with the type of hormones. Some have increased secretions during specific hours of the day while others, such as luteinizing hormone and follicle-stimulating hormone have longer rhythms during the menstrual cycle. There is not yet a comprehensive understanding of the role endocrines may play in the causation of psychiatric illness. However, symptoms in psychiatric patients are often exacerbated when there is also endocrine pathology (Goldman, 1992).

Psychoimmunology

Studies of the effects of natural and induced stress on the immune system of animals have generated interest in the relationship of emotional states and the human immune system. The immune system regulates the body's defenses against infection and is known to influence the pathological manifestation of autoimmune disorders and malignancies. Antibodies and white blood cells, *leukocytes,* circulate through a separate lymphatic vessel system that takes excess fluid from tissue spaces and returns it to the blood stream. *Phagocytes,* containing many white blood cells, are able to surround and digest bacteria, debris from cells, and foreign substances. *Lymph nodes,* small oval clumps of lymphatic tissue located at various points along the vessels, become swollen in the presence of an inflammation or infection. They produce *lymphocytes,* a type of white blood cell involved with immunity, which act to filter out microorganisms and foreign particles from entering the blood stream.

Although poorly understood, there is a known relationship between the nervous system and the lymphatic system, as lymphocytes have receptors for substances like acetylcholine and norepinephrine. Acetylcholine and norepinephrine were identified previously as important neurotransmitters. The mechanisms include neuroendocrine pathways involving, but not limited to, the adrenal axis and the autonomic nervous system. A number of investigators have observed changes in the body's immunologic activity in response to stress. However these changes have not been clearly shown to cause or exacerbate an illness (Rogers and Reich, 1988). Research

on this fascinating aspect of human response to stress continues, seeking to understand the effects of the nervous system and emotions on other body systems.

Examinations for Biologic Assessment in Mental Disorders

With current advances in radiologic technology and imaging, there are a variety of noninvasive imaging techniques available with which to visualize brain structure, functions and metabolic activity in clients experiencing mental disorders, brain injury or disease. While some procedures are more clinically significant than others, nurses play a major teaching role in describing these sophisticated examinations to clients and their families, whenever appropriate. Nurses may also explain the relevance of these tests to the mental disorder in question, in accordance with client and family needs, level of knowledge and anxiety states. Whenever possible, it is a function of the nurse to demystify these relatively safe procedures and explain their purpose in clear, basic terms to clients and families.

Procedures used to assess and examine brain structure and activity include:

- Electroencephalography (EEG)
- Computerized Tomography (CT)
- Magnetic Resonance Imaging (MRI)
- Positron Emission Tomography (PET)
- Brain Electrical Activity Mapping (BEAM)
- Cerebral Blood Flow (CBF)

EEG: This examination maps the brain's electrical activity via a monitoring system from which a set of electrodes are attached to strategic areas of the client's head and scalp, using a conducting substance. EEG's are used with sleep disorders, seizure disorders, Alzheimer's disease, and schizophrenia.

CT: This examination is one method of visualizing gross pathology in the brain by taking very fine photographs of specific areas of the brain. The CT scan reveals slices or segments of the brain that allow the examiner to make a very precise and complete study of brain structures and density, and compare their findings with those of normal brains. The CT scan shows ventricular enlargement, density changes in various areas of the brain, and cortical atrophy in clients with schizophrenia, ventricular changes and decreased cerebellar mass in some clients with the dual diagnosis of alcoholism and bipolar disorder, and a reduced density in the brain of clients with dementia.

MRI: This examination yields images of portions of the brain that are superior to those images observed in CT scans. Images are formed by placing the client's body within a stationary magnetic field that causes nuclei to align in the direction of the field. A radio frequency pulse is then applied that results in an electronic signal which

Summary of theoretical approaches

	Psychoanalytic	TA	Gestalt	Client-Centered	Behavioral	RET	Cognitive	Strategic	Psychobiology
BASIC ORIENTATION	All behavior is meaningful. Behavior is influenced by unconscious impulses and conflicts.	Life stance reflected in changing communication patterns. Can enhance effectiveness and decrease dysfunction by clarifying communication.	Intrapsychic conflicts arise from interactions with society.	Human beings move toward constructive change and integration.	Behavior is learned.	Individuals can choose thoughts and behaviors which promote or limit self acceptance.	Individual's affect and behavior are determined by his or her organization of world through thoughts and assumptions.	Reality is created through communication with others.	Anatomy and physiology are the structural bases.
CONCEPTS	Id, ego, superego. Unconscious and preconscious.	Ego states: parent, adult, child. Games. Script analysis.	Organism; top dog and underdog. Figure-background formation.	Interpersonal relationships are basis for health and neurosis.	Conditioning. Separation of client from problem.	ABCs of interaction.	Cognitive triad. Schemas. Faulty information processing.	Attempted solutions. Position.	Biology is the primary influence of psychologic changes.
GOAL	Uncover unconscious conflict and empower the ego to deal with it.	Interact from role-appropriate ego state.	Mutual acknowledgment and integration of organisms top dog and underdog through completion of unfinished situation.	Bring aspects of self into awareness and acceptance.	Modify observable behavior.	Provide skills to scientifically challenge irrational premises and change behavior.	Develop balanced cognitions and self-statements.	To decrease pain person is experiencing as a result of his or her view of a situation.	Psychologic balance is achieved through biologic manipulation.
TECHNIQUES	Dream analysis. Free association.	Structural analysis. Transactional analysis. Game analysis. Script analysis.	Chair work. Dream work.	Unconditional and positive regard. Therapeutic relationships. Alter ego.	Systematic desensitization. Relaxation training.	Cognitive approach. Behavioral: • role playing • progressive tasks • questioning	Cognitive: • questioning • reattribution Behavioral: • activity schedule • cognitive rehearsal	Reframing. Symptom prescription.	Chemical and technological interventions.

yields an image. MRI scans reveal pathologic lesions or tumors, enlarged ventricles and white matter changes in clients with Alzheimer's disease, and ventricular changes in clients with schizophrenia.

PET: This examination is a method of scanning physiologic and biochemical functions as they occur in live tissue. A compound is inhaled or injected which contains a radioactive "Tag" that is able to trace compounds such as glucose, and observe its use in the brain. Glucose is directly related to functional activity in certain regions of the brain. PET scans show decreased use of glucose in the frontal lobes of unmedicated clients with schizophrenia, less use of glucose in the left cortex of select clients with schizophrenia, and reduced uptake of glucose in frontal, temporal, and parietal lobes of clients with Alzheimer's disease.

BEAM: This examination is a form of electrical activity mapping that enhances the clinical usefulness of the EEG. It records spontaneous brain activity and the data at each electrode site are characterized via spectral properties. Spatial power maps are then calculated for each of the standard frequency bands, e.g., delta, theta, etc. Thus, for each client, a topographic map of power in each frequency band is generated (Orrison et al, 1995). It is then possible to compare data of a particular client with the normal data base and identify significant abnormal sites. This revolutionary neurometric examination is useful in the early identification and categorization of persons with a wide range of neurologic and psychiatric disorders. Current opinion is that the BEAM may be of significant clinical use in the future.

CBF: This examination explores the relationship between brain dysfunction, cerebral blood flow and metabolism of oxygen and glucose in the brain. Current opinion is that its future use may not be as clinically significant as the BEAM.

Summary of Key Concepts

1. Theories of human behavior are developed with the goal of producing frameworks that enhance understanding of the complexities of human behavior and somehow define them or interpret them and thus base effective interventions.

2. The psychoanalytic approach to treatment is based on the belief that all behavior is meaningful and is influenced by unconscious impulses and conflicts represented by id, ego, superego, unconscious, and preconscious.

3. Transactional analysis treatment is based on the belief that life stance is reflected in communication and that dysfunction can be decreased by clarifying the communication in the specified ego state.

4. Gestalt therapy treatment is based on the belief that intrapsychic conflicts arise from interactions with society and that only integration of all the organisms can offer completion.

5. The client-centered approach to mental health is based on the belief that human beings move toward constructive change and integration and that interpersonal relationships are the bases for health and neurosis.

6. The behavioral approach maintains that behavior is learned; therefore, conditioning and separation of the client from the problem through systematic desensitization and relaxation training can modify undesirable behavior.

7. Rational emotive therapy is based on the belief that individuals can choose thoughts and behaviors and thus select to sometimes promote or limit self-acceptance. Through cognitive tasks, a therapist can provide the skills to scientifically challenge irrational premises and change behavior.

8. Cognitive (Beck's) therapy is based on the belief that an individual's behavior is influenced by the way he or she structures the world, through thoughts and assumptions. Through cognitive and behavioral activities, one can develop balanced thoughts and self-statements.

9. Strategic therapy assumes that reality for each person is created through communication with others, affecting his or her view of every situation.

10. Each theory outlines various techniques for promoting desirable behavior.

11. There are four major lobes of the brain on each hemisphere: the frontal, parietal, temporal, and occipital lobes.

12. The basic structures of interest in genetics are the chromosomes, genes, deoxyribonucleic acid (DNA), and ribonucleic acid (RNA).

13. The peripheral nervous system refers to all parts of the nervous system that lie outside the brain and spinal cord; it includes twelve pairs of cranial nerves and the thirty-one pairs of spinal nerves and their branches.

14. The autonomic nervous system, subdivided into the sympathetic and the parasympathetic systems, is important to the maintenance of equilibrium in the face of external and internal challenges to the organism.

15. A number of neurologic and psychiatric symptoms are caused by problems in the activity of neurotransmitters as they interact at critical sites in the brain.

16. A number of neurologic and psychiatric disorders, including Parkinson's disease, schizophrenia, mood disorders, and Tourette's syndrome, are linked to the dysfunction of the neurotransmitter dopamine.

17. Family studies, twin and adoptive studies, high-risk studies, segregation and pedigree analyses, linkage analysis, and molecular approaches are all strategies used by investigators to uncover genetic and familial correlates to mental illness.

18. Evidence has led clinicians and researchers to consider possible connections between the endocrine system and psychiatric disorders.

19. There is a known relationship between the nervous system and the lymphatic system; a number of investigations have observed changes in the body's immunologic activity in response to stress.

20. Modern brain-imaging techniques can help nurses understand and explain to clients their use in diagnosing psychiatric disorders.

REFERENCES

American Nurses Association: *Psychiatric mental health nursing psychopharmacology project,* Washington, D.C., 1994, American Nurses Publishing.

Baldessarini RJ, Cole JO, Nicholi, AM Jr, ed 5.: Chemotherapy, *The new Harvard guide to psychiatry,* Cambridge, 1988, The Belknap Press of Harvard University Press.

Beck AT: *Depression: Causes and treatment,* Philadelphia, 1971, University of Pennsylvania Press.

Beck AT: *Depression: clinical, experimental and theoretical aspects,* New York, 1967, Harper & Row.

Beck AT: *The diagnosis and management of depression,* Philadelphia, 1973, University of Pennsylvania Press.

Beck AT et al: *Cognitive therapy of depression,* New York, 1979, Guilford Press.

Berne E: *Games people play,* New York, 1964, Ballantine.

Berne E: *What do you say after you say "Hello"?* New York, 1972, Grove Press.

Buckle VJ, Fujita N, Rider-Cook AS: Chromosomal localization of GABA D receptor subunit genes: Relationsip to human genetic disease, *Neuron,* 3:647–654, 1989.

Cutting J, Yudofsky SC, Hales RE, eds.: Neuropsychiatric aspects of attention and consciousness: Stupor and coma, *Textbook of neuropsychiatry* 2 ed, 277–290, Washington, D.C., 1992, American Psychiatric Press.

Daly JM, Salloway S: Dopamine receptors in the human brain, *Psychiatric times,* 11(5) 27–32, 1994.

Dollard J, Miller NE: *Personality & psychotherapy,* New York, 1950, McGraw-Hill.

Dubovsky S, Yudofsky SC, Hales RE, eds.: Psychopharmacological treatment in neuropsychiatry, *Textbook of neuropsychiatry* 2 ed, 663–701, Washington, D.C., 1992, American Psychiatric Press.

Ellis A: *Handbook of rational-emotive therapy,* New York, 1977, Springer Publishing.

Ellis A: *The practice of rational-emotive therapy,* New York, 1987, Springer Publishing.

Ellis A: *Humanistic psychotherapy,* New York, 1973, McGraw-Hill.

Fisch R, Weakland J, Segal: *The tactics of change,* San Francisco, 1986, Jossey-Bass Publishers.

Fitzgerald MJT: *Neuroanatomy basic and clinical,* ed 2, Philadelphia, 1992, Bailliére Tindall.

Freud A: *Introduction to psychoanalysis for teachers,* London, 1931, George Allen.

Freud A: *The writings of Anna Freud,* New York, 1967, International Universities Press.

Freud A: *Psychoanalysis for teachers and parents—Introductory lectures,* New York, 1979, Norton.

Freud S: *The ego and the id,* New York, 1960, Norton Library.

Gallagher W: *The power of place,* New York, 1993, Poseidon Press.

Goldman MB; Yudofsky SC, Hales RE, eds.: Neuropsychiatric features of endocrine disorders, *Textbook of neuropsychiatry* 2 ed, 519–540, Washington, D.C., 1992, American Psychiatric Press.

Goulding M, Goulding R: *Changing lives through redecision therapy,* New York, 1979, Grove Press.

Greene RL: Brief strategic treatment: The tactical promotion of change, *Newsletter, Academy of San Diego Psychologists,* May 1991, 1–4.

Keltner, NL, Callwood GB: Neurosciences: Developing a basic science foundation for psychiatric nurses, *Psychiatric mental health nursing psychopharmacology project,* 22–24, Washington, D.C., 1994, American Nurses Publishing.

Kety SS, Matthysse S, Nicholi AM Jr, eds.: Genetic and biochemical aspects of schizophrenia, *The new Harvard guide to psychiatry,* 139-151, Cambridge, 1988, The Belknap Press of Harvard University Press.

Klerman GL, Nicholi AM Jr, eds.: Classification and DSM-III-R, *The new Harvard guide to psychiatry,* 70-87, Cambridge, 1988, The Belknap Press of Harvard University Press.

Kovel J: *A complete guide to therapy from psychoanalysis to behavior modification,* New York, 1976, Pantheon Books.

Malaspina D, Qutkin AB, Kaufmann CA, Yudofsky SC, Hales RE, eds.: Epidemiology and genetics of neuropsychiatric diseases, *Textbook of Neuropsychiatry* 2 ed, 187-226, Washington D.C., 1992, American Psychiatric Press.

Mesulam M; Nicholi AM Jr, ed: Neural substrates of behavior: The effects of brain lesions upon mental state, *The new Harvard guide to psychiatry,* 91-128, Cambridge, 1988, The Belknap Press of Harvard University Press.

Nemiah JC, Nicholi AM Jr, eds.: Psychoneurotic disorders, *The new Harvard guide to psychiatry,* 91-128, Cambridge, 1988, The Belknap Press of Harvard University Press.

Orrison WW, Jr, Levine JD, Sanders JA, and Hartshorne MF: *Functional Brain Imaging,* St. Louis, 1995, Mosby.

Rawlins RP, Williams SR, Beck CK: *Mental health-psychiatric nursing,* ed 3, St. Louis, 1993, Mosby.

Rogers CP: *Client centered therapy,* Boston, 1951, Houghton Mifflin.

Rogers CP: *On becoming a person,* Boston, 1961, Houghton Mifflin.

Rogers CR: *Person to person, the problem of being human,* Walnut Creek, Calif., 1967, Real People Press.

Rogers P, Reich R, Nicholi AM Jr, eds.: Psychosomatic medicine and consultation-liaison psychiatry, *The new Harvard guide to psychiatry,* 387-417, Cambridge, 1988, The Belknap Press of Harvard University Press.

Skinner BF: *Science & human behavior,* New York, 1953, MacMillan Co.

Snyder SH: *The new biology of mood,* New York, 1988, Roerig.

Stevens O, ed: *Gestalt is—Addresses, essays, lectures,* Moab, Utah, 1975, Real People Press.

van Praag HM, Bruinvels J, eds.: *Neurotransmission and disturbed behavior,* New York, 1978, SP Medical & Scientific Books.

Watzlawick P, Weakland J, Fisch R: *Change,* New York, 1974, WW Norton.

Watzlawick P: *How real is real?* New York, 1977, Vintage Books.

PART TWO

Dynamics of Nursing Practice

Tree of Life
ANCIENT BABYLONIA

This symbol represents a tree of life and knowledge and appears throughout the world in various forms. It signifies the perpetual nature of life, knowledge, and learning. Part Two presents key concepts in the application of psychiatric nursing principles to life situations as perpetuated through the nursing process and principles of communication.

CHAPTER 6

The Nursing Process

Katherine M. Fortinash

Analysis Taking apart collected data to examine and interpret each piece and identify variations from typical behaviors or responses. Discovering patterns or relationships in the data that may be cues or clues that require further investigation. One cognitive process involved in diagnostic reasoning.

Clinical pathway A standardized format used to provide and monitor client care and progress by way of the case management, interdisciplinary health care delivery system. (Also known as a critical pathway, care path, or Care Map.)

Insight Ability to perceive oneself realistically and understand oneself.

Intuition Insight into a situation without the benefit of critical analysis. (Also known as intuitive reasoning.)

Synthesis Combining several parts of relevant data into a single piece of information. Comparing behavioral patterns to learned theories or typical patterns of behavior in order to identify strengths and seek explanations for symptoms. One cognitive process involved in diagnostic reasoning.

Taxonomy A classification of known phenomena under a hierarchical structure.

- Discuss the roles of intuition, expertise, and critical thinking and their application to the nursing process in mental health.

- Describe the cyclical nature of the American Nurses Association six-step nursing process.

- Compare and contrast nursing and medical assessment frameworks, with particular focus on the NANDA taxonomy.

- Differentiate actual, risk, and wellness diagnoses with emphasis on the most current NANDA labels, etiologies, risk factors, and defining characteristics.

- Identify outcomes that accurately measure clients' achievable behaviors based on their nursing diagnoses.

- Formulate nursing interventions that are prescriptive and directive, for both actual and risk diagnoses.

- Construct rationale statements for each proposed nursing intervention.

- Develop evaluations for outcomes that effectively measure client progress within an appropriate time frame.

- Design a clinical pathway for a client with a DSM-IV diagnosis or psychiatric symptoms, using appropriate outcomes, processes, and length of stay.

T he nursing process is a time-honored method that consists of a series of planned steps and actions whereby nurses treat and evaluate human responses to actual or potential health problems. Once a five-step process, the nursing process has been revised to a six-step process in recent years, according to the American Nurses Association Standards of Practice (ANA, 1991). See comparison below:

Five-Step Process
Standard I–Assessment
Standard II–Nursing Diagnosis
Standard III–Planning
Standard IV–Implementation
Standard V–Evaluation

Six-Step Process
Standard I–Assessment
Standard II–Nursing Diagnosis
Standard III–Outcome Identification
Standard IV–Planning
Standard V–Implementation
Standard VI–Evaluation

117

In order to maintain the most current practice standards, the six-step process is used throughout this text, although the authors recognize the merits of the five-step process and realize it is still in use. In the six-step process, outcome identification is featured as a separate step, as some believe it may be useful to list outcomes directly after nursing diagnoses and prior to the planning phase. They contend that the planning phase incorporates measures that assist clients in achieving outcomes, and this can be done more readily if outcomes have been already selected. In the five-step process, the planning phase exists, in part, to plan outcomes, so that outcomes are actually part of the planning phase and therefore not singled out as a separate step.

In recent times, outcomes, whether client centered or organizational, have emerged as a major focus for accrediting bodies and managed care companies. The current trend toward cost-effective quality outcomes and methods of achievement is a major component of health care delivery systems.

Regardless of the method used, the nursing process remains a forceful, systematic, problem-solving method that encompasses all the significant components necessary to care for clients, with attention given to families, significant others, and the community. Many nursing theorists concur that the nursing process is even more than an organized, systematic approach to clinical problems. Unlike most episodic or linear problem-solving methods, in which a problem is identified, diagnosed, treated, and resolved (thus the problem ends with a resolution), the nursing process is an ongoing, multidimensional, cyclical

approach in which data are continually collected, critically analyzed, and incorporated into the treatment plan according to the client's fluctuating responses to health and illness. Figure 6-1 shows the cyclical nature of the nursing process.

The steps in the nursing process are not necessarily taken in strict sequence (beginning with assessment and ending with evaluation). They may be taken concurrently, since nurses may be evaluating their assessment or even their plan of action at any given time.

Since the client's health status is dynamic rather than static, so too is the nursing process. This challenges the seasoned nurse to make sound, clinical judgments and decisions, and guides the novice toward practicing and mastering clear, analytical thinking and keen organizational skills. The steps of the nursing process create a circular pattern of continuous interpretation of data and management of client care.

Kritek (1978) states that the phases of the nursing process are interactive as well as continual. Thus, the phases influence each other and the client at the same time. There are points throughout the process in which the phases converge. The nurse can attend the client at any point throughout this interactive, fluid process.

For psychiatric nurses, whether students, new graduates, or seasoned clinicians, the use of the nursing process presents significant challenges that can be mastered. In the world of mental health, the nursing process focuses primarily on the client's behavior and its meaning beyond the spoken word, including psychosocial stressors. A client's psychic strength, vulnerability, cop-

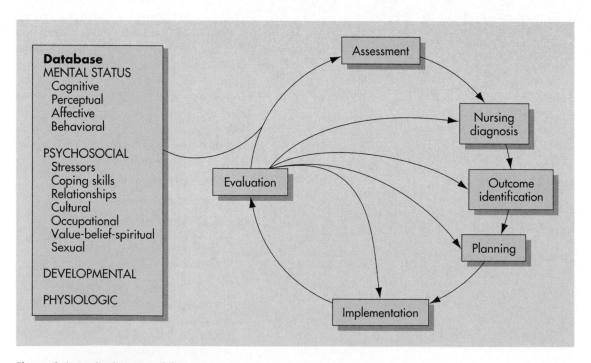

Figure 6-1 Cyclical nature of the nursing process.

From Fortinash K, Holoday-Worret P: *Psychiatric nursing care plans*, ed 2, St. Louis, 1995, Mosby.

ing skills, and ego defense mechanisms are among the major components that are the psychiatric nurse's primary focus for the nursing process.

The psychiatric-mental health component of holistic client assessment includes the Mental Status Examination and psychosocial criteria (Box 6-1), which consist of an organized collection of data that reflects an individual's functioning at the time of the interview. It is a basis for subsequent medical and nursing diagnoses and management of care by all disciplines that interface with psychiatric nursing.

Components of the Mental Status Examination, such as mood, affect, thoughts and perceptions, become the psychiatric nurse's major focus, in contrast to the familiar multisystem assessment most often used in the medical-surgical setting. This does not mean that psychiatric

---

Box 6-1 Components of Assessment: Mental Status and Psychosocial Criteria

MENTAL STATUS EXAMINATION

Appearance

Dress, grooming, hygiene, cosmetics, apparent age, posture, facial expression

Behavior/activity

Hypoactivity or hyperactivity, rigid, relaxed, restless or agitated motor movements, gait and coordination, facial grimacing, gestures, mannerisms, passive, combative, bizarre

Attitude

Interactions with the interviewer: cooperative, resistive, friendly, hostile, ingratiating

Speech

Quantity: poverty of speech, poverty of content, voluminous
Quality: articulate, congruent, monotonous, talkative, repetitious, spontaneous, circumlocutory, confabulations, tangential, pressured, stereotypical
Rate: slowed, rapid

Mood and affect

Mood (intensity, depth, duration): sad, fearful, depressed, angry, anxious, ambivalent, happy, ecstatic, grandiose
Affect (intensity, depth, duration): appropriate, apathetic, constricted, blunted, flat, labile, euphoric, bizarre

Perceptions

Hallucinations, illusions, depersonalization, derealization, distortions

Thoughts

Form and content: logical versus illogical, loose associations, flight of ideas, autistic, blocking, broadcasting, neologisms, word salad, obsessions, ruminations, delusions, abstract versus concrete

Sensorium/cognition

Levels of consciousness, orientation, attention span, recent and remote memory, concentration; ability to comprehend and process information; intelligence

Judgment

Ability to assess and evaluate situations, make rational decisions, understand consequences of behavior, and take responsibility for actions

Insight

Ability to perceive and understand the cause and nature of own and others' situations

Reliability

Interviewer's impression that individual reported information accurately and completely

PSYCHOSOCIAL CRITERIA

Stressors

Internal: psychiatric or medical illness, perceived loss, such as loss of self-concept/self-esteem
External: actual loss, e.g., death of a loved one, divorce, lack of support systems, job or financial loss, retirement, dysfunctional family system

Coping skills

Adaptation to internal and external stressors; use of functional, adaptive coping mechanisms and techniques; management of activities of daily living

Relationships

Attainment and maintenance of satisfying, interpersonal relationships congruent with developmental stage; includes sexual relationship as appropriate for age and status

Cultural

Ability to adapt and conform to prescribed norms, rules, ethics, and mores of an identified group

Spiritual (value-belief)

Presence of a self-satisfying value-belief system that the individual regards as right, desirable, worthwhile, and comforting

Occupational

Engagement in useful, rewarding activity, congruent with developmental stage and societal standards (work, school, recreation)

From Fortinash K, Holoday-Worret P: *Psychiatric nursing care plans,* ed 2, St. Louis, 1995, Mosby.

nurses ignore physical problems. They are well prepared to make holistic assessments given that most clients present with multiple symptomatology that affects both the mind and body. It is not likely, however, that psychiatric clients will be attached to intravenous tubing, oxygen, or a cardiac monitor, yet their wounds are equally painful and just as profoundly debilitating. It is the nurse's challenge to discover the source of these wounds by applying critical thinking and decision-making generated through the familiar guidelines of the nursing process and combined with a uniqueness of self and experiential wisdom.

Even with the help of the nursing process, there will be times when psychiatric nurses are unsure of which approach to take for certain client behaviors. Unlike the medical-surgical field, there are not always specific interventions for specific client behaviors, and clients may not always respond predictably to standard approaches. As such, mental health clients may be resistant to even the most carefully designed treament plan, whereby a variety of treatment approaches is generally applied before a response is elicited.

The nursing process, like other decision-making methods, does not guarantee instant improvement of symptoms. Psychiatric clients seldom leave the hospital completely symptom-free, given the complex nature of mental illness. But it is hoped that clients will achieve a higher level of functioning because of nurses who are willing to try a variety of acceptable approaches, with patience, understanding, and hope. In the final analysis, it is the nurse and his or her unique spirit that adds a critical dimension to the nursing process and brings it to life.

HISTORY AND PERSPECTIVES OF THE NURSING PROCESS

The nursing process is the long-standing method by which nurses make critical decisions for clinical care. It is influenced by such important elements as intuition, expertise, and critical thinking.

Intuition and the Nursing Process

Intuition, also known as "intuitive reasoning," is an individual's insight into a situation without the benefit of critical analysis. A strong "hunch" and a "gut feeling" are examples of intuition. It is often proposed that a person operating on intuition needs little data to support his or her insights (Wescott, 1968). It is generally acknowledged that, in the past, nurses relied strongly on intuition for their nursing assessments and actions. With the advent of nursing as a science, intuitive reasoning fell into disfavor as a method by which to make critical decisions. Intuitiveness came to be viewed as unscientific. As technology grew and the pendulum swung toward scientific reasoning as a method of knowing, and away from the in-

tuitive approach, intuition was devalued (Munhall and Oiler, 1993).

As a result of this scientific revolution, nursing resisted using intuitive terms and instead opted for a more concrete, linear problem-solving method considered to be gender neutral and relatively safe. More recently, intuition has appeared in nursing journals as a valid component of the complex nature of clinical reasoning. Some now consider intuition as a component of critical thinking.

Benner's significant work, *From Novice to Expert: Excellence and Power in Clinical Nursing Practice* (1984), described the role of intuition in critical care nurses and concluded that many of them were not consciously aware of the higher-level reasoning processes they used to assess and deliver client care. Yet the nursing interventions based on these intuitive forces reflected superior insights and sound judgments. Smith (1988) noted that these nurses somehow had the ability to sense impending deterioration in their clients before such crises actually occurred.

Given this information, it makes sense that in the psychiatric-mental health arena where clients' fluctuating behaviors are the main focus for nursing assessment, diagnosis, and interventions, nurses inevitably incorporate judgments based on intuitive reasoning to make clinical decisions. It seems obvious, then, that intuition has a role in influencing the phases of the nursing process and has strongly resurfaced as a major force in clinical reasoning. Although the mental mechanisms by which intuition works remain in part mysterious and elusive, the results as measured by client outcomes have nonetheless been impressive. Intuitive reasoning most decidedly has a place in the future of clinical nursing research and practice.

Example of a nurse's use of intuition: A nurse retreats from an intense interview with a client and focuses on less volatile topics. When asked about her strategy, she stated that she experienced a "gut" feeling that prompted her to change the topic. When questioned later about his feelings during the interview, the client stated that he experienced a buildup of anger, although he wasn't fully aware of it at the time.

Expertise and the Nursing Process

Expertise is another component necessary for sound clinical judgments. Only through clinical experience can nurses develop expertise in selected specialty areas of practice (Benner, 1984). Expertise, like intuition, influences the phases of the nursing process. Although it is said that intuition cannot be taught, it can nonetheless be learned through clinical practice. The exact process by which this occurs, however, remains elusive and complex. Both expertise and intuition are worthwhile goals that nurses should continue to develop and pursue throughout their professional lives. Expertise can incorporate intuitiveness in clinical practice.

Critical Thinking in the Nursing Process

Critical thinking is most important in the nursing process and contains many of the components of keen judgment, intuition, and expertise. Critical thinking skills enhance and become a part of the nurse's continually expanding knowledge base and help the nurse decide which data are meaningful and which take priority.

When using the nursing process, the nurse incorporates experience and knowledge from nursing and other courses to apply theories and principles in practice. Knowledge of basic human needs; anatomy and physiology; disease processes; growth and development; sociologic patterns and trends; and various cultures, religions, and philosophies are all crucial components of the critical thinking framework. The following critical thinking skills are used in all phases of the nursing process (Wilkinson, 1992):

- *Observing* (observations should be planned and ongoing versus casual and singular)
- *Distinguishing* relevant from irrelevant data
- *Validating* data through observations and communication
- *Organizing* data into meaningful parts
- *Categorizing* data for efficient retrieval and communication

ASSESSMENT

Assessment, the initial phase of the nursing process, is perhaps the most critical component because it is the phase in which nurses collect enormous amounts of data about clients' holistic health status. Holistic assessment provides nurses with relevant data from which to accurately formulate and prioritize nursing diagnoses, the crux of treatment planning, according to clients' needs or immediate conditions. Throughout the assessment phase, nurses collect data through learned, time-proven, interactive and interviewing skills, and observations of verbal and nonverbal behaviors, based on a broad biopsychosociocultural background and knowledge of functional and dysfunctional behaviors (Fortinash and Holoday-Worret, 1995).

In psychiatric-mental health nursing, assessment takes place in a number of settings, e.g., inpatient, outpatient, or community and home environments. This gives the nurse many opportunities to observe the client and modify assessment data in accordance with the client's continued adjustment to the milieu and progress made throughout hospitalization. Ideally, the client is the primary source of information during the assessment phase. Occasionally, however, the client may be unable to offer a complete or accurate health history, given the acuity of his or her illness. In such cases, a reliable source may be interviewed on the client's behalf, with the understanding that such information will be evaluated in terms of that person's relationship with the client (Fortinash, 1990).

Assessment of the individual includes the following criteria: physical, psychiatric, psychosocial, mental status, developmental, cultural, spiritual, and sexual. The method of assessment includes the client's subjective report of symptoms and problems, and the nurse's objective findings (Fortinash, 1990; Fortinash and Holoday-Worret, 1995). Box 6-1 details mental status and psychosocial criteria that should be covered during assessment.

A major focus of a client's mental status is identification of his or her strengths and capabilities for interaction with and within the environment. This includes the ability to initiate interactions, sustain meaningful communication and relationships, and attain satisfaction congruent with his or her developmental and sociocultural lifestyle. Knowledge and appreciation of the psychodynamics and psychopathology of human behavior are essential for effective assessment of the individual's adjustment or maladjustment to internal and external life stressors (Fortinash and Holoday-Worret, 1995).

The Nurse-Client Interview

The interview is the most critical process involved in gathering information related to the overall health status of clients with psychiatric disorders. It is a more meaningful, flexible method of collecting important data than are questionnaires or computers, and it allows the examiner to use all the senses to explore specific topics and key themes or concerns expressed by the client through verbal and nonverbal responses. Box 6-2 lists samples of some general questions that can be asked during the nurse-client interview.

In assessing a client's mental status, the primary instrument or "tool" of evaluation is the nurse interviewer. The success of the interview depends in large part on the development of trust, rapport, and respect between the nurse and the client, and between the nurse and the family. Keen therapeutic communication skills such as active listening and reflective questioning are used throughout the interview in an effort to determine the client's immediate needs and actively engage him or her in treatment (Fortinash, 1990; Fortinash and Holoday-Worret, 1995). See Chapter 7 for more information on development of good communication skills.

Assessment Frameworks

Assessment frameworks are not new or unique to nursing. As a result of nursing's orientation and commitment to holistic assessment, nurses collect large amounts of data about a client's biopsychosociocultural health status. Assessment frameworks are organizational systems by which to store data for easier access to information.

Box 6-2   The Nurse-Client Interview—Sample General Questions

Presenting problem

- Tell me the reason you are here (in treatment).

Present illness

- When did you first notice the problem?
- What changes have you noticed in yourself?
- What do you think is causing the problem?
- Have you had any troubling feelings or thoughts?

Family history

- How would you describe your relationship with your parents?
- Did either of your parents have emotional or mental problems?
- Were either of your parents treated by a psychiatrist or therapist?
- Did their treatment include medication or ECT?
- Were they helped by their treatment?

Childhood/premorbid history

- How did you get along with your family and friends?
- How would you describe yourself as a child?

Medical history

- Do you have any serious medical problems?

Psychosocial/psychiatric history

- Have you ever been treated for an emotional or psychiatric problem? Have you been diagnosed with a mental illness?

- Have you ever been a patient in a psychiatric hospital?
- Have you ever been in counseling/therapy for an emotional or psychiatric problem?
- Have you ever taken prescribed medications for an emotional problem or mental illness? Did you ever have ECT?
- If so, did the medication ECT help your symptoms/problem?
- How frequently do your symptoms occur? (about every six months? once a year? every five years? first episode?)
- How long are you generally able to function well in between onset of symptoms? (weeks? months? years?)
- What do you feel, if anything, may have contributed to your symptoms? (nothing? stopped taking medications? began using alcohol? street drugs?)

Recent stressors/losses

- Have you had any recent stressors or losses in your life?
- What are your relationships like?
- How do you get along with people at work?

Education

- How did you do in school?
- How did you feel about school?

Legal

- Have you ever been in trouble with the law?

Such frameworks can also serve as guides for assessment since their compartments consist of categories that correspond to those qualities accepted by nurses as constituting the nature of humans, health, illness, and nursing. Table 6-1 depicts three separate assessment frameworks. The traditional medical framework model is now considered insufficient for the holistic assessment required in psychiatric-mental health nursing and, most likely, in other nursing specialty areas. The other two columns describe the two frameworks most commonly used in today's nursing practice, which are discussed below.

FUNCTIONAL HEALTH PATTERN FRAMEWORK

Developed by Marjory Gordon, functional health patterns are categories of human, biologic, physiologic, psychologic, developmental, cultural, social, and spiritual assessments. Health patterns related to these categories are assessed over a time sequence as either functional or dysfunctional. Functional patterns reflect the client's strengths and adaptive coping strategies, while dysfunctional patterns form the basis for client problems and nursing diagnoses (Gordon, 1994). Functional health patterns are currently widely accepted framework methods in both educational and practice settings.

NANDA TAXONOMY

At the seventh conference of the North American Nursing Diagnosis Association (NANDA) in 1986, a classification system for nursing diagnoses was officially formulated. It is currently called Taxonomy I-Revised. This system is NANDA's conceptual framework. It replaces the previously used alphabetized list of diagnoses (a collection of names) as a method of categorizing.

A **taxonomy** classifies phenomena under a hierarchical structure and also helps guide new phenomena. Both the taxonomy and the diagnostic terminology guide nurses toward building a solid scientific foundation for the profession. It also provides nursing with a standard-

---

Box 6-2   The Nurse-Client Interview—Sample General Questions—cont'd

Marital history

- How do you feel about your marriage (if client is married)?
- How would you describe your relationship with your children (if client has children)?
- What kinds of things do you do as a family?

Social history

- Tell me about your friends, your social activities.
- How would you describe your relationship with your friends?

Support systems

- Who would you turn to if you were in trouble?
- Do you feel you need someone to turn to now?

Insight

- Do you consider yourself different now than before your problem began? In what way?
- Do you think you have an emotional problem or mental illness?
- Do you think you need help for your problem?
- What are your goals for yourself?

Value-belief system

- What kinds of things give you comfort and peace of mind?
- Will those things be helpful to you now?

Special needs

- How can staff help you during your treatment?
- What kinds of things will be most helpful to you now?

Discharge goals

- How do you want to feel by the time you're ready for discharge?
- What do you think you can do to help yourself reach that goal?
- What things will you do differently than you did before?
- What things can you do to help prevent your symptoms from reoccurring and stay out of the hospital?
- What are your goals for daily medication compliance?
- How will you manage your leisure time?

From Fortinash K, Holoday-Worret P: *Psychiatric nursing care plans,* ed 2, St. Louis, 1995, Mosby; Fortinash K: Assessment of mental states. In Malasanos L, Barkauskas V, Stoltenberg-Allen K, editors: *Health assessment,* ed 4, St. Louis, 1990, Mosby.

TABLE 6-1   Comparison of medical and nursing assessment frameworks

Medical model		Nursing models	
BODY SYSTEMS	**NANDA TAXONOMY I-REVISED**	**FUNCTIONAL HEALTH PATTERNS (GORDON, 1987)**	
Cardiovascular	Exchanging	Health Perception/Health Management	
Respiratory	Communicating	Nutritional/Metabolic	
Neurologic	Relating	Elimination	
Endocrine	Valuing	Activity/Exercise	
Metabolic	Choosing	Sleep/Rest	
Hematopoietic	Moving	Cognitive/Perceptual	
Integumentary	Perceiving	Self-Perception/Self-Concept	
Gastrointestinal	Feeling	Role/Relationship	
Genitourinary	Knowing	Sexuality/Reproductive	
Reproductive		Coping/Stress Tolerance	
Psychiatric		Value-Belief	

From Davie JK: The nursing process. In Thelan L et al, editors: *Critical care nursing: diagnosis and management,* ed 2, St. Louis, 1994, Mosby.

---

ized, more efficient method of communication (NANDA, 1994).

Frameworks are necessary tools with which to process the large amount of data collected by nurses in assessing clients. Frameworks form a basis for diagnostic reasoning (discussed later) by gathering assessment in-formation and organizing it into manageable pieces. An organized collection system assures easier retrieval of critical client information and shows important relation-ships among the data. The selection of one framework over another is an individual choice (Fortinash and Holo-day-Worret, 1995).

NURSING DIAGNOSIS

The formulation of nursing diagnoses involves the interpretation of data collected in the assessment phase and the application of standardized labels to clients' health problems and responses to illness and life events. Nursing diagnoses are written as statements that describe an individual's health state or an actual or potential alteration (known as a "risk" diagnosis) in a person's life process. The nursing diagnosis statement may reflect one's biologic, psychologic, sociocultural, developmental, spiritual, or sexual process (Table 6-2). At NANDA's ninth conference (1990), nursing diagnosis was defined as ". . . a clinical judgment about individual, family, or community responses to actual or potential health problems/life processes. Nursing diagnoses provide the basis for selection of nursing interventions to achieve outcomes for which the nurse is accountable."

The development and refinement of nursing diagnoses are still in the early stages and are continuously being revised. This challenging task is evident in the 19 newest diagnostic labels endorsed at NANDA's tenth conference in 1994. A list of the most current NANDA diagnoses is found on the inside front cover of this book.

Nursing diagnoses provide nurses with a vocabulary that is distinctive to nursing. Nursing diagnosis language enhances communication among nurses and clarity of purpose to other health care disciplines, in relation to the problems nurses assess and treat. By using its own vocabulary, nursing grows as a profession and gains respectability. Carpenito states that NANDA's attempt to upgrade nursing's status as a profession by its unifying vocabulary, which enhances communication among nurses, is as much for purposes of a social policy as it is for "clarifying nursing for nurses" (1996).

Diagnostic Reasoning

Once the data have been collected and recorded, the next step is interpretation of what the data actually mean in terms of the client's health-illness status. Critical thinking in diagnostic reasoning consists of the following two major cognitive processes:

TABLE 6-2 Nursing diagnosis statements in relation to life processes

Nursing diagnoses	Life processes
Altered nutrition	Biologic
Self-esteem disturbance	Psychologic
Impaired social interaction	Sociocultural
Altered growth and development	Developmental
Spiritual distress	Spiritual
Sexuality pattern alteration	Sexual

Analysis: Taking apart the collected data to examine and interpret each piece and identify variations from typical behaviors or responses. Also includes discovering patterns or relationships in the data that may be cues that require further investigation.

Synthesis: Combining several parts of relevant data into a single piece of information. Also involves comparing behavioral patterns to learned theories or typical patterns of behavior in order to identify strengths and seek explanations for symptoms (Wilkinson, 1992).

The term *inference,* as defined by Webster's Collegiate Dictionary, is ". . . the process of arriving at a conclusion by reasoning from evidence." However, inherent in the use of inference is a tendency to assume if the evidence is slight or has not been fully examined. Therefore, in order to avoid (as much as possible) a rush to judgment or an "inferential leap," the nurse reaches conclusions and formulates diagnoses on logical and factual data. This can be achieved by limiting the amount of bias that can influence the diagnostic process and by remaining as objective as possible (Benner, 1984; Carnevali, 1993; Tanner, 1987).

Definitions of Health Problems

Nearly all approved diagnoses are accompanied by definitions that more clearly describe or explain the health problem. This feature is useful for students who may need more specific clarification of the problem than the label alone conveys. The following examples present definitions for two sets of similar diagnoses that are often confused with one another:

Fear: "Feeling of dread related to an identifiable source which the person validates" (NANDA, 1994, p. 87).

Anxiety: "A vague, uneasy feeling whose source is often non-specific or unknown to the individual" (NANDA, 1994, p. 86).

Powerlessness: "Perception that one's actions will not significantly affect an outcome; a perceived lack of control over a current situation or immediate happening" (NANDA, 1994, p. 77).

Hopelessness: "A subjective state in which an individual sees limited or no alternatives or personal choices available and is unable to mobilize energy on own behalf" (NANDA, 1994, p. 76).

Qualifying Statements

For additional clarity, some nursing diagnoses require qualifying statements based on the nature of the health problem as it is manifested in each particular client response or situation. Table 6-3 gives examples of nursing diagnoses and qualifying statements.

TABLE 6-3 Examples of nursing diagnoses and qualifying statements

Nursing diagnoses	Qualifying statements
Altered Nutrition	Less than body requirements
Self-Care Deficit	Bathing, grooming, feeding
Noncompliance	Medication, milieu activities
Knowledge Deficit	Illness, medication, treatments
Altered Parenting	Response to child's mental illness
Caregiver Role Strain	Difficulty caring for relative with Alzheimer's disease
Potential for Effective Coping	Increased knowledge of mental illness
Risk for Loneliness	Increased social isolation

TABLE 6-4 Examples of nursing diagnoses and etiologies

Nursing diagnoses	Etiologies (related to):
Anxiety	Threat to biologic, psychologic, and/or social integrity
Ineffective Individual Coping	Situational crisis, maturational crisis, personal vulnerability
Hopelessness	Long-term stress or illness, prolonged spiritual distress
Powerlessness	Lifestyle of helplessness, illness-related regimen, prolonged hopelessness
Impaired Verbal Communication	Psychological barriers, e.g., psychosis, mania, panic state

From Fortinash K, Holoday-Worret P: *Psychiatric nursing care plans,* ed 2, St. Louis, 1995, Mosby.

Guidelines for Etiologies

Etiologies, also known as related factors or "related to," are the source from which the nursing diagnoses emerge. They are also known as factors that are associated with the diagnosis, contribute to the diagnosis, or may be considered a probable cause of the diagnosis to the extent that the cause can be determined. Nursing diagnoses are often accompanied by several etiologies that interact to produce the health problem (diagnosis). Etiologies may be psychologic, biologic, relational, environmental, situational, developmental, or sociocultural, yet they are all in some manner associated with the problem. Examples of nursing diagnoses and etiologies are presented in Table 6-4.

As noted in Table 6-4, many etiologic factors are broad categories or examples that require more specific information based on the nature of the problem and the client who is the focus of treatment. For example, the first etiology listed is a threat to biologic, psychologic, or social integrity. Considering the source of anxiety in a particular client, the nurse needs to be more precise in delineating which aspects of biologic, psychologic, or social integrity are threatened, for example, recent illness (biologic); loss of job or status (psychologic); divorce, separation (social).

Etiologies may be treated by nurses independently or in collaboration with other health care professionals, as determined by the client's needs. However, the nurse is primarily responsible for constructing the client's treatment plan and formulating etiologies that are both specific to the client's identified problem and largely managed and treated by nurses. Therefore, the treatment plan for any given nursing diagnosis must include interventions aimed at managing or resolving etiologic factors as well as the health problem (nursing diagnosis).

Nursing diagnoses can also be appropriately used as etiologies for other nursing diagnoses. The use of nursing diagnoses as etiologies can be very effective in resolving or reducing the problem. Nurses tend to focus their interactions on diagnostic labels, so it is logical that they focus on the diagnosis that serves as the etiology. Also, if nurses can manage or modify the etiologic factors as well as address the nursing diagnosis, the client is more likely to benefit from the overall impact of these focused interventions because the etiologies most closely represent the core of the problems as defined by nursing. Some examples are the following:

1. Anxiety—related to Powerlessness

2. Impaired Social Interactions—related to Self-Esteem Disturbance

3. Ineffective Individual Coping—related to Anxiety

4. Spiritual Distress—related to Dysfunctional Grieving

5. Altered Parenting—related to Knowledge Deficit

It is considered inadvisable to cite medical diagnoses as etiologies for nursing problems. It is more difficult for nurses to treat an etiology that is stated as a medical diagnosis, such as schizophrenia, since that type of label suggests a whole array of treatment strategies which are not uniquely nursing.

However, many symptoms and behaviors resulting from mental disorders and medical conditions are of great concern to nurses and require management and treatment by nurses. Some examples are:

Altered thought processes as a result of the schizophrenic process

Altered nutrition—less than body kilocalorie requirements as a result of anorexia nervosa

Impaired verbal communication as a result of bipolar disorders

In such situations, the nurse isolates those aspects that contribute to the symptoms that can be treated by nursing interventions and cite them as etiologies. Some examples are the following:

Altered thought processes. Related to:
   internal and external stressors
   impaired ability to process internal and external stimuli

Altered nutrition (less than body kilocalorie requirements). Related to:
   inadequate intake and hypermetabolic need
   loss of appetite secondary to constipation

Impaired verbal communication. Related to:
   rapid thought processes secondary to manic state

The above-cited etiologic factors that accompany the nursing diagnoses more clearly specify the focus of care for nursing interventions.

Guidelines for Defining Characteristics

Defining characteristics, also known as signs and symptoms and labeled "As Evidenced By" (AEB) in the nursing care plan, are the observable, measurable manifestations of clients' responses to the identified health problems (nursing diagnoses). As with diagnoses and etiologies, defining characteristics are generally in nonspecific terms and often need to be modified to reflect the particular situation or response presented by the client. For example, the diagnosis Ineffective Individual Coping has as one of its defining characteristics "ineffective problem solving" (NANDA, 1990). The nurse can clarify the defining characteristic statements by quoting the client. Examples of ineffective problem solving:

- "I can't decide if I should stay with my family or move to a board and care home."

- "I can't decide what to do first—get a job or begin day treatment."

Therefore, defining characteristics, when applicable, should be present in the nurse's assessment criteria to give some validity to the health problem that is being diagnosed. Some examples of defining characteristics used to define the diagnosis Chronic Low Self-Esteem are the following:

- Self-negating verbalization
- Expression of shame or guilt
- Evaluation of self as unable to deal with events
- Hesitancy to try new things or situations

Risk Diagnoses[†]

Risk factors are used in assessing potential health problems. They describe existing risk states that may contribute to the potential problem becoming actual. There are no defining characteristics in a risk diagnosis since the actual problem has not been manifested. Also, there are no etiologies in a risk or potential problem, since etiologies reflect causality, and cause cannot exist without effect. Thus, a risk diagnosis carries a *two-part* statement, whereas an actual nursing diagnosis consists of a three-part statement. Box 6-3 presents the two types of nursing diagnosis formats, using two examples of each type (NANDA, 1994).

The prediction of a risk problem in a particular client requires an estimation of probability of occurrence. Risk problems can be assigned to almost any individual in a compromised health state. For example, a client taking a tricyclic antidepressant medication may be at risk for several potential problems as a result of the actions of these drugs on many of the body systems, such as risk for injury (hypotension, dizziness, blurred vision); risk for constipation; risk for urinary retention; risk for altered mucous membranes (dry mouth).

Examples of a risk diagnosis:

PART 1 Nursing Diagnosis:	Risk for constipation
PART 2 Risk Factors:	Tricyclic antidepressant medications
	Refusal to drink water, juice, etc.
	Noncompliance to high-fiber foods

Several of the approved diagnoses address potential dysfunctional states and cite risk factors. The following are examples of such diagnoses:

- Risk for Violence
- Risk for Injury

[†]Currently NANDA terminology; formerly known as High Risk Diagnoses.

Box 6-3   Format of Nursing Diagnoses

TWO-PART STATEMENTS

Risk problem (two-part statement):

PART 1   **Nursing Diagnosis**
Risk for Violence; directed at others

PART 2   **Risk Factors (Predictors of Risk Problem)**
History of violence
Hyperactivity secondary to manic state
Low impulse control
Aggressive verbal remarks

Risk problem (two-part statement):

PART 1   **Nursing Diagnosis**
Risk for Loneliness

PART 2   **Risk Factors (Predictors of Risk Problem)**
Social isolation
Deprivation of love/affection
Physical isolation
Long-term institutionalization

THREE-PART STATEMENTS

Actual problem (three-part statement):

PART 1   **Nursing Diagnosis**
Post-Trauma Response

PART 2   **Etiologic Factor(s) (Related to)**
Overwhelming anxiety secondary to:

- Rape or other assault
- Catastrophic illness
- Disasters
- War

PART 3   **Defining Characteristics**
Reexperience of traumatic event (flashbacks)
Repetitive dreams or nightmares
Intrusive thoughts about traumatic event
Excess verbalization about traumatic event

Actual problem (three-part statement):

PART 1   **Nursing Diagnosis**
Chronic Confusion

PART 2   **Etiologic Factors (Related to)**
Disorientation secondary to Alzheimer's
  disease
Psychosis secondary to Korsakoff's syndrome
Trauma secondary to recent head injury
Memory loss secondary to dementia

PART 3   **Defining Characteristics**
Altered interpretation/response to stimuli
Progressive long-standing cognitive impairment
No change in level of consciousness
Impaired socialization
Impaired short-term memory

- Risk for Trauma
- Risk for Altered Parenting

In addition to those diagnoses formally listed as "risk" types, any actual diagnosis from the approved list can be stated as a "Risk" diagnosis if it meets the criteria for an "at-risk" problem. For example, Self-Esteem Disturbance can be written as "Risk" for Self-Esteem Disturbance by virtue of the presence of risk factors but not as yet the existence of the actual health problem (NANDA, 1990).

Guidelines for Wellness Diagnoses

Wellness nursing diagnoses represent clinical judgments about an individual, family, or community in transition from a specific level of wellness to a higher level of wellness or functioning.

The diagnosis Potential for Enhanced Coping is the designated diagnostic label of a wellness diagnosis. Most wellness diagnoses are one-part statements; for example, Potential for Enhanced Coping and Potential for Enhanced Parenting. Some of the latest (NANDA, 1994) wellness diagnostic statements, however, are accompanied by either defining characteristics or both defining characteristics and etiologic factors; for example, Potential for Enhanced Spiritual Well-Being and Poten-

tial for Enhanced Community Coping (NANDA, 1994). (See NANDA listing on inside front cover of this book.)

OUTCOME IDENTIFICATION

Outcome statements consist of highly specific, measurable indicators that are used by nurses in the evaluation phase as criteria to illustrate the following:

The actual nursing diagnosis has been resolved or reduced.

The risk diagnosis has not occurred.

Outcomes derive from nursing diagnosis statements and are projections of the expected influence that the nursing interventions will have on the client, in relation to the identified diagnosis. Figure 6-2 shows the nursing process depicting actual and risk diagnosis format of the six-step process. Outcomes are often confused with client goals or nursing goals, but they are more specific, descriptive, and measurable. Outcomes also do not describe nursing interventions. Box 6-4 lists examples of outcome statements.

Outcome criteria for an actual diagnosis are generally considered the opposite of the defining characteristics. In other words, the signs and symptoms discovered in

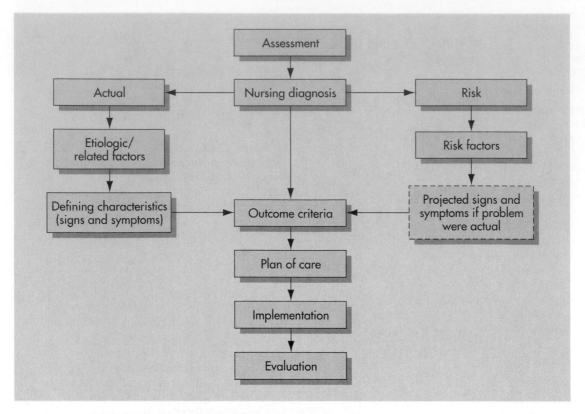

Figure 6-2 Nursing process depicting actual and risk diagnosis format of the six-step process.

Adapted from Fortinash K, Holoday-Worret P: *Psychiatric nursing care plans,* ed 2, St. Louis, 1995, Mosby.

Box 6-4   Examples of Outcome Statements

Client will:

* Verbalize absence of suicidal thoughts and plans
* Demonstrate absence of self-mutilation and other self-destructive behaviors
* Interpret environmental stimuli accurately
* Interact socially with clients and staff
* Participate actively in group discussions
* Seek staff when experiencing troubling thoughts and feelings
* Comply with treatment and medication regimen

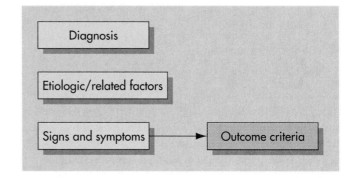

Figure 6-3 Developing outcome criteria for an actual diagnosis.

Adapted from Davie JK: The nursing process. In Thelan LA et al: *Critical care nursing: diagnosis and management,* ed 2, St. Louis, 1994, Mosby.

---

the assessment phase to help establish the nursing diagnosis are also used to identify outcomes for improvement or resolution (Figure 6-3). For example:

Nursing Diagnosis	**Outcome Criteria**
Self-Care Deficit: Grooming/Hygiene	Neat, clean appearance Grooms and cleans self

Related to: Psychotic state

As evidenced by:

Disheveled appearance

Poor grooming/hygiene

Outcome criteria for a risk diagnosis are developed from the risk factors that replace the defining characteristics found in an actual diagnosis. Clinical symptoms are absent in a risk diagnosis since it is a two-part statement (Figure 6-4). For example:

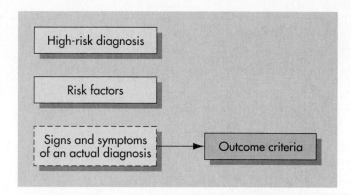

Figure 6-4 Developing outcome criteria for a risk diagnosis.
Adapted from Davie JK: The nursing process. In Thelan LA et al: *Critical care nursing: diagnosis and management,* ed 2, St. Louis, 1994, Mosby.

Nursing Diagnosis	Outcomes
Risk for Violence: Self-Directed	Verbalizes absence of suicidal intent
	Absent demonstration of suicidal gestures/acts

Risk Factors:

History of Suicide Attempts

Verbalizes Suicidal Intent

Measurable outcomes should include client statements, behaviors, and/or psychosocial or physical conditions or parameters that are observable. This presents a challenge to psychiatric nurses, however, since concepts such as anxiety, hopelessness, powerlessness, ineffective coping, or self-concept disturbance require the client's subjective perceptions and often resist measurability. Outcome statements such as "reduced anxiety," "more hopeful," or "copes effectively" offer minimal criteria for measuring client outcome achievements. Therefore, when measuring client behaviors, the challenges for the psychiatric nurse include the following:

* Phrase the outcomes so that they clearly describe client behavioral activity

* Use the client's own words to describe feelings and thoughts whenever relevant

* Incorporate some type of measurement tool or parameters by which to quantify client progress or resolution of problem/symptoms

See Table 6-5 for examples of correct and incorrect outcome statements.

In some instances, nurses place a specific target date for each outcome criterion as a means of predicting the evaluation time for each outcome attainment. Designated dates ensure that certain problems do not exceed specified, acceptable time periods. The outcome criteria throughout this text do not include projected target dates or time lines, since this practice is better applied to actual situations, not hypothetical client symptoms and behaviors. Developing clear, measurable outcomes assists the nurse in managing, resolving, preventing, and improving clients' multiple health and illness states. Effective client outcomes also justify reimbursement for nurses and assure quality client care (Olsen et al, 1995).

PLANNING

The planning phase consists of the total planning of the client's overall treatment in order to achieve quality outcomes in a safe, effective, timely manner. Nursing interventions with rationales are selected in the planning phase, based on the client's identified risk factors and defining characteristics. The process of planning includes the following:

* Collaboration by the nurse with clients, significant others, and treatment team members

* Identification of priorities of care

* Critical decisions regarding the use of psychotherapeutic principles and practices

* Coordination and delegation of responsibilities according to the treatment team's expertise as it relates to client needs

TABLE 6-5   Correct and incorrect outcome statements

Nursing diagnosis	Incorrect outcome	Correct outcome
Anxiety	Exhibits decreased anxiety; engages in stress reduction	Verbalizes feeling calm, relaxed, with absence of muscle tension and diaphoresis. Practices deep breathing.
Hopelessness	Expresses increased feelings of hope	Makes plans for the future, for example, to continue therapy after discharge. States "my kids need me to be well."
Ineffective Individual Coping	Demonstrates effective coping abilities	Makes own decisions to attend groups. Seeks staff for interactions versus isolating in room.

Planning client care builds on the prior phases of the nursing process and is vital for the ultimate selection of relevant nursing interventions by which to achieve successful client outcomes.

Interdisciplinary Treatment Team Planning

A typical method used to plan and monitor a client's treatment is known as *interdisciplinary treatment team planning*. The treatment plan is generally constructed on a standard form and consists of various sections in which to document diverse information relevant to client care, such as strengths, legal status, discharge plans, medical and nursing diagnoses, therapies, and social work data.

The treatment plan is implemented the first time the treatment team meets to discuss the client (ideally, no later than three days following the client's admission). The team is generally represented by nursing, social work, occupational and recreational therapy, and the client's physician. The client may also be present during a portion of the meeting unless contraindicated. Each team member is given an opportunity to discuss the client from the perspective of his or her own discipline and expertise. The treatment plan may be updated after the initial treatment team meeting as each discipline has more opportunity to spend time with the client and elaborate on its specific criteria.

The interdisciplinary treatment plan for a client with bipolar disorder in Figure 6-5 was developed in conjunction with the sample standard care plan in Figure 6-6. The information on each form should be reflected on the other. For example, the nursing diagnoses identified during the treatment team meeting should be the same diagnoses initiated on the client's standard care plan. Thus, client assessment and treatment will flow from one document to the other, illustrating consistency and reliability. Treatment plans are generally updated as often as the team meets to discuss a particular client. Ideally, the second team meeting should occur not later than three to four days after the first meeting. With the current trend toward shorter lengths of stay for all acute care clients, treatment team planning needs to occur in a timely fashion in order to effectively address each client's specific needs.

Standardized Care Planning

One method used to plan and measure client care is known as standardized care planning (Figure 6-6). In this type of documentation, NANDA diagnoses, client outcomes, and interventions are formulated according to the identified DSM-IV diagnostic categories in a standardized format. This standard format style is gaining popularity with nurses for the following reasons:

- The need to create new care plans for each client is reduced or eliminated.

- Consistency of care is encouraged through standardized guidelines.

- It requires a minimum of writing, thus freeing the nurse to spend more time interacting with clients.

- Standards of care are upheld, assuring safe, effective treatment over time.

- It addresses managed care criteria for quality outcomes and length of stay.

- Problems are primarily initiated, evaluated, and resolved by nursing.

Standardized care plans do not preclude individualized treatment for each client, nor do they replace relevant narrative documentation.

Clinical Pathways

A **clinical pathway** (also referred to as a *critical pathway, care path,* or *Care Map*) is a standardized format used to provide and monitor client care and progress by way of the case management, interdisciplinary health care delivery system. Although nursing is a primary proponent of the clinical pathway method, other disciplines responsible for client care in the psychiatric setting are actively involved in the development of each individualized clinical pathway. Such disciplines include social services, occupational therapy, therapeutic recreation, and dietary services, with strong collaborative input from psychiatrists. Consultations may be provided by psychologists, family practice physicians, or other professionals, depending on the special needs of the client.

A clinical pathway refers primarily to a written clinical process that identifies projected caregiver behaviors and interventions and expected client outcomes, based on the client's mental disorder as defined in the Diagnostic and Statistical Manual of Mental Disorders, edition 4 (DSM-IV). The pathway is mapped out along a continuum that depicts chronologic milestones, generally the number of days that reflects the client's estimated length of stay for each specific diagnosis.

The pathway is a projection of the client's entire length of treatment, detailing interdisciplinary interventions or processes and client outcomes each day, from admission through discharge. A pathway may be extended to include the client's transfer to home care or another type of treatment facility. The pathway would then continue for as long as necessary. Clinical pathways may originate for clients in a home care situation and would then be developed by the interdisciplinary home care team.

VARIANCES

Variances (also known as outliers) occur when a client's response to interventions is different from what is typically expected. A variance may therefore be considered

Text continued on p. 135

BEHAVIORAL HEALTH INTERDISCIPLINARY TREATMENT PLAN

THIS PLAN WAS FORMULATED AT THE INTERDISCIPLINARY TREATMENT MEETING:

DATE _1/1/96_   REVIEW DATES _1/4/96, 1/7/96_

RECORDER _Roseann Giordano, R.N. BSN_

ATTENDING PHYSICIAN _Dr. Jones_

Present at Meeting: MD _Dr. Jones_   RN _Mary Webster, MS, RN, CS_

Social Worker _Maggie Barker, LCSW_   Therapy

Other _John Clark, Student Nurse_   Services _Beth Trottier, OTR_

PRIMARY CONTACT

Name _Jane Smith_   Relationship _temporary conservator_   Tel. # _123-4567_

REASON FOR ADMISSION: _Striking out at   LEGAL STATUS: [√] Voluntary   [√] 72°h   Exp. Date _____
other clients and staff at Board and Care_   [ ] 14 d.h. Exp. Date _____
facility. Has refused to take meds X 3 days.   Conservator [√] Temp. [ ] Perm.
PATIENT STRENGTHS   Date filed _1/1/96_   Name _Jane Smith_

[√] Verbal   [√] Adequate Financial Resources   [ ] Supportive Family
[√] Intelligent   [ ] Recognizes Own Problems   [ ] Employed
[√] Intact Physical Health   [√] Supportive Friends
[ ] Consistent Work History   [ ] Resourceful   [√] Other _Cooperative and functional_
[ ] Compliant with Treatment   [√] History of Independent Functioning   _when taking medications regularly_

PRELIMINARY DISCHARGE PLAN
Admission Date _12/30/95_   ADDRESSOGRAPH
Anticipated Length of Stay _8 days_
Anticipated Services Required: _Patient name: B. Brown_

[ ] Financial Counseling   [ ] Payee   [√] Conservatorship
[√] Board & Care [ ] SNF Placement [√] Partial Hospitalization Referral
[ ] Home Health Nurse   [ ] Psychotherapy, Marital/Family
[ ] Crisis House   [√] Medication Monitoring
[ ] Recovery Home/Sober Living [ ] Other
[√] Self-Help Group

Continued

Figure 6-5 Example of an interdisciplinary treatment plan for a client with bipolar disorder.

Developed by and reprinted with permission from Tri-City Medical Center Mental Health Department, Oceanside, California

PATIENT NAME: B. Brown

PHYSICIAN: SIGNATURE:

DIAGNOSIS

AXIS I   Bipolar Disorder I
      II Deferred
      III None known
      IV mod-sev. (3-4)
      V   30/60

DATE	PROBLEMS	PATIENT OUTCOME	INTERVENTION	GOAL DATE	DATE REVIEWED	DATE MET
12/30	Risk for Violence	Demonstrates absence of aggression	Provide safety by least restrictive means	12/30	12/31	12/31
12/30	Altered Thought Processes	Verbalizes clear realistic thoughts	Orient to reality in brief contacts	1/3	12/31	1/3
12/30	Self Care Deficit	Demonstrates improved grooming; hygiene	Assist in grooming; hygiene as needed	1/3	1/1	1/3
12/30	Knowledge Deficit (disorder)	States understanding of diagnosis	Teach signs/symptoms of diagnosis	1/5	1/3	1/6

NURSING: SIGNATURE:

NURSING ADMISSION DATA BASE Completed On _____

STANDARD NURSING PATIENT CARE PLAN (Title): _____

Additional Nursing Diagnosis:

1. Non compliance, medications   4.
2. Ineffective Individual Coping   5.
3. Self-Esteem Disturbance   6.

The complete and individualized Standards of Patient Care are located in the Nursing section of the Patient Care Record.

THERAPY SERVICES   O.T. SIGNATURE: _____   T.R. SIGNATURE:

PROBLEMS	PATIENT OUTCOME	INTERVENTION	GOAL DATE	DATE REVIEWED	DATE MET
	OT/TR: - Demonstrates logical thought processes	[√] Task Skills Group Helps perform tasks	1/3	1/1	1/3
[√] Impaired Cognitive Skills:		[√] Living Skills Group Engages in living skills	1/2	1/2	1/5
[√] Attention Span	Demonstrates increased attention span	[ ] Creative Arts	1/2		
[√] Concentration	Concentrates on unit tasks/activities	[√] Coping Skills Assists with coping skills	1/3	1/3	1/5
[√] Reality Testing	Tests reality appropriately	[ ] ADL Training	1/4		
[√] Disorganization	Structures and organizes routine ADLs	[√] Goal Setting Assists with simple goals	1/4	1/2	1/4
[√] Safety/Judgment	Utilizes safe judgment/behaviors	[√] 1:1 Engages in 1:1 interactions		12/30	12/31
[ ] Orientation		[√] Leisure Education Engages in leisure ed	1/3	1/2	1/3
[√] Decreased Participation in Functional Activities	Increased participation in tasks/groups	[√] Communication Skills Helps in group interactives	1/5	1/2	1/3
[√] Ineffective Coping Skills	Demonstrates effective coping skills	[ ] Sensory Motor			
[ ] Social Withdrawal		[ ] Hygiene/Grooming			
[√] Self-Destructive Behavior	Demonstrates absence of self-harm	[√] Community Outings Accompany on outings	12/31		
[√] Low Self-Esteem	Verbalizes positive self-qualities	[ ] Other:	1/5	1/3	1/3
[ ] Other _____		___ 1-2X wk ___ Frequency			
ACL Score: _____		___ 30-45 min ___ Duration			

SOCIAL WORK

SIGNATURE: _____

PSYCHOSOCIAL DATA BASE

Appearance   *SL. disheveled; hyperactive; inappropriate dress for age*

Age   42   Marital Status   [ ]S   [ ]M   [√]D   [ ]W

Children   (N)/ Y

Status of Current Family   *Former spouse remarried; moved out of state; no contact*

Parents elderly – unwilling or unable to help. Ø other known family.

Religion   [ ] Catholic   [√] Protestant   [ ] Jewish   [ ] Other

Military Service   N /(Y)

Place of Birth   *U.S.A.*

Family of Origin   *American*

Occupation   *Unemployed*   Employer _____

Financial Support: Rep. Payee _____

   Manages Own Funds _____

   √   Receives Assistance   Type: *SSI*

Living Arrangement   [ ] Home   [ ] Apt.   [ ] Hotel   [ ] Shelter

[√] Board & Care   [ ] S.N.F.   [ ] None Known   [ ] Other: _____

Pt. Cooperative   N / Y

Lives   [ ] By Self   [ ] W/Family   [ ] W/Friends

Case Manager/Conservator   N /(Y)   Name   *Jane Smith*

    Tel. # _____

Education: [ ] Did not complete high school   [ ] College degree

    [√] High school degree   [ ] Graduate degree

    [√] Some college

Primary Language   *English*

Requires Interpretation Services   (N)/ Y

Past Psychiatric Hospitalizations   N /(Y)

Dates _____   Locations _____

Contact: Name(s)   *Jane Smith, Conservator*

   Tel. # _____

Patient's Goal for this Admission

1. *To maintain control over aggressive impulses*
2. *To comply with medication regimen*
3. *To utilize effective coping skills & solve problems*
4. *To increase self-esteem*
5. *To return to baseline or higher level of function*

Discharge Plan: *D/C to Board and Care with partial hospitalization referral*

Tentative D/C Date: 1/7/96

ROOM	NAME	AGE	ADMIT DATE	DOCTOR
10-A	B. Brown	42	12/30/95	J. Jones

IDENTIFIED NEEDS/PROBLEMS

	DATE REVIEWED	DATE MET
[√] Family Dysfunction		
[ ] Placement		
[ ] Financial		
[ ] Employment		
[ ] Daily Structure		
[ ] Substance Abuse		
[√] Limited Functioning		
[ ] Spiritual		
[√] Inadequate Coping		
[√] Inadequate Support System		
[ ] Other		

REFERRALS/INTERVENTIONS

	DATE REVIEWED	DATE MET
[√] Family Contact *(Family resistant to help)*		
[ ] Family Session		
[ ] Social Service Group		
[ ] CPS/APS		
[√] Board & Care		
[ ] SNF		
√ PHP/Day Treatment *(To increase support base)*		
[ ] AA/NA/Alanon		
[ ] Home Health		
[ ] Clergy		
[ ] Voc. Rehabilitation		
[ ] MediCare/MediCal/SSI		
[ ] Other _____		
[√] Extended Psychosocial Assessment *(See SW notes)*		

Assessment/Recommendations:

Attend all groups; interactions q shift

Continued

BEHAVIORAL HEALTH SERVICES
PATIENT CARE PLAN

TITLE: **STANDARD OF CARE ON PATIENTS**

BIPOLAR DISORDER

| INITIATED | | NURSING DIAGNOSIS | PATIENT OUTCOMES | EVALUATION Documentation | INTERVENTIONS | RESOLVED | | NOT RESOLVED | |
Date	RN					Date	RN	Date	RN

12/30	RG	1. Alteration in thought processes R/T Psychosis, paranoia, or delusions.	Patient will demonstrate logical, goal-directed speech and behaviors with an absence of psychosis, paranoia, or delusions.	q shift	1. Assess patient for:
					  a. Nature and content of thought processes.
					  b. Risk for harm to self or others.
					  c. Ability to participate in groups/milieu.
					  d. Ability to perform ADLs.
					2. Report to physician:
					  a. Actual or escalating risk for harm to self or others.
					  b. Refusal to eat/drink.
					  c. Refusal to take medication.
					3. Record assessments in the Progress Notes on Patient Care Record.
					4. Implement the following interventions:
					  a. Frequent supportive contacts with gentle reality orientation as tolerated.
					  b. Limit-setting to control inappropriate sexual, financial, or potentially harmful interpersonal behaviors.
					  c. Encourage participation in milieu groups consistent with patient's attention span.
					5. Implement the following protocols:
					  a. Hallucinations/Delusions Management
					  b. Lithium Management
					  c. Antipsychotic Medication Therapy Management
					6. Validate that outcome is met when patient has demonstrated goal-directed/logical speech and behaviors x 48°.
						1/3	RG		

12/30	MW	2. Risk for Violence: Self-directed or directed at others. Risk Factors: Delusions, hyperactivity, irritability	Patient will not harm self or others.	q shift	1. Implement the following protocols in increasing order of restrictiveness:
					  a. Agitated/Assaultive Behavior Management
					  b. Time-out
					  c. Seclusion
					  d. Restraint Management (only when it is least restrictive measure.)
					2. Validate that outcome is met when patient demonstrates freedom from behaviors harmful to self/others x 72°.
						12/31	MW		

Figure 6-6 Example of the first page of a care plan for a client with bipolar disorder.

Developed by and reprinted with permission from Tri-City Medical Center Mental Health Department, Oceanside, California.

an unexpected client response that "falls off" the pathway, requiring separate documentation and further investigation by the interdisciplinary team. Causes of pathway variances may be related to client/family, caregivers, hospital, community, and payer (including insurance companies, health maintenance organizations, or managed care organizations).

A variance may be positive or negative and affect the client's length of stay and/or outcomes. An example of a positive variance would be a client who responds more rapidly to medication or other forms of treatment than expected and leaves the hospital prior to the estimated length of stay. An example of a negative variance would be a client who fails to achieve the desired nonmanic state or therapeutic lithium level in accordance with the time line designated on the clinical pathway continuum (generally by date of discharge), and whose length of stay is therefore prolonged.

Clinical pathways help ensure timely lengths of stay, prevention of complications, cost effectiveness, and continued quality assurance. Also, overall coordinated management of each client's care and progress by the RN case manager and the interdisciplinary team is assured.

Figure 6-7 is an example of a clinical pathway describing a client with bipolar disorder mania, with a length of stay of 8 days. The upper columns on the far left list client outcomes. The larger lower columns consist of categories of care known as processes. Evaluation of client progress is measured daily along the pathway time lines. Clinical pathways continue to be developed, improved, and instituted in a variety of health care settings and are expected to reflect the changing trends and complexities of current health care delivery systems.

IMPLEMENTATION

In the implementation phase, the nurse actually sets in motion the interventions prescribed in the planning phase. Some general nursing considerations directed toward clients and families during this phase include the following:

- Promote health and safety.
- Monitor medication regimen/effects.
- Provide adequate nutrition/hydration.
- Facilitate a nurturing, therapeutic environment.
- Build self-esteem, trust, and dignity.
- Engage in therapeutic groups/activities.
- Develop strengths/coping methods.
- Enhance communication/social skills.
- Use family/community support systems.
- Educate according to identified learning needs.
- Prevent relapse through effective discharge planning.

Nursing Interventions

Interventions represent the heart of nursing and are critical action components of the implementation phase. Nursing interventions are also termed *nursing orders* or *nursing prescriptions* and are the most powerful pieces of the nursing process. They comprise the management and treatment approach to an identified health problem. Interventions are selected to achieve client outcomes and to prevent or reduce problems. Some flaws noted in nursing interventions, both in the literature and in clinical practice, are that they are often weak, vague, and nonspecific.

For nursing interventions to be prescriptive, they must prescribe a course of action and not simply support the existing regimen. The interventions listed throughout this text reflect both actual and typical nursing responses and behaviors derived from educational preparation and a wide range of clinical experience.

In the psychiatric-mental health setting, treatment frequently incorporates verbal communication skills, a major source of psychosocial interventions. Such treatments are intended to effect a change in the client's present condition, not merely to maintain the problem in its present state. Nursing interventions should explicitly describe a course of therapeutic activity that helps mobilize the client toward a more functional state. Here are some descriptive examples:

Gradually engage client in interactions with other clients, beginning with individual contacts, progressing to informal gatherings, and eventually structured group activities.

Teach client and family/significant other that therapeutic effects of antidepressant medications may take up to two weeks, and uncomfortable effects may begin immediately.

Praise the client for attempts to seek out staff and other clients for interactions and activities, and to respond to others' attempts to engage the client in interactions and activities.

Nondescriptive examples include:

Assist the client to interact with others.

Teach client and family about medications.

Praise the client for socializing.

Note the clarity and substance demonstrated in the descriptive examples, as opposed to the weaker, more vague statements in the nondescriptive examples.

Nursing interventions that simply repeat physician's orders are not substantive enough to treat or manage the health problem effectively. Here are nonsubstantive examples:

Monitor the client's progress.

Check lithium levels.

Clinical Pathway: Mania
DRG #430 - LOS - 8 Days

Interval		Day of Admit	Day 2	Day 3	Day 4
	Location				
O U T C O M E S	Physiologic	*Takes adequate nutrition, fluids with assistance *Complies with lithium level evaluation	*Demonstrates increased sleep/rest time *Demonstrates adequate elimination	*Takes adequate nutrition/fluid with reminders *Demonstrates adequate elimination	*Sleeping 4–6 hours *Demonstrates adequate elimination
	Psychologic	*Involved in stimulation-reducing activities with staff supervision	*Oriented to person and place	*Demonstrates reduction in: movement racing thoughts grandiosity/euphoria irritability	*Demonstrates increased attention span *Reality tests with staff *Oriented to person, place, time, and situation
	Functional Status/Role	*Tolerated orientation to the unit *Refrains from harming self/others with assistance	*Interacting with staff as told *Attends to hygiene/grooming needs with assistance *Refrains from harming self/others with assistance	*Engages in unit activities with staff supervision	*Maintains impulses with reminders *Complies with meds with reminders
	Family/Community Reintegration		*Identifies significant others to staff	*Attends community meetings with staff supervision	*Significant others involved in treatment/discharge planning
P R O C E S S E S	Discharge Planning	*SW Assessment *Identify DC Placement *ELOS, contact family/SO *Nursing Assessment *Identify H/O chronicity *Med compliance, strengths, needs, knowledge deficit	*Team: Involved in D/C Planning Discuss with MD *UR notify managed care ( )	*SW eval completed *Treatment Team meeting #1 ( ) *Specific D/C plans, placement facility identified ( )	*Involve family/SO in DC plans *Review DC plans with patient
	Education	*Orient to unit *Inform of patient's rights *Assess patient's and family's/SO knowledge of disorder/meds	*Assist with symptom recognition and importance of compliance *Teach family/SO as needed	*Continue with symptom recognition *Continue assessing patient and family/SO learning needs	*Assist in linking symptoms with precipitating events
	Psychosocial/ Spiritual	*Assess: Safety ( ) *Mental status ( ) Spiritually ( ) *Legal status: Vol ( ) 72 hour hold ( ) *Reise Writ ( ) Payor ( ) Conservator ( )	*Continue to assess: Safety issues Mental status Spiritual needs Legal status	*Continue to assess: Safety issues Mental status (e.g. racing thoughts, grandiosity, euphoria, irritability) Spiritual/Legal needs	*Continue to assess: Safety issues Mental status (e.g. racing thoughts, grandiosity, euphoria, irritability) Spiritual/Legal needs
	Consults	*Physical exam within 24 hours	*Other consults as needed	*Other consults as needed	*Other consults as needed
	Tests/ Procedures	*Lithium level ( ) *Tegretol level ( ) *Drug screen ( ) *Thyroid function ( ) *CBC/SMAC ( ) *Other ( )	*Tests/Procedures as ordered	*Tests/Procedures as ordered	*Tests/Procedures as ordered
	Treatment	*Monitor: I&O *Sleep/Rest patterns *Level A ( ) *Reduce milieu stimulation *S&R yes( ) no( ) *Other	*Monitor: I&O *Sleep/Rest patterns *Level A ( ) *Reduce milieu stimulation *S&R yes( ) no( ) *Other	*Move to level B ( ) *Continue with treatment plan: Monitor: I&O Sleep/Rest Other	*Move to level B ( ) *Continue with treatment plan: Monitor: I&O Sleep/Rest Other
	Medications (IV & Others)	*Medications as ordered *See relevant protocols: Lithium *Other *Monitor side effects *Toxicity	*Medications as ordered *Continue to monitor side effects/toxicity	*Medications as ordered *Continue to monitor side effects/toxicity	*Medications as ordered *Continue to monitor side effects/toxicity
	Activity	*OT assessment *1:1 brief contacts *Reality orientation *Intervene to manage impulses: prevent harm to self/others	*Engage in stimulation-reducing activities as tolerated *Assist with hygiene, grooming, ADLs *Prevent harm to self/others during activities	*OT eval completed *Encourage hygiene, grooming, ADLs with reminders *Prevent harm to self/others during activities	*Engage in 2 groups per day *Increase group stimulation as tolerated *Prevent harm to self/others during activities
	Diet/Nutrition	*Offer adequate nutrition and fluids; normal salt intake	*Provide simple meals, finger foods, easy to carry drinks	*Encourage meals in patient community as tolerated with staff supervision	*Encourage meals in patient community as tolerated with staff supervision

Figure 6-7 Clinical pathway for a client with bipolar disorder mania.

Reprinted with permission from Sharp HealthCare Behavioral Health Services, San Diego, California.

Interval		Day 5	Day 6	Day 7	Day 8
Location					
O U T C O M E S	Physiologic	*Takes adequate nutrition/fluid *Sleeps 4–6 hours *Lithium level in therapeutic range *Other drug level in therapeutic range	*Sleeps 5–8 hours *Absence of drug toxicity	*Sleeps 5–8 hours	*Sleeps 5–8 hours *Able to manage food and activity requirements independently
	Psychologic	*Demonstrates more reality based thoughts *Able to focus on one topic x5–10 minutes	*Demonstrates enthymic mood *Able to focus on one topic x5–10 minutes	*Able to complete activities and unit assignments	*Able to complete activities and unit assignments independently *Able to plan and structure day
	Functional Status/Role	*Demonstrates less intrusive behaviors	*Able to interact with peers *Able to make simple decisions	*Demonstrates safe appropriate activities/behaviors *Independently complies with medical regimen	*Verbalizes need for ongoing medication compliance
	Family/Community Reintegration	*Identifies discharge needs	*Identifies discharge needs	*Identifies discharge needs *Able to identify supports and their appropriate use	*Able to utilize supports and lists ways to access them *States specific plans to manage symptoms, comply with medications, and aftercare
P R O C E S S E S	Discharge Planning	*Assist patient/family/SO to identify discharge needs *UR contact managed care as needed ( )	*Continue to problem-solve discharge needs with patient, family/SO	*Treatment team meeting #2 ( ) *Transition to Day Treatment if indicated *Assist patient, family/SO in finalizing discharge plans	*Discharge to least restrictive environment completed *UR inform managed care as needed ( )
	Education	*Teach patient/family/SO about medication effects on symptom management *Instruct in medication, diet, exercise regimen	*Emphasize importance of compliance with meds after discharge *Teach about drug-to-drug effects on symptom management	*Develop aftercare plan to manage symptoms and contact supports	*Reinforce aftercare teaching plan with patient, family/SO as needed
	Psychosocial/ Spiritual	*Continue to assess: Safety issues Mental status Spirituality Voluntary status	*Continue to assess: Safety issues Mental status Spirituality Voluntary status	*Continue to assess: Safety issues Mental status Spirituality Voluntary status	*Complete assessments confirm: Safety Mental status Spirituality Legal status
	Consults	*Complete consults as ordered *Arrange for aftercare consults as ordered	*Complete consults as ordered *Arrange for aftercare consults as ordered	*Complete consults as ordered *Arrange for aftercare consults as ordered	*Complete consults as ordered *Arrange for aftercare consults as ordered
	Tests/ Procedures	*Check lithium level for therapeutic range *Check other drug levels for therapeutic range as needed *Tests/Procedures as needed	*Check lithium level for therapeutic range *Check other drug levels within therapeutic range as needed *Tests/Procedures as needed	*Check lithium level for therapeutic range *Check other drug levels within therapeutic range as needed *Tests/Procedures as needed	*Confirm lithium level for therapeutic range *Confirm other drug levels within therapeutic range as needed *Tests/Procedures as ordered aftercare
	Treatment	*Move to level C ( ) *Continue with treatment plan I&O Sleep/Rest Other	*Move to level C ( ) *Continue with treatment plan I&O Sleep/Rest Other	*Transfer to open unit ( ) *Aftercare treatment instructions reviewed with patient, family/SO as needed	*D/C with aftercare treatment instructions
	Medications (IV & Others)	*Medications as ordered *Contact managed care if any change in medication regimen	*Medications as ordered *Contact managed care if any change in medication regimen	*Medications as ordered *Review of medications with patient, family/SO as needed	*D/C with medications and instructions as ordered
	Activity	*Encourage: Independent hygiene and grooming Independent ADLs Increased participation in groups	*Engage in all unit activities and groups *Encourage independent decision-making	*Reinforce active participation in all unit activities and groups; independent decision-making	*Confirm: Ability to complete activity assignments independently Ability to make decisions independently
	Diet/Nutrition	*Teach family/SO importance of adequate foods/fluids/salt intake	*Teach family/SO importance of adequate foods/fluids/salt intake	*Reinforce adequate nutrition fluids and normal salt intake	*Confirm patient/SO/family knowledge of adequate foods/fluids/salt intake

Notify social services.

Obtain client's consent form.

Report changes in mood and affect.

Effective nursing interventions should have the capability of moving the client to a more functional health state by virtue of their clarity, substance, and direction. In the psychiatric-mental health setting, nurses constantly assess, diagnose, and treat clients' health states. Therefore, the challenge for nurses is to formulate strong, effective nursing interventions that address and modify the client's health problem, based on researched, independent nursing therapies.

Interventions' Impact on Etiologies

Interventions have the greatest impact when focused toward etiologies (related factors) that accompany the nursing diagnosis or, if the problem is a risk nursing diagnosis, when they are aimed at the risk factors. (Figure 6-8 illustrates the former, Figure 6-9 the latter.) This suggests that nursing can modify or affect the etiologies of a problem. It makes sense considering that etiologies are in some respects causal factors that greatly impact or provoke the health problem (nursing diagnosis). By the same token, risk diagnoses are less likely to become actual, if interventions are aimed primarily at their accompanying risk factors. To achieve the most favorable client outcomes, etiologic factors associated with the problems (nursing diagnoses) should be examined meticulously and interventions carefully selected to modify each of them.

Interventions and Medical Actions

Interventions can include medically focused actions, such as the administration of medications. *But the major focus of nursing interventions should emphasize nursing actions, judgments, treatments, and directives.* Examples of nontherapeutic, medically focused interventions include:

Administer antipsychotic medications as prescribed.

Observe for extrapyramidal effects.

Initiate Cogentin as ordered.

Note in the above examples the obvious absence of any prescribed nursing actions that would influence the client's health state.

Rationale Statements

A rationale statement is the reason for the nursing intervention. Rationales are not usually listed as part of a written care plan in clinical practice, however, they are generally part of the overall discussion of interventions in treatment team meetings. Rationales reflect nurses' accountability for their actions. Clear, descriptive rationale statements (in italics following the interventions) are provided in the disorders chapters in this text to enhance the reader's overall understanding of the selected interventions. For example:

- Actively listen, observe, and respond to client's verbal and nonverbal expressions *to let the client know he or she is worthwhile and respected.*

- Initiate brief, frequent contacts with the client throughout the day *to let the client know he or she is an important part of the community.*

- Praise client for attempts to interact with others and participating in group activities *to increase self-esteem and reinforce repetition of healthy, functional behaviors.*

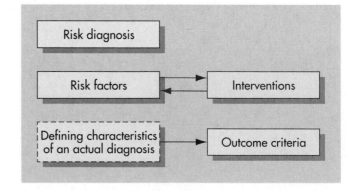

Figure 6-8 Developing interventions for an actual diagnosis. The red arrow indicates interventions for an actual diagnosis, while the blue arrow indicates the impact of the interventions on etiologies.

Adapted from Davie JK: The nursing process. In Thelan LA et al: *Critical care nursing: diagnosis and management,* ed 2, St. Louis, 1994, Mosby.

Figure 6-9 Developing interventions for a risk diagnosis. The red arrow indicates interventions for a risk diagnosis, while the blue arrow indicates the impact of the interventions on risk factors.

Adapted from Davie JK: The nursing process. In Thelan LA et al: *Critical care nursing: diagnosis and management,* ed 2, St. Louis, 1994, Mosby.

EVALUATION

Evaluation of achieved expected client outcomes must occur at various intervals as designated in the outcome criteria, with the capability and health state of each client as a primary consideration. There are two steps in the evaluation phase:

1. *The nurse compares the client's current mental health state or condition with that described in the outcome criteria.* Is the client's anxiety reduced to a tolerable level? (For example, can the client sit calmly for 10 minutes, attend a simple recreational activity for 10 minutes, and engage in one-to-one interaction with staff for 5 minutes without distractions? Is there a significant reduction in pacing, fidgeting, scanning? Were these outcomes attained within the times originally projected?) The degree to which client outcomes are achieved or not achieved is also an evaluation of the effectiveness of nursing.

2. *The nurse considers all the possible reasons why nursing outcomes were not achieved, if this is the case.* For example, perhaps it's too soon to evaluate, and the plan of action needs further implementation. (For example, the client needed another two days of one-to-one interactions before attending client group activities). Or maybe the interventions were too forceful and frequent or too weak and infrequent? It may be that the outcomes were unattainable, impractical, or just not feasible for this client, or perhaps they were not within the client's scope and capabilities on a developmental or sociocultural level. What about the validity of the nursing diagnosis? Was it developed with a questionable or faulty database? Are more data required? What were the conditions during the assess-ment phase? Was it too hurried? Were conclusions drawn too quickly? Were there any language, cultural, or other communication barriers?

Specific recommendations are then made based on conclusions drawn from the above questions. They include either continuing implementation of the plan of action or review of the previous phases of the nursing process (assessment, nursing diagnosis, outcome identification, planning, or implementation). Evaluation of the client's progress and the nursing activities involved in the process are critical because they require that nursing be accountable for the standards of care defined by its own discipline. Informal evaluation of the client's progress, much like that of the nursing process, takes place continuously.

Figure 6-10 and Figure 6-11 show how evaluation is determined according to the identified outcomes and is also the measurement tool used to appraise outcome attainment for both actual and risk diagnoses, respectively.

THE NURSING PROCESS IN COMMUNITY AND HOME SETTINGS

In the past, the nursing process and its multistep format have been most associated with the care of hospitalized clients. Current trends in health care delivery systems have shifted from inpatient facilities to community and home-based settings and provide yet another important avenue for use of the nursing process. Home health care is a primary alternative to hospitalization, and the nursing process continues to be a major factor in the effective management of home client care.

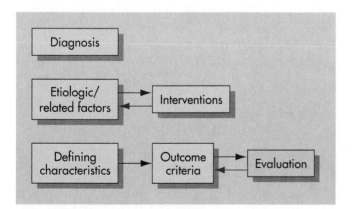

Figure 6-10 Evaluation process in an actual diagnosis. The arrows show how evaluation is determined according to identified outcomes.

Adapted from Davie JK: The nursing process. In Thelan LA et al: *Critical care nursing: diagnosis and management,* ed 2, St. Louis, 1994, Mosby.

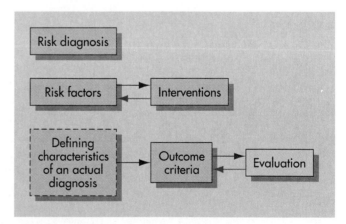

Figure 6-11 Evaluation process in a risk diagnosis. The arrows show how evaluation is determined according to identified outcomes.

Adapted from Davie JK: The nursing process. In Thelan LA et al: *Critical care nursing: diagnosis and management,* ed 2, St. Louis, 1994, Mosby.

Psychiatric Home Health Care Case Management System

The changes in today's health care delivery system have resulted in several trends in health care reform designed to bring about cost-effective quality care. Although the case management concept has existed for years in acute care settings and public health arenas, only recently has the private home health model subscribed to total case management, and only more recently has psychiatric home care been incorporated under the case management umbrella.

Psychiatric home care case management is a method by which a client is identified as a candidate for home care and treated on a health care continuum in the familiar surroundings of the home. The interdisciplinary home care team, facilitated by a registered nurse, coordinates all available resources to meet its goals for treatment and to achieve the client's expected outcomes in a quality and cost-effective manner. At one end of the continuum is the highest degree of independent wellness within the client's capacity, and at the other end of the continuum is death, with varying levels of wellness-illness in between.

Critical to successful use of case management is the accurate placement of the client at the entry point on the continuum, and a clear understanding of the team's best estimate for the date of termination of home care services (Provancha and Hurst, 1994).

Summary of Key Concepts

1. The nursing process is a decision-making method used by nurses for clinical care. As defined by the ANA it has six steps: assessment, diagnosis, outcome identification, planning, implementation, and evaluation.

2. The nursing process is an ongoing, multidimensional, cyclical approach in which data are continually collected, analyzed, and incorporated into a treatment plan.

3. Intuition, expertise, and critical thinking are important elements in the nursing process.

4. The two most common nursing assessment frameworks are the NANDA taxonomy and Gordon's Functional Health Patterns.

5. Nursing diagnoses provide nurses with a vocabulary that is distinctive to its own discipline and encourage nursing's theory and science-building efforts. NANDA diagnoses are the most common and accepted diagnoses used in nursing.

6. Nursing diagnoses can have two formats: two-part statements that describe potential or risk problems and three-part statements that describe an actual problem.

7. Outcome statements are highly specific, measurable indicators derived from nursing diagnoses and used to evaluate client progress.

8. The planning phase consists of the total planning of the client's treatment regimen. Nursing interventions are selected in the planning phase.

9. A clinical pathway is an interdisciplinary standardized format used to provide and monitor client care and progress.

10. The implementation phase involves the actual setting into motion of the interventions that have been prescribed in the planning phase.

11. Evaluation of the achieved expected client outcomes as designated by the outcome criteria should occur at various levels.

REFERENCES

American Health Consultants: Monthly update on hospital-based care planning and critical pathways, *Hospital Case Management* 1(10):173, 1993.

American Nurses Association: *Diagnostic and statistical manual of mental disorders*, ed 4, Washington, D.C., 1994, ANA.

American Nurses Association: *Nursing, a social policy statement*, Kansas City, Mo., 1990, ANA.

American Nurses Association: *Standards of clinical nursing practice*, Kansas City, Mo., 1991, ANA.

Benner P: *From novice to expert: excellence and power in clinical nursing practice*, Menlo Park, Calif., 1984, Addison-Wesley.

Carnevali DL, Thomas MD: *Diagnostic reasoning and treatment decision-making in nursing*. Philadelphia, 1993, JB Lippincott.

Carpenito LJ: *Nursing diagnosis: application to clinical practice*, ed 6, Philadelphia, 1996, JB Lippincott.

Davie JK: The nursing process. In Thelan L et al, editors: *Critical care nursing: diagnosis and management*, ed 2, St. Louis, 1994, Mosby.

Fortinash K: Assessment of mental status. In Malasanos L, Barkauskas V, and Stoltenberg-Allen K, editors: *Health assessment*, ed 4, St. Louis, 1990, Mosby.

Fortinash K, Holoday-Worret P: *Psychiatric nursing care plans*, ed 2, St. Louis, 1995, Mosby.

Kaplan H: *The comprehensive textbook of psychiatry*, ed 6, Baltimore, 1995, Williams and Wilkins.

Kaplan H, Sadock B: *Synopsis of psychiatry-behavioral science-clinical psychiatry*, ed 7, Baltimore, 1994, Williams and Wilkins.

Kritek PB: Generation and classification of nursing diagnoses: toward a theory of nursing, *Image J of Nursing Scholarship* 10:73, 1978.

Medina L: Clinical pathways: sharp home health, *Home Care,* October 1995.

Munhall PL, Oiler CJ: *Nursing research*, ed 2, New York, 1993, National League for Nursing.

North American Nursing Diagnosis Association: *NANDA, nursing diagnoses: definitions and classification, 1995-1996*, Philadelphia, 1994, The Association.

North American Nursing Diagnosis Association: *Taxonomy I-revised-1990, with official diagnostic categories*, St. Louis, 1990, NANDA.

Olsen DP, Rickles H, Travlik K: A treatment team model of managed mental health care, *Psychiatric Services* 46(3):252, 1995.

Provancha LE, Hurst S: Home health case management: an old approach to a new system, *NSI Home Health Newsletter Services*, 1994, Newsletter.

Smith SK: An analysis of the phenonemon of deterioration in the critically ill, *Image J of Nursing Scholarship* 20:12, 1988.

Southwick K et al: Strategies for health care excellence: care paths for psychiatric patients, *COR Health Care Resources, 1995*, 8(2):1, 1995.

Tanner C et al: Diagnostic reasoning strategies of nurses and nursing students, *Nursing Research* 36:358, 1987.

Wescott MR: *Antecedents and consequences of intuitive thinking. Final report to U.S. Department of Health, Education and Welfare*, Poughkeepsie, N.Y., 1968, Vassar College.

Wilkinson J: *Nursing process in action: a critical thinking approach*, Redwood City, Calif., 1992, Addison-Wesley.

CHAPTER 7

Principles of Communication

Susan Fertig McDonald

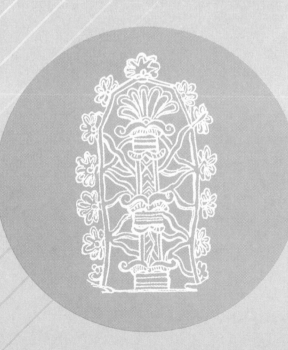

Boundary violations Going beyond the established therapeutic relationship standards.

Communication A reciprocal process of sending and receiving messages between two or more people and their environment; the vehicle for establishing a therapeutic relationship.

Congruence Consistency or agreement between verbal and nonverbal behavior.

Confidentiality The right of the psychiatric client to keep information from people outside the health care team.

Countertransference The nurse's unconscious and inappropriate responses to a client who is associated with a significant person in the nurse's life.

Empathy Projecting sensitivity and understanding of another's feelings and communicating the understanding in a way the client comprehends.

Feedback The measure by which the effectiveness of the message is gauged.

Genuineness A quality of an effective nurse that encompasses openness, honesty, and sincerity.

Interpersonal communication Communication between two or more persons containing both verbal and nonverbal messages.

Intrapersonal communication Communication occurring within oneself that can be functional or dysfunctional.

Medium Method by which a message is sent, which can be written, verbal, or tactile.

Message The information (feelings or ideas) being sent and received.

Nonverbal communication Nonverbal behaviors displayed by individuals during the process of an interaction.

Positive regard Acceptance of and respect for a client.

Receiver The individual who both receives and interprets the message.

Resistance The inability, whether conscious or unconscious, to accept change; denial of new problems.

Sender The individual who initiates the transmission of information.

Therapeutic communication Communication that takes place between the nurse and client; the content has meaning and focuses on the client's concerns.

Transference An unconscious response whereby a client associates the nurse with someone significant in his or her life and acts on those feelings.

Verbal communication Spoken or written words that comprise the symbols of language.

- Describe the components of communication.
- Discuss factors that influence communication.
- Compare and contrast social, intimate, collegial, and therapeutic communication.
- Describe the characteristics of effective helpers.
- Discuss the core qualities of the nurse and the various roles the nurse plays in interacting therapeutically with clients.
- Explain the principles of therapeutic communication.
- Compare and contrast the communication techniques that enhance and hinder therapeutic communication.
- Examine therapeutic communication in the context of the nursing process.
- Discuss three special communication challenges and their implications for the future.

Communication is a dynamic, two-way, circular process in which all types of information are shared between two or more people and their environment. Since we learn how to communicate at an early age, it might be thought of as quite simple. However, communication is a complex process requiring much practice in order to do it effectively.

Communication is the most powerful tool a psychiatric nurse can have. It is the basic component of the therapeutic nurse-client relationship and the medium through which the nursing process occurs. Communication is critical to the successful outcome of nursing interventions, for without effective communication, a therapeutic nurse-client relationship would not be possible. Therefore, the nurse must understand and master the general principles of communication as well as the specific principles of therapeutic communication.

COMPONENTS OF COMMUNICATION

Communication consists of several components: the stimulus (reason for communication), the sender, the message, the medium, the receiver, and feedback. Usually there is a stimulus, a need or reason for the communication to occur. The individual who initiates the transmission of information is the **sender.** Each transmission is both verbal and nonverbal. The information being sent and received, such as feelings or ideas, is the **message.** The method by which the message is sent is the **medium,** which can be written (seen), verbal (heard), or tactile (felt). For example, a note or letter is *sent;* a shout, scream, or whisper is *heard;* a hug or pat on the back is *felt.*

The **receiver** both receives and interprets the message which has been sent. Ideally, the receiver interprets the message exactly how the sender meant to give it, thus producing effective communication. The **feedback** that the receiver gives back to the sender is the measure by which the effectiveness of the message is gauged. Feedback is a continual process because it is a response to the message and provides a new stimulus to the sender, whereupon the original sender then becomes the receiver. Therefore, in any interaction, the sender and receiver continually reverse roles. Figure 7-1 shows a model of the communication process.

FACTORS THAT INFLUENCE COMMUNICATION

Communication is a learned process influenced by several factors including the environment, the relationship between the sender and the receiver, the content of the message, and the context in which the message takes place. Other factors include one's own attitude, ethnic background, socioeconomic status, family dynamics, other life experience, knowledge level, the ability to relate to others, and one's own value perceptions.

Environmental factors that control the effectiveness of communication include time, place, noise, privacy, comfort, and temperature. Timing of interaction can be very important. The phrase "counting to ten" describes a waiting or "cooling off" period necessary for some individuals to ensure that they can rationally discuss a "hot" topic or understand a critical concept. Consider the nurse who chooses to wait for an appropriate period of time to begin teaching a client about medications, since the client has just experienced an emotional outburst in the medication-teaching group, and is unable to concentrate in that environment. A carefully chosen time can mean the difference between successful and unsuccessful client learning. The place of the interaction can be instrumental in conveying the sincerity or importance of communication. Consider the man who wishes to propose marriage to a woman and chooses a mutually predetermined, romantic place in which to do it. A carefully chosen location could mean the difference between a yes, maybe, or no. If the location is noisy and other people are present, messages in the conversation may not be heard, resulting in ineffective communication. Therefore, the type, quality, and perceived importance of the specific message conveyed depend in part on the general comfort of the environment.

The *relationship* between two people in a conversation greatly influences the communication. For example, a casual friend can give the same message to an individual as an intimate friend, but the receiver may react quite differently to each person due to the nature of each relationship.

The context as well as the content of the message also influences the receiver's response. The *context,* or

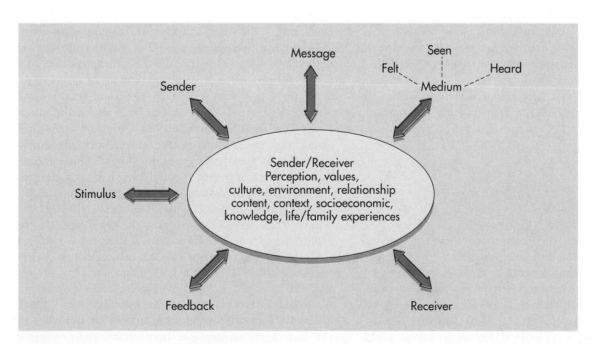

Figure 7-1 Model of the communication process

circumstances in which the message is given, must be appropriate to the type of interaction. Individuals need to feel safe in their environment in order to disclose highly personal information.

Interaction is also affected by attitude. *Attitude* determines how one person generally responds to another person and includes one's biases, past experiences, and levels of openness and acceptance. Also, people from one socioeconomic class, ethnic background, or family background often have difficulty communicating with individuals from a different background or class, due to possible language or knowledge barriers.

Communication is greatly influenced by one's upbringing and those aspects of communication that were encouraged, modeled, and discouraged by significant others. Boys in traditional households are often taught that "boys don't cry" and may grow up unable to easily express sad emotions. A teenager who is continually told to "shut up" for "talking too much" may develop a quiet or nonassertive style of communication as an adult.

Knowledge differences can create a deficiency in understanding during communication. If the sender has a greater knowledge of the subject matter than the receiver, it is the responsibility of the sender to ensure that the receiver understands the message. This is always one of the challenges in teaching students or clients important concepts. Some people have an ability to relate with ease to a variety of people and can explain complex information in simple, concrete terms. Some have a great deal of difficulty with this task and are easily intimidated by others. People can learn to communicate more easily and clearly and feel secure about it, with knowledge about communication techniques, with practice, and with feedback about their efforts.

Perception is an individual's subjective experience that influences how the message is interpreted. Because misperceptions create problems in communication, the sender must be certain that the receiver has a clear understanding of the message. Thus, effective communication depends on understanding what is being communicated, interpreting the message as it was meant to be given, and providing feedback that supports the correct interpretation.

MODES OF COMMUNICATION
Written Communication

Written communication is primarily for the purpose of sharing information. The reader reads for knowledge, pleasure, and understanding. The reader who is able to understand the written word as it appears and comprehend its meaning, is prepared to absorb the meaning. It is important that the nurse be able to clearly convey ideas on paper through documentation in the medical record, on statistical reports, and through use of computers (e.g., computerized reports). The ability to write legibly, spell correctly, use proper grammar, and organize ideas clearly are critical skills for the nurse and cannot be replaced by technology.

Verbal Communication

Verbal communication commonly refers to the spoken words that encompass the symbols of language. Precise verbal communication is important because spoken words often mean different things to different people. Many words or phrases have slang meanings or have developed new meanings. Words or phrases may also have different meanings for different groups. Figures of speech, jokes, cliches, colloquialisms, and other terms or special phrases have a variety of meanings. For example, "It is a blue Monday" could mean it is a sad day to one person, but to a client with schizophrenia who interprets concretely and literally, it could mean that the sky is blue. "Don't rain on my parade" means "don't spoil my fun" to one person but to the client with psychosis, it prompts the question regarding whether a parade is actually occurring and whether it will rain.

When interacting with individuals from different cultures, slang phrases and idioms such as "double dipping," "making good bread," "rad," "cool," and "let's party" would not be understood, and therefore, misinterpreted. It is easy to assume that other people understand intended meanings. So it is necessary to periodically check their interpretation, including examining the cues obtained from their nonverbal responses.

It is increasingly important for nurses to develop a greater sensitivity to the cultural aspects of communication. It is clearly a challenge to learn how to communicate effectively with psychiatric clients who not only have difficulty communicating in a clear, logical, or reasonable manner due to their mental disorder, but are also from another culture. (Chapter 4 further discusses issues of communication with those from cultural groups different from one's own.)

Nonverbal Communication

Nonverbal communication is believed by many communication theorists to be the most important part of any message. It includes elements such as tone of voice, hand and body movements, facial expressions, auditory noises that do not involve actual words, and other movements and expressions. Nonverbal cues involve all five senses. They add to the meaning of verbal messages by performing several functions such as expression of feelings, the contradiction or validation of verbal messages, and the preservation of both the ego and the relationship. As a general rule, nonverbal behavior is more revealing and truthful than verbal communication. Therefore, it is important for the nurse to observe and consider the client's entire message, both verbal and nonverbal, prior to arriving at a conclusion.

Ninety percent of a communication is thought to be nonverbal. To have effective communication, nonverbal cues should be **congruent,** or consistent, with the verbal message.

An example of congruent communication follows:

Verbal: I have been waiting a long time and was worried about you.
Nonverbal: concerned facial expression, warm, friendly, outstretched hand.

An example of incongruent communication follows:

Verbal: I have been waiting a long time and was worried about you.
Nonverbal: frowning, cold, sarcastic voice, no physical contact.

Nonverbal cues are grouped into four categories: body cues (kinesics), space (proxemics), touch, and appearance (Northouse and Northouse, 1992).

BODY CUES

Body cues comprise facial expressions, reflexes, body posture, hand gestures, eye movement, mannerisms, touch, and other body motions. Body posture and facial expressions, including eye movements, are two of the most important cues to determine how a person is responding to the message. When a client who is frowning, with clenched teeth and fists, wide eyes, and a red face says "I really enjoy my mother visiting me," there is a contradiction between verbal and nonverbal cues that needs to be addressed. A slumped or stooped posture can mean a client is depressed or, at the very least, feeling sad or dejected. A closed posture with arms folded may indicate a client is withdrawing or possibly feeling some anger or angst. An erect posture with shoulders back can mean that the client feels more confident or may be attempting to portray confidence. The gait of an individual as it relates to posture can also indicate one's self-concept. The person who bounces along in a self-assured manner may be perceived as more "upbeat" than the individual who walks at a slow-moving pace.

Nurses should carefully observe hand gestures as they may also signal anger, restlessness, frustration, giving up, relaxation, or apathy. The nurse needs to be aware of impending anger so that early interventions can be implemented to prevent a situation from becoming quickly out of control. Remember the old adage "when in doubt, observe what people do, not only what they say." This is especially important when dealing with psychiatric clients, because what they say and what they do may often be incongruent.

Paralinguistics (paralanguage) behavior includes any audible sound which is not a spoken word. It includes voice tone, inflection, word spacing, rate, emphasis or intensity, groans, coughing, laughing, crying, grunting, moans, and other audible sounds. Along with the silent cues, these audible nonverbal cues are very important in assessing clients.

SPACE

The use of *space* is another nonverbal cue. Each person has a "comfort zone," or space boundary, which invisibly surrounds him or her when interacting with others. The boundary becomes larger or smaller depending on the nature of the relationship. *Intimate space* is the closest distance between two individuals. *Personal space* is for close relationships within touching distance. *Consultive space* is farther apart than personal space, requiring louder speech. *Public space* is used for public gatherings such as speeches and is usually seen in a large hall or auditorium.

Space as a concept of boundaries and safety is important to understand because the nurse and the client need to respect the distance each one needs. For successful communication to occur, both parties need to feel comfortable. Some clients have problems with their boundary and may "invade" other clients' own "safe zone." Clients who perceive this as threatening may react aggressively to such boundary violations. At such times the nurse may need to help the client understand the appropriate distance by actually stating the boundary for the client in inches or feet, as needed. When the client violates the nurse's own comfortable space, the nurse may need to set a limit for the client after the initial intrusion.

TOUCH

Touch is a nonverbal message that involves both action and personal space. Touch typically conveys a message to connect with another person. In nursing, touch has been used to convey messages of concern and empathy. The nurse must be careful when deciding whether to touch a psychiatric client. Not all clients want to be touched. They may perceive it as a threat and respond with aggression, or interpret it as an intimate move and respond by withdrawal or inappropriate sexual response. Touch as communication is discussed in more detail later in the chapter.

APPEARANCE

Appearance communicates a particular image as well as a clue to one's mental status. Appearance refers to the way an individual uses clothing, makeup, hairstyle, jewelry, and other items such as hats, purses, glasses, etc., as well as grooming and hygiene. These nonverbal cues often disclose how the person wishes to be viewed by others. For example, a female who wears overtly masculine clothes with very short hair may be giving a message of her sexual identity, exhibiting the gender-neutral popular dress of the times, or simply showing her preferred, unique fashion style.

Another example is an individual who came in for a supervisory job interview wore shorts, a wrinkled knit shirt, and sandals; his hair was uncombed and his beard untrimmed. On first glance, the employer wondered if the job candidate was serious about being hired, since his appearance was sloppy and projected an unfavorable image. A third example is an elderly woman who was admitted to the hospital wearing dirty, wrinkled clothing. She was found by the home health nurse in a filthy apartment and had not bathed in several weeks. On further assessment, it was revealed that her husband had died two months ago, and she was subsequently diagnosed as depressed. Therefore, her appearance was a result of her obvious unresolved grief reaction which incapacitated her.

Nurses must try to interpret a client's nonverbal behavior when evaluating the verbal content. They then need to incorporate this evaluation into the assessment and plan of care.

Finally, nurses need to be aware of their own nonverbal cues. For effective communication to occur, these nonverbal messages should communicate genuine interest and respect.

TYPES OF COMMUNICATION

Intrapersonal Communication

In **intrapersonal communication,** self-talk occurs. Individuals give themselves all types of positive and negative messages. Self-talk can be helpful if the messages one gives oneself are helpful or positive. Intrapersonal communication can be functional or dysfunctional.

For example, a 45-year-old client spends a session with the nurse developing a realistic set of goals for her hospital stay. The client subsequently tells herself she is pleased that she has finally accomplished a useful task and is clear about what she needs to do before she leaves the hospital. In this situation, she gives herself positive messages that assist her in her recovery.

An example of dysfunctional self-talk occurs if this same individual persists in giving herself negative, self-defeating messages, e.g., "I can never do anything right," "I'll never get well." This type of self-talk can impede recovery.

In another example, a client with a diagnosis of schizophrenia continually hears many internal voices which tell him he is cursed, evil, and that he must kill himself as the only way out. These internal voices, displayed through auditory hallucinations, are considered dysfunctional self-talk.

Interpersonal Communication

Interpersonal communication occurs between two or more individuals and contains both verbal and nonverbal messages. It is a complex process consisting of a variety of factors affecting its outcome. The nurse communicates on an interpersonal level with a variety of individuals and groups throughout the day. Emphasis is placed on *therapeutic* and *collegial* communication when the nurse is at work. *Social communication,* primarily used away from work, will be discussed only briefly. The characteristics of social and therapeutic communication are listed in Table 7-1.

SOCIAL COMMUNICATION

Social communication occurs in everyday situations, usually away from the work setting. This type of interaction may include discussions regarding family business, social activities, family issues, vacations, school, and church.

TABLE 7-1   Characteristics of social and therapeutic communication

	Social	Therapeutic
Who	Friends, family, acquaintances	Helper and client
Setting	Home, away from work, any type of setting	Clinical setting; private, quiet, confidential, safe environment
Purpose	Maintain relationships; mutual sharing of information, thoughts, beliefs, ideas, feelings	Promote growth and change in clients
Content	Social talk, focus on children, vacations, family, leisure, church, doing a favor, giving advice	Therapeutic talk, client expresses thoughts, beliefs, feelings, anxieties, fears, problems; client identifies needs
Characteristics	Superficial, light, not necessarily goal-directed; spontaneous, enjoyable. Two-way, focusing on both sender and receiver; giving suggestions, advice; personal or intimate relationship occurs	Learned skill; purposeful, client-focused, client sets goals; planned, difficult, intense; disclosure of personal information by client; meaningful and personal, but not intimate relationship occurs
Skills	Uses a variety of resources during socialization	Uses specialized professional skills, primarily therapeutic interpersonal communication

Much of this interaction is superficial, light, and may not have a goal. The purpose of much social communication is to maintain a relationship and for enjoyment, and it is primarily done for the mutual benefit of all involved.

Varying levels of intimacy exist in social communication. Communication between parent and child carries a level of intimacy different from communication between parent and teacher. Self-disclosure occurs at varying levels, but superficiality is more the norm, since there are no real expectations of help. When help is the expected outcome of social communication, it is typically given in the form of suggestions and advice by friends and family. This differs dramatically from the help given to the client in therapeutic communication.

COLLEGIAL COMMUNICATION

Collegial communication occurs among colleagues in the professional work setting. An example is when psychiatric nurses interact with members of the interdisciplinary treatment team.

The nurse may also be involved in professional nursing groups within the work setting and in the community. This type of collegial communication is called intradisciplinary. The purpose of collegial communication is professional collaboration. Within the interdisciplinary team the purpose is to discuss client treatment. Within a nursing professional group, the intent is to share knowledge, collaborate on a project, or in other ways enhance or improve upon the profession itself.

Effective collaboration has the advantage of breaking through power issues and competition that arise when teams of professionals are brought together. In the collaborative process, no member is more important than another member or the group as a whole. Each member's contribution is important to the success of the project, purpose, or goal.

The nurse, therefore, communicates in the collegial arena with supervisors, coworkers, physicians, outside consultants, and other members of the treatment team. These relationships exist within the profession of nursing and outside it. Simultaneously, the psychiatric nurse communicates on a therapeutic level with clients and their family members or significant others.

THERAPEUTIC COMMUNICATION

Therapeutic communication occurs between the nurse (helper) and the client (recipient). It is the psychiatric nurse's single most important tool. The art of interacting therapeutically is a learned skill involving both nonverbal and verbal communication; its purpose is to promote client growth. It is the medium through which health promotion interventions occur.

Therapeutic communication is client-focused, whereas social communication consists of sharing information equally between two or more individuals. Even though the nurse may engage in some social interaction with the client, such as greeting the client at the begin-

ning of the shift, the progress toward a greater level of health occurs through the therapeutic interaction between the nurse and client.

This therapeutic interaction involves the disclosure of personal information by the client. It may include hurtful memories and situations that stir up painful emotions. Sharing such feelings can be extremely beneficial for the client because it allows him or her to identify and discuss experiences and accompanying feelings in a safe, therapeutic setting. The nurse provides a confidential and quiet setting in which the interaction takes place; encourages the client to openly discuss thoughts and feelings; and practices active listening, acceptance, and empathy.

Therapeutic communication can be intimidating not only for the client, but also for the nurse. Intense negative feelings are not easy to discuss. Many clients have not previously discussed them for fear of undesired responses such as a lack of understanding on the part of the listener, retaliation, feeling unworthy, and inadequacy in explaining them. The intensity of the client's feelings or verbal responses may frighten or catch the new nurse off guard—especially when a client openly discusses such issues as wanting to die because life is not worth living. The nurse may also feel uneasy when a client discusses an emotion or feeling similar to the nurse's personal experience. The nurse's own anxiety level may rise if she or he has not dealt with personal problems effectively.

In summary, therapeutic communication has three essential purposes:

1. To allow the client to express thoughts, feelings, behaviors, and life experiences in a meaningful way in order to promote healthy growth.

2. To understand the significance of the client's problem(s) and the role the client and the significant people in his life play in perpetuating those problems.

3. To assist in the identification and resolution processes of the client's problem areas.

The nurse's therapeutic use of communication is the mechanism by which clients can achieve successful outcomes to the problems currently preventing them from achieving optimum health.

PERSONAL ELEMENTS IMPORTANT FOR THERAPEUTIC COMMUNICATION

The nurse's use of self as the primary tool in psychiatric nursing is similar to the singer's use of voice as an instrument to create music. All the elements essential to helping another individual are within the nurse. This is both exciting and challenging.

The therapeutic use of self begins with *knowing oneself*. Nurses will not be able to help others unless they are first able to help themselves. Knowing the self is a complex and life-long learning process. It is essential to have self-knowledge prior to the use of the therapeutic self.

At the core of self-knowledge is the nurse's ability to correctly identify negative or unresolved issues of the self. Nurses need to know what values and beliefs they hold. It is also important for them to know and understand their own family background, including dynamic, cultural and social issues, values, biases, and prejudices.

Nurses also need to be aware of unresolved family life issues and make every effort to resolve them as soon as they are recognized. For example, consider a female nurse who has a long-held belief regarding men and alcohol dependency. She believes they can stop drinking if they really want to. Her belief developed because her maternal grandfather had died from alcohol-related liver disease. The nurse may be unaware that she holds this belief until the first alcohol-dependent male client is assigned to her. It is only when the nurse understands and resolves her issues that she can truly succeed in the necessary separation of her own issues from the client's.

Since therapeutic communication occurs for the purpose of helping others, it is vital that nurses understand *what motivates them to help others*. Nurse's emotional needs must be recognized so that they do not interfere with the ability to relate therapeutically to clients. Since clients do not take care of nurse's emotional needs, nurses must meet their own emotional needs outside of work. A well-balanced, multifaceted lifestyle satisfies one's emotional needs. When the nurse's needs are met, he or she can better assist the client through therapeutic communication.

Nurses who are *in control of their own lives and emotions* can engage the client in effective communication while maintaining therapeutic control of the conversation, especially when a client is attempting to be intimidating, manipulative, or threatening.

Also, nurses who are comfortable with themselves will be able to put the client's needs first by listening attentively and recognizing emotions in the client that may hinder a therapeutic exchange. For example, high anxiety can produce "tunnel vision" in a client which can impair communication.

Finally, the nurse needs to be able to *conduct a periodic self evaluation of his or her responses to the client*. Questions to ask oneself may include:

- Am I open- or closed-minded regarding this issue?

- Am I accepting? Am I rejecting?

- Am I being supportive? Nonsupportive?

- Am I being objective? Or am I allowing my biases to interfere with the interaction?

- Am I remaining calm and in control of my own feelings? Or am I allowing my anxiety, sympathy, anger to surface?

- What are my true feelings? Do my nonverbal cues match my verbal communication? (Shives, 1994)

ROLES OF THE NURSE IN THERAPEUTIC COMMUNICATION

Nurses assume many roles during therapeutic communication with clients, such as the professional role and the model role. In the professional role, the nurse acts as teacher, socializer, technician, advocate, parent, counselor, and therapist.

Clients learn about their illnesses and treatment modalities from the teacher nurse. The nurse socializer brings clients together for activities to prevent social isolation during hospital treatment. In the technician role, the nurse changes the I.V., administers medications, or takes vital signs. As an advocate, the nurse informs the client of his or her rights and responsibilities, and supports the client in decision making. The advocate nurse also serves as a liaison between the client and other members of the mental health team, ensuring that the client's rights, either legal or human, are not violated (Fontaine and Fletcher, 1995). The nurse in the parent role does not mean that the nurse becomes the parent, but rather performs traditional nurturing tasks such as feeding, bathing, or comforting. As a counselor, the nurse can assist the client with personal problems, such as a disagreement between the client and a family member. With advanced education, the nurse can take on the role of a therapist, conducting individual, group, or family therapy sessions in the hospital, clinic, or community setting.

In any relationship with a client, the nurse may take on part or all of these roles. The number of roles the nurse assumes will vary according to the type and length of the individual nurse-client relationship as well as the setting of the interactions.

TRAITS OF THERAPEUTIC COMMUNICATION

The following are traits of effective therapeutic communication: genuineness, positive regard, empathy, trustworthiness, clarity, responsibility, and assertiveness. These characteristics allow the nurse to influence growth and change in others because they incorporate verbal and nonverbal behaviors as well as attitudes, beliefs, and feelings behind the communication. Thus, they are necessary for therapeutic communication to take place.

Genuineness

Genuineness is demonstrated by congruency between the nurse's verbal and nonverbal behavior. Consistent verbal and nonverbal behavior implies that the nurse is open, honest, and sincere. Genuineness is necessary for clients to develop trust in the nurse. Trust is built when the nurse does not appear mechanical but rather responds with sincerity. Genuine interaction does not mean the nurse must disclose personal information or relate to the client in a social manner. Rather, the nurse remains focused on the client and responds therapeutically. Nurses cannot expect a client to be open and honest if they do not display these characteristics themselves.

Positive Regard

Positive regard refers to respect and acceptance. Nurses can show that they view their clients as worthy, for example, by addressing clients by names they prefer. Nurses accept clients for who they are and do not expect them to change except in a therapeutic way.

Positive regard is communicated in a variety of ways. It can be conveyed by sitting and listening to a client, by expressing appropriate emotion about events affecting a client, by validating the client's feelings, or by effectively responding to a client's inappropriate behavior. For example, a client who has just been through the admission process is found on his bed openly masturbating. After assessing the situation and understanding that this activity is not harmful to others, the nurse explains to the client that this behavior should be private. The nurse closes the door to allow the client to continue, but out of the view of others.

Part of positive regard is being nonjudgmental. The nurse should avoid harsh judgment or evaluation of a client's behavior and feelings because both are real and cannot be argued with, discounted, or criticized. The client must not be made to feel wrong. Labeling behaviors as bad or good based on one's own value system is not useful. Instead, the nurse needs to help clients explore their behavior by discussing the thoughts and feelings which determine the behavior. When clients realize they are not being judged, they may feel free to express their most intimate thoughts and feelings. A nonjudgmental attitude in the nurse relaxes the client by removing fears of being misunderstood or rejected. This open relationship can occur only when nurses identify their own thoughts and feelings regarding the client's behavior.

Empathy

Empathy or *empathic understanding* is the nurse's ability to see things from the client's viewpoint and to communicate this understanding to the client. There are two types of **empathy.** The first type—*natural, trait,* or *basic* empathy—implies it is an inherent human trait apparent in varying degrees in everyone. Some research suggests that trait empathy is a naturally inherited potential that matures during growth. This viewpoint suggests that we all have an instinctual sensitivity that unfolds in a person like other characteristics of human development (Alligood, 1992).

The second type, *trained* or *clinical empathy*, is said to build on the nurse's own natural level of empathy. Natural empathy is a tool or skill used consciously to achieve a therapeutic intervention (Pike, 1990). Some researchers suggest that nursing students should be tested for their level of basic or natural empathy prior to being

taught the clinical empathy techniques to determine potential problematic levels which are either too low or too high (Alligood, 1992; Wheeler, 1988; Williams, 1990). Testing would give a baseline indicator prior to any empathy to determine effectiveness of the instruction. High levels of natural empathy may indicate that the nurse has a tendency to overidentify and thus become too involved with clients' problems. Low levels may indicate that the nurse may not be able to demonstrate enough genuine concern for clients.

Empathy should not be confused with sympathy. Sympathy is overinvolvement and sharing one's own feelings after hearing about another person's similar experience. It is not objective, and its primary purpose is to decrease one's own personal distress.

An empathic response involves an appreciation and awareness of the client's feelings and keeps focus on the client. For example, a client reveals to the nurse that her father died in an automobile accident one month prior to her arrival at the hospital. The nurse responds sympathetically by saying that her own mother died in a small plane crash, and that made the nurse feel sad for a year afterward. Here the focus is on the nurse, and the client may not know how to respond. An empathic response by the nurse would be: "I can understand how difficult that would be for you. Tell me how it made you feel and how you have been coping with the loss." Now the focus is on the client, and the client is better able to reply.

The development of empathy poses a challenge for the psychiatric nurse in the hospital setting who typically has a brief time frame with clients and who must primarily use crisis intervention principles. Lower levels of empathy from the nurse are healthier for clients in the beginning stage of the relationship. However, it has been shown through research that empathy is clearly related to positive outcomes; if expressed early in a relationship, it predicts later success.

Empathy consists of two stages. If a client shares important and uncomfortable emotions, nurses should first be receptive to and understand the client's communication by putting themselves in the client's place. This does not mean nurses need to have had the same problem or feeling. Then, after stepping back into the professional role, nurses must be able to communicate understanding, which demonstrates objectivity and sensitivity to the client. This understanding mirrors the client's identity and is the process by which the client makes changes to achieve positive outcomes. The following skills help nurses develop greater empathic responses:

- Attending to the client physically, by sitting in front of the client, at a slight angle, leaning slightly forward with hands and arms in an open stance.

- Attending to the client emotionally by clearing one's mind of other personal or work-related business and focusing one's full attention on the client.

- Listening and providing response to each of the client's verbal and nonverbal communications.

- Focusing on the client's strengths.

- Conveying caring, warmth, interest, and concern through nonverbal behaviors.

- Picking out the most important point of what the client is trying to say.

- Demonstrating congruence between one's own nonverbal and verbal communication.

- Checking whether or not one's empathic responses are effective by looking for verbal and nonverbal clues.

Closely aligned with empathy is *active listening* because it incorporates both nonverbal and verbal behaviors necessary for therapeutic communication. Nonverbally, the nurse leans slightly forward facing the client, uses comfortable, intermittent eye contact, nods, and uses verbal phrases such as "uh huh" or "I hear you." Active listening results in articulation of the client's feelings, specifically providing the client with the knowledge that the nurse accepts how the client is feeling and attempts to understand this (Smith, 1990). A nurse who listens actively also displays interest. A client trying to work through problems needs to know the nurse is there to help and wants to help.

Trustworthiness

Another essential characteristic of an effective nurse is *trustworthiness*. Being trustworthy means nurses are responsible and dependable. They adhere to commitments, keep promises, and are consistent in their approach and response to clients. Clients need to learn they can rely on the nurse so that trust can be built. Trustworthy nurses respect the client's privacy, rights, and the need for confidentiality. Clients need to be convinced that the information they share will not go beyond the health care team.

Clarity

Nurses must communicate *clearly*. Often, psychiatric clients have difficulty processing information. If the nurse is specific and detailed, there will be less room for miscommunication. Clear communication involves selecting concise words when speaking, and asking questions to clarify meaning. Although using medical jargon is part of the nurse's way of life, the nurse should remember that clients might not speak the same language. Everyday terms such as "taking your vitals," "NPO after midnight," or "take these meds," could be misunderstood, especially by psychiatric clients who may not be thinking clearly as a result of their disorders. Problems may arise if instructions or information are relayed in a highly technical manner, because the client may be too embarrassed to ask for clarification.

A study conducted at the University of Alberta Hospital revealed that clients frequently do not understand or often misunderstand professional jargon (Cochrane, 1992). For two weeks, several nurses listened to themselves and other nurses in conversation with clients. Each time a word or phrase considered to be medical jargon was used, it was recorded. Thirty-four of the most common medical words or phrases were selected for the study. One hundred one adult clients, both newly admitted and those on their fourth day of hospitalization, were surveyed. The results of the study showed that most of the words were defined correctly by more than half of the respondents. For example, 98% of the respondents knew what "OR" meant. But words that had one meaning in everyday terminology and another in the nursing profession were often misinterpreted. The newly admitted clients did not do better or worse than clients hospitalized for four days or those who had been hospitalized prior to this admission.

Thus, nurses need to make a conscious effort to speak at a level the client will understand. Avoidance of abstract, lengthy explanations is also necessary.

Responsibility

Responsible communication involves being accountable for the outcome of one's professional interactions. When nurses communicate, they need to be responsible for their part in the interaction and assure that all messages are received and interpreted correctly. Nurses who communicate responsibly enhance growth in others.

Assertiveness

Assertive communication is the ability to express thoughts and feelings comfortably and confidently in a positive, honest, and open manner that demonstrates respect for self while respecting others (Balzer-Riley, 1996). An assertive nurse should control negative feelings which is important not only in communication with clients, but also with supervisors, employees, physicians, and colleagues. The nurse who communicates assertively makes a conscious choice about how to communicate with others. Communicating assertively is a style choice and can be implemented in any situation at any time. Box 7-1 lists behaviors of assertive communication.

RESPONDING TECHNIQUES THAT ENHANCE THERAPEUTIC COMMUNICATION

Techniques of responding therapeutically are methods used to encourage clients to interact in a manner that promotes their growth and moves them toward their treatment goals. These strategies create an atmosphere that promotes communication for problem solving. (See Table 7-4 for examples of many of these techniques.)

Silence is an important listening skill for psychiatric nurses to develop. It is not the absence of communica-

---

Box 7-1   Behaviors of Assertive Communication

Assertive: Stands up for rights and respects those of others. Uses expressive, directive, self-enhancing speech. Chooses appropriate words and actions.

Aggressive: Stands up for rights but abuses those of others. Speaks in demeaning or attacking manner. Fails to monitor or control words or actions.

Acquiescent: Does not stand up for own rights and accepts the domination and bullying of others. Performs unwanted tasks and feels victimized.

Examples of assertive behaviors

1. "I" messages, e.g., "I need," "I feel," "I will."
2. "Eye" contact, e.g., looking directly into the eyes of the person while making or refusing a request.
3. Congruent verbal and facial expressions, e.g., making certain that the facial expression matches the intent of the spoken message. A serious message accompanied by laughter could negate the credibility of the message.

Example of assertive plan for change

1. Target the behavior that one desires to change. For example, how to say no and mean it.
2. List approximately ten situations in which it is difficult to say no, and order them from least to most difficult.
3. Practice saying no, using the least threatening method

first and working up to more challenging situations, for example, imagery, tape recorder, feedback, role playing, and practice in actual situations.

4. Say no as the first word in the practice response, as it is a clear message without excuses or apologies.
5. Follow with a clear, concise, declarative statement, for example, "I will not rearrange my schedule; I need my day off."
6. Use eye contact appropriate to the intent of the verbal message.

Assertiveness training is most often done in small group sessions and has been described in detail in a variety of textbooks.

From Fortinash K and Holoday-Worret P: *Psychiatric nursing care plans,* ed 2, St. Louis, 1995, Mosby.

---

tion, but rather a useful and purposeful communication tool to give the client time to feel comfortable and respond when ready to do so. Silence must be used to serve a particular function and not to frighten or discomfort the already anxious client. A successful interview is largely dependent on the nurse's ability to remain silent long enough to allow the client to share relevant information. Silence gives the client an opportunity to consider what is being said, weigh alternatives, and formulate an answer.

Support and reassurance are provided in a genuine and honest manner. Clients need to be in an atmosphere where they can safely disclose information that may be of a sensitive nature. Nurses can offer both verbal and nonverbal support so the client feels free to share thoughts and feelings, which is necessary for progress toward mental health to occur.

Sharing observations made by the nurse is important in order to increase the client's self-understanding. It also demonstrates to the client that the nurse is actively listening.

Acknowledging feelings is a form of client support. It is important to let the client know his or her feelings are valid and important. There are no right or wrong answers when it comes to feelings. They cannot be taken away, or argued with, or discounted.

Broad, open-ended statements allow the client to assume some control over topics to be discussed. However, the nurse should not allow the client to discuss only nonrelevant topics or engage in a conversation with a superficial or social content. The nurse should frequently ask the client questions that will not produce one-word answers. Open-ended questions result in fuller, more revealing answers which typically stimulate further questions by the nurse.

Information giving is an ongoing process for the nurse. Information is provided to enhance the client's knowledge about a variety of topics on his or her illness and treatment. Information may decrease fears and anxiety and increase the client's fund of resources and support for his or her problem. Examples may include information regarding the client's disorder, medication, aftercare support groups, structured living options, or treatment alternatives. Information should be given according to the client's level of understanding and willingness to receive it.

Interpretation of what is being shared by clients is useful to help them see the real meaning behind their message. Helping clients *focus* to pursue a particular topic allows them to spend their time discussing subjects of most importance. *Identification of themes* is necessary to help clients see what they repeatedly bring up in the conversation. *Placing events in order and time* is also important to help clients develop a greater perspective on events in their lives.

Clients often need to be encouraged to *describe their perceptions* regarding their thoughts and feelings. For example, some psychiatric clients hear imaginary voices telling them to hurt themselves or others. The nurse asks such clients to tell the staff when this occurs in order to intervene and prevent clients' attempts to harm themselves or others. Treatment strategies can then be introduced to reduce this perception and therefore minimize the client's dysfunctional behavior.

To develop a sense of clients' past and current behavior, the nurse may ask clients to *compare* their present anxiety to that of their last hospitalization. Or the nurse may ask clients if they have ever experienced before what they are telling the nurse now.

Restating what clients say lets them know the nurse heard and understands them. It is an active listening technique.

Reflecting is a technique used to turn a question around to obtain a response from the client. Forcing clients to answer a question best answered by clients themselves helps them accept their own ideas and feelings regarding an important event or behavior.

Clarifying is a method used to ask the client to elaborate or restate something just said. It serves to increase the nurse's understanding and to allow the client to rethink and restate the thought or feeling.

Confrontation in an accepting manner is necessary for the client to be more aware of incongruent thoughts, feelings, and behaviors. This helps to bring the issue into focus and is used only after rapport has been established (Fortinash and Holoday-Worret, 1995). When a client is struggling to explore and solve a problem but can only see one or two solutions, the nurse may *offer alternatives*. Suggesting to the client other possible solutions to the problem is not the same as giving advice. It uses introductions such as "Have you thought of," "Other clients have solved it using this solution," and "Other alternatives may be." The nurse avoids phrases such as, "You should do," and "I think you need to solve it the way I did (giving advice)."

Voicing doubt is a technique to use when the client is having difficulty relating in a way that sounds believable. Voicing some doubt may help the client to be more realistic about perceptions and conclusions of events.

On a regular basis the nurse will need to *summarize* the information the client provides. Summarizing the main points of what a client has been discussing helps focus on the most important issues related to the client's life situation. After the summary is provided, the client can agree or disagree with any point, and then together the nurse and client will agree on a final summary.

Role-playing provides a place for the client to act out a particular event, problem, or situation in a safe environment. The nurse can play the other part or role. He or she can also provide feedback to the client on a variety of components within the dialogue, such as voice tone, use of assertive language, identification of feelings, emotion expressed, and nonverbal behavior exhibited (Fortinash and Holoday-Worret, 1995).

SPECIAL COMMUNICATION TECHNIQUES
Self-Disclosure

Self-disclosure is opening up of oneself to another and can be an effective therapeutic skill if fully understood and used carefully. Nurses reveal their thoughts, feelings, and life events to demonstrate to the client that they understand what the client is going through.

Disclosing one's own personal beliefs, views, and life experiences occurs in social relationships on a continual basis. In intimate relationships, what is revealed is very personal. In social relationships, the individuals reveal information about themselves until both parties decide how much is too much and then reach a certain level acceptable to both.

Guidelines are necessary for the use of self-disclosure in therapeutic relationships. Because a professional nurse-client relationship exists for the purpose of helping the client, whatever the nurse discloses needs to be for the client's benefit. Therefore, it is important to explore the what, where, why, and when of self-disclosing to see what purpose it serves (Balzer-Riley, 1996).

Since self-disclosures are subjectively true personal statements about the self, they must be carefully thought out before being revealed. Criteria have been developed to help the nurse discern appropriate use of self-disclosure. The purpose of the self-disclosure should be one or more of the following:

1. To model and educate: Will clients learn more about themselves and be able to deal better with the problems in their lives?

2. To build the therapeutic partnership: Will disclosure foster a greater nurse-client alliance by obtaining a greater amount of cooperation?

3. To validate reality: Will clients be supported in their natural feelings in response to an event?

4. To foster clients' autonomy: Will the disclosure help clients to express previously held feelings on their own? (Stricker and Fisher, 1990).

The use of self-disclosure requires that the nurse and client have a therapeutic relationship. The rationale for using self-disclosure comes from the belief that in doing so, the client will in turn self-disclose. Both the amount and the relevance of the nurse's own self-disclosure need to be monitored. If the self-disclosure is too lengthy, it may decrease the time the client has for disclosure and may result in a breakdown in the interaction.

TABLE 7-2 Self-Disclosure	
Therapeutic	**Nontherapeutic**
Client: "I'm real upset that I have to leave the hospital today." *Nurse:* "I have enjoyed working with you. I realize endings can be sad. It is important for you to use the tools you have learned when you go home." *Discussion*: The nurse is using self-disclosure in the termination phase of the relationship. She is validating the client's feelings and is also validating the alliance with the purpose of encouraging the client to transfer what has been learned after care.	*Client:* "That jerk of a husband had to leave me with three children to support, and it is hard." *Nurse:* "I know how you feel because my husband was just like that, leaving me 10 years ago with one small child, when he ran off with another woman. He gives me no support and doesn't see his daughter. I get angry a lot too." *Discussion*: The nurse is using self-disclosure in the admission interview or beginning phase of the relationship. It revealed too much personal information. Also, it occurred 10 years ago and was much too lengthy. It served the nurse's purpose, rather than the client's, to share the incident.

If the disclosure is irrelevant to the client's problem, the client may become distracted and feel alienated from the nurse. It is important to emphasize that disclosing as a therapeutic tool must always be to benefit the client, never the nurse. Table 7-2 compares an example of therapeutic versus nontherapeutic self-disclosure.

Both research and literature have indicated that self-disclosure can be an important tool for client growth; however, it remains a tool that can produce uncomfortable feelings for the nurse. The nurse must realize that not all self-disclosure is revealing personal information. It can simply be sharing a feeling. Genuine, open communication that creates a therapeutic alliance can be achieved without the use of self-disclosure. Self-disclosure can enhance that alliance only when the nurse feels comfortable with its use and when it will benefit the client.

Touch

Touch is a nonverbal method of communication that may convey many messages. Handshaking, holding hands, hugging, and kissing all demonstrate positive feelings for another human being. Nonessential touch is purposeful physical contact with the client other than the touch necessary for a procedure. Nonprocedural touches range from a light touch on the arm or a handshake, to holding the hand or a full embrace. For touch to convey warmth, the nurse must be comfortable with it.

Touch carries a different meaning for each person. Several variables influence the intended message of the touch, including the length of the touch, the part of the body touched, the way in which the client is touched, and the frequency of the touch.

The nurse must use caution when touching clients in a psychiatric setting. Reactions to touch are influenced by the age and gender of the client, the client's interpretation of the gesture, the client's cultural background, and the appropriateness of the touch.

The nurse needs to take potential reactions into consideration when deciding which clients to touch and what type of touch to use, if any. For example, the depressed client may respond positively to touch as a gesture of concern. An elderly frail client or a client who is dying, may be equally comforted by the nurse's touch. However, a paranoid, hostile client may misinterpret touch to mean confrontation, and may strike out at the nurse. The abused client may pull away and feel frightened by a hand on the shoulder.

Procedural touch may include positioning the arm of a client when taking a blood pressure or drawing lab work, turning a client to change a dressing or diaper, lifting or assisting a client from the bed to a wheelchair, or performing a seclusion or restraint procedure on a highly agitated and hostile client. *Nonprocedural touch* may include holding an elderly client's hand as she is conveying sadness over her husband's death, hugging an adolescent client as he leaves the hospital, shaking the hand of new clients as they are introduced by another nurse during their transfer to your unit, or giving a back rub to a long-term, bedridden client (Figure 7-2).

The use of touch is an individual preference by the nurse because not all practitioners feel comfortable doing it. Much depends on the nurse's comfort level, the ability to correctly interpret the situation, and the appropriate use of touch. Using touch can be highly beneficial to the client's progress by enhancing the nurse-client relationship and promoting health (see Understanding and Applying Research on page 157).

Humor

Humor can be a useful tool in psychiatric nursing. Humor is defined as the quality that makes something seem funny, amusing, or ludicrous. It is the ability to perceive, appreciate, and express what is funny, amusing, or absurd. Use of humor has been controversial in psychiatric settings and is seen by some as unprofessional and inappropriate. Healthy humor elicits laughter between people;

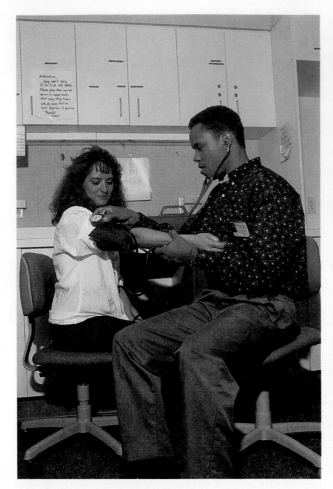 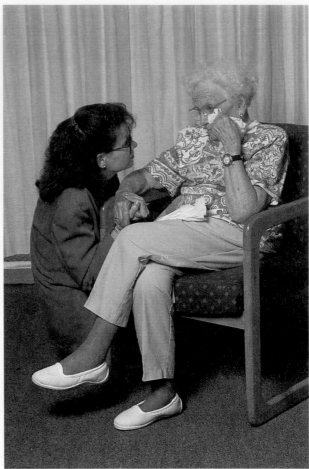

Figure 7-2 A. Positioning the arm of a client when taking blood pressure is an example of procedural touch. B. Comforting an elderly client as she grieves over her husband's death is an example of nonprocedural touch.

(Copyright Cathy Lander-Goldberg, Lander Photographics.)

it encourages laughing *with* others and not at them. It includes others, is appropriate to the situation, respects others, and preserves their dignity. Harmful humor excludes others. It singles out people from a group and ridicules them.

A good sense of humor is considered to be a mature coping mechanism and can help the nurse adequately handle difficult situations. It also assists in gaining a different perspective on the problem by lightening a serious mood for a few moments.

Physiologically, humor has been known to improve the circulatory system, stimulate the respiratory system, and increase blood oxygen levels and heart rate. These changes result in a rise in the epinephrine levels which make one feel more alert and offer a sense of well-being. Laughing and having positive social interactions during mealtimes has been reported to aid digestion. The psychological benefits of laughter decrease fears and anxiety, lessen negative emotions, and decrease stress and tension (Ferguson and Campinha-Bacote, 1989).

The nurse should assess the degree to which a client has a sense of humor. In depressed clients, the outward expression of laughter and pleasure is usually missing.

Clients with paranoid features are unable to laugh. In fact, they may view others' laughter as a personal attack. This is important to remember. For example, nurses in the nursing station may choose not to laugh and joke behind a glass partition where paranoid clients can see them and interpret the behavior as a personal affront. On the other hand, manic clients may laugh at everything, whether or not it is actually humorous. This exaggerated sense of well-being demonstrates a lack of judgment on the part of the client that can turn into biting sarcasm which can hurt others.

Clinicians who have studied humor as an important indicator of a person's health believe that asking the client simple questions, such as what their favorite joke is, how often they laugh, and how their patterns of laughter change offers the nurse new insights into their illness (Ferguson and Campinha-Bacote, 1989).

The psychiatric nurse can use humor as a therapeutic tool in a variety of ways. For example, it can be used to teach the client the difference between hurtful and healthy humor, to encourage healthy humor on the unit by role modeling, and to introduce humor in formal and informal groups and individually. The use of humor can

Understanding and Applying
RESEARCH

Tommasini N: The use of touch with the hospitalized psychiatric patient, *Arch Psych Nursing* 4(4)213, August 1990.

The purpose of this study was to identify and describe the ways and reasons registered nurses use nonprocedural touch in the inpatient psychiatric setting. Natural setting observation and nurse interviews were used to examine the nurses' reasons for touch.

Twenty-six incidents of nonprocedural touch initiated by 13 registered nurses with 17 psychiatric clients were recorded over 27.5 hours of observation. Observations were made on one adolescent unit and two adult psychiatric units in a large university teaching hospital.

Of the 30 nurses who agreed to participate in the study, 24 were observed. Of those 24, 13 touched clients.

Several elements went into the decision to touch. Both the client and the nurse were taken into account. Client characteristics such as age, gender, needs, and the nurse's knowledge of the client were involved in the decision to touch. Also, the nurses' feelings, beliefs, intuition, style, and role expectations were acknowledged.

Ninety-two percent of the touches recorded were used in a purposeful, therapeutic manner. The nurses' intentions for using touch were establishing contact with the client, enhancing communication, conveying warmth and caring, interest and recognition, offering reassurance and comfort. Nonprocedural touch can be very effective in conveying therapeutic messages, and nurses should use touch whenever therapeutically appropriate.

increase the flexibility of interactions and create a more relaxed milieu. It can enhance insight and facilitate the type of interaction that is difficult for the client, in a safe, low-keyed environment.

OBSTACLES TO THERAPEUTIC COMMUNICATION

Certain obstacles can occur in the client-nurse relationship that affect the nature of the communication. Some obstacles are due to the client's pathology or lack or knowledge; some have to do with the nurse's own inability to be effective due to inexperience, lack of knowledge, or personal problems. For the relationship to grow in a healthy manner, these obstacles must be overcome.

Four key therapeutic obstacles are introduced here for discussion: resistance, transference, countertransference, and boundary violations.

Resistance

Resistance occurs in clients who consciously or unconsciously maintain a lack of awareness of problems they are having to avoid anxiety. It can take the form of a natural and short-lived reservation about accepting a problem, or a long-term, firmly stated denial that there are problems. This resistance to change is a part of human nature but must be addressed and dealt with by both the client and the nurse for positive growth to occur. Nurses can help clients overcome resistance by pointing out their progress and strengths.

For example, a nurse can assure a client who resists impending discharge because of fear of failure, abandonment, or loneliness that such fears are not uncommon at the time of termination or discharge. The nurse can then remind the client of progress made, e.g., "You've been a big part of the success of the activities, and you even facilitated a few groups; these are accomplishments you didn't believe possible when you first arrived at this facility." Such observations build the client's confidence and offer hope which will counteract resistance.

Transference

Transference is the unconscious response whereby clients associate the nurse with someone significant in their lives. Feelings and attitudes about the other person are transferred to the nurse. For example, a male client sees a female nurse as a mother figure because she has a similar mannerism to his own mother. The client may have negative feelings about his mother and, without provocation, becomes angry or bothered by the nurse's interaction with him because of the resemblance. Oftentimes, the client's intense response does not match the situation or the content of the interaction. The interaction will come to a standstill if the nurse does not address and examine the client's reasons for transference.

The nurse can deal with both resistance and transference by being prepared to hear a client's irrational and highly charged responses to the nurse. The nurse must truly listen to the client and then use the therapeutic techniques of clarifying and reflecting to begin problem solving. The goal is for the client to gain awareness and recognition of what lies behind the resistance.

Countertransference

Countertransference is initiated by the nurse's emotional response to a specific client. The response is irrational, inappropriate, highly charged, and is generated by certain qualities of the client. It is simply the nurse's own transference. Nurses have a natural response to each client and will like or dislike some more than others. Countertransference occurs when the feelings are intense—either positive or negative—and are not based on reality. Because it will impede the nurse's ability to be therapeutically effective, the nurse must always observe for signs of its occurrence.

From time to time, countertransference issues are bound to surface. Even though it is natural, it is destructive if ignored by the nurse as insignificant. The nurse most often encounters countertransference when the client is displaying disruptive, aggressive, irritating, or resistive behaviors. If the nurse remains angry with the client as a result of these behaviors, the degree of objectivity needed to promote healthy change is lost. Nurses may also find themselves attracted positively to clients in excessive ways, and must recognize and take steps to avoid countertransference.

Countertransference can also occur as a group phenomenon. This occurs when the entire psychiatric nursing staff becomes upset by a particular client's behavior and does not obtain the information necessary to understand the client's problems. This type of client is typically seen as manipulative and demanding and generates strong negative feelings from the staff who may then become engaged in a power struggle with the client.

To deal with countertransference, the nurse must conduct an honest self-appraisal throughout the course of the therapeutic relationship while gaining a good understanding of the client's background and issues. If the self-appraisal reveals any problems, the nurse must explore why these feelings are occurring. This work needs to be done as soon as the problem is recognized. The nurse may not be able to handle these feelings alone and may need some clinical supervision time to deal with them. If countertransference occurs in a group, the team may need to meet with an impartial psychiatric consultant or clinical instructor to review the issues.

Boundary Violations

Boundary violations occur when the nurse goes beyond the established therapeutic relationship standards and enters into a social or personal relationship with the client. Violations can also occur if the nurse treats the client at odd hours or in an unusual setting, if the nurse accepts compensation or gifts for treatment, if the nurse's language or clothing are inappropriate, or if the nurse's self-disclosure or physical contact lack therapeutic value (Stuart and Sundeen, 1995).

RESPONDING TECHNIQUES THAT HINDER THERAPEUTIC COMMUNICATION

In a previous section, therapeutic skills that have enhanced the communication process were presented. There are also many responses which are counterpro-

ductive to healthy outcomes and are therefore considered nontherapeutic.

There are several reasons why nurses fail to interact effectively. The inexperienced nurse's insecurity is one factor. A certain amount of experience and maturity greatly helps the nurse deal effectively with the difficult and complex behaviors psychiatric clients often display.

Other explanations for nontherapeutic communication are that the nurse has allowed necessary skills to stagnate or diminish. Or the nurse may have developed personal problems that have not been dealt with sufficiently and are thus interfering with his or her ability to focus on the client and the client's needs (Table 7-3).

It is important that nurses build on the knowledge they possess by continually practicing and perfecting skills, attending skills-building classes and therapeutic communication inservices to refresh and enhance skills they already possess, and know when to obtain outside help for their own life problems so those problems do not interfere with work.

There are other potential instances for a nurse's ineffective responses. A nurse may display anger toward the client for not behaving in a socially acceptable manner or for not doing what is asked. Or the nurse may take personally what the client says. A client may be angry, delusional, and display out-of-control behavior, and may say something to the nurse that hurts his or her feelings. For example, a client may say to the overweight nurse placing him in seclusion, "Get out of here, you big fat. . ." The nurse, upset by the client's statement, may respond angrily or defensively if he or she is not able to detach from the statement and realize that the client is angry at his own behavior, and is projecting it to the nurse in the form of a personal statement.

COMMUNICATION AND THE NURSING PROCESS

There are many opportunities to communicate therapeutically throughout the nursing process. Each step of the nursing process—assessment, nursing diagnosis, outcome identification, implementation, planning, and evaluation—corresponds with the three phases of the therapeutic relationship—orientation, working, and termination. Therapeutic responding techniques unique to each step and phase are used throughout.

The nurse's first communication task is to greet the client on admission. The nurse communicates the nature of his or her role. This orientation phase begins with the initial contact, continues with the admission interview and assessment, and ends with the formulation of a nursing diagnosis. This phase can last one or more sessions because much of highly personal data must be collected, and it occurs when the client is in most need of help and may be displaying highly dysfunctional behavior.

In the working phase of the relationship when the care plan with outcome criteria is being developed and

TABLE 7-3 Ineffective responses that hinder therapeutic communication

Response	Discussion	Nontherapeutic response	Therapeutic response
Offering false reassurance	The nurse, in an effort to be supportive and to make the client's pain disappear, offers reassuring cliches. This response is not based on fact. It brushes aside the client's feelings and closes off communication. Often, it is due to the nurse's inability to listen to the client's negative emotions. No one can predict the outcome of a situation.	"Don't worry, everything will be o.k." "Things will be better soon; you'll see."	"I know you have a lot going on right now. Let's make a list and begin to discuss them one at a time. Working toward solutions will assist you to get through this."
Not listening	The nurse is preoccupied with other work that needs to be done, is distracted by noise in the area, is thinking about personal problems.	"I'm sorry, what did you say?" "Could you start again? I was listening to the other nurse."	"That is interesting. Please elaborate." "I really hear what you are saying . . . it must be difficult."
Offering approval	It is most important how a client feels about what he or she said or did. The client ultimately must approve of his or her own actions.	"That's good." "I agree—I think you should have told him."	"What do you think about what you said to him?" "How do you feel about it?"
Minimizing problem	The nurse may use this when it is difficult to hear the enormity of a particular problem. This is used in an effort to try to make the client feel better. It cuts off communication.	"That's nothing compared to that other client's problem." "Everyone feels that way at times, it's not a big deal."	"That is a very difficult problem for you." "That sounds pretty important for you to deal with."
Offering advice	This response undermines clients' ability to solve their own problems. It serves to render them dependent and helpless. If the solution provided by the nurse does not work, the client may blame the outcome on the nurse. Clients do not take responsibility for developing outcomes. The nurse maintains control and at the same time devalues the client.	"I think you should..." "In my opinion, it would be wise to..." "Why don't you do..." "The best solution is..."	"What do *you* think you should do?" "There can be several alternatives—let's talk about some. However, the final decision must be yours. I will listen to your problem and help you see it clearly. We can develop a pros and cons list which may assist you in solving the problem."
Giving literal reponses	The nurse feeds into a client's delusions or hallucinations, denies client the opportunity to see reality. This does not provide a healthy response toward growth.	C: "That TV is talking to me." N: "What is it saying to you?" C: "There is nuclear power coming through the air ducts." N: "I'll turn off the A/C for a while."	N: "The TV is on for everyone." N: "There is cool air blowing from the vents. It is the A/C system."
Changing the subject	The nurse changes the topic at a crucial time because the discussion is too uncomfortable. It negates what the client seems interested in discussing. Communication will remain superficial.	C: "My mother always puts me down." N: "That's interesting, but let's talk about..."	N: "Tell me about that."

Continued

TABLE 7-3 Ineffective responses that hinder therapeutic communication—cont'd

Response	Discussion	Nontherapeutic response	Therapeutic response
Belittling	The nurse puts down client's expressed feelings to avoid having to deal with painful feelings.	C: "I don't want to live anymore now that my child is gone." N: "Anyone would be sad, but that's no reason to want to die."	N: "The death must be very difficult for you. Tell me a little more about how you are feeling."
Disagreeing	The nurse criticizes the client who is seeking support.	"I definitely do not agree with your view." "I really don't believe that."	"Let's talk about the way you see that." "It seems hard to believe. Please explain further."
Judging	The nurse's responses are filled with his or her own values and judgments. This demonstrates a lack of acceptance of the client's differences. It will provide a barrier to further disclosures.	"You are not married. Do you think having this baby will solve your problems?" "This is certainly not the Christian thing to do." "You are thinking about divorce when you have three children?"	"What will having this baby provide for you?" "What do you think about what you are attempting to do?" "Let's discuss this option," or "Let's discuss other options."
Excessive probing	Serves to control the nature of the client's responses. The nurse asks many questions of clients before they are ready to provide the information. This is self-protective to the nurse by avoiding the anxiety of uncomfortable silences. The client feels overwhelmed and may withdraw.	"Why do you do this?" "What do you think was the real cause?" "Do you always feel this way?" "Why do you think that way?"	"Tell me how this is upsetting to you." "Tell me what you believe to be the cause." "Tell me how you feel when that happens." "Explain your thinking on this if you can."
Challenging	This stems from the nurse's belief that if clients are challenged regarding their unrealistic beliefs, they will be coerced into seeing reality. The client may feel threatened when challenged, holding onto the beliefs even more strongly.	"You are not the Queen of England." "If your leg is missing, then why can you walk this hall?"	"You sound like you want to be important." "It seems to you like you are missing a leg. Tell me more about that."
Superficial comments	The nurse gives simple or meaningless responses to clients. It suggests a lack of understanding regarding the client as an individual. The interactions remain superficial, maintaining distance between nurse and client. Nothing of significance gets communicated.	"Great day, huh!" "You should be feeling good; you are being discharged today." "Keep the faith; your doctor should be coming anytime now."	"What kind of day are you having?" "How are you feeling about leaving the hospital today?" "You look worried. Your doctor called and said he would be here within the hour."
Defending	The nurse may believe she or he must defend herself or himself, the staff, or the hospital. The nurse may not take the time to listen to the client's concerns. Efforts need to be made to explore the client's thoughts and feelings.	"Your doctor is a good doctor. He would never say that." "We have a very experienced staff here. They would not ever do that."	"What has you so upset about your doctor?" "Tell me what happened on the evening shift."

TABLE 7-3 Ineffective responses that hinder therapeutic communication—cont'd

Response	Discussion	Nontherapeutic response	Therapeutic response
Self-focusing	The nurse focuses attention away from the client by thinking about sharing his or her own thoughts, feelings, problems. The focus is taken away from the client who is seeking help. The nurse is more interested in what to say next instead of actively listening to the client.	"That may have happened to you last year, but it happened to me twice this month, which hurt me a great deal and ..." "Excuse me but could you say that again? I have a response to make, but I want to be sure of what you said."	"Tell me about your incident and how it might relate to your sadness now." "If I heard you accurately, you said ..."
Criticism of others	The nurse puts down others.	C: "The staff members on the day shift let me smoke two cigarettes." N: "The day shift is always breaking the rules. On this shift, we follow the one cigarette policy." C: "My daughter is hateful to me." N: "She must be just awful to live with."	N: "The policy is one cigarette, which we must follow." N: "It sounds like you are having a rough time right now with your daughter."
Premature interpretation	The nurse does not wait until the client fully expresses thoughts and feelings related to a particular problem. This rushes the client and disregards his or her input. The nurse may miss what the client wants to explain.	"I think this is what you really mean." "You may think that way consciously, but your unconscious believes. . ."	"What do you think this means?" "So you think..."

implemented with the client and treatment team, many therapeutic responding techniques can be used. The therapeutic communication skills the nurse uses during this phase are designed to help clients deal with the issues that brought them into the hospital.

During the termination phase, both evaluation and discharge planning are predominant. The nurse uses communication techniques associated with assisting the client toward discharge and aftercare. Table 7-4 presents examples of therapeutic responding techniques that relate to each nursing process step and therapeutic relationship phase. The phases of the therapeutic relationship are discussed in greater detail in Chapter 22.

CHALLENGES IN COMMUNICATION

Legal Issues

Confidentiality and informed consent are legal issues that impact nurse-client communication. They are discussed briefly here as they relate to this relationship. They are discussed in detail in Chapter 3.

CONFIDENTIALITY

All client information the nurse obtains is protected by the client's right to privacy. Information can be shared with the health care team so that the most effective plan of care can be developed. However, the nurse must fiercely protect the client's right to privacy and the right to keep that information from people outside the health care team.

All communication is therefore considered **confidential** or privileged. In the initial interview the nurse has the responsibility to inform the client of the confidential nature of the disclosure. The client also has the right to know with whom the nurse will share the disclosed information. The nurse needs to explain that the information may be shared with team members such as the social worker, the physician, and other nursing staff, but not the client's family members or friends. If information is to be shared with them, it is usually done by the physician with express permission from the client.

Often, clients with mental illness have difficulty trusting. To encourage clients to confide in the nurse, he or she must gain the client's trust through honest, open, and congruent communication, and in doing what he or she says will be done. However, the client may wish to confide something that the nurse needs to share. It is the nurse's responsibility to tell the client that secrets cannot be kept. Therefore, it is most important for the nurse to inform the client that shared information essential to the client's own or others' safety or treatment plan will be discussed with various members of the health care team.

For example, a client shares with a nursing student that he wishes to gain access to a sharp object to cut himself when everyone has gone to bed because he is feeling even more depressed than on the previous day. The student explains that this type of disclosure must be shared

with the charge nurse. The client then begs the student not to tell the doctor. The student replies that the charge nurse must communicate to the client's physician all disclosures that reveal behavior harmful to the client.

LEGAL STATUS AND RIGHTS

There is much opportunity for the nurse to communicate with clients regarding their legal status. For example, a client is brought into the hospital by the police who have placed the client on a legal "hold." A client may not understand this term, which can seem confusing. It is often the nurse who communicates to the client the exact nature of his or her legal status, explaining the implications and rights associated with the status. Clients' specific legal rights are discussed in Chapter 3.

INFORMED CONSENT

Informed consent simply means that a legal document must outline any procedure to be conducted or specific types of medication to be given to the client. The client must be informed fully in an understandable manner so that he or she can decide whether to have the procedure or take the specific medication considered helpful to treatment. Effective nurse-client communication is extremely helpful in processing legal paperwork, especially with clients who have difficulty trusting. The nurse must be honest, open, congruent, and clear in all messages given to the client regarding all communication of a legal nature, thus preparing a client to be well-informed and to consent to treatment.

Length of Stay

Another communication challenge comes with brief hospital stays. For the chemically dependent client, for example, the length of stay could be as short as three days. For the client with schizophrenia, it could be a seven- or eight-day stay. Communication must then be geared toward a crisis intervention style of relating where the initial phase of the relationship takes on a new meaning. The data gathering must be accomplished within hours. Thus the nurse needs to quickly establish rapport. If the client's behavior is not conducive to working quickly, then rest and medication can be provided to calm the client so that the preliminary interview and data gathering can occur.

Physical Impairments

Other issues affecting communication are special client care needs. Consider, for example, the client with hearing impairment. If the client reads lips or the nurse "signs," then communication is possible. The nurse must sit in a manner that facilitates the communication. The nurse may wish to inform the other clients what is being done and why. This is especially helpful in a group setting.

TABLE 7-4 Therapeutic responding techniques as related to steps of the nursing process and phases of the therapeutic relationship

Therapeutic relationship phase	Nursing process step	Technique	Examples
Orientation	Assessment and Nursing Diagnosis	*Introducing* self when the client is admitted.	"Hi, my name is Susan. I will be your nurse today."
		Offering self. The nurse demonstrates an honest, open posture, making self available to demonstrate concern, interest.	"I have some information to gather. Let's sit here so we can begin your admission."
		Active listening is practiced by using both verbal and nonverbal skills that show the nurse is giving full attention to the client.	The nurse faces the client and takes an open position, maintains eye contact, uses verbal and nonverbal messages to demonstrate client has nurse's full attention. "Go on. I hear what you are saying."
		Questioning. The nurse skillfully asks open-ended questions during the initial admission. Interviewing skills are necessary to avoid asking too many personal questions in one session. Questions are geared to achieve relevance and depth. Closed questions are used to gather factual information.	"How many children do you have?" "Has this ever happened before?" "How come you stopped taking your medications?" "What is that all about?" "Tell me how you feel now."
		Waiting in silence is used frequently so the client has time to verbalize thoughts and feelings. It is planned and used to draw out the client. Silence should be comfortable for both client and nurse.	Sit quietly, maintain comfortable eye contact, demonstrate interest using nonverbal nods and expressive facial movements.
		Empathizing. The nurse demonstrates warmth and acknowledges the client's feelings.	"I know how hurt you must have felt. It sounds like that made you sad."
		Reality orienting/providing information. The nurse explains to the client the type of unit, gives a brief tour, and provides client with unit information, admission paperwork.	"John, here is a copy of the unit rules. Let's go over a few important items." "You are on the locked unit now." "Today is Friday. You were admitted yesterday afternoon."
		Restating. The nurse repeats what the client says to show understanding and to review what was said.	"You say you are saddened by your friend's death." "You became depressed soon after the accident?"
		Clarifying. The nurse asks specific questions to help clear up a specific point a client makes.	"Did it help when you tried any of the techniques you mentioned?" "Which technique helped the most?" "So your mother remarried soon after you were born?"
		Offering reality. The nurse presents a realistic view to the client in a reasonable manner.	"I know you think people are out to get you. I do not think that. You are safe here, and we are here to help you. This medication will help decrease those thoughts."

Continued

TABLE 7-4 Therapeutic responding techniques as related to steps of the nursing process and phases of the therapeutic relationship—cont'd

Therapeutic relationship phase	Nursing process step	Technique	Examples
Orientation	Assessment and Nursing Diagnosis	*Stating observations.* The nurse offers a view of what is seen or heard to increase verbalization.	"I see you are quite anxious." "I noticed you had trouble sleeping last night."
		Fostering description of perceptions. The nurse requests clients to describe their situation.	"Help me to understand how this is affecting you right now." "What is the voice telling you?"
		Placing event in time and order. The nurse asks questions to determine the relationship among events and helps to put events in perspective.	"Was the birth of your first child before or after your mother came to live with you?" "Did your alcohol abuse begin immediately after your divorce?"
		Voicing doubt. The nurse discusses uncertainty of the client's perceptions.	"I find it hard to believe that you felt no joy on hearing that she survived." "Are you sure you were in bed for one full year after that?"
		Identifying themes. The nurse voices issues which arise again and again in the course of conversation.	"It sounds like that is very important to you. You've mentioned it a few times." "When this happens over and over, how do you feel?"
		Encouraging comparisons. The nurse asks for similarities and differences among feelings, thoughts, behaviors, and various life situations.	"Is this feeling the same as or different from what you felt the last time it happened?"
		Summarizing. The nurse verbalizes a compilation of what has been expressed on a particular subject or event.	"Let me see if I understand your panic..." "From what you describe, your family..."
		Focusing zeroes in on a subject until the important points come into clear view for both the client and the nurse.	"When you talk about loss, tell me more about the losses you've experienced." "You touched upon his drinking. Tell me more about that."
Working	Outcomes, Planning and Implementation	*Evaluating.* The nurse encourages the client to express the importance of an event.	"What does this type of behavior mean to you?" "After thinking about it all, how does it affect you?"
		Encouraging plan formulation helps the client develop steps to make changes and solve problems.	"What are the steps you'll need to take to achieve that?"
		Assisting in goal setting encourages client to set goals during hospitalization and after hospitalization.	"I will help you set some achievable goals during your hospital stay. What are your ideas?"
		Providing information offers data that will help the client in setting goals and developing a plan of action.	"This list and description of crisis houses may help you decide on which one will be best for you after discharge." "I have a problem-solving guide that helps people go through the necessary steps to follow in solving big problems."

TABLE 7-4 Therapeutic responding techniques as related to steps of the nursing process and phases of the therapeutic relationship—cont'd

Therapeutic relationship phase	Nursing process step	Technique	Examples
Working	Outcomes, Planning, and Implementation	*Fostering decision-making* encourages client to work on arriving at healthy, growth-producing decisions.	"Looking over these pros and cons, which alternative would be best for you?" "What would be your best choice, given this situation?"
		Role playing. The nurse plays the part of a person the client needs to say something to, in order to help the client practice what she/he wants to say.	"Let's go over what you want to say to her." "I'll play your father and you play yourself." "Sometimes it helps to say it in the mirror a few times before the real encounter."
		Providing feedback. The nurse provides client with supportive comments in reaction to behaviors or statements made.	"Tell me what you want to say; I'll listen and give you my honest reaction." "When you walked away I felt..." "You may anger some people with a response like that."
		Confronting. The nurse supports but directly challenges inaction on the part of the client.	"I know this is hard to do but I believe it will help you to make a decision." "I understand your concerns; however, you have to take some action now."
		Setting limits. The nurse provides client with external boundaries to an expressed thought, feeling, or behavior.	"You became very angry again. In order to stay in the Day Room you'll need to act calmer. You can walk in the hallway if you need to get up."
Termination	Evaluation	*Evaluating actions* encourages clients to look at their behavior and the outcomes it produces.	"When you tried to do that, how well did it work?" "When you told her to leave, how did she react?" "Was that useful for you?"
		Reinforcing healthy behaviors offers positive responses to the client who is trying out new growth-producing behaviors and making helpful decisions.	"It sounds like you have made a healthy choice." "Standing up for yourself is new." "You've successfully tried it, so now keep practicing it."
		Encouraging post-hospital transition helps the client see that new thoughts and actions can be accomplished after discharge.	"I know you will continue to practice being assertive." "What situations will you run into that will make this new action necessary?" "How can that stress reduction plan assist you at home?" "Which techniques will be useful to you after you return home?"

With clients who are visually challenged, the nurse must physically assist the clients to and from activities, groups, and their rooms. These actions communicate caring and concern, as does sitting near the client when speaking. When approaching the visually impaired client, the nurse must proceed slowly and speak in soft tones to avoid startling the client. Communicating is challenging but it can be effective with the help of the client and the nurse's own sensitivity.

Language and Cultural Differences

People from other cultures experience problems in both verbal and nonverbal communication. Nonverbal communication can create a problem when the observed behavior does not fit the spoken words. Many people from other cultural backgrounds who do not speak English may understand nonverbal behaviors much more easily than those who speak English. Sometimes explicit and suggested meanings of words may differ, causing problems for those from other backgrounds. The use of slang or medical terminology presents many communication problems. When clients are unable to understand a conversation, they may feel cut off or alienated.

If a language barrier exists, the nurse may need to locate an interpreter to help with communication during the client's treatment. Most hospitals have lists of local interpreters who offer their services. For nontechnical, uncomplicated translation, the nurse can usually locate a hospital staff member who communicates in the client's own language. (Chapter 4 discusses this in greater detail.)

Difficult Clients

Nurses may find it difficult to communicate with clients who are aggressive, unpopular, or distressed.

Clients who exhibit *aggressive* behaviors are hostile, verbally or physically abusive, rejecting, and manipulative. These are unpleasant behaviors that are difficult to be around. This attacking style of behavior demonstrates a general lack of consideration and respect for others, and the natural response is to protect the self and reject the client. Even though the nurse's self-esteem and personal safety are under attack, they must meet the aggression assertively by setting firm limits that do not embarrass themselves or the client.

Unpopular clients have a variety of characteristics. Nurses naturally have likes and dislikes regarding client behaviors. The behavior that one nurse enjoys working with may be another nurse's displeasure. Some general characteristics of unpopular clients are shown in Box 7-2.

When dealing with unpopular clients, nurses often feel frustrated, angry, or fearful. These clients may be ignored, labeled as troublemakers or problems, medicated more often admonished, and generally given less care than other clients.

Box 7-2   General Characteristics of Unpopular Clients

- Claim they are more ill than nurses believe
- Complain about their dislike of hospital
- Take up much of the nurse's time and attention
- Misuse hospitalization
- Uncooperative and argumentative
- Have severe, complicated problems and poor prognosis
- Have problems brought on by self, for example, alcohol-related disease
- Have low morals, social stigmas
- Produce feelings of incompetence in nurse

Distressed clients express their emotional pain both verbally and nonverbally, sometimes continuously. Becoming too involved with a client's distress can overwhelm the nurse and interfere with effective communication. Often, the nurse feels inadequate dealing with severe emotional distress. It is important for the nurse to remain clear-headed and to responsibly communicate understanding and concern without becoming judgmental.

Not only must the nurse deal effectively with clients who are distressed, aggressive, and unpopular, but there are also times when the nurse has to deal with health care professionals exhibiting this same behavior. Health care can be emotionally and physically demanding, which produces stress and conflict in the health care environment. There are times when colleagues become irritated, angry, and argumentative, and occasionally even verbally abusive.

The nurse can use similar effective communication techniques when dealing with conflict in professional relationships. Conflict in health care settings has to do with responsibility conflicts, role differences and uncertainty, power issues and beliefs, and value differences. Effective communication skills are necessary in order to deal with a variety of conflicting professional relationships. Win-win solutions are necessary for a growth-producing outcome. Thus, both parties must employ creative problem-solving techniques. Communication efforts are geared toward understanding the other person and the issues involved, employing compromise and collaboration, and avoiding competition. In these situations, nurses should communicate both assertively and responsibly, owning their part of the conflict (Northouse, 1992).

The nurse not only has the skills necessary to communicate therapeutically with clients and their families but also the responsibility to communicate effectively with other health professionals and throughout the health care setting using some of these same learned skills.

Summary of Key Concepts

1. The components of communication are: the stimulus (reason), the sender, the message, the medium, the receiver, and feedback.

2. Communication can be influenced by environmental factors; the relationship between the sender and receiver; the context of the communication; and the individuals' attitudes, knowledge, and perception.

3. Nonverbal communication cues involve all five senses. Ninety percent of communication is thought to be nonverbal. Verbal and nonverbal communication must be congruent for the communication to be effective.

4. Interpersonal communication—communication between two or more people—can be collegial, social, or therapeutic.

5. The three purposes of therapeutic communication are to allow the client self-expression to promote healthy growth, to understand the significance of the client's problems, and to assist in the identification and resolution of the problems.

6. Empathy is an important quality of therapeutic communication and necessary to the success of the nurse-client relationship.

7. Some responding techniques that enhance therapeutic communication are silence, support and reassurance, giving information, interpretation, restating, reflecting, clarifying, and role playing.

8. Self-disclosure by the nurse can be an effective technique if used for the right reasons.

9. Resistance, transference, countertransference, and boundary violations can be obstacles to therapeutic communication.

10. Certain therapeutic responding techniques correspond to specific steps of the nursing process and phases of the nurse-client relationship.

11. Effective communication can be challenged by issues relating to a client's stay in treatment, a client's physical impairments, or language and cultural differences.

REFERENCES

Alligood MR: Empathy: the importance of recognizing two types, *J Psychosoc Nurs* 30:3, 1992.

Armstrong MA, Kelly AE: Enhancing staff nurses' interpersonal skills: theory to practice, *Clin Nurse Specialist* 7:6, 1993.

Balzer-Riley J: *Communications in nursing,* ed 3, St. Louis, 1996, Mosby.

Cochrane DA et al: Patient education: do they really understand us?, *Am J Nurs,* July, 1992.

Edelstein J: A study of nursing documentation, *J Psychosocial Nsg* 21(11):40, 1990.

Ferguson MS, Campinha-Bacote J: Humor in nursing, *J Psychosocial Nsg* 26(4):29, 1989.

Fontaine, KL, Fletcher JS: Essentials of mental health nursing, ed 2, Reading, Mass., 1995, Addison-Wesley.

Fortinash K, Holoday-Worret P: *Psychiatric nursing care plans,* ed 2, St. Louis, 1995, Mosby.

Kemper BJ: Therapeutic listening: developing the concept, *J Psychosocial Nsg* 30:7, 1992.

Morse J et al, Exploring empathy: a conceptual fit for nursing practice?, *Image: J Nsg Scholarship* 24:4, 1992.

Northouse PG, Northouse LL: *Health communication: strategies for health professionals,* ed 2, East Norwalk, Conn., 1992; Appleton & Lange.

Pike AW: On the nature and place of empathy in clinical nursing practice, *J Prof Nsg* 6(4):235, 1990.

Rowland-Morin PA, Carroll JG: Verbal communication skills and the patient satisfaction survey, *Evaluation and the health professions* 13:2, 1990.

Shives LR: *Basic concepts of psychiatric mental health nursing,* ed 3, Philadelphia, 1994, JB Lippincott.

Smith J: Privileged communication: psychiatric mental health nurses and the law,

Perspectives in Psychiatric Care 26:4, 1990.

Stern SB: Privileged communication: an ethical and legal right of psychiatric clients, *Perspectives in Psychiatric Care* 26:4, 1990.

Stricker G, Fisher M: *Self-disclosure in the therapeutic relationship,* New York, 1990, Plenum Press.

Stuart GW and Sundeen ST: *Principles and practice of psychiatric nursing,* ed 5, St. Louis, 1995, Mosby.

Tommasini NR: The use of touch with the hospitalized psychiatric patient, *Arch Psych Nsg* 4:4, 1990.

Wheeler K: A nursing science approach to understanding empathy, *Arch Psychiatric Nurs* 2:96, 1988.

Williams C: Biopsychosocial elements of empathy: a multidimensional model, *Issues Mental Health Nurs,* 11:155, 1990.

Developmental Aspects Across the Life Span

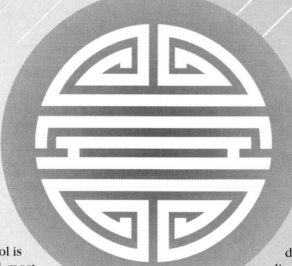

Shou
CHINA

The Chinese Shou symbol is one of the oldest and most frequently used symbols for longevity. Included in the representation is quality of life, from birth to death. The chapters in Part Three discuss developmental issues related to children and adolescents, adults, and the elderly.

CHAPTER 8
Children and Adolescents

Diane Podsedly Oran

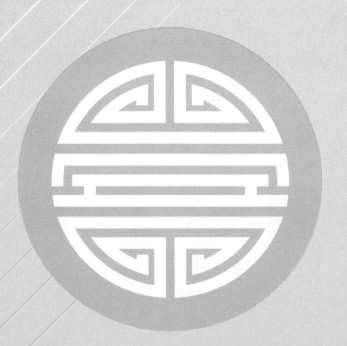

Behavioral reorganization A view of development emphasizing that new developmental capabilities are fitted together and organized into previous capabilities in an orderly, patterned, and predictable fashion and build in a cumulative manner from earlier capabilities toward greater complexity.

Trust vs. mistrust Erikson's term for the first developmental crisis that the child tries to resolve. Consistent, predictable, and continuous care results in developing a sense of trust in oneself, others, and the world. Inconsistent, unpredictable, or discontinuous care results in the polar opposite, or mistrust of oneself, others, and the world.

Autonomy vs. shame and doubt Erikson's term for the second developmental crisis. Parental encouragement toward self-sufficiency in basic tasks of toileting, dressing, and feeding, foster autonomy. Thwarted efforts by under- or overcontrolling parents result in the polar opposite, or shame and doubt. Shame is rage turned against the self. Doubt is an internal feeling of badness.

Initiative vs. guilt Erikson's term for the third developmental crisis. Self-sufficiency allows the child to undertake and plan tasks and join with others in cooperative effort resulting in increased initiative. If the child's desire to show initiative causes excessive conflict in the family, guilt results.

Industry vs. inferiority Erikson's term for the fourth developmental crisis. From the initiative achieved in the previous stage the child develops an ability to master learning and develop peer relationships, which leads to self-assurance or industry. Failure to master academic and social pursuits leads to inferiority and hinders attempts to try new things.

Identity vs. role confusion Erikson's term for the fifth developmental crisis. Self-assurance of the previous stage leads to the adolescent's gaining a self-identity and the ability to determine where the adolescent fits in society. Failure to develop a self-identity leads to role confusion, poor self-confidence, and alienation.

Self-system Sullivan's term for the system that infants develop to cope with anxiety associated with the interpersonal process of need satisfaction and security. The individual develops self-appraisal as a result of significant others' responses to actions from the individual. Actions that cause anxiety result in "bad me" self-appraisals. Actions that cause no anxiety result in "good me" self-appraisals. Actions of disapproval cause severe anxiety, emotional withdrawal, and "not me" self-appraisals.

Sensorimotor period Piaget's term for the first stage of cognitive development, in which children use their senses and motor skills to manipulate the environment and develop the ability to differentiate self from objects.

Preoperational period Piaget's term for the second stage of cognitive development, in which the child remains egocentric, is oriented in the present, and only guesses about cause and effect.

Concrete operations period Piaget's term for the third stage of cognitive development, in which the child begins to think and reason in logical ways about the present and past.

Formal operations period Piaget's term for the fourth stage of cognitive development, in which the child learns to think in abstract and hypothetical ways about future events and learns to develop strategies for solving complex problems.

Adaptation The adjustment of an individual to changing life conditions.

Social learning The process by which children acquire the behaviors they need to survive and function in society. The behaviors result from repeated interactions in their environments.

Preconventional morality Kohlberg's first stage of morality, in which moral decisions are self-centered and the child's behavior is first based on avoidance of punishment and later based on a desire to gain rewards or benefits.

Conventional morality Kohlberg's second stage of morality, in which moral decisions consider the perspective of the victim and are first based on a desire for approval from others to avoid guilt and later based on defined rights, assigned duty, rules of the community, and respect for authority.

Postconventional morality Kohlberg's third stage of morality, in which moral decisions reflect underlying ethical principles that consider societal needs and are first based on a sense of community respect and disrespect and later based on principles of justice, the reciprocity and quality of human rights, and respect for the dignity of human beings as individuals.

Developmental contexts The necessary circumstances that must exist for development to occur. Some circumstances are related to nature (genes, inheritance), and others are related to nurture (environment).

LEARNING OBJECTIVES

- Examine the process of developmental change and the factors that influence development.

- Discuss important historical perspectives that have influenced modern ideas about development.

- Compare and contrast developmental theories and use them in trying to understand developmental progression.

- Describe the difference between normal, abnormal, resilient, and vulnerable developmental pathways.

- Discuss the effects of both genetics/nature and environment/nurture on developmental change.

This chapter will discuss development from birth through adolescence, focusing on both traditional theories of child development and emerging new theories from current research. Developmental theory is important to understand for two reasons. First, nurses must have a knowledge base of normal development to recognize deviations from normal that result in mental disorders that are defined in the *Diagnostic and Statistical Manual of Mental Disorders,* 4th edition (DSM-IV). Second, without knowledge of child development it is impossible to apply the nursing process in safely caring for children and adolescents. Data cannot be collected without a systematic knowledge base that allows one to differentiate normal from abnormal development. This assessment data will in turn affect the accuracy of nursing diagnosis, outcome identification, planning, implementing the plan and carrying out interventions, and evaluating child and adolescent responses to nursing care. Faulty knowledge can lead to unrealistic or improper treatment, which has the potential to cause harm.

THEORETICAL AND HISTORICAL PERSPECTIVES OF DEVELOPMENT

A developmental perspective includes several views of the ways in which children grow and change over time. At any one time children are expected to achieve certain tasks called milestones. In addition to milestones, developmental theorists have identified stages or life periods when changes in emotional, cognitive, and social development emerge. Understanding how children develop involves more than knowing what a child should be achieving at a particular time. Developmental changes occur in an orderly fashion building in a cumulative manner from the capacities that the child accrued earlier in a direction of greater complexity. The rate and manner in which the individual develops and changes is coherent and remains relatively consistent. The 1-year-old child who walked and began pointing at an early age will probably be running in a coordinated manner and talking with more sophisticated sentences earlier than another child who may have been generally slower. Through a process called **behavioral reorganization,** the toddling of a 1-year-old paves the way for the running of the same child at age 3. The 1-year-old's pointing builds up to the 3-year-old's more complex communication of using sentences. The threads of continuity over time are as much a part of development as is change (Stroufe et al, 1992).

Development has been observed to occur with remarkable consistency and orderliness through generations of observations. Developmental change depends on three factors: (1) a preexisting developmental plan built into the organism, (2) the individual's prior developmental history, and (3) supportive environmental conditions (Stroufe et al, 1992). Each individual has a set of genes that are expressed in a time frame that has been set in motion since birth. The exact moment specific genes are expressed in observable developmental changes (phenotype) depends on current environmental support (i.e., nutrients, opportunity, challenges, encouragement, circumstances). Scar (1992) described examples of gene-environment interactions: "Feeding a well-nourished but short-statured genotype will not give them the stature of a basketball player. Feeding a below-average intellect more information will not make them brilliant. Exposing a shy child to socially demanding events will not make them feel less shy. The child with below-average intellect and the shy child may gain some specific skills and helpful knowledge of how to behave in specific situations, but their enduring intellectual and personality characteristics will not be fundamentally changed."

The mechanism by which genetics and environment interact to produce developmental change is still not fully understood; however, important clues can be traced back to the evolutionary theory of Charles Darwin.

Darwin's work focused on evolution of various animal species. Two views of human development regarding heredity and environment can be traced to the philosophies of John Locke and Jean-Jacques Rousseau. Locke saw the human infant as a *tabula rasa,* a blank slate to be written on by life's experiences. Rousseau saw children as individuals from birth and believed that human development unfolds naturally. Rousseau believed that maturation takes a natural course without much need for shaping from parents or caretakers. Locke's work can be traced to contemporary social learning theory, which stresses the importance of rewards and punishments in shaping development. Rousseau's work can be traced to modern maturational theories, which focus on stage-specific development (Stroufe et al, 1992).

There has been and continues to be a debate regarding how much of development is related to nature vs. nurture and biology vs. culture (Scar, 1993; Baumrind, 1993; Jackson, 1993). This debate will be discussed under Developmental Contexts.

THEORIES OF DEVELOPMENT

There are several theories that try to explain how and why children develop. Several theories of development are presented below.

Psychosexual Theory

The psychosexual theory of development was formed by Sigmund Freud (1856–1939). Freud's ideas of development resulted from his work with adult clients who suffered from hysterias and unexplained paralyses. In trying to understand the cause of his adult clients' illnesses, he encouraged clients to talk about and explore childhood experiences using various techniques such as asking them to talk freely about childhood memories, and hyp-

TABLE 8-1 Psychosexual Theory—Freud

Development results from sexual aim or biological need for tension reduction. The goal of development is maximizing need gratification while minimizing punishment and guilt, using defenses to control anxiety.

Stage	Age (yr)	Basic concepts	Developmental issues
Oral	0–1	Id	Internalized, selfish, unable to delay gratification of needs. Primary activities: receiving and taking. Major conflict: feeding
Anal	2–3	Ego	Develops ability to delay gratification of impulses, and self-control; responds to external limits. Primary activity: giving and withholding. Major conflict: bowel training.
Phallic	3–5	Superego	Learns values and rules from parents; development of guilt and self-esteem. Primary activity: heterosexual interactions. Major conflicts: Oedipus/Electra in male and females respectively.
Latency	6–12	Sexuality repressed	Mastery of learning: focus is on relationship with same-sex peers.
Genital	13	Mature sexuality	Combines learning of pregenital stages, develops ability to love and work.

nosis. Freud suspected that the root of their problems could be traced to early childhood traumas. He believed that early trauma caused intense feelings, but because the child was immature these feelings could not be expressed.

In describing how the personality developed, Freud believed that the infant begins life in a selfish, internal, uncivilized state with basic instincts that are aimed at self-preservation and self-gratification. Through interactions with parents the infant learns that selfish behaviors are not always tolerated, which causes conflict.

Within the first few years of life, according to Freud, the ego evolves and is the individual's sense of reality. The ego serves as mediator between the id (primitive drives) and the superego (conscience and values). Freud's psychoanalytic theory is described in Chapter 5.

According to Freud's early theory, all behavior is motivated by a desire to satisfy biological needs and release tension. The amount of frustration or gratification the child wishes to release is expressed through different body zones during the course of development. Freud described development in terms of psychosexual stages (Maddi, 1972). A summary of Freud's theory is found in Table 8-1.

Freud (1923) believed that conflict shapes a person's life. Man is caught in opposition of the two great forces, one force being the selfish, evil individual, the other force being the good society. Life, according to Freud, is at best a compromise. In attempting to maximize instinctual gratification while minimizing punishment and guilt, the individual employs defenses. Whenever an instinct (need) becomes strong enough to make a difference, an alarm reaction occurs in the form of anxiety. This anxiety reaction represents the anticipation of punishment and guilt based on remembrance of past punishment and guilt, and triggers the defensive process (Freud, 1923). The defensive process balances the two

conflicting forces, thereby leading to tolerance of life.

When the inevitable conflict encountered at each psychosexual stage is minimal in intensity, the stage is successfully passed through. However, when the parents or caretakers intensify the conflict by depriving or indulging the child unduly or inconsistently, growth is arrested, or stopped, through the occurrence of massive defensiveness aimed at avoiding anxiety through avoiding conflict. Therefore, conflict in manageable doses encourages maturation, whereas conflict in massive doses arrests development and causes immaturity or fixation at that level of development. If growth is fixated at one particular stage of development, the individual will operate and adapt to the defenses at the stage in which they are fixated. The stage in which one becomes fixated determines the character one carries through life.

The oral character has as its major defenses projection (attributing to others an objectionable quality that the individual possesses), denial (failing to perceive some threatening object in the external world), and introjection (becoming like another person in order to avoid threats posed by them or one's own needs).

The anal character has as its major defenses intellectualization (making socially acceptable excuses for one's wishes or actions), reaction formation (substituting for one's true wishes or feelings the directly opposite wishes or feelings), isolation (severing the links between thoughts and feelings to enable one to consciously tolerate an unpleasant or threatening situation), and undoing or restitution (certain thoughts and actions are used to cancel out or atone for previous thoughts or actions).

The phallic character has as its major defense repression (the active removal from consciousness of instinctual wishes and actions that are threatening). The genital character has as its major defense sublimation (socially unacceptable impulses are channeled into socially acceptable activities).

TABLE 8-2	Psychosocial Theory—Erikson

Development results from social aims or conflicts arising from feelings, parent-child interaction, and social relationships.

Stage	Age (yr)	Virtue	Developmental issues
Trust vs. mistrust	0–1	Sense of hope	Satisfying basic oral and sensory needs: feeding, cuddling, bowel relaxation. Develops trust in self and world. Inconsistent, unpredictable, discontinuous care develops mistrust in self and world.
Autonomy vs. shame and doubt	1–3	Sense of willpower	Satisfying needs for autonomy and free choice: child develops impulse control; mastery of toileting, dressing, feeding, separation from parents. Under- or overcontrolling parental behavior results in shame and doubt in abilities.
Initiative vs. guilt	3–6	Sense of purpose	Learns to plan tasks, join with others in cooperation and pretend play. Accepts responsibility and is enthusiastic about helping. If desire to show initiative causes excessive conflict in family, guilt results.
Industry vs. inferiority	7–11	Sense of competence	Focus on learning and mastery of skills. Success in peer interactions leads to self-assurance. Failure to master academic and social pursuits leads to inferiority and hinders attempts to try new things.
Identity vs. role confusion	12–18	Sense of fidelity	Concerned with how others view him or her. Begins to make occupational choices and fit in society. Development of self-identity leads to making long-term goals, self-esteem, and emotional stability. Failure to develop self-identity leads to role confusion, poor self-confidence, alienation, acting out, and no occupational choice.

Psychosocial Theory

Unlike Freud, who believed that the personality is completely formed in childhood, Erik Erikson (1963) believed that development continued throughout the life span. Whereas Freud attributed development to a sexual aim or biological need for tension reduction expressed through different body zones, Erikson attributed development to social interactions and relationships. Erikson rejected Freud's belief that a child was fixated in a developmental stage as a result of not having his or her needs met. Erikson, instead, described a series of developmental tasks or lessons that all individuals must face and resolve. Failure to resolve the task at a particular stage of the life cycle results in an extension of the developmental period but allows for a gradual movement toward later developmental issues. Furthermore, Erikson placed more emphasis on the quality of parent-child interaction and the responsiveness and dependability of parents in fostering development, rather than merely emphasizing the quantity of gratification or lack of gratification. Erikson described development in terms of eight psychosocial crises or stages. Along with each stage, Erikson associated a specific psychosocial strength or basic virtue that emerges from the struggles that occur during each stage (Erikson, 1982). Erikson's psychosocial theory is summarized in Table 8-2.

Trust vs. mistrust occurs during the first year of life. Through satisfying basic oral and sensory needs, the infant's ability to demonstrate social trust is noted in the ease in feeding, depth of sleep, and relaxation of the bowels (Erikson, 1963). Infants who receive outer predictable, consistent, and continuous care develop a sense of trust and feelings of inner goodness, or beginnings of self-worth. Infants who receive inconsistent, unpredictable, or discontinuous care may grow to mistrust themselves and the people in their world. The infant's first social achievement is the willingness to let the primary caretaker out of sight without undue anxiety or rage because of the inner conflict that develops from the outer predictability of consistent care. This is the beginning of the development of the ego, or self. The psychosocial strength that emerges from a basic trust in the world is a sense of hope. If children do not resolve the issue of basic trust in themselves and the world, they will have a mistrustful disposition toward the challenges that must be confronted in the next stage of development.

Autonomy vs. shame and doubt occurs during the first through the third year of life. The child's ability to develop muscular maturation (including anal) sets the stage for experimentation in the social area of holding on and letting go. Children learn a sense of impulse control and conforming to social rules if they are provided with parental guidance in the areas of autonomy and free

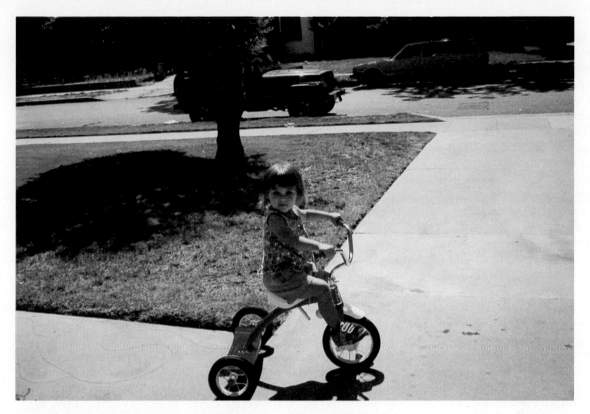

Figure 8-1 Self-sufficiency in mastering basic tasks autonomously allows the 3-year-old to initiate new tasks and take pleasure in being active.

choice. These opportunities for parent-supported autonomy lead to self-sufficiency in mastering tasks such as toileting, dressing, and feeding themselves, and a gradual ability to separate from their parents. Children whose efforts toward autonomy are thwarted by under- or overcontrolling parental behavior are not allowed to develop mutual regulation in the parent-child relationship. This lack of child autonomy results in feelings of shame and doubt for the child. Erikson (1963) described shame as rage turned against the self. A shamed child does not wish to be seen. Doubt is the internal feeling of badness that accompanies shame. This stage, according to Erikson, becomes important for the child's development in the ability to develop a balance between love and hate, cooperation and willfulness, and freedom of expression or suppression. The psychosocial strength that emerges from a sense of self-control and autonomy without loss of self-esteem and shame and doubt is a sense of willpower.

Initiative vs. guilt occurs during the third to sixth year of life. At this stage, children have a burst of energy. This energy allows them to add initiative to the autonomy gained in the previous stage (Fig. 8-1). Initiative involves the ability to undertake and plan tasks, the ability to take pleasure in being active, and the development of a sense of purpose. Children take pleasure in attack and conquest, which leads to developing sexual identity and roles. The child's developing conscience helps to control

initiative. The child learns to join with other children in a cooperative effort through pretend play, and begins to identify with adults and imitate adult-desired behaviors. They recognize adult roles, functions, and responsibilities, and they begin to develop a work identification by showing interest in adult occupations. For example, children at this stage generally show excitement in the presence of a police officer, fire fighter, physician, or nurse. The child begins to accept responsibility and has an enthusiastic desire to help with household chores. Sometimes the child's desire for initiative creates conflicts with other family members, and these conflicts can create guilt. For instance, a 3-year-old child may show an intense interest in wanting to help a parent wash expensive china after a holiday meal. This desire may conflict with the parent's concern that the china may get broken. A parent who wishes to foster the child's initiative might allow the child to simultaneously wash unbreakable dishes. Excessive guilt inhibits initiative. Children resolve the crises by learning to balance initiative against parental demands (Stroufe et al, 1992). The psychosocial strength that develops from initiative without excessive guilt is a sense of purpose.

Industry vs. inferiority occurs during the seventh through the eleventh year of life. From the initiative and budding interest in work identification of the earlier stage, children are able to focus on the tasks of learning and of preparation for a career. In all cultures, at this stage, children receive systematic instruction. The major task achieved is industry, or the ability to master increasingly difficult skills. Because industry involves doing things with others, it is a decisive and important stage in the development of social interaction with peers (Erikson, 1963). Children whose industry enables them to succeed in peer interactions and academic performance develop a sense of mastery and self-assurance. Children who fail to master academic and social pursuits develop a sense of inferiority and inadequacy, which hinders their attempts to try new activities. The psychosocial strength that develops from industry rather than inferiority is a sense of competence.

Identity vs. role confusion occurs during the twelfth through the eighteenth year. With the mastery of social and academic skills of the previous stage and the onset of puberty, childhood ends and adolescence begins. Adolescents are primarily concerned with how they are perceived in the eyes of others compared with how they feel about themselves (Erikson, 1963). They also begin to apply the skills learned at earlier stages and connect them to occupational choices. The task of the adolescent is to develop an identity, which involves finding one's place in society, committing to a career, and developing a confident sense of self. Developing a strong self-identity results in an ability to work toward long-term goals and the development of self-esteem and emotional stability. In their search for an identity, adolescents may temporarily overidentify with cliques and crowds. They can be remarkably petty, clannish, and cruel in their exclusion of others who are different in color, manner, or dress, and they tend to develop in and out crowds (Erikson, 1963). Adolescents who fail to develop a self-identity or who already have self doubts as to where they fit in society run the risk of role confusion, and they may lack self-confidence, feel alienated, display acting-out behaviors, and feel confused regarding occupational choices and the roles they must perform as adults. The psychosocial strength that emerges from the development of identity rather than role confusion is fidelity or loyalty.

Erikson's psychosocial theory can be visualized as a bucket. At each stage, new developmental achievements are added to the bucket. If trust is added to the bucket, it is fuller than if mistrust is added, but the bucket can still be added to. If there is trust, the bucket will likely be filled fuller with autonomy, initiative, industry, and identity. If there is mistrust, the bucket will likely be filled with shame and doubt, guilt, inferiority, and role confusion. This is an important concept in psychosocial theory. Although children may experience developmental stalls, they do not necessarily get fixated at any one stage; they still move on, but their developmental bucket may not be as full if each developmental challenge is not resolved. Unsuccessful resolution of each developmental challenge may present difficulties for the child in accomplishing the positive tasks of the next stage.

Interpersonal Theory

The interpersonal theory was developed by Harry Stack Sullivan (1882–1949). Sullivan was one of the first prominent American-born psychiatrists. Much of his work in understanding development came from his work with adult clients with schizophrenia and neuroses. He believed individuals' development resulted from their interpersonal relationships with others. Whereas Freud viewed development in terms of an intrapersonal process of maximizing instinctual gratification while minimizing punishment and guilt, Sullivan believed that an individual's development resulted from interpersonal relationships in which satisfaction of needs were maximized while insecurity was minimized (Maddi, 1972). According to Sullivan, satisfaction included biological needs such as food, water, air, sex, and excretion, and psychological needs such as desire for power and physical closeness. In trying to meet individual or selfish needs, there is an unavoidable interpersonal conflict from others in the form of disapproval. A fear of disapproval threatens the individual's sense of security, creating anxiety. The individual develops mechanisms to cope with anxiety. Thus an individual's development is motivated by a need for social conformity and a desire to satisfy biological and psychological needs with minimal disapproval from others and minimal loss of security. Rather than describing development in terms of stages, Sullivan described development in six eras. Sullivan's eras are summarized in Table 8-3.

The *infancy era* occurs during the first 2 years of life and ends with maturation of language capacity. Infants are essentially dependent on others for meeting biological survival needs. Infants are in a *prototaxic mode* (unable to differentiate themselves from the outside world). The parents' moods are communicated to the child by an empathetic process in which the child feels anxiety when the parents are annoyed by the infant's neediness or crying, and feels good when the parents show approval in the form of tenderness. Gradually the infant learns to differentiate self from others and determines that comfort and discomfort are connected to the caregiver. Sullivan termed this differentiation the *parataxic mode*. The infant develops a **self-system** to cope with anxiety surrounding need gratification. When the "good mother" meets the infant's needs and shows a positive mood and approval, the child develops a sense that Sullivan called "the good me." When needs are not met and the caregiver shows a negative mood and mild disapproval, the child develops a sense that Sullivan called "the bad me" with accompanying anxiety. The infant is trained through repeated interactions (trial and error) to avoid negative parental mood and the accompanying anxiety it carries for the infant. For example, during toilet training, at first the infant has no control over the bowels. Gradually as the child shows signs of an ability to toilet (physical maturation and motor skills of being able

TABLE 8-3　Interpersonal Theory—Sullivan

Development results from interpersonal relationships with others in maximizing satisfaction of needs while minimizing insecurity.

Era	Age (yr)	Basic concepts	Developmental issues
Infancy	0–2	Trial and error learning from parental interactions of tenderness, or annoyance molds development. Ends with language development.	Infant learns to differentiate self from others and that comfort and discomfort are connected to caregiver: parataxic mode. Develops self-system: "good me" from positive parental mood, "bad me" from negative parental mood with mild anxiety, and "not me" from extreme parental disapproval with severe anxiety and emotional withdrawal.
Childhood	2–6	Language development allows child to be educated, not trained	Language takes on symbolic function of communication. Self-system continues to develop with sublimation (expression of impulses in socially acceptable ways) or develops malevolent transformation (a feeling of living among enemies).
Juvenile	6–10	Relations with peers allow children to see themselves objectively	Increased peer interactions help to give child feedback from others and widen sphere of interactions to include society. Develops conscience. Self-system develops internalized reputation and cultural stereotypes. Able to distinguish fantasy and reality and develop syntaxic communication (a mature method of communicating): their own behavior is connected to others' opinions of them.
Preadolescent	10–13	Develops same-sex chums	Transition from egocentrism to love. Development of chumships helps to validate personal worth through collaboration and mutual satisfaction of needs. Able to work with peers toward a common goal and develop sense of oneness. All for one and one for all.
Adolescent	13–17	Lust: interest in sexual activity	Sexual attractions allow adolescent to test the waters of intimacy. If attractions are severely discouraged or thwarted by adults the adolescent will feel insecure and lonely.
Late adolescent	17–19	Personality integration	Able to become genuinely intimate with others by integrating needs of society without excessive insecurity or anxiety. Inability to achieve personality integration results in regression and egocentrism for life.

to pull their pants up and down), parents introduce toileting and praise the child for desired toileting. When inevitable accidents occur, most parents show a mild level of frustration with having to change soiled clothes. This parental mood is transformed into anxiety for the child. In an attempt to avoid anxiety and relieve the tension of excretion, the child learns that "potty makes Mommy happy and me too." This mild form of anxiety helps to train the child. On the other hand, if the child experiences extreme disapproval and parental frustration and unrealistic or excessively punitive responses, the child may develop a sense that Sullivan termed the "not me." This causes severe anxiety and emotional withdrawal. Without either good or bad emotions the infant is confused and does not know what to do.

If potty training begins too early or the child receives excessively punitive responses to soiling, the child's anxiety will interfere with training, and the child will not be able to associate the parent's mood with release of excretion or any other form of relief.

The *childhood era* begins in the second year with the onset of language development and ends around the sixth year or when the child develops a need for peers. With language development, the child can be educated rather than merely trained through trial and error. Language takes on a symbolic function of communication. The self-system ("good me," "bad me," "not me") continues to develop under the influence of the caregivers. If relations with caregivers are in the range of tenderness and mild disapproval ("good me" and "bad me") without continuous extreme disapproval ("not me"), the child develops the unconscious defense mechanism of sublimation (expression of impulses in socially acceptable ways). One especially important negative development, which Sullivan termed *malevolent transformation* (a feeling of living among enemies), can occur during the childhood era. With the continued development in the self-system via parental influence, the child develops feelings of fear of disapproval, anger, and resentment. If these feelings become too strong, the child is unable to respond positively to the affectionate advances of others (Maddi, 1972). Sullivan (1953) described these children as mischievous, who progress to become the potential bully who takes out their anger and resentment on younger family members, pets, or other children. Parental-communicated malevolence educates the child to become malevolent (malicious, spiteful, ill-willed).

The *juvenile era* begins around age 6 years with the emergence of a need for peers and lasts through most of the grammar school years; it ends around the tenth year when there is a need for close relationships. During this era the child is surrounded by peers and adults other than their parents, such as teachers and neighbors. With this widening social sphere of experience, juveniles are able to look at themselves more objectively, develop a conscience, and begin to function in society. Along with increased peer interaction comes the development of rivalry, competition, and compromise. School-age children develop "in groups" and "out groups" and engage in various forms of ostracism among their group members. Now, security is not based solely on parental approval but also involves a reputation in a broader social sense (Maddi, 1972). In the juvenile era cultural stereotypes with relation to the self-system develop. The youngster begins to see the self in terms of being a Protestant, Jew, a tough guy, or a nice guy (Maddi, 1972; Sullivan, 1953). The juvenile also learns to distinguish more clearly between fantasy and reality and develops the mature mode of communicating and experiencing, termed *syntaxis*. This mode is characterized by a full appreciation of the logical interrelatedness of various symbols, and the recognition and acceptance of their consensual meaning. The child realizes that similar behaviors result in similar opinions about their behavior, from parents and other adults as well as peers.

Sullivan described what he called supervisory patterns that emerge from the self-system and the developing personality during the juvenile era. The first supervisory pattern Sullivan termed *the hearer.* The hearer judges the approval of what one says to others. The hearer develops an internal sense of the extent to which others want to listen to what the juvenile has to say. The second supervisory pattern is *the spectator.* The spectator pays attention to what is shown to others and done with others. It warns the self-system when interactions are not right or if there is a need to cover up for breaches in relating. The third supervisory pattern is *the reader.* This pattern pays attention to others' responses to what one writes. Sullivan believed that he was a poor writer and thus wrote almost nothing. Most of Sullivan's work came through others' interpretations of what he lectured or taught. Sullivan (1953) felt that these supervisory patterns, developed in the juvenile era, remain (with some refinements) with each individual from then on.

The *preadolescent era* begins around age 10 and ends with the onset of puberty and beginning interest in the opposite sex around the age of 12 or 13. The preadolescent transitions from egocentrism to love (Maddi, 1972). The basis for the transition comes from the need to develop relationships with same-sex friends. These friendships help validate personal worth through collaboration. The collaborative relationship is based on a process of learning to adjust to the needs of others as well as one's own needs and reaching mutual satisfaction of needs. The preadolescent is able to work with peers toward a common goal and develop a sense of oneness (e.g., the success of our team or dislike of our teacher) (Sullivan, 1953). The peer relationships of this era are marked by equality, mutuality, and reciprocity. (See Understanding and Applying Research, p. 179.) From these peer experiences, the preadolescent is able to transcend the stereotypes of the juvenile era (Maddi, 1972).

The early *adolescent era* begins with puberty, genital interest, and sexual attractions. Sullivan termed this attraction *lust*. Sullivan believed that lust was often on a collision course with other needs for personal security, freedom from anxiety, and intimacy. Lust, according to Sullivan, is extremely powerful and creates anxiety in connection with the adolescent's newfound motivation toward sexual activity. If attractions are not met or are severely prevented by parents, there may be a loss of self-esteem and personal worth, thereby threatening one's personal security and needs for intimacy. For example, the early adolescent has lustful attractions; however, parents may severely ridicule and prohibit interactions because of their fears of sexually transmitted diseases or pregnancy. Without opportunities to "test the waters" of intimacy, the adolescent is left feeling lonely. Sullivan also described the collision between lust and needs for personal security, freedom from anxiety, and intimacy when the early adolescent is labeled a "good" or "bad" girl in regard to sexual experimentation. For example, the young girl may be viewed as "good" by adults if she does not experiment sexually. On the other hand, she may be viewed unfavorably or "bad" by peers who have had sexual experiences, and therefore be made to feel she does not meet their expectations, due to her sexual inexperience.

The *late adolescent era* begins when the adolescent is able to integrate the needs of society without being overwhelmed with anxiety. The adolescent who does not experience extreme opposition during the previous eras is able to become genuinely intimate with others. The adolescent who is presented with problems in personality integration that are extremely difficult to solve may regress to the juvenile era, thereby losing the values of the preadolescent era. This results in a personality that is essentially egocentric for life (Maddi, 1972). An individual with an egocentric perspective would have difficulty meeting the need for social conformity, which Sullivan felt was at the core of developing satisfactory interpersonal relationships. Sullivan believed that human devel-

Understanding and Applying
RESEARCH

Shields A, Cicchetti D, Ryan R: The development of emotional and
behavioral self-regulation and social competence among maltreated
school-age children, *Dev Psychopathol* 6:57–75, 1994.

Behavioral and emotional self-regulation are important areas of competence in school-age children. In this study maltreated and nonmaltreated 8- to 12-year-old children were rated at a summer day camp on measures of aggression, defiance, noncompliance, impulsivity, antisocial acts, fearfulness, anxiety, prosocial behavior, withdrawn behavior, and social competence. The results showed that maltreated children were deficient in behavioral and emotional self-regulation compared with nonmaltreated children. Maltreated grade-schoolers were less socially competent. In addition, maltreated children's interactions during play reflected maladaptive patterns of emotional regulation by being inflexible and situationally inappropriate in their affective displays. Because a similar process was observed in prior studies of toddlers and preschoolers, this study suggests that emotional and behavioral deficits may be enduring, placing maltreated children at ongoing risk through childhood. The authors suggest that although emotional and self-regulatory processes are interrelated, each appears to represent a distinct developmental path that affects children's competence. Because emotional regulation was related to a variety of behavioral difficulties that impaired children's ability to interact with peers, the authors believe that interventions should target specific behaviors themselves first in priority and in addition target self-regulation of emotions insofar as they promote and support behavioral difficulties. In so doing, clinicians may foster more effective self-regulatory strategies in children, which would in turn help establish positive relationships with peers.

opment primarily results from the learning that individuals gain from their interpersonal relationships within the context of their environments.

Cognitive Theory

Jean Piaget (1896–1980) was a Swiss psychologist whose work centered mainly on how humans develop intelligence in terms of structure and function. Unlike Freud, who studied adult clients, Piaget directly observed how infants and children develop intelligence, which he believed then allowed them to have increasingly effective and more organized interactions with the environment. Piaget believed that all individuals are born with a tendency to organize and adapt to the environment, and he described the basic organizational units of learning as schemas, or schemata. A *schema* is a mental image or action pattern. Schemata may be simple, such as an innate reflex, or complicated, such as a task requiring several steps. Piaget believed that environmental adaptation occurs in observable periods through the complementary processes of assimilation and accommodation. Assimilation occurs when new experiences are incorporated into preexisting experiences. Accommodation occurs when a new experience requires some new way of thinking or a modification of preexisting experiences. For instance, when a child who has been fed solely baby formula is introduced to apple juice, the child may assimilate the introduction of apple juice (a new experience) into the preexisting experience of formula. However, when the child is introduced to solid food, the child must accommodate to the new experience because a spoon and a different texture are introduced. Piaget defined cognitive development in four general periods, with each period building cumulatively from the one before. Piaget believed that a complete mastery of period-specific achievements was not necessary for development to progress into the next period. He was more interested in the process of development of cognitive skills than time frames. Piaget's cognitive theory is summarized in Table 8-4.

The **sensorimotor period** occurs from birth to 2 years. Initially the infant is unable to differentiate self from others or objects and shows only innate, preprogrammed reflexes such as grasping and sucking. Intelligence emerges when the baby begins to recognize objects and grasp for them and begins to suck on a nipple or pacifier for need gratification rather than from a reflex action (Fig. 8-2, page 181). The discovery of how actions can lead to outcomes develops through trial and error. Piaget termed this discovery *instrumentality.* By the end of the sensorimotor period, the infant is able to differentiate self from objects, a term called *decentering,* and develops *object permanence,* a term that means the child realizes an object is in a given area even when it is thrust out of the child's visual field. Thus if a toy is hidden or dropped from a high chair, the 2-year-old child will look for the object. Where the infant operated under the assumption of "out of sight, out of mind," the 2-year-old child begins to hold mental representations when objects or people are out of sight.

The second period is the **preoperational** one, which occurs from ages 2 through 7. During this period the child is able to use mental symbols and words to represent objects and actions, and people and places not present. The child can now engage in pretend (symbolic)

TABLE 8-4   Cognitive Development—Piaget

Development results from a tendency to organize and adapt to the environment. Intelligence development allows children to have increasingly effective and more organized interactions with the environment.

Stage	Age (yr)	Basic concepts	Developmental issues
Sensorimotor	0–2	In-the-moment thinking: ability to differentiate self from objects	Child moves from reflexive action to instrumentability: actions lead to outcomes through trial and error. Develops decentering: ability to differentiate self from objects. Develops object permanence: ability to hold mental representations when objects or people are out of sight.
Preoperational	2–7	Here-and-now thinking: uses symbols and words to represent objects, actions, people, and places not present	Engages in pretend (symbolic) play. Remains egocentric: unable to take another's point of view. Cannot distinguish reality from fantasy. Acquisition of language. Only intuitive guesses about cause and effect. Time oriented in present only. Can only focus on one emotion at a time. Beginning development of self-system. Noncontested respect for authority.
Concrete operational	7–11	Past and present thinking	Able to conserve: understands that physical properties such as volume and length remain the same when there are changes in shape, group, or position. Able to reverse operations. Able to decenter: relates two classifications at one time. Able to think about past and present events but not future. Begins to appreciate perspective of others.
Formal operational	11–16	Future thinking	Able to think in abstract and hypothetical terms. Able to ponder what might be rather than just what is. Can think of future events and develop strategies for solving complex problems.

play. The child remains egocentric and is unable to take another's point of view, and he or she has difficulties distinguishing reality from fantasy. There is an acquisition of language. Intelligence is intuitive, and the child only guesses about cause and effect. The child is unable to relate two classifications at one time (centrality). Time is oriented in the present only. Emotional states fluctuate, and the child can only focus on one emotion at a time (e.g., either love or hate). One minute the child loves his or her parents, and the next minute hates them. The child's ability to symbolically represent enables the child to remember emotions longer in the absence of provocative conditions. There is a beginning ability to experience feelings of inferiority and superiority toward the self (self-esteem). A noncontested respect for authority begins to emerge.

Concrete operations occur during ages seven to eleven. The child is able to understand the concept of conservation and can recognize that manipulation of objects is reversible. The child is able to decenter (focus on and coordinate) two or more concepts, such as height and width or longer and shorter, at one time. The child can recognize that a dimension such as narrowness compensates for the dimension of height. The child is able to imagine a series of events and think about past and present events, but cannot envision future events or what might be. He or she is unable to think logically or ab-

stractly. The child begins to appreciate the perspective of others and develops moral sentiments such as feelings of justice, honesty, and camaraderie. He or she develops an ability to integrate and experience more than one emotion at the same time.

Formal operations emerge around age 11 and fully develop by age 16, although some adults never completely develop formal operations (Sternberg, 1990). During formal operations, the child learns to think in abstract and hypothetical terms rather than merely concretely. The child develops an ability to understand ideas about what might be rather than simply what is (Stroufe et al, 1992). The child learns to think of future events and can develop systematic strategies for solving abstract and complex problems. Teenagers learn to take on the role of devil's advocate and are able to construct logical arguments and see errors in others' logic.

Adaptation Theory

John Bowlby (1908–1990) was an English psychiatrist who was influenced by Freud and Meyer. Bowlby gave credit to Freud for his ideas that an individual's internal world influences the way people learn to think, feel, and behave in terms of how they perceive, construe, and structure events and situations they encounter (Bowlby, 1988). In addition to Freud's theory of internal drives in-

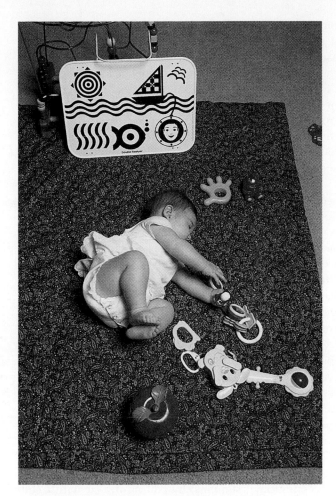

Figure 8-2 Intelligence emerges when the baby starts to recognize objects and reach for them.

(Copyright Cathy Lander-Goldberg, Lander Photographics)

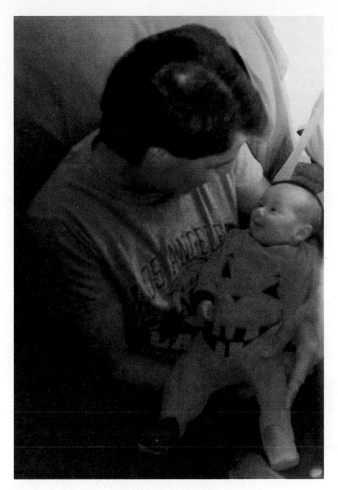

Figure 8-3 The crux of human development lies in the strength of the infant's attachment to the caretaker and in the strength of the caretaker's bond to the infant.

fluencing development, Bowlby gave credit to Adolf Meyer for Meyer's emphasis on the role of events and situations people experience and how environment can influence development.

Bowlby believed that the crux of human development lies in the strength of the infant's attachment to the caretaker and in the strength of the caretaker's bond with the infant (Fig. 8-3). Bowlby was also influenced by Darwin's evolutionary theory and believed that the infant and caretaker are preprogrammed. The infant gives out signals of distress, and the caretaker responds in relation to the intensity of the infant's signal. Sometimes the signal is of low intensity, and the caretaker's response of coming closer to the infant will generally satisfy the infant. At other times the signal is of high intensity, and nothing but a prolonged cuddle will do. The biological function of this signal response pattern was postulated to be protection, especially protection from predators (Bowlby, 1988). Through hours of repeated interactions of signals and responses, the infant develops a generalized expectation about caretaker responses and the infant's own role in producing these reactions. Bowlby called these

expectations internal working models of self and parent and believed that, once formed, they guide future social interactions (Stroufe et al, 1992). When parenting behavior is consistent and responsive, the infant develops a sense that he or she has a secure base, or attachment. When parenting is inconsistent, nonresponsive, or over-responsive, an insecure attachment results. Bowlby believed that secure or insecure attachments are profoundly influenced by the way parents treat the child. Bowlby's (1988) central concept of parenting was that both parents need to provide a secure base from which a child or an adolescent can travel into the outside world, and to which he or she can return, knowing that he or she will be welcomed when returning home, nourished physically and emotionally, comforted if distressed, and reassured if frightened. The parenting role is one of being available, ready to respond when asked to encourage and perhaps assist, but to intervene actively only when clearly necessary. Without a secure attachment and feeling of security, the individual develops anxiety about exploring the world, or feels that he or she will be rebuffed or rejected.

Bowlby described securely attached children as cheerful, cooperative, popular, resilient, and resourceful, and insecurely attached children as hostile, antisocial, impulsive, passive, helpless, or attention-seeking.

Although Bowlby considered the security of the child's base as central to normal development, he recognized that developmental pathways could be influenced by changing life conditions. For instance, an insecurely attached child who had an internal working model of helplessness and defeatism could be positively influenced by a caring teacher whose encouragement, support, and nurturing would help promote a healthy developmental pathway. Conversely, a child with a secure base who loses a parent through death may select a vulnerable pathway. Bowlby termed this process of life **adaptation.**

A recent example of the adaptation theory can be seen in the life of Olympic figure skating gold medal winner Oksana Baiul. Oksana's father abandoned her when she was young, and she was raised as an only child by her mother, who helped form a secure base for Oksana. When Oksana was 16 her mother died of ovarian cancer. Oksana was left vulnerable without a secure base. Her developmental pathway had the potential to deviate from normal. However, her life situation changed, and her base became secure again when her figure skating coach assumed the role of "mother." Oksana's resiliency (obtained from her early secure base with her natural mother) allowed her to face extreme adversity (losing her mother) and become an Olympic champion. After winning her gold medal, she said that through all the stress of competition and loss, her mother was always with her. Oksana, according to Bowlby's theory, was able to adapt because she had an inner working model that promoted resiliency even during periods of vulnerability. Bowlby (1988) believed that a person's degree of vulnerability to stressors is strongly influenced by their development and the current state of their intimate relationships.

Social Learning Theory

From birth, parents try to help infants learn what they will need to survive and function in society. An important aspect of human development, called *socialization,* occurs when parents help to mold the children's behaviors to make them effective members of society. The process by which children acquire these behaviors is called **social learning** (Fischer and Lazerson, 1984). Social learning theorists believe that behaviors are gradually learned and modified as a result of repeated interactions with the environment. Children are socialized not because of an inner developmental mechanism but from environmental responses. According to social learning theory, behaviors that are rewarded will be repeated and behaviors that have been punished will be avoided. This includes desirable and undesirable behaviors. A 4-year-old child who wants a toy from another child can ask for it politely or grab it rudely from the child and get the same result—possession of the desired toy. However, there may be undesirable consequences for rudely grabbing a toy, such as severe emotional reactions in the form of crying from other children, and unwanted reprimands from adults. Social learning theorists would argue that the child would gradually opt for the more rewarding behavior of asking for the toy to avoid the undesirable consequences of crying and reprimands.

CLASSICAL CONDITIONING

Social learning theory was influenced by the work of American psychologist John B. Watson (1878–1958). Watson believed that psychologists could not measure introspective processes such as thoughts and feelings and should limit themselves to the study of observable behavior. Using an experimental technique developed in the early 1900s by Russian physiologist Ivan Pavlov, Watson tried to establish that new human behaviors could be learned through a process called *classical conditioning.* In his original experiment, Pavlov produced a salivation reflex in dogs by giving them food and ringing a bell at the same time. Eventually the bell alone made the dogs salivate. Pavlov conditioned the dogs to salivate in response to a stimulus (bell) that normally would not produce a salivation response. Watson replicated the classical conditioning experiment with an 11-month-old child named Albert. Watson conditioned Albert to fear a white rat (conditioned stimulus) by pairing the rat with a sudden loud noise (unconditioned stimulus). Eventually Albert became fearful whenever he saw a white rat (conditioned response). Watson demonstrated that the behavioral change in Albert (fear in response to a white rat) was due to learning and not to some extraneous factor or innate internal mechanism.

OPERANT CONDITIONING

B.F. Skinner (1904–1990), another American psychologist, further influenced social learning theory by demonstrating that learning was due less to classical conditioning and more to what Skinner called *operant conditioning.* Skinner believed that behavior was influenced most strongly in response to its consequences. Skinner defined operant behavior as voluntary action. Classical conditioning demonstrated that an antecedent event could influence a developmental outcome. Operant conditioning expanded this idea with an emphasis on consequences of behaviors in learning.

There are three basic outcome controls in operant conditioning: reinforcement, punishment, and extinction. *Reinforcement,* a pleasant or favorable response, increases the future frequency of behaviors. *Punishment,* an unpleasant or unfavorable response, decreases the future frequency of behaviors. *Extinction* eliminates a behavior by decreasing reinforcement to a point where its frequency gradually stops. Skinner believed that behav-

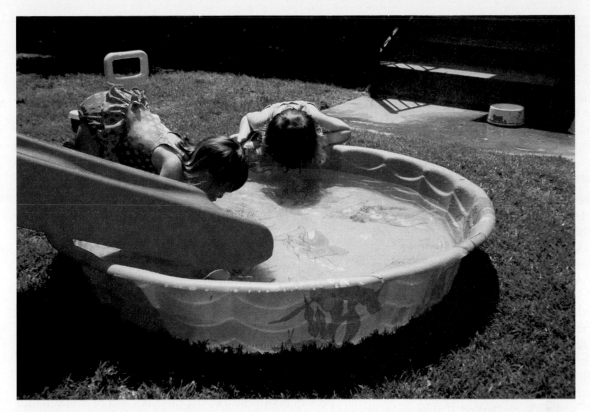

Figure 8-4 Learning for the very young child is initially limited primarily to spontaneous imitation. Later, when the child develops increased symbolic ability, delayed modeling of complex behaviors emerges.

iors could be modified or shaped by varying the schedule of reinforcement. Continuous reinforcement refers to rewarding the behavior each time it occurs. Intermittent or partial reinforcement refers to occasional reinforcement that is given once the behavior is learned. For example, a 5-year-old child can learn to comply with adult requests when adults reinforce the compliance with positive responses such as praise or hugs each time he or she demonstrates correct behavior. Conversely, when the child does not comply, the child could be punished by scolding, being sent to his or her room, or being made to sit quietly in a corner. Both reinforcing the desired behavior and punishing the undesired behavior result in increased compliance by the child. Eventually compliance will need only to be rewarded occasionally for it to continue, and noncompliance will be extinguished.

MODERN COGNITIVE CONDITIONING

Albert Bandura (1986) expanded classical and operant conditioning approaches by stating that learning and development proceeded not merely from reinforcement or consequences but more from the influence that modeling plays in learning. Rather than viewing development as a series of trial-and-error events that are either strengthened or weakened by reinforcement or consequences, Bandura believed that much of social learning is fostered by observing the actions of others and the consequences of their actions. Therefore people could learn

by one-trial learning through observation without ever having been reinforced. Like Piaget, Bandura believed that observational learning depends on one's developmental level. Very young children are limited mostly to spontaneous imitation, whereas delayed modeling of complex behaviors requires the development of the ability to use symbols (Fig. 8-4). Unlike Piaget, he believed that new learning is not restricted by preexisting mental schemes but rather is more a function of attentional, retention, motor, and motivational processes. People, according to Bandura, cannot learn much by observation unless they attend to, and accurately perceive, the relevant aspects of modeled activities. People cannot be influenced by observation if they do not remember or retain modeled behavior in a symbolic form that can be retrieved. They cannot model behaviors if they do not have the motor capabilities to carry out the behavior. People are also more motivated to exhibit modeled behavior if it results in valued outcomes than if it yields unrewarding or punishing effects. More recently, Bandura (1989) has focused on the cognitive factors of self-efficacy or reinforcement. He believes that if one thinks of oneself as capable and effective, one is more likely to overcome failures and master and exercise control over potential threats and challenges. An example of Bandura's approach can be seen in a preschool child whose baby sibling is crying in the playpen. Without being told, the preschooler runs to the refrigerator, gets a bottle of formula, and gives it to the baby. The mother is surprised when she returns from another room to see the baby with the bottle. The preschooler smiles and says that "the baby was crying and now is not." The mother says, "How nice of you to help the baby." In this instance, the preschooler attended to the parental modeling, retained and retrieved the information, had the motor ability to get the bottle, and was rewarded by the mother's praise and the baby's comfort.

Moral Development

The main theorists who have studied the development of moral judgment or reasoning are Jean Piaget, Lawrence Kohlberg, Carol Gilligan, and Robert Coles. The development of moral judgment or reasoning is the process of thinking and making judgments about right and wrong courses of action in a given situation (Stroufe et al, 1992).

Piaget's model begins with an *amoral* stage and lasts until age 7. With the emergence of concrete operations, the child moves to the stage of *moral realism.* At this stage behavior is seen in concrete terms as either totally right or totally wrong. When asked whether an action is right or wrong, children at this stage base their answers on the consequences of the action and ignore the intentions behind the action. When asked if it is right or wrong to take something that does not belong to them, children may say it is wrong because they will get in trouble. Children in the moral realism stage also believe in imminent justice. If they break a moral precept, they think that God or some moral authority will provide retribution. The next stage is called *autonomous morality* and is usually attained during late middle childhood or early adolescence. During this stage, children are able to consider consequences and intentions when making moral judgments. They begin to consider rules as the result of social agreement rather than as absolute right or wrong. Rather than viewing theft as wrong merely because they will get in trouble, children in this stage know that they may make another person feel bad or that others might view them as untrustworthy.

Piaget believed that moral development occurred as a result of both cognitive development and increased social experience. For instance, as children move into concrete operations they are able to appreciate the perspectives of others, which allows them to make moral judgments based on social agreement. The child who has developed formal operations has an ability to think in hypothetical and future terms, which allows him or her to look critically at different moral viewpoints regarding the same situation (Stroufe et al, 1992).

Lawrence Kohlberg also identified stages of moral development. He empirically studied how morality develops at different ages by presenting hypothetical moral dilemmas to children at various ages. Kohlberg (1983) identified three levels of moral development: preconventional, conventional, and postconventional. Kohlberg's

stages are summarized in Table 8-5. At the **preconventional** level the first stage is the punishment-obedience orientation stage. Moral decisions are based on avoiding punishment by authority. The second stage is hedonistic and instrumental orientation. Moral decisions are motivated by a desire for rewards or benefits rather than to avoid punishment. There is also a belief in helping others to get help in return: "You scratch my back and I'll scratch yours." At the **conventional** level, the third stage is good boy/nice girl orientation. Actions at this stage are motivated by a sense of wanting approval from others. Disapproval is avoided not because of a fear of punishment but by guilt that is experienced by not doing the right thing. When asked why stealing is wrong, a child at this stage might say "because people would think you were bad and did not come from a good family." The fourth stage is the law-and-order orientation. In this stage, the moral judgments are defined by rights, assigned duty, and rules of the community. At this stage, when asked about stealing, the child would likely say "you'd be mad too if you worked for something and someone just came along and stole it." At both stages of the conventional level, the child is able to see the perspective of the victim; however, the good girl/boy expresses disapproval of the thief as a bad or unloved individual, whereas the child at the law-and-order stage expresses a sense that the victim's rights as a community member have been violated. At the **postconventional** level individuals move beyond conventional reasoning and begin to focus on more abstract principles underlying right and wrong rather than moral rules. The child at the postconventional level is able to accept the possibility of conflict between norms. The fifth stage is *social contract orientation.* Moral judgments are motivated by a sense of community respect and disrespect. Even if a person does not believe in a rule or sees the rule as arbitrary, he will follow the rule to maintain community harmony. The sixth stage is the *hierarchy of principles orientation.* The hallmark of this stage is that moral principles are abstract and ethical. Moral judgments are based on principles of justice, the reciprocity and quality of human rights, and respect for the dignity of human beings as individual persons. Examples of stage six principles are the Golden Rule (do to others as you would have them do to you), the utilitarian principle (the greatest good for the greatest number), and Kant's categorical imperative (a moral principle is an ideal rule of choice between legitimate alternatives, rather than a concrete prescription of action) (Kohlberg, 1983). Kohlberg believed that moral development was influenced by three important factors: (1) the child's motivation or need, (2) the child's opportunity to learn social roles, and (3) the forms of justice that the child encounters in the social institutions where he or she lives.

Carol Gilligan also studied moral development; however, she focused on the perspective of women and moral development. Kohlberg believed that women

TABLE 8-5 Moral Development—Kohlberg

Moral development is influenced by a child's motivation or need, the child's opportunity to learn social roles, and from the forms of justice the child encounters in the social institutions where he or she lives.

Level	Age (yr)	Stage	Development issues
I. Preconventional (self-centered orientation)	4–10	1. Punishment-obedience orientation	Moral decisions based on avoidance of punishment
		2. Hedonistic and instrumental orientation	Moral decisions motivated by desire for rewards rather than avoiding punishment, and belief that by helping others they will get help in return
II. Conventional (able to see victim's perspective)	10–13 but can go into adolescence	3. Good boy/girl orientation	Moral decisions based on desire for approval from others and on avoiding guilt experienced by not doing the right thing
		4. Law and order orientation	Moral decisions defined by rights, assigned duty, rules of community, and respect for authority
III. Postconventional (underlying ethical principles are considered that take into account societal needs)		5. Social contract orientation	Moral decisions based on a sense of community respect and disrespect. Rules should be followed to maintain community harmony.
		6. Hierarchy of principles orientation	Moral judgments are based on principles of justice, the reciprocity and quality of human rights, and respect for dignity of human beings as individual persons: Golden rule—do to others as you would have them do to you.

reach stages five and six (postconventional) less often than men. Gilligan (1982) suggested that this observation may reflect social roles ascribed to women less than full realization of moral development. Women, according to Gilligan, are more likely to respond to moral dilemmas based on concepts such as caring, personal relationships, and interpersonal obligations—concepts that are scored according to Kohlberg at stage three. Men, in contrast, are more likely to appeal to abstract concepts such as justice and equity—concepts that are scored at stage five or six. Further research has shown no consistent sex differences on Kohlberg's dilemmas, and when there are differences, women actually tend to score higher than men (Stroufe et al, 1992).

Robert Coles (1986) also studied the moral lives of children. He observed numerous children in stressful life situations. He believed that the moral lives of children may not follow a prescribed developmental sequence but may result more from unique life experiences. He observed that even very young children can express advanced moral development in unique and stressful situations. Coles believed that unique experiences that foster moral and ethical development depend heavily on the models to which the child is exposed.

DEVELOPMENTAL CONTEXTS

Spring in California begins in March. The tulips and daffodils are in full bloom by Easter. To a native Californian who recently moved to Maine, spring was a long overdue event. The winter thaw in Maine starts nearly 2 months later than in California, and spring erupts in its magnificent beauty in May. It is hard to imagine the beauty that lies beneath the frozen cover, but it is there waiting for the right circumstances to make the springtime greenery burst. There must be just the right conditions for spring to emerge. The sun melts the snow away and supplies the energy for budding and blossoming, and the soil must supply nutrients. **Developmental contexts** are like spring. A child must be given the right circumstances to grow and blossom in the process of development. These necessary circumstances are called developmental contexts. Some of these circumstances are related to nature (genes, inheritance), and some are related to nurture (environment). The significance of both nature and nurture is a topic of continuous discussion.

The nature vs. nurture debate is alive and well. In her presidential address to the Society for Research in Child Development (SRCD), Sandra Scar (1992) proposed that developmental research during the past 25 years supports the idea that normal genes and normal environments promote species-typical development and that, given a wide range of opportunities, individuals make their own environments on the basis of their own inherited characteristics. Scar (1992) cited the example that smiling, cheerful infants who evoke positive social interactions from parents and other adults seem likely to form positive impressions of the social world and its attractions. Conversely, infants who are fussy and irritable and who experience negative or neutral interactions with their caregivers and others are less likely to interpret social interactions as a positive source of reinforcement. Therefore, Scar supported the idea that an individual's inherited temperament (genotype) influences their social world and ultimately the environment in which they will grow. The central theme here is that individuals create their own environments based on the inherited characteristics they are dealt from birth.

In response to Scar's address, Baumrind (1993) provided a lively response. Baumrind believes that Scar's assertion that individuals create their own environment undermines parents' belief in their own effectiveness as nurturers. She believes that caretakers construct the external environment to which the young child must then accommodate. Baumrind cited Piaget's work to counter Scar's assertions. Piaget contended that the child assimilates and accommodates to environmental input. For Piaget, children's construction of their world is based on experiences that the caregiver provides. Baumrind (1993) also contends that "parent's denial of responsibility for child outcomes is associated with negative child outcomes." She believes that an environmentalistic perspective helps to empower parents to reinforce their sense of responsibility to their children. In addition, Baumrind (1993) cites Patterson's (Patterson and Capaldi, 1991) demonstrations that parents can be taught how to respond in more constructive ways to difficult children or those with special needs. According to Baumrind (1993), negative, hostile, and coercive responses by parents to their difficult children, although natural, are neither inevitable nor helpful.

Ecological Systems Model

Urie Bronfenbrenner's (1989) ecological systems model describes developmental contexts in a way that identifies factors that help shape development and their relationships to each other. The ecological systems model contains four contexts in concentric rings, with each ring influencing those inside. As can be seen in Fig. 8-5, the child is placed in the center of the ring and brings to development the *biological context* that he or she inherited. Surrounding the child's biological context is the child's *immediate environment,* which contains all the settings, people, and objects that touch the child in a direct way. For example, the immediate environment contains the child's home. The home may be a single house, an apartment, a battered women's shelter, or housing project. The immediate environment also includes the family. In the family there are parents, siblings, and perhaps other relatives. The family may be a single-parent family, a blended family, or a traditional family. Other examples of immediate environments are the child's toys, school (teachers, classroom, library), neighborhood (peers, playgrounds), and pets. Each of these different immediate environments provide different opportunities and challenges that influence development.

The people, settings, and objects of the immediate environment are found within a larger *social and economic context.* The home may be indirectly influenced by the parents' employment situation in terms of economic resources for the family or demands placed on the parent at work. A parent who is stressed at work may bring the stress from the social and economic context to the immediate home environment. The parent who is stressed from work may be tired and emotionally unavailable or irritable and impatient. A single teenage mother may have less economic resources to share than a two-income intact family. The child's school is influenced by the finances and policies of the local school board. If the child's school district has limited resources, the child may not get the exposure to a wide variety of educational tools with which to enhance development. The neighborhood is part of the larger city, county, or state context. There may be high levels of unemployment in a city or state that have an influence on social situations such as poverty and crime. The toys in the home may have been subject to regulatory standards for safety. The child's dog may be regulated by animal control standards and must have a rabies vaccination.

At the outer rung of the ring in Fig. 8-5 is the *cultural context.* It contains all the beliefs, values, and guidelines that people in society share. For instance, most adults in the United States share the belief that mothers are important in shaping a child's development; however, some believe that fathers should take an active role too. Most adults believe that children should be able to grow up free from abuse and neglect and that children should be protected. The contexts of development provide the foundation and support for development to continue in an orderly, cumulative, directional, and coherent manner.

Summary of Key Concepts

1. Psychosexual, psychosocial, interpersonal, cognitive, adaptation, social learning, and information-processing are all theories that try to explain how and why children develop.

2. Freud's psychosexual theory holds that the root of adult problems can be traced back to childhood trauma.

3. The stages in Freud's psychosexual theory include the oral, anal, phallic, latency, and genital stages.

4. Erikson's psychosocial theory states that all individuals must face and resolve a series of developmental tasks or issues during the life span including trust vs. mistrust, autonomy vs. shame and doubt, initiative vs. guilt, industry vs. inferiority, and identity vs. role confusion.

5. Sullivan believes that development results from interpersonal relationships in the infancy, childhood,

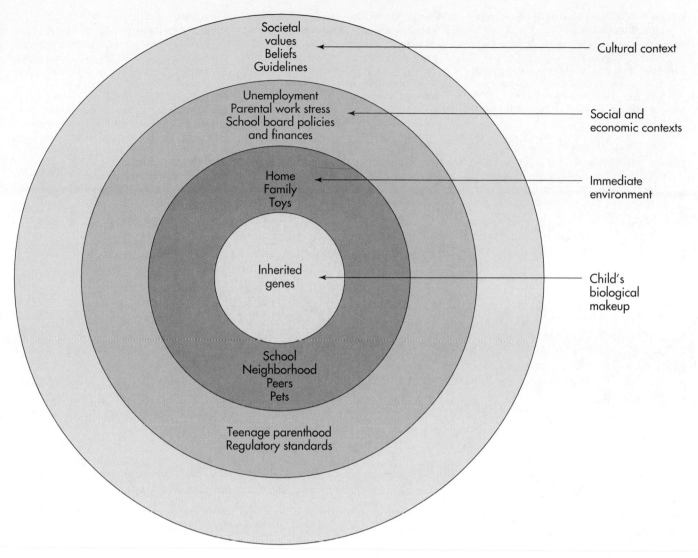

Figure 8-5 Developmental contexts.

juvenile, preadolescent, adolescent, and late adolescent eras.

6. Piaget's cognitive theory includes four periods that build on each other during the life span: sensorimotor, preoperational, concrete operational, and formal operational.

7. Bowlby's adaption theory states that the crux of human development lies in the strength of an infant's attachment to the caretaker, and the strength of the caretaker's bond with the infant.

8. The social learning theory states that behaviors are gradually learned and modified as a result of repeated interactions with the environment.

9. The moral development theory by Kohlberg includes three levels: preconventional (self-centered), conventional (victim awareness), and postconventional (society awareness).

REFERENCES

Bandura A: *Social foundations of thought and action: a social cognitive theory,* Englewood Cliffs, N.J., 1986, Prentice-Hall.
Bandura A: Human agency in social cognitive theory, *Am Psychol* 44:1175–1184, 1989.

Baumrind D: The average expectable environment is not good enough: a response to Scar, *Child Dev* 64:1299–1317, 1993.
Bowlby J: Developmental psychiatry comes of age. *Am J Psychiatry* 145:1–10, 1988.

Bowlby J: *A secure base,* New York, 1988, Basic Books.
Coles R: *The moral life of children,* Boston, 1986, Atlantic Monthly Press.

Erikson E: *Childhood and society,* New York, 1963, WW Norton.

Erikson E: *The life cycle completed,* New York, 1982, WW Norton.

Fischer K, Lazerson A: *Human development from conception through adolescence,* New York, 1984, WH Freeman.

Freud S: *The ego and the id,* New York, 1923, WW Norton.

Gilligan C: *In a different voice,* Cambridge, Mass., 1982, Harvard University Press.

Jackson J: Human behavioral genetics, Scar's theory, and her views on interventions: a critical review and commentary on their implications for African-American children, *Child Dev* 64:1318–1332, 1993.

Kohlberg L: The development of children's orientations toward a moral order. In Damon W, editor: *Social and personality development essays on the growth of the child,* New York, 1983, WW Norton.

Maddi S: *Personality theories: a comparative analysis,* Illinois, 1972, Dorsey Press.

Patterson G, Capaldi D: Antisocial parents: unskilled and vulnerable. In Cowan PE, Hetherington M, editors: *Family transitions,* Hillsdale, N.J., 1991, Erlbaum.

Scar S: Developmental theories for the 1990s: development and individual differences, *Child Dev* 63:1–9, 1992.

Scar S: Biological and cultural diversity: the legacy of Darwin for development, *Child Dev* 64:1333–1353, 1993.

Shields A, Cicchetti D, Ryan R: The development of emotional and behavioral self-regulation and social competence among maltreated school-age children, *Dev Psychopathol* 6:57–75, 1994.

Sternberg R: *Metaphors of the mind: conceptions of the nature of intelligence,* New York, 1990, Cambridge University Press.

Stroufe A, Cooper R, DeHart G: *Child development: its nature and course,* New York, 1992, McGraw-Hill.

Sullivan H: *The interpersonal theory of psychiatry,* New York, 1953, WW Norton.

CHAPTER 9

The Adult

Margaret T. Barker

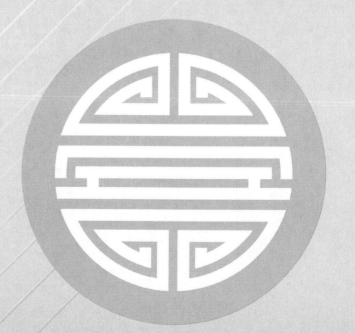

Defense A means or method of protecting oneself; an unconscious mental activity or mental structure (e.g., defense mechanism) that protects the ego from anxiety.

Defense mechanism A structure of the psyche that protects the ego against anxiety, unpleasant feelings or impulses. Defense mechanisms are unconscious and deny, falsify, or distort reality.

Generativity In Erikson's personality theory, the positive outcome of one of the stages of adult personality development; the ability to do creative work or to contribute to the raising of one's children. The opposite of stagnation.

Metaneed The need for belonging and love that emerges as physiological and safety needs are met.

Psychosocial stages Erikson's eight stages in a person's social development, each stage marked by a particular type of crisis resulting from the ego's attempt to meet the demands of social reality.

Rites of passage Rituals such as puberty, marriage, birth, death that facilitate maturational development, associated with life transition. These rites commonly consist of three stages: separation, transition, and incorporation.

Self-actualization A concept developed by Maslow as an ongoing actualization of potentials, capacities, and talents as fulfillment of a mission, and as a greater knowledge and acceptance of one's own intrinsic nature.

- Discuss early and contemporary theories of adult development.
- Recognize and apply Erikson's psychosocial stages in client assessment and care.
- Identify the major life-span transitions.
- Discuss life-span transitions and their biological, psychological, and social aspects.
- Compare and contrast mature and immature developmental defense mechanisms for success in transitional crises.

ADULT DEVELOPMENT OVERVIEW

It is essential for the psychiatric nurse to have a clear understanding of child and adult developmental stages, because many mental health crises result from life-span issues or transitions and are impacted by the individual's developmental maturity. Furthermore, many mental health disorders characteristically develop or are detected at certain stages of life. For example, schizophrenia generally begins in the late teens and early adulthood and rarely occurs after age 50. Although depressive disorders may occur anytime, they generally begin between the ages of 20 and 50, with 40 as the mean age of onset for depression.

Throughout the ages humans have needed to have an understanding of life, its meaning, and their place in the universe. "Where are we going? And what is our purpose?" are questions that have always been asked. Confucius (511–479 BC) saw his own life as representative of man's journey. At 15 came learning; at 30, Confucius established stability (planting one's feet on the ground); at 40, he no longer suffered from his perplexities; at 50, he knew the bidding of heaven; and at 60, he could "follow the dictates of his own heart, for what [he] desired no longer overstepped the boundaries of right." The relevant central themes of ancient writings can be summarized as follows (Colarusso and Nemiroff, 1981):

1. A comprehensive, chronological life cycle can be described.

2. Adulthood is not static; the adult is in a constant state of dynamic change and flux, always "becoming" or "finding the way."

3. Development in adulthood is contiguous with that in childhood and old age.

4. There is continual need to define the adult self, especially with regard to the integrity of the inner person vs. his or her external environment.

5. Adults must come to terms with their limited span and individual mortality. A preoccupation with time is an expression of these concerns.

6. The development and maintenance of the adult body and its relationship to the mind is a universal preoccupation.

7. Narcissism, that is, love of self, vs. responsibility to the society in which one lives, and the individuals in that society toward whom one bears responsibility as an adult, is a central issue in all civilized cultures.

The study of adult development has lagged in contrast to the study of infancy, childhood, and adolescence. Stevens-Long (1992) believed that the lag is attributable to economic, social, and psychological issues. With the introduction of compulsory education it became imperative to study child development to provide the optimum teaching methods and environment. Biologists and psychologists stressed the relevance of child development study as an important source of information regarding the evolution of the species.

The average life span has increased from 45 years at the turn of the century to well beyond 70 years in the 1990s. Longitudinal child studies and gerontological studies are now meeting in the middle (Neugarten, 1979), providing a much-needed focus on the adult years.

ADULT DEVELOPMENTAL THEORISTS
Pioneer Adult Developmentalists

Prior to this century there was little written on a scientific level regarding adult changes and development. It took the writings of four men—Arnold Van Gennep, Sigmund Freud, Carl Gustav Jung, and Erik H. Erikson—to stimulate this discourse. Three of these—Freud, Jung, and Erikson—became the main theorists on adult development, and their work became the cornerstone of later work. The fourth, Van Gennep, in his landmark text *The Rites of Passage* (1908), described the importance and meaning of the rituals surrounding life-span transitions (e.g., pregnancy, childbirth, menarche, betrothal, marriage, death).

Freud's developmental ideas form the bases for psychoanalysis and much subsequent theoretical work. Prior to Freud, issues of adult development were viewed essentially as the "unwinding meaning of hidden springs" within an organism. Freud was both a biologist and a neurologist; he emphasized the interaction of biological and psychological variables and described development as the interaction between focus within the biological organism and the individual's world, which is the psychological experience.

Whereas Freud focused on the developmental sequences in childhood, Carl Jung, a disciple of Freud's, was the first psychoanalyst to study the second half of life. Jung viewed adult development as continuous throughout the life cycle. Jung wrote that adults in their twenties and thirties continue to work on separation and personality individuation from their primary families at the same time that they are trying to establish a family. Jung was one of the first to write a psychological description of midlife transition, with its often growing awareness of the masculine and feminine aspects of personality.

To support Jung's view, there are many women who have awakened to social responsibility and assertiveness, and men in their forties and fifties who have become more aware of their nurturing sides. Often, the reversal of the individual's ego identity is accompanied by questions and ego dissonance "when the husband discovers his tender feelings, and the wife, her sharpness of mind."

PSYCHOSOCIAL STAGES

Erik Erikson was the first to define a developmental outlook for the life span. His eight stages of development were a significant theoretical advance, as it was the first time developmental concepts were validated for the entire life span (Fig. 9-1). Prior to this, development was thought to be complete after adolescence. Contemporary developmentalists base their hypotheses on Erikson's concepts. Erikson continues to have enormous influence in many fields, including nursing, psychology, psychiatry, psychoanalysis, the social sciences, and the humanities.

Erikson and later contemporary developmentalists believed that development is lifelong and that adulthood is a time of dynamic growth and change. Each of Erikson's **psychosocial stages** is organized around a critical developmental issue for the individual self in its relation to the social world. The issue is described as a polarity, that is, two opposites on a continuum, creating intrapsychic tension that results in a unique growing experience for the individual. Each human being must pass eight great tests. Chapter 8 deals in depth with the first five psychosocial stages. At this point it is relevant to touch on the earlier stages to reinforce that the resolution of each stage is interlinked and dependent upon the prior stages.

At the first stage (Freud's oral stage), the crisis is one of basic trust or mistrust, the source of "both primal hope and doom throughout life" (Erikson, 1963). This critical stage is a steppingstone for successful resolution of subsequent stages. The mature, postadolescent personality is a combination of successful or unsuccessful outcomes of the preceding crisis. At worst, a person would be completely mistrustful, full of shame and doubt, riddled with guilt and feelings of failure, confused about his/her roles, and isolated from humanity. At the

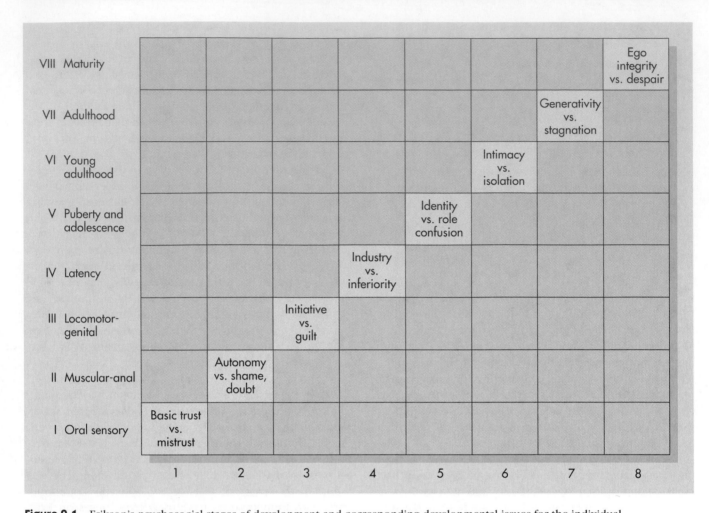

Figure 9-1   Erikson's psychosocial stages of development and corresponding developmental issues for the individual.

(Adapted *Childhood and Society* by Erik H. Erikson, with the permission of W. W. Norton & Company, Inc. Copyright 1950, © 1963 by W. W. Norton & Company, Inc., renewed © 1978, 1991 by Erik H. Erikson)

other extreme, a person would be completely trusting, autonomous, able to initiate, competent, and intimate with humanity. Most people's personalities reflect experiences of both success and failure. In his sixth, seventh, and eighth stages, Erikson discussed key crises of young adulthood, adulthood, and old age. Erikson took psychology and psychiatry beyond a constricted view of the life span to a more comprehensive lifelong view of development.

ADULT DEVELOPMENT WITHIN THE PSYCHOSOCIAL STAGES

Adult developmental stages incorporate the sixth and seventh stages of life. During the sixth, or young adult stage, individuals struggle with issues of intimacy vs. self-absorption. As in each of the other stages, how one resolved the preceding crisis plays an important role in the individual's approach to and resolution of the current task. Successful resolution of the earlier developmental tasks is particularly important for the achievement of intimacy vs. self-absorption. To achieve true intimacy the individual must experience another person's needs and concerns as equally important to his or her own. To have

genuine concern for another, one needs a cohesive sense of personal self and little fear or anxiety about losing oneself in giving to another, whether in the emotional, intellectual, or sexual sphere.

Intimacy requires near-fusion of one's identity with that of another, and to achieve that in any relationship, whether it is sexual, between parent and child, with friends, or in marriage, one must be able to face the threat of ego loss. If one cannot allow oneself to experience another individual on this level, one faces isolation and self-absorption (Colarusso and Nemiroff, 1981).

During the seventh stage, or the midlife period, the conflict between **generativity** and stagnation emerges. For Erikson, successful generativity is simply the concern for establishing and guiding the next generation. This is the midlife, the generation between developing adolescents and aging parents. As early adulthood is terminated and middle adulthood begins, there is a new and necessary awareness of the generational sequence. As children become more independent, aging parents become more dependent; therefore, the adult at midlife is faced with new generational roles, responsibilities, and conflicts.

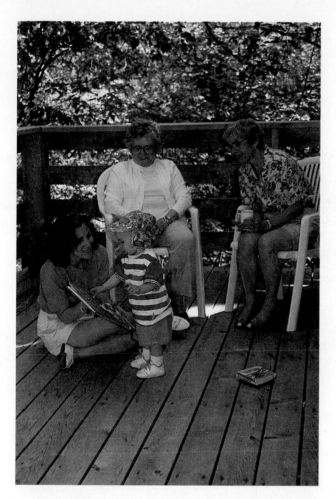

Each generation faces unique roles, responsibilities, and conflicts. Generativity is the concern for establishing and guiding the next generation, something that adults face at midlife.

(Copyright Cathy Lander-Goldberg, Lander Photographics.)

Erikson addresses this as the seventh stage of ego development, the stage of generativity vs. stagnation. Generativity includes the ability to evaluate and appreciate one's past life, embrace the future, assume new responsibilities and new relationships, and acknowledge and utilize one's creativity, in contrast to stagnation in a life of unfulfilling sameness and emotional isolation. When such enrichment and emotional self-knowledge is absent, the individual can regress to an obsessive need for pseudointimacy, stagnation, boredom, and interpersonal impoverishment.

The eighth and final psychosocial stage, ego integrity vs. despair, is covered in Chapter 10. Briefly, those individuals who have taken care of people and have effectively adapted themselves to life's triumphs and disappointments will not be threatened with the despair of an empty, fruitless old age. Truly, such individuals personify the healthy, cumulative outcome of the previous seven stages.

The possessor of integrity is ready to defend the dignity of his own lifestyle against all physical and economic threats. Without successful accomplishment of the earlier developmental tasks, the individual lacks this accumulated ego integration, and may be beset by fear of death and/or a sense of bitterness owing to an unfulfilled life. With the inevitability of death, feelings of despair and worthlessness ensue, rather than satisfaction in a life well-lived. Time is generally too short to try alternatives, and the individual is stagnated in despair.

Contemporary Theorists

In adult life, developmental issues of childhood continue as central themes, but the adult's developmental focus is on the ability of the person to interact with transitional aspects of the life span and the environment. A central theme in childhood is the development of trust, autonomy, and individuation. Integral to adult development in middle and later life is the recognition and acceptance of the finiteness of time and the inevitability of death.

Daniel Levinson, a psychosocial theorist, and associates, in *The Seasons of a Man's Life*, looked at life from the aspect of stages that move from early into middle and late adulthood. The stages are broadly based on Erikson's stages of ego development, but Levinson's group focused less on changes occurring within the person, and more on the interface between the self and the interpersonal world. This requires an assessing of one's self within the world, the functioning of the individual self, and one's relationship to one's world (Newton and Levinson, 1979).

Levinson's psychosocial theory of adult development proposes a universal life cycle consisting of specific eras in a set sequence from birth to old age. The basic unit of the life cycle is the era, which lasts about 20 years, for example: preadulthood, 0-20 years; early adulthood, 20-40 years; middle adulthood, 40-60 years; late adulthood, 80 years-death (Fig. 9-2).

In systematic sequential alternation, stable periods of 6 to 7 years are followed by transitional intervals of 4 to 5 years, each with its specific tasks to be met and mastered. Clinicians find the concept of stable periods followed by transitional periods useful, because internal conflict during the transitional epochs is, for many individuals, an impetus for seeking treatment.

The Harvard Grant Longitudinal Study has followed the life course of 268 undergraduate students from 1939 to the present. The current director of the Grant study, George Vaillant, has used this data to study adaptation in adulthood, particularly in terms of ego **defense mechanisms.** The interviews and collected data supported Erikson's concept of the life cycle. The study examined the qualities that distinguished effective adaptation and how problems were resolved, rather than the absence of problems.

Vaillant's study focused on the intrapsychic styles of adaptation first described by Freud. These ego mechanisms of defense are major means of managing instinct and affect. They are unconscious, discrete from one an-

Developmental Periods

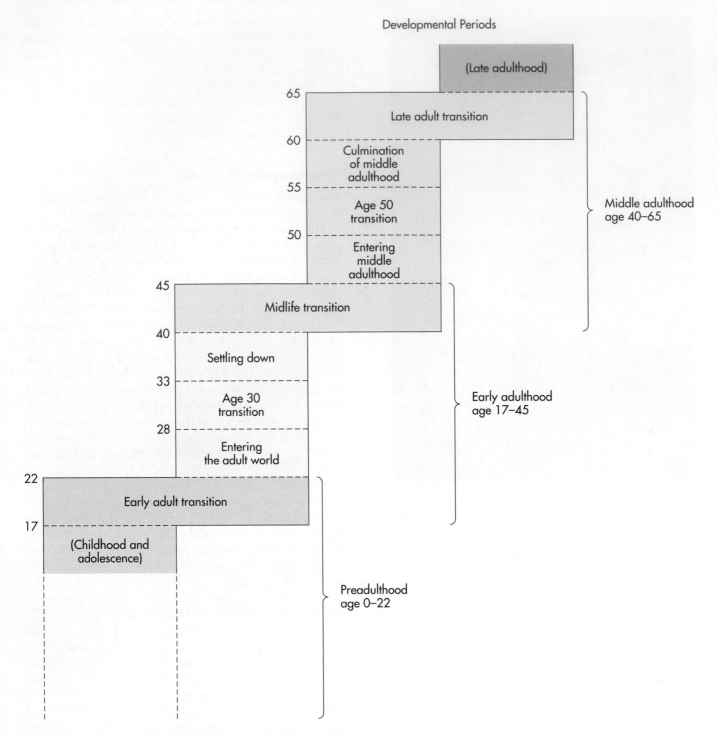

Figure 9-2 Levinson's psychosocial theory of adult development.
(From Levinson DJ et al: *The seasons of a man's life*, New York, 1986, Ballantine.)

other, dynamic, and reversible, and can be adaptive as well as pathologic. Building on Freud's work and using data collected from the Harvard study, Vaillant devised a theoretic hierarchy, grouping eighteen defenses according to their relative maturity and pathology (Box 9-1).

Central to Vaillant's work is the thesis that if individuals are to master conflict gracefully, and are to be successful and efficient in their life choices, ego defense mechanisms must change and mature throughout the life cycle. What distinguished effective adaptations was how problems were dealt with, not the absence of problems.

In looking at the change in specific **defenses** over time, Vaillant's group traced the decline of the defense mechanisms of fantasy and acting out, with the emergence of maturity and an accompanying increase in suppression. Dissociation, repression, sublimation, and altruism increase in midlife, while projection, hypochondriasis, and masochism are most common in adoles-

Box 9-1   Vaillant's Hierarchy of Adaptive Mechanisms

Level I: Psychotic mechanisms (common in psychosis, dreams, childhood)

Denial (of external reality)
Distortion
Delusional projection

Level II: Immature mechanisms (common in severe depression, personality disorders, and adolescence)

Fantasy (schizoid withdrawal, denial through fantasy)
Projection
Hypochondriasis
Passive-aggressive behavior (masochism, turning against the self)
Acting out (compulsive delinquency, perversion)

Level III: Neurotic mechanisms (common in everyone)

Intellectualization (isolation, obsessive behavior, undoing, rationalization)
Repression
Reaction formation
Displacement (conversion, phobias, wit)
Dissociation (neurotic denial)

Level IV: Mature mechanisms (common in "healthy" adults)

Sublimation
Altruism
Suppression
Anticipation
Humor

From Vaillant GE: *Adaptation to life*, Boston, 1974, Little, Brown.

cence. Vaillant points out that the decade from 25 to 35 years is a guilty period, in which defenses of reaction formation and repression are used with greater frequency.

Vaillant compared men who were considered generative, that is, more psychosocially mature in Eriksonian terms, with a group of "perpetual boys," men who retained immature qualities. Over time, the perpetual boys failed to show any significant shift in their adaptive patterns, unlike the pattern seen in the generative men (Vaillant, 1977).

Vaillant described the association between adult maturity and external adjustment. He contrasted the subjects with the best and worst outcomes in negotiating Erikson's psychosocial stages of development. Vaillant was able to document that difficulties for those with worst outcomes began in childhood, with events seen as traumatic and interfering with the establishment of basic trust, autonomy, and initiative.

Those men who had difficulty with the earlier psychosocial stages appeared to be less well integrated in adolescence, and, subsequently, their identities were less secure as adults. They were also less likely to have internalized their fathers as role models and still seemed dependent on their mothers. Finally, both at age 30 and 50, these individuals were still having trouble with intimacy. Their marriages and friendships were more likely to be problematic, and they seemed to be considerably less generative in the sense of being willing to assume responsibility for other adults.

PERSONALITY DISORDERS: AN ADULT DEVELOPMENT PERSPECTIVE

Many mental health professionals have little interest in exploring the relationship between personality, behavior, and early childhood influences. The roles of heredity and environmental factors continue to be subject to disagreement. But despite the different viewpoints, psychoanalytic and psychosocial experts do concur that the child's earliest years critically affect subsequent development and behavior. It is understood that later experiences and environmental conditions can either reinforce or reverse early influences as they interact with the personality (Blanck and Blanck, 1974, 1979; Millon, 1987).

The inflexible, maladaptive life patterns that are the hallmark of personality disorders can be viewed as originally developing as defensive survival patterns. However dysfunctional the personality style, it seems safe to observe that, at one time, such behavior was the individual's safeguard against intolerable anxiety, self-hate, helplessness, and insecurity created by the early developmental environment. These behaviors and personality styles were a means for warding off unacceptable sexual or hostile impulses. At the time these defensive styles are developed, to protect against inner and outer threats, they may be the most adaptive alternatives available to the young person unconsciously creating them.

Defensive life patterns can prevent the development of healthy defense mechanisms. For example, the individual with a dependent personality disorder or dependent traits may never have developed defenses against separation anxiety, which is necessary for autonomy, individuation, and the ability to deal effectively with reality (Millon, 1987; Bowlby, 1988).

Defensive personality traits may be converted into assets. Many nurses have strong caregiving qualities, which may have been defensive adaptations in early life. Perhaps as a young child, the nurse defended against feelings of insecurity by eventually becoming a protective caregiver for dependent, vulnerable, mentally or physically frail adults.

A thorough overview of the literature regarding personality disorders is beyond the scope of this chapter. See Chapter 14 for more comprehensive information.

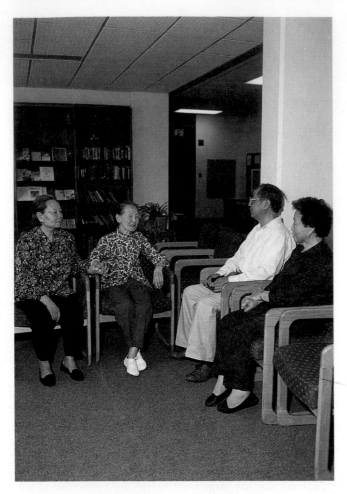

A normal adult life transition is providing support and care for one's parents as they age.

(Copyright Cathy Lander-Goldberg, Lander Photographics.)

LIFE-SPAN TRANSITIONS
Transitions

Normative adult life transitions consist of leaving one's original family, forming new relationships, starting a family, having and raising children, children leaving home, reforming as a couple, becoming adult caregivers for the older generation, and retirement. Throughout these normal life stressors, an individual's ability to use learned coping strategies and unconscious ego defense mechanisms to resolve crises or transitions depends on earlier accomplishment of developmental tasks. Any of the above can become extraordinary life stressors if they occur out of sequence to life's expected developmental pattern. Individuals who seek help often have a combination of poor mastery of developmental tasks and a life stressor that is unexpected (e.g., an out-of-sequence life event such as the premature death of a parent or child), which results in ego dissonance and crisis. All individuals need added support at these times, and individuals with fragile ego development tend to need more intensive support, perhaps even hospitalization, during these crises.

Midlife Transitions

The term *midlife crisis* is a misnomer, because many changes that occur at midlife are not crises. Transitions generate a range of feelings and events in individuals, from a private, low-key introspection to a more obvious transition, but few experience a dramatic midlife change and possibly a crisis. Levinson et al (1978) prefer the term *midlife transitions* because it includes aspects of crisis, process, and change. According to Levinson et al, approximately 80% of individuals experience the period of midlife—the years crossing the third and fourth decade—as marked by tumultuous struggles within the individual and the external world.

During the years between the late thirties or early forties and continuing at an individual-specific rate throughout the life span, the beginnings of expected midlife biological changes occur. These include alterations in strength and endurance, skin and muscle tone, hearing, and vision. Reaction time may also be affected, as well as graying or loss of hair and sexual function. These changes affect individuals differently, often depending on how each person has achieved the earlier developmental tasks, and one's level of knowledge and self-acceptance. Integral to acceptance and mastery of these changes is the individual's ability to incorporate the concept of death and perception of time in such a way as to accept it as part of life. Neugarten (1975) described a shift in thinking from asking oneself "How long have I lived?" to "How long do I have left?"

Rites of Passage: Meaning and Purpose

Although much of our socialization takes place gradually, during certain transitional periods the shaping of adult development within the context of the social structure is accelerated, often creating a feeling of anxiety and crisis. Some of these transitions may be closely associated with biological developments like menstruation and menopause, and others are influenced by sociocultural factors, such as school graduation, marriage, or retirement.

Transitions are frequently occasions for ceremonies that focus on the importance of the person's change in status and affirm his or her new place in society. Rituals can contribute to a person's identity and make change manageable. Rituals are steppingstones toward resolving conflict and facilitating maturational development and change through such life transitions as puberty, marriage, birth, and death. The rituals associated with these transitions are called **rites of passage**. These rites commonly comprise three stages: separation, transition, and incorporation (Van Gennep, 1960).

The marriage ceremony in many Western cultures provides a clear example of the stages of a rite of passage. In the first stage the bride is separated physically from the groom until the ceremony, where she prepares herself for her change in status; she is separated symbolically by the veil over her face, which shields her against the external world. The transitional stage is the ceremony, or ritual, in which the bride and groom are suspended between the old existence and the new. During the ceremony, spiritual leaders often offer guidance for the new life that is to follow. Vows and rings are exchanged to bind the couple as a unit. Finally, the newly married couple is reintroduced to the wedding party and guests as husband and wife, which indicates their new beginning. Parents and friends deliver speeches at the celebration following the ceremony, offering words intended to help them as they enter the world in their new status. The honeymoon follows, where the couple has a chance to adapt to their new status and new roles before they return.

Rites of passage are cross-cultural. Van Gennep (1960) described these rites as necessary to facilitate the transition from group to group and from one social situation to the next. They are viewed as critical to an individual's and to a society's existence. In all cultures, men and women's lives are made up of a succession of stages with similar ends and beginnings: birth, social puberty, marriage, parenthood, advancement to a higher social class, occupational specialization, and death. For each of these events, there are ceremonies whose essential purpose is to enable the individual to pass from one defined position to another equally defined position.

Many contemporary social scientists and clinicians believe that with each life transitional crisis, these unique social rituals help an individual achieve his or her potential and obtain group support in the transition. With the decline in sacred rituals and ceremonies, individuals and social groups are forced to accomplish their life tasks during transitional periods, essentially alone, often failing or not completing the needed maturational development. As a result, their individual potential and development may be compromised, and the family and society may also be adversely impacted (Colarusso and Nemiroff, 1981).

GENDER DIFFERENCES IN ADULT DEVELOPMENT

There are important basic similarities between adult male and adult female development, but there are also significant differences. These differences have only recently been recognized, because all early studies on adult development were carried out with male subjects. Only recently have studies included women or examined gender differences.

Psychological Differences

In analyzing the responses of both men and women to four natural transitions (i.e., leaving one's primary family, starting a family, children leaving home, and retiring),

there are significant differences in how the two genders deal with each transition (Lowenthal, Turner, and Cheroboga, 1975). These differences become more apparent with age, indicating that the development parallels throughout adolescence and early adulthood, but diverges through the late twenties. At 30, when most people reassess their life structure, women seem to struggle between two major life choices: whether to marry and start a family or work on a career first. Those who attempt to do both at the same time may deal with consequences such as guilt, anxiety, and fatigue. Those who postpone either the family or the career may fear that time is running out and that one of their life choices will be sacrificed.

Hormonal Differences

Hormonal differences and their relationship to mood have been studied extensively. Postpartum psychosis and postpartum depression have been related to the precipitous postpartum reduction, in chorionic gonadtropins (Vandeburgh, 1989). Bardwick (1976) hypothesized that premenstrual depression is related to low levels of estrogen, which has been shown to induce high levels of monoamine oxidase (MAO). Estrogen appears to be the most potent of the gonadal hormones affecting MAO levels. High levels of MAO at the synapse are associated with low levels of catecholamines, a state associated with certain types of depression. An increase in estrogen, which elevates mood, may act to decrease the quantity of MAO or to increase the levels of catecholamines. It is important for the psychiatric nurse to be aware of this, especially with clients who are postoophorectomy, who have total hysterectomy, or who are in their late thirties through early fifties. Certainly with a first-time depression during this age range, the possibility of a hormonal imbalance should be ruled out. Studies have shown that:

The rate of depression is twice as high for women as for men in the United States and in Western societies. Depression resembles grief because feelings of loss and sadness dominate the emotions. Depression has components involving self-esteem, cognition, sleep, appetite, energy level, and behavior (DSM-IV, 1994; Bardwick, 1976).

As mood and the endocrine system are interrelated, so is the gender response to the tricyclic antidepressants. Women not only become depressed more often than men, but also demonstrate slower response to tricyclic antidepressants. Women are most affected by losses involving close relationships, whereas men tend to become depressed with the loss of an ideal, an achievement-related goal, or a performance issue. Many middle-aged women experience the loss of their youth by becoming painfully preoccupied with the physical signs of aging. Society's overvaluation of the youthful female body results in fears of being "unsexed" by the aging process and losing love as a consequence. Men generally are not faced so brutally with this issue, because male sexuality is depicted by society as continuing well beyond midlife.

Social Differences

Women appear to be more pressured and restricted than men by what Neugarten (1973) terms a *socially defined sense of time*, or a sense of the temporal appropriateness of major events. Such socially defined standards are based on the male life cycle, which places career as the dominant component. Women who have raised a family are viewed as out of synchrony with current standards. Often where there is a shift between one's career goals and the desire to start a family, this change in goals can result in a serious midlife reappraisal of career, marriage, goals, life, and an individual's essential values.

Depression occurring at this stage, as in any other transitional phase, requires a mourning period to enable the individual to move and grow beyond the confusion of the developmental crisis.

HIERARCHY OF NEEDS

The construct of human need satisfaction has played an important role in nursing theory, education, and practice. A chapter on adult development would be incomplete without a review of Maslow's theory of the hierarchy of needs (Maslow, 1968, 1970) (Table 9-1). The existence of unmet needs and the desire to achieve optimum self-potential are fundamental sources of human motivation. Essential needs constitute an inexact hierarchy of relative predominance, beginning with the most urgent physiological necessities and culminating in the search for self-actualization.

Physiological needs include the somatically based drives of hunger, thirst, sexual desire, and the need for activity, exercise, sleep, rest and sensory pleasure. With the gratification of these most basic needs, other higher needs emerge, such as more socially oriented goals and the predominance of the need for safety and security, including stability, protection, and freedom from fear, anx-

iety, and chaos. People with unmet safety needs experience their world as hostile or threatening. Individuals with met safety needs perceive their world as trustworthy and are more self-directed, autonomous, and interested in others.

Metaneeds

As the physiological needs are met, the need for belonging and love emerges; these **metaneeds** include the yearnings for affection, intimacy, and establishing relationships with others to find a place in one's peer group. The person with unmet love and intimacy needs is likely to experience feelings of desolation, alienation, and rejection.

The fourth level of Maslow's hierarchy describes the need for self-esteem, and respect and esteem from others. Self-esteem needs include a desire for adequacy, self-respect, competence, independence, and freedom. The need to acquire esteem or respect from others includes the desire for recognition, dignity, and appreciation. When any of these four human needs is frustrated, a deficiency in one's motivation predominates. Individuals with deficient motivation experience feelings of threat, anxiety, and tension, and they tend to use immature defense mechanisms, such as projection, in an effort to gratify the prevailing need. In contrast, individuals whose physiological and safety needs have been met, are characterized by a predominance of growth, maturation, and an appreciation of challenge (Maslow, 1970).

The final need to emerge, when all prior needs are relatively satisfied, is the desire for **self-actualization**. This is defined as an ongoing actualization of potentials, capacities, and talents, as fulfillment of a mission (or call, fate, destiny, or vocation), and as a greater knowledge and acceptance of the individual's intrinsic nature. Therefore this need is not environmentally dependent. Rather, it is a process of growth and development from within that is considered rewarding and exciting. Although this higher-level need develops only as lower needs are satisfied, the need for self-actualization can become relatively independent of those fundamental de-

TABLE 9-1 Maslow's hierarchy of needs

Need	Characteristic
1. Physiological	Satisfying needs for oxygen, water, food, shelter, sleep, relief of sexual tension
2. Safety	Avoiding harm and achieving security and physical safety
3. Love and belonging	Giving and receiving affection, developing companionship, and gaining acceptance by a group
4. Esteem and recognition	Achieving recognition by others, leading to self-esteem and feelings of prestige; achieving success in work
5. Self-actualization	Achieving one's own unique potential in all dimensions

Understanding and Applying
RESEARCH

Anderson-Whiting S: A Delphi study to determine defining characteristics of interdependence and dysfunctional independence as potential nursing diagnoses, *Ment Health Nurs* 115:37-47, 1994.

The focus of this study was on the patterns of individual behaviors that influence relationships and interactions. Behavioral patterns studied were dependence, independence, and interdependence. The purpose of the study was to:

1. Determine the defining characteristics for interdependence and dysfunctional independence.
2. Determine the prevalence of the behavior patterns according to gender and race.
3. Generate questions for hypothesis testing.
4. Add to the nursing taxonomy.

Over 100 certified psychiatric-mental health clinical nurse specialists who encounter these behaviors in their clients, participated in three rounds of a Delphi study. The Delphi technique was used because it has been found useful for generating, analyzing, and synthesizing expert opinions about controversial or intangible content. From a collection of judgments, this technique achieves a uniform opinion through repetition and controlled feedback.

The results suggest there is agreement on the behavior patterns and characteristics of dependence, independence, and interdependence. It confirmed a set of defining characteristics for interdependence and dysfunctional independence. Nurses can use these defining characteristics as criteria to measure client behaviors against, and to establish client goals.

tion. He wrote that from the stages of life come faith, willpower, purposefulness, competence, fidelity, love, care, and wisdom— all criteria of vital individual strength that also flow into the institutions. Without these strengths, institutions wilt; but without the spirit of institutions and training, no strength can emerge for the next generations. Psychosocial strength depends on a total process that regulates the individual's life cycles, the sequence of generations, and the structure of society simultaneously (Erikson, 1974).

Summary of Key Concepts

1. Freud believed that development is the result of biological and psychological interactions.
2. Jung viewed adult development as continuous throughout the life cycle.
3. Erikson's eight psychosocial stages and developmental tasks are the following: oral sensory, basic trust/mistrust; muscular-anal, autonomy/shame, doubt; locomotor-genital, initiative/guilt; latency, industry/inferiority; puberty and adolescence, identity/role confusion; young adulthood, intimacy/isolation; adulthood, generativity/stagnation; and maturity, ego integrity/despair.
4. Successful resolution of earlier crises determines the likelihood of resolution of current crises.
5. Generativity, the task of the seventh psychosocial stage, includes the ability to evaluate and appreciate one's past life, embrace the future, assume new responsibilities and relationships, and acknowledge and utilize one's creativity.
6. Modern theorists view adult development as an ongoing dynamic process.
7. Adult development is concerned with the continued evolution of that structure previously developed in childhood.
8. Vaillant's theory holds that if individuals are to master conflict gracefully, and to be successful and efficient in their life choices, ego defense mechanisms must change and mature throughout the life cycle.
9. Defensive personality traits may prevent the development of healthy defense mechanisms and/or be converted into assets.

sires, as the sense of satisfaction develops through the self-actualization process and becomes well established (Maslow, 1970).

Most individuals are partially satisfied and partially unsatisfied in their basic needs at any given time. An individual can be helped to meet the basic and metaneeds through support, reassurance, acceptance, education, and protection. These actions are the therapeutic essence of nursing practice and the core of many nursing theories. (See the box Understanding and Applying Research above.)

Optimum Growth

Erikson put it well when he wrote about optimum opportunity for growth, and a person's ability to continue to grow and mature, individually and within an institu-

REFERENCES

Bardwick J: Psychological correlates of the menstrual cycle and oral contraceptive medication. In Sachar E, editor: *Hormones, behavior, and psychopathology,* New York, 1976, Raven.

Blanck G, Blanck R: *Ego psychology: theory and practice,* New York, 1974, Columbia University Press.

Blanck G, Blanck R: *Ego psychology,* ed. 11, New York, 1979, Columbia University Press.

Bowlby J: *A secure base: clinical applications of attachment theory,* London, 1988, Routledge.

Colarusso CA, Nemiroff RA: *Adult development,* New York, 1981, Plenum Press.

Diagnostic and Statistical Manual of Mental Disorders, ed. 4, Washington, DC, 1994, American Psychiatric Association.

Erikson EH: *Childhood and society,* ed. 2, New York, 1974, WW Norton.

Erikson EH: *Dimensions of a new identity: Jefferson lectures,* New York, 1974, WW Norton.

Erikson EH: *Eight stages of man in childhood & society.* New York, 1963, WW Norton.

Levinson DJ et al: *The seasons of a man's life,* New York, 1978, Alfred A. Knopf.

Lowenthal MF, Turner M, Cheroboga D: *Four stages of life: A comparative study of men and women facing transitions.* San Francisco, 1975, Jossey-Bass.

Maslow AH: *Motivation & personality.* New York, 1954, Harper & Row.

Millon T: *Millon clinical multi axial inventory manual* 3ed.) Minneapolis, 1987, National Computer Systems.

Neugarten BL: Time, age, and the life cycle, *Am J Psychiatr* 136:887, 1979.

Newton PM, Levinson DJ: Crisis in adult development. In Lazare A, editor: *Outpatient. Psychiatry, diagnosis and treatment,* Baltimore, 1979, Williams and Wilkins.

Stevens-Long J: *Adult life: developmental processes,* 4, Palo Alto, Calif, 1992, Mayfield.

Vaillant GE: *Adaptation to life,* Boston, 1977, Little, Brown.

Vandenbergh RL: Postpartum depression, *Clin Obstet Gynocol* 23:1105-1111, 1980.

Van Gennep A: *The rites of passage,* Chicago, 1960, University of Chicago Press.

CHAPTER 10
The Elderly

Linda Hollinger-Smith

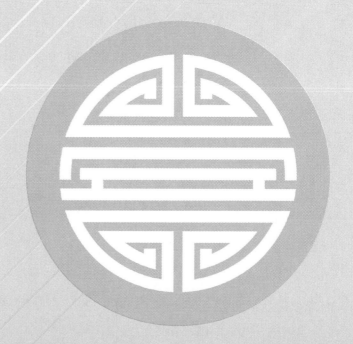

Activities of daily living (ADL) Categories of personal care (e.g., bathing, grooming, toileting, etc.)

Activity theory Theory that supports that maintaining an active lifestyle and social roles offsets the negative effects of aging

Ageism Systematic stereotyping and discrimination against the elderly

Cohort A group having one or more factors in common

Continuity theory Theory that promotes the premise that people become "more like themselves" as they age, maintaining continuity of habits, beliefs, and values

Dependency ratio The number of individuals under age 18 and over age 64 who are dependent on persons age 18 to 64 years

Disengagement theory Process of mutual withdrawal between the aging individual and society

Dystonic Pertaining to unstable states or to some disorder

Gerontology The study of the aging process involving multiple disciplines and settings

Instrumental activities of daily living (IADL) Activities required of an individual to function in the community (e.g., shopping, preparing meals, getting around)

Intraphysic Pertaining to the mind or mental processes

Locus of control An aspect of personality that deals with the degree of control an individual perceives over one's own destiny. *Internal locus of control* refers to the ability to actively control one's destiny. *External locus of control* refers to the inability to control one's destiny.

Metamemory One's self-perceptions of memory changes

Psyche The mind as the center of thought processes, emotions, and behavior

Selective attention The ability to discriminate and focus on relevant information

Syntonic Pertaining to a state of stability

Vigilance The ability to sustain attention

- Describe characteristics of the biologic, social, and psychologic theories of aging from a developmental perspective.
- Distinguish between normal and abnormal physical and psychosocial processes of aging.
- Discuss the process of functional assessment as related to the elderly client.
- Explore the meaning of health and wellness for the elderly.
- Examine how negative attitudes toward the elderly have influenced others' behaviors.
- Compare the developmental tasks of aging with tasks of younger cohorts.

A ging is a complex process of continual development and change. Biologic, psychologic, social, and environmental factors influence how an individual adapts to the process of aging. Many theories have attempted to explain aging and its effects from a developmental perspective, but no single theory has successfully explained the complexities of the aging process. Growing research programs, such as psychoneuroimmunology, may hold promise for the discovery of a unified biopsychosocial theory of aging.

The process of aging is defined in terms of physiologic and psychosocial changes. It is imperative that psychiatric nurses have an understanding of normal and abnormal aging changes and their effects on the functional and mental processes of the elderly. Additionally, the nurse must consider the elderly person's perceptions of health and wellness as part of the assessment process and in the management of care. The psychiatric nurse also needs to be aware of his or her own attitudes toward the elderly. Ageist stereotypes, past experiences with the elderly, and culture influence one's beliefs, values, attitudes, and behaviors.

The psychiatric nurse is in a key position to facilitate the developmental tasks of aging. Several developmental tasks are important across the life span, and those that are unique to the elderly include adjusting to retirement, reminiscing/life review, and preparing for death.

OVERVIEW OF THE ELDERLY POPULATION

Since over 75% of all health care and resources are used by those 65 years and older, an imperative for all health care professionals is an understanding of basic gerontology. *Gerontology* is defined as the study of the aging process across multiple disciplines and settings. Gerontologists, who receive specialized training and education in the field of aging, may be found in many disciplines, including nursing, medicine, psychiatry, social services, pharmacology, biology, and the humanities.

Demographics of the Elderly Population

According to the United States Bureau of the Census (1992), the percentage of the population age 65 and older is 12.6%. This is compared with 1980 census data that reported the elderly population to be 11.3% of the total population. A marked increase in the proportion of elderly is anticipated. By 2030 elderly persons will represent over 13% of the U.S. population. Minority groups, including African-Americans, Pacific Islanders, Native Americans, and Asian-Americans, are expected to have population growths that will double and possibly triple over the next thirty to forty years (U.S. Bureau of the Census, 1992).

The most rapidly growing group of elderly are those age 85 and older. Currently, 1.3% of the U.S. population is 85 years of age and older. By 2050 this group will represent 5% of the entire population (U.S. Bureau of the Census, 1991). Proportionally, the group over age 85, termed *the oldest old,* will be growing at the most rapid rate in comparison with the 65 to 74 and 75 to 84 age groups. Table 10-1 presents the percentage distribution of those over age 65 for 1970-1991.

Health Status of the Elderly Population

Overall, the elderly report that their health is good to excellent (Fries et al, 1992). Socioeconomic status and availability of social support have direct effects on reports of health. Minority groups and those with low incomes consistently report poorer health, even when age is controlled. Because both males and females are living longer, a greater proportion of couples are surviving into old age. The elderly of today are more educated, with a greater portion having completed some college. Over 22% of persons age 65 years and older completed at least 1 year of college, compared with 12.5% in 1970. The elderly also maintain better health care practices than some of their younger-age cohorts. The most recent data from the U.S. Department of Health and Human Services (1993) reported that elderly persons had better dietary habits and smoked and consumed alcohol to a lesser extent than those less than 65 years of age. Only in the area of physical exercise did the elderly report less activity than younger age groups.

TABLE 10-1   Percentage distribution of population 65 years old and over by age group and sex: 1970–1991

Age group/sex	Distribution (%)			
	1970	**1980**	**1990**	**1991**
ALL PERSONS				
65-69 years	35.0	34.3	32.4	31.6
70-74 years	27.3	26.6	25.7	26.0
75-79 years	19.2	18.8	19.6	19.8
80-84 years	11.4	11.5	12.6	12.7
85 years and over	7.1	8.8	9.7	10.0
MALES				
65-69 years	37.3	37.8	36.1	35.1
70-74 years	27.7	27.7	27.2	27.6
75-79 years	18.7	18.0	19.1	19.4
80-84 years	10.5	9.9	10.9	11.0
85 years and over	5.8	6.6	6.7	6.9
FEMALES				
65-69 years	33.4	31.9	29.9	29.2
70-74 years	27.0	25.9	24.6	24.8
75-79 years	19.6	19.3	20.0	20.0
80-84 years	12.1	12.6	13.7	13.9
85 years and over	7.9	10.3	11.7	12.0

Adapted from United States Bureau of the Census: *Current population reports,* series P-25, Nos. 917 and 1045.

Although a majority of the elderly across all settings suffer from at least one chronic condition, illness in itself does not appear to influence individual perception of health status, if functional abilities are not impaired. Functional ability is categorized as activities of daily living (ADL) and instrumental activities of daily living (IADL). Physical and psychosocial functions are included in a functional assessment. Assessing functional abilities of the elderly is discussed later in this chapter.

LIFE EXPECTANCY VERSUS LIFE SPAN

Life expectancy and life span are terms that require differentiation. *Life expectancy* is defined as the expected number of years of life. Several factors affect life expectancy, including gender, race, and environmental conditions.

The average life expectancy in the United States is 75 years (Centers for Disease Control, 1990). Females outlive males by about 6.9 years, and this difference is not expected to change dramatically over the next 30 years. Both male and female African-Americans have a shorter life expectancy than whites.

Researchers disagree about the possibility of significant increases in life expectancy. Some researchers predict that life expectancy will increase an additional 10 years by the year 2040 as a result of medical advancements and decreased mortality. The primary focus of all health care providers must be to provide comprehensive and affordable medical care to this growing population.

Life span refers to the maximum length of survival that is genetically fixed for each species. Most scientists consider 100 to 115 years as the maximum verified human life span. Increases in life expectancy are a result of increases in survival rates of infants and children to a much greater extent than increases in survival rates for those over age 50.

Dependency ratio is another measure used to describe the demographic characteristics of a population. Dependency ratio is defined as the number of individuals under age 18 and over age 64 who are dependent on persons age 18 to 64 years. The ratio is an estimate of the main workforce required to provide health, education, social, and recreational resources to the young and old.

Any factors that cause shifts in the population, such as an increased or decreased birthrate, will alter the dependency ratio. A major decrease in the dependency ratio will occur in the early part of the twenty-first century due to the Social Security Amendment of 1983, which adjusts the retirement ages to 66 years of age by the year 2000 and to 67 years of age by the year 2027.

A LIFE SPAN PERSPECTIVE OF AGING

Gerontologists in a variety of scientific fields have attempted to explain the developmental processes of aging from biologic and behavioral perspectives. A variety of theories on aging exist because scientists do not agree on a single definition of aging. Chronological, biologic, psychologic, and social definitions of aging have been extensively described in the literature but are inadequate in describing the process of aging. Therefore, scientists and philosophers have developed theories to explain the meaning, causes, and factors related to the aging process.

Biologic Theories of Aging

Biologic theories of aging are classified into various categories based on causative factors. Most biologic theories view the process of aging as either a normal, gradual wearing down of all systems or as an abnormal series of cellular damage or mutations eventually leading to the body's inability to make repairs (Schneider and Rowe, 1990).

One method to classify biologic theories of aging relates to categorizing predisposing factors as intrinsic or extrinsic to the organism. Intrinsic or genetic theories focus on the process of aging as internal to the organism. It is estimated that up to 80% of one's life expectancy is genetically determined, although researchers do not have a clear understanding of which genes control aging. Several changes within cells also occur with aging, such as cellular compositions and the ability of cells to divide, synthesize protein, and transport waste materials.

Extrinsic or nongenetic theories propose that aging occurs as a result of environmental factors acting on the organism, such as radiation, ozone, drugs, and toxic substances, which have been theorized to damage cellular structures, leading to aging and death.

Researchers have not agreed on any single biologic theory to explain the aging process. A combination of genetic and environmental factors may best explain why individuals age differently. Four of the biologic theories of aging most examined by researchers follow.

GENETIC THEORY

The genetic theory of aging represents a group of intrinsic aging theories, all of which focus on an internal genetic code that drives the aging process. The premise of the theory is that genes are categorized as juvenescent or senescent. *Juvenescent* genes promote and maintain growth and vigor through the adult years, while *senescent* genes become active in middle adult and later years and initiate a process of decline and deterioration. Empirical evidence to support the theory of this "aging" gene is lacking.

Another popular genetic theory is known as the *biologic clock theory* (Schneider and Rowe, 1990) and suggests that an organism's development and subsequent decline are regulated by some programmed internal genetic clock. This internal clock runs down over a predetermined length of time. Supporters of this theory point to certain normal physiologic changes in humans that appear to be correlated with time, such as hair greying and menopause.

Although the biologic clock theory gives dramatic evidence for boundaries of human life span, there are limitations to this theory. One limitation is the inability to generalize in vitro to in vivo studies. Second, the theory does not explain what factor triggers the end of cellular replication and the beginning of cellular degeneration. Finally, the theory does not explain extreme cases of longevity.

A final genetic theory, *error theory,* has been suggested to explain the development of harmful genes that interfere with biologic processes such as protein synthesis (Hayflick, 1985). Damage to biologic synthesis results in the development of damaged cells that interfere with normal biologic functions. The proliferation of cancerous cells is an example of a process in which normal cells become aberrant through some error process.

IMMUNOLOGIC THEORY

Most biologists agree that changes in the immunologic system after puberty impact the process of aging. Antibody production declines, and autoimmune responses change in response to the decline. The result is that the body's ability to differentiate normal and abnormal or foreign substances fails. This response is sometimes seen in cases of tissue rejection in organ transplantation.

Immune function significantly declines with aging. By age 85, an individual's immune system functions at 5% to 10% of the system's level at puberty. Rheumatoid arthritis and mature onset diabetes are two diseases commonly experienced in older age and are caused by alterations to the immune system. Although it's not exactly known how or why the immune system exhibits a functional decline with aging, the appearance of autoantibodies in the serum of elderly persons is common. Autoantibodies are antibodies particular to an individual's own normal serum or tissue. It is hypothesized that their appearance signals declines in immune system function.

CROSS-LINKAGE THEORY

Collagen tissue, an important component of connective tissue that maintains the structure of cells, tissues, and organs, undergoes changes with aging. Collagen provides the elasticity necessary in many types of tissue such as cardiac and muscle. With age, the combination of chemical changes and external stimuli cause the formation of molecular bonds in collagen called *cross-links,* which tend to stabilize the collagen fibers resulting in rigid, fragile tissue. Scientists do not understand the mechanism that triggers the formation of cross-links, but it is believed that the most active period of cross-link development is between 30 and 50 years of age.

Cross-links also form in elastin in connective tissue. Elastin is similar to collagen in that it maintains tissue flexibility and permeability. The effects of cross-linking in elastin fibers are most pronounced in the changes in fa-

cial skin with aging. Skin becomes brittle, dry, saggy, and appears translucent. The formation of cross-links is probably not the sole cause of aging, but structural and functional changes associated with aging are impacted by collagen alterations at the cellular level.

FREE RADICAL THEORY

Biologists theorize that some environmental stimuli, such as radiation, ozone, and certain chemicals, interfere with cellular activity, resulting in the production of *free radicals,* which are compounds produced in cells as a result of environmental stimuli. They may interact with various cellular structures, causing damage to normal cellular function. Free radicals are also formed during the normal process of cellular oxygenation when the cell removes waste products. Although the cell is capable of neutralizing and removing such by-products, it is theorized that over time the cell loses its capacity to eliminate waste and repair itself. Researchers are continuing to study the potential effectiveness of antioxidants, such as vitamins A, C, and E, in protecting cellular structures (Packer and Glazer, 1990).

Sociological Theories of Aging

Sociologists have observed that an individual's role, relationships, and social experiences change as one ages. Sociologic theories of aging attempt to explain the social aspects of the aging process. Three of the earliest theories were developed in the 1960s. These three theories, *disengagement, continuity,* and *activity* all take a different approach to the social aspects of aging. Common to the three theories is the focus on action and adaptation by the individual—that is, the aging person needs to change or adjust to new situations. Relocation to a nursing home is often traumatic for the elderly person who cannot adjust to the highly structured institutional routines. Social theories that focus more on the interaction between the aging individual and the environment have evolved.

DISENGAGEMENT THEORY

The **disengagement theory** was the first sociologic aging theory developed by social gerontologists. In 1961 Cumming and Henry published the results of their exploratory study of 275 healthy, financially stable persons, age 50 to 95, who lived in Kansas City. They theorized that a process of mutual withdrawal naturally occurs between the aging individual and society which is inevitable and universal in its occurrence. The retirement process is an example of this disengagement. Society clearly identifies the age of 65 years as the time for retirement. Identifying a retirement marker, or target, is also a mechanism for society to open the opportunity for a young person to enter the work force. According to Cumming and Henry (1961), if the older person is prepared for retirement, he or she will have an easier time "disengaging" from society. The elderly person's social ties continue to shrink, perpetuating the individual's further withdrawal into self.

The disengagement theory has been the most controversial of the social aging theories. Most of the criticism focuses on its presumed universality and on the fact that it does not allow for biologic or personality differences between individuals. Additionally, the initiator (i.e., individual or society) of the disengagement also seems to influence the person. The effect on the elderly person may be positive or negative, depending on the degree of preparedness and acceptance by the individual.

Havighurst, Neugarten, and Tobin (1968) reexamined the original data used to formulate the disengagement theory and arrived at different conclusions in support of disengagement. For example, they found that individual personality traits and past experiences influence how an individual in society adapts to aging. A person who is withdrawn early in life will probably continue to withdraw and adapt if his or her social ties also support withdrawal behaviors. Society today is less insistent that elderly persons completely disengage. For example, some industries are hiring retired persons on a part-time or per diem basis or using them as expert consultants. It is more of a combination of one's personal preferences and the needs of society that dictates the degree and pattern of disengagement rather than personal preference or societal needs alone.

CONTINUITY THEORY

The **continuity theory** was developed out of Havighurst's reformulation of the disengagement theory (1968). The basic premise behind the continuity theory is that people adapt best when they are allowed to be who they are and that, with aging, people become "more like themselves;" that is, as one ages, he or she attempts to maintain continuity and consistency of habits, beliefs, norms, values, and other aspects of personality. If a person is having difficulties adjusting to changes such as retirement or relocation, the continuity theory holds that it is not the process of aging that interferes with adaptation, but rather personality factors or one's social environment that influences adaptation. The continuity theory allows for individual differences in the aging process, and theorizes that each individual's personality contains a self-maintaining component, meaning that one's long-standing behavior patterns enhance coping and adjustments to new situations across the life span (Atchley, 1989).

ACTIVITY THEORY

The supporters of the **activity theory** believe that maintaining an active lifestyle and social roles offsets the negative effects of aging (Fig 10-1). By retaining a high level of participation in one's socioenvironment, activity theorists postulated that the elderly individual would report a higher level of overall life satisfaction and a more positive

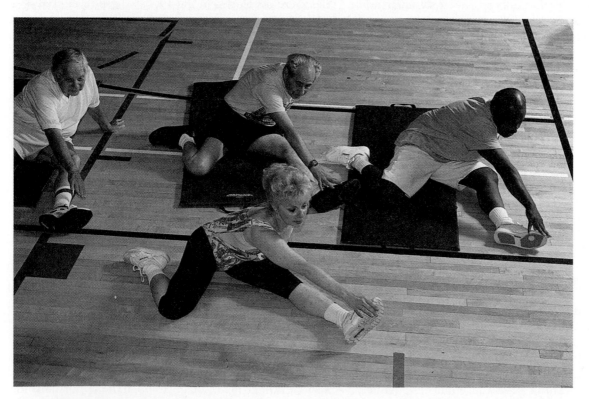

Figure 10-1 Physical exercise is good for the elderly, as it is for any age group, and would be viewed by an activity theorist as possibly offsetting the negative effects of aging.

(Copyright Cathy Lander-Goldberg, Lander Photographics.)

self-concept. Four propositions were initially identified in the conceptualization of the activity theory (Lemon et al, 1972):

1. The greater the loss in social roles (both formal and informal), the less the activity participation.

2. The more activity maintained, the greater the social role support for the older person.

3. Maintaining stability of social roles supports one's positive self-concept.

4. The more positive the person's self-concept, the greater the degree of life satisfaction experienced.

Wider acceptance of the activity theory is hindered by the lack of empiric evidence to support these postulates. The importance, type, and availability of a particular activity as perceived by the elderly person is an important consideration affecting self-concept and life satisfaction. The activity theory may only apply to those elderly who enjoy and have the opportunity to participate in meaningful activities and social interactions.

Psychologic Theories of Aging

Studying human behavior and attempting to explain why persons act the way they do have been the focus of developmental psychologists since Freud, the founder of psychoanalysis. Because in many cases the elderly do not exhibit the same patterns of behavior as their younger counterparts, theorists developed psychologic theories and models of aging. Whereas sociologic theories of aging focus more on the interaction between the aging individual and his or her socioenvironment within an age **cohort** (group with one or more factors in common) or a culture, developmental psychologists examine human development from an **intrapsychic** or mental viewpoint. Few of the human development theories address characteristics of developmental change in the elderly. Most of the developmental theories focus on a single area of one's **psyche.** Psyche refers to the mind as the center of thought processes, emotions, and behavior. For example, Freud's theory and practice focused on sexual aspects across the human life span. A focus on cycles or stages during which key developmental tasks or events are carried out is apparent in most of the developmental theories.

LIFE STAGE THEORIES

Several life stage theories have been advanced over the past several years. These theories divide the life span into a series of sequential transitions. Individuals who are adjusted and happy are able to achieve age-appropriate developmental tasks at each stage.

Levinson's life stage theory of human development focused on an individual's shift from one stage to another being guided by a *mentor* who was usually at least 10 years older than the individual. The mentor may be any-one significant to the individual, not necessarily a blood relative. Levinson's theory is limited in its application to the elderly, as the last shift described is that of ages 35 to 45 years. Levinson described the 35- to 45-year-old shift as comprising midlife crises and the end of youthful dreams.

Carl Jung's life stage theory (1971) was based on psychoanalytic theory that states that as one goes through life he or she develops inner exploratory abilities that add meaning to life. He also postulated that personality differences between males and females become less distinct as people age. The final life stage deals with maintaining a balance between wisdom and senility in old age. The elderly person who is successful in life does not attempt to compete with youth, but rather is able to deal with age changes.

Erikson, a social psychoanalyst, is the most well known of the life stage theorists and identified eight stages of psychological development. Each stage of development involves maintaining a balance between the **syntonic** (state of stability) and **dystonic** (state of disorder) (Erikson et al, 1986) to adjust and move forward to the next level. In describing the final stage of life, Erickson stated that "the process of bringing into balance feelings of integrity and despair involves a review of and a coming to terms with the life one has lived thus far" (Erikson et al, 1986).

HUMAN MOTIVATION AND DEVELOPMENT THEORY

Maslow's motivation and development theory (1962) is widely viewed as a valuable framework to understand human needs and values from a holistic point of reference. Maslow's theoretic construct is described as a hierarchy of needs and is diagrammed in the form of a pyramid. Five levels of needs are identified, the most basic representing the base of the pyramid. From the most basic (1) to the highest (5) level, these needs include the following:

1. biologic and physiologic;

2. safety and security;

3. affiliation or sense of belonging;

4. self-esteem; and

5. self-actualization.

Ebersole and Hess (1994) have conceptualized Maslow's hierarchy of needs and applied his theory to identification of special needs of the elderly at each level. Table 10-2 identifies some of these specific needs of the older adult and potential strategies to meet those needs.

ADAPTATION THEORY

The adaptation theory as described by Vaillant (1977) is more of a conceptual model that categorizes the changes brought about by aging. Vaillant identified a series of shifts and trade-offs that occur during the aging process. What is critical to successful adaptation is the ability of the individual to let go of parts of the past, while pursuing

TABLE 10-2 Special needs of the elderly according to Maslow's Hierarchy of Needs

Needs of the elderly	Maslow's Hierarchy of Needs	Strategies to meet needs
Finding meaning in life and death Transcendence over aging processes Creativity and mastery	Self-actualization	Identify value and contributions of the individual Encourage continuity of participation in decision making processes Reminisce about past in relation to present and future
Responsible roles Social supports Locus of control Cognitive awareness	Self-esteem	Maintain aspects of roles important to the individual Facilitate socialization Promote physical appearance Facilitate decision making
Relationships Intimacy Affiliations	Belonging	Identify impact of loss on individual Support needs for intimacy and sexuality Facilitate changes in lifestyle
Sensory awareness Environmental safety Legal and economic issues	Safety and security	Obtain necessary equipment or supplies for home independence Assist with obtaining legal or financial help Educate the elderly person and family regarding home safety
Biologic needs Comfort needs	Biologic integrity	Provide for physical comfort Provide for nutritional needs

From Ebersole P, Hess P: *Toward healthy aging: human needs and nursing responses,* ed 4, St. Louis, 1994, Mosby.

quality of life components. For example, the elderly person often experiences sensory losses, especially in the areas of vision and hearing and adapts to such losses by facilitating the quality of the remaining sensory perceptions. For instance, the use of large-print books, direct lighting, or hearing aids would enhance the older person's remaining sight and hearing. Encouraging the use of other sensory perceptual systems such as touch or taste would be another way for the older individual to gather pertinent information from the environment.

LIFE STRUCTURE THEORY

Lowenthal (Lowenthal and Chiriboga, 1973) described a human developmental theory based on organizational life cycles and transitions. His theory was based on clinical observations of the ability of individuals to cope with transitions such as college, marriage, and retirement. Transitions may be categorized as occupational, familial, economic, and life cycle (e.g., infancy, childhood, adolescence). Each transition may bring on a period of stress, depending on the degree of preparation, type of transition, and the individual's coping mechanisms. Although life structure transitions may be gradual, others may be sudden or unexpected, resulting in severe role reversals in some cases.

PSYCHOANALYTIC MODEL

Gould (1977) developed and described a model of human development that was based on his psychoanalytic practice, that combined some basic premises of psychoanalysis with Maslow's hierarchy of needs. Gould believed that human development begins as an internal process of reflection. One must give up lower-level needs, such as biologic and safety, to achieve self-actualization during mature adulthood. He believed that old age should be a period of individuality and continued self-development through such means as recreational or creative activities.

PROCESS OF AGING

The process of aging incorporates physiologic and psychosocial changes within the individual. As described in several of the biologic and psychosocial theories of aging, external or environmental factors impact aging in many ways. The physiologic changes that come with aging are universal and irreversible and usually indicate decreases in functioning. Because the changes that characterize normal physiologic aging mirror pathologic changes, normal and abnormal aging processes are often confused.

Psychosocial changes during aging in the areas of cognition, personality, social interactions, sexuality, and roles are even less distinct. Personality and socioenvironmental factors play a huge role in determining psychosocial aging changes. Particular aspects of such processes as cognition and memory may decline with aging, while other aspects may remain the same or even be enhanced with advanced age.

Physiologic Aging

The physiologic aging changes considered part of normal aging affect all body systems, but not necessarily at the same rates. It is important to have an understanding of the common physiologic aging changes, as some of these changes may indicate the development of pathologic conditions. Many of these changes begin as early as the fourth and fifth decades of life. There are also individual differences in the rates of aging of some biologic systems due to factors such as heredity, environment, lifestyle, and nutrition (Steinberg, 1983).

MUSCULOSKELETAL SYSTEM

Aging changes occur in bone and muscle mass, tendon and joint flexibility, and cartilage structure (Meier, 1988). It appears that bone continues to grow up to the eighth decade in some bony structures, but the reabsorption of the interior of flat and long bones occurs at a greater rate than bone growth. Also, bone minerals and proteins are lost from the bone matrix. Loss of bone mass, commonly termed *osteoporosis,* and loss of minerals, especially calcium, increase the possibility of fractures and subsequent immobility. Women are affected by osteoporosis twice as often as men.

Changes in joints begin about the third decade and continue throughout the remainder of the life span. With severe loss of cartilage and fluids, bones may begin to rub together, resulting in painful, slow movements. Changes in the vertebral column combined with osteoporosis cause a loss of sitting height with aging.

CARDIOVASCULAR SYSTEM

Changes in the cardiovascular system as a result of aging are complex. Some of the changes that have been attributed to disease may be part of normal aging, so it is difficult for researchers to separate normal vs. abnormal cardiovascular changes to a great extent (Lakatta, 1988).

With normal aging, the size of the heart may decrease slightly due to a loss of muscle cells. In the heart, muscle cells are replaced with fat cells and connective tissue that causes rigidity in the heart muscle. This results in a slower heart rate and decreased cardiac output. A decrease in oxygen consumption by the heart reflects decreased effectiveness of the heart. Changes in the structure of the heart muscle fibers may result in changes in the heart rhythm. Atrial dysrhythmias, including atrial fibrillation and atrial flutter, are common.

Blood pressure may increase to compensate for changes in atrial circulation. The structure of arteries changes with aging. Collagen fibers, lipids, and minerals increase in the walls of arteries and in veins. These arterial changes also affect the baroreceptors that are important in moderating blood pressure during postural changes. This is reflected in the elderly person's complaint of dizziness when standing quickly.

RESPIRATORY SYSTEM

The respiratory system exhibits changes in its structure and function with aging (Kumpe et al, 1985). The diameter of the chest wall increases with age due to a loss of lung resiliency and muscle strength, giving the appearance of a "barrel" chest. Lung compliance increases with aging, but the work of breathing increases because the chest wall compliance decreases. The ability to remove secretions through ciliary movement and coughing decreases with aging. The lungs of older adults stay partially inflated at rest due to an increase in residual volume. It is believed that changes in lung tissue with aging decrease pulmonary diffusion capacity, which results in decreased oxygen saturation. Under normal circumstances, the older person puts less stress on the lungs, so a slight decrease in oxygen use balances out the decrease in oxygen availability.

GASTROINTESTINAL SYSTEM

Changes in the gastrointestinal system with aging are not well understood. Most of the gastrointestinal changes are primarily due to disease rather than to aging alone.

Decreased motility of the esophagus may lead to spasm and reflux. Delayed emptying of stomach contents may occur as a result of decreased motility and acid secretion. Decreased absorption of vitamins, nutrients, and water also results from diminished muscle tone and changes in vascular perfusion (Bowman and Rosenberg, 1983).

The size of the liver decreases with age and results in decreased blood flow, protein synthesis, and metabolism of some drugs. The potential for serious toxic effects of drugs that are metabolized in the liver should be closely monitored through blood levels.

The formation of stones in the gallbladder increases with aging. It is believed that the absorption of cholesterol is less efficient as one ages, resulting in stone production. Changes in the pancreas with aging primarily affect enzyme production, but not to a degree that significantly affects normal digestive processes in the absence of disease.

INTEGUMENTARY SYSTEM

Changes in the skin, hair, and nails are most pronounced with advancing age. A loss of subcutaneous fat, thinning of the dermis and epidermis, and loss of elastin flexibility are responsible for the wrinkling and saggy appearance of the skin. Fragility of the dermal vasculature causes "senile purpura," a condition that appears as bruises under the skin.

Sometimes the loss of skin turgor in the elderly is mistaken for dehydration. Decreased skin turgor results from a combination of less body water and subcutaneous fat and a loss of flexibility of the skin's elastin. Dryness of the skin also increases with aging, due to a loss in the number and size of sweat glands and reduced hormonal levels.

Changes in hair production and appearance occur with aging. Decreased melanin production results in the appearance of grey hair. Genetics influence the onset of grey hair. Hair also grows more slowly with aging and becomes coarse and thick in such areas as nose, ears, and eyebrows, while general body hair thins.

The growth of nail tissue also decreases with aging. Years of use or injury may cause changes in the appearance of nails. Yellowing, formation of ridges, or thickening of the nails may be observed in older individuals.

IMMUNE SYSTEM

The ability of the body to form antibodies to some antigens such as pneumococcal and influenza vaccines is greatly reduced in the elderly. Delays in hypersensitive reactions also come with aging. Across the life span, the elderly individual's immune system was required to fight off exposure to many pathogens, with the additive effect resulting in more frequent and severe infections in the elderly.

The thymus, a small organ above the heart, is important to the development of the immune system. The thymus produces hormones that assist with the maturation of *T lymphocytes,* which are one type of lymph cell that may ward off cancer cells. The actual number of T lymphocytes does not decline with aging, but their ability to proliferate in the presence of particular viruses decreases significantly. Therefore the elderly person has a more difficult time developing defense mechanisms to infections such as pneumonia, bronchitis, and bloodstream infections.

RENAL SYSTEM

The renal system is critical in the removal of a variety of waste products and drugs and in the regulation of fluid volume in extracellular space. With normal aging, the functioning of the renal system decreases significantly, although the remaining kidney functions are usually adequate. Changes to the kidney as a result of aging include loss of glomeruli, loss of total kidney tissue mass, and decreased glomerular filtration rate. Glomeruli are small structures in the kidney made up of clusters of blood capillaries. The rate and degree of changes to the kidneys are highly variable; therefore, researchers believe that aging is not the chief cause for the structural and functional changes. Because cardiac output decreases as a result of aging, the elimination of waste products is affected.

NERVOUS SYSTEM

Unlike cells of other body systems, the cells of the nervous system do not reproduce. There is a loss of nerve cells with normal aging, but the degree of loss differs, depending on the structure of the nervous system. The aging pigment, lipofuscin, is deposited in nerve cells, and neurofibrillary plaques and tangles form in the aging brain. These plaques and tangles may indicate Alzheimer's disease but are found in normal aging brains in the absence of dementia. (See Chapter 16.)

The amount of neurotransmitters also decreases with normal aging. Changes in cognitive functioning such as memory storage may be affected by a decrease in acetylcholine and epinephrine. Because of the redundancy of nerve cells, it is impossible to generalize that all elderly have diminished memory or cognitive abilities. Decreases in another neurotransmitter, serotonin, is also part of normal aging. Serotonin is important in the regulation of activities such as sleeping, drinking, and breathing. Serotonin also affects temperature regulation, heart rate, and affect. Reductions in the amount of serotonin results in the elderly person's inability to respond to physical and psychologic stressors in an appropriate manner. (See Chapters 11 and 22.)

Sleep cycle is influenced as a result of the normal aging process. The elderly usually complain of frequent periods of restlessness or insomnia. They may go to the bathroom often during the night and, as a result, they may nap during the day to make up for the loss of night sleep. Periods of rapid eye movement (REM) sleep are also decreased with aging.

REPRODUCTIVE SYSTEM

In females, *menopause,* or the permanent cessation of menses, occurs at around age 51 years. Ovarian estrogen ceases to be produced, but adrenal estrogens continue to be manufactured. Menopausal women commonly complain of hot flashes, or intermittent sensations of warmth and palpations in the upper body. Hot flashes lessen in frequency with aging. There is a narrowing of the vagina and a decrease in vaginal secretions. The uterus, ovaries, and cervix also decrease in size due to vascular and muscular changes.

In males, the production of androgen hormones decreases with aging. The consequences of reductions in androgen to aging are not yet known. Androgens may affect libido and nocturnal erections, but they do not appear to influence erections due to the presence of erotic stimuli. The changes in testosterone levels with aging are not agreed upon at this time. Although not well studied, the production of sperm, or *spermatogenesis,* seems to be sustained well into old age in the absence of disease. Physically, the testes and penis may decrease in size while the scrotal sac becomes pendulous.

Many health caregivers erroneously believe that the physiologic changes to the reproductive system due to aging mean that the elderly person's sexuality is also impaired. This has become a self-fulfilling prophecy for some elderly individuals who think that sexual pleasures are taboo in the later years. Many elderly do enjoy various forms and degrees of intimacy, and caregivers need to encourage such feelings. (See Chapter 18.)

ENDOCRINE SYSTEM

Changes in the endocrine organs and the hormones they secrete vary with aging. The endocrine organs are highly interrelated, so a change in one system usually impacts the others. Researchers believe that focusing on preventing some endocrine changes may hold the greatest promise for reducing the occurrence of disabilities and disorders of the aged.

The endocrine system is made up of the following organs:

- adrenal glands
- thyroid gland
- parathyroid glands
- pancreas
- pituitary gland

The adrenal glands appear to decrease in size with aging. The major hormones secreted by the adrenal glands (i.e., cortisol, aldosterone, and the adrenal androgens) decrease in amounts, but the functional implications of these reductions are not well understood.

The thyroid gland atrophies with aging and undergoes some structural changes such as the development of fibrotic tissue and nodules. Thyroid hormonal production decreases with aging, but the impact appears to be minimal, as there is less need for these hormones into old age. The parathyroid hormone may decrease or increase with aging. It appears that the parathyroid hormone increases in the presence of osteoporosis, as it is a factor stimulating bone demineralization.

The secretion of the hormone insulin by the pancreas appears to decrease with aging, resulting in a decreased ability of the elderly to metabolize glucose. Insulin is nec-

essary to the metabolism of blood sugars, or glucose, and for maintenance of normal blood sugar levels in the body. Recent studies have demonstrated that the amount of total insulin produced by the body remains the same across the life span, so the problem for the elderly may be that release of the available insulin is delayed in some still-unknown manner.

The pituitary gland, which secretes several hormones, undergoes structural changes with aging in its cellular and vascular components. With aging there is a decline in growth hormone and an increase in levels of follicle-stimulating and luteinizing hormones. Alterations in mechanisms that regulate the secretion of thyroid-stimulating hormones, adrenocorticotropic hormones, and antidiuretic hormones are believed to occur with aging, but further research is needed before determining the significance of these changes for the elderly.

SENSORY SYSTEM

The senses of vision and hearing decline with aging. Everyone experiences some visual changes as a part of the normal aging process. The lens of the eye continues to grow throughout aging, but the appearance of the lens changes. The lens becomes rigid and transparent and loses the ability to accommodate or adjust to changing distances, commonly termed *presbyopia.* The pupil decreases in size and becomes less responsive to light. Ability to discriminate color in the blue, green, and violet hues becomes less distinct (Carter, 1982). Decreases in the lacrimal secretions result in feelings of dryness in the eyes. *Arcus senilus,* a condition that appears as a white circle around the iris, is due to lipid deposits and is considered a definite normal result of aging.

Hearing loss is gradual with aging and occurs in about one third of individuals age 75 years and older (Olsho et al, 1985). Diminished ability in hearing acuity related to perception of tones is known as *presbycusis.* Increases in earwax in the ear canal and external noise also contribute to presbycusis.

It is believed that taste sensation is not markedly changed as a result of normal aging and that changes in taste sensation may be due to individual perceptions. The sense of smell appears to have minor decreases with aging, although environmental exposures to smoke or chemicals influence changes in the sense of smell over the life span.

Changes in the sense of touch during aging is complex and highly individualized. There are few changes to tactile nerve endings, but dermal changes may decrease touch sensation acuity in the elderly. Although some elderly experience a decreased pain threshold, others experience an increased pain threshold, and it appears that past experiences with pain are an influential factor in pain perception.

The sense of proprioception, or *kinesthetics,* refers to the individual's sense of balance and orientation in space. Due to skeletal and inner ear structural changes with aging, the person's sense of orientation, and especially of balance, may be severely compensated. The older person also has difficulty regaining a sense of balance.

Functional Assessment

In view of all the physiologic changes the elderly experience throughout the life span, most individuals are able to cope with the minor aches and pains attributed to normal aging. It is when the elderly person's ability to function and carry out activities of daily living independently is hindered that coping mechanisms may fail. Most situations that bring the elderly person to the primary care practitioner involve an inability to carry out specific functional tasks. Therefore it is important to assess the elderly person's functional status and its effect on one's daily life (Table 10-3).

Functional assessment usually consists of evaluating two areas. The first, the **activities of daily living (ADL)**, includes categories of personal care such as bathing, grooming, toileting, and transferring. The second, **instrumental activities of daily living (IADL)**, addresses activities important for the individual to function in the community. IADL include shopping, preparing meals, and getting around. Table 10-4 on page 214 highlights the major categories of ADL and IADL assessment.

ACTIVITIES OF DAILY LIVING

ADL focus on the physical skills necessary to function from day to day. A recent study by the U.S. Department of Health and Human Services (1993) reported that 12.9% of the total population age 65 years or older reported having at least one ADL problem. The elderly reported having the greatest amount of difficulty bathing, walking, and transferring between the bed and chair.

Several ADL assessment instruments are available. A good ADL instrument should be able to discriminate between physical and cognitive sources of the limitations. ADL scales typically categorize activity limitations in one of two ways. One type of ADL scale classifies limitations as present or absent. This scale fails to differentiate degrees of ADL limitations. The value of an ADL assessment tool is in its ability to identify areas for interventions. The *Katz Index of ADL* is a valid, objective tool which measures six areas of function: (1) bathing, (2) dressing, (3) toileting, (4) transferring, (5) continence, and (6) feeding. The degree of limitation in each category is measurable. For example, in assessing transfer ability, the caregiver selects from one of the following three choices:

1. Moves in and out of bed or chair without assistance (may be using object for support such as cane or walker).
2. Moves in or out of bed or chair with assistance.
3. Does not get out of bed.

The Katz Index of ADL was developed and tested with elderly subjects across a variety of settings and is considered a reliable measure of function in the aged.

INSTRUMENTAL ACTIVITIES OF DAILY LIVING

The ability of the individual to function in the community is an important aspect of the functional assessment. Approximately 17.5% of the elderly report difficulty with at least one IADL (U.S. Department of Health and Human Services, 1993). Transportation, or getting around in the community, was most often identified as a problem area, followed by difficulty with shopping and light household chores.

There is a subjective as well as objective component of IADL. Assessing the ability of the older person to perform daily skills needed to function in the community is important. Additionally, the meaning of the activity to the individual needs to be assessed. For example, taking care of shopping needs may not be as important as housekeeping or meal preparation to an individual. An older individual who fears going out into the community because of safety issues may essentially become isolated. Another elderly person may have difficulty with chewing and swallowing, so meal preparation seems like a difficult task.

Both aspects of the functional assessment, ADL and IADL, are relevant indicators for identifying outcomes of illness, both physical and mental. Often, changes in ADL and IADL may be the forerunner of a new illness. Individuals respond differently to physical aging changes, so the ability to function independently is more predictive of outcomes of aging than physical aging change alone.

Psychosocial Aging

Psychosocial aging changes typically focus on an individual's responses to particular events across the life span. Past coping mechanisms may not be effective in adjusting to stressful events in later life. The reason adaptation may be more difficult for the elderly is that the life events of old age differ from those of younger ages. Miller (1995) distinguished the life events of the elderly as follows:

1. They are viewed as losses, rather than gains.
2. They are most likely to occur close together with less time to adjust to each event.
3. They are more intense and demand greater energy in the coping process.
4. They are longer lasting and often become chronic problems.
5. They are inevitable and evoke a feeling of powerlessness.

Preparing for some life events may facilitate adjustment in old age. For instance, some employers offer preretirement counseling for older employees in preparation for retirement. Psychosocial aging changes are reflected in several areas including cognition and memory, personality, social support, sexuality, and role status. From a developmental perspective, the meaningfulness of life events is important in determining patterns of psychosocial aging in these particular areas. There is a great

TABLE 10-3 Functional assessment of common physiologic aging changes

System	Normal aging changes	Areas for functional assessment
Musculoskeletal	↓ muscle strength ↓ body mass ↑ fat deposit ↓ bone mass ↓ joint mobility ↓ sitting height	Activity/exercise tolerance Joint pain on movement Gait, balance, and posture Susceptibility to falls Ability to perform ADL and IADL
Cardiovascular	↓ cardiac output ↓ basal metabolic rate ↓ cardiac performance ↓ arterial circulation ↑ peripheral resistance ↑ systolic blood pressure	Adaptation to stress Activity/exercise tolerance Orthostatic hypotension
Respiratory	↓ elasticity of chest walls ↑ anteroposterior diameter of chest ↓ intercostal muscle strength ↑ rigidity of lung tissue ↑ residual capacity ↓ cough reflex	Cough reflex Ability to blow out candle with open mouth Use of accessory muscles
Gastrointestinal	↓ saliva production ↓ motility ↓ gastric acid production ↓ absorption of nutrients ↓ drug metabolism	Condition of teeth/denture fit Dental hygiene Swallow reflex Frequency/size of meals Pattern of elimination Drug blood levels (metabolized by liver) History of constipation
Integument	↑ wrinkling of skin ↑ dryness of skin ↓ skin turgor ↑ thinning, greying body hair ↓ nail growth ↑ nails thicken, yellow	Assess for skin breakdown, especially over bony prominences Assess hydration status Susceptibility to infection
Immune	↓ size of thymus gland ↓ antibodies ↑ healing time	Assess for secondary infections History of allergies
Renal	↓ mass of kidney ↓ nephrons ↓ glomerular filtration rate ↓ nitrogen waste removal	Criterion for renal function is creatinine clearance Maintain adequate hydration Assess for incontinence
Nervous	↓ nerve cells ↓ neurotransmitters ↓ blood flow to CNS ↑ lipofuscin ↑ plaques and tangles ↓ REM sleep	Response to pain is highly individualized Diminished deep tendon reflexes Complaint of restlessness/frequently go to bathroom May have memory changes
Reproductive	↓ estrogen production ↓ size of clitoris, cervix, uterus and ovaries ↓ free testosterone ↓ penis and testes size	Support need for intimacy/sexuality Hormonal replacement
Endocrine	↓ production of adrenal gland hormones ↓ insulin release ↓ thyroid structure ↓↑ mixed changes to pituitary hormones	Response to stressors may be diminished
Sensory	↓ vision (loss of depth perception, accommodation, and visual acuity; increased glare) ↓ hearing (loss of sound conduction) ↓ odor recognition ↓↑ changes in pain threshold ↓ sense of balance	Need for increased illumination Need for corrective appliances Avoidance of night driving Assess tolerance to pain Assess thresholds for hot/cold Safety precautions

TABLE 10-4 ADL and IADL functional assessment categories

ADL categories	IADL categories
Bathing	Shopping
Dressing	Meal preparation
Hair care	Transportation
Mouth care	Use of telephone
Nutrition/assist with feeding	Medication usage
Ambulation/mobility	Housekeeping
Mental status	Laundry
Elimination	Financial management

deal of research needed before any conclusion may be drawn regarding normal vs. abnormal psychosocial aging. The following section explores the current state of knowledge on psychosocial aging from a developmental perspective.

COGNITION AND MEMORY

There is probably no other area of aging research that has been studied to such an extent as cognition, especially in the areas of intelligence and memory. Yet, researchers have no conclusive evidence on the development of cognitive functions into old age. During the 1960s and 1970s most researchers believed that decline in cognitive abilities, intelligence, and memory were part of the normal aging process (Botwinick, 1977). In the 1980s researchers began to change their views, realizing that earlier researchers used some measures of intelligence that were not appropriate for the elderly. Depending on the type of cognitive function being measured and the instrument used, not all aspects of cognitive functioning decline with aging (Denney et al, 1991). Some aspects of intelligence may become more refined into old age. Most recently, researchers are finding that intellectual decline is avoidable or possibly reversible in healthy elderly, with interventions focusing on development of cognitive skills (Baltes et al, 1992; Hatfield and Hatfield, 1992).

Cognitive behaviors are divided into several interrelated processes including intelligence, memory, attention, reaction time, and problem solving. These divisions are arbitrary and are based on the ways researchers typically study cognitive behaviors.

Studies of intelligence during the 1940s reported that the elderly experience declines in all aspects of intelligence including knowledge acquisition, calculating, vocabulary, and abstract thought. The problem with these early studies was that the cross-sectional method was used to collect the data with younger-age cohorts being compared to elderly cohorts in these studies. The younger-age cohorts consistently had higher intelligence scores on the various tests, prompting researchers to conclude that intelligence declines with aging

(Woodruff, 1983). Later longitudinal studies, which followed the same older subjects over a period of time, found that intelligence showed little or no decline in healthy aging persons. Declines that occurred were in the oldest age cohorts (Schaie and Willis, 1991).

Horn and Cattell (1967) theorized that age-related differences in intelligence may be due to distinctions between two types of intelligence that seem to develop from birth. *Crystallized intelligence* develops from knowledge gained through the accumulation of experience and education. Crystallized intelligence may decline slightly, remain the same, or even increase with aging, depending on one's life experiences. On the other hand, *fluid intelligence* is affected by neurophysiologic processes across the life span. Declines in the nervous system with aging that affect one's attention span or reaction time reflect a loss of fluid intelligence. Instruments that measure intelligence using performance standards show declines in intelligence with aging (Birren and Schaie, 1985); and even these conclusions have been questioned by some gerontologists. The increased reaction time by the elderly in intelligence performance tests may be because they are more cautious and take additional time to make correct choices.

Much aging research is devoted to the study of memory processes during aging. It is unfortunate that society equates aging with memory loss. Elderly are often portrayed on television or in movies as forgetful. A common joke is, "There are three telltale signs you are getting old. The first is loss of memory, and the other two . . . I forget." There is much that is still unknown about the process of memory perception, storage, and retrieval.

Most of the early theories of memory focused on the three components of memory (i.e., perception or encoding, storage, and retrieval). Memory was categorized as short or long term, or as primary, secondary, or tertiary. These categorizations were based on the length of storage time and the process of retrieval.

Other memory theories focused on the encoding processes, which yield different types of information in various ways. For instance, information that is processed in a more complex manner, such as algebraic equations, is stored in a deeper area of memory and will last longer. Information that is easily recognized requires less attention, so tasks such as starting a car are performed almost automatically. It is believed that automatic processing of information does not change with aging (Botwinick, 1984). Offering cues to the elderly may help them recall information stored in deeper areas of memory.

Contextual theory of memory was developed from the information processing model. This expands the information processing model by including individual factors that may impact memory, such as learning behaviors, past experiences, personality, degree of motivation, physical health, and socioeconomic status (Perlmutter et al, 1987).

Self-perception of memory changes and self-efficacy also influence memory performance (Ryan, 1993; Ryan and See, 1992). The concept of **metamemory** refers to one's self-perceptions of memory changes and their effect on memory processes (Hertzog et al, 1990). For example, an elderly person may falsely believe that memory loss is part of aging and perceive that forgetfulness indicates the start of memory decline. In reality, forgetting information may be due to a lack of attention to detail in a particular situation. Further study is needed to determine whether an individual can mentally control or influence the development of memory across the life span.

Attention span refers to the ability to concentrate throughout performance of some task. With aging, the ability to maintain attention span through completion of complex tasks diminishes. This is due to the fact that complex tasks require dividing one's attention among several tasks at the same time. Some of these normal aging changes with attention span are misinterpreted as dementia. Two other segments of attention also show some decrements in aging. **Vigilance,** or the ability to sustain attention over longer periods of time, and **selective attention,** the ability to discriminate and focus on relevant information, are less acute in the elderly.

Decreases in reaction time and speed of performance on intelligence tests is one of the most agreed-upon changes in normal aging and its mechanism is not well understood. Unfamiliarity with performance tests or increased cautiousness due to a fear of failure resulting in test anxiety may impact reaction time in the elderly.

Problem-solving ability is considered a higher cognitive function. Complexity of the problem, past experiences, the amount of information that is irrelevant to a situation, and level of education are factors that influence problem solving. There is little known about changes in higher cognitive functioning during aging. Most elderly persons are able to live and function effectively in the community.

PERSONALITY

Personality traits develop over the life span and are influenced by internal and external environmental factors. Personality is molded by an individual's ability to cope with stress and adapt to change. It is reflected in how individuals perceive themselves and is referred to as *self-concept.* In general, most personality traits remain stable during the aging process. Personality influences how an individual interacts and reacts within the socioenvironment. (See Chapter 14.)

Personality theorists have attempted to identify specific traits that predict successful aging. Individuals described as introverted are more self-centered and internalize behaviors and responses. Extroverted personalities focus more on the outside world and are described as outgoing. Certain personality traits may assist individuals to adapt to aging better than others. Successful aging is determined more by the individual's ability to adapt to change than by a particular category of personality traits.

Some traits may intensify with aging, such as that of cautiousness, which may be an effective safety mechanism for the elderly. For example, the elderly person may tend to drive a car with more caution, drive only in daylight hours, or avoid high speeds. In unfamiliar situations or when several choices are available, the elderly tend to act more cautiously. They also tend to prefer familiar tasks, places, or situations.

Early research studies concluded that the elderly demonstrate rigidity in such things as psychomotor performance and adjusting to new situations and new habits. Later studies that followed the same group of subjects through aging proposed that individuals who demonstrate rigidity in younger years continue to behave in the same manner or intensify these responses in old age.

Locus of control is another aspect of personality that remains stable over time. Individuals with an *internal locus of control* perceive that they actively control their own destiny. On the other hand, individuals with an *external locus of control* believe they have no control over their destiny and think their behaviors have no effect on any outcomes. Another phenomenon, that of *secondary locus of control,* describes individuals with an external locus of control who learn to adapt to their beliefs. This has also been termed *learned helplessness.* These individuals learn dependency and prefer others to decide for them.

SOCIAL SUPPORT AND INTERACTIONS

In an extensive review of the literature, Broadhead et al (1983) presented Kahn and Antonucci's comprehensive definition of social support as interpersonal transactions that include one or more of the following behaviors: (1) expression of positive affect between individuals, (2) affirmation or endorsement of another person's behaviors, and (3) providing direct aid or assistance to another. Different individuals within one's social network may provide different types of support.

Hyde (1988) suggested that the quality rather than the quantity of social relationships is significantly related to life satisfaction among older adults. The quality of social support is a key area for interventions in the training of health care providers. Social support has been conceptualized as a communication process, in which facilitation of communication skills improves the quality of support (Albrecht and Adelman, 1984).

Social networks are generally viewed as the web of social ties that surround a person and include several characteristics important in the study of health and well-being of the elderly, including size of the social network, frequency of social contacts, density of the interactions, intimacy or closeness among members, durability of ties, geographic dispersion of members, and reciprocity of assistance.

Social networks and social supports are different concepts. Considering the network as the web or structure, social support refers to the emotional or tangible assistance obtained from the social resource network. Not all

TABLE 10-5   Social relationship components and characteristics

Component	Characteristics	Sample questions
Social network Structure and composition	Marital status/confidant	Are you married? Is there any one special person that you feel very close and intimate with?
	Number, kinship	How many children do you have?
	Proximity	How many live within an hour's drive?
	Frequency and type of contact	How many do you have phone or letter contact with at least once per month?
Type and amount of social support function	Emotional	How frequently did someone try and make you feel better about your illness in the past month?
	Tangible aid	How frequently did someone help you get your medications in the past month?
	Guidance	How frequently did someone suggest that you call the doctor in the past month?
Perceived adequacy of social support	General	In the past year could you have used more help with daily tasks than you received?
	Specific	How helpful was it for your children to try and make you feel better about your illness?

From Oxman T, Berkman L: Assessment of social relationships in elderly patients, *Int J Psychiatry Med* 20: 69, 1990.

social ties are supportive, and not all social supports come from the closest social network such as a son or daughter living near elderly parents. Oxman and Berkman (1990) proposed a three-component model of social relationships that incorporates the quantitative and qualitative nature of social relationships. Because social relationships have been associated with subsequent physical and mental illness in the elderly, an assessment tool that addresses the multidimensional aspects of social relationships is important. An example of some of the questions according to the dimensions being assessed is presented in Table 10-5 (Oxman and Berkman, 1990).

SEXUALITY AND INTIMACY

Physical aging changes related to the reproductive system occur in men and women. Psychologic aspects of sexuality and intimacy in the elderly are influenced by several factors including past experiences, attitudes toward intimacy, societal views about sexuality in the elderly, and functional status.

Many elderly feel a newfound freedom in their sexual behaviors because they no longer need to focus on concerns regarding pregnancy. Hindering such feelings may be the unavailability of an acceptable partner, stereotypes that elderly are asexual, or fears of inability to initiate and maintain sexual performance. Elderly women probably experience the greatest effects because many become widowed or there may exist long-standing values about sexual taboos.

It has only been in recent years that elderly persons, and especially those over 80 years, have been subjects of studies of sexuality. Bretschneider and McCoy (1988) reviewed the available studies of psychosocial aspects of sexuality and aging. The following summarizes some of their findings:

1. The frequency of sexual activity decreases with aging, but the interest and ability in sexual function does not necessarily decline with aging. Older individuals in normal health and functioning have the ability to maintain sexual activity.

2. Declines in sexual activity are mostly related to lack of a partner, especially for women.

3. Psychosocial factors that may impede sexual activity by the elderly include stereotypic beliefs, attitudes, and personality factors.

4. Sexual behaviors and beliefs generally remain stable across the life span.

5. Men remain more sexually active than women across the life span.

ROLE TRANSITIONS

Accompanying aging changes are changes in roles for the older person. Some of these role changes are more obvious than others, and individuals adapt to role changes in different ways. The degree of importance attributed to a particular role by the individual influences how well the older person is able to cope with a role transition. From a developmental perspective, roles contain various tasks one must carry out in life. Each role carries with it different life tasks. Some tasks may be new to the person if the role is a completely new one, and other tasks may be similar to ones carried out early in life, as in role reversals.

Retirement implies a major role transition for many individuals. As individuals live longer and retire earlier, the retirement period may last for 30 to 40 years. Only recently have researchers begun to explore gender differences in adaptation to retirement. Adaptation to retirement appears to be affected more by the life events surrounding retirement than by the retirement process itself (Szinovacz and Washo, 1992). Particular life events may even precipitate retirement. For instance, a middle-age woman may take an early retirement because she needs to care for her elderly mother at home who has Alzheimer's disease. This individual's adjustment to retirement may be negatively affected due to a conflict between the woman's role in the workforce and her caregiver role.

A major role transition occurs after loss of one's spouse when adaptation requires the survivor to assume tasks previously performed by the partner. Couples who have shared responsibilities across the life span have less difficulty with the role changes. Personality traits seem to influence adjustment to widowhood. For example, the husband who lost his wife may not have learned how to cook or clean, but if the husband can adapt to change he will rapidly adjust and learn these tasks. The widower may also find himself the center of attention by family members who want to assist him, as well as by widows looking for male companionship.

The role of the grandparent is another transition. The grandparent who adjusts successfully can provide grandchildren with a viewpoint that may differ from the parents although be equally positive. Many grandparents take on the role of full- or part-time surrogate parents.

In the presence of physical or mental deterioration, the roles of the parent and child may be reversed. Most often the oldest female child, on reaching middle age, may need to provide care for the incapacitated elderly parent. This is an especially difficult transition for the female middle-age child who has just completed raising her own children and who was planning her own retirement in a few years. If the caregiver is a middle-age male, it is often an awkward situation, because his wife is called upon to adapt to a role for which she may have no emotional connection in caring for the elderly parent-in-law. Supporting the caregiver is as important as supporting the care receiver under these circumstances. Table 10-6 summarizes some normal aging changes discussed in this section and areas for functional assessment.

TABLE 10-6 Functional assessment of common psychosocial aging changes

Area	Normal aging changes	Areas for functional assessment
Cognition and memory	Normal crystallized intelligence ↓ fluid intelligence (slight, gradual) ↑ reaction time ↓ divided attention ↓ vigilance ↓ selected attention ↑ information processing time ↑ cautiousness	Degree of external stimulation Environmental distraction Assess barriers to learning (e.g., sensory impairments, relevancy/level of information, learning environment) Assess factors influencing memory process (e.g., education level, learning style, past experiences, physical/mental health, motivation)
Personality	Stability of most personality traits ↑ cautiousness ↑ rigidity (slight)	Adaptive coping mechanisms Decision making processes Adjustment to change (e.g., retirement, relocation, loss)
Social support and interactions	Perceived social support impacted by several factors (personality, health status, past experiences, coping style, etc.) Changes in social network (size, intimacy, geographic dispersion, reciprocity of assistance, etc.) Changes in source of social support with aging	Attitude/perception of social support Past experience with social support Social network ties Types of social support needed Sources of social support
Sexuality and intimacy	Sexual behaviors/interests maintained across life span in absence of physical/mental disorders ↓ sexual activity in males ↓ intensity of sexual responses Lack of partner is greatest factor impacting sexual activity	Attitudes toward expressions of sexuality and intimacy Means to maintain sexual behaviors/interests Availability of privacy in environment Risk factors impeding sexual behaviors
Role transitions	Retirement Widowhood Grandparenting	Importance of past roles/tasks Responses to retirement Relation of life events to retirement Effects of retirement on spouses Impact of loss of spouse Ability to take on new tasks in ADL/IADL Social supports/network Relationships with children/grandchildren Parenting role

Mental Assessment

Assessment of mental status and cognitive functioning is an area in which gerontologists are attempting to develop adequate standardized tests specifically for the elderly. Designing reliable instruments for the elderly continues to be a challenge because of the interrelationships among several factors including health status, physical/mental aging changes, socioenvironmental variables, and life events. Thus the context of what is considered normal development for an elderly individual should be the focus of any mental status assessment.

Several mental status assessment instruments have been designed to evaluate mental and cognitive functions. Most instruments examine mental status in view of the individual's ability to function in daily living activities. However, the mental status assessment is not sufficient to provide a diagnosis of a disorder. Other sources of information, such as the health history, physical examination, diagnostic/laboratory tests, and psychosocial factors are required for diagnosing. (See Chapters 6 and 16.)

The mental status assessment of the elderly includes the following areas: appearance, mood, communication, thought processes, perceptual motor abilities, attention, memory, consciousness, and orientation. Appearance, behaviors, and responses of the elderly client should be areas for attention by the health caregiver performing the assessment. For instance, the older person may state that he or she has no suicidal ideations, but appearance may indicate self-neglect, and behaviors may include withdrawing from social networks and accumulating drugs. Such discrepancies are important to identify.

Several screening instruments are available for the health caregiver to provide a quick assessment of mental status. Each instrument addresses different areas of the mental status examination. Often, these brief instruments provide an initial baseline of cognitive functioning, to be used for further in-depth assessment and screening for diagnosis and subsequent interventions.

The Mini-Mental State (MMS) examination is one of the most commonly used instruments to screen for cognitive disorders in the elderly (Folstein, Folstein, and McHugh, 1975) (Fig. 10-2). Several dimensions of cognitive function are assessed, including orientation, memory, attention, and speech. Out of a total score of 30, normal persons score 25 and above, while individuals diagnosed with dementia score lower than 20 points.

Another commonly used instrument is the Short Portable Mental Status Questionnaire (SPMSQ) (Pfeiffer, 1975). Though not adequate to provide a diagnosis of dementia, this tool provides a rapid assessment of mental status. Areas of cognitive function assessed by the SPMSQ include orientation, immediate and remote memory, thought processes, and attention span. The scoring also allows for differences in education and race (Figure 10-3).

MEANINGS OF HEALTH AND WELLNESS FOR THE ELDERLY

Perceptions of health and wellness develop across the life span and affect attitudes and behaviors related to health care practices. For the elderly, their present physical and mental health represent the summation of health care beliefs and practices across the years. Imogene King (1981), a well respected nursing theorist, defined health from a developmental perspective and considered it the "dynamic life experiences of a human being, which implies continuous adjustment to stressors in the internal and external environment through optimal use of one's resources to achieve maximum potential for daily living."

According to King, the meaning of health and wellness differs among individuals, that is, for each elderly person, health and wellness are determined by the importance given to aspects of physical and psychologic functions. Describing health in respect to functional capacity has more meaning for the elderly than does discussing health in relation to disease. Overall, the elderly have great ability to adapt to many diseases as long as their capacity to function is not jeopardized to a significant extent. When older persons are asked what health means to them, they invariably respond that health means the ability to get around, to be active and social, or to remain independent. Health and wellness also may be defined by many elderly as the ability to continue to be a contributing member of society. For example, an elderly woman in a nursing home who was confined to a wheelchair because of a stroke and heart disease considered herself healthy. She could use her creative talents all day in knitting various items that would be sold in the nursing home gift shop to residents and visitors. Ebersole and Hess (1994) remarked that "even in chronic illness and dying there is an optimal level of wellness and well-being attainable for each individual."

Ebersole and Hess (1994) present a five-dimensional model of health and wellness for the elderly based on a developmental perspective. This model is summarized in Table 10-7 on page 221.

ATTITUDES TOWARD THE ELDERLY

The majority of attitudes in society toward the elderly tend to be negative. Nurses' attitudes toward the elderly have been the subject of many studies, but findings are inconsistent. Some researchers report that nurses hold negative attitudes toward the elderly across a variety of settings, and other researchers report positive or mixed attitudes of nurses depending on previous experience with the elderly.

Nurses' education and experience in caring for the elderly do not necessarily provide them with greater positive attitudes toward the aged (Downe-Wamboldt and Melanson, 1985). It is also believed that the work setting influences caregivers' attitudes, but researchers do not

Mini-Mental State Examination

Maximum Score	Score	
		Orientation
5	( )	What is the (year)(season)(date)(day)(month)?
5	( )	Where are we (state)(country)(town or city)(place)(floor)?
		Registration
3	( )	Name three random objects, taking one second to say each one. Then ask the patient to name all three objects (apple, table, penny) after you have said them.
		Give 1 point for each correct answer. Count the number of trials and record the number. (number of trials _____).
		Attention and Calculation
5	( )	Begin with 100, and count backward by 7 (stop after 5 answers): 93, 86, 79, 72, 65. Score one point for each correct answer.
		If the patient will not perform this task, ask the patient to spell "world" backwards (dlrow). Record the patient's spelling. Score 1 point for each correctly placed letter.
		Recall
3	( )	Ask the patient to repeat the names of the objects learned in the Registration section. Give one point for each object correctly named.
		Language – Naming
2	( )	Show a pencil and a watch, and ask the patient to name them.
		Repetition
1	( )	Ask the patient to repeat, "No ifs, ands, or buts."
		Three-stage Command
3	( )	Have the patient follow a three-stage command: "Take this paper in your right hand, fold the paper in half, and put the paper on the table."
		Reading
1	( )	Ask the patient to read and obey the following command: **CLOSE YOUR EYES.**
		Writing
1	( )	Have the patient write a sentence of his or her choice. The sentence should contain a subject and an object and should make sense. Ignore spelling errors when scoring.
		Construction/Copying
1	( )	Enlarge the design given below to 1.5 cm per side and have the patient copy it. Give one point if all sides and angles are preserved and if the intersecting sides form a quadrangle. 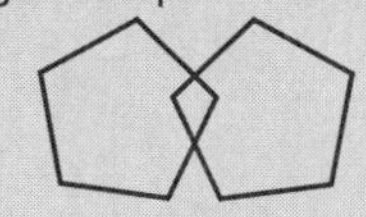
30	___	**Total**

Scoring: 0–12 (severe), 13–22 (moderate), 23–24 (mild), 25–30 (none). These ranges vary

Reprinted with permission from *J Psychiatric Research*, Vol. 12, p. 189–198, Folstein MF, Folstein SE, and McHugh PR, Mini-mental state examination: A practical method of grading the cognitive state of patients for the clinician, 1975, Elsevier Science Ltd., Pergamon Imprint, Oxford, England.

Figure 10-2 Mini-mental state examination.

(From Folstein M, Folstein S, McHugh P: Mini-mental state: A practical method of grading the cognitive state of patients for the clinician, *J Psychiatr Res* 12: 189, 1975.)

Instructions:

Ask questions 1–10 in this list, and record all answers. Ask question 4A only if patient does not have a telephone. Record total number of errors based on ten questions.

1. What is the date today? (month, day, tear)

2. What day of the week is it?

3. What is the name of this place?

4. What is your telephone number?

4a. What is your street address? (Ask only if patient does not have a telephone.)

5. What is your street address?

6. When were you born? (month, day, year)

7. Who is the president of the United States now? (last name)

8. Who was president just before him? (last name)

9. What was your mother's maiden name?

10. Subtract 3 from 20 and keep subtracting 3 from each new number, all the way down.

Scoring

For Caucasian subjects with at least some high school education, but not more than high school education, the following criteria have been established:

0–2 errors	Intact intellectual functioning
3–4 errors	Mild intellectual impairment
5–7 errors	Moderate intellectual impairment
8–10 errors	Severe intellectual impairment

Allow one more error if subject has only grade school education.

Allow one more error for African = American subjects, using identical education criteria.

Allow one less error if subject has education beyond high school.

Figure 10-3 Short portable mental status questionnaire (SPMSQ).

(From Pfeiffer E: A short portable mental status questionnaire for the assessment of organic brain deficit in elderly, *J Am Geriatr Soc* 23: 433–441, 1975.)

agree on the effect on attitudes. Several researchers found that in settings with a high degree of contact with the elderly, the health professionals held more negative attitudes toward the aged (Campbell, 1971; Fielding, 1979; Taylor and Harned, 1978). In contrast, other researchers found a higher degree of positive attitudes by health caregivers in nursing home settings (Brower, 1985; Brower, 1981). The differences in results may have been due to differences of level of experience, education, and motivational factors of the staff in each study. There is a lack of research in the area of relating attitudes to actual behaviors of nurses who work with the elderly. Other factors that influence attitudes toward the elderly include stereotyping, myths on aging, and culture.

TABLE 10-7 Five-dimensional model of health and wellness for the elderly

Dimension	Characteristics of the dimension
Self-responsibility	Self-help strategies Assume responsibilities and accountability for own health care practices Educated consumer Extends along entire health care continuum (e.g., preventative, acute, chronic, maintenance, and terminal care)
Nutritional awareness	Education about foods and food groups for healthy living Identification of barriers to good nutrition (e.g., economic, transportation, ethnic dietary habits) Nutritional supplements
Physical fitness	Individualized programs of exercise based on physical abilities Elements of fitness: aerobic capacity, body structure, body composition, balance, muscle flexibility, and muscle strength
Stress management	Effects of stress are additive across the life span in some situations Returning to a state of balance is more difficult with aging (physical and psychological stressors) Stress management activities may include relaxation, exercise, meditation, biofeedback, and autogenic training
Environmental sensitivity	Physical and social components of the environment influence one's health Environmental factors affecting elderly's health and well-being include pollution, smoking, safety, transportation, social network, economics

Compiled from Ebersole P, Hess P: *Toward healthy aging: human needs and nursing responses*, ed 4, St. Louis, 1994, Mosby.

Ageism and Stereotyping the Elderly

Levin and Levin (1980) remarked that "ageism can be regarded as an attitude, a negative evaluation that serves to orient individuals toward old people as a group." **Ageism** is defined as "a process of systematic stereotyping and discrimination against people because they are old, just as racism and sexism accomplish this for skin color and gender" (Butler, 1987). Ageism takes on many forms in society. Ageism often leads to stereotyping that may result in discriminative behaviors toward the elderly. Buschmann et al, (1981) stated that these stereotypic beliefs or myths may be a factor in some of the studies that report negative attitudes of nurses toward the elderly.

Ageism may be expressed in the daily language of a society. Adjectives such as *crotchety, grumpy, old-fashioned, feebleminded,* and *doddering* are frequently used to describe the appearance, behaviors, and demeanor of the elderly. This terminology is demoralizing to elderly persons, and may result in the elderly believing and behaving according to these terms.

Ageism also may take the form of stereotypic beliefs or images. The myths of aging are one form of stereotypic belief. Believing that myths of aging represent reality affects attitudes and behaviors. Table 10-8 summarizes some common age myths and the subsequent realities of aging.

Myths of the Golden Years

A contributor to *Reader's Digest* wrote about his feelings on retirement, when no longer tied to a 7-day work week. The children were all raised and graduated from college and now he could relax, sleep as long as he wished, go wherever and whenever he wanted. He was "free at last" (Lee, 1983), or was he? Rosenkoetter (1985) remarked that the popular view of retirement is one of "full-time leisure: playing golf, traveling, fishing, and in general, doing whatever one wishes." The lay literature on the subject of retirement depicts retirement as the endless vacation, representing an example of a "Golden Years" myth.

The myths of the golden years stemmed from supporters of the activity theory of aging, stating that the elderly substitute a host of activities to fill the void caused by retirement. Such an active, "carefree" lifestyle is often costly and therefore may not be available for everyone.

Cultural Impact

Cultural beliefs also influence one's attitudes toward the elderly. Culture influences the responses of the elderly to health, illness, and treatment. Some cultures subscribe to health care practices or home remedies that may be in direct opposition to modern health care practices. The health caregiver needs to examine his or her own feelings toward differing cultural beliefs and health care practices of elderly clients. The incorporation of some home remedies into the elderly client's care plan may increase compliance, given that these remedies are not in conflict with treatment.

Various cultures hold different views regarding aging. Since ancient times, the contributions of the elderly to a

TABLE 10-8 Myths/stereotypes and realities of aging	
Myth/stereotype	**Reality**
Elderly people are all the same as a group.	As people age, they become more heterogeneous among individuals, due to an accumulation of varied life events.
Chronologic, biologic, and psychosocial aging occur at the same rate.	People age differently. One's chronologic, biologic, and psychosocial ages may not be the same. Overall, perceptions of health status and ability to function are better indicators of aging than number of years.
Old age is a period of ongoing losses.	Old age need not be a downhill course. Many elderly contribute to society in many ways well into old age. The loss of what is meaningful to an individual seems to have the greatest negative effect.
Senility and old age are synonymous.	Senility is not an accurate term to describe dementia. Dementia is due to pathologic conditions and is not a part of normal aging.
Elderly cannot learn new skills.	Elderly are capable of learning a great deal of new information and skills. Skills requiring psychomotor coordination or speed may be more difficult and take more time to learn by the elderly.
Elderly are generally more depressed.	The rates of depression in the elderly are somewhat greater than other age cohorts. The number of young adults experiencing depression is growing at a much more alarming rate than depression in the elderly.

society affect the status of the aged within a particular cultural group. For example, Far Eastern cultures value the wisdom of their elders and thus hold the aged in high esteem. In contrast, some primitive cultures may have considered the elderly a burden, unable to hunt and provide for the tribe. Such cultures have been known to banish the elderly from the tribe.

In the current Western culture, there is greater support for views of successful aging. The focus on age has presented the public with potential issues that future elderly persons will experience, related to functional, economic, and political issues. The situation of today's elderly may be the most optimistic in terms of availability of social and economic resources, but future generations of elderly may face difficult resource issues (Conrad, 1992). The costs may outweigh the contributions by future elderly in society, and cultural values toward the elderly may change.

Summary of Key Concepts

1. The elderly population is growing in number and proportion of the entire U.S. population, especially those in minority groups, so health care providers need to have an understanding of biologic, social, and psychologic aging processes.

2. The process of aging is a period of decreases in function, but the elderly have great reserves to adapt to loss and change.

3. The major theories that attempt to explain developmental processes of aging can be divided into biologic, sociologic, and psychologic theories of aging.

4. Many physiologic and psychosocial changes occur as a result of aging.

5. Most elderly perceive their overall health as good to very good.

REFERENCES

Albrecht T, Adelman M: Social support and life stress: new directions for communication research, *Hum Communication Res* 11: 3–32, 1984.

Atchley R: A continuity theory of normal aging, *Gerontologist* 29: 183–190, 1989.

Baltes M, Kuhl K, Sowarka D: Testing for limits of cognitive reserve capacity: a promising strategy for early diagnosis of dementia?, *J Gerontol* 47: 165–167, 1992.

Bennett N, Garson L: Extraordinary longevity in the Soviet Union: fact or artifact? *Gerontologist* 26: 358–361, 1986.

Birren J, Schaie K: *Handbook of the psychology of aging*, ed 2, New York, 1985, Van Nostrand Reinhold.

Botwinick J: *Aging and behavior*, ed 3, New York, 1984, Springer Publishing.

Botwinick J: Intellectual abilities. In Birren J, Schaie K, editors: *Handbook of the psychology of aging*, New York, 1977, Van Nostrand Reinhold.

Bowman B, Rosenberg I: Digestive function and aging, *Human Nutrition: Clinical Nutrition*, 27C: 75–89, 1983.

Bretschneider J, McCoy N: Sexual interest and behavior in healthy 80 to 102 year olds, *Arch Sex Behav* 17: 109–129, 1988.

Broadhead W et al: The epidemiologic evidence for a relationship between social support and health, *Am J Epidemiol* 117: 521–537, 1983.

Brower H: Do nurses stereotype the aged?, *J Gerontol Nursing* 11: 17–28, 1985.

Brower H: Social organization and nurses' attitudes toward older persons, *J Gerontol Nursing* 7: 293–298, 1981.

Buschmann M, Burns E, Jones F: Student nurses' attitudes towards the elderly, *J Nurs Educ* 20: 7–10, 1981.

Butler R: Ageism. In Maddox G, editor: *The encyclopedia of aging*, New York, 1987, Springer Publishing.

Campbell M: Study of the attitudes of nursing personnel toward the geriatric patient, *Nurs Res* 20: 127–151, 1971.

Carter J: The effects of aging upon selected visual functions: color vision, glare sensitivity, field of vision, and accommodation. In Sekuler R, Kline D, Dismukes K, editors: *Aging and human visual function*, New York, 1982, Oxford University Press.

Centers for Disease Control: *Life expectancy in 33 developing countries*, Atlanta, April 7, 1990.

Conrad C: Old age in the modern and post-modern western world. In Cole T, Van Tassel D, Kastenbaum R, editors: *Handbook of the humanities and aging*, New York, 1992, Springer Publishing.

Cumming E, Henry W: *Growing old: the process of disengagement*, New York, 1961, Basic Books.

Denney N et al: An adult development study of contextual memory, *J Gerontol* 46: 44–50, 1991.

Ebersole P, Hess P: *Toward healthy aging: human needs and nursing responses*, ed 4, St. Louis, 1994, Mosby.

Enloe C: Managing daily living with diminishing resources and losses. In Carnevali D, Patrick M, editors: *Nursing management for the elderly*, ed 3, Philadelphia, 1993, JB Lippincott.

Erikson E, Erikson J, and Kiunick H: *Vital involvement in old age: the experience of old age in our time*, New York, 1986, WW Norton.

Fielding P: An exploratory investigation of self concept in the institutionalized elderly, and a comparison with nurses' conceptions and attitudes, *Int J Nurs Stud* 16: 345–354, 1979.

Folstein M, Folstein S, McHugh P: "Mini-mental state": a practical method of grading the cognitive state of patients for the clinician, *J Psychiatr Res* 12: 189, 1975.

Fries J, Williams C, Morfeld D: Improvement in intergenerational health, *Am J Public Health* 82: 109–112, 1992.

Hatfield T, Hatfield S: As if your life depended on it: promoting cognitive development to promote wellness, *J Counseling Development* 71: 164–167, 1992.

Havighurst R, Neugarten B, Tobin S: Disengagement and patterns of aging. In Neugarten B, editor: *Middle age and aging*, Chicago, 1968, University of Chicago Press.

Hayflick L: Theories of biological aging. In Andres R, Bierman E, Hazzard W, editors: *Principles of geriatric medicine*, New York, 1985, McGraw-Hill.

Hertzog C, Dixon R, Hultsch D: Relationships between metamemory, memory predictions, and memory task performance in adults, *Psychol Aging* 5: 215–227, 1990.

Hollinger L, Buschmann M: Factors influencing the perception of touch by elderly nursing home residents and their health caregivers, *Int J Nurs Stud* 30: 445–461, 1993.

Horn J, Cattell R: Age differences in fluid and crystallized intelligence, *Acta Psychologica* 26: 107–129, 1967.

Hyde R: Facilitative communication skills training: social support for elderly people, *Gerontologist* 28: 418–420, 1988.

Jung C: The stages of life. In Campbell J, editor: *The portable Jung*, New York, 1971, Viking Press.

Kumpe P, et al: The aging respiratory system. *Clin Geriatr Med* 1: 143–175, 1985.

Lakatta E: Cardiovascular system aging. In Kent B, Butler R, editors: *Human aging research: concepts and techniques*, New York, 1988, Raven Press.

Lee H: Why I won't retire, *Reader's Digest* 122: 61–64, 1983.

Lemon B, Bengston V, Peterson J: An exploration of the activity theory of aging: activity types and life satisfaction among inmovers to a retirement community, *J Gerontol* 27: 511, 1972.

Levin J, Levin W: *Ageism: prejudice and discrimination against the elderly*, Belmont, Calif, 1980, Wadsworth.

Levinson D, Darrow C, Klein E: *The seasons of a man's life*, New York, 1978, Knopf.

Lowenthal M, Chiriboga D: Social stress and adaptation: toward a life course perspective. In Eisdorfer C, Lowton M, editors: *The psychology of adult development and aging*, Washington, D.C., 1973, American Psychological Association.

Maslow A: *Toward a psychology of being*, New York, 1962, Van Nostrand.

Meier D: Skeletal aging. In Kent B, Butler R, editors: *Human aging research: concepts and techniques*, New York, 1988, Raven Press.

Miller C: *Nursing care of older adults: theory and practice*, Glenview, Ill., 1990, Scott, Foresman & Co.

Olsho L, Harkins S, Harmon B: Aging and the auditory system. In Birren J, Schaie K, editors: *Handbook of the psychology of aging*, ed 2, New York, 1985, Van Nostrand Reinhold.

Oxman T, Berkman L: Assessment of social relationships in elderly patients, *Int J Psychiatry Med* 20: 65–84, 1990.

Packer L, Glazer A: *Oxygen radicals in biological systems. Part B, oxygen radicals and antioxidants*, San Diego, 1990, Academic Press.

Perlmutter M et al: Aging and memory, *Annu Rev Gerontol Geriatr* 7: 57–92, 1987.

Pfeiffer E: A short portable mental status questionnaire for the assessment of organic brain deficit in elderly patients, *J Am Geriatr Soc* 23: 433–441, 1975.

Rosenkoetter M: Role change after retirement, *J Gerontol Nurs* 11: 21–24, 1985.

Ryan E: Beliefs about memory changes across the adult life span, *J Gerontol* 47: 41–46, 1992.

Ryan E, See S: Age-based beliefs about memory changes for self and others across adulthood, *J Gerontol* 48: 199–201, 1993.

Schaie K, Willis S: *Adult development and aging*, Boston, 1986, Little, Brown.

Schneider E, Rowe J: *Handbook of the biology of aging*, ed 3, San Diego, 1990, Academic Press.

Smith L: Retirement options: pack up or stay put, *Grandparents*, Spring: 62–74, 1987.

Steinberg F: The aging of organs and organ systems. In Steinberg F, editor: *Care of the geriatric patient*, ed 6, St. Louis, 1983, Mosby.

Szinovacz M, Washo C: Gender differences in exposure to life events and adaptation to retirement, *J Gerontol* 47: 191–196, 1992.

Taylor K, Harned T: Attitudes toward old people: a study of nurses who care for the elderly, *J Gerontol Nurs* 4: 43–47, 1978.

U.S. Bureau of the Census: Census of population: general population characteristics (1990). Washington, D.C., 1992, U.S. Department of Commerce, Economics, and Statistics Administration.

U.S. Bureau of the Census: How we're changing: demographic state of the nation, 1990. In *Current Population Reports*, series P-23, No. 170. Washington, D.C., 1991, U.S. Department of Commerce, Economics, and Statistics Administration.

U.S. Bureau of the Census: Population profile of the United States. In *Current Population Reports*, series P-23, special studies. Washington, D.C., 1991, U.S. Department of Commerce, Economics, and Statistics Administration.

U.S. Department of Health and Human Services, Public Health Service: *Healthy People 2000*, DHHS Publ. No. (PHS) 91-50213, 1990.

U.S. Department of Health and Human Services: Health data on older Americans. Hyattsville, Md., Public Health Service, Centers for Disease Control and Prevention, National Center for Health Statistics, No. PHS93-1411, 1993.

Vaillant G: *Adaptation to life*, Boston, 1977, Little, Brown.

Woodruff D: A review of aging and cognitive processes, *Res Aging* 5: 139–153, 1983.

Mental/Emotional Disorders

False Face Mask
IROQUOIS

The highly organized Iroquois Indians carved masks into trees that were alive and growing and then cut them away from the tree. The masks were used in ceremonies to heal individuals' mental, emotional, or physical disorders, or to protect the entire tribe from illness. Part Four discusses the major mental disorders and treatment according to an interdisciplinary process.

CHAPTER 11

Anxiety and Related Disorders

Monica Ann Molloy

CHAPTER OUTLINE

Anxiety A vague, subjective, nonspecific feeling of uneasiness, tension, apprehension, and sometimes dread or impending doom. It occurs as a result of a threat to one's biologic, physiologic, or social integrity arising from external influences.

Compulsion A continual, repetitive impulse to perform a behavior (for example, hand washing, counting, or checking) or mental acts (for example, praying, counting, or repeating words silently), the goal of which is to prevent or reduce anxiety or distress and not to provide pleasure or gratification. In most cases the person feels driven to perform the compulsion to reduce the distress that accompanies an obsession or to prevent some dreaded event or situation.

Dissociation The separation of an overwhelming event or experience from an individual's conscious awareness.

Humanistic nursing A view of nursing as an interactive process that occurs between two people, one needing help and one willing to give help; developed by nursing theorists Patterson and Zderad.

Obsessions Persistent ideas, thoughts, impulses, or images about death, sexual matters, religious matters, or any themes that lead to efforts to resist them, are associated with marked distress or interference, and result in marked anxiety or distress.

Phobias Group of disorders primarily characterized by avoidance of a specific situation or escape, if that situation is unexpectedly encountered.

Repression Involuntary exclusion of a painful, threatening experience. It begins in infancy and continues throughout life. It underlies all other defense mechanisms but also operates as its own defense mechanism.

Stress The nonspecific response of the body to any demand made upon it, regardless of whether the demand is pleasant or unpleasant (Seyle, 1956).

- Employ two of the etiologic models to explain the four stages of anxiety.

- Use the defining characteristics in the NANDA diagnosis *anxiety* to differentiate between circumscribed and pervasive anxiety disorders.

- Design a teaching plan for family members of clients with obsessive-compulsive disorder.

- Appraise the coping mechanisms of trauma victims in order to evaluate risk for posttraumatic stress disorder.

- Apply a cost-benefit approach to weigh the advantages of inpatient and outpatient treatment of dissociative identity disorder.

- Evaluate the advantages of the humanistic nursing model in providing care to clients experiencing varying levels of anxiety.

- Discuss the usefulness of clinical rating scales in evaluating collaborative treatment outcomes of inpatients with anxiety disorders and obsessive-compulsive disorder.

- Relate the biologic models to target symptoms and therapeutic agents for psychopharmacologic intervention in anxiety and related disorders.

Anxiety is an integral part of the universal human experience. For most people, most of the time, it is a vague, subjective, nonspecific feeling of uneasiness with no identifiable object, resulting from an external threat to one's integrity. The function of anxiety is to warn the individual of impending threat, conflict, or danger.

Anxiety is also a state of tension, dread, or impending doom, arising from external influences that threaten to be overwhelming. When an individual receives a signal of approaching danger, he or she is motivated to action: flee the threatening situation or attempt to control dangerous impulses. The person may also freeze to the spot, immobilized.

Defense mechanisms are the primary methods the self uses in an attempt to control or manage anxiety. Defenses protect the individual from threats to biological, psychological, and social aspects of self.

Anxiety responses exist on a continuum. Most individuals are more or less successful at using various methods, including adaptive use of defense mechanisms, to control their own experiences of anxiety. Those who are less successful or rely primarily on less adaptive or rigid use of defense mechanisms (for example, dissociation in the case of dissociative identity disorder, or projection in the case of paranoid schizophrenia), develop the defining characteristics of the anxiety disorders.

HISTORICAL AND THEORETICAL PERSPECTIVES

Hildegard Peplau, a pioneer of psychiatric-mental health nursing, identified four stages of anxiety on a continuum in *Interpersonal Relations in Nursing* in order to illustrate Sullivan's view of anxiety and tension (Peplau, 1952). These stages are expanded on in Figure 11-1. Optimally functioning people generally function in the mild range of anxiety. This level of anxiety facilitates learning, creativity, and personal growth. Occasional movement to the moderate level is also an adaptive mechanism to cope with situational stressors, whether they are pleasant or unpleasant. When the stressor is managed, the adapted person moves back along the continuum to mild anxiety. Moderate and severe anxiety can be acute or chronic. In severe anxiety, energy is focused primarily on reducing anxiety rather than on coping with the environment. Consequently the individual's level of function is impaired. In panic anxiety the individual is disorganized, with increased motor activity, distorted visual perceptual field, loss of rational thought, and decreased ability to relate to others. Responses to anxiety are more fully explained in Table 11-1.

Rollo May distinguishes between fear and anxiety by differentiating anxiety from all other affects. Fear is a threat to the periphery of an individual's existence, but anxiety is a threat to the foundation and center of existence. The experience of anxiety confirms the existence of a measure of freedom (Hall and Lindzey, 1978).

In addition to describing anxiety by degree, anxiety can also be differentiated by types. *Signal anxiety* is experienced when a precipitant is identified; it is a learned anxiety response. Although signal anxiety is learned, it results from situations that have been successfully repressed or coped with using another defense mechanism. Consequently, the precipitant is successfully excluded from consciousness. Signal anxiety is the predominant etiologic factor in phobic disorders.

Trait anxiety is a function of personality structure. As a part of developmental processes or events, some individuals have more traumatic experiences or have less success in coping with them, resulting in unresolved

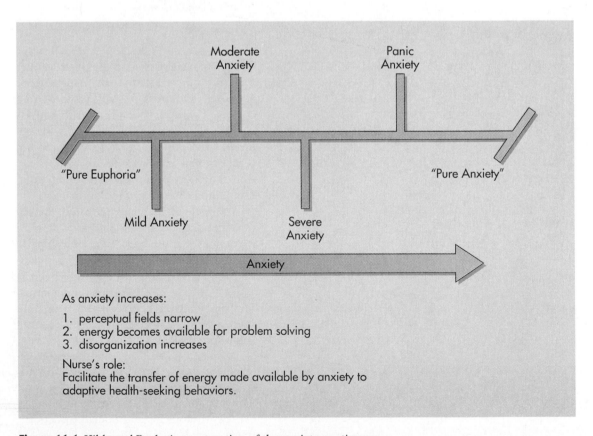

Figure 11-1 Hildegard Peplau's construction of the anxiety continuum.

(Adapted from Peplau H: *Interpersonal relations in nursing: a conceptual frame of reference for psychodynamic nursing,* New York, 1991, Springer Publishing Co. Used with permission.)

TABLE 11-1	Responses to anxiety		
Anxiety level	**Physiologic**	**Cognitive/perceptual**	**Emotional/behavioral**
Mild	Vital signs normal. Minimal muscle tension. Pupils normal, constricted.	Perceptual field is broad. Awareness of multiple environmental and internal stimuli. Thoughts may be random, but controlled.	Feelings of relative comfort and safety. Relaxed, calm appearance and voice. Performance is automatic, habitual behaviors occur here.
Moderate	Vital signs normal or slightly elevated. Tension experienced, may be uncomfortable or pleasurable (labeled as "tense" or "excited").	Alert; perception narrowed, focused. Optimum state for problem solving and learning. Attentive.	Feelings of readiness and challenge; energized. Engage in competitive activity and learn new skills. Voice, facial expression interested or concerned.
Severe	Fight or flight response. Autonomic nervous system excessively stimulated (vital signs increased, diaphoresis increased, urinary urgency and frequency, diarrhea, dry mouth, appetite decreased, pupils dilated). Muscles rigid, tense. Senses affected; hearing decreased, pain sensation decreased.	Perceptual field greatly narrowed. Problem solving difficult. Selective attention (focus on one detail). Selective inattention (block out threatening stimuli). Distortion of time (things seem faster or slower than actual). Dissociative tendencies; vigilambulism (automatic behavior).	Feels threatened, startles with new stimuli; feels on "overload." Activity may increase or decrease (may pace, run away, wring hands, moan, shake, stutter, become very disorganized or withdrawn, freeze in position/unable to move). May seem and feel depressed. Demonstrates denial; may complain of aches or pains; may be agitated or irritable. Need for space increased. Eyes may dart around room or gaze may be fixed. May close eyes to shut out environment.
Panic	Above symptoms escalate until sympathetic nervous system release occurs. Person may become pale, blood pressure decreases, hypotension. Muscle coordination poor. Pain, hearing sensations minimal.	Perception totally scattered or closed. Unable to take in stimuli. Problem solving and logical thinking highly improbable. Perception of unreality about self, environment, or event. Dissociation may occur.	Feels helpless with total loss of control. May be angry, terrified, may become combative or totally withdrawn, cry, run. Completely disorganized. Behavior is usually extremely active or inactive.

From Fortinash K, Holoday-Worret P: *Psychiatric nursing care plans,* ed 2, St. Louis, 1995, Mosby.

conflict or confusion. These people are described as having an *anxiety diathesis,* a predisposition to anxiety when stressed. Situations that re-create or represent the original conflict or experience evoke a more severe anxiety response in people with a higher level of trait anxiety. For example, a woman whose mother was chronically ill for much of her childhood may worry excessively about her own children being injured or catching colds. As a result she limits their activity and is anxious and overprotective.

State anxiety develops in a situation identified as stressful or conflictual, and in which the individual experiences limited control. This is often perceived as anxiety that has occurred before. For example, the "butterflies" a student experiences before an important exam is mild state anxiety. The increased heart rate a person who has been bitten by a dog may experience when confronted by a Great Dane is a more moderate form of state anxiety. A woman with a strong family history of cancer who delays making an appointment with her primary health care provider after noticing a lump in her breast demonstrates severe and maladaptive state anxiety. Free-floating anxiety is characterized by a pervasive sense of dread or doom that cannot be attached to any idea or event.

State and trait anxiety are important concepts for nurses because they can be differentiated and estimated by a rating scale, the State/Trait Anxiety Inventory. Persons with high levels of trait anxiety can be expected to experience higher levels of state anxiety when confronted with significant stressors. Nurses who can estimate their client's level of trait anxiety during the assessment process are better able to promptly institute interventions directed at facilitating the client's coping with high state anxiety responses to identified stressors.

Anxiety in Psychiatric Practice

Descriptions of anxiety as a phenomenon of concern in mental health are relatively recent. Psychiatry as a medical specialty had its origins in the late eighteenth century. Prior to that time, care for the insane (lunatics) fell to the law or to the church. Foucault (1965) asserts that madness replaced death as a major theme in human experience.

During the Age of Reason and into the nineteenth century, early psychiatric practitioners concerned themselves with the psychoses, those mental disorders thought to pose the greatest risk to society. However, in the second half of the nineteenth century as the roots of psychoanalytic theory developed, anxiety (neuroses) emerged as a source of a variety of emotional and behavioral disturbances.

Anxiety in the Context of Psychiatric-Mental Health Nursing

The term *anxiety* is used in such a variety of contexts that it is important to be precise in its usage. One definition for anxiety is the inability to choose among potentials (May, 1979). Facilitating the discovery of meaning or becoming, as well as facilitating choices through a relationship, is one way to conceptualize the process of psychiatric-mental health nursing. All relationships are not nursing, but the basis for all nursing is a relationship. The phenomenon of relationship as applied to nursing does not imply equal participation or responsibility on the part of the nurse and client but merely the nurse's intention to establish a connection. Caring for an unconscious, anesthetized, or psychotic individual establishes a connection; therefore, it is a relationship. For psychiatric nurses, the primary goal of the nurse-client relationship is to become available to the individual. Through establishing a relationship, both the client and the nurse have the opportunity to develop their potentials as human beings. Managing anxiety by recognizing and learning to make choices is critical to both the nurse and the client in this process.

Humanistic Nursing

Hildegard Peplau's anxiety continuum is a nursing theory widely used in the treatment of anxiety disorders. Humanistic nursing theory can also be applied to treating anxiety disorders. Patterson and Zderad developed a theory of **humanistic nursing** based on existential theory and the phenomenological method.

The cornerstone of their theory is that nursing is an interactive process that occurs between two persons, one needing help and one willing to give help. Nurses and clients interact. The client "calls," and the nurse "responds." Humanistic nursing differs from Peplau's interpersonal nursing in that the nurse is clearly identified as a participant in the process. The nurse strives to be fully present in the process and is described in relationship "with" the client. The nurse's availability to the client is critical to the process of nursing.

ETIOLOGY
Biologic Model

Roots of the biologic model for anxiety disorders date back to the nineteenth-century writings of Charles Darwin. Darwin postulated that emotional expression and anatomical structures both changed in the course of evolution to enable the species to adapt to its environment. He further postulated that certain emotions are universally demonstrated through expression, using motor and postural changes. In the early twentieth century, investigators linked the endocrine system with emotions, initially by establishing the relationship of the adrenal medulla in production of epinephrine, resulting in the fight or flight response theory.

Seyle built on this work after World War II, using observations of stress and anxiety demonstrated by soldiers who served in combat. A new conceptualization of stress replaced the former "psychic trauma." Seyle expanded the notion that the endocrine system and the central nervous system (CNS), particularly the hypothalamus and pituitary gland, have a reciprocal relationship. At the same time, important investigations were conducted in the neuropharmacology of the autonomic nervous system (ANS) in regulating cardiovascular, gastrointestinal, and motor responses. The ANS, particularly the sympathetic nervous system, was shown to be responsive to environmental stimuli, including emotional states. These biological investigations accept the continuity between normal states of fear and anxiety and the clinical disorders (Klerman in Ballenger, 1990). Today, psychopharmacological interventions target the serotonin, noradrenergic, and GABA systems primarily. (For a more detailed discussion see the section on psychobiology in Chapter 5.)

Psychodynamic Model

In psychoanalytic terms, anxiety is viewed as a warning to the ego that it is in danger from an internal or external threat. Anxiety is involved in the development of personality, personality functioning, and in the development and treatment of neuroses and psychoses. Freud's work is the basis for anxiety neurosis existing as a separate classification.

There are three types of anxiety identified in psychoanalytic theory: reality anxiety, moral anxiety, and neurotic anxiety. Reality anxiety is a painful emotional experience resulting from the perception of danger in the external world. Fear is the response to external danger; consequently, anxiety parallels fear. Moral anxiety is the ego's experience of guilt or shame. Neurotic anxiety is the perception of a threat from one's instincts (Hall, 1954).

In his theory of signal anxiety, Freud postulated that anxiety was a signal of impending emergence of threatening unconscious mental content. Neurotic symptoms developed in an attempt to defend against anxiety—including hysterical symptoms, obsessions, compulsions, and phobias.

Interpersonal Model

The interpersonal model views anxiety as a response to the individual's external environment, rather than the relatively simple psychoanalytic view of a response to instinctual drives. Interpersonal theorists, particularly Sullivan, regarded symptom formation as a result of expectations, insecurities, frustrations, and conflicts between individuals and primary groups. Primary groups include families, work colleagues, and social associates.

Like psychoanalytic theorists, interpersonal theorists place a great deal of emphasis on the impact of early development and experiences on later mental health. Sullivan marks the individual's first experience of anxiety as the infant's perception of the anxiety of the mothering person. The self system develops in the context of approval or disapproval from significant others. Disapproval results from a threat to the self system, a fear of rejection; in other words, anxiety.

Interpersonal theorists define anxiety broadly. Sullivan believed that anxiety is the first great educative experience in living. Sullivan believed that one of the great tasks of psychology is to discover the basic vulnerabilities to anxiety in interpersonal relations rather than to try to deal with the symptoms of anxiety.

Behavioral Model

In behavioral models, based on learning theory, the etiology of anxiety symptoms is a generalization from an earlier traumatic experience to a benign setting or object. For example, an awkward child, ridiculed by parents while bowling, pairs embarrassment and shame with sports events in indoor facilities and develops panic attacks during basketball games. The same kinds of cognitive operations that link embarrassment with sporting events link cognitions of the expectation of embarrassment with the idea of a sporting event, and the individual begins experiencing panic attacks while reading the sports page. Consequently, in this model, anxiety occurs when an individual encounters a signal that "predicts" a painful or feared event.

Early behavioral therapists directed their efforts at the anxiety disorders. In 1958, Wolpe, a South African physician working with soldiers experiencing symptoms now classified as post-traumatic stress disorder, reported success using systematic desensitization applied to simple phobia (1973). Systematic desensitization is a method derived from learning theory in which the deeply relaxed client is exposed to a graded hierarchy of phobic stimuli. This method was refined further into a method termed *in vivo desensitization* where the individual is exposed to progressively more anxiety-provoking situations, often accompanied by a therapist. These live exposure treatments can take a variety of forms, including graded practice, participant modeling, and prolonged or brief duration.

Continuum Model

Until the 1980 publication of the DSM-III and the subsequent epidemiological data obtained in the Epidemiological Catchment Area (ECA) study, the most prevalent view of the anxiety disorders was a continuum of neurotic states, increasing in severity. Disorders characterized by delusions, hallucinations, and dementia clearly were outside of ordinary experiences. But the experiences of anxiety and depression were common to most people, and the line between normal variance and pathology was blurred.

This continuum model was consistent with social agendas aimed at destigmatizing mental illness and eliciting compassion and concern for persons with mental illness. As more and more research conflicting with the continuum model was conducted and disseminated, it was abandoned in favor of several distinct paradigms. These formulations are better suited to some of the disorders described in this chapter than others, and no single model is comprehensive enough to explain the etiology of all anxiety, somatization, and dissociative disorders. The biological and behavioral paradigms or models are the most recent and have the most convincing evidence to explain pathogenesis and treatment strategies to date. The models relating to anxiety are summarized in Box 11-1.

Box 11-1   Etiology Models of Anxiety and Related Disorders

Biological: Involves dysregulation of neurotransmitter system. Provides framework for symptom development and pharmacotherapeutic intervention.

Psychodynamic: Involves unconscious conflict. Provides framework for continuum of anxiety responses as individual attempts to defend against anxiety.

Interpersonal: Involves interaction. Provides framework to explain anxiety responses experienced in relation to other individuals.

Behavioral: Involves cognition. Provides framework to explain anxiety as physiological and cognitive responses to external stimuli.

EPIDEMIOLOGY

Sex Ratio

The Environmental Catchment Area (ECA) study has recently emphasized the extensiveness of the anxiety disorders in terms of short-term and lifelong prevalence. According to Ross et al (1988), the six-month prevalence of anxiety disorders in the general population ranges from 6%–8%, with a phobic anxiety rate of about 1.5%. Lifetime prevalence of anxiety disorders is estimated to exceed 15%. The rates of panic disorder were higher in women, in persons ages 24–44, and in the separated and divorced (APA, 1994).

Almost all clients presenting with agoraphobia in clinical samples have a current diagnosis or history of panic disorder. In contrast, epidemiological samples identify more clients with agoraphobia without history of panic disorder. Agoraphobia is diagnosed more often in women than men.

Simple phobia is common in the general population, with reported lifetime prevalence rates of 10%–12% (APA, 1994). Overall, the prevalence of simple phobia is higher for women than men. However, among fear of heights and blood injection injury, the percentage of males is higher, from 30%–45% as compared with 10%–25% in other categories.

In contrast to other anxiety disorders, in clinical samples, equal numbers of men and women seek treatment for social phobia. However, in community-based samples, social phobia is more common among women. Lifetime prevalence rates vary from 3%–13% (APA, 1994). In outpatient treatment settings, rates of social phobia range from 10%–20% of persons seeking treatment for anxiety disorders. Similarly, obsessive-compulsive disorder is equally common in men and women; lifetime prevalence is estimated at 2.5% (APA, 1994).

Estimates for prevalence of post-traumatic stress disorder range from 3%–58% of at-risk individuals, with this wide variability due to both sampling methods and the population assessed. Community-based samples for prevalence range from 1%–14% (APA, 1994).

The prevalence of dissociative disorders is difficult to estimate. The diagnosis is usually made after an individual seeks treatment. There is still substantial controversy surrounding dissociative disorders. The lack of epidemiological data reflects both case-finding difficulty as well as clinician bias. The disorder is more commonly diagnosed among women.

Age of Onset

In general, anxiety disorders develop during adolescence and early adulthood. The typical age of onset for panic disorder varies from late adolescence to the mid-30s. Rare cases have an onset in childhood, and a small number develop symptoms after age 45. Acute and post-traumatic stress disorders can develop at any age.

Age of onset for specific phobias, situational type, is bimodally distributed. There is a peak of onset in childhood and another peak in early adulthood. Other types of phobias usually have an onset in childhood.

Cultural Variance

Most of the research supporting the development of the DSM-IV was done in the United States; consequently, symptoms defining disorders are representative of that culture. However, care should be taken to establish cultural norms when evaluating clients for anxiety and related disorders. For example, some cultures restrict women's participation in public activities, thus agoraphobia is less commonly diagnosed. Fears of magic or spirits are present in many cultures and should only be considered pathological when the fear is excessive in the context of that culture. Many cultures prescribe rituals to mark important events in peoples' lives. The observation of these rituals is not considered indicative of obsessive-compulsive disorder unless it exceeds norms for that culture, is exhibited at times or places inappropriate for that culture, or interferes with social functioning.

It seems that with the exception of obsessive-compulsive disorder and social phobia, anxiety and related disorders exhibit a higher prevalence among women than men. This observation may represent a cultural variation. Overall, women are more likely to present for treatment or come in contact with health care providers than men.

Comorbidity

Anxiety disorders do not exist in a clinical vacuum. In one study of a general medical practice, Katon et al (1986) determined that 13% of clients presenting for treatment met criteria for panic disorder. In the same sample, another 25% had past histories of panic disorder or less severe anxiety syndromes.

An early estimate of the comorbidity between anxiety and depression was offered by Rosh in 1959 who estimated that half of the clients suffering from the phobic-anxiety depersonalization syndrome experienced varying degrees of depression (Stein and Uhde, 1990). ECA risk ratios were not quite as high. Clients with major depression had an 18.8%-fold increased risk of panic, and a 15.3%-fold increased risk of agoraphobia. There is substantial comorbidity between substance abuse disorders and anxiety disorders.

Obsessive-compulsive disorder (OCD) exists with other anxiety disorders, as well as substance abuse, major depression, and eating disorders. In Tourette's disorder, 30%–50% of clients also have OCD; however, the rate of Tourette's among OCD clients is lower, with estimates from 5%–7%.

Acute and post-traumatic stress disorders are associated with increased risk for major depression, other anxiety disorders, somatization disorder, and substance

Box 11-2   Epidemiology of Anxiety and Related Disorders

- Anxiety disorder manifests for six months in 6%–8% of the general population, as phobia in 1.5%, and for life in more than 15%.

- Women are diagnosed with anxiety disorder more often in the 24–44 age group and in the separated/divorced group.

- 10%–12% of the general population have simple phobia.

- Women are diagnosed more often with simple phobia except for fear of heights and blood injection injury.

- Lifetime prevalence rates for social phobia are from 3%–13%.

- Obsessive-compulsive disorder, equally common in men and women, has a lifetime prevalence rate of 2.5%.

- Prevalence of post-traumatic stress disorder ranges from 3%–58%.

- Most anxiety disorders develop during adolescence and early adulthood.

- Differences in cultures affect manifestation of anxiety disorders.

- Except for obsessive-compulsive disorder and social phobia, anxiety disorders are more common among women.

- Clients with major depression have an 18.8% increased risk for panic disorder and a 15.3% increased risk for agoraphobia.

- While 30%–50% of clients with Tourette's disorder have obsessive-compulsive disorder, only 5%–7% of clients with obsessive-compulsive disorder have Tourette's.

- Obsessive-compulsive disorder exists with anxiety disorders, substance abuse, major depression, and eating disorders.

abuse disorders. Because of the nature of the disorder and its presentation after a significant event, it is difficult to determine whether the comorbid condition developed before the stress disorder or as a consequence of it. The epidemiology of anxiety disorders are summarized in Box 11-2.

CLINICAL DESCRIPTIONS
Anxiety Disorders

The anxiety disorders as they are described in this chapter are categorized by whether they have circumscribed or limited symptom complexes, or whether their symptoms are pervasive.

PANIC

Freud first named panic attacks as occurring when "the connection between anxiety and threatened danger is entirely lost from view . . . spontaneous attacks . . . represented by intensely developed symptoms . . . tremor, vertigo, palpitations of the heart" (Freud, 1917, 1963). Freud also noted the comorbidity of the anxiety disorders and depression.

Following World War II, neuropsychiatrists identified a similar symptom complex and named it anxiety neurosis. The neuropsychiatrists were describing what is today called panic disorder.

Panic anxiety refers to anxiety symptoms that occur during panic attacks. Panic anxiety is differentiated from generalized anxiety by the sudden onset of distressing physical symptoms, combined with thoughts of dread, impending doom, death, and fear of being trapped. However, despite the gains made in describing the condition, the analytical conceptualization of anxiety neurosis remained intact until 1980.

PANIC ATTACK

Panic attacks are not codeable as psychiatric illnesses on the axes of the DSM-IV system. Panic attacks are symptoms that meet some of the defining characteristics of many of the disorders described in this chapter.

Panic attacks are sudden, spontaneous episodes accompanied by symptoms such as racing heart or palpitations, dizziness, dyspnea, and a feeling that death is imminent.

In order to be described as a panic "attack," four of the symptoms defining a panic attack must be present. Episodes of panic anxiety with fewer than four symptoms are termed *limited symptom attacks*. Panic attacks occur in a variety of the anxiety disorders, including panic disorder, social phobia, simple phobia, and post-traumatic stress disorder. Panic attacks can occur in specific, cued situations (as with simple phobias) or in uncued (unexpected) situations (APA, 1994). The DSM-IV Criteria box on page 234 lists the defining symptoms of a panic attack.

PANIC DISORDER

DSM-IV criteria state that an individual may be diagnosed with panic disorder who has both of the following criteria: (1) recent and unexpected panic attacks, and (2) at least one of the attacks has been followed by a month or more of (a) persistent concern about having additional attacks; (b) worry about the implications of the attack or its consequences (for example, losing control, having a heart attack, "going crazy"); or (c) a significant change in behavior related to the attacks.

In panic disorder without agoraphobia, the individual must be free from agoraphobic symptoms, the panic attacks must not be related to direct effects of a substance (for example, drugs of abuse, medication) and must not

DSM-IV CRITERIA

Panic Attack

A discrete period of intense fear or discomfort in which four or more of the following symptoms developed abruptly and reached a peak within 10 minutes.

1. Palpitations, pounding heart, accelerated heart rate
2. Sweating
3. Trembling or shaking
4. Sensations of shortness of breath or smothering
5. Feeling of choking
6. Chest pain or discomfort
7. Nausea or abdominal distress
8. Feeling dizzy, unsteady, lightheaded, or faint
9. Derealization or depersonalization
10. Fear of losing control or going crazy
11. Fear of dying
12. Parasthesias
13. Chills or hot flashes

Reprinted with permission from *Diagnostic and statistical manual of mental disorders,* ed 4, Washington, D.C., 1994, American Psychiatric Association.

be due to a physiological condition (for example, hyperthyroidism). In addition, the anxiety is not better accounted for by another mental disorder—obsessive-compulsive disorder (for example, fear of contamination) or post-traumatic stress disorder (for example, in response to stimuli associated with a severe stressor). To be diagnosed with panic disorder with agoraphobia, the individual must meet the criteria for panic disorder specified above, as well as experience debilitating agoraphobic symptoms (APA, 1994).

PHOBIAS

The prominent features of **phobias,** or phobic disorders, are that the patient experiences panic attacks in response to particular situations or learns to avoid the situations that evoke panic attacks.

Agoraphobia. Agoraphobia is defined as anxiety about being in places or situations from which escape may be difficult (or embarrassing), or in which help might not be readily available in the event of having an unexpected or situationally predisposed anxiety or panic attack. Agoraphobic fears typically involve characteristic clusters of situations that include being outside the home alone, being in a crowd or standing in line, being on a bridge, and traveling in a bus, train, or car. Agoraphobic situations are avoided, endured with distress or with anxiety about having a panic attack, or require the presence

of a companion. Agoraphobia can exist with or without panic attacks. If panic attacks are present, they are not due to the direct effects of a substance or a general medical condition. The individual may develop panic-like symptoms if panic attacks are not present. In addition, the anxiety or phobic avoidance is not better accounted for by another mental disorder, as described in the panic disorder section (APA, 1994).

If the individual has a comorbid medical condition, the fear described must be clearly in excess of that usually associated with the medical condition.

Specific phobias. The DSM-IV criteria define specific phobia as a marked and persistent fear that is excessive or unreasonable, cued by the presence or anticipation of a specific object or situation. Exposure to the phobic stimulus, such as animals or heights, invariably provokes an anxiety response that may take the form of a cued panic attack (see DSM-IV Criteria for a panic attack at left).

Children with specific phobia may express their anxiety by crying, tantrums, freezing, or clinging. Adults with simple phobia recognize that their fear is excessive or unreasonable. They avoid phobic situations or endure them with distress. The avoidance, anticipatory anxiety, or distress interferes significantly with the person's routine or occupational or social functioning. Or there is marked distress about having the phobia. The condition cannot be better accounted for by another AXIS I mental disorder (APA, 1994).

Social phobia. Social phobia or social anxiety disorder is characterized by a marked and persistent fear of one or more social or performance situations in which the person is exposed to unfamiliar people or to possible scrutiny by others. The individual fears that he or she will act in a way (or show anxiety symptoms) that will be humiliating or embarrassing. To make this diagnosis in a child, the child must demonstrate the capacity for social relationships with familiar people, and the anxiety must occur in interactions with peers. In addition, the exposure to the feared social situation almost invariably provokes anxiety, which may take the form of a situationally bound panic attack. Children may express their fear by crying or tantrumlike behavior. Adults acknowledge that their fear is excessive or unreasonable. Individuals with social phobia avoid social or performance situations or endure them with intense anxiety or distress (APA, 1994).

POST-TRAUMATIC STRESS DISORDER

Persons diagnosed with post-traumatic stress disorder (PTSD) must have experienced a traumatic event prior to the onset of symptoms. The individual may have experienced the event, witnessed it, or have been confronted with an event that involved actual or threatened death or serious injury, or a threat to the physical integrity of oneself or others. The individual's response involved intense fear, helplessness, or horror. Children may express their response with agitated or disorganized behavior.

The second group of defining criteria for PTSD involve various mechanisms of reexperiencing the event. One of the following must be present: (a) recurrent and intrusive disturbing recollections of the event, including thoughts, images, or perceptions; (b) recurrent dreams of the event; (c) acting or feeling that the event was recurring; (d) the experience of psychological distress when internal or external cues resemble the event; and/or (e) physiological reactivity on exposure to internal or external cues that resemble the event.

Further, the individual avoids stimuli associated with the trauma and experiences a numbing of general responsiveness that was not present before the trauma. This numbing and avoidance are marked by at least three of the following: (a) efforts to avoid thoughts, feelings, or conversations about the trauma; (b) efforts to avoid persons or places that evoke memories of the trauma; (c) an inability to remember an important aspect of the trauma **(repression)**; (d) diminished interest or participation in significant activities; (e) a feeling of estrangement or detachment from others; and (f) restricted range of affect and/or a sense of a foreshortened future (no expectation of a career or normal life span).

The fourth criterion is concerned with symptoms of increased arousal that were not present before the trauma. Two of the following must be present: (a) sleep disturbances; (b) irritability or angry outbursts; (c) difficulty concentrating; (d) hypervigilance; and (e) exaggerated startle response. The symptoms must persist for more than one month and cause significant impairment in social or occupational or other significant areas of functioning.

PTSD can be further defined as acute if symptoms have occurred from between one to three months, or chronic if the symptoms have persisted for at least three months or more. When the onset of symptoms is more than six months after the traumatic event, the further definition of delayed onset is specified (APA, 1994).

ACUTE STRESS DISORDER

Acute stress disorder is differentiated from PTSD in three ways: the individual experiences at least three symptoms indicating dissociation, the time frame of development and duration of symptoms is shorter, and the dissociative symptoms may prevent the individual from adaptively coping with the trauma.

Three of the following indications of **dissociation** must be present: (a) subjective sense of numbing or detachment; (b) reduced awareness of surroundings (being in a daze); (c) derealization; (d) depersonalization; and (e) dissociative amnesia.

In terms of time, the symptoms may last from two days to a month. The onset of the dissociative experience may occur during the trauma experience or develop immediately afterward. The defining characteristic of causing significant distress or impairment in social and occupational functioning is that the individual is prevented from pursuing some necessary task, such as obtaining necessary medical or legal assistance.

GENERALIZED ANXIETY DISORDER

Generalized anxiety disorder is characterized by excessive anxiety and worry (apprehensive expectation) that occurs more days than not for at least six months. This anxiety involves concerns about a number of events and activities. The individual finds it difficult to control the worry. Three of the following six symptoms must be present to some degree for a period of at least six months: (a) restlessness or feeling on edge; (b) being easily fatigued; (c) difficulties with concentration; (d) irritability; (e) muscle tension; and (f) sleep disturbance. The focus of the anxiety and worry is not confined to features of another AXIS I disorder (for example, worry about having a panic attack, as in panic disorder; or fear of contamination, as in obsessive-compulsive disorder), and is not a part of post-traumatic stress disorder. The anxiety or worry interferes with normal social or occupational functioning; it is not due to the direct effects of a substance or a general medical condition and does not occur exclusively in the presence of another AXIS I disorder (for example, mood disorder, psychotic disorder, or pervasive developmental disorder).

OBSESSIVE-COMPULSIVE DISORDER

Obsessive-compulsive disorder is characterized by the presence of either obsessions or compulsions. **Obsessions** are recurrent and persistent ideas, impulses, or images experienced at some time during the disturbance as intrusive and inappropriate and cause marked anxiety or distress.

The ideas, thoughts, impulses, and images are not simply excessive worry about real problems. The individual attempts to suppress or ignore them, or to neutralize them with some other thought or action. Finally, the individual recognizes the obsessional thoughts are a product of his or her own mind and not imposed from without, as in thought insertion.

Compulsions are repetitive behaviors that the person feels driven to perform in response to an obsession. Examples are repeated hand washing in response to thoughts of contamination and checking over and over again to ensure that appliances are unplugged before leaving the house. The behaviors or mental acts are an attempt to prevent or reduce the distress occasioned by the obsession, or to prevent some dreaded threatening situation (such as a fire in the example of checking appliances). However, these behaviors or mental processes are either not connected in a realistic way with what they are designed to prevent, or they are clearly excessive.

Except in children, individuals have recognized that the obsessions or compulsions are excessive or unreasonable at some point in the disorder. The obsessions or compulsions cause marked distress, are time-consuming,

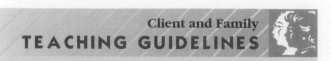

Client and Family
TEACHING GUIDELINES

Obsessive-Compulsive Disorder

Teach the client's family:

1. Obsessive-compulsive disorder is a chronic anxiety disorder that responds to different treatment strategies.

2. Thoughts, impulses, and images are involuntary and may worsen with stress.

Teach the client:

1. Behavioral and cognitive strategies to manage anxiety and reduce the symptoms of the disorder.

2. Medication management is an effective treatment modality and usually involves treatment with a drug in the antidepressant category.

3. Different classes of drugs have different side effect profiles; recognizing and reporting side effects is an important part of managing client's drug therapy.

4. Achieving symptom control through pharmacotherapy may take months.

---

or significantly interfere with the person's normal routine or occupational functioning. The Client and Family Teaching Guidelines above list management tips. If another AXIS I disorder is present, the content of obsessions or compulsions is not restricted to it (for example, food rituals in anorexia and hair pulling in trichotillomania). The disorder must not be due to the direct effects of a substance or a general medical condition.

Somatoform Disorders

The common focus of somatoform disorders is physical symptoms in the absence of clinically significant organic disease.

BODY DYSMORPHIC DISORDER

This disorder is characterized by a preoccupation with an imagined defect in appearance. If the person has a slight physical anomaly, his or her concern is excessive. This preoccupation causes clinically significant distress or impairment in social or occupational functioning. Finally, the preoccupation is not better accounted for by another mental disorder.

PAIN DISORDER

The predominant focus of the clinical presentation in pain disorder is pain in one or more anatomical sites. This pain is of sufficient severity to warrant clinical at-

tention and causes major impairment in one or more areas of functioning. Psychological factors are judged to have an important role in the onset, severity exacerbation, or maintenance of the pain. Finally, the pain is not better accounted for by a mood, anxiety, or psychotic disorder and does not meet the criteria for dysparenuria.

The disorder can further be defined as a pain disorder associated with psychological factors if an associated medical condition does not play a major role in onset, severity, and maintenance of the symptoms. If a general medical condition does play a major role in the maintenance of the syndrome, the disorder is termed pain disorder associated with both psychological factors and a general medical condition. Both disorders can be specified acute (if the duration is less than six months) or chronic.

SOMATIZATION DISORDER

The characteristic pattern of clients presenting with somatization disorder is one of frequently seeking and obtaining medical treatment for multiple clinically significant somatic complaints. The complaints must begin before age 30 and cannot be adequately explained by any general medical disorder or the direct effects of a substance. For example, clients with multiple sclerosis, systemic lupus erethematosis, or other chronic debilitating diseases that have an onset in early adulthood frequently present with multisystem complaints would not also be diagnosed as having somatization disorder because a general medical condition better explains their symptom complex.

The distribution of symptoms in somatization disorder requires that they have a distinct pattern that can be differentiated from general medical conditions if the following three criteria are met: (1) there is an involvement of multiple organ systems (gastrointestinal, sexual/reproductive, and/or neurological); (2) the symptoms exhibit an early onset and chronic course, without development of physical signs or structural abnormalities (for example, degenerative changes in bones and joints associated with complaints of pain); and (3) the absence of the clinical laboratory abnormalities expected to be associated with general medical conditions. The specific diagnostic criteria are detailed in the DSM-IV Criteria box on page 237. Nurses in general hospital or clinic practices are more likely to encounter clients with somatization disorder than those working in inpatient psychiatric units.

CONVERSION DISORDER

Clients who present with conversion symptoms exhibit one or more symptoms or deficits that affect voluntary motor or sensory function and that appear to be related to a neurological or general medical condition. As in somatization disorder, however, the symptom or deficit cannot be fully accounted for by a general medical condition, the direct effects of a substance, or as a culturally

DSM-IV CRITERIA

Somatization Disorder

A. A history of many physical complaints beginning before age 30 years that occur over a period of several years and result in treatment being sought or significant impairment in social, occupational, or other important areas of functioning.

B. Each of the following criteria must have been met, with individual symptoms occurring at any time during the course of the disturbance:

   (1) *four pain symptoms:* a history of pain related to at least four different sites or functions (e.g., head, abdomen, back, joints, extremities, chest, rectum, during menstruation, during sexual intercourse, or during urination)

   (2) *two gastrointestinal symptoms:* a history of at least two gastrointestinal symptoms other than pain (e.g., nausea, bloating, vomiting other than during pregnancy, diarrhea, or intolerance of several different foods)

   (3) *one sexual symptom:* a history of at least one sexual or reproductive symptom other than pain (e.g., sexual indifference, erectile or ejaculatory dysfunction, irregular menses, excessive menstrual bleeding, vomiting throughout pregnancy)

   (4) *one pseudoneurological symptom:* a history of at least one symptom or deficit suggesting a neuro-logical condition not limited to pain (conversion symptoms such as impaired coordination or balance, paralysis or localized weakness, difficulty swallowing or lump in throat, aphonia, urinary retention, hallucinations, loss of touch or pain sensation, double vision, blindness, deafness, seizures; dissociative symptoms such as amnesia; or loss of consciousness other than fainting)

C. Either (1) or (2):

   (1) after appropriate investigation, each of the symptoms in Criterion B cannot be fully explained by a known general medical condition or the direct effects of a substance (e.g., a drug of abuse, a medication)

   (2) when there is a related general medical condition, the physical complaints or resulting social or occupational impairment are in excess of what would be expected from the history, physical examination, or laboratory findings

D. The symptoms are not intentionally produced or feigned (as in Factitious Disorder or Malingering).

Reprinted with permission from *Diagnostic and statistical manual of mental disorders,* ed 4, Washington, D.C., 1994, American Psychiatric Association.

---

sanctioned behavior or experience. The symptom is not intentionally produced or feigned, is not limited to pain or sexual dysfunction, and does not occur exclusively in the context of somatization disorder. As in other somatoform disorders, the symptom causes clinically significant distress or impairment in social or occupational or other important areas of functioning.

The critical defining characteristic of conversion disorder is that psychological factors are identified as being related to the onset or exacerbation of the symptom. Specifically, identifiable conflicts or stressors precede the development of the conversion symptoms.

HYPOCHONDRIASIS

There are six major criteria associated with hypochondriasis. First, the individual is preoccupied with fears of having—or the idea of having—a serious medical disorder based on his or her misinterpretation of bodily symptoms. Second, this misinterpretation of symptoms persists despite appropriate medical evaluation and reassurance. Third, the individual's preoccupation with symptoms is not as intense or distorted as would be found in delusional disorder, nor is it as restricted as found in body dysmorphic disorder. Fourth, as in the other somatoform disorders, the preoccupation causes clinically significant distress or impairment in social, occupational, or other major areas of functioning. Next, the duration of the disturbance must be at least six months. Finally, as in other AXIS I diagnoses, the condition is not better accounted for by another anxiety disorder, somataform disorder, or major depressive episode.

Dissociative Disorders

Dissociative disorders are characterized by a disruption in the usually integrated functions of consciousness, memory, identity, and perception of the environment (APA, 1994).

DISSOCIATIVE AMNESIA

In persons with dissociative amnesia, the defining symptom is one or more episodes of inability to recall important personal information, usually of a traumatic or stressful nature, that is too extensive to be explained by ordinary forgetting. In addition, the disturbance does not occur exclusively during the course of dissociative identity disorder, and is not due to the effects of a substance (blackouts during alcohol intoxication) or as a result of a general medical condition (amnesia following head trauma).

DISSOCIATIVE FUGUE

Dissociative fugue is characterized by sudden, unexpected travel away from one's home or customary place of work, with an inability to recall one's past. The individual demonstrates confusion about personal identity or assumes a new identity, which may be partial ("filling in the blanks"). As in dissociative amnesia, the disturbance does not occur in the context of a dissociative identity disorder, and is not due to the effects of a substance or to a general medical condition.

DISSOCIATIVE IDENTITY DISORDER

Dissociative identity disorder (formerly Multiple Personality Disorder) is diagnosed according to the following criteria in DSM-IV. First, the individual must demonstrate two or more distinct identities or personality states, each with its own relatively enduring pattern of perceiving, relating to, and thinking about the environment and self. Second, at least two of these personality states recurrently take control of the person's behavior. The individual is unable to recall important personal information that is too extensive to be accounted for by ordinary forgetting. Third, these phenomena are not due to the effects of a substance (for example, blackouts or chaotic behavior during alcohol intoxication), or a general medical condition (for example, complex partial seizures). In children the symptoms are not attributable to imaginary playmates or other fantasy play.

PROGNOSIS

The prognosis for anxiety and associated disorders is related to factors specific to the disorder, the client, and the clinician. Clients treated for panic disorder with or without agoraphobia are typically described as chronic. Follow-up studies indicate that 6–10 years after treatment, 30% of clients are well, 40%–50% are improved but still symptomatic, and the remaining 20%–30% are the same or slightly worse (APA, 1994).

Specific phobias that persist into adulthood generally do not remit. The course of social phobia is often continuous with onset or reemergence after stressful or humiliating experiences. The prognosis for obsessive-compulsive disorder is similar to the other anxiety disorders, with waxing and waning symptoms related to stressors. However, 15% of clients demonstrate a chronically deteriorating course with progressive compromise of social and occupational functioning.

For acute and post-traumatic stress disorders, prognosis is closely related to individuals' exposure to the stressful event, as well as their premorbid functioning and support systems. Persons with acute stress disorder by definition either recover in four weeks or are diagnosed with PTSD. Approximately half of those diagnosed with PTSD recover in three months; half continue to experience symptoms persisting for longer than a year after the trauma.

The somatoform disorders, with the exception of conversion disorder, are chronic and fluctuating and rarely remit fully. Conversion disorders usually remit within two weeks; however, there is recurrence in 20%–25% of cases. A recurrence of symptoms once is predictive of future episodes. Factors that have been identified with a good prognosis are identifiable stressors at the time symptoms develop, early treatment, and above-average intelligence.

The dissociative disorders have varying prognoses, ranging from a rapid, complete recovery (fugue) compared to both episodic and continuous chronic courses (dissociative identity disorder). Dissociative identity disorder frequently reemerges during periods of stress or relapse of substance abuse (APA, 1994).

DISCHARGE CRITERIA

The client:

- identifies situations and events that trigger anxiety and ways to prevent or manage them
- identifies anxiety symptoms and levels of anxiety
- discusses connection between anxiety-provoking situation or event and anxiety symptoms
- discusses relief behaviors openly
- identifies adaptive, positive techniques and strategies that relieve anxiety
- demonstrates behaviors that represent reduced anxiety symptoms
- uses learned anxiety-reducing strategies
- demonstrates ability to problem-solve, concentrate, and make decisions
- verbalizes feeling relaxed
- sleeps through the night
- uses appropriate supports from nursing and medical community, family, and friends
- acknowledges inevitability of occurrence of anxiety
- discusses ability to tolerate manageable levels of anxiety
- seeks help when anxiety is not manageable
- continues postdischarge anxiety management, including medication and therapy

THE NURSING PROCESS ■ ■ ■ ■ ■ ■ ■ ■ ■ ■ ■ ■ ■ ■ ■ ■ ■ ■ ■

■ ASSESSMENT

New treatment modalities have markedly improved the quality of life and level of participation in activities for people with anxiety disorders. Nurses no longer expect to encounter clients with psychiatric disorders only in traditional psychiatric settings. It is important for all nurses to identify dysfunctional manifestations of anxiety so that treatment can be implemented promptly.

Panic disorders are primarily seen in ambulatory settings. Nurses are among the first health care providers to come in contact with clients who are experiencing their first symptoms of panic disorder, either in a clinic or physician's office or, more typically, in a hospital emergency department. The sudden onset of physical symptoms and the pervasive feelings of impending doom are frightening, and the client often responds by seeking reassurance from a caregiver. It is these physical symptoms that bring clients to the emergency room.

The client with agoraphobia may come to the attention of a nurse when preparing a client for diagnostic testing that includes a CT scan or an MRI. The client who becomes visibly anxious at the prospect of entering a confined space when the nurse describes the procedure and the equipment may be agoraphobic.

Most often clients with anxiety symptoms do not present with anxiety as their reason for seeking treatment. Anxiety by definition is a vague, nonspecific feeling of discomfort. Nurses who use an assessment tool that addresses each identified human response pattern will obtain cues from the client experiencing anxiety that indicate further assessment is needed. The guidelines for a comprehensive nursing assessment, listed in Box 11-3, are adaptable for any practice setting. When thought of as a list of questions, an "admission interview" becomes a task for nurses, and consequently an ordeal for clients. As the nurse becomes more experienced, assessment is integrated into the continuing nursing process, and inquiring about human response patterns evolves into a less threatening interaction between client and nurse.

■ ■ NURSING DIAGNOSIS

To determine which nursing diagnoses will most effectively guide treatment for clients with anxiety and related disorders, the nurse relies on information obtained in the assessment process. The nurse identifies defining characteristics for the target diagnoses from the client, and the nurse and client jointly identify etiologic factors.

Etiologic factors influence selection of intervention. It is impossible to anticipate each potential diagnosis for all of the disorders discussed in this chapter. Typical diagnoses for clients with anxiety and related disorders are listed below.

NANDA Diagnoses for Anxiety and Related Disorders

Activity intolerance
Alered family process
Altered nutrition: more or less than body requirements
Altered role performance
Altered thought process
Anxiety
Body image disturbance
Chronic pain
Decisional conflict
Fatigue
Fear
Hopelessness
Impaired adjustment
Impaired physical mobility
Impaired social interaction
Ineffective individual coping
Knowledge deficit
Noncompliance
Post-trauma response
Powerlessness
Rape-trauma syndrome
Rape-trauma syndrome: compound reaction
Rape-trauma syndrome: silent reaction
Relocation stress syndrome
Risk for impaired skin integrity
Risk for self-mutilation
Risk for violence: self-directed or directed at others
Self-care deficits
Sensory/perceptual alterations
Sexual dysfunction
Situational low self esteem
Sleep pattern disturbance
Social isolation
Spiritual distress

■ ■ ■ OUTCOME IDENTIFICATION

Outcome criteria will differ according to the characteristics that define each client's nursing diagnoses and collaborative (DSM-IV) diagnoses. Determining outcomes before implementation of the plan will guide both nursing interventions and evaluation. The following nursing diagnoses are associated with outcomes (goals) to serve as a guide in outcome development. In practice, outcomes are generally determined by the patient's presentation of clinical manifestations.

Box 11-3   Nursing Assessment Guidelines According to Human Response Patterns

- *Exchanging: a pattern involving mutual giving and receiving*

  Assess eating and elimination patterns. *Clients with anxiety disorders and somatization disorders have frequent appetite disturbances and such gastrointestinal complaints as gas, constipation, and diarrhea. Urinary frequency is another associated symptom.*

- *Communicating: a pattern involving sending messages*

  Observe for tics, stuttering, or other unusual speech patterns. Note whether client maintains eye contact throughout the interview, and whether there are any instances of blushing. *There is comorbidity between Tourette's syndrome and obsessive-compulsive disorder; blushing and difficulty communicating with those the client perceives as authority are common in social phobia.*

- *Relating: a pattern involving established bonds*

  In taking a social history be particularly attentive to the client's affect in describing roles and role-related problems, including occupational function, financial issues, and role in the home. Ask about client's role satisfaction and what contributes to it. Note whether client presented alone for appointment with provider. If client was accompanied, what is the client's relationship to the accompanying individual? *Clients with multiple roles are at risk for role strain, and role strain is often characterized by anxiety symptoms. Alternatively, if the individual describes an isolated existence, probe gently for contributing factors to this isolation. Clients with severe obsessive-compulsive disorder are*

  isolated in part because their degree of involvement with rituals is a competing demand on their time available for social and occupational functioning. Clients with dissociative identity disorder also have poor role functioning, or one of the personality states may be unable to articulate its role functioning. Chronic worry about children or parents as a defining characteristic of anxiety disorders also may be expressed in exploring this pattern.

- *Valuing: a pattern involving the assigning of relative worth*

  Inquire about cultural background and values. *Be particularly attentive when assessing a client with a cultural experience different from your own. In addition to various culture-bound syndromes that are related to anxiety, somatization, and dissociative disorders, clients may exhibit behaviors and cognitive patterns that are adaptive and syntonic in one culture yet labeled pathological in another.*

- *Choosing: a pattern involving the selection of alternatives*

  Assess client's usual methods of coping with stressors. What aspects of client's life are stressful? If the individual is part of a family unit, how does the family cope with change? Does the individual use alcohol to cope with stressful situations or public appearances? *Social phobia is often diagnosed only after a maladaptive substance use disorder is identified.* What is the client's usual method of decision making? Does the individual usually follow recommendations? What strategies does the person use to enhance success? *Clients with obses-*

Outcome Identification for Selected Anxiety and Related Disorders Diagnoses

Generalized Anxiety Disorder
Client will:

1. Demonstrate significant decrease in physiologic, cognitive, behavioral, and emotional symptoms of anxiety

2. Demonstrate effective coping skills

3. Exhibit enhanced ability to make decisions and problem-solve

4. Demonstrate ability to function adaptively in mild anxiety states

Obsessive-Compulsive Disorder
Client will:

1. Participate actively in learned strategies to manage anxiety and decrease obsessive-compulsive behaviors

2. Describe increasing sense of control over intrusive thoughts and ritualistic behaviors

COLLABORATIVE DIAGNOSES

DSM-IV Diagnoses*	NANDA Diagnoses**
Generalized Anxiety Disorder	Anxiety
Obsessive-Compulsive Disorder	Impaired social interaction
Post-traumatic Stress Disorder	Rape-trauma syndrome
Somatization Disorder	Constipation, perceived
Dissociative Identity Disorder	Personal identity disturbance

*Reprinted with permission from *Diagnostic and statistical manual of mental disorders*, ed 4, Washington, D.C., 1994, American Psychiatric Association.

**Reprinted with permission from *NANDA, nursing diagnoses: definitions and classifications, 1995–1996*, Philadelphia, 1994, North American Nursing Diagnosis Association.

Box 11-3 Nursing Assessment Guidelines According to Human Response Patterns—cont'd

sive-compulsive disorder most often experience a disturbance in this pattern. Obsessional thinking and ritualistic behaviors are developed to cope with perceived threats (that range from intrusive thoughts to adaptive motor responses that become overgeneralized). If the nurse suspects symptoms of obsessive-compulsive disorder, the client should be asked quite frankly if she or he has any particular ways that tasks should be performed and if interruptions during the performance of these are stressful. Clients with other anxiety disorders, particularly generalized anxiety disorder, often express difficulties in coping and making choices, fearing they will make the wrong decision.

- **Moving: a pattern involving activity**
  In inquiring about an individual's history of physical disability, remember to ask about any episodes of motor dysfunction that may indicate conversion symptoms. If the client indicates past traumatic injury, ask about the circumstances. *Although post-traumatic stress disorder develops after combat situations, sexual abuse, and disasters, it also can follow less dramatic events such as automobile accidents.* Questions about traveling, sports activities, and hobbies may yield content suggesting agoraphobic symptoms.

- **Perceiving: a pattern involving the reception of information and Knowing: a pattern involving the meaning associated with information**
  These two patterns together compose the traditional mental status examination, formerly a touchstone for psychiatric and mental health nurses. Orientation and memory questions are key to identifying anxiety, somatization, and dissociative disorders. *Look for signs of hesitation in answering questions about an individual's history that may indicate periods of dissociation. Listen carefully as the client describes past medical treatment for clusters of illnesses that suggest somatization disorder.* When asking about self-perception and self-concept, be alert for responses that indicate a negative body image. *Clients with body dysmorphic disorder may seek reassurance about a perceived defect if offered the opportunity and the subject is opened in a nonthreatening manner.*

- **Feeling: a pattern involving the subjective awareness of information**
  Ask directly about experience of pain and fears. Anxiety symptoms are more easily identified if the nurse prompts the client for actual phenomena, for example, "Are your muscles tight from time to time, is your mouth dry, do you perspire a lot—particularly when you're expecting something unpleasant?" "Have you had more difficulty concentrating lately?" "Have you ever had these feelings come out of nowhere?" *Endorsement of several of the defining characteristics of panic attack warrants a more thorough evaluation for panic disorder and agoraphobia.* Explore the client's experiences of guilt and shame for signs of social phobia.

---

3. Demonstrate ability to cope effectively when ruminations or rituals are interrupted

4. Spend less time involved in anxiety-binding activities and instead use time gained to complete tasks of daily living and in social/recreational activities

5. Successfully manage times of increased stress by integrating knowledge that thoughts, impulses, and images are involuntary, thus reducing sense of responsibility and consequent anxiety

Post-traumatic Stress Disorder
Client will:

1. Demonstrate concern for personal safety by beginning to verbalize worries

2. Participate actively in support group

3. Identify and involve significant support system

4. Assume decision-making role for own health care needs

5. Acquire and practice strategies for coping with anxiety symptoms such as breathing techniques, progressive relaxation exercises, thought, image and memory substitution, and assertive behaviors

Somatization Disorder
Client will:

1. Increase level of exercise to walking one mile four times a week

2. Accurately describe the potential consequences of laxative dependence

3. Meet with a dietitian to evaluate eating habits

4. Keep an intake log to document fluid and fiber intake

Dissociative Identity Disorder
Client will:

1. Respond to name when addressed by a member of the treatment team

2. Refer to self in the first-person pronoun form: "I think"

3. Identify periods of increasing anxiety

4. Inform others of dissatisfaction in a nonthreatening manner

5. Use assertive behavior to meet needs

CASE STUDY

Social Phobia

Neil is a 19-year-old freshman at a local college. He is brought to the emergency room from a fraternity party one Saturday night with acute alcohol intoxication. He is referred to the college health service.

During his initial evaluation, the nurse asks Neil about his patterns of drinking. He reports that he began drinking at age 14 when one of his friends suggested having a beer or two before attending a school dance. He reported that ever since he started school he was unable to participate in the easy banter, the "social chit-chat" common among fellow students. However, he did not have the same experience with family members. He was afraid that he wouldn't have anything to contribute to the conversation. He began to worry about his appearance, and his tendency to trip over his own feet.

When Neil reached high school, he found that this uneasiness was beginning to isolate him from others in his age group. At home his parents usually began dinner parties with a glass of wine or a cocktail, so when his friend suggested a beer before the dance, Neil eagerly accepted. To his surprise he found that once he arrived at the dance, he was relaxed and able to interact. He was even able to ask two girls to dance!

He continued to drink before arriving at parties, dances, football games, and just about any other social activity. He was worried that he was an alcoholic. The clinical specialist at the health service talked with Neil at length about social phobia and prescribed imipramine. Neil also began attending a group focused on behavioral strategies to cope with anxiety.

Critical Thinking and Nursing Diagnosis

1. What cues does Neil offer that will lead to the most appropriate nursing diagnoses for him?

1. List two beliefs Neil may have formed that led to his experience at the fraternity party.

2. Using information in this chapter and information in Chapter 15, Substance Related Disorders, what would be the prognosis for Neil?

3. Identify an alternative pharmacologic choice for Neil (see Chapter 23, Psychopharmacology and Other Biologic Therapies).

4. How would you describe the advantages of group therapy to Neil?

CASE STUDY

Obsessive-Compulsive Disorder

Mark is a 31-year-old accountant who has been disabled from his job with a national firm for eight months. He reports that he has been hospitalized for treatment of depression, which he has experienced since college. Despite his depression, he graduated with honors, obtained certification as a Public Accountant, and finished graduate school.

Mark first was treated for OCD two years later when he began experiencing trouble with his supervisor. A number of the firm's clients had complained that Mark was unable to either give them completed tax forms or file for the necessary extensions in a timely manner.

Mark received some relief from his counting and checking behaviors with treatment with clomipramine, but presently spends his time preoccupied with thoughts about killing himself. He is unable to decide on a method of suicide that will not endanger his family's entitlement to his accidental death insurance policies. Mark is admitted to an inpatient facility to begin a course of ECT.

Critical Thinking and Planning

1. Identify 3 inpatient treatment outcomes for Mark.

2. What are three collaborative treatment approaches that are important in Mark's long-term therapy?

3. Which methods can be used to measure outcomes achieved as a result of Mark's treatment?

structured behavioral programs. Treatment for dissociative identity disorder also occurred in special units with a protracted hospitalization.

Today, both clinicians and administrators in inpatient facilities are struggling to balance effective treatment with the high costs associated with these specialty units. Increasingly, inpatient hospitalization is available only for short periods of time for clients at imminent risk to themselves or others. Rather than their traditional roles of providing direct care to clients in inpatient facilities, nurses are increasingly involved as case managers. Among other responsibilities, as case managers nurses provide information on treatment alternatives to clients and families.

■ ■ ■ ■ ■ IMPLEMENTATION

The role of a nurse in the implementation of a care plan for clients with anxiety and related disorders depends on the setting in which the client is treated. The following interventions are useful for clients with anxiety symptoms, regardless of diagnosis or treatment setting. Specific issues community nurses may face are found in Nursing Care in the Community on page 243.

■ ■ ■ ■ ■ PLANNING

Treatment planning for the client with anxiety and related disorders in the current health care environment is complex and varied. Clients with severe obsessive-compulsive disorder were formerly hospitalized for

Nursing Care in the Community

Anxiety and Related Disorders

Anxiety disorders are seldom found in pure form. Clients who call for help or are found at home in a highly anxious state are usually reacting to a situational crisis that may be physical or psychological. They can benefit from a brief intervention, such as reassurance or a reality check.

Often, older adults become extremely anxious about somatic complaints ranging from worries about constipation to sensations of having a heart attack. The nurse should not assume these complaints are psychogenic because they have been verbalized before. Proper tests should be performed to rule out a medical condition before psychiatric intervention begins. Anxious clients who do not have a medical condition usually respond to cognitive interventions or psychoactive medication. They may benefit from increased, unsolicited attention from, and involvement in, a community-based support system, such as the family, visiting nurse, and/or social worker.

Clients with chronic mental illness, such as paranoid schizophrenia, have a low threshold of apprehension and may seek repeated reassurance from the nurse. Generally, kindness and simple self-care suggestions for stress reduction will be enough to return clients' attention to normal functioning, but an adjustment in medication may also be needed.

Occasionally the nurse will encounter clients who cannot identify a current stressor but are experiencing severe anxiety verging on panic. Daily functions are seriously impaired, and a family member or friend must intervene to call for help or drive the client to a care site. These individuals may respond to anxiolytic medications but will generally not respond to immediate cognitive therapy. They will usually continue to experience overwhelming apprehension despite reassurance and reality testing.

It is essential to recognize that clients' sensations are beyond rationality. The nurse should maintain a calm manner, in spite of client or personal impatience, until the appropriate medications act to decrease pathological activity in the brain and allow resumption of reasonable response patterns. Clients should not be expected to supply information in a state of panic. If information is needed, situation permitting, it should be accessed from a significant other. As the client becomes calmer, the nurse can establish a more therapeutic relationship and fill in gaps in the client's history.

If the intensity of the anxiety is not mitigated by a standard dose of medication within a reasonable time, the nurse working in the community must consider hospitalizing the client. Hospitalization will relieve the client of the pressures of family and daily maintenance until rational abilities are restored. It also provides a safe environment with reduced stress and therapeutic suggestions for more positive coping activities.

Nursing Interventions

1. Assess own level of anxiety and make a conscious effort to remain calm. *Anxiety is readily transferable from one person to another.*

2. Recognize the client's use of relief behaviors (pacing, wringing of hands) as indicators of anxiety *to intervene early in managing anxiety and prevent escalation of symptoms.*

3. Inform the client of the importance of limiting caffeine, nicotine, and other central nervous system stimulants *to prevent/minimize physical symptoms of anxiety, such as rapid heart rate and jitteriness.*

4. Teach the client to distinguish between anxiety that can be connected to identifiable objects or sources (illness, prognosis, hospitalization, known stressors) and anxiety for which there is no immediate identifiable object or source. *Knowledge of anxiety and its related components increases the client's control over the disorder.*

5. Instruct the client in the following anxiety-reducing strategies:

   progressive relaxation technique

   slow deep-breathing excercises

   focusing on a single object in the room

   listening to soothing music or relaxation tapes

   visual imagery

   Strategies help reduce anxiety in a variety of ways and distract the client from focusing on anxiety.

6. Help the client build on previously successful coping methods to manage anxiety symptoms. *Coping methods that were successful in the past are generally effective in subsequent situations.*

7. Help the client identify support persons who can help him or her perform personal tasks and activities that present circumstances (such as hospitalization) make difficult. *A strong support system can help circumvent anxiety-provoking situations/activities.*

8. Help the client gain control of overwhelming feelings and impulses through brief, directive verbal interactions. *Individual interactions executed at appropriate intervals can help reduce/manage client's anxious feelings/impulses.*

9. Help the client structure the environment so it is less noisy. *A less-stimulating environment can create a calming, stress-free atmosphere that reduces anxiety.*

10. Assess the presence and degree of depression and suicidal ideation in all clients with anxiety and related disorders *to prevent self-harm and intervene in depression early.*

11. Employ anxiolytic medication as least restrictive measure to reduce anxiety. *Appropriate medicine may be an effective adjunct to other psychosocial therapeutic interventions, when necessary, to manage stress.*

Additional Treatment Modalities

Biological

Pharmacological interventions alone or in combination with cognitive behavioral interventions are among the most successful treatments for anxiety and related disorders. Since the early 1960s, benzodiazepines have been widely used in the treatment of anxiety disorders. They are relatively safe and effective for short-term use in controlling debilitating symptoms of anxiety. Longer-term treatment raises issues of abuse and dependence.

Tricyclic antidepressants, monoamine oxidase inhibitors, and benzodiazepines are effective in the treatment of panic disorder. Selective serotonin reuptake inhibitors are currently being investigated in double-blind clinical trials to evaluate their efficacy in panic disorder.

Clients with obsessive-compulsive disorder have been sucessfully treated with tricyclics and MAOIs, and recent development of SSRIs have widened treatment options. Although other TCAs have been used to treat OCD, Clomipramine (Anafranil) has demonstrated significant anti-obsessional activity in large clinical trials. Fluvoxamine (Luvox) has recently been approved for use in the United States. Dosage of antidepressant drugs required for control of symptoms of OCD may be higher than those traditionally used for depression.

Pharmacological treatment for post-traumatic stress disorder and dissociative identity disorder is largely symptomatic. Varying combinations of antidepressants, antipsychotics, and to a lesser extent benzodiazepines are used. Psychopharmacological management of the somatoform disorders includes tricyclic antidepressants, used adjunctively for pain management (Arana and Hyman, 1991). For more specific information about dosages and side effect profiles see Chapter 23, Psychopharmacology and Other Biologic Therapies.

Electroconvulsive Therapy

The primary indication for electroconvulsive therapy (ECT) is depression. However, it is used for anxiety disorders when other treatments are too high a risk or have failed. For example, in clients with obsessive-compulsive disorder who have only a partial response to Anafranil and who are suicidal, ECT is a reasonable treatment alternative. The mechanism of ECT is unknown, but it is thought to be related to improving transmission of dopamine, norepinephrine, and serotonin, and release of hypothalamic and pituitary hormones (Keltner and Folks, 1993).

Psychotherapy

Psychotherapeutic intervention can take place in group or individual settings. One advantage of group therapy is the opportunity for the client to learn from the successes and failures of others with similar symptoms.

Behavioral Therapy   Behavioral treatments, including systematic desensitization, are among the most effective treatments for panic disorder with agoraphobia. First, the phobic stimulus is defined. Clients are assisted in defining a hierarchy for the phobic stimulus. The client and therapist then expose the client to events on the hierarchy that increase the client's degree of anxiety. As the client and therapist move through the hierarchy, the client experiences progressive mastery of increasing levels of anxiety until the phobic stimulus is encountered.

Cognitive Behavioral Therapy   Cognitive behavioral therapy is widely used in the treatment of anxiety disorders. The success of this approach centers on the client's understanding that symptoms are a learned response to thoughts or feelings about behaviors that occur in daily life. The client and therapist identify the target symptoms and then examine circumstances associated with the symptoms. Together they devise strategies to change either the cognitons or the behaviors. Cognitive behavioral therapy is short-term and demands active participation on the part of both client and therapist.

Addititonal treatment modalities and collaborative interventions may include consultation with occupational therapists, vocational rehabilitation counselors, and psychologists, depending on the particular treatment needs of a patient. A summary of additional treatment modalities appears below. See Understanding and Applying Research on page 245 for discussion of an intensive partial hospitalization program used to treat anxiety disorders.

ADDITIONAL TREATMENT MODALITIES

Biologic
Pharmacologic

- Benzodiazepines
- Tricyclic Antidepresessants
- MAOIs
- SSRIs

Electroconvulsive Therapy (ECT)
Psychotherapy

- Behavioral Therapy
- Cognitive Therapy

Understanding and Applying
RESEARCH

Waddell KL, Demi AS: Effectiveness of an intensive partial hospitalization program for treatment of anxiety disorders, *Archives of Psychiatric Nursing*, vol 7, no 1, 1993: pp. 2–10.

The purpose of this study was to evaluate the outcome of an intensive partial hospitalization program (IPHP), integrating biological, psychological, and social modalities for the treatment of anxiety disorders.

The 5-week treatment program consisted of an integrated theoretical approach, using medications to treat the biological basis of the disorder, and behavioral and cognitive approaches to deal with avoidant behaviors and phobias. Each of the 32 participants was treated as a unique individual and this philosophy was reflected in individualized treatment plans.

Each client admitted into the program underwent a thorough psychiatric assessment. Most of the clients (84%) had a primary diagnosis of panic disorder with agoraphobia. Other primary diagnoses were agoraphobia without panic attacks, major depression, and obsessive-compulsive disorder.

Using Neuman's systems model as the theoretical framework, treatment was aimed at addressing three types of stressors: extrapersonal (outside stressors), interpersonal (stressors occurring between one or more persons), and intrapersonal (stressors occurring within the individual).

The study concluded that intensive partial hospitalization was effective in reducing the cognitive, emotional, and behavioral manifestations of agoraphobia. Spontaneous panic attacks were absent, anticipatory panic attacks were reduced, and anxiety that resulted from this program was managed adequately.

Because psychiatric nurses play a key role in the development and implementation of treatment programs for persons with agoraphobia and other anxiety disorders, they should be aware of the potential benefits of an IPHP of this kind. This particular treatment model is very adaptable for use in nursing practice. Nurses can use the educational components (cognitive restructuring, relaxation techniques, information regarding the disease process) and the behavioral interventions when working with clients. The psychotherapeutic individual and group therapy components of the program are also areas in which nurses work very well.

■ ■ ■ ■ ■ ■ EVALUATION

One of the most difficult aspects of applying the nursing process to psychiatric-mental health nursing, in particular, nursing care of clients with anxiety and related disorders, is generating measurable outcomes. Outcome criteria for clients with the more concrete nursing diagnoses, such as hyperthermia, decreased cardiac output, or even altered thought processes as evidenced by auditory hallucinations, seem clear and straightforward when compared with the more vague concept of anxiety. Fortunately, there are a number of valid, time-tested tools available that will yield such reliable information for anxiety-related disorders. Although not developed by and for nurses specifically, clinical rating scales offer a method to track changes in symptoms over time with a numerical value. These changes can be correlated with discrete interventions (such as instituting a behavioral program or a change in medication). Two rating scales commonly used with clients exhibiting anxiety disorders are the Yale-Brown Obsessive-Compulsive Scale and the Hamilton Anxiety Scale.

Ideally, nurses evaluate client progress toward identified outcomes at every interaction with the client. If satisfactory progress is not made, the nurse either modifies the expected outcome or the intervention. The nurse examines all factors that relate to the outcome, including the role of the nurse in setting the expectation, the clarity of communication about the goal with the client, and other intervening events since the objective was set.

NURSING CARE PLAN

Sarah, a 47-year-old woman, presented to the employee health department of a teaching hospital after walking there from her office, complaining of chest pain and shortness of breath. The staff instituted the standard cardiac work-up for new onset chest pain clients. Sarah's medical history included psoriasis. Her vital signs were remarkable for a pulse of 116; her EKG and lab work were within normal limits.

Sarah mentioned to the staff that her son had died three months ago. She was referred to a research team conducting a study on panic disorder and was seen by a clinical specialist in psychiatric nursing. Sarah participated in the research protocol after giving informed consent. During the course of the interview, she revealed that her deceased son, an only child, had been an alcoholic whose death was a suicide. She was presently considering separating from her husband of 27 years who was involved in a long-term extramarital affair. Her screening was positive for limited-symptom panic attacks that were increasing in frequency. She agreed to an extended evaluation after her initial interview.

During her evaluation, Sarah and the nurse explored her symptoms of anxiety and depression, the exacerbation of her psoriasis, and her chronic headaches which had become worse since her son's death. On moving back from the west coast, Sarah obtained her first job in 24 years. In addition to concern about financial matters and her son's alcoholism, she now worried frequently about her performance at work. She revealed that her husband's extramarital affair had been ongoing for several years, and related his behavior to their sexual difficulties. The nurse recommended a medication trial. Sarah refused medication because of her fears of addiction and loss of control.

DSM-IV Diagnoses

AXIS I	Generalized Anxiety Disorder (with limited-symptom panic attacks)
	Bereavement
	Partner Relational Problem
AXIS II	Dependent/Avoidant Traits
AXIS III	Psoriasis
	Headaches
AXIS IV	Coded above as being a primary focus of treatment
AXIS V	60 presently, 75 past year

Nursing Diagnosis: Anxiety, related to change in role functioning, recent loss of son, (dysfunctional grieving), threat to socioeconomic status, stressors exceed ability to cope, as evidenced by uncertainty, intermittent sympathetic nervous system stimulation, restlessness, and exacerbation of medical condition (psoriasis).

Client Outcomes	*Nursing Interventions*	*Evaluation*
• Sarah will identify common situations that provoke anxiety.	• Assign "homework" to patient, for example, keeping a panic attack and headache diary. *Documenting anxiety responses helps client link symptoms with precipitating events.* • During weekly sessions, review with Sarah her patient log of panic symptoms. *Discussing the linking of events/situations with anxiety symptoms teaches Sarah which stressor events provoke anxiety so she can learn to manage/avoid them.*	• Sarah identifies returning home after work as a critical time for symptoms to develop. Reports that she visits mother or does errands daily.
• Sarah will describe early warning symptoms of anxiety.	• Assist Sarah in associating her panic attack symptoms with thoughts about separation from her husband *to illustrate to Sarah specific situations in her life that result in panic anxiety.*	• Sarah reports that she doesn't experience headaches when husband is traveling.
• Sarah will report willingness to tolerate mild-to-moderate levels of anxiety.	• In weekly sessions explore with Sarah the advantages and disadvantages of separation and divorce *to help Sarah problem-solve viable options that may offer some control over her anxiety.*	• Sarah reveals unwillingness to live alone.
• Sarah will demonstrate adaptive coping mechanisms.	• During weekly sessions discuss options that will allow Sarah maximum control over her choices. *Increased choices over life situations tend to minimize anxiety responses to some degree.*	• Sarah informs husband she wants a trial separation. He moves into son's former room.

NURSING CARE PLAN ■ ■ ■ ■ ■ ■ ■ ■ ■ ■ ■ ■ ■ ■ ■

Nursing Diagnosis: Dysfunctional grieving, related to son's death, as evidenced by anxiety on returning home, alteration in sleeping patterns, expression of guilt, sadness, and crying, difficulty in concentration.

Client Outcomes	*Nursing Interventions*	*Evaluation*
• Sarah will return to her home directly after work, without going immediately to bed.	• Explore with Sarah her usual patterns of behavior before son's death. Identify possible modifications of those behaviors *to help Sarah focus on alternative activities/behaviors that would minimize dysfunctional grieving patterns and increase coping skills.*	• Sarah describes cooking dinner for son. Identifies other constructive activities she could perform to modify that routine.
• Sarah will be able to talk with family and significant others about son's death.	• Promote recognition that others also experience the loss of Sarah's son *to help Sarah understand that others share her grief, which can be comforting at such times.*	• Sarah is able to visit with her mother and talk about son without experiencing panic symptoms.
• Sarah will be able to use son's former bedroom as a functional part of the house.	• Initiate discussion of ways Sarah and husband can plan for disposal of some of son's possessions without feeling disloyal to his memory *to expedite functional grieving process via discussion of feelings.*	• As part of trial separation agreement, Sarah's husband moves into son's room.

Nursing Diagnosis: Decisional conflict, related to unclear personal values and beliefs, as evidenced by delayed decision making and physical signs of distress.

Client Outcomes	*Nursing Interventions*	*Evaluation*
• Sarah will make an informed decision about her relationship with husband.	• During weekly sessions explore with Sarah her expectations of marriage, how her relationship with her husband has changed over the course of their marriage, and what part she played in the changes *to help Sarah clarify values and expectations and her role in marriage, which can assist her in making critical life choices.*	• Sarah describes increasing involvement with her son as his substance abuse worsened and consequent discord in an already strained marriage. Reports frequent conflict with husband over his own drinking.
• Sarah will identify potential outcomes of separation and divorce and prioritize them according to social, financial, and interpersonal values.	• Review with Sarah some of the important relationships in her life. Support her considerations in the values clarification process. *It is critical that the nurse be aware of his or her own values and choices and maintain clear distinctions between his or her worldview and the client's.*	• Describes parental relationship as conflict-ridden, with father frequently abusing alcohol. Is critical of mother's domination of father. Acknowledges long-standing differences with husband over sexual issues, and feelings of disgust toward husband when he smells of beer.

NURSING CARE PLAN ▪ ▪ ▪ ▪ ▪ ▪ ▪ · · ▪ ▪ ▪ ▪ ▪ ▪

Nursing Diagnosis: Chronic low self-esteem, related to unresolved developmental issues as evidenced by self-negating verbalizations, evaluation of self as unable to deal with decisions, and passive dependence on marital partner.

Client Outcomes	Nursing Interventions	Evaluation
• Sarah will exhibit a more positive self-evaluation.	• Suggest use of diary *to record interactions with husband that result in anxiety symptoms.* • During weekly sessions, role-play other responses that seem more satisfactory to Sarah *to help Sarah distinguish anxiety-producing interactions and modify responses through role-play and other teaching strategies.*	• Sarah reports fewer episodes of headaches and limited-symptom panic attacks. • Frequently describes reinitiating discussions with husband that she previously identified as being unsatisfactory to her.
• Sarah will demonstrate assertive behaviors and positive interpersonal relationship.	• Provide feedback to Sarah about behaviors observed *to give her information about her responses/ behaviors so she can begin to modify/manage them.* • Help Sarah identify and label angry feelings *so she can begin to process feelings correctly and not misinterpret feelings or their meaning.*	• Initiates subject of marital therapy with nurse. • Requests that husband join her in weekly sessions to deal with issues involving husband's use of alcohol, his extramarital affair, and their sexual difficulties.

Nursing Diagnosis: Sexual dysfunction, related to values conflict, as evidenced by alteration in relationship with husband and inability to achieve desired satisfaction.

Client Outcomes	Nursing Interventions	Evaluation
• Sarah will demonstrate ability to attain ongoing intimate relationship with husband.	• Provide an open, neutral atmosphere where Sarah and her husband can discuss their differences regarding the level of interest in intimate relations and achievement of satisfaction *to open up sound discussion in a nonthreatening environment.*	• Sarah and husband report increased mutually satisfying sexual encounters.

Summary of Key Concepts

1. Anxiety and related disorders encompass a wide variety of illnesses that share the common symptoms of anxiety.

2. Etiologic models for anxiety include biologic, psychosocial, psychodynamic, and social theories.

3. Anxiety disorders have high comorbidity with depression and substance abuse.

4. Anxiety disorders are more commonly diagnosed and treated among women, although obsessive-compulsive disorder is a notable exception.

5. Treatment of anxiety and related disorders is multidisciplinary, and usually combines more than one modality.

6. Inpatient treatment of anxiety disorders is increasingly rare and is generally confined to managing acute exacerbations.

7. The nursing role in the treatment of clients with anxiety symptoms varies. Common to all treatment settings is the nurse's role in client and family education about the disorders and their treatment.

8. Nursing care plans for clients with symptoms of anxiety reflect the understanding that managing anxiety effectively is part of daily living.

9. Nurses actively participate in behavioral interventions structured to decrease phobic responses.

10. Rating scales are an effective means for nurses to measure success of strategies implemented to reduce anxiety.

REFERENCES

American Psychiatric Association: *Diagnostic and statistical manual of mental disorders,* ed 4, Washington, D.C., 1994, APA.

Arana G, Hyman S: *Handbook of psychiatric drug therapy,* ed 2, Boston, 1991, Little Brown.

Bailey K, Glod CA: Post-traumatic stress disorder; a role for psychopharmacology, *J Psychosocial Nursing & Mental Health Services* 29(9):42–45, 1991.

Fortinash K, Holoday-Worret, P: *Psychiatric nursing care plans,* ed 2, St. Louis, 1995, Mosby.

Foucault M: *Madness and civilization,* New York, 1988, Vantage.

Freud S: *The standard edition of the complete psychological works,* London, 1963, Hogarth Press.

Freud S: Introductory lectures on psychoanalysis. In *The standard edition of the complete psychological works,* London, 1963, Hogarth Press (originally published in 1917).

Gellengarg A et al: *The practitioner's guide to psychoactive drugs,* ed 3, New York, 1991, Plenum.

Hall C, Lindzey G: *Theories of personality,* New York, 1978, Wiley.

Hall CS: *A primer of Freudian psychology,* Cleveland, 1954, World.

Heidegger M: *Being and time,* New York, 1962, Harper & Row.

Katon W et al: Panic disorder epidemiology in primary care, *J Fam Prac* 23(3):233–239, 1986.

Keltner NL, Folks DG: *Psychotropic drugs,* St. Louis, 1993, Mosby.

Kierkegaard S: *The concept of anxiety,* Princeton, 1980, Princeton University Press.

Kim M et al: *Pocket guide to nursing diagnosis,* ed 6, St. Louis, 1995, Mosby.

Klerman G: Modern concepts of anxiety and panic. In Ballenger J, editor: *Clinical aspects of panic disorder,* New York, 1990, Wiley-Less.

Kluft, RP: Enhancing the hospital treatment of dissociative disorder patients by developing nursing expertise in the application of hypnotic techniques without formal trance induction, *Am J Clin Hypnosis* 34(3):158–167, 1992.

May R: *The meaning of anxiety,* New York, 1979, Pocket Books.

Meleis A: *Theoretical nursing, development and progress,* Philadelphia, 1985, JB Lippincott.

North American Nursing Diagnosis Association: Classification of nursing diagnosis. In *Proceedings of the ninth conference,* Philadelphia, 1991, JB Lippincott.

Patterson JG, Zderad, LT: *Humanistic nursing,* New York, 1976, Wiley.

Peplau H: *Interpersonal relations in nursing,* New York, 1952, Putnam.

Ross, CA et al: Management of anxiety and panic attacks in immediate care facilities, *Gen Hosp Psych* 10(2):120–131, 1988.

Seyle H: *The stress of life,* New York, 1956, McGraw-Hill.

Stein M, Unde T: Panic disorder and major depression: lifetime relationship and biological markers. In Ballenger J, editor: *Clinical aspects of panic disorder,* New York, 1990, Wiley-Less.

Swenson RP, Kuch K: Clinical features of panic and related disorders. In Ballenger J, editor: *Clinical aspects of panic disorder,* New York, 1990, Wiley-Less.

Wolpe J: *The practice of behavior therapy,* ed 2, New York, 1973, Pergamon Press.

CHAPTER 12

Mood Disorders: Depression and Mania

Bonnie Hagerty

Affect the external manifestation of an emotional feeling tone

Anhedonia loss of pleasure and interest in activities previously enjoyed, or in life itself

Atypical depression depression with features that include hypersomnia, weight gain, mood reactivity, and sensitivity in interpersonal relationships

Bipolar disorder a mood disorder characterized by episodes of mania and depression

Dysphoric depressed, sad mood

Dysthymia chronic, low-level depression lasting more than 2 years that may lead to more severe depression if untreated

Euthymia mood that is normal and level

Flight of ideas rapid shifting from one idea to another without completion of the preceding idea, commonly manifested in mania

Hypomania mood of elation with higher than usual activity and social interaction, not as expansive as full mania

Kindling creation of electrophysiologic sensitivity in the brain from stress, altering neural functioning

Learned helplessness perception that events are uncontrollable, leading to apathy, helplessness, powerlessness, and depression

Mania elevated, expansive, or irritable mood accompanied by hyperactivity, grandiosity, and loss of reality

Melancholic depression severe depression characterized by anhedonia, feeling worse in the morning, weight loss, and psychomotor retardation

Mood a feeling state reported by the client that can vary with external and internal changes

Neurotransmission process by which electrochemical signals are sent throughout the brain

Nihilism belief that existence is senseless and useless

Psychomotor agitation agitated motor activity

Psychomotor retardation the slowing of physiologic processes resulting in slow movement, speech, and reaction time

Seasonal affective disorder (SAD) type of mood disorder that occurs at a regular time each year

Schemata the cognitive set of the self and world through which situations are perceived, coded, and interpreted

Unipolar depressive disorder characterized by episodes of depression with no mania

- Describe biologic and psychosocial theories about the etiology of mood disorders.

- Compare and contrast the DSM-IV groupings of depressive disorders and bipolar disorders.

- Discuss the epidemiology and life course of depressive and bipolar disorders.

- Apply the nursing process (i.e., assessment, diagnosis, outcome identification, planning, implementation, and evaluation) for clients with mood disorders.

- Describe collaborative interventions and interventions used by nurses and other mental health professionals for clients with mood disorders.

- Examine personal feelings, thoughts, and reactions to clients with mood disorders that may affect the therapeutic relationship and management of client care.

M ood disorders, previously known as affective disorders, are a group of common psychiatric disorders characterized by disturbances in regulation of emotion, ranging from intense elation or irritability to severe depression. These disorders often result in personal suffering, family distress, interpersonal and occupational impairment, and untold social costs. Over the past decade, considerable research has shown the recurrent and cyclical nature of mood disorders and the disabling outcomes associated with repeated episodes of depression and mania. Indeed, mood disorders are a major public health problem both in terms of economic costs and personal suffering. Some estimates indicate that depression alone costs the United States over $16 billion a year (Depression Guideline Panel, 1993).

While everyone experiences mood fluctuation, depression, and elation, normal variations tend not to be prolonged or incapacitating. Mood fluctuation is often a normal response to experiences and events that influence the human capacity for feeling. Grief and sadness in response to loss of a loved one, or excitement at the thought of a long awaited vacation are normal, adaptive responses. Most people experience sadness and depression with losses (e.g., loved ones, jobs, status, possessions). This sadness may persist for days, weeks, or longer as the individual grieves the loss (see Chapter 26). Mood states become maladaptive, however, when they persist, become pervasive, and interfere with usual functioning. At that point, the mood dysregulation is accompanied by a pattern of signs and symptoms affecting cognitive, behavioral, spiritual, social, and physiologic functioning.

HISTORICAL AND THEORETICAL PERSPECTIVES

Disturbances in mood have been recognized for many years. It is thought that the term *melancholia* was first coined by Hippocrates when he described changing temperament. In 1896 Kraepelin distinguished between dementia praecox (now known as schizophrenia) and manic depression. He described dementia praecox as a chronic illness with progressive deterioration in the client's functioning. Kraepelin (1913, 1921) saw manic depression as cyclical abnormalities of mood, marked by a family history of similar disorders and caused by innate physical factors. This differentiation served as a primary underpinning for modern approaches to understanding and diagnosing mood disorders.

Since Kraepelin, attempts have been made to describe nuances of both depression and mania. Freud (1957) differentiated between maladaptive depression and grief in his famous paper "Mourning and Melancholia," detailing the psychodynamic genesis of depression. Leonhard, a German psychiatrist, proposed the separation of manic-depressive illness into two types: bipolar (history of depression and mania) and monopolar (history of depression only). This differentiation is the basis for the current clinical depiction of bipolar and unipolar mood disorders.

Throughout much of the twentieth century, various forms of bipolar and unipolar disorders have been described. Unipolar depression, for example, has been considered to be one of two types: reactive (exogenous) depression or endogenous depression. Reactive depression was believed to be caused by external stressors and was considered less severe than endogenous depression, which was believed to be due to physiological dysregulation. Mental health professionals currently recognize various forms of bipolar disorders and unipolar depression. Researchers and clinicians continue to document a broad spectrum of mood disorders with varied features and clinical characteristics.

In recent years, mood disorders have commanded more public attention as a result of their pervasiveness. New treatments, including use of the drug Prozac, have created social controversy. Famous persons, such as Patty Duke, William Styron, and Dick Cavett, have acknowledged publicly their struggles with mood disorders, and it is now recognized that many other prominent persons, including Abraham Lincoln, Winston Churchill, Vincent Van Gogh, Ernest Hemingway, Sylvia Plath, and Herman Melville, have experienced one of the mood disorders.

ETIOLOGY

Various theories have been presented to explain the development of mood disorders, but their exact cause remains unknown. Many researchers and clinicians support the premise that mood disorders have multicausal origins, in which biologic, psychologic, social, and cognitive factors converge to promote the development of depression and mania. Others contend that specific types of mood disorders may be related more to certain, specific etiologic factors. Each theoretical perspective helps to explain some aspect of mood disorders, but none fully accounts for their development. In general, these etiologic factors can be grouped primarily as neurobiologic or psychosocial. These factors are summarized in Box 12-1.

Neurobiologic Factors

Over the past decade, research on the etiology of mood disorders has focused on the biologic mechanisms that may be related to their development. While this research has been able to identify physiologic correlates of depression and mania, direct cause and effect relationships

---

Box 12-1   Etiologic Factors Related to Mood Disorders

Neurobiologic factors

- Altered neurotransmission
- Neuroendocrine dysregulation
- Genetic transmission

Pyschosocial factors

- Psychoanalytic theory
    Depression is a result of loss.
    Mania is a defense against depression.
- Cognitive theory
    Depression is a result of negative processing of thoughts.
- Learned helplessness
    Depression is a result of a perceived lack of control over events.
- Life events and stress theory
    Significant life events cause stress, which results in depression or mania.
- Personality theory
    Personality characteristics predispose an individual to mood disorders.

have not been established. For example, a strong relationship between low mood and low systolic blood pressure was found in a study conducted in Great Britain, but no direct causal relationship was identified (Pilgrim, 1992). The more common biologic theories include those related to altered neurotransmission, neuroendocrine dysregulation, and genetic transmission.

NEUROTRANSMISSION

Current research on the biology of mood disorders is dominated by the role of neurotransmitter disturbances. Interest in neurotransmission was sparked initially by investigating the action of antidepressant drugs. In 1954 it was discovered that clients treated with reserpine for hypertension developed depression. Several years later isoniazid was found to have an antidepressant effect on persons being treated for tuberculosis. Imipramine was introduced as an antidepressant in 1958, and research began on its mechanisms of action in the brain. The discoveries resulting from this line of research became the basis for the monoamine hypothesis of mood disorders.

Monoamine or biogenic amine neurotransmitters are crucial for sending electrical signals throughout the brain. While there are hundreds of neurotransmitters in the brain, the biogenic amine neurotransmitters include the catecholamines of epinephrine, norepinephrine, dopamine, and acetylcholine, and the indolamine of serotonin. To accomplish **neurotransmission,** these chemicals are released from the presynaptic neuronal terminal into the synaptic cleft. Once in the synaptic cleft, the neurotransmitter diffuses until it reaches its specific receptors on the postsynaptic membrane of the adjacent neuron, is reabsorbed through special receptors on the presynaptic membrane, or is degraded by another chemical, such as the enzyme monoamine oxidase. When the neurotransmitter locks into its receptors on the postsynaptic membrane of an adjacent neuron, it triggers a series of chemical actions that electrically depolarize the cell and sends an electrical impulse throughout that neuron, thus continuing the process of transmission of nerve impulses. Specialized neurons of each of the neurotransmitters project to various parts of the brain that control a wide range of functions, including appetite, sleep, and arousal.

It is believed that monoamine neurotransmitter systems, especially those of norepinephrine and serotonin, their metabolites, and their receptors are somehow altered during episodes of depression and mania. More recent research on neurotransmission has focused on the altered sensitivity of neuronal receptors and properties of neuronal membranes in mood disorders. In response to a decrease or increase in availability of neurotransmitters, it appears that, over time, there is a change in the sensitivity or density of presynaptic and postsynaptic receptors specific to a particular neurotransmitter. This results in delayed postsynaptic receptor-mediated responses.

Availability and receptor change theories propose that there is an underactivity of neurotransmission in depression and an overactivity in mania. Support for this comes from the administration of monoamine oxidase inhibitors (MAOIs) to clients with depression. MAOIs inhibit the monoamine oxidase enzyme from breaking down neurotransmitters, thus resulting in an increased supply of neurotransmitters and an accompanying decrease in clinical depression. Additional support is evident through recent research that demonstrates how medications, such as Prozac, Paxil, and Zoloft (selective serotonin reuptake inhibitors, or SSRIs), selectively block serotonin reabsorption in their presynaptic neuronal receptors, thus increasing the supply of serotonin in the synaptic cleft (Fuller, 1991). It can be argued that therapeutic responses to most antidepressant medication usually take several weeks, because of the delayed sensitization or change in quantity of receptors.

Post (1992) has postulated that a phenomenon called **kindling** occurs, in which neurotransmission is altered initially by stress, resulting in a first episode of depression. This initial episode creates an electrophysiologic sensitivity to future stress, requiring less stress to evoke another depressive or manic episode. In essence, kindling creates new "hardwiring" of the brain or long-lasting alterations of neuronal functioning. It appears as though this alteration influences many cellular processes, including changes in DNA, RNA, and, ultimately, selective gene expression. The kindling model is consistent with the cyclical and progressive nature of mood disorders and suggests that clients remain on medication for extended periods to avoid physiologic deterioration over time.

Recent technological advances in studying the brain provide additional support for disturbances in brain functioning during depression. The PET (positron emission tomography) scanner enables researchers to examine brain physiology of depressed persons vs. normal controls as well as comparison of brain functioning in individuals both during depression and after recovery. Fig. 12-1 depicts the differences that are apparent using PET scanning of depressed, recovered, and normal control brains. Fig. 12-2 indicates increased blood flow in components of the brains of persons with major depression. PET scanning has found that the prefrontal cerebral cortex and the limbic system (including the amygdala) appear to have physiologic disruptions in the brains of persons experiencing depression.

While research continues on the biochemical theories described above, these theories concerning the relationships between neurotransmission and mood disorders continue to be somewhat speculative. The investigation is hampered by inconsistent definitions and criteria for depression and mania, and the difficulties of measuring concentrations of specific neurotransmitters in selected sites in the brain. Peripheral indicators of neurotransmitters and their metabolites, such as those in the blood,

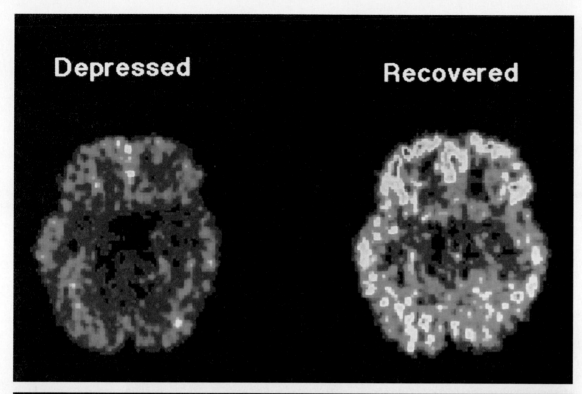

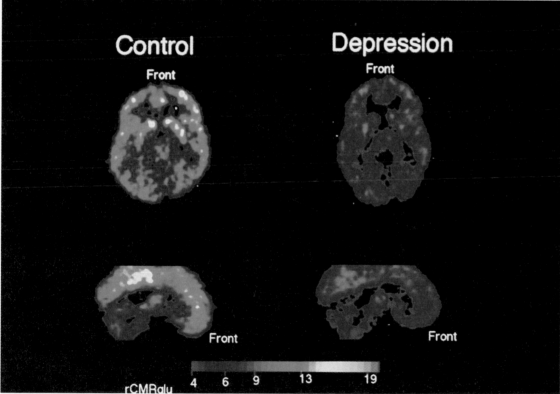

Figure 12-1 A. PET (positron emission tomography) scans of the same depressed individual's brain when depressed (left) and after recovery through treatment with medication (right). Several brain areas, particularly the prefrontal cortex (at top), show diminished activity (darker colors) during depression.

(Courtesy Mark George, MD, National Institute of Mental Health Biological Psychiatry Branch, U.S. Dept. of Health and Human Services.)

B. PET scans of a normal subject (left) and a depressed subject (right) reveal reduced brain activity (darker colors) during depression, especially in the prefrontal cortex. A form of radioactively tagged glucose was used as a tracer to visualize levels of brain activity.

(Courtesy Mark George, MD, National Institute of Mental Health Biological Psychiatry Branch, U.S. Dept. of Health and Human Services.)

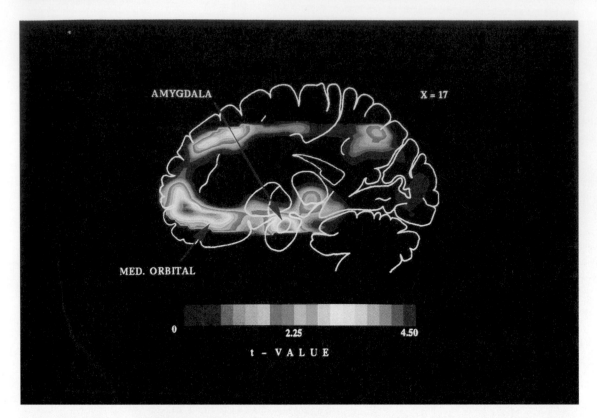

Figure 12-2 PET (positron emission tomography) scan indicates increased blood flow in the amygdala and prefrontal cortex in persons with major depression of the familial pure depressive disease subtype. Scan is a composite of images of thirteen individuals.

(Courtesy Wayne C. Drevets, MD, Dept. of Psychiatry, Washington University School of Medicine, St. Louis, Missouri.)

urine, or central spinal fluid, may not be related to amounts in various parts of the brain. In addition, neurotransmission is a complex activity, and many of its aspects, such as neurotransmitter synthesis and release, receptor sites, interactions among the various neurotransmitters and hormones, and their action on genetic material, can be related to the role of altered neurotransmission in mood disorders.

NEUROENDOCRINE DYSREGULATION

Another area of research on the biologic basis of mood disorders is the role of the endocrine system. Studies indicate that dysregulation of the *hypothalamic-pituitary-adrenal (HPA) axis* is associated with depression. The HPA axis comprises the hypothalamus, pituitary, and adrenal glands and controls physiologic responses to stress. The hypothalamus regulates endocrine functions and the autonomic nervous system and is involved in behaviors related to fight, flight, feeding, and mating. In response to stress, the hypothalamus releases corticotropin-releasing hormone (CRH), which stimulates the anterior pituitary to secrete corticotropin. In turn, corticotropin causes the adrenal cortex to release cortisol into the blood. Through an elaborate feedback mechanism, levels of cortisol signal the hypothalamus to increase or decrease CRH production. The specific physio-

logic ways that stress signals for this process to begin are not well understood, although stress-input signals may come from the brain stem, autonomic nervous system, or cerebral cortex (Young et al, 1993).

Hyperactivity of the HPA axis is often evident in depression. Up to 50% of the clients with moderate to severe depression exhibit elevated serum cortisol levels. This phenomenon led to the creation of the *dexamethasone suppression test* (DST), which was hoped to be a potential biologic diagnostic indicator of endogenous depression. The DST is based on the premise that when clients are given dexamethasone (synthetic cortisol) at night, a signal is sent to the hypothalamus to shut down production of CRH, leading to decreased output of corticotropin and, subsequently, cortisol by the following morning. For many clients with severe depression, measurement of this blood cortisol level the following morning revealed continued excessive amounts of cortisol production. Subsequent research regarding the DST has revealed problems with its selectivity and specificity. It is not consistent with regards to its results in persons with depression, may be affected by other variables (e.g., age, gender), and is evident in other disorders, such as alcoholism and anorexia nervosa (Zimmerman et al, 1986).

The functioning of the HPA axis is related to the 24-hour cycle of *circadian rhythms* that control physiologic processes. With mood disorders, many normal, cyclical patterns are disrupted. Blood cortisol is normally at a low level in the early morning and highest in late afternoon, though constant increases are often apparent in depression. Sleep-wake cycles are disrupted in mood disorders, and during depression, clients experience decreased REM latency and decreased shallow, slow delta wave sleep, thus fragmenting the sleep/wake cycle. Even seasonal patterns appear to have some relationship to mood disorders, with episodes of depression often occurring during periods of decreased light. Ehlers et al, (1988) proposed an interaction between behavior and environment and posited that zeitgebers (cues or stimuli from the environment) altered physiology that in turn affected mood. Research on HPA axis dysfunction continues, with special interest in the relationships between mood disorders and stress.

GENETIC TRANSMISSION

Mood disorders tend to run in families, and it is commonly believed that, to some extent, genetic transmission is responsible for their manifestation. Data regarding the genetic transmission of mood disorders are derived from family, twin, and adoption studies.

In *family studies,* families who exhibit mood disorders are selected, and the morbid risk for developing these disorders in relatives is compared with the general population. Results of these studies consistently demonstrate that first-degree relatives of persons with bipolar disorder and unipolar depression have a greater risk for developing a mood disorder. This risk is particularly high for relatives of persons with bipolar disorder, possibly indicating a greater genetic component than that of unipolar depression (McGriffin and Katz, 1989).

Twin studies are based on the assumption that monozygotic twins share the same genes and dizygotic twins have about 50% of their genes in common. Results of twin research provide additional evidence for the genetic transmission of mood disorders. If one monozygotic twin suffers from bipolar disorder, there is a high rate of concordance, ranging to 100% in some studies, whereby the other twin will also develop a mood disorder, usually bipolar illness. Although there are high rates of concordance for dizygotic twins, they tend to be less than those for monozygotic twins. For unipolar disorders, the concordance rates continue to be higher for monozygotic twins, and both twin types have a higher concordance than the general population.

Using *adoption studies,* researchers can examine the contributions of both the environment and genetic transmission. In general, adoption studies also support the role of genetic factors in mood disorders. Most studies have focused specifically on bipolar disorder and have found that the biologic parents of adult adoptees diagnosed with bipolar disorder have a much higher incidence of the disorder than parents of adoptees with no mood disorder.

Although all of the above information supports the role of genetics in the development of mood disorders, particularly bipolar disorders, this research does not reveal the specific genes or genetic mechanisms involved in transmission. Early scientific reports describing the location of genetic markers on specific genes have not been replicated. The search for the specific genetic basis of mood disorders continues with special emphasis on genetic location and genetic processes, including the role of selective gene expression and neuromodulation (Barondes, 1993).

Psychosocial Factors

Psychosocial explanations for the development of mood disorders represent a range of theoretical positions, including psychoanalytic theory, learned helplessness, cognitive theory, life events (stress) theory, and personality theory.

PSYCHOANALYTIC THEORY

The basic premise of psychoanalytic theory is that unconscious processes result in expression of symptoms, including depression and mania. Freud (1957) distinguished between depression and normal grief, citing both as a response to real or symbolic loss. He noted that in depression, the loss generated intense, hostile feelings toward the lost object that were turned inward onto the self (anger turned inward), creating guilt and loss of self-esteem.

Thus depression is viewed together with loss and aggression. The loss of an object either physically or emotionally is compounded by the development of anger. Struggling with feelings of rejection, the child is unable to direct anger and hostility toward the lost love object for fear of more rejection and loss and because of a strong, punitive superego. The child experiences ambivalence, or both love and hate for the lost love object. Feelings of anger and aggression are repressed, and the child interprets the loss as rejection and a reflection of his or her own lack of self-worth. As a result, patterns of low self-esteem, depression, and helplessness become established and endure as the person confronts future loss. This scenario occurs early in childhood, creating a vulnerability to real or perceived loss throughout adulthood that results in periods of depression.

Psychodynamically, mania is explained as a defense against depression. The client denies feelings of anger, low self-esteem, and worthlessness and reverses the affect such that there is a triumphant feeling of self-confidence. Mania represents a conquered superego with little inclination to control id impulses. Yet, over time, this distorted view of reality waivers, and the client demonstrates outward hostility toward others, often focusing on the weaknesses of others that are similar to the internal weaknesses being avoided.

There are few data that support the psychodynamic theories of depression and mania, but there is some evidence that clients with depression have experienced more early childhood loss and deprivation than persons without depression (Boulby, 1969; Brown and Harris, 1978). Clinicians also note that anger is often associated with depression, although the relationship between anger and depression remains obscure. Many people who experience early childhood loss and anger never experience depression, while many who do not experience a visible or acknowledged loss do experience depression. The psychoanalytic theory is only one of many explanations that attempt to explain the internal dynamics of depression and mania.

COGNITIVE THEORY

The cognitive model of depression points to errors of logical thinking as causative factors for depression. It assumes that mood is influenced by underlying cognitive structures, some of which are not fully conscious. These cognitive structures are shaped by early life experiences and are predisposed to negative processing. In a diatheses-stress model, when persons predisposed to depression with negative schemata encounter stress, the negative processing is activated, resulting in depressive thinking (Beck, 1967).

Beck (1967) differentiated among levels of cognition that influenced depression: automatic thoughts, schemata or assumptions, and cognitive distortions. Automatic thoughts are those that can be brought into awareness, although they appear fleetingly and are usually unrecognized. They form the person's perception of a situation, and it is this perception, rather than the objective facts about the situation, that results in emotional and behavioral responses. If the perceptions are distorted, inferences and responses will be maladaptive. For example, a client expressed anger that his wife was picking vegetables from his garden and giving them to her friends. He interpreted this as an attempt to get rid of his belongings and was surprised at the suggestion that she may have been proud of his vegetables and wanted to share his accomplishment with others who appreciated good food.

Schemata are internal representations of the self and the world. They facilitate information processing because they are used to understand, code, and recall information. Beck (1967) proposed a triad of thinking (schemata) that gives rise to the development of depression:

1. negative, self-deprecating views of self

2. pessimistic views of the world so that life experiences are interpreted in a negative way

3. the belief that negativity will continue into the future promoting a negative view of future events

These mind-sets result in the misinterpretation of events and situations so that the client's cognitive schema of self

as worthless and the world and future as hopeless are supported. This faulty cognitive processing leads to assumptions and continued errors of logic that result in depressive symptoms and an ongoing negative view of life. This was evidenced by a client who began each meeting with the nurse by saying, "There is no point to this. I know things will never be better."

Cognitive distortions link schemata and automatic thoughts. Faulty information processing includes cognitive distortions, such as overgeneralization (drawing general conclusions based on isolated incidents), dichotomous thinking (perceiving events and experiences in only one of two opposite categories), and magnification (placing a distorted emphasis on a single event or error). Mary, a 32-year-old female, presented with each of these types of distortion. She reported that her supervisor had not spoken directly to her at two recent company meetings. She concluded that he must be unhappy with her performance (overgeneralization). Mary stated that there were only two types of employees, good and bad, and that bad ones lost their jobs (dichotomous thinking). Mary's concern began after she forgot to give her supervisor an important message. In spite of a good work history, she was convinced that she had demonstrated what a poor employee she was (magnification).

There is considerable research support for the cognitive model of depression (Robins and Hayes, 1993). It has led to the development of specific treatment for depression using cognitive techniques. These techniques are short-term and focus on changing the client's faulty negative cognition.

LEARNED HELPLESSNESS THEORY

The learned helplessness theory is actually a variant of cognitive theory, tracing the determinants of depression to altered cognition. The term **learned helplessness** was used first to describe the lack of motivation exhibited by dogs to laboratory shocks that they were unable to control. Seligman (1975) originally proposed that stressful events that were experienced as uncontrollable resulted in the development of helplessness, apathy, powerlessness, and depression.

This perspective was somewhat modified when Abramson et al (1978) posited that the primary issue was the person's expectation (cognition) that external events were uncontrollable. This causal attribution regarding current events, combined with the person's perceptions of past uncontrollable experiences, yields the expectation that the event or situation cannot be controlled. This, in turn, results in helplessness, passivity, and sadness, which lead to other symptoms of depression, such as decreased appetite and low self-esteem.

More recently, the reformulated model of learned helplessness was revised to become the hopelessness theory of depression (Abramson et al, 1989). This theory presents hopelessness as a sufficient cause of depression, and the individual's inferred negative outcomes and negativity about self as key elements of depression. Helplessness is viewed as one component of hopelessness; perceived lack of control over events assumes a less central role. With the occurrence of an unpleasant event, persons prone to depression attribute stability (vs. instability), globalization (vs. specific), and importance (vs. unimportance) to those events.

This is exemplified by John, who perceived that his unemployment would be long-lasting (stability), that his entire life had been ruined (globalization), and that his former job had been the major focus of his life (importance). Symptoms of depression relating to apathy and motivation (helplessness expectancy) and depressed, sad affect (negative outcome expectancy), as well as other symptoms of depression, are believed to flow from this condition of hopelessness. **Affect** is the external manifestation of an emotional feeling tone. Unfortunately, the specific mechanisms by which these conditions and attributions are converted into the specific symptom pattern of depression (or mania) remain elusive.

LIFE EVENTS AND STRESS THEORY

It is widely acknowledged that there appears to be some type of relationship between life events and the onset of unipolar depression. It is unclear, however, to what extent external social determinants and negative life circumstances contribute to the development and course of mood disorders, particularly bipolar disorders (McPherson et al, 1993). Some episodes of depression and mania occur in the absence of any notable stressor, while others are clearly associated with life events. The role of life events in the onset of depression is stronger in nonendogenous depression and dysthymia. There is less evidence regarding the role of life events in the development of bipolar disorders. It appears that life events are often major precipitants of bipolar disorder only for the first episodes. This supports Post's theory of electrophysiological sensitization, or kindling, and suggests that there may be subtypes of depression and mania related to some etiologies (e.g., biologic vs. psychosocial) more than others.

In studying depression, researchers have been interested in the quantity and nature of life events and the size and perceived supportiveness of the client's social network in relation to the initial onset and recurrence of mania and depression. Paykel (1979), for example, found that clients with depression reported three times as many life events in the 6 months prior to the onset of depression as persons without depression. Brown and Harris (1978) reported that stressful social factors (e.g., lack of an intimate, confiding relationship with a significant other, having three or more children at home, being unemployed, and loss of mother before age 11) contributed significantly to vulnerability for depression. Additional evidence suggests that events involving social loss, such as death of a loved one, have potent effects on the onset of depression. Cornelis et al (1989) suggested that the emotional evaluation of an event is as important as the change it causes in daily life, and that life events evoke various degrees of stress. The effect of an event is influenced by mechanisms such as social support and the person's perception of that event. Life events most likely influence the development and recurrence of depression through the psychologic and, ultimately, biologic, experiences of stress.

PERSONALITY THEORY

For many years, psychiatric clinicians have described a depressive personality that encompasses personality traits and characteristics often seen in clients with depression. The term *depressive personality* has been used broadly to describe personality traits that (1) exist prior to, during, or after a depressive episode, (2) modify depression, (3) are variants of normal personality rather than reflective of a mood disorder, or (4) are indicative of enduring character and temperament (Phillips et al, 1990). Personality characteristics commonly associated with depression include negativity, pessimism, low self-worth, prone to worry and anxiety, tendency to be hypercritical toward self and others, self-denying, serious and overly responsible, dependent on other's love and affection, demanding, feeling bored and empty, hypochondriasis, quietness, incapacity for enjoyment and relaxation, and interpersonal sensitivity to rejection.

According to personality theory, these characteristics are long-standing, structural components of the person's psyche. The extent to which they predispose an individual to mood disorders, are outcomes of having had a depressive or manic episode, or are consistent, ongoing elements is unclear. There is some evidence that certain traits, such as interpersonal rejection sensitivity and neuroticism (worry), do increase vulnerability for depression (Boyce et al, 1991). It appears, however, that these traits interact with other variables, such as age, social factors, and stressors. For example, in one prospective study, personality variables did not differentiate between subjects who did and did not develop depression in those under age 30. However, there was a differentiation for those over age 30, including drive and emotional strength, increased dependency, and increased reflection and thoughtfulness in the group that had depression (Hirshfeld et al, 1989).

While there are advocates who support depressive personality as a DSM-IV, Axis II personality disorder, caution must be exercised not to attribute these traits to all with depression. The experience of depression or mania can shape behavioral characteristics or strengthen preexisting personality features.

EPIDEMIOLOGY

Mood disorders, particularly depression, are common. Recent data suggest that the lifetime prevalence of developing any affective disorder is 19.3%, 14.7% for men and

23.9% for women (Kessler et al, 1994). Since the lifetime prevalence of bipolar disorder is about equal for men and women (1.4% and 1.3%, respectively), much of this difference is due to unipolar depression. Women have a 21.3% lifetime prevalence of major depression and 8.0% for dysthymia, while men have a lifetime prevalence of only 12.7% and 4.8%, respectively. These gender differences for depression have not been adequately explained, and additional research is needed to determine why female gender is a high-risk factor for depression.

The first episode of a mood disorder seems to be occurring at younger ages. The average age for onset of bipolar illness is the mid to late twenties. Although the average age of onset for unipolar depression has been considered the middle thirties, there is some evidence that onset is occurring in younger cohorts (Lewinsohn et al, 1993). While the most frequent age of onset for depression is the 25 to 44 year age group, people in younger age groups have an ever-increasing risk of developing depression. Data indicate that the onset of depression at an early age (teens or early twenties) or at age 55 and over predicts a more protracted, chronic course (Klerman and Weissman, 1992). Rates of depression do not significantly increase during menopause. Risk of developing depression and mania is also increased if there is a positive family history for mood disorders (Akiskal, 1989).

Sociocultural factors may be related to the onset of depression and mania. Depression seems to occur less frequently in African-Americans than in either white or Hispanic groups in the United States. It also appears that depression may be more frequent in lower socioeconomic groups, while bipolar disorders are more frequent in higher socioeconomic groups. While depression and mania occur throughout the world, the expression of symptoms are influenced by ethnicity and culture.

Asians, for example, describe more somatic symptoms of depression, whereas people from Western cultures describe more mood and cognitive changes.

In an increasingly stressful society characterized by mobility, family disruptions, and economic stressors, women and younger persons are manifesting depression more than in previous generations. Unfortunately, the relationships among biologic, psychologic, developmental, and sociocultural factors and their influence on the development of mood disorders are still unclear. Epidemiology data for mood disorders are summarized in Box 12-2.

CLINICAL DESCRIPTION

Mood is defined as a feeling state reported by the client that can vary with external and internal changes. Mood disorders are defined by a pattern of episodes over time and by a pattern of symptoms in each episode. Mood disorders are classified in the DSM-IV as depressive disorders, bipolar disorders, or other mood disorders. The signs and symptoms of these disorders are described in the following sections.

Depressive Disorders

Persons diagnosed with a depressive disorder have experienced only episodes of depression with no manic or hypomanic episodes. This is also referred to as **unipolar** depression. The DSM-IV box on page 261 lists criteria for a major depressive episode. The clinical symptoms of depressive disorders are summarized in the box on page 262.

MAJOR DEPRESSIVE EPISODE, SINGLE OR RECURRENT

An episode of major depression can be indicative of a first episode or of a recurrent episode of depression. Symptoms occur as a result of the disorder and not from the effects of a substance, medical condition, or loss of a loved one within the previous 2 months.

Emotional Symptoms.   Two primary symptoms of major depression are depressed mood and **anhedonia,** or loss of interest and pleasure in activities. In order for clients to be diagnosed with major depression, one of these symptoms must be present most of the day, nearly every day, for at least 2 weeks. Clients may describe their mood as depressed, sad, empty, or numb. They may report difficulty experiencing pleasure or satisfaction from their usual activities, including eating and sex. Feelings of sadness may be accompanied by frequent crying. Anxiety, irritability, or anger may also be present. Clients may report feelings of loneliness, helplessness, or hopelessness. The affect of a person with depression is often flat and constricted, with minimal expression.

Cognitive Symptoms.   Cognitive criteria for major depression include the diminished ability to think, concentrate, or make decisions; recurrent thoughts of death, and excessive focus on self-worthlessness and guilt.

Box 12-2   Epidemiology of Mood Disorders

- 19.3% of the general population develop a mood disorder.

- 21.3% of women and 12.7% of men develop major depression.

- Average age of onset for bipolar illness is mid to late twenties.

- Average age of onset of depression is mid thirties.

- Depression occurs more frequently in whites and Hispanics than in African-Americans.

- Depression occurs more frequently in lower socioeconomic groups.

- Bipolar disorders occur more frequently in higher socioeconomic groups.

DSM-IV CRITERIA

Major Depressive Episode

A. Five (or more) of the following symptoms have been present during the same 2-week period and represent a change from previous functioning; at least one of the symptoms is either (1) depressed mood or (2) loss of interest or pleasure.

Note: Do not include symptoms that are clearly due to a general medical condition, or mood-incongruent delusions or hallucinations.

1. depressed mood most of the day, nearly every day, as indicated by either subjective report (e.g., feels sad or empty) or observation made by others (e.g., appears tearful). **Note:** In children and adolescents, can be irritable mood.

2. markedly diminished interest or pleasure in all, or almost all, activities most of the day, nearly every day (as indicated by either subjective account or observation made by others)

3. significant weight loss when not dieting or weight gain (e.g., a change of more than 5% of body weight in month), or decrease or increase in appetite nearly every day. **Note:** In children, consider failure to make expected weight gains.

4. insomnia or hypersomnia nearly every day

5. psychomotor agitation or retardation nearly every day (observable by others, not merely subjective feelings of restlessness or being slowed down)

6. fatigue or loss of energy nearly every day

7. feelings of worthlessness or excessive or inappropriate guilt (which may be delusional) nearly every day (not merely self-reproach or guilt about being sick)

8. diminished ability to think or concentrate, or indecisiveness, nearly every day (either by subjective account or as observed by others)

9. recurrent thoughts of death (not just fear of dying), recurrent suicidal ideation without a specific plan, or a suicide attempt or a specific plan for committing suicide

B. The symptoms do not meet criteria for a Mixed Episode.

C. The symptoms cause clinically significant distress or impairment in social, occupational, or other important areas of functioning.

D. The symptoms are not due to the direct physiologic effects of a substance (e.g., a drug of abuse, a medication) or a general medical condition (e.g., hypothyroidism).

E. The symptoms are not better accounted for by bereavement, i.e., after the loss of a loved one, the symptoms persist for longer than 2 months or are characterized by marked functional impairment, morbid preoccupation with worthlessness, suicidal ideation, psychotic symptoms, or psychomotor retardation.

Reprinted with permission from *Diagnostic and Statistical Manual of Mental Disorders*, ed 4, 1994: Washington, D.C. American Psychiatric Association.

Many clients describe difficulty attending to and concentrating on a task or conversation. Reading a newspaper or following the train of thought in a lecture may be overwhelming. Clients may be unable to make decisions about routine concerns, such as what clothing to put on in the morning or what to buy at the grocery store. Recurrent thoughts of death are often evident, including thoughts of suicide, death from natural causes, or existential thoughts about dying. At times, these thoughts may occupy a large portion of the client's waking hours. Negative thinking is often apparent with feelings of worthlessness and excessive guilt. Clients ruminate about past deeds and their negative view of themselves and the world. Clients with severe depression can become delusional with fixed beliefs that cannot be changed by logic, focusing on persecution, punishment, **nihilism** (belief that existence is senseless and useless), or somatic concerns.

Behavioral Symptoms. Behavioral symptoms that are criteria for major depression are significant weight loss or gain or change in appetite, insomnia or hypersomnia, psychomotor agitation or retardation, and fatigue. Weight gain or weight loss is considered to be significant when it represents a 5% change in body weight in one month. Sometimes the weight change is not apparent but the client reports a major change in appetite. Sleep disturbances are common, and clients report not being able to sleep or sleeping too much. **Psychomotor agitation** is evident when the client appears to be restless, paces, fidgets, or is irritable. With **psychomotor retardation,** the client appears to be slowed down in movement and in speech. Persons with depression may appear listless and disheveled. They may not carefully attend to their dress, appearance, or hygiene. They may exhibit a stooped posture and make little eye contact. Many clients report feelings of fatigue and loss of energy, citing their inability to accomplish tasks and their increased need for naps. This symptom may cause many clients to visit their family physician or nurse practitioner, believing that the fatigue is indicative of a physical problem.

CLINICAL SYMPTOMS

Depressive disorders

Major depression

EMOTIONAL
   Anhedonia
   Depressed mood
COGNITIVE
   Diminished ability to think, concentrate, or make
      decisions
   Recurrent thoughts of death
   Excessive focus on self-worthlessness and guilt
BEHAVIORAL
   Significant weight loss or gain or change in appetite
   Insomnia or hypersomnia
   Psychomotor agitation or retardation
   Fatigue
SOCIAL
   Withdrawal from family and social interactions
   Problems at work in organizing, initiating, and com-
      pleting work

Dysthymic disorder

EMOTIONAL
   Depressed mood
   Anhedonia
   Irritability or angry mood
COGNITIVE
   Feelings of low self-esteem and inadequacy
   Feelings of guilt and brooding about the past
   Difficulty with concentration, memory, and deci-
      sion-making
   Attitudes of pessimism, despair, and hopelessness
BEHAVIORAL
   Chronic fatigue
SOCIAL
   Social withdrawal

Thus depression is often diagnosed first during a visit to the primary care provider.

Social Symptoms. To diagnose major depression, the convergence of symptoms must cause personal distress and significant impairment in social and occupational functioning. Clients may withdraw from family and social interactions. They may have problems at their job, including inability to organize, begin, and complete their work. While some are able to function at work with relatively little impairment, this often comes at great personal and family expense as their energy for social interaction is depleted. Family members begin to feel confused, angry, guilty, abandoned, and sad.

Marital distress is often a cited stressor at least six months before the onset of a depressive episode (Schmaling and Becker, 1991). During an episode, the client's er-

ratic behavior, mood, and cognition can alienate a loved one, who may become frustrated about how to help the partner. Unfortunately, it appears as though marital distress continues even after the acute episode subsides. Continued marital strain has been cited as a factor in episode recurrence (Schmaling and Becker, 1991).

DYSTHYMIC DISORDER

Dysthymic disorder differs from major depression because it is a chronic, low-level depression. To receive this diagnosis, the client must have had depressed mood and at least three of the following symptoms for most of the day, nearly every day, for at least 2 years (one year for children and adolescents): poor appetite or overeating, insomnia or hypersomnia, low energy, low self-esteem, poor concentration or difficulty making decisions, and feelings of hopelessness. There cannot have been a manic or hypomanic episode. The client may have experienced an episode of major depression before the onset of dysthymia, provided there were at least 6 months with no signs or symptoms of depression. After 2 years of dysthymia, the client may be diagnosed with major depression superimposed with dysthymia if symptoms increase in severity. The dysthymic disorder is not due to the effects of a substance or medical condition. Psychotic features are usually not present in this disorder.

Cognitive Symptoms. Cognitive symptoms of **dysthymia** include low self-esteem and inadequacy; guilt and brooding about the past; difficulty with concentration, memory, and decision-making; and negative thinking evidenced by pessimism, despair, and hopelessness. Clients with dysthymia often have little regard for themselves and are plagued by a sense of inadequacy and a lack of self-confidence. They reflect on past actions and attribute personal guilt to their circumstances. Negativity pervades much of what they do and say; life seems hopeless, and situations are bounded by pessimism and despair. Clients often report poor memory and decreased concentration on tasks. They may have problems making decisions, but the impairment is usually not as severe as impaired decision-making during major depression.

Emotional Symptoms. The predominant symptom that must be present for the diagnosis of dysthymia is depressed mood. Clients report feeling chronically "down, gloomy, sad." Many are unable to remember a time when they felt their usual self. Another symptom indicative of dysthymia is a generalized loss of interest or pleasure in activities, but unlike major depression, anhedonia is not a primary emotional symptom. Another symptom is irritability or angry mood. Clients may find themselves feeling impatient with family members or coworkers and demonstrating angry outbursts. Many feel bad about their irritable state but find themselves unable to control it.

Behavioral Symptoms. Clients with dysthymia commonly complain of chronic fatigue. They are exhausted from usual activities and often believe that they have a physical illness or chronic fatigue syndrome. Clients may take repeated trips to their health care provider, hoping to determine the cause of their fatigue. In conjunction with the fatigue, clients display decreased activity and productivity. Everything becomes a chore, and it becomes difficult to complete tasks in the usual amount of time.

Social Symptoms.   Social withdrawal is common with dysthymia. Clients are tired, irritable, and depressed and no longer get satisfaction from outings or activities with family and friends. Clients' mood states and negativity may prevent people from wanting to be with them, increasing their isolation from others.

DEPRESSIVE DISORDERS NOT OTHERWISE SPECIFIED

There are types of depression that do not meet the criteria for the depressive disorders presented thus far. Some of these include premenstrual **dysphoric** disorder, minor depressive disorder, recurrent brief depressive disorder, and the postpsychotic depression of schizophrenia. **Dysphoria** refers to a depressed, sad mood. The reader is referred to the DSM-IV for more extensive descriptions of these diagnoses.

Bipolar Disorders

Bipolar disorders occur when the client experiences episodes of depression and episodes of mania or hypomania over time. Bipolar disorders are defined by the pattern of manic, hypomanic, and depressed episodes over time. The depressed and manic episodes are not due to the effects of a substance, including antidepressant medication, electroconvulsive therapy, or light therapy. Clients may be diagnosed with a Bipolar I or a Bipolar II disorder. The DSM-IV criteria box on this page describes these bipolar patterns. Although the public continues to refer to bipolar disorders as manic depression, this term connotes a single, polarized disorder. A bipolar disorder encompasses the range of possible disturbances in mood. The clinical symptoms of bipolar disorders are summarized in the box on page 264.

MANIC EPISODE

Manic episodes occur when there is an abnormally and persistently elevated, expansive, or irritable mood for at least 1 week. At least three of the following symptoms must also be present: inflated self-esteem, decreased need for sleep, more talkative than usual, racing thoughts, distractibility, increase in goal-directed activity, and excessive involvement in pleasurable activities.

Emotional Symptoms.   To be diagnosed as having a manic episode, the client must exhibit an abnormally and persistently elevated, expansive, or irritable mood for at least 1 week. The client appears euphoric, with periods punctuated by irritability and anger. Some clients report minimal euphoria but describe irritability as their primary mood. Emotional lability, fluctuating between euphoria and anger, is common.

DSM-IV CRITERIA

Bipolar I and Bipolar II Disorders

Type	Characteristics
Bipolar I, Single Manic Episode	• only one manic episode • no past major depressive episodes
Most Recent Episode Hypomanic	• current hypomania • at least one previous manic episode
Most Recent Episode Manic	• current mania • at least one previous depressive, hypomanic, or manic episode
Most Recent Episode Mixed	• meets criteria for both manic and depressive current episode • at least one past major depressive or hypomanic episode
Most Recent Episode Depressed	• current depressive episode • at least one past manic episode
Bipolar II Disorder	• must never have had full, manic episode • at least one past major depressive and past hypomanic episode

Adapted From American Psychiatric Association: *Diagnostic and Statistical Manual of Mental Disorders*, ed. 4, Washington, D.C, 1994.

Cognitive Symptoms.   Inflated self-esteem and grandiosity are common symptoms of **mania.** Clients report that they are confident, capable, and can do things better than others. As the mania becomes more intense, clients describe themselves in glowing terms and may even believe that they are capable of amazing feats and achievements. Delusions of grandeur may be evident during severe episodes of mania as clients believe that they possess extraordinary gifts and talents or that they are someone famous. These delusions of inflated self-worth and ability represent mood-congruent psychotic features of mania. Cognitively, clients with mania also experience thought flow disturbance with racing thoughts and flight of ideas. **Flight of ideas** is a type of thought disorder, in which somewhat connected thoughts occur quickly, resulting in little elaboration and rapid changing of subjects. It becomes difficult to block out incoming stimuli, and the client becomes distractible, responding to irrelevant stimuli. Clients with mania often deny the

CLINICAL SYMPTOMS

Bipolar disorders

Manic episode
EMOTIONAL
  Abnormally and persistently elevated, expansive, or irritable mood
COGNITIVE
  Feelings of inflated self-esteem and grandiosity
  Thought-flow disturbance with racing thoughts and flight of ideas
BEHAVIORAL
  Increased talkativeness
  Increased goal-directed behavior or agitation
  Excessive involvement in activities thought to be pleasurable
SOCIAL
  Increased sociability
  Intrusive, interruptive, and disruptive during conversations or activities
  Fluctuations between euphoria and anger
PERCEPTUAL
  Distractibility
  Hallucinations

Cyclothymic disorder
BEHAVIORAL
  Periods of hypomania
  Periods of depressed mood and anhedonia

seriousness of their status and lack judgment regarding personal, social, and occupational needs and activities.

Behavioral Symptoms. Increased talkativeness, increased goal-directed behavior or agitation, and excessive involvement in pleasurable activities are notable symptoms of mania. As the mania progresses, clients become more talkative and their speech is pressured (delivered with urgency.) The rate of speech may increase and become rapid. Clients may exhibit extremes in appearance, wearing bright colors, unusual dress, and heavy makeup. Clients begin and engage in more activities, taking on additional tasks and initiating new projects. Productivity may appear to increase as the client delves into more tasks, but as the mania becomes more intense, actual productivity decreases as clients become more distractible, disorganized, and agitated. They begin to physically move faster—pacing, fidgeting, rarely letting their body stand still. As insight and judgment become more impaired, clients become involved in activities that they perceive as pleasurable, but that may carry a high risk for harm or negative consequences. Clients often report engaging in extramarital affairs, promiscuity, spending sprees, gambling, wild driving, and unwise business deals.

Social Symptoms. At first, mania seems to promote sociability, and clients become more outgoing and active; however, before long, insight and judgment fail, and these same clients become intrusive—interrupting others conversations and activities, fluctuating from euphoria to anger, disrupting social interactions. Clients with mania find it difficult to set both physical and emotional boundaries, infringing on the physical space and personal issues of others. The funny, witty client becomes angry and isolated as the mood escalates and intensifies.

Perceptual Symptoms. One symptom of mania is distractibility, in which attention is easily and frequently drawn to irrelevant external stimuli. Clients appear unable to screen out peripheral stimuli (e.g., noises, other voices, and visual attractions) that are not necessary or relevant to the task at hand. Distractibility interferes with attention, concentration, and memory. Perceptual disturbances can also occur in the form of hallucinations. Manic hallucinations can occur in any sensory mode, but are usually auditory, with themes that pertain to grandiosity, power, and, occasionally, paranoia. These indicate manic psychosis.

HYPOMANIC EPISODE

Manic and hypomanic episodes share symptom criteria and are differentiated primarily by their severity and duration. Hypomanic episodes are not severe enough to cause significant impairment in social and occupational functioning or to require hospitalization. However, it must be evident that the mood and behavioral disturbances of **hypomania** represent a definite change in the person's usual functioning for at least 4 days. During a hypomanic phase, clients may appear extremely happy and congenial, at ease with social conversation, and offering humorous input. Although the moments of elevated mood appear to be desirable, they represent dysfunctional affective states during which the client is not fully in control of moods and accompanying behavior.

CYCLOTHYMIC DISORDER

Cyclothymic disorder is a chronic mood disturbance of at least 2 years' duration (1 year for children and adolescents), with many periods of hypomanic symptoms, depressed mood, and anhedonia. Clients with cyclothymic disorder have not been without the symptoms for more than 2 months over a period of 2 or more years; however, these symptoms are less severe or intense than those in major depressive or manic episodes.

Additional Types of Mood Disorders

The DSM-IV also provides diagnostic criteria for mood disorders due to general medical conditions and to substance use. In these instances, the depressed or elevated mood and accompanying symptoms can be attributed to some general medical condition or to the ingestion of or

---

> **Box 12-3 Medical Conditions and Substances Associated with the Development of a Mood Disorder**
>
> | **Medical conditions** | **Substances** |
> | --- | --- |
> | hypo/hyperthyroidism | digitalis |
> | mononucleosis | thiazide diuretics |
> | diabetes mellitus | reserpine |
> | Cushing's disease | propranolol |
> | pernicious anemia | anabolic steroids |
> | pancreatitis | oral contraceptives |
> | hepatitis | disulfiram |
> | HIV | sulfonamides |
> | multiple sclerosis | alcohol |
> | | marijuana |

withdrawal from medications or other substances. Box 12-3 lists examples of the types of medical conditions and substances commonly associated with the development of mood disorders.

Additional Symptom Features of Mood Disorders

The DSM-IV recognizes that there are features of mood disorders that may indicate various subtypes of unipolar and bipolar disorders. Persons experiencing an episode of major depression, whether it is part of a unipolar or bipolar pattern, may demonstrate melancholic, atypical, or seasonal features. Postpartum onset represents another type of mood disorder.

Features of **melancholic depression** include anhedonia and a lack of reactivity to any pleasurable stimulus; distinct quality of mood, in which the depression is perceived as different from the feeling felt after death of a loved one; depression that is worse in the morning; sleep disturbance of early morning, awakening at least 2 hours before usual time; marked psychomotor retardation or agitation; significant weight loss or loss of appetite; and excessive guilt.

Features of **atypical depression** include mood reactivity; the ability to react to positive stimuli; significant weight gain or increase in appetite; hypersomnia; leaden paralysis or a heavy feeling in the arms and legs; and a long-standing pattern of being sensitive to interpersonal rejection.

A seasonal pattern occurs when there is a regular, temporal relationship between the onset and the remission of an episode of major depression (unipolar or bipolar) at a particular time of the year. This pattern must be evident for 2 consecutive years with no intervening, nonseasonal episodes. Seasonal episodes of altered mood must outnumber any nonseasonal episodes over a lifetime. This pattern is commonly called **seasonal affective disor-**

> ## CLINICAL SYMPTOMS
>
> **Additional mood disorders**
>
> ***Melancholic depression***
>
> EMOTIONAL
> > Anhedonia
> > Increased depression in the morning
>
> COGNITIVE
> > Excessive feelings of guilt
>
> BEHAVIORAL
> > Waking at least 2 hours before normal and being unable to fall back asleep
> > Psychomotor retardation or agitation
> > Significant weight loss
>
> ***Atypical depression***
>
> EMOTIONAL
> > Mood reactivity
> > Ability to react to positive stimuli
>
> COGNITIVE
> > Sensitivity to interpersonal rejection
>
> BEHAVIORAL
> > Significant weight gain or increase in appetite
> > Hypersomnia
> > Leaden paralysis
>
> ***Seasonal affective disorder***
>
> EMOTIONAL
> > Depression between October/November and March/April

der, or SAD. Clients with SAD often develop depression during October or November and find it remitting in March or April. Atypical features may also be associated with SAD. A seasonal pattern can also occur with bipolar disorder, particularly bipolar II disorder, in which increased light triggers manic or hypomanic episodes.

Women may experience a postpartum mood disorder, including depression or mania, following the birth of a child. This usually occurs within 4 weeks of the birth and consists of symptoms of depression or mania described earlier.

A summary of clinical symptoms of these additional types of mood disorders is in the box above.

PROGNOSIS

Recently, more attention has been given to understanding the life course of mood disorders. The bipolar disorders have historically been perceived as recurrent, with cycles of mania and depression interspersed with periods of euthymia. The pattern of cycles varies from person to person, with episodes of depression, mania, and euthymia varying widely in length. The bipolar disorders have a high rate of recurrence and relapse. Factors that contribute to relapse include number of and recovery from previous episodes; family history of bipolar disorder; functional incapacity associated with episodes; past psychotic episodes; and past suicide attempts (Consensus Development Panel, 1985). Many recurrences, however, can be controlled with proper treatment and monitoring (Keller, 1988).

Major depression, historically viewed as a single, acute occurrence, is now understood to be recurrent and chronic for the majority of persons with major depression (Greden, 1993). Research indicates that 50%—85% of clients with unipolar depression experience a subsequent episode and that recurrent episodes tend to be increasingly intense with shorter time periods between episodes (Angst, 1988). There are more episodes of recurrent depression than first-time episodes (Thase, 1992). Twenty percent of persons with depression are not fully recovered from an episode after 1 year (Sargeant et al, 1990). Adverse, long-term effects impair self-care, productivity, social functioning, occupational functioning, and physical health (Tweed, 1993).

These data depict the need for lifetime monitoring and maintenance treatment for depression. The prognosis for major depressive disorder is good; it can be well-controlled with medications, psychotherapy, and self-help strategies. However, clients need to be made aware of the recurrent nature of their disorder and educated about the importance of recognizing symptoms and seeking help early when depression begins. Unfortunately, less than a third of the people who experience depression seek help, putting them at risk for future, more severe depression.

Dysthymia often continues for years before individuals seek assistance for their symptoms. Many people are unaware that the chronic, low-level depression that is depleting their energy can be treated. Unfortunately, over 50% of persons with dysthymia go on to develop major depression (Horwath et al, 1992).

With proper treatment, the prognosis for maintaining individual functioning with a mood disorder is favorable. Inevitably, failure to seek help, lack of adherence to treatment, or resistance of the symptoms to usual treatments means that some persons will become so impaired that their daily functioning will diminish for long periods.

DISCHARGE CRITERIA

Client will:

- Verbalize plans for the future, including absence of suicidal intent or behavior.
- Demonstrate ability to manage self-care needs, or verbalize strategies to acquire assistance.
- Describe mood and any changes from euthymic mood.
- Verbalize realistic perceptions of self and abilities.
- Verbalize realistic expectations for self and others.
- Set realistic, attainable goals.
- Identify psychosocial stressors that may have negative influences.
- State positive methods to cope with threats and stressors.
- Identify signs and symptoms of disorder.
- Contact appropriate sources for validation and/or intervention when necessary.
- Use learned techniques and strategies to prevent or minimize symptoms.
- Verbalize knowledge about medication treatment and necessary self-care strategies.
- Engage family or significant other as sources of support.
- Structure life to include appropriate activities.

THE NURSING PROCESS ■ ■ ■ ■ ■ ■ ■ ■ ■ ■ ■ ■ ■ ■ ■ ■

■ ASSESSMENT

The prevalence and incidence of mood disorders demand that nurses be alert for symptoms of depression and mania. Most persons experiencing a mood disorder, particularly depression, never seek psychiatric care. More often, these individuals present to family practitioners, clinics, or emergency departments reporting symptoms of fatigue or lack of activity, or vague physical complaints. Many do not realize that they are experiencing a mood disorder.

Clients with mood disorders pose a challenge because their primary symptom is one of depression or emotional elation. Their affective dysregulation often evokes emotional responses in nurses who find themselves feeling depressed, anxious, or angry while caring for the individual. The negativity of depression, or the expansive euphoria, hyperactivity, and grandiosity of mania, may also promote fatigue, irritability, and negativity in the nurse. Therefore, when caring for clients with mood disorders, it is important that nurses maintain awareness of their own personal reactions to the client and the ways in which these reactions can affect the nurse-client relationship and subsequent care.

Clients experiencing mood disorders are in emotional pain. They are unable to change their emotional state at will. Yet, many have heard people close to them make comments such as, "Pull yourself up by your bootstraps . . . get a hold of yourself." These clients need validation that this is not their fault, that they are experiencing a psychiatric illness. They should be approached with acceptance and respect.

It is important that nurses appear confident, straightforward, and hopeful. Reassuring comments such as, "I know you'll feel better soon," are usually not helpful because this may be false reassurance. It is appropriate to convey hope with comments such as, "I've known many clients with depression, and they have felt better within several weeks of starting on their medications."

Communication with the person with depression depends on the severity of the depression. Clients with severe depression may be physically and cognitively slowed down and have problems with attention, concentration, and decision-making. Simple, clear communication is most helpful in this situation. The nurse may need to be more directive if the person is having a difficult time making decisions, for example, "It's time for lunch. I'll go with you," rather than "Would you like to go to lunch?" As clients' conditions improve, they can cognitively process more complex information and make decisions more easily.

Communication with clients experiencing mania also can be difficult. Their hyperactivity, expansive or irritable mood, and inability to filter stimuli are barriers to effective communication. Nurses need to be simple, clear, direct and firm. Clients need to know that the nurse cares about them and is concerned about their behavior. Acute episodes of mania are not appropriate times for the nurse to delve into the client's feelings and motives. Interactions should be brief and direct, with minimization of unnecessary stimuli. It is also important not to threaten or challenge a client in the turmoil of a manic episode, because the client might respond with rage.

Information from the client may be minimal or inaccurate due to their cognitive impairment, altered mood, or behavioral disturbances. A significant other can be an important source of information when the client is not reliable. Interviews may need to be short and more directive if the client is having behavioral or cognitive difficulty.

Assessment of the client with depression or mania includes information about his or her presenting problem and mental status, past psychiatric history, social and developmental history, family history, and physical health history. Assessment instruments can assist with the specificity of data collection. These instruments include the Beck Depression Inventory, Carroll Rating Scale for Depression, and the Zung Self-Rating Depression Scale.

CASE STUDY

Jack, a 55-year-old single man, arrived at the public health clinic for his annual flu shot. He appeared tired and sad. He moved slowly and frequently sighed deeply. He reported that he was having difficulty getting out of bed in the morning and felt physically ill. He reported a lack of energy. The nurse noted that Jack's weight had dropped from 165 lbs to 140 lbs over the past 2 months. Jack told the nurse that he was worried that he might be fired from his job of 20 years because the company was downsizing. He reported that he had also stopped golfing with his friends.

Critical Thinking and Assessment

1. Which data indicate that Jack is experiencing a mood disorder?

2. What other types of information about Jack would be important for the nurse to assess at this point?

3. Which type of mood disorder might Jack be experiencing?

4. What are three relevant assessment criteria for Jack?

Nurses can also ask clients to assess their own level of depression or mania by having them rate it on a 10-point scale, for example, "If 0 represents feeling fine and 10 represents the worst depression you have ever experienced, how would you rate your depression now?" This allows for daily comparisons of mood.

Physiological Disturbances

Body physiology is altered during episodes of depression and mania. During moderate or severe depression, body processes frequently slow down. The client with depression may report and exhibit neurovegetative signs of depression, which include psychomotor retardation fatigue, constipation, anorexia (loss of appetite), weight loss, decreased libido (sex drive), and sleep disturbances. These symptoms relate to changes in body processes that cause disruption and slowing of normal physiology. Clients may also describe vague physical symptoms, such as headache, backache, gastrointestinal pain, and nausea. Clients may seek assistance from their family health care provider, thinking that they are experiencing some physical illness that is causing fatigue and loss of energy. Sleep disturbance is a common problem. Clients describe initial insomnia (the inability to fall asleep after going to bed), middle insomnia (waking up in the middle of the night and unable to return to sleep easily), and terminal, or late, insomnia (waking up in the early hours of the morning and unable to return to sleep). Another type of sleep disturbance seen in depression is hypersomnia, in which the client sleeps excessively but never feels rested. Clients with depression may have decreased or increased appetite with corresponding changes in weight. Food is often described as tasteless.

The client experiencing mania also has difficulty sleeping. Not feeling the need for sleep, the client may sleep only a few hours a night or not at all and yet feel rested afterward. Hyperactive behavior and the inability to attend to tasks often preclude the client from eating properly, resulting in dehydration and inadequate nutrition. As the client becomes increasingly stimulated, metabolic activity increases, and vital signs may become elevated. Without proper intervention, clients with mania may be at physical risk for dehydration, hypertension, and cardiac arrest, which can lead to death.

■ ■ NURSING DIAGNOSIS

The nurse uses objective and subjective data obtained during the assessment of clients with mood disorders to arrive at relevant nursing diagnoses. Data from all sources, including the client, significant others, and other professionals, are organized into a pattern of relationships that reflect the client's major areas of health care needs. The following nursing diagnoses are relevant to clients experiencing a mood disorder.

NANDA Diagnoses for Depression

Risk for violence, self-directed or other directed
Self-care deficit (bathing/hygiene, dress/grooming, feeding)
Sleep pattern disturbance
Fatigue
Constipation
Sexual dysfunction
Impaired social interaction
Hopelessness
Powerlessness
Spiritual distress
Knowledge deficit (depression/mania, treatment)

Nursing Assessment Questions

Mood Disorders

How would you describe your mood? (to assess client's insight into feeling state)

Have you noticed a change in your behavior within the past month? (to determine client's awareness of behavioral changes)

Do you feel that people are noticing a change in your behavior, such as irritability or hyperactivity? (to determine client's sensitivity to others' observations of behavioral changes)

What activities have you found enjoyable over the past month? Did you enjoy them as much as you previously did? Can you imagine an event or situation that would give you pleasure? Have you been able to enjoy food and/or sex over the past month? (to determine client's current quality of life)

When did you first begin to feel depressed or elated? Did others comment that your mood seemed more depressed (or higher) than usual? Have you ever felt this way before? When? What was it like? (to establish behavioral patterns)

How has your sleep been? Are you able to fall asleep at night? Stay asleep? Do you find yourself waking up early and being unable to return to sleep? Are you sleeping more than usual in a 24-hour period? How much? (to determine sleep patterns)

How has your appetite been in the past month? How much weight have you lost or gained in the past month? (to determine nutritional/metabolic status)

How has your energy level been? Do you feel tired every day? Do you ever feel as though your limbs are heavy? (to assess fatigability)

How has your concentration been? Are you able to attend to things such as reading the newspaper? Can you concentrate on projects or activities to finish them? What has your decision-making been like? (to evaluate cognitive abilities)

How have you felt about yourself lately? Have you felt guilty more than usual about things you have done? (to determine client's level of self-worth/self-esteem)

Have you felt particularly slowed down, or have others told you that you seemed to move or speak more slowly than usual? (to determine presence of sensorimotor retardation)

Have you felt particularly "speeded up" to the point where you noticed it or someone told you this? (to evaluate presence of mania/hypermania)

Have you had thoughts of death or suicide? How often? What specifically have you thought about doing to harm yourself? (to determine suicidal intent/plans)

What have you been doing lately to manage your feelings? Has it helped? (to assess for effective coping mechanisms/strategies)

How has your mood affected your job? Your family? Your social life? (to assess pervasiveness of client's present mood state)

COLLABORATIVE DIAGNOSES

DSM-IV Diagnoses*	NANDA Diagnoses**
Major Depressive Episode	Risk for violence, self-directed or other directed
Dysthymic Disorder	Self-care deficit (bathing, hygiene, dress/grooming, feeding)
Bipolar I Disorder, Manic or Hypomanic	Altered nutrition Sleep pattern disturbance Constipation Fatigue
Bipolar II Disorder	Impaired verbal communication Altered thought processes Sensory/perceptual alterations
Cyclothymic Disorder	Sexual dysfunction
Mood Disorder Due to General Medical Condition	Impaired social interaction Altered family processes Ineffective individual coping
Substance-Induced Mood Disorder	Defensive coping Self-esteem disturbance Hopelessness Powerlessness Spiritual distress Knowledge deficit Noncompliance

*From American Psychiatric Association: *Diagnostic and Statistical Manual of Mental Disorders*, ed. 4, Washington D.C., 1994.

**From North American Nursing Diagnosis Association: *NANDA Nursing Diagnoses: definitions and classifications* 1995-1996, Philadelphia, 1994.

Nursing Diagnoses for Mania

Altered nutrition, more or less than body requirements
Impaired verbal communication
Altered thought processes
Sensory/perceptual alterations
Altered family processes
Ineffective individual coping
Self-esteem disturbance
Defensive coping
Noncompliance (therapeutic regimen)

■ ■ ■ OUTCOME IDENTIFICATION

Outcome criteria for clients with mood disorders include short- and long-term client behaviors and responses that indicate improved functioning. These criteria are based on nursing diagnoses and are achieved through implementation of planned nursing care. Outcome criteria provide the nurse with direction for evaluating client response to treatment.

Outcome Identification for Mood Disorders

Client will:

1. Remain safe and free from harm.
2. Verbalize suicidal ideations and contract not to harm self or others.
3. Verbalize absence of suicidal or homicidal intent or plans.
4. Express desire to live and not harm others.
5. Make plans for self for the future, verbalizing feelings of hopelessness.
6. Engage in self-care activities in accordance with ability, health status, and developmental stage.
7. Develop a plan to manage or correct causes of inadequate sleep.
8. Establish a pattern of rest/activity that enables fulfillment of role and self-care demands.
9. Make decisions based on examination of options and problem solving.
10. Report absence of hallucinations/delusions.
11. Initiate satisfying social interactions with significant others, peers.
12. Demonstrate participation in milieu, group, and community activities.

CASE STUDY

Mrs. Myers is a 50-year-old mother of two, admitted to the inpatient psychiatric unit and given the diagnosis of Major Depressive Disorder, recurrent. She was brought to the hospital by her 28-year-old son. He had been calling her home for 2 days with no response. Upon arriving at her home, he found his mother lying in bed, crying. The house had not been cleaned for weeks, and Mrs. Myers appeared disheveled and unkempt. He noticed that she had lost a lot of weight since he had seen her a month ago. Her movements and verbalizations were slow. Mrs. Myers told her son that she just wanted to be left alone, that she was "waiting for God to take me."

Critical Thinking and Outcome Identification—Depression

1. What additional information would be helpful for the nurse to know about Mrs. Myers to develop nursing diagnoses and goals?
2. Which nursing diagnoses would be relevant for Mrs. Myers?
3. What long- and short-term outcomes, based on the nursing diagnoses, might be established with Mrs. Myers?

CASE STUDY

Edward, a 40-year-old district manager for an insurance company, was admitted to an inpatient psychiatric unit, diagnosed with Bipolar I Disorder, manic episode. This was his sixth episode of mania since the onset of his disorder 18 years ago. He admitted himself after spending the night in his yard cutting down all of his trees with a chainsaw. He had become increasingly active over the past week, driving all over the state to visit insurance colleagues, ordering new office furniture, and announcing that he would be appointed the next president of this national insurance company. Edward's wife was able to convince him to be hospitalized. Edward has been pacing in the unit, unable to sit during a meal, intruding in other's conversations, and writing memos to his employees.

Critical Thinking and Outcome Identification— Mania

1. What specific information would be assessed by the nurse immediately upon Edward's admission to the unit?

2. Which nursing diagnoses are most relevant for Edward according to the data?

3. What long- and short-term outcomes might be reasonable to establish with Edward?

13. Report increased communication and problem solving among family members regarding issues related to client's disorder.

14. Describe alternative coping strategies, strengths and limitations.

15. Report increased feelings of self-worth and confidence.

16. Engage in activities and behaviors that promote confidence, belonging, and acceptance.

17. Describe information about disorder, including course of illness and personal symptom patterns, resources.

18. Identify medications, including action, dosage, side effects, therapeutic effects, self-care issues.

19. Adhere to prescribed professional and self-care treatment strategies.

■ ■ ■ ■ PLANNING

Recent information about the epidemiology and recurrent course of depression and mania provides the basis for caring for clients with mood disorders in the hospital and in the community. Nursing care addresses the acute episodes of the disorder and the client's risk for recur-

rent episodes. Interventions during the acute depressive or manic episodes can be effective, but too often the client is left with little understanding of the importance of long-term management and self-care strategies. Interventions must be planned for each client based on his or her particular behaviors and concerns. Planning care involves not only the client but may also include the client's significant others and additional health care providers. Using nursing diagnoses derived from assessment data, interventions that facilitate achievement of desired client outcomes are planned.

■ ■ ■ ■ ■ IMPLEMENTATION

The plan of action for clients with mood disorders varies depending on whether the client is depressed or manic. In the short-term, nursing and collaborative interventions are available, which are effective in reducing the acuity of the episode and promoting more optimal functioning. With the current trend of short-term hospitalizations, nurses in the hospital setting probably do not have the opportunity to watch the client recover from the episode. Treatment responses should, however, be evident prior to discharge. Nurses who care for clients in the community are able to see treatment responses over time. (See Nursing Care in the Community on page 273).

Mood disorders, although primarily a disturbance in emotional regulation, affect the whole person—physically, cognitively, socially, and spiritually. Short-term interventions in the hospital or community address priority issues, such as preventing self-harm, promoting physical health (e.g., adequate nutrition, bathing, grooming, sleep), monitoring effects of medications, and assisting with altered thought flow and impaired communication. Other concerns to be addressed include promoting social interaction, self-esteem, knowledge of the disorder and its treatment, treatment compliance, and planning for discharge or discontinuation of services. Because episodes of depression and mania affect the entire family, involving the client's significant others provides an opportunity for them to understand the disorder and to support clients in their recovery. Clinical pathways for mood disorders, which specify collaborative interventions, can be found in Fig. 6-8 in Chapter 6 and in Appendix D.

Nursing interventions for clients with mood disorders span a wide range of biopsychosocial areas, with consideration of the effects of depression and mania on the physiologic, cognitive, psychologic, behavioral, and social spheres. Intervention for clients experiencing depression and mania requires that nurses maintain self-awareness and boundaries regarding their own reactions to clients, because client depression, irritability, anger, negativity, euphoria, and hyperactivity can influence nursing response. It is potentially difficult and exhausting to interact with clients who provoke personal feelings and reactions during emotional encounters. Initiating and maintaining a therapeutic connection with

NURSING CARE PLAN ■ ■ ■ ■ ■ ■ ■ ■ ■ ■ ■ ■ ■ ■ ■

June is a 40-year-old mother of three children. Her husband recently divorced her and married another woman. June also just learned that her mother had been diagnosed with advanced breast cancer. June had two previous episodes of manic behavior in her thirties, including grandiosity, hyperactivity, spending sprees, and decreased need for sleep. During those times, June believed that she had special abilities for financial matters and would someday manage a major corporation. She also had three previous episodes of depression, the first when she was 22. During the episodes of depression, June was unable to work at her job as an accountant, slept 14 to 16 hours a day, lost weight, and considered suicide. For the past 3 weeks, June has become increasingly depressed, sleeping 14 to 16 hours a day, losing 16 pounds from her usual weight of 115 pounds, not caring for her personal appearance and looking disheveled, moving and talking more slowly than usual, and missing work. She was taken to the hospital by her ex-husband after she told him she wanted to die. The children went to live with their father upon June's hospital admission. She admits that she has not been taking her medications of Lithium and Prozac. She is being treated with Azmacort inhaler for her asthma. In the hospital, she was placed on lithium 300 mg qid and Pamelor (nortriptylene) 25 mg qid.

DSM-IV Diagnoses

AXIS I:	Bipolar I Disorder, Current Episode Depressed
AXIS II:	Deferred
AXIS III:	Asthma
AXIS IV:	Severity of Psychosocial Stressors, Severe=4
	Divorce, Mother's serious illness
AXIS V:	GAF=70 (highest in past year)
	GAF=40 (current)

Nursing Diagnosis: Risk for violence, self-directed. Risk factors: depressed mood, hopelessness, and suicidal ideation.

Client Outcomes	Nursing Interventions	Evaluation
• June will remain safe from self-harm.	• Assess suicidal thinking, including frequency, plan, opportunity, past attempts *to determine suicidal risk and intent.* • Provide close observation as indicated *to ensure June's safety.* • Monitor safety of environment for potentially harmful items, such as sharp objects, hoarded medications, and belts *to provide a safe, nonthreatening environment.* • Observe for behaviors and statements that may be indicators of self-harm intent, such as hopeless statements, giving away possessions, sudden calmness or change in behavior *because such behaviors may be signals of suicidal thoughts and intent.*	• June remained safe from self-harm.
• June will verbalize any suicidal ideations and contract not to harm self.	• Contract with June to tell someone if her suicidal thinking increases or if she feels as though she might act on a plan. *Contracting establishes an expectation of behavior between nurse and client.*	• June discussed her suicidal thoughts with staff when they occurred and contracted not to harm herself. • June reported the absence of suicidal intent upon discharge.
• June will be able to discuss feelings about her situation. June will be able to describe reasons to live.	• Encourage June to express her feelings rather than suppress them *to relieve pent-up feelings and allow them to be validated.* • Encourage June to focus on people and things that are important to her, such as her children *to reinforce client's strengths and positive resources.*	• June willingly discussed her feelings with staff. • June described reasons important to her for living.

NURSING CARE PLAN

Client Outcomes	Nursing Interventions	Evaluation
• June will describe resources and options available to her if she begins to feel suicidal in the community.	• Encourage June to problem-solve about alternatives to self-harm, such as talking with friends *to promote activation of alternative coping mechanisms that increase client's self-control.* • Provide June with information about community resources available if she begins to feel suicidal, including community mental health, or a crisis line, *to provide resources available for assistance.*	• June identified resources, including people and activities that are available to her if she begins to feel suicidal in the community.

Nursing Diagnosis: Impaired social interaction, related to low self-esteem, psychomotor retardation, hypersomnia, fatigue, depressed mood, actual and perceived loss, as evidenced by self-imposed seclusion, failure to initiate interaction, divorce, and concern regarding mother's potential death.

Client Outcomes	Nursing Interventions	Evaluation
• June will participate in unit activities while in the hospital	• Encourage June to attend group and unit activities *to promote social interaction; clients will gain support from others.* • Arrange to spend time with June at regular, prearranged time for interaction. *Nurse provides supportive presence and encourages interaction.*	• June participated in most unit activities in the hospital.
• June will initiate social interaction with family, friends, and peers.	• Help June identify opportunities for social interaction with family, friends, and peers both in the hospital and after discharge *to strengthen client's social support network.* • Provide positive reinforcement to June for engaging in social interactions *to reinforce rewarding, supportive interactions.*	• June initiated contact with family and friends while in the hospital. • June described a plan for continued social interaction with family and friends after discharge.

Nursing Diagnosis: Noncompliance, related to belief that medication was not helpful, as evidenced by self-reported failure to take medications.

Client Outcomes	Nursing Interventions	Evaluation
• June will adhere to her treatment regimen, including taking her medications as prescribed.	• Teach June about her medications, including their value and success in treating depression and mania, their actions, their therapeutic and side effects, and usual dosage. *Knowledge allows the client to make informed choices about medications and promotes adherence to prescribed medications.* • Review the potential side effects of the medications and develop with June strategies to address those *to allow client sense of control with medications and ability to initiate self-care strategies that minimize side effects.* • Discourage June from stopping her medication without input from her mental health provider. *Client can experience withdrawal symptoms and relapse of depression.* • Provide opportunities for June to discuss her feelings about her disorder and the need to be on medication. *Expression of values and feelings provides validation for client's experience.*	• June was able to discuss the rationale for her medication therapy and the action, side effects, and damage of the medications. • June was able to describe self-care strategies useful to address the side effects of her medications. • June's lithium and nortriptyline levels were within normal therapeutic ranges.

clients is accomplished through consistency, caring, concern, empathy, and genuineness on the part of the nurse. Clients with mood disorders often have a difficult time developing a therapeutic alliance and avoid interpersonal connection with others. A knowledgeable, consistent, and matter-of-fact (but genuine and caring) presentation is reassuring to clients and promotes their confidence in the nurse.

Nursing Interventions

1. Conduct a suicide assessment as necessary *to ensure the client's safety and prevent harm to self or others.*

2. Maintain a safe, harm-free environment through close and frequent observations *to minimize the risk of violence.*

3. Establish a trusting relationship with the client *to facilitate the client's willingness to communicate thoughts and feelings.*

4. Assist the client to verbalize feelings *to promote a healthy, expressive form of communication.*

5. Identify the client's social support system and encourage the client to use it *to minimize isolation and loneliness as possible precursors to hopelessness.*

6. Praise the client for attempts at alternate activities and interactions with others *to encourage socialization.*

7. Monitor the client's fluid intake and output, food intake, and weight *to ensure adequate nutrition and hydration and adequate weight for body size and metabolic need.*

Nursing Care in the Community

Mood Disorders

Working with persons experiencing mood disorders can be challenging for the community mental health nurse. The nurse must deal with a wide range of behaviors and may find his or her recommendations minimized by the client, if not negated entirely. A person manifesting a manic episode may be grandiose, express pleasure in his increased activity level, and become irritable when confronted about problematic behavior. In contrast, the person with depression also often rejects help, because, in their view, nothing seems to matter or is effective. In either case the client may see the process of assessment as intrusive, and efforts to engage him or her in treatment may be rejected. The nurse must work carefully through the assessment process to determine if hospitalization is indicated.

Context and timing are significant when assessing a person with depression in the community. The nurse should consider the following questions:

- Have situational stressors caused the sadness?
- Has a grief process evolved into a depressed state?
- Have vegetative signs developed? Is the person sleeping and eating?
- Are nonverbal signs, such as posture and affect, consistent with expressed emotion?
- Is there a history of suicidal behavior, current suicidality, or a plan for suicide?
- Has the person ever been successfully treated for depression?
- Is the person willing to accept treatment now?

The nurse must maintain an objective, unbiased attitude, neither trying to superficially cheer the client, nor offering situational advice. The nurse may suggest treatment options and assess the client's response. Screening tests for depression may be used to facilitate diagnosis. Some facilities offer free community screening for depression.

Assessing a person experiencing a manic episode is often dramatic and can be frustrating for the nurse. The manic individual reiterates that he is fine, does not need help from anyone, and resents the nurse's "interrogation." If possible, it is best to enlist members of the client's support system, as well as the client, in order to identify an apparent manic episode. Members of the client's support system can comment on behavioral changes in the client, such as changes in spending patterns, sexual activity, or sleep patterns. It is easier to influence the client to seek help early in the episode, rather than wait until sleep deprivation and increased tension have made the client so irritable or fatigued that he becomes psychotic and needs involuntary hospitalization.

Monitoring the intake of medications and their effects is another critical element for the nurse caring for clients with mood disorders in the community. Antidepressants sometimes cause clients to feel more physically energized, but still depressed enough to be at high risk for suicide. The added strength can make the suicidal act easier. Antimanic medications, especially lithium and tegretol (an anticonvulsant used to treat manic behavior), can be life-threatening if excesses build up in the client's system. These medications may also produce symptoms that are difficult to perceive without the use of blood tests. Such symptoms may even resemble an increasing disease process, and more medication may be administered if evaluation is not timely and insightful. The nurse must encourage the client to discriminate between feeling states and pathologic or physiologic symptoms, so that he can seek assistance before he is out of control.

8. Promote self-care activities, such as bathing, dressing, feeding, and grooming *to ascertain the client's level of functioning and increase self-esteem.*

9. Assist the client to establish daily goals and expectations *to minimize confusion/anxiety.*

10. Plan self-care activities around those times when the client may have more energy *to increase activity tolerance and minimize fatigue.*

11. Reduce choices of clothing and tasks *to make decision-making easier.*

12. Assess the client's cognitive/perceptual process *to ascertain the existence of hallucinations/delusions that may be troubling or harmful for the client.*

13. Assist the client in identifying negative, self-defeating thoughts and modifying them with realistic thoughts *to promote more accurate, positive thoughts about self.* (See the cognitive therapy discussion in Chapter 5).

14. Encourage the client in therapeutic groups that provide feedback regarding thinking *to reframe thinking with the support of others.* (See Chapter 5).

15. Provide simple, clear directives/communication in a low-stimulus environment *to assist the focus and attend with minimal distractions.*

16. Teach the client and significant others about the disorder and treatment *to minimize guilt and remorse in clients and families about the disorder.*

17. Gradually increase levels of activity and exercise *to minimize fatigue and increase activity tolerance.*

18. Identify sources of external stress and assist the client to cope with them in a more effective manner *to minimize stressors and promote adaptive coping mechanisms.*

19. Educate the client with depression about the disorder and symptoms as appropriate *to lessen feelings of inadequacy, minimize guilt, and increase the knowledge base about the effects of the illness.*

20. Educate the client with mania about the disorder and symptoms as appropriate *to lessen feelings of inadequacy, minimize guilt, and increase the knowledge base about the effects of the illness.*

Additional Treatment Modalities

Psychopharmacology

Over the past 30 years, there have been major advances in the use of medications to treat symptoms of mood disorders. Investigation of the neurobiology of depression and mania has provided directions for development of these new medications. These are discussed in Chapter 23. Because there are multiple types of medications that seem to work with various individuals and their types of depression and mania, selecting the drug and the dosage that is effective for any individual is often a difficult process. Clients who do not respond to one type of medication may do well on another.

CLINICAL ALERT !

The nurse must be alert to suicidal ideation and intent with clients with depression, and clients with mania who are cycling into depression or whose insight and judgment are impaired. A particularly high-risk time is 1 to 6 weeks after the initiation of antidepressant therapy, prior to its full therapeutic effect.

CLINICAL ALERT !

Foods containing tyramine must be avoided while taking MAOI antidepressants. These include avocados, yogurt, aged cheese, smoked or pickled fish, meat, poultry, processed meats, yeast, overripe fruit, chicken or beef liver pate, red wine, beer, liqueurs, and fava beans. Foods to use in moderation include caffeine beverages, cottage and cream cheese, soy sauce, chocolate, and sour cream. **Medications** to avoid include over-the-counter cough and cold medicines, appetite suppressants, muscle relaxants, allergy remedies, hay fever remedies, narcotics, and analgesics. The nurse should ask the client to contact the physician or nurse *before* taking any over-the-counter medication.

Various types of antidepressant medications are used to treat persons with episodes of major depression, and some persons with dysthymia. These include tricyclics, heterocyclics, monoamine oxidase inhibitors (MAOIs), selective serotonin reuptake inhibitors (SSRIs), and, most recently, serotonin and norepinephrine reuptake inhibitors. These medications exert powerful effects not only on mood, but also on the entire syndrome of depression symptoms, including the neurovegetative symptoms. Not surprisingly, medications also create side effects that can create discomfort and even danger. Taken in large quantities, many are toxic, even lethal. In addition, these medications usually have a lag period of 1 to 6 weeks for initiation of therapeutic effects, during which time the side effects are often the most pronounced. As the medication begins to exert its therapeutic effect, the side effects often diminish. In view of recent data regarding the recurrent nature of depression and how it impairs functioning over time, many clients are now taking these medications for years, or for an entire lifetime.

Mood stabilizers have been demonstrated to be effective in treating mania in clients with bipolar disorders. The primary, most widely used mood stabilizer is lithium, although anticonvulsants (e.g., carbamazepine, valproate) also appear to promote mood stabilization. Lithium acts as a salt within the body, and its blood levels are closely linked to the client's hydration and sodium intake. The side effects of lithium include neuromuscular and central nervous system effects (tremor, forgetfulness, slowed cognition), gastrointestinal effects (nausea, diarrhea), weight gain and hypothyroidism, and renal effects (polyuria). Blood levels are monitored to ensure an adequate, but not toxic, level. Usually blood levels of 0.5 to 1.0 mEq/L are appropriate for maintenance therapy, whereas in the treatment of acute mania, levels of up to 1.5 mEq/L are required. The therapeutic-range blood level for lithium is narrow; toxicity can occur quickly and is marked by vomiting, oversedation, ataxia, and, finally, seizures. Lithium blood levels approaching 2.0 are considered toxic. Lithium is excreted through the kidneys and should be used with caution for clients with renal disease. Clients on lithium should use diuretics only with extreme caution and under close supervision, because diuretics can elevate lithium blood levels quickly.

Other medications prescribed for clients during episodes of depression or mania may include benzodiazepines for associated anxiety symptoms, sedative-hypnotics for sleep regulation, and antipsychotics for relief from hallucinations, delusions, and extremely agitated behavior. While antidepressants and mood stabilizers can assist with minimizing and regulating symptoms related to anxiety and sleep, their therapeutic effects take longer to occur than those of the medications mentioned above.

Although medications are prescribed by physicians or advanced practice nurses, the nursing care related to administration of psychopharmacologic agents is extensive. The nurse needs to understand the mechanisms of action, dosages (therapeutic), side effects, and self-care considerations of each medication. This enables the nurse to explain the medication to clients and to observe for intended and unintended effects of the drugs. Through teaching clients more about their medications, the nurse promotes and encourages adherence to the treatment regimen, and the minimization of negative effects. Clients are able to discuss their concerns and to make informed decisions about their treatments.

Many of these medications require special considerations that clients must understand to ensure efficacy and safety. Nurses teach clients specific self-care activities associated with medication, such as the required dietary restrictions for MAOIs, precautions regarding hydration and salt intake for lithium, and management of anticholinergic effects of the tricyclics. The Client and Family Teaching Guidelines on this page and page 276 present teaching plans for clients on lithium and selective serotonin reuptake inhibitors.

Biological Interventions

Electroconvulsive Therapy   Electroconvulsive therapy (ECT) involves the use of electrically induced seizures to treat severe depression or, less frequently, intense mania not controlled with lithium or antipsychotics. Research has demonstrated it to be the most effective treatment for psychotic depression (Depression

---

Client and Family
TEACHING GUIDELINES

Selective Serotonin Uptake Inhibitors

Teach the client:

- The purpose of SSRIs is to treat depression. The medication alters brain nerve cells, thus increasing the availability of serotonin. A deficiency of serotonin in the brain is believed to be related to the onset of depression.

- It is important to take the medication as prescribed; changing the dosage or missing a dose can prevent it from helping the depression.

- Common side effects of SSRIs include nausea, increased anxiety, and insomnia. These side effects often diminish once the medication begins to exert its therapeutic effect.

- The medication usually does not immediately improve symptoms of depression. It may take 1-6 weeks before you feel the effects of the medication. At first, you may still feel depressed, but have more energy and look less depressed. These medications often work "from the outside inward."

Guideline Panel, 1993). Although ECT was introduced in the 1930s, its use decreased after the discovery of antidepressants and lithium. In recent years, procedures have been developed for ECT that make it a safe and effective treatment for many individuals who have not achieved a treatment response with medication or other types of treatment. The exact mechanism by which ECT alleviates depression and mania is unknown, but it is believed to be related to alteration of neurotransmission. A complete discussion of ECT is presented in Chapter 23.

Phototherapy   Seasonal affective disorder (SAD) has been identified as a type of mood disorder, and its features are recognized in the DSM-IV. Phototherapy is one type of treatment that has effectively lessened symptoms of this recurrent, seasonal disorder. The exact mechanism of action remains unclear, although it is believed that exposure to morning light causes a circadian rhythm shift (phase advance) that regulates the normal relationships between sleep and circadian rhythms.

Clients are referred for phototherapy after a careful and complete psychiatric history that documents the occurrence of SAD. Phototherapy consisting of a minimum of 2500 lux is usually administered upon waking in the morning. Clients sit or lie in front of the light box for 30 minutes to several hours, depending on the strength of the light source. An antidepressant effect is usually seen within 2 to 4 days and is complete after 2 weeks. Maintenance therapy consists of sitting in front of the lights for

Client and Family
TEACHING GUIDELINES

Lithium

Teach the client:

- Lithium is a mood stabilizer for persons with mania and depression.

- Lithium alters brain neurotransmission, changes cell-membrane function, and inhibits release of thyroid hormone. It is not clear how lithium specifically stabilizes mood.

- Before starting lithium, lab tests are done to ensure adequate functioning of the heart, kidneys, thyroid gland, and electrolytes.

- It is important to take lithium daily as prescribed in order to maintain a steady blood level of the medication. Do not take extra to make up for missed doses.

- Lithium may take a week to begin working and to develop a steady blood level. Your health care provider will have you get your blood drawn, to check lithium blood levels. Blood for the lithium level must be drawn about 12 hours after the last dose of lithium, e.g., if you take your dose at 8 PM, your blood level must be drawn at 8 AM.

- Common side effects of lithium include increased urine output, increased thirst, fine tremors, muscle weakness, nausea, weight gain, and diarrhea.

- Lithium levels can be increased rapidly, leading to toxicity. Signs of toxicity included nausea and vomiting, marked tremors, muscle weakness, muscle twitching, lack of coordination, sluggishness and drowsiness, confusion, seizures, and coma. Toxicity can occur as blood levels approach 2.0.

- It is important to maintain a stable blood level of lithium. You should not change the amount of sodium (salt) in your diet, because decreasing salt may increase the amount of lithium in the blood.

- Any activity or situation that can affect your fluid and salt intake or output can change the level of lithium in your blood. Exercise, sunbathing, and the flu are examples of situations in which you may perspire and lose salt and fluid, increasing your lithium level. It is important to contact your health care provider if you believe that your lithium level may be changed or if you experience any side effects or early toxic signs.

- Other drugs can affect your lithium level. Medications (e.g., diuretics, ibuprofen, verapamil) can raise lithium levels. Be sure to check with your health care provider before taking any new prescribed or over-the-counter medications.

- Lithium can cause birth defects if taken during the first trimester of pregnancy. Tell your health care provider if you intend to become pregnant or are pregnant.

about 30 minutes each day. Side effects are rare, although some clients do report irritability, headaches, or insomnia. Phototherapy is not effective for everyone with a diagnosis of SAD; some fail to respond, and others experience only a partial response. Because phototherapy requires a large amount of time each day, research is in progress that examines alternative methods to acquire the additional light, including the use of light visors and lights that shine onto the bed in early morning prior to awakening.

Family Intervention

Mood disorders affect the entire family, not just the client who is experiencing the depression or mania. Most often, the family or significant others become known to the nurse during the client's acute episode of depression or mania. Conflicts and communication problems, which may have existed in the family network prior to the onset of the episode, become intensified, and usual role functioning is disrupted.

Nurses in both the hospital and the community interact with the client's family, who often appreciate the opportunity to vent feelings of confusion, anger, concern or frustration. Teaching family members about the client's disorder, including the biologic components, allows them to reframe the situation and minimize blame on the client. Many are relieved to hear that their loved one's behavior has an explanation and can be managed. They also find it helpful to know that the client's behavior (e.g., irritability, inability to accept love, and negativity) is not necessarily a personal affront to other family members but may be part of the symptomology of depression or mania. Nurses run family education groups in the hospital and in the community, inviting family and clients to learn more about the disorder and its impact on the family.

Nurses also collaborate with other mental health professionals, including advanced practice nurses, regarding assessing the need for family therapy. Nurses observe client-family interactions, listen to their concerns, and identify potential problem areas. Referrals are made for marital therapy or family therapy that also includes the children.

Interventions that include preparing the family for the client's discharge can facilitate the client's return to functioning in the community. Recent data suggest that even after abatement of symptoms, the client who has experienced affective episodes continues to have difficulty in his or her interpersonal and occupational functioning (Klerman and Weissman, 1992).

Group Intervention

Group intervention can provide multiple benefits to clients with mood disorders, including socialization, education about their disorder and more useful coping mechanisms, venting feelings, establishing personal goals, and realizing that others have similar problems, thus reducing isolation and hopelessness. (See Understanding and Applying Research at right.) Nurses assess clients' ability to participate in groups based on their behavior, mental status, psychologic readiness in view of the nature of the particular group, and physiologic status. For example, clients with mania who are hyperactive and extremely agitated are not able to attend to the group discussion and may become overstimulated and disruptive in the group. Clients with severe depression with psychomotor retardation and cognitive impairment may have a difficult time and become overwhelmed by a formal group. Certain types of groups (e.g., a unit community meeting or activities groups) may be less structured and less imposing to clients than formal group therapy.

In addition to assessing client's readiness for groups, nurses encourage their attendance at the appropriate functions. Some clients may need to be directed with statements such as, "It's time for group now. I'll walk there with you." Others require only encouragement or reminders.

Nurses who are qualified may conduct groups in conjunction with other nurses or therapists. Nurses may initiate and lead groups, such as social skills training and educational groups. Clients often need to debrief or discuss their experiences and reactions after the completion of a group. Nurses listen, allow ventilation of feelings, and reinforce new insights or perceptions experienced by the clients.

Psychotherapeutic Intervention

While the effectiveness of antidepressant and mood stabilizing medications is undisputed, psychotherapeutic interventions are also important in the treatment of mood disorders. Psychopharmacologic agents pose a number of problems for many clients. These medications have major side effects that create discomfort, interfere with usual functioning, and promote noncompliance. Twenty to thirty percent of persons with mood disorders do not respond to medications and require alternative treatment. And although mood disorders represent alterations in neurobiologic functioning, numerous psychologic, social, and interpersonal issues that warrant psychotherapeutic intervention are associated with episodes of depression and mania.

Types of psychotherapy that have been used to treat mood disorders and associated psychosocial issues include cognitive therapy, behavioral therapy, interpersonal relationship therapy, and psychodynamic therapy. While each of these differs with respect to underlying theoretical framework, goals, and approach, there are some commonalities. Therapeutic success is related to several factors: the nature of the relationship between therapist and client; provision of understanding, support, help, and hope; establishing a framework for understanding and interpreting clients' problems; and providing the opportunity to explore and try out new coping strategies.

Cognitive Therapy Cognitive therapy, as outlined by Beck (1976), addresses systematic errors in the client's thinking that maintain negative cognitive processing. The goal of the therapy is to identify underlying cognitive schemata and specific cognitive distortions. Schemata are internal models of the self and the world that individuals use to perceive, code, and recall information. Clients are asked to identify their automatic thoughts, silent assumptions, and arbitrary inferences so that negative thoughts and assumptions can be examined logically, challenged against realistic attributes and subsequently validated or refuted.

Cognitive therapy has been demonstrated to be effective in treating outpatients with unipolar, mild to moderate depression. In studies that have investigated the effectiveness of medication vs. cognitive therapy, findings indicate that both appear to be equally effective with outpatients with depression and may provide some modest gain when used in combination. In addition, use of cognitive therapy also may increase the rate of symptom improvement in depression, although longer-term follow-up studies fail to find differences over time. The use of cognitive therapy with inpatients experiencing severe depression has not been extensively explored, although there are indications that it may be useful for symptom reduction (Stravynski and Greenberg, 1992).

Behavioral Therapy Behavioral therapy, often used in conjunction with cognitive therapy for treating mild to moderately depressed outpatients, is an effective treatment for depression, comparing favorably to medication and cognitive therapy (Stravynski and Greenberg, 1992). There is less information about its usefulness with persons experiencing mania (Freeman et al, 1990).

Understanding and Applying
RESEARCH

Maynard CK: Comparison of effectiveness of group interventions for depression in women, *Arch Psych Nsg* 7:277-283, 1993.

Using an experimental three-group pretest and posttest design, Maynard evaluated the effectiveness of a structured cognitive-behavioral group intervention, designed by Gordon, to reduce depression in women. Women reporting depression were assigned randomly to one of three groups: a cognitive-behavioral group (experimental group), a supportive, feeling-oriented group, and a control group, which did not receive treatment. Subjects were administered the Beck Depression Inventory (BDI), the Beck Hopelessness Scale (BHS), and the Speilberger State-Trait Anxiety Inventory (STAI) prior to intervention and after 12 group sessions. Results indicated that women in the structured, cognitive-behavioral group reported significantly less depression, hopelessness, and anxiety, and more self-esteem than those in either the support or untreated control group. Nurses can consider cognitive-behavior therapy for depressed clients as appropriate.

The behavioral approach is based on learning theory. Abnormal behaviors, such as the symptoms of depression and mania, represent behaviors acquired as the result of aversive (negative) environmental events. These are reinforced by positive environmental responses to the maladaptive behaviors or by avoidance of negative consequences. The behavioral therapist works with clients to determine specific behaviors to be modified and to identify the factors that evoke and reinforce these behaviors. Using role modeling, role playing, and situational analysis, clients are assisted to learn and practice different adaptive behaviors that elicit positive environmental reinforcement. The therapy is not concerned with understanding underlying issues or pathopsychology, only those discrete behaviors that can be modified. Behavioral therapy has several advantages (e.g., shorter treatment duration than other types of therapy, focus on specific behaviors that can be modified) and is applicable to various types of clients.

Interpersonal Therapy   The therapist utilizing interpersonal therapy views depression as developing from pathologic, early interpersonal relationship patterns that continue to be repeated in adulthood. The emphasis is on social functioning and interpersonal relationships, with emphasis on the milieu. Life events, including change, loss, and relationship conflict, trigger earlier relationship patterns, and the client experiences a sense of failure, decreased importance, and loss. The goal of the therapy is to understand the social context of current problems based on earlier relationships and to provide symptomatic relief by solving or managing current interpersonal problems. The client and the therapist select one or two current interpersonal problems and examine new communication and interpersonal strategies for more effective management of relationships.

Interpersonal therapy has been demonstrated to be effective for clients with mild to moderate depression, although not more so than other types of psychotherapy. Some research suggests that, when used in combination with medications, interpersonal therapy may help clients adhere to medication treatment and may lengthen the time between the recovery period and recurrence of a major depression episode (Klerman, 1990).

Psychodynamic Therapy   This type of therapy is derived from Freud's psychoanalytic model. Depression is viewed as the result of early childhood loss of a love object, ambivalence about the object, introjection of anger onto the ego resulting in blockage of libido, and unresolved intrapsychic conflict during the oral or anal stage of psychosexual development. Thus self-esteem is damaged and eroded, with repetition of the primary loss pattern occurring throughout life. Through the relationship with the therapist, the client is helped to uncover repressed experiences, experience catharsis of feelings, confront defenses, interpret current behavior, and work through early loss and cravings for love.

ADDITIONAL TREATMENT MODALITIES

Psychopharmacologic

- Antidepressants
- Mood stabilizers
- Anxiolytics
- Sedatives
- Antipsychotics

Electroconvulsive Therapy
Family Intervention
Group Intervention

- Formal groups
- Activity groups
- Community groups

Somatic/Biologic Intervention

- Phototherapy

Psychotherapeutic Intervention

- Cognitive
- Behavioral
- Interpersonal
- Psychodynamic

There has been little research on the effect of psychodynamic psychotherapy on depression or mania. Techniques used in this therapy have been modified over time, and there have been problems with standardizing the approach for research purposes. For some clients, psychodynamic psychotherapy assists in developing insights that promote behavioral change. However, many clients, including those with severe depression, may be unable or unmotivated to participate in this type of therapy. For these clients, problems such as self-care deficits, psychomotor retardation, and fatigue assume priority. Refer to Chapter 5 for additional discussion of psychodynamic therapy. A summary of all additional treatment modalities for mood disorders is above.

■ ■ ■ ■ ■ ■ EVALUATION

Nurses evaluate clients' progress by measuring their achievement of identified outcomes. Data that support or refute achievement of outcomes are collected from personal observations, clients, clients' family and friends, and other health care providers. Evaluation occurs throughout hospitalization, and may be continued by community mental health providers after clients have been discharged. Nurses working in community settings, such as psychiatric home care, may be evaluating outcomes for clients who have never been admitted to an inpatient setting.

NURSING CARE PLAN

Yvonne is a 50-year-old woman diagnosed with bipolar disorder since she was 26. She is an English professor at the local university and is on summer break. Three weeks ago, Yvonne began to stay up all night writing a novel. Her speech had become more rapid and pressured, and she described her thoughts as racing. Her home study was becoming increasingly cluttered, and no one was able to walk into it because of the piles of books, articles, and papers in the floor. She would write for several minutes, pace around the house, then write for several more minutes. She began calling *The New York Times,* telling them that they would want to read the book she was finishing, because it was the best novel ever written. Yvonne began telling people that she was Louisa May Alcott reincarnated. She spent more than $5,000 on new books to build her library. She had not slept more than 2 hours a night for several weeks and had not eaten for 2 days. Yvonne's husband, Rob, brought her to the psychiatric emergency room for admission. She was angry with him, insisting that he interfered with her work. On admission to the unit, she exhibited pacing, flight of ideas, pressured speech, and angry, rude, and intrusive behavior. She was dressed in a short red skirt, pink low-cut blouse, and a yellow straw hat, and had bare feet. Yvonne wore heavy, bright make-up and changed her clothes up to 15 times each day. She was given lithium (300 mg qid) and haloperidol (Haldol) (5 mg bid). She had been on a regimen of lithium, but stopped taking the medication 4 months ago after becoming concerned about its long-term effects.

DSM-IV Diagnoses:

AXIS I: Bioplar I Disorder, Current Episode, Manic

AXIS II: Deferred

AXIS III: R/O Dehydration

AXIS IV: Severity of Psychosocial Stressors
Deferred

AXIS V: GAF = 78 (highest in past year)
GAF = 25 (current)

Nursing Diagnosis: Self-care deficit (grooming, dressing, feeding), related to manic hyperactivity, difficulty concentrating and making decisions, as evidenced by inappropriate dress, and dysfunctional eating patterns.

Client Outcomes	Nursing Interventions	Evaluation
• Yvonne will dress self appropriately for age and status.	• Offer assistance for selecting clothing and for grooming *to provide input and direction for appropriateness of dress and hygiene to preserve self-esteem and avoid embarrassment.*	• Yvonne dresses self appropriately and maintains hygiene.
• Yvonne will eat and drink adequately to sustain fluid balance and proper nutrition.	• Encourage and remind Yvonne to drink fluids and eat nutritious food *to focus the client on necessary feeding activities to prevent dehydration and starvation.*	• Yvonne eats and drinks fluids necessary to maintain physical health.
	• Offer Yvonne beverages in easy-to-carry containers, and nutritious, high-protein, high-calorie finger foods *to provide important nutrients and fluids in a way that the client is able to eat and drink, because she is unable to sit and complete a meal.*	
	• Reduce environmental stimulation, such as noise or presence of other people, during self-care times, e.g., have client eat meals alone in room rather than in dining room. *Decreased stimulation allows for better concentration on tasks.*	
	• Provide recognition and positive reinforcement for feeding and dress/grooming accomplishments *to reinforce appropriate behaviors and enhance self-esteem.*	

With decreasing lengths-of-stay in hospitals, nurses in inpatient psychiatric units may not see dramatic changes in client's symptoms. However, they must see some clear progress related to priority short-term outcomes, such as absence of suicidal intent, plan for addressing potential return of suicidal ideation after discharge, ability to conduct self-care activities, alleviation of neurovegetative symptoms of depression (sleep, loss of appetite, fatigue, psychomotor retardation), alleviation of severe hyperactive behavior of mania, absence of hallucinations and

NURSING CARE PLAN

Nursing Diagnosis: Defensive coping, related to impaired self-concept, unrealistic perceptions of self, secondary to manic episode, as evidenced by intrusive and disruptive behavior, grandiosity, anger, impulsivity, and excessive use of make-up and clothing.

Client Outcomes	*Nursing Interventions*	*Evaluation*
• Yvonne will refrain from interrupting and disrupting activities and conversations of others.	• Continue to state the rules and expectations of the unit in a calm, matter-of-fact way. *Nonthreatening manner is better tolerated by a client with mania, and repetition of rules and expectations may be needed due to impaired concentration and impulsivity.*	• Yvonne stated unit rules and expectations.
• Yvonne will adhere to established limits and expectations.	• Praise client for statements about realistic self-appraisal and adherence to expectations *to provide support, positive reinforcement, and learning.* • Establish any necessary limits in calm, matter-of-fact, nonpunitive way *to prevent alienation from client and assist in regaining control.* • Provide opportunities for client to interact with others in ways that are manageable, such as short activities *to help client to focus, prevent overstimulation, and provide opportunity for support and reality-testing.*	• Yvonne stopped intrusive, disruptive behaviors and adhered to expectations and unit rules.
• Yvonne will realistically discuss her thoughts, feelings and behaviors.	• As client improves, encourage expression of feelings, beliefs, and actions *to assist client to gain insight and appropriately express feelings.*	• Yvonne was able to discuss her self-perceptions in a nongrandiose manner, and related feelings she was experiencing.

Nursing Diagnosis: Altered thought processes, related to psychomotor hyperactivity, ineffective processing of internal and external stimuli, anxiety, psychosocial stresses, secondary to biologic disruption of neurotransmission, as evidenced by flight of ideas, grandiosity, impaired judgment and decision-making.

Client Outcomes	*Nursing Interventions*	*Evaluation*
• Yvonne will demonstrate logical and coherent flow of thoughts, with the absence of delusion of grandeur.	• Demonstrate concern and acceptance of client's underlying feelings while not overtly agreeing with delusion of grandeur *to promote trust and self-esteem, but not reinforce the delusion.*	• Yvonne was able to express herself logically and clearly, acknowledging that she was not a famous author (e.g., Louisa May Alcott).
• Yvonne will demonstrate appropriate decision-making and judgment.	• Listen for themes, feelings, meanings behind the client's words and reflect on those *to build trust, demonstrate understanding, and reinforce reality and expression of feelings.* • Redirect client to here-and-now activities and topics *to provide reality-oriented focus.* • Praise client for expressing doubt about delusion and attempting to focus thoughts in more logical, relevant manner *to promote self-esteem and reality-based thinking.* • Relate to client with simple, concrete, here-and-now words and interactions, avoiding abstractions. *Simple, direct, clear communication can be better understood.* • Teach client about lithium, including action, therapeutic effects, side effects, dosage, and importance in controlling mood *because information promotes compliance.*	• Yvonne expressed desire to remain in the hospital until her mania was better controlled, and stated that she understood why her husband brought her to the hospital.

NURSING CARE PLAN ■ ■ ■ ■ ■ ■ ■   ■ ■ ■ ■ ■ ■

Nursing Diagnosis: Noncompliance with medication regimen, related to knowledge deficit, belief system, as evidenced by failure to continue lithium as prescribed.

Client Outcomes	*Nursing Interventions*	*Evaluation*
• Yvonne will adhere to medication regimen, taking medications as prescribed.	• Teach client about bipolar disorder and the need for lifelong management *because information promotes compliance.* • Teach client about lithium and other medications as needed *because information promotes adherence.*	• Yvonne expressed the importance of taking her lithium and agreed to stay on the medication.
• Yvonne will discuss her feelings about lithium and her bipolar disorder.	• Discuss with client her feelings about lithium and having a lifelong disorder requiring medication management *to provide opportunity to express feelings and beliefs about medication and bipolar disorder.*	• Lithium blood level 2 weeks after discharge was 0.95. • Yvonne discussed her feelings about lithium and her disorder.

delusions, improvement in cognitive functioning and communication, and initial understanding of the disorder and its treatment, including necessary self-care management. Referrals are made to therapists, psychiatrists, home care and community mental health agencies, and partial hospitalization programs for continued care in the community.

Nurses working with the clients in the community see improvement in longer-term outcomes such as improved socialization, return to usual activities, reduction in negative thinking, increased self-esteem, use of new coping strategies, resumption of family/work roles, continued improvement in cognitive processes (e.g., attention and concentration), decrease or absence of fatigue, and adherence to regimens. For some clients, these outcomes become evident within weeks of starting psychotherapy or somatic treatment regimens. For others, improvement may require months before longer-term outcomes are achieved. Recent data suggest that return to previous levels of functioning after an episode of depression takes longer than previously thought, particularly if clients have had multiple episodes (Klerman and Weissman, 1992).

Clients with mania present a unique evaluative situation, because episodes of mania may be followed by episodes of depression. Therefore, although clients may have returned to a hypomanic or euthymic state at the time of hospital discharge, the nurse should be alert to any indications of depression. Careful follow-up after discharge into the community is imperative for clients with bipolar disorders.

CASE STUDY

Andrew is a 55-year-old widowed male. He lives alone in an apartment and has a 32-year-old married daughter who lives 1000 miles away. Three months ago, Andrew was forced to take early retirement from his job in middle management at a computer firm. Over the past month, he has exhibited depressed affect and has become so withdrawn that he no longer attends church or his weekly evening out with his friends. He reports difficulty falling asleep and staying asleep, agitation, loss of 15 pounds in 1 month, difficulty concentrating and making decisions, and ruminations and guilt about his wife's death 10 years ago. He was admitted to the hospital after his neighbor brought him to the emergency room. There, Andrew admitted plans to kill himself with a handgun he kept at home. He had one previous episode of major depression at age 45, about the time of his wife's death. He has never made an actual suicide attempt. Andrew has been in the hospital for 13 days. He has been taking Zoloft (100 mg qd) and trazodone hydrochloride (100 mg hs), and is being considered for discharge.

Critical Thinking and Evaluation

1. Which specific indicators would the nurse use to evaluate Andrew's self-destructiveness in view of his impending discharge?

2. What outcome criteria are appropriate for evaluation of Andrew's response to medication?

3. What outcomes might be evaluated by the nurse that would best demonstrate Andrew's progress for a community mental health referral?

Summary of Key Concepts

1. Mood disorders are a major public health problem and result in billions of dollars in health care costs and lost productivity each year.

2. Major depression is currently occurring at younger ages, and those most at risk are women with a family history of mood disorders.

3. Mood disorders are usually recurrent and require lifetime management.

4. Two major types of mood disorders include unipolar depressive and bipolar disorders.

5. Mood disorders are explained by multiple theories, including cognitive, psychodynamic, personality, and biologic theories. Mood disorders are probably caused by the interaction of multiple factors.

6. Mania and depression are manifested by symptoms involving the affective, cognitive, physical, social, and spiritual aspects of the individual.

7. The nursing care of persons experiencing depression or mania consists of thorough assessment and subsequent planning and interventions for an array of nursing diagnoses related to physical, psychosocial, and spiritual needs.

8. Nurses collaborate with other mental health care providers for care related to somatic, family, and group interventions.

REFERENCES

Abramson LY, Melalsy GI, Alloy LB: Hopelessness depression: a theory based type of depression, *Psychol Rev* 93: 358–379, 1989.

Abramson LY, Seligman MEP, Teasdale JD: Learned helplessness in humans: critique and reformulation, *Abnorm Psychol* 87: 49–74, 1978.

Akiskal HS: New insights into the nature and heterogeneity of mood disorders, *J Clin Psychiatry* 50: 6–10, 1989.

American Psychiatric Association: *Diagnostic and Statistical Manual of Mental Disorders*, ed. 4, Washington, D.C., 1994, The Association.

Angst J: Clinical course of affective disorders. In Helgason T, Daly, R, editors: *Depressive illness: prediction of course and outcome*, Berlin, Germany, 1988, Springer-Verlag.

APA Task Force: The dexamethasone suppression test: an overview of its current status in psychiatry, *Am J Psychiatry* 144: 1253–1262, 1987.

Barondes S: *Molecules and mental illness*, New York, 1993, Scientific American Library.

Beck AT: *Depression: clinical, experiential, and theoretical aspects*, New York, 1967, Hober.

Boulby J: *Attachment*, New York, 1969, Bask Books.

Boyce P et al: Personality as a vulnerability factor to depression, *Br J Psychiatry* 159: 106–114, 1991.

Brown GW, Harris T: *Social origins of depression*, New York, 1978, The Free Press.

Consensus Development Panel: Mood disorders: pharmacological prevention of recurrences, *Am J Psychiatry* 142: 469–476, 1985.

Cornelis CM, Ameling EH, Delonghe F: Life events and social network in relation to the onset of depression, *Acta Psychiatr Scand* 80: 174–179, 1989.

Depression Guideline Panel: *Depression in primary care. Volume I. Detection and diagnosis.* Washington D.C., 1993, U.S. Department of Health and Human Services, AHCPR.

Diehl DJ, Gershon S: The role of dopamine in mental disorders, *Compr Psychiatr* 33: 115–120, 1992.

Ehlers CL, Frank E, Kupfer DJ: Social Zeitgebers and biological rhythms: a unified approach to understanding the etiology of depression, *Arch Gen Psychiatry* 45: 948–952, 1988.

Freeman A et al: *Clinical applications of cognitive therapy*, New York, 1990, Plenum Press.

Freud S: Mourning and melancholia. In *The complete psychological works of Sigmund Freud*, London, 1957, Hogarth Press.

Fuller RW: Role of serotonin in therapy of depression and related disorders, *J Clin Psychiatry* 52: 52–57, 1991.

Greden JF: Recurrent depression, Indianapolis, 1993, Dista Products Co.

Hirshfeld RMA et al: Premorbid personality assessments of first onset of major depression, *Arch Gen Psychiatry* 46: 345–350, 1989.

Horwath E et al: Depressive symptoms as relative and attributable risk factors for first onset major depression, *Arch Gen Psychiatry* 49: 817–823, 1992.

Keller MB: The course of manic-depressive illness, *Clin Psychiatry* 49: 4–6, 1988.

Kessler RC et al: Lifetime and 12-month prevalence of DSM-IIIR psychiatric disorders in the U.S., *Arch Gen Psychiatry* 51: 8–19, 1994.

Klerman GL: Treatment of recurrent unipolar major depressive disorder, *Arch Gen Psychiatry* 47: 1158–1162, 1990.

Klerman GL, Weissman MM: The course, morbidity, and costs of depression, *Arch Gen Psychiatry* 49:831–833, 1992.

Kraepelin E: *Lectures in clinical psychiatry*, London, 1913, Bailliere, Tindall, & Cox.

Kraepelin E: *Manic-depressive insanity and paranoia*, Edinburgh, 1921, E & S Livingstone.

Leonard BE: Biochemical aspects of treatment-resistant depression, *Br J Psychiatry* 152: 453–459, 1988.

Leonhard K: Aufteilung der endogenen Psychosen. As quoted in Buher J: *Depression: theory and research*, New York, 1974, Winston Wiley.

Lewinsohn PM et al: Age cohort changes in the lifetime occurrence of depression and other mental disorders, *J Abnorm Psychiatry* 102: 110–120, 1993.

McGriffin P, Katz R: The genetics of depression: current approaches, *Br J Psychiatry* 155: 18–26, 1989.

McPherson H, Herbison P, Romans S: Life events and relapse in established bipolar affective disorder, *Br J Psychiatry* 157: 381–385, 1993.

Paykel ES: Recent life events in the development of the depressive disorder, in Depue RA, editor: *The psychobiology of the depressive disorders: implications for the effects of stress*, New York, 1979, Academic Press.

Phillips KA et al: A review of the depressive personality, *Am J Psychiatry* 147: 830–837, 1990.

Pilgrim JA, et al: Low blood pressure, low mood? *Br Med J*, 304:75, 1992.

Post RM: Transduction of psychosocial stress in the neurobiology of recurrent affective disorders, *Am J Psychiatry* 149: 999–1010, 1992.

Robins CJ, Hayes AM: An appraisal of cognitive therapy, *J Consult Clin Psychol* 61: 205–214, 1993.

Sargeant JK et al: Factors associated with 1-year outcome of major depression in the community, *Arch Gen Psychiatry* 47: 519–526, 1990.

Schmaling K, Becker J: Empirical studies of the interpersonal relations of adult depressives, in Becker J, Kleinman (editors): *Psychosocial aspects of depression,* Hillsdale, N.J., 1991, Laurence Erlbaum Associates.

Seligman MEP: *Helplessness: on depression development and death,* New York, 1975, WH Freeman.

Stravynski A, Greenberg D: The psychological management of depression, *Acta Psychiatr Scand* 85: 407–414, 1992.

Thase ME: Long-term treatment of recurrent depressive disorders, *J Clin Psychiatry* 53: 32–44, 1992.

Tweed DL: Depression-related impairment: estimating concurrent and lingering effects, *Psychol Med* 23: 373–386, 1993.

Young EA et al: Dissociation between pituitary and adrenal suppression to dexamethasone in depression, *Arch Gen Psychiatry* 50: 395–403, 1993.

Zimmerman M, Coryell W, Pfohl B: The validity of the DST as a maker for endogenous depression, *Arch Gen Psychiatry* 43: 347–355, 1986.

CHAPTER 13

The Schizophrenias

Marjorie F. Bendik

Affect Outward, bodily expression of emotions, ranging through joy, sorrow, anger, etc. **Blunted affect:** Restricted expression of emotions. **Flat affect:** Lack of outward expression of emotions. **Inappropriate affect:** Affect that is not congruent with the emotion being felt (for example, laughing when sad). **Labile affect:** Rapid changes in emotional expression.

Agnosia Inability to recognize familiar environmental stimuli such as sounds or objects seen or felt.

Ambivalence Simultaneously holding two different attitudes, emotions, thoughts or feelings about a person, object, or situation.

Autistic thinking Disturbances in thought due to the intrusion of a private fantasy world, internally stimulated, resulting in abnormal responses to people and events in the real world.

Delusions False beliefs that are fixed and resistant to reasoning.

Derealization The feeling that the world around one is not real or is distorted.

Dereism A loss of connection with reality and logic that occurs just prior to autistic thinking. Thoughts become private and idiosyncratic. Dereism is seen in schizophrenia.

Double-bind A situation in which contradictory messages are given to one person by another, demanding a response or choice between two opposing alternatives.

Flight of ideas Abrupt change of topics in a rapid flow of speech. It may be seen in schizophrenia but is more common in the manic phase of bipolar disorder. It is more reality based than L.O.A. and can be a response to stressful stimuli.

Hallucination A subjective disorder of perception in which one of the five senses is involved, in the absence of external stimulation.

Loosening of associations (L.O.A.) Thought disturbance in which the speaker rapidly shifts expression of ideas from one subject to another in an unrelated manner.

Negative symptoms Syndrome that includes flat affect, poverty of speech, poor grooming, withdrawal, and disturbance in volition.

Perseveration A disturbance in thought association in which there is a persistent repetition of the same idea in response to different questions.

Positive symptoms Syndrome that includes hallucinations, increased speech production with loose associations, and bizarre behavior.

Poverty of thought A psychopathologic thought disturbance in schizophrenia. The client's inability to think logically and sequentially is reflected in **Poverty of Content of Speech,** which is vague, repetitious, and disconnected.

Premorbid Period just preceding the onset of a mental illness. Characteristics of the personality may indicate the type of disorder that may occur.

Primary process thinking Prelogical thought that aims for wish fulfillment. It is associated with the pleasure principle characteristic of the *Id* portion of the personality.

Prodromal symptoms Early symptoms, such as a deterioration in functioning, that may mark the onset of a mental illness.

Psychosis Inability to recognize reality, bizarre behaviors, and to deal with life's demands.

Residual symptoms Minor disturbances that may remain after an episode of schizophrenia but do not include delusions, hallucinations, incoherence, or gross disorganization.

Thought blocking Abrupt interruption in the flow of thoughts or ideas due to a disturbance in the speed of associations.

- Explain the various theories and models that evolved over the years to describe the schizophrenic disorders.
- Describe the epidemiologic factors and symptom profiles related to schizophrenia.
- Discuss the various assessment tools currently available for medical diagnosis of the schizophrenias, and use rating scales and observational and subjective data available to nurses in formulating accurate nursing diagnoses.
- Demonstrate the application of the nursing process to clients suffering negative symptomatology and those displaying positive symptoms.
- Engage in collaborative treatment for schizophrenia with other members of the health care team.
- Differentiate the nursing responsibilities in the care of clients with schizophrenia from those of the other health care professionals; compare and contrast the approaches.
- Evaluate the effectiveness of various treatment modalities in the clinical setting.
- Appraise the situation of persons with schizophrenia and their families in the community, developing plans for nursing involvement in prevention, aftercare, and research.

Schizophrenia is a condition that exists in all cultures, and in all socioeconomic groups (Betemps and Ragiel, 1994; Kaplan and Sadock, 1994). Despite their prevalence, the schizophrenias have not had the benefit of a scientific approach until the mid-nineteenth century.

HISTORICAL AND THEORETICAL PERSPECTIVES

If space is the last frontier in exploration of the universe, then schizophrenia is the last frontier in medical science discoveries. Until recently, little was known about the cognitive functioning of the brain. The term *schizophrenia* has been used to describe a particular form of mental illness only since the mid-1800s (Arieti, 1974).

Clients with schizophrenia are particularly troubling for society because of their overt **psychosis,** an impaired ability to recognize reality, bizarre behaviors, and an inability to deal with life's demands. The earliest knowledge about recognition and treatment of psychotic disorders comes from artifacts and cave drawings from the Stone Age, a half a million years ago. The earliest writings on the subject date to the Sanskrit (an ancient Indo-European language) of 1400 B.C. The notion of possession by demons persisted as early civilizations developed, as noted in the early writings of the Hebrews, Egyptians, Chinese, and Greeks.

Two prominent psychiatrists in the nineteenth century made progress related to symptoms now associated with the schizophrenias. The first was Emil Kraepelin (1856–1926), who described the syndrome *dementia praecox,* characterized by **hallucinations** (a subjective disorder of perception involving any one of the five senses in the absence of external stimulation) and **delusions** (false beliefs that are fixed and resistant to reasoning).

The second major psychiatrist, Eugen Bleuler (1857–1939), saw the inconsistency between emotion, thought, and behavior noted in the client with schizophrenia. He introduced the term *schizophrenia,* which means split-minded. The "split," however, refers only to emotion, thought, and behavior, not to personality, and should not be confused with dissociative identity disorder (see Chapter 11). He also further refined the description by calling it a *thought disorder* with fundamental symptoms which are Bleuler's 4 A's:

- **loosening of associations (L.O.A.):** thought disturbance in which the speaker rapidly shifts expression of ideas from one subject to another in an unrelated fragmented manner

- disturbances of **affect:** observable, outward, bodily expression of emotions, such as joy, sorrow, anger, etc.

  blunted affect: restricted expression of emotions

  flat affect: lack of expression of emotions

  inappropriate affect: affect that is not congruent with the emotion being felt (for example, laughing when sad)

  labile affect: rapid changes in emotional expression

- **ambivalence:** simultaneously holding two different attitudes, emotions, thoughts, or feelings about a person, object, or situation

- **autistic thinking:** Disturbances in thought due to the intrusion of a private fantasy world, internally stimulated, resulting in abnormal responses to people and events in the real world

In addition, Bleuler named hallucinations and delusions as accessory symptoms to the syndrome (Kaplan and Sadock, 1994).

Sullivan, a social learning theorist, emphasized the importance of interpersonal relationships and believed that social isolation was the key in schizophrenia. Schneider described first-rank symptoms as various delusional and hallucinatory experiences, and second-rank, less decisive symptoms such as perceptual disturbances, confusion, mood changes, and emotional impoverishment (Kaplan and Sadock, 1994).

ETIOLOGY

The foremost etiology of schizophrenia today is the biologic perspective. This includes not only the traditional medical model that stresses chemical control (medication) but also the new discoveries of genetic influences; the role of neuroanatomy, endocrinology, and immunology in producing symptoms; and the issues of trauma and disease in causation. Declaring brain research as one of the truly great frontiers of science, Congress designated the decade beginning January 1, 1990, as the "Decade of the Brain." This designation has renewed interest in schizophrenia as a disease. The research being generated in this decade presents a strong challenge for nurses, who now must integrate the biologic sciences with the caring concepts of the psychosocial models. Box 13-1 lists etiologic factors.

Biologic Factors

Several early twentieth-century theorists favored biologic factors as causes for schizophrenia. Hans Selye (1936) was a successful pioneer with his work on the general adaptation syndrome (GAS). Selye demonstrated that the phases of alarm, resistance, and exhaustion following stress were related in a causal manner to several physiologic disease states, for example, hypertension and peptic ulcer (McCain and Smith, 1994). Extensive research on the neuroendocrine mechanisms underlying the stress response also influenced the psychiatrists as a possible explanation of several forms of psychotic states. This foundation remains a part of the theoretical framework explaining psychopathology even today, and a part of the stress and adaptation theories used in psychiatric nursing (for example, Roy's Adaptation Model).

Five biologic models have been expanded or changed, due to recent research:

- the heredity/genetic model
- the neuroanatomic and neurochemical model
- neurotransmitters and the dopamine hypothesis
- the immunologic model
- the stress/disease/trauma causation model

HEREDITY AND GENETIC INFLUENCES

There are two ways of looking at a possible connection between heredity and schizophrenia. One is related to the well-known twin study by Kallmann (1953), an early

Box 13-1   Etiologic Factors

Biologic factors

- Heredity and Genetics
- Neuroanatomics and Neurochemicals

   structure and function of nervous system

   teratogenic drug exposure

   neuroanatomical differences in the brain

- Neurotransmitter function

   abnormal neurotransmitter-endocrine interactions

- Immunologic Factors

   viral exposure in pregnancy

- High arousal levels from Stress, Disease, Trauma, and Drugs

   Stress such as a bombardment of stimuli from life events

   Diseases such as prenatal virus exposure, encephalitis

   Trauma from obstetrical complications, head trauma, childhood accidents

   Drugs such as cannabis and cocaine

Psychoanalytic and developmental factors

- Distortions in mother-child relationship
- Ego disorganization
- Faulty reality interpretation

Familial factors

- Repressed unhappiness
- Double-bind patterns
- Marital schism of parents
- Destructive, expressed emotion communication patterns

Cultural and environmental theories

- Low socioeconomic status
- Lessened social support of family and community, changes in social roles

Learning theories and behavioral models

- Irrational problem-solving methods, distorted thinking, deficient communication patterns learned from parents
- Generalized social interactions

Theories of psychophysiologic effects of the environment

- Toxic substances (selenium) in the atmospheric pollution

example of the epidemiologic potential for the occurrence of schizophrenia among related individuals. Kallmann's statistics have been challenged, and later studies have shown a lower incidence of schizophrenia among first-degree relatives than the 86% that Kallmann predicted. However, the lifetime risk of developing schizophrenia when one has a parent, identical twin, or sibling with schizophrenia is much higher (46% for an identical twin of a person with schizophrenia and 10% for a sibling) than in the population at large (1% for an unrelated person). In Figure 13-1, MRI scans compare the size of brain ventricles in identical twins, one who has schizophrenia and one who does not.

Recent studies in genetic epidemiology support the theme of familial transmission, although how it occurs is not known (Malone, 1990; Shore, 1989). Evidence shows that there are multiple correlated risk factors that are important in susceptibility, although inheritance is regarded as the most important component.

The search for a major gene or gene sites consistent with schizophrenia (Tsuang, 1994) is another area of study. A major goal at the Salk Institute for Biological Studies in La Jolla, California, is to produce a map of the human genetic structure that will isolate and identify all of the genes (50,000–100,000) in the human cell nucleus.

Currently, about 5,000 genes have been identified, with about 2,000 mapped on the chromosomes. Although a linkage to schizophrenia was established by one researcher from a genetic anomaly on chromosome 5, the finding was controversial because further analyses failed to support inheritance of schizophrenic tendencies through a single major gene.

NEUROANATOMIC AND NEUROCHEMICAL FACTORS

There have been many recent advances in the study of neuroanatomic and neurochemical factors as they relate to schizophrenia. Starting with the work of Plum (1972), Crow (1980), and others, the field has expanded to include the study of the human nervous system, from the prospectives of physiology, chemistry, and endocrinology (Hemsley et al, 1993; Joseph, 1993). Also, the immune system may be involved in schizophrenia (Lieberman and Koreen, 1993; Tsuang, 1994).

Structural and functional factors. The structure of the nervous system may include both gross and microanatomic defects, possibly resulting from a congenital developmental condition (Benes, 1993; Bogerts, 1993; Cannon and Marco, 1994). Other researchers have called attention to teratogenic drug exposure in utero or to birth trauma, leading to gradual deteriorative changes that seem to affect many clients with chronic schizophrenia. Both of these notions may be part of a faulty developmental pattern.

With the help of electroencephalograms (EEG) and the new brain imaging techniques available today, it has been found that ventricular enlargement, prominence of

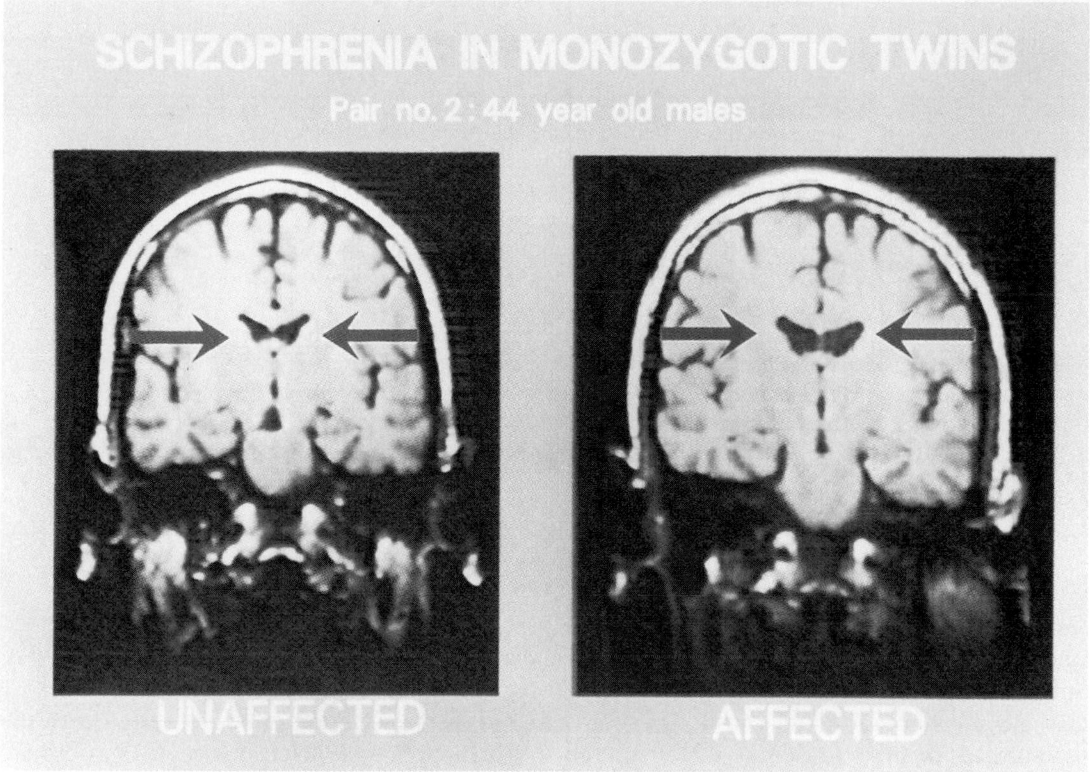

Figure 13-1 Loss of brain volume associated with schizophrenia is clearly shown by magnetic resonance imaging (MRI) scans comparing the size of ventricles (butterfly-shaped, fluid-filled spaces in the midbrain) of identical twins, one of whom has schizophrenia (right). The ventricles of the person with schizophrenia are larger.

(Courtesy National Institute of Mental Health Biological Psychiatry Branch, U.S. Dept. of Health and Human Services.)

cortical sulci, defects in limbic brain structures, and cortical atrophy occur, usually more pronounced in the left hemisphere. Smaller cerebrums and frontal lobes are noted in clients with chronic schizophrenia. Specifically, there are subtle neuroanatomical differences in parts of the thalamus, septum, hypothalamus, hippocampus, amygdala, and cingulate gyrus in the brains of these clients, when compared with the brains of unaffected persons (Bogerts, 1993; Cannon and Marco, 1994; Joseph, 1993). (See Figure 5-6 in Chapter 5.

Physiologically, there is a decrease in metabolic activity and slower brain waves in the frontal lobes (Malone, 1990). At the micro level, changes in neurotransmitter activity at the synaptic junctions between the nerve cells lead to abnormalities in the brain circuits (Benes, 1993; Cannon and Marco, 1994). It is difficult to establish the relationship between neuron damage and functional impairment, but Previc (1993) maintains that the visuoperceptual and visuomotor functions of the brain, situated in the posterior parietal lobes, are affected in individuals with schizophrenia. Consequently, they manifest poor audiovisual integration, spatial orientation difficulties, prolonged reaction-time responses, accommodation problems, and distortions in perceived body image. Some clients with schizophrenia cannot tell whether another person is looking at them or not, and then always think they are, due to eye tracking dysfunctions (Clementz et al, 1994). To cite another specific relationship, Hemsley et al, (1993) believe that hippocampal lesions can cause learning failure and an inability to differentiate between meaningless and meaningful information. These are only two examples of the functional difficulties encountered by clients, due to damage in neuron structures.

NEUROTRANSMITTERS AND THE DOPAMINE HYPOTHESIS

Although there are many neurotransmitters involved in brain and body activity, seven are known to be of special importance in schizophrenia: dopamine, serotonin, acetylcholine, norepinephrine, cholecystokinin, glutamate, and gamma-aminobutyric acid (GABA). Their types and functions are shown in Table 13-1.

Theories about schizophrenia and the role of neurotransmitters include:

- A serotonin deficiency may be responsible for some forms of schizophrenia

- Norepinephrine may be insufficient in clients with schizophrenia displaying anhedonia

- The dopamine hypothesis, explained below

TABLE 13-1 Neurotransmitters in schizophrenia: type and function

Neurotransmitter	Type	Function
Dopamine	Catecholamine	Regulates motor behavior and also transmits in the cortex
		Increases vigilance; may increase aggressive behavior
Serotonin	Indolamine	Brain-stem transmitter
		Modulates mood, lowers aggressive tendencies
Acetylcholine	Cholinergic	Transmits at nerve-muscle connections (CNS and ANS)
		A deficiency may increase confusion and acting-out behavior
		Controls EPS
Norepinephrine	Catecholamine	Transmits in the sympathetic nervous system; induces hypervigilance: "fight or flight" syndrome
Cholecystokinin	Peptide	Excites limbic neurons; a deficiency is related to avolition and flat affect
Glutamate	Amino Acid	Excitatory neurotransmitter
Gamma-aminobutyric acid (GABA)	Amino Acid	Inhibitory neurotransmitter (predominant brain transmitter)

The dopamine hypothesis is the major neurotransmitter hypothesis for schizophrenia. Dopamine affects mood, affect, thoughts, and motor behavior. Too much dopamine could result in psychosis and not enough could cause movement disorders. Recently this theory has been challenged as being limited in scope. There is evidence that other neurotransmitters are also involved, either alone or in interactions with dopamine neural systems. (Joseph, 1993; Kaplan and Sadock, 1994; Lieberman and Koreen, 1993; Previc, 1993). The dopamine theory states that there is too much dopamine in schizophrenia. This is supported by postmortem data showing that in schizophrenia the numbers of dopamine receptors are increased by two-thirds. Also, the positive effects of the older antipsychotic drugs was due to their action as dopamine antagonists, blocking the dopamine receptors (Figure 13-2) so that less dopamine was available, thus reducing the client's psychosis.

One of the newer antipsychotic drugs, clozapine, is more selective in which receptors it blocks. It also decreases psychosis but does not produce movement disorders as the older drugs do (Lieberman and Koreen, 1993). Other dopamine receptors, have been investigated in recent years but were not found to be associated with the presence of schizophrenia (Macciardi et al, 1994; Sabate et al, 1994). In all studies, there is no clear evidence of dopamine abnormalities, but the refined hypothesis continues to generate interest in researching the involvement of the neurotransmitters and neuroendocrine systems in schizophrenia (Joseph, 1993; vanKammen et al, 1994).

Neurotransmitter-endocrine interactions. Human behavior, thoughts, and feelings are also influenced by a much larger and more complex component, the endocrine system. Schizophrenia has been linked to abnormal neurotransmitter and neuroendocrine interactions (Benes, 1993; Hemsley et al, 1993; Lieberman and Koreen, 1993; Malone, 1990). For example, although direct evidence of serotonal dysfunction has not been obtained, the antipsychotic drugs clozapine and risperidone owe their unique therapeutic effects to their influ-

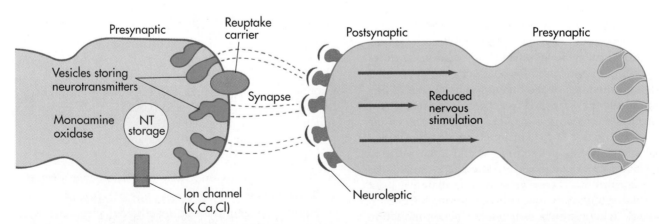

Figure 13-2 Neuroleptic action. Neurotransmitter action at the synapse is modified by neuroleptics, which block postsynaptic receptor sites to reduce nervous stimulation.

ence on dopamine and the serotonin receptors in the frontal cortex. The role of GABA in schizophrenia promotes a balance of dopamine and glutamate and thus inhibits impulsive behaviors.

Several recent studies have examined not only neurotransmitter interactions but also the effect of interactions between hormones and neurotransmitters in schizophrenia. Patterns of dopamine-thyroid interactions and dopamine–pituitary hormone secretions were found to be consistent with schizophrenia symptoms. Other patterns involved beta endorphins and other opioid compounds, cholecystokinin and other neuropeptides, in interaction with dopamine. In addition, abnormal composition and structure of neuronal membranes may also contribute to schizophrenic symptoms (Lieberman and Koreen, 1993).

Presently, the studies of neurochemistry and neuroendocrinology are fragmentary, but show promise. It is clear that the patterns and balance between the neurotransmitter and neuroendocrine systems in schizophrenia are distinctly different from those of unaffected individuals.

Immunologic Factors

Viral exposure, particularly exposure to influenza during pregnancy, is a risk factor for schizophrenia. It is theorized that the influenza virus may create maternal antibodies. In the fetus, these become autoantibodies, which are an external source of developmental change (Cannon and Marco, 1994; Malone, 1990; Takei et al, 1994; Tsuang, 1994). There are few immunological studies of schizophrenia, and they depend on epidemiologic data for their hypotheses.

STRESS, DISEASE, TRAUMA, AND DRUG ABUSE

In Selye's stress model, the individual was seen as interacting with the environment, being bombarded by various stimuli in the form of life events. This created stress, which differed in magnitude and meaning for each individual.

For clients with chronic schizophrenia, environmental stressors of events and situations are always present. They increase dopaminergic transmission and precipitate a high level of arousal, leading to episodic recurrences of the disease. The high level of arousal results in intense hallucinatory experiences (Hemsley et al, 1993). Several of the nursing theories (King's, Levine's, and Neuman's, for instance) examined the relationship between stress and illness (physical or mental) using this notion.

Some recent studies support the idea that schizophrenia may be developmentally related to disease and trauma occurring during the prenatal period or in early childhood. Takei and his associates (1994) studied the effect of prenatal exposure to the influenza virus. They concluded that exposure in the second trimester of pregnancy was a significant risk for adult schizophrenia, especially for females. Thus, there are observed gender differences in the presentation of the disease.

With regard to trauma, a few studies have focused on obstetrical complications or childhood accidents that could cause minimal brain damage and hinder development of the cerebral cortex. Obstetrical complications studied included preeclampsia, antepartum hemorrhage, premature rupture of the membranes, prolonged labor, umbilical cord prolapse, unusual or uncommon presentations (such as breech births), prematurity, and postmaturity.

Studies of childhood included encephalitis, found to be a risk factor for schizophrenia. Also, studies of head trauma requiring hospitalization for the child under 10 years of age indicated there was a significant difference in the later occurrence of schizophrenia between persons who had suffered prenatal or childhood head trauma and a comparison group. The injuries included hemorrhage into the ventricles and ischemic damage to the cortex in areas commonly associated with schizophrenia (Gureje et al, 1994).

The relationship between drugs of abuse and schizophrenia has also been studied. Cannabis abuse may be a precipitant of schizophrenia or may promote relapse, according to Linszen et al (1994). Also, the extreme stimulating effect of cocaine, which generates impulsivity, induces relapse in persons with schizophrenia (Stirling et al, 1994). Cocaine initiates neurochemical changes in the brain by substituting for the natural endorphins, creating an intense craving for the drug. Eventually, the long-term user experiences apathy, depression, and anhedonia, as often seen in clients with chronic schizophrenia. In addition, there is accumulating evidence that certain drugs, taken in pregnancy, are linked with later schizotypal illnesses in childhood and adolescence. For example, cocaine used by a pregnant woman is linked to later schizotypal illness in the child victim (Scherling, 1994).

Psychodynamic Theories

Many biologic factors may predispose one to schizophrenia; however, psychosocial considerations are significant as well. Most causative models postulate that vulnerability interacts with stressful environmental influences to produce the symptoms of schizophrenia (Kaplan and Sadock, 1994). The theories that deal with psychosocial and environmental factors are psychoanalytic, family, and sociocultural/environmental. Systems theory has also been used to explain the reciprocal interactions among the theories.

PSYCHOANALYTIC AND DEVELOPMENTAL THEORIES

Psychoanalytic theory states that there are distortions in the mother-child relationship, brought on by anxious mothering, so that the child is unable to progress beyond dependence. This affects the ego organization and the interpretation of reality in the developing child. Being unable to interpret reality, the individual is susceptible to a fantasy world in which hallucinations and delusions attempt to create a reality of wishful thinking or to express inner fears. Inner drives, such as sex and aggression, are not brought under the person's control, and self-object differentiation is not achieved. Thus, the person's sense of identity is weak, and his or her personality is vulnerable to stress (Kaplan and Sadock, 1994).

THE FAMILY THEORY MODEL

According to the family theory model, the child is assumed to have been raised in an atmosphere of unhappiness and tension, which may not be apparent to others or even to the family members themselves. Families make great attempts to conceal or repress unhappiness, resulting in psychological insensitivity. However, no studies have demonstrated that family attributes are *causally* related to schizophrenia. Considering the reciprocal nature of interactions, one cannot say whether stressful relationships would precede or follow an episode of schizophrenia.

Several family patterns have been cited as being particularly damaging to the developing child. The first pattern is the **double-bind,** in which the child is forced to make a choice between two unreasonable perceptions, thus producing confusion, anxiety, and fear in the child's mind. For example, a verbal message may differ from a nonverbal one; a parent may insist that he or she is not angry at the child's behavior but expresses obvious anger in aggressive, hostile, and destructive behavior.

The second family pattern seen as destructive involves marital problems between the parents. This pattern results in the children being asked to support one parent against the other. Such a situation causes guilt feelings in the children because of divided loyalties. Often a power struggle begins between the parents, with one parent emerging as dominant and authoritative. This authoritative stand is likely to suppress the child's drive toward independence. In addition, the spouse forced to submit may displace his or her anger onto the children, or scapegoat (blame) one child in particular.

The third serious family disturbance arises from destructive expressed emotion (EE) communication patterns within the family. At times there is a false agreement about family rules that is not communicated directly but produces explosive behavior when violated. There is also an air of pseudohostility that forces some family members into emotional isolation. The constant criticism and hostility destroy the family functions of support and protection.

CULTURAL AND ENVIRONMENTAL THEORIES

Although schizophrenia exists in all socioeconomic groups, it is disproportionately represented in the lower socioeconomic group. Various explanations have been advanced for this condition, one having to do with a "downward drift hypothesis" (Kaplan and Sadock, 1994). According to this hypothesis, the client with schizophrenia who possesses low social skills either moves into a lower socioeconomic group or fails to rise to a higher group.

On the other hand, some social scientists believe that the stress of living in a lower socioeconomic group is often enough to trigger schizophrenia in the vulnerable population (Fortinash and Holoday-Worret, 1995). Individuals with schizophrenia who are under psychological stress manifest low levels of self-esteem and self-efficacy perception (view of the self as a normally functioning, partially functioning, or a dysfunctioning member of society) and may have limited resources to cope with their situation. In addition, the family networks of mentally ill persons are often not able to be supportive (Bendik, 1992).

Low socioeconomic status affects not only the psychologic, but also the biologic functioning of an individual, adding to chronic symptom profiles (Cohen, 1993). For example, clients with schizophrenia are more likely than other persons in the lower socioeconomic group to get an infectious disease, particularly tuberculosis. Living in heavily populated rural areas, in poverty, adversity, and fear due to rising crime rates, is conducive to psychopathology (Betemps and Ragiel, 1994).

Learning Theory

According to learning theory, the irrational ways of handling situations, the distorted thinking, and the deficient communication patterns of schizophrenics are a result of poor parental models in early childhood. Children learn what they are exposed to on a daily basis, from parents who have their own significant emotional problems. Thus, the child does not learn skill in forming good interpersonal relationships (Fortinash and Holoday-Worret, 1995; Kaplan and Sadock, 1994).

Sullivan was a principal proponent of learning theory, believing that the developing individual was shaped by social interactions. Therefore, the complex of feelings, thoughts, and behavioral expressions grew out of the individual's experiences with those closest to him or her. For example, if the child's father was perceived as mean and dictatorial, this perception may have generalized to other men in positions of authority, such as teachers, policemen, and employers, and colored the interpersonal relationships with these individuals. Or, if the child's mother coped with problems by projecting blame onto others, the child learned this pattern of behavior and alienated others by putting it into practice.

THEORIES OF PSYCHOPHYSIOLOGIC EFFECTS OF ENVIRONMENT

Recent studies have also looked at the physical environment and its relationship to schizophrenia. Since toxic substances that cause a variety of illnesses may come to people through atmospheric pollution or through the food chain (for example, lead and mercury), researchers have compared the geographic distribution of selenium and other trace elements to the prevalence of schizophrenia in the same area. The hypotheses were formulated according to an assumption that either an excess or a deficiency of certain substances in the environment can cause the disease (Brown, 1994).

EPIDEMIOLOGY

The incidence of schizophrenia, or the frequency of newly diagnosed cases in a specified population during a certain time period, is between 0.3% and 0.6% per 1000 persons per year in the United States (see Box 13-2). Lifetime prevalence, or the total number of cases in the U.S. population, is about 1.5%. The prevalence and prognosis of the disease vary according to socioeconomic, geographic, and cultural factors; schizophrenia presents itself in different ways, depending on the clients' situations and demographic characteristics (Betemps and Ragiel, 1994; Kaplan and Sadock, 1994). Family, twin, and adoption studies have consistently found varying rates of inheritance patterns, according to the closeness of the genetic relationship (Kaplan and Sadock, 1994; Kendler and Diehl, 1993).

Age and Gender

Two demographic characteristics that have been extensively studied with regard to schizophrenia are age and gender. These variables have an interactive effect. For ex-

ample, the age of onset of the disease in females is significantly greater than the age of onset in males.

Subtypes of schizophrenia tend to appear at different times. In males, the paranoid type, in which prominent delusions or auditory hallucinations of a persecutory nature are present, appears earlier than in females. On the other hand, the disorganized type, which features confusion in speech, disorganization in behavior, and inappropriate affect, appears earlier in females (Castle and Murray, 1993; APA, 1994). Over the course of time, however, there is no difference in the prevalence of schizophrenia between males and females (Kaplan and Sadock, 1994).

In a recent incidence study of the age of onset, the oldest group ranged in age from 66 to 77 years, and composed about one-third of the prevalence rate. This is contrary to earlier beliefs that schizophrenia rarely occurs after age 50. Clients in the older age of onset group tended to be females exhibiting paranoid symptoms (Castle and Murray, 1993).

When the fetus is exposed to the influenza of the mother during the second trimester, it is the female child who is at greatest risk for schizophrenia in her adult years (Takei et al, 1994). Males, on the other hand, show significantly more structural brain abnormalities than females as a result of perinatal or early childhood trauma (Gureje et al, 1994). In all, gender differences in age of onset, physiological deficits, prognosis, and response to treatment give evidence of a gender difference in the expression of schizophrenia.

Marital Status, Rates of Reproduction, and Mortality

Since the introduction of psychotherapeutic drugs, people with schizophrenia have been freed from continual care in a state mental institution. Free of much of their symptoms and allowed access to rehabilitation programs where available, many with schizophrenia have gone on to live reasonably normal and even productive lives, including marrying and having a family. Thus, the marriage and fertility rates among people with schizophrenias, once low, are nearly on a par with the larger population aggregate (Fortinash and Holoday-Worret, 1995; Kaplan and Sadock, 1994).

However, schizophrenia still carries with it the high rates of suicide in those who cannot cope with the demands of society. Despite the relief of some of their symptoms, many people with schizophrenia are prone to episodic decompensation when the pathology is exacerbated. During these times they may attempt suicide, become accident-prone, or neglect their health, raising their morbidity rates and accounting for the lifetime 50% suicide attempt figure in the schizophrenic population.

Socioeconomic Class

The portion of schizophrenia that can be attributed to the social problems endured by the lower class remains controversial (Betemps and Ragiel, 1994; Fortinash and

---

Box 13-2   Epidemiology

- New diagnoses of schizophrenia occur between 0.3% and 0.6% per 1000 persons per year in the United States

- 1.5% of the U.S. population has been diagnosed with schizophrenia

- Age of onset is greater in females than in males

- Paranoid-type schizophrenia occurs earlier in males than in females

- Disorganized-type schizophrenia occurs earlier in males than in females

- Prevalence is equal for males and females

- The oldest age of onset group is between 66 and 77 years old

- A female fetus exposed to influenza has a higher risk for schizophrenia than a male fetus

- Males show significantly more structural brain abnormalities from perinatal or early childhood trauma than females

- 50% of persons with schizophrenia attempt suicide

Holoday-Worret, 1995; Kaplan and Sadock, 1994). However, the population density of the slums and the homeless mentally ill persons who receive poor follow-up care add to the stress on this vulnerable population. In economic terms, schizophrenia is the costliest of all mental disorders.

Culture, Geography, and Seasonal Influences

The manifestations of schizophrenia and the prognosis vary in different cultures. In less-developed nations, the prognosis for schizophrenia is better than in the technologically advanced cultures. Clients in the developing countries tend to have a more acute onset, fewer episodic occurrences, and less frequent problems with affect. Severe cognitive impairment is rare in Western nations. However, after an acute episode, the person with schizophrenia in the developing countries is more readily reintegrated into family and community (Betemps and Ragiel, 1994; Kaplan and Sadock, 1994).

Variations in the prevalence of schizophrenia in different geographical regions have been studied. In some climates, seasonality of birth is a factor. More babies who later become schizophrenic are born in the winter months. There are two possible explanations for this phenomenon. One is that schizophrenia may be related to prenatal exposure to viral infections. The other is that there is a seasonal release of overripe ova in the winter, with consequent anomalies in the fetus at fertilization (Kaplan and Sadock, 1994).

CLINICAL DESCRIPTION

Schizophrenia, according to DSM-IV, has the following criteria: (1) it lasts at least six months, at least one month of which includes "active-phase symptoms," and (2) the active-phase symptoms include at least two of these manifestations: hallucinations, delusions, disorganized or catatonic behavior, or disorganized speech.

There are five major subtypes of schizophrenia, and several closely related disorders. The five subtypes of schizophrenia are:

- paranoid
- disorganized (formerly called hebephrenic)
- catatonic
- undifferentiated
- residual

The closely related disorders are:

- schizophreniform
- schizoaffective
- delusional
- brief psychotic disorder
- shared psychotic disorder

- psychotic disorder due to a general medical condition
- substance-induced psychotic disorder
- pervasive developmental disorder (autism and others)
- simple schizophrenia
- postpsychotic depressive disorder of schizophrenia
- psychotic disorder not otherwise specified (NOS)

PARANOID SCHIZOPHRENIA

Paranoid schizophrenia results in less neurological and cognitive impairment and a better prognosis for the individual. However, in the active phase of the disorder, the afflicted individual is extremely ill, and the symptoms may constitute a danger to the self or others.

Delusions tend to be persecutory or grandiose and have a coherent theme. The persecutory delusions may generate anxiety, suspiciousness, anger, hostility, and violent behavior. Auditory hallucinations are common and are related to the delusionary theme. Interactions with others are rigid, intense, and controlled (APA, 1994; Fortinash and Holoday-Worret, 1995; Kaplan and Sadock, 1994).

According to the DSM-IV criteria for schizophrenia opposite, a diagnosis of paranoid schizophrenia must meet two of criteria A: the presence of delusions and hallucinations.

The other diagnostic criteria for paranoid schizophrenia—disorganized speech, behavior, and other negative symptoms—are not prominent. The delusions and hallucinations must be present for a significant portion of time, over a period of one month. This time period can be shorter if the condition is successfully treated. Also, if delusions are unusually bizarre, or if the hallucinations involve commanding or commenting voices, then only one of the criteria needs to be met. Paranoid schizophrenia often has a sudden onset, sometimes triggered by severe stressors (Fortinash and Holoday-Worret, 1995; APA, 1994). The individual with paranoid schizophrenia is sometimes referred to as a Type I, productive client, with positive symptoms.

Crow (1980) proposed that symptoms in schizophrenia could be classified as **positive** (the syndrome includes hallucinations, increased speech production with loose associations, and bizarre behavior) or **negative** (the syndrome includes flat affect, poverty of speech, poor grooming, withdrawal, and disturbance in volition) as a guide to establishing prognosis (Andreasen and Carpenter, 1993). Table 13-2 defines positive and negative symptoms.

Prognosis. The course of paranoid schizophrenia is varied but tends to be more hopeful than the courses of other subtypes. Of all the schizophrenias, paranoid schizophrenia is the most responsive to proper treatment and the most likely to qualify for the course of a single episode in full remission (APA, 1994; Kaplan and Sadock, 1994).

DSM-IV CRITERIA

Schizophrenia

A. *Characteristic symptoms:* Two (or more) of the following, each present for a significant portion of time during a 1-month period (or less if successfully treated):

    (1) delusions

    (2) hallucinations

    (3) disorganized speech (e.g., frequent derailment or incoherence)

    (4) grossly disorganized or catatonic behavior

    (5) negative symptoms, i.e., affective flattening, alogia, or avolition

Note: Only one Criterion A symptom is required if delusions are bizarre or hallucinations consist of a voice keeping up a running commentary on the person's behavior or thoughts, or two or more voices conversing with each other.

B. *Social/occupational dysfunction:* For a significant portion of the time since the onset of the disturbance, one or more major areas of functioning such as work, interpersonal relations, or self-care is markedly below the level achieved prior to the onset (or when the onset is in childhood or adolescence, failure to achieve expected level of interpersonal, academic, or occupational achievement).

C. *Duration:* Continuous signs of the disturbance persist for at least 6 months. This 6-month period must include at least 1 month of symptoms (or less if successfully treated) that meet Criterion A (i.e., active-phase symptoms) and may include periods of prodromal or residual symptoms. During these prodromal or residual periods, the signs of the disturbance may be manifested by only negative symptoms or two or more symptoms listed in Criterion A present in an attenuated form (e.g., odd beliefs, unusual perceptual experiences).

D. *Schizoaffective and Mood Disorder exclusion:* Schizoaffective Disorder and Mood Disorder with Psychotic Features have been ruled out because either (1) no Major Depressive, Manic, or Mixed Episodes have occurred concurrently with the active-phase symptoms; or (2) if mood episodes have occurred during active-phase symptoms, their total duration has been brief relative to the duration of the active and residual periods.

E. *Substance/general medical condition exclusion:* The disturbance is not due to the direct physiological effects of a substance (e.g., a drug of abuse, a medication) or a general medical condition.

F. *Relationship to a Pervasive Developmental Disorder:* If there is a history of Autistic Disorder or another Pervasive Developmental Disorder, the additional diagnosis of Schizophrenia is made only if prominent delusions or hallucinations are also present for at least a month (or less if successfully treated).

Classification of longitudinal course (can be applied only after at least 1 year has elapsed since the initial onset of active-phase symptoms):

Episodic With Interepisode Residual Symptoms (episodes are defined by the reemergence of prominent psychotic symptoms); *also specify if:* **With Prominent Negative Symptoms**

Episodic With No Interepisode Residual Symptoms

Continuous (prominent psychotic symptoms are present throughout the period of observation); *also specify if:* **With Prominent Negative Symptoms**

Single Episode In Partial Remission; *also specify if:* **With Prominent Negative Symptoms**

Single Episode In Full Remission

Other or Unspecified Pattern

Reprinted with permission from *Diagnostic and statistical manual of mental disorders,* ed 4, Washington, D.C., 1994, American Psychiatric Association.

DISORGANIZED SCHIZOPHRENIA

The disorganized type of schizophrenia, formerly known as hebephrenic schizophrenia because of its early, insidious onset and silly, childish affect, is characterized by a severe disintegration of the personality. Speech is disorganized and may include word salad (communication that includes both real and imaginary words, in no logical order), incoherent speech, and clanging (rhyming). Behavior is odd, encompassing grimacing, grunting, sniffing, posturing, rocking, stereotyped behaviors, and uninhibited sexual behaviors such as masturbating in public. Socially, the client with disorganized schizophrenia is withdrawn and inept. There may be many cognitive and psychomotor defects, such as concrete thinking, the literal interpretation and use of language or inability to abstract, **primary process thinking,** prelogical thought that aims for wish fulfillment and is associated with the pleasure principle characteristic of the *Id* portion of the personality, and poor coordination (APA, 1994; Fortinash and Holoday-Worret, 1995).

The client with disorganized schizophrenia has poor personal grooming and is often unable to complete activities of daily living (ADLs) without constant structural reminders, because the behavior is aimless and without

TABLE 13-2   Symptoms of schizophrenia classified according to Type I (positive) or Type II (negative)

Type I	Type II
• Delusions, persecutory or grandiose	• Flat or inappropriate affect
• Delusions of being controlled	• Poor eye contact
• Mind reading or thought insertion ideas	• Anhedonic attitude and asocial behavior; withdrawal
• Hallucinations, auditory or other sensory modes	• Poverty of speech; blocking and lack of inflection
• Bizarre dress and behavior	• Poor grooming and hygiene
• Thought disorganization and tangential speech	• Decreased spontaneity in behavior
• Aggressive, agitated behavior	• Lack of expressive gestures
• Pressured speech	• Lack of volition; apathy
• Suicidal ideation may be present	• Severely disturbed relationships with family, friends, peers
• Ideas of reference	• Inattentiveness

goals (Kaplan and Sadock, 1994). Many Type II symptoms are present. Development seems to have been impaired and held to about the age of seven or eight.

Prognosis. Prognosis for the client with disorganized schizophrenia is poor, stemming from an early premorbid history of impaired adjustment that continues after the active phase of the disorder. **Premorbid** refers to the period just preceding the onset of the mental illness. This individual may or may not hallucinate or have delusions, but, if they exist, they are disorganized and fragmented.

Of all the subtypes, paranoid schizophrenia and disorganized schizophrenia have the most clearly defined clinical criteria and have been studied the most. However, according to Andreasen and Carpenter (1993), insufficient attention has been paid to the negative symptoms by both the medical and the pharmacologic communities. It is, after all, the residual negative symptoms that prevent former clients from holding jobs and forming normal relationships.

CATATONIC SCHIZOPHRENIA

Catatonic schizophrenia has, as its predominant feature, intense psychomotor disturbance. This disturbance may take the form of stupor (psychomotor retardation) or excitement (psychomotor excitation). Manifestations of psychomotor disturbance include posturing, immobility, catalepsy (waxy flexibility), mutism, and negativism. There may be automatic obedience on the one hand, and excessive and purposeless movement on the other. Other symptoms include echopraxia (imitating the movements of others), echolalia (repeating what was said by another), grimacing, and stereotypical movements. Often there is rapid alteration between these extremes (APA, 1994; Fortinash and Holoday-Worret, 1995; Kaplan and Sadock, 1994).

The onset of catatonic schizophrenia often occurs with dramatic suddenness. Catatonic stupor may be preceded by an earlier withdrawal, carried to the extreme. It reflects the individual's reduced neurologic ability to fil-

ter out stimuli. There is no significant difference of age, sex, or education in the incidence of catatonic schizophrenia. To meet the DSM-IV criteria for catatonic schizophrenia, the client must exhibit two of the following behaviors: motor immobility or excessive motor activity; extreme negativism (resistance to all instructions and attempts to be moved); peculiar voluntary movements such as grimacing, stereotyped movements, or posturing; and echolalia or echopraxia (APA, 1994).

The person with catatonic schizophrenia presents a nursing challenge. While in a state of psychomotor excitement, the client may develop hyperpyrexia or collapse from extreme exhaustion. Close watch is indicated to prevent harm to self or others. Conversely, while in a stuporous state, the disease can be life-threatening because the person approaches a vegetative condition, will not eat, and is in danger of malnutrition or even starvation. Other complications may include pressure sores from lack of mobility or strange posturing, constipation, or even stasis pneumonia in the older client.

Delusions often persist throughout the withdrawn state. For example, a client may believe that he has to hold his hand out flat in front of him because the forces of good and evil are warring on the palm of his hand, and he will upset the balance of good and evil if he moves his hand. Oddly enough, although this individual may seem not to be attending to the environment around him, when he later returns to a normal state of consciousness he will remember in detail what has occurred. Nurses need to be aware of this factor and not say or do anything within the stuporous client's hearing that they would not say or do when the client is in a normal state of consciousness.

Prognosis. The prognosis for catatonic schizophrenia varies, depending on the age of onset, which is often in the early 20s to 30s. It tends to begin with an acute episode having an identifiable precipitating factor. If the client has developed a good support system before the illness, he or she will probably recover from the acute phase and have a partial or complete remission. More research is indicated for this particular type of illness, especially since it seems to have subsided in Western nations but is more prevalent in undeveloped nations where remission is usually complete.

UNDIFFERENTIATED SCHIZOPHRENIA

Undifferentiated schizophrenia meets Criterion A for schizophrenia but cannot be classified as paranoid, disorganized, or catatonic. It does not clearly meet the criteria necessary for a diagnosis in any of these conditions, but has some aspects of each type. The psychotic manifestations are extreme, including fragmented delusions, vague hallucinations, bizarre and disorganized behavior, disorientation, and incoherence (Fortinash and Holoday-Worret, 1995; Kaplan and Sadock, 1994). Affect is usually inappropriate rather than flat, and catatonic symptoms are not present.

The onset can be acute, with excited behaviors such as aggressive hitting or biting. Or the client may have chronic schizophrenia, with behavior that no longer fits a specific type but is a mixture of positive and negative symptoms. Usually the prodromal symptoms have developed over a period of years. Growth and development milestones may have been delayed. Thought processes are fragmented and have a high fantasy content (primary process thinking). The individual has few or no friends, and family relationships are strained because of odd and restless behaviors. Dress and grooming are careless, and the individual seems bored with life. Sleep patterns are disturbed by nightmares and early morning awakening.

Prognosis. The prognosis for the client with undifferentiated schizophrenia is generally poor, and the course is usually a chronic one. There are periods of exacerbation and remission where many negative symptoms prevent the patient from doing productive work, pursuing normal relationships, or enjoying life (Kaplan and Sadock, 1994).

RESIDUAL SCHIZOPHRENIA

If an individual has had at least one acute episode of schizophrenia and is now free of prominent positive symptoms but has some negative symptoms, he or she is diagnosed as suffering from residual schizophrenia. In some clients, this pattern may persist for years, with or without exacerbations. In others, it seems to taper down to a complete remission. The usual signs of the illness that may persist for the chronic or subchronic individual are mild loosening of associations, illogical thinking, emotional blunting, social withdrawal, and eccentric behavior. Diagnostic criteria for the client with residual schizophrenia are (1) absence of prominent delusions, hallucinations, disorganized speech, and disorganized or catatonic behavior; and (2) continuing evidence of the presence of negative symptoms or attenuated positive symptoms.

Prognosis. Prognosis is varied and unpredictable. It depends largely on premorbid history and the adequacy

of support systems (APA, 1994; Kaplan and Sadock, 1994).

Symptom Profiles

Neuropsychiatrists have tried to find common threads that link the schizophrenias, or areas of differentiation that separate them. There is a common, underlying dimension in schizophrenic disorder that gives rise to certain symptom profiles of a perceptual, cognitive, emotional, behavioral, or social nature. They are displayed in Table 13-3.

PERCEPTUAL DISTURBANCES

Hallucinations can occur in any of the five receptive senses (auditory, visual, tactile, olfactory, or gustatory), but the most common are auditory. It is believed that a left hemisphere brain abnormality may precipitate hallucinations because the left hemisphere contains Broca's area, the language processing center. From assessment procedures, it was determined that the left hemisphere responded to hallucinations as if it were hearing real voices. There is an indication that the hallucinations are a reflection of the actual delusional thinking of the person with schizophrenia (Green et al, 1994; Lewandowski, 1991).

Another aspect of perception that has been explored in the individual with schizophrenia is self-perception (Fortinash, 1990). One way in which the nurse can assess the severity of perceptual disturbances is by using art forms that indicate how the person with schizophrenia perceives the world or the self. Individuals with schizophrenia, because of their tendency to generalize, often report an overall negative self-perception (Evans et al, 1994). However, Dzurec (1990) revealed that clients with schizophrenia who lived in a satisfactory setting saw themselves as mentally well, although they were disabled to the extent that they were not able to live independently.

COGNITIVE DISTURBANCES

According to D'Angelo (1993), thought disorders can begin in children at risk for schizophrenia because of their heredity. Children of parents with schizophrenia tend to be conceptually disorganized, possibly because they do not correctly categorize information as other children do, in the childhood learning process. Also, children are very distractable (Smothergill and Kraut, 1993). Implications for the psychoeducation of persons with schizophrenia include:

- using times when symptoms are relatively stable
- simplifying instructions and reducing distractions
- providing both visual and verbal information
- using direct, clear terms
- teaching in small segments with frequent reinforcement
- not offering choices, which often confuse

TABLE 13-3 Clinical symptoms of schizophrenia

Perceptual	Cognitive	Emotional	Behavioral	Social
Hallucinations: 1) auditory: may be commanding; content matches delusions 2) visual 3) tactile: for example, may feel like being surrounded by spider webs 4) olfactory and gustatory: client may refuse to eat because food seems to smell or taste bad **Illusions:** false perceptions due to misinterpretations of real objects **Altered internal sensations:** 1) formication: sensation of worms crawling around inside one 2) chill: feelings of chills in the marrow of one's bones **Agnosia:** perceptual failure to recognize familiar environmental stimuli such as sounds or objects seen or felt; sometimes called "negative hallucinations" **Distortion of body image:** with respect to size, facial expression, activity, amount and nature of detail, exaggeration or diminution of body parts **Negative self-perception:** with respect to ability and competence	**Delusions:** unusual ideas, not reality based: 1) omnipotence 2) persecution 3) controlling or being controlled **Derealization:** loss of ego boundaries; cannot tell where own body ends and environment begins; feeling that the world around one is not real or distorted **Ideas of reference:** notion that other people or the media are talking to or about one **Errors in recall of memory:** due to incorrect categorization **Difficulty sustaining attention:** 1) unable to complete tasks 2) errors of omission **Incorrect use of language:** 1) neologisms (invented words) 2) incoherence 3) echolalia and word salad 4) concrete, restricted vocabulary 5) comprehension difficulties 6) looseness of associations **Flight of ideas:** abrupt change of topic in a rapid flow of speech	**Labile affect: range of emotions:** 1) apathy, dulled response 2) flattened affect 3) reduced responsiveness 4) exaggerated euphoria 5) rage **Inappropriate affect:** laughing at sad events, crying over joyous ones **Disruption in limbic functioning:** inability to screen out disruptive stimuli and loss of voluntary control of response	**Little impulse control:** 1) sudden scream as a protest of frustration 2) self-mutilation, to substitute physical for emotional pain 3) injury to a body part believed to be offensive 4) response to command hallucinations **Inability to cope with depression:** 1) depressed client has a 50% risk for suicide 2) frequent exacerbations and remissions in one who has insight 3) lack of social support to help **Inability to manage anger:** anger and lack of impulse control lead to violence: verbal aggression, destruction of property; injury to others, homicide **Substance abuse as coping:** dulls painful psychological symptoms **Noncompliance with medication:** may feel it is not needed or has too many side effects	**Poor peer relationships:** 1) few friends, as a child or adolescent 2) preference for solitude **Low interest in hobbies and activities:** 1) daydreamer 2) not functioning well in social or occupational areas 3) preoccupied and detached 4) behavioral autism **Loss of interest in appearance:** 1) careless grooming 2) introversion **Not competitive in sports or academics:** 1) poor adjustment to school 2) withdrawal from activities **May suffer from:** 1) attention deficit disorder 2) somatic symptoms

As a result of thought disturbance, speech is affected. Subtle forms of speech disorders are *circumstantiality,* in which the person digresses to unnecessary details, and *tangentiality,* or responding in a manner irrelevant to the topic at hand. If the person is less impaired, listening for themes may help to identify client concerns (Hoffman, 1994; Kaplan and Sadock, 1994).

The process of thought in schizophrenia fluctuates with the clinical status and may venture into the world of fantasy, with autistic thinking, **perseveration** (persistent repetition of the same idea, in response to different questions), or **poverty of thought** (lack of ability to produce thoughts, loose associations) (Gundel and Rudolf, 1993). In the client who is chronic, there is a general decline in intellectual functioning over the years.

Memory in adult-onset schizophrenia is usually intact. But in persons with chronic schizophrenia, it is affected by emotion; the client remembers less and forgets rapidly over time. However, negative emotional experiences and concepts are remembered more readily than positive ones, perhaps reflecting a depressed and negative outlook on the world (Calev and Edelist, 1993). Clients with chronic schizophrenia have little insight into their illness and suffer impaired judgment.

EMOTIONAL DISTURBANCES

Although emotional disturbance is a primary sign of all forms of schizophrenia, affect flattening and poor eye contact are most associated with undifferentiated schizophrenia. Persons with schizophrenia cannot adapt their thinking to the common reality; they block whatever does not fit into their own inner reality (Gundel and Rudolf, 1993).

Biologically, the individual with schizophrenia may be unable to screen out disruptive stimuli because of an imbalance in neurotransmitters. A deficiency in GABA, for example, may result in a rush of conflicting stimuli and labile or inappropriate emotional expression, while a deficiency in cholecystokinin is related to avolition and flat affect (see Table 13-1). Developmentally, it was found that in children at risk for schizophrenia, neuromotor dysfunction due to trauma or other causes indicated the later appearance of flat affect (Dworkin et al, 1993).

BEHAVIORAL DISTURBANCES

The behavioral disturbance of greatest concern that is seen in schizophrenia is the possibility of violence. The incidence and type of violence largely depend on certain factors: diagnostic type of schizophrenia, degree of psychopathology, history of violent behavior in the past, abuse of substances, and noncompliance with medications (Kennedy, 1993; Mulvey, 1994). In terms of diagnostic type, there is a significant difference between paranoid schizophrenia and other types of schizophrenia; the client with paranoia is higher in physical aggression toward other people (Kennedy, 1993; Mulvey, 1994).

However, although the *relative risk* for violence is higher in the mentally ill population (of any diagnosis) than in the general population, the *absolute risk* is very small (Mulvey, 1994). Whether or not the inclination for violence is expressed depends on other factors, as indicated above.

SOCIAL COMPETENCE PROFILES

Typically, the individual with schizophrenia has a history of a schizoid or schizotypal personality. Dworkin et al (1994) maintain that poor social competence may be important in the development of schizophrenia. Once again, the issue of nature versus nurture arises, and there is speculation that children raised by parents with schizophrenia may emulate their parents in socialization behavior (Turner, 1993). There is a detachment from the environment and an autistic relationship to reality (Gundel and Rudolf, 1993; Kaplan and Sadock, 1994).

Of all of the diagnostic profiles, however, the two still commonly used to describe schizophrenia were derived from the early work of Bleuler (1911) and Schneider (1934), as presented in Table 13-4.

BIOLOGIC PROFILES

Symptom profiles are supported by neurologic examinations, neuropsychologic tests, and various brain-scanning techniques (neuroimaging), particularly relevant for clients with schizophrenia. Some of these examinations are presented in Table 13-5. (See Chapter 5 for an explanation of relevant brain-scanning techniques.) In general, the tests verify findings that schizophrenia has diffuse, nonlocalizable areas of dysfunction. Evidence of generalized impairment can be found in persons with first-episode as well as chronic schizophrenia, although the degree of impairment may differ with subtypes. Individuals with schizophrenia seem to have impairments in the stimulus inhibition (gating) circuitry of the brain, sometimes leading to stimulus overload. They are thus handicapped in sorting out and paying attention to the information necessary to solve a problem.

Modern brain-scanning technology has enabled scientists to assemble not only a structural image of the brain, active or inert, but also a functional image that indicates activity in various areas. Figure 13-3 shows a BEAM of a client with schizophrenia.

PROGNOSIS

In addition to the general statements about prognosis to be expected for each subtype of schizophrenia, there is recent evidence for specific relationships between symptom profiles and predictions for prognosis. For example, Goldman et al (1993) looked at the interrelationship between neuropsychological functioning and treatment response and found that the ability to encode, process information, and interact with the environment depends

---

TABLE 13-4 Diagnostic profiles of Bleuler and Schneider

Bleuler	Schneider
Characteristics of schizophrenia: • incongruence between feelings and thoughts • incongruence in the behavioral expression of feelings and thoughts Four primary symptoms of schizophrenia: • affect is disturbed • autism is present • ambivalence is common • associations are loosened Assessory symptoms: • hallucinations • delusions	First-rank symptoms of schizophrenia: • hallucinations • thought withdrawal (belief that one's thoughts have been removed from one's head) • thought broadcasting (belief that one's thoughts are broadcast from one's head) • delusions • somatic experiences Second-rank symptoms of schizophrenia: • perceptual disorders • perplexity • mood changes • feelings of emotional impoverishment

---

TABLE 13-5 Biologic profiles in schizophrenia

NEUROLOGIC EXAMINATIONS

Test	Function
Apgar Rating of the Newborn	To rate functioning of the newborn nervous system
Physiologic and Anatomic Testing of the Nervous System (General)	To discover infections, lesions, or metabolic problems that may affect the nervous system

NEUROPSYCHOLOGIC TESTS

Test	Function
Halstead-Reitan Battery	To test higher cortical functioning To detect early signs of memory and cognitive dysfunction To design and evaluate remediation programs (Osmon, 1991)
Luria-Nebraska Test Battery	To predict behavior by examining neurologic functioning (Meador and Nichols, 1991) To assess client progress in various areas
Eye-Tracking and Auditory Tests	To discover information-processing deficits (Perry and Braff, 1994)

ELECTRICAL IMPULSE TESTING

Test	Function
Electrodermal Activity Test (EDA)	To indicate the extent of negative symptomatology present in the client with schizophrenia (Fuentes et al, 1993)
Electroencephalogram (EEG)	To detect electrical activity in seizure disorders, sometimes associated with schizophrenia

---

on being able to attend, focus, and remember. When these abilities are compromised by frontal lobe impairment, negative symptoms tend to remain and interfere with daily living.

Unfortunately, although there are many drugs on the market that have helped some clients with schizophrenia, the drugs do not seem to be effective for all. Those clients having positive symptoms are most helped by drugs. However, clozapine, discussed later in this chapter, does seem to relieve some negative symptoms as well (Breier et al, 1994). A better adjustment to the community is thus made possible for more clients with schizophrenia. Specific issues a community nurse faces are discussed in Nursing Care in the Community on page 302.

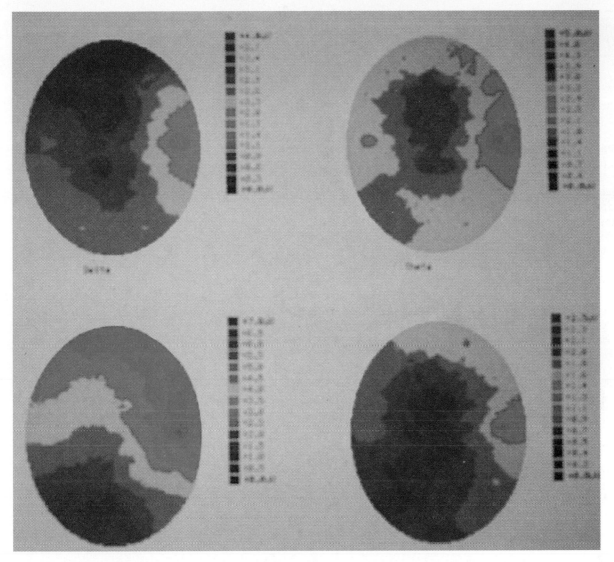

Figure 13-3 BEAM (Bio-Electron Activity Measure) of a client with schizophrenia. The differences in topography in the various brainwave bands indicate differences in metabolism. When compared with BEAMs of individuals without the disorder, variations can confirm symptoms such as hallucinations or emotional withdrawal.

(From WW Orrison, JD Lewine, JA Sanders, MF Hartshorne, *Functional brain imaging,* St. Louis, 1995, Mosby.)

DISCHARGE CRITERIA

For the client with schizophrenia to be discharged to the community, the following criteria need to be met. The client will:

- Verbalize absence or control of hallucinations

- Identify events or episodes of increased anxiety that promote hallucinations

- Have family or significant other willing to serve as a support network

- Accept referral of self or significant other to a physician, therapist, or agency for help and monitoring

- Accept responsibility for own actions and self-care

- Verbalize ways of coping with anxiety, stress, and problems encountered in the community

- Have access to safe living environment in the community: own home, board and care, or halfway house

- Use known community resources such as support groups, day care centers, and vocational or rehabilitation programs

- Explain the following about medication: importance, expected effects, adverse effects, prescribed dose and time of taking the medication, effects of the interaction of the medication with other substances such as food or alcohol

Nursing Care in the Community

Schizophrenia

The community mental health nurse often works with a continuum of clients with schizophrenia. This clientele includes young persons newly diagnosed with schizophrenic illnesses and persons with schizophrenia who have been functioning adequately for a few years on neuroleptic medications. Older adults with long-standing diagnoses may be taking medications but are socially isolated because their support systems have been exhausted as family members withdraw, die, or move away. The former and the latter may be the most problematic for the nurse providing support in the community; the first requires support due to increased family involvement, the second due to diminished family care.

When a young person who has been hospitalized and diagnosed with schizophrenia returns to the community, his or her family has already been disrupted by the individual's bizarre behavior. Family members may need increased help to adjust to this frightening diagnosis. The nurse is an important liaison with the medical community and may also provide a reality check when family interactions seem out of control. The nurse may make referrals to community service organizations and support groups, while serving as the "gatekeeper" or contact to the hospital.

For the adult client diagnosed with schizophrenia, the community mental health nurse is also an important contact. The nurse can help with problems of medication management, give support when stressful situations arise, and advise the psychiatrist when the client's behavior indicates that the current regimen is not effective. The goal is to maintain the client at an optimal, satisfying level of life activities, to be determined together with the client's expressed desire. The cooperative nature of the interaction must be emphasized.

Many older adults who have had schizophrenia for much of their life may be isolated because many of their family of origin are either dead or remote. Their most important contacts may be either in mental health agencies or in secondary support systems, such as board and care operators, hotel managers, store owners in the local community, or employers. They may need not only guidance about medications but also help with financial management and basic ADLs, such as nutrition, clothing, and cleanliness. Sometimes planning a periodic special outing could promote increased interest in appearance and behavior.

The problems of street drug abuse and homelessness are also concerns of mental health nurses in the community. Many of the more socially isolated individuals with schizophrenia have found the society of the streets tolerable and the use of street drugs an acceptable alternative to prescribed medications. The mental health nurse who attempts to intervene in this cycle may encounter much resistance from the community, as well as from the client. Often it will require the support of not only a trained mental health team but also the education and participation of the entire community to break this cycle. Mental health nurses must be prepared to work with the political system to help their clients on the edge of the system.

THE NURSING PROCESS ■ ■ ■ ■ ■ ■ ■ ■ ■ ■ ■ ■ ■ ■ ■

■ ASSESSMENT

Assessment of the individual with schizophrenia is complicated because of the different symptom profiles for the various subtypes of the condition. Subjective data are obtained through symptom reporting and by the behavioral descriptions of significant others. Objective assessment is done by observation, rating scales, and by checking biologic indicators, as described in earlier sections. For psychiatric-mental health nurses, it is important not to lose sight of the biologic focus so prevalent in the other specialties. For example, ataxia may indicate extrapyramidal side effects of medication. And, just as with

any patient, vital signs, nutrition, exercise, and sleep assessment are important (Trygstad, 1994).

Although the nursing assessment includes certain biologic indicators, it relies largely on psychological data and may use the Mental Status Examination rating scale to organize the data (see Chapter 6, The Nursing Process). The Mental Status Examination considers the categories of appearance, behavior, orientation, memory, thought processes, perceptual processes, intellectual functioning, feelings (mood) and affect, insight, and judgment. Four of these categories are particularly important in schizophrenia: disturbances in perception, thought, feelings, and behavior.

Nursing Assessment Questions

The Schizophrenias

1. "What problems have you been having recently? How do you feel differently now than before?" (to determine client's perception of problem)

2. "Do you now or have you ever in the past used alcohol or drugs? If so, when and how often?" (to determine client's use of substances)

3. "Have you heard (sounds, voices, messages), seen (lights, figures), smelled (strange, bad, good odors), tasted (strange, bad, good tastes), or felt (touching, warm, cold sensation) anything that others who were present did not?" (to determine if the client is having hallucinations)

4. "What are the voices that you hear like? What do they say? Are they troubling for you?" (to determine if they instruct client to harm self or others)

Questions to determine if client is experiencing delusions:

1. "Do you feel that someone or something outside of you is controlling you in some way? Are you able to control other people?"

2. "Do you feel you are being watched? Followed?"

3. "Are people talking about you? If yes, explain how you know this."

4. "Are you experiencing guilt? Do you have anything to feel guilty about? Do you think you are a bad person? If yes, what makes you believe this?"

Things to observe for during assessment:

- Cognitive changes, e.g., concrete thinking, delusions, fantasies, or autistic communication
- Hallucinations
- Depersonalization
- Somatization
- Unusual gestures, posture, tone of voice, mannerisms
- Flat affect
- Disheveled, unkempt physical appearance
- Reaction to the interviewer (receptive, distant, resistant)

For children and adolescents, the assessment of positive and negative symptoms must take into consideration the developmental status of the individual. Measures of thought disturbances in children must consider that their normal patterns of thinking are concrete; abstract thought is not a part of normal thinking in the child. Likewise, since impulse control is developmental in the adolescent, the measures of impulse control must be adjusted in consideration of the client's age (Fields et al, 1994).

■ ■ NURSING DIAGNOSIS

Nursing diagnoses are formulated from the information obtained during the assessment phase of the nursing process. The accuracy of the diagnosis depends on a careful in-depth assessment. The following is a listing of some of the more common diagnoses applicable to schizophrenia.

NANDA Diagnoses for Schizophrenia

Sensory/Perceptual Alteration
Altered Thought Processes
Impaired Verbal Communication
Ineffective Individual Coping
Altered Family Processes
Social Isolation
Self-Care Deficit
Risk for Violence

■ ■ ■ OUTCOME IDENTIFICATION

Outcome identification is an estimate of the behavioral change anticipated following interventions and is influenced by the severity of the symptoms, the cultural milieu,

---

COLLABORATIVE DIAGNOSES

DSM-IV Diagnoses*	NANDA Diagnoses**
Schizophrenia, Paranoid	Sensory/perceptual alteration
Schizophrenia, Catatonic	Altered thought processes
Schizophrenia, Disorganized	Impaired verbal communication
Schizophrenia, Undifferentiated	Ineffective individual coping
Schizophrenia, Residual	Altered family processes

*Reprinted with permission from *Diagnostic and statistical manual of mental disorders,* ed 4, Washington, D.C., 1994, American Psychiatric Association.

**Reprinted with permission from *NANDA nursing diagnoses: definitions and classifications, 1995–1996,* Philadelphia, 1994, North American Nursing Diagnosis Association.

and the prognosis for the particular diagnosis. Thus, the outcomes of schizophrenia may reflect complex interactions.

Client will:

1. Demonstrate significant reduction in hallucinations and delusions.
2. Demonstrate absence of self-mutilating, violent, or aggressive behaviors.
3. Demonstrate reality-based thinking and behavior.
4. Engage in own hygiene, grooming, and ADL skills.
5. Socialize with peers and staff and participate in all groups.
6. Comply with medication regimen and verbalize an understanding of the role of medications in reducing psychotic symptoms.
7. Demonstrate more functional coping and problem-solving methods.
8. Participate in discharge planning with family.

CASE STUDY

Henry, a 40-year-old man living on Social Security payments in a single-room occupancy (SRO) facility, was never quite able to budget his meager income to last the whole month. An individual with chronic schizophrenia, Henry had a fixed delusion that he owned the hotel where he lived but that the manager and the town government were defrauding him of his rental money. When he was short of cash at the end of the month, he became abusive and aggressive. Fearing assault, the manager would call the police, and Henry would be readmitted to the psychiatric hospital. In about 10 days he would be discharged to the same SRO, where he lived quietly for a while, helping the manager with tasks. This was a repetitive pattern.

Critical Thinking and Outcome Identification

1. What is the significance of Henry's delusion, given his low socioeconomic status?
2. Henry received good care at the psychiatric hospital. Standard outcome criteria for discharge were always met. If this continues, what are the chances Henry will hold his delusion? Why might a staff attempt to break it be risky?
3. What are some teaching strategies that nurses could try with this client? In what form would they best be implemented?
4. If you were a community mental health nurse, how would you do follow-up care on Henry? What signs of rising anxiety would you look for?

PLANNING

Planning nursing interventions and treatment geared to the whole person and his or her social environment, including the family, is challenging. Since behavioral problems come from many sources, and may range from less serious to much more serious, interventions at a variety of levels also need to be considered. Medical interventions generally are focused on underlying biologic factors and involve diagnostic procedures such as neuroimaging, somatic strategies, and treatment with medication. The nurse's role at this level is to prepare the client and family by explaining the rationale for the interventions and assisting with compliance. The nurse can also use nursing measures at this level, based on his or her knowledge of basic biologic functioning and needs.

Interpersonally and socially, clients with schizophrenia are disadvantaged by being unable to view things from the perspectives of others. Because of the inability to abstract and correctly interpret, the individual with schizophrenia sees others as unpredictable, as being competitors for attention, and as being in control of what is "right" or "wrong" in an absolute sense. Role-playing scenarios, which help clients to see things from another person's perspective, are helpful. Socialization should be a focus of the treatment plan by including the clients in activities that are supportive, nonthreatening, and provide helpful feedback on how the client presents to others. Activities that do not include competition are useful in quelling aggressive tendencies. Nurses must be alert to avoid power struggles.

Family interactions may be particularly difficult for the client with schizophrenia. If the family (or foster family) does not understand what the treatment team is trying to accomplish and how they are structuring the treatment plan, clients who have been discharged from an acute psychotic episode are more likely to experience recidivism. The closer the kinship, the stronger the tension created by ambivalent emotions, which often confuse the client whose insight may be poor (McEnvoy et al, 1993).

IMPLEMENTATION

First and most important is the involvement of the client and family in the treatment process, with explanations and rationales given for all interventions. Interventions may be well planned but challenging for the nurse if there are misunderstandings about what is expected; resistance from client, family, or others; or financial or environmental constraints. As much as possible, clients should set their own goals and pace for treatment and progress.

In the beginning, a client may be so ill that he or she cannot understand or accept an appropriate effort to help. In that case, the nurse may need to work on establishing a therapeutic relationship first before the well-meaning interventions will be accepted.

NURSING CARE PLAN ■ ■ ■ ■   ■ ■ ■ ■   ■ ■ ■ ■ ■ ■

Michael, a studious 16-year-old boy, was picked up at his home by the police because a neighbor had accused him of burglary. He spent the night at the local jail because his distraught parents were unable to obtain his release. The next day the matter was cleared up in court as a case of mistaken identity, and Michael was released. However, he appeared to be terrified by the experience and stayed in his bed, unmoving and unresponsive, completely neglecting self-care and feeding. This continued for several days. His worried parents spoke to the school psychologist, who recommended hospitalization. His admission was another frightening experience. He became very agitated, accused the staff of plotting against him, and watched everyone in the room. He yelled at the television set, threw a chair at it, and complained that bugs were coming out of it and crawling all over him. Michael appeared markedly dehydrated and disheveled.

DSM-IV Diagnoses

AXIS I   Schizophrenia, Paranoid Type

AXIS II   (Personality disorders) No diagnosis

AXIS III (Medical diagnosis) None

AXIS IV   (Severity of Psychosocial Stressors) Severe = 7
Frightened by police
False accusation of burglary
Embarrassed by arrest procedure
Spent the night in jail
Having to explain to parents
Traumatic experience in courtroom
Having to face peers and teachers at school

AXIS V   GAF: Serious Impairment = 10 on admission

Nursing Diagnosis: Risk for violence: self-directed and directed at others. Risk factors: history of violence, agitated behavior patterns, paranoid delusion, vigilance and scanning, and hallucinations.

Client Outcomes	Interventions	Evaluation
• Michael will demonstrate absence of violent or aggressive behaviors.	• Continue to assess and monitor risk factors *to prevent violence and promote safety of client and others.* • Provide frequent "time outs," brief, low-key interactions and PRN medications *to calm Michael by providing opportunities for rest and relaxation, ventilation of feelings, and decreased agitation.*	• Michael demonstrates calmer behavior patterns with reduced episodes of "yelling" and absence of violent outbursts.
• Michael will state that he no longer feels the urge to throw objects and will cease to pace.	• Reduce environmental stimulation and offer PRN medications *to promote a quiet, soothing milieu that may reduce Michael's impulsivity, agitated pacing, and increase safety.*	• Michael verbalizes fewer urges to engage in compulsive outbursts and ceases to throw objects.
• Michael will show absence or reduction of psychosis. He will no longer believe others are plotting against him. He will no longer see or feel bugs. He will stop vigilance and scanning.	• Present nonthreatening reality; reassure Michael that others in environment are clients, staff, and visitors, and offer PRN medications *to minimize psychosis, enforce reality, and prevent violent episodes.*	• Michael says he no longer believes people are plotting against him, does not see or feel bugs, and is able to watch T.V. without incident.
• Michael will manifest calm, cooperative behavior and comply with medication regimen.	• Praise Michael for efforts made to refrain from impulsive, angry outbursts and comply with medication regimen *to encourage positive feedback that tends to reinforce functional behaviors.* • Continue to support, monitor and teach the merits of prescribed medications and psychosocial interventions *to engage Michael and his family in the treatment plan and prevent aggressive episodes.*	• Michael and his parents express a basic understanding of the role medication plays in reducing or eliminating Michael's troubling thoughts and feelings that may provoke violent or impulsive behaviors.

NURSING CARE PLAN

Nursing Diagnosis: Sensory perceptual alterations related to psychosocial stressors that exceed Michael's ability to cope, possible biologic factors, anxiety as evidenced by withdrawal from the environment, seeing and feeling bugs, and experiencing fear and terror, guardedness, and self-care deficit.

Client Outcomes	Interventions	Evaluation
• Michael will report absence or reduction in experiences of fear and terror.	• Continue to monitor etiologies *to prevent further increase in symptoms.* • Establish trust with Michael through brief, frequent interactions. *The client must first trust the nurse in order to talk about fears, hallucinations, and other concerns.*	• Michael appears calmer, and seeks nurses when troubled by sensory-perceptual disturbances and other fears and concerns.
• Michael will demonstrate a reduction in anxiety to a tolerable level, and will cease to withdraw from the environment.	• Approach Michael in a calm, nonthreatening manner with low to moderate voice tone *to reduce Michael"s guardedness, anxiety, and fear, and increase his ability to interpret reality.*	• Michael is no longer guarded and begins to interact with others in the milieu in a calm manner.
• Michael will attend to self-care needs (hygiene, grooming, eating).	• Assist and encourage Michael to attend to self-care needs *to increase self-esteem, provide structured routine, and encourage peer acceptance.*	• Michael appears clean and adequately groomed, feeds himself and eats with peers in client dining area.
• Michael will express absence or reduction in hallucinations (bugs, possible voices) and will participate in unit activities.	• Continue to present a nonthreatening reality to Michael, engaging him in reality-based topics and activities *to increase Michael's awareness of actual versus irrational events, and to promote socialization.*	• Michael engages in reality-based conversations with staff, peers and family, and participates in unit groups and activities.
• Michael will comply with the medication regimen and express an understanding of the role medications play in reducing or eliminating hallucinations.	• Offer Michael PRN medications and teach the importance of medications in establishing a biochemical balance that reduces hallucinations and restores clear realistic perceptions *to encourage and reinforce Michael's compliance with his medication regimen.*	• Michael and his family verbalize understanding of how medications work to reduce hallucinations and promote functional, realistic behaviors.

Nursing Diagnosis: Altered thought process, related to anxiety, psychosocial/environmental stressors, biologic factors, impaired ability to process and synthesize information, as evidenced by exaggerated responses of fear and terror following traumatic experience, increased agitation, guarding and scanning, pacing, and paranoid delusion.

Client Outcomes	Interventions	Evaluation
• Michael will display a calm, low-key demeanor versus agitated, anxious or pacing behaviors.	• Approach Michael in a calm, low-key manner *to avoid increasing Michael's anxiety which could foster altered thoughts and perceptions.*	• Michael appears calm and seeks out staff for help when he feels anxiety rising due to excessive stimulation.
• Michael will cease to display hypervigilant, scanning, or guarding behaviors.	• Reduce environmental stimulation that distracts Michael *to decrease his suspiciousness and guardedness.*	• Michael ceases to scan his environment and is less guarded and suspicious.

NURSING CARE PLAN ▪ ▪ ▪ ▪ ▪ ▪ ▪ ▪ ▪ ▪ ▪ ▪ ▪ ▪ ▪

Client Outcomes	Interventions	Evaluation
• Michael will manifest absence of delusions (bugs coming out of the television set; staff plotting against him).	• Present reality to Michael in a calm, nonthreatening manner with statements such as, "Michael, those people are on the nursing staff. They are discussing the clients' daily schedule of activities. I don't see any bugs," *to assist Michael in correcting misinterpretations and reduce paranoia, without challenging his belief system, which is tied in with his self-esteem.*	• Michael states, "It seems like a bad dream. It was really frightening to me at the time, but I know now that there were no bugs coming out of the television set." • Michael recognizes and acknowledges staff, other clients on the unit, and visitors for who they are and the roles they have in reality.
• Michael will socialize with others and participate in group activities.	• Engage Michael in group activities, beginning with the more structured, less threatening ones first, and gradually incorporating more informal, spontaneous activities *to increase Michael's socialization skills and expand his reality base in a nonthreatening way.*	• Michael states that he enjoys the activities in arts and crafts, where he made a drawing for his mother, and the recreation sessions, where he played volleyball with other clients.
• Michael will use judgment, insight, and problem-solving abilities and demonstrate reality-based thinking with absence of paranoia.	• Continue to assess Michael's ability to think logically and use realistic judgment and problem-solving abilities *to determine the extent of Michael's cognitive impairment and progress made in use of logical thinking.* • Offer Michael praise as soon as he begins to differentiate reality-based and nonreality-based thinking. *Positive reinforcement increases Michael's self-esteem and encourages him to identify and continue reality-based thoughts and appropriate behaviors.*	• Michael interacts logically in client community meetings, bringing reality-based problems and reasonable suggestions to the group. He participates willingly in the activities of the unit.

Nursing Diagnosis: Risk for altered parent/child attachment, related to parents' and client's responses to client's psychosis and acting out episodes, as evidenced by parents' concern, fear, and bewilderment regarding their son's dysfunctional behavior.

Client Outcomes	Interventions	Evaluation
• Michael and family will respond favorably to client's treatment plan and family will participate in Michael's care.	• Listen actively to Michael's parents' concerns, allowing them to express fears and anxieties about their son's mental illness, giving them support, empathy, and information. *Listening allows the parents to express pent-up emotions and realistic concerns, while it lessens critical fears and strengthens parent-child bonding.*	• Michael's parents express understanding of their son's mental disorder and willingness to engage in his treatment plan.
• Michael's parents will express realistic hope in their son's rehabilitation and recovery.	• Discuss Michael's strengths and accomplishments with his parents *to show that his previous accomplishments and strengths can work to overcome current setbacks.*	• Michael's parents express their love for their son and hope for his recovery.

NURSING CARE PLAN ▪ ▪ ▪ ▪ ▪ ▪ ▪ ▪ ▪ ▪ ▪ ▪ ▪ ▪ ▪ ▪

Client Outcomes	*Interventions*	*Evaluation*
• Michael and his parents will comply with his medication and psychosocial regimens.	• Educate Michael and his family about the importance of both medication and therapeutic interventions in treating Michael's debilitating symptoms *to assist them in understanding the importance of all aspects of treatment.*	• Michael and his parents are able to explain the actions of and importance of medication and other interactions before Michael is discharged home.
• Michael will be discharged home to parents after one week on the unit and resume school and home activities one week after returning home.	• Educate Michael and his parents about the importance of follow-up care and making appointments with therapist *to prepare Michael and family for transition to home and school and promote parent/child relations at highest possible level.*	• Michael and his family express satisfaction at the discharge planning arrangements. They are observed leaving the hospital smiling. Michael is between his parents and his arms are linked with theirs.

An existing therapeutic relationship between client and nurse will later be expanded to include the client's family or significant other, for lasting effectiveness of the proposed interventions. In some cases, the interventions will need to be made at yet another level, the level of the school or the workplace. Everyone must be made aware of the what, why, and how of the therapeutic plan so that they can work as a team. The client's cultural background must also be considered when planning interventions.

The family's economic situation also deserves attention. Health care personnel are not usually thinking of the cost of implementing a care plan, which may involve psychotherapy, medication, diet, transportation access to outpatient care, or other factors creating unplanned expenses. It is important to assess for such expenses, problem-solve the issues, and include the solutions with the plan.

Nursing Interventions

1. Assess and monitor risk factors *to prevent violence and promote safety of client and others.*

2. Reduce/minimize environmental stimulation *to promote a quiet, soothing milieu that may lessen client's impulsivity and agitation and prevent accident or injury.*

3. Provide frequent "time-outs" and/or brief, low-key interactions *to calm client by providing opportunities for rest, relaxation, and ventilation of impulsive feelings, which will reduce risk of acting-out behavior.*

4. Support and monitor prescribed medical and psychosocial interventions *to encourage client and family in the treatment plan and prevent client's behavior from escalating to violence.*

5. Use clear, concrete statements versus abstract, general statements. *The client may not be able to understand complex messages, and, as such, they may exacerbate misperceptions and/or hallucinations. Individuals with schizophrenia generally respond better to concrete messages during the acute phase.*

6. Attempt to determine precipitating factors that may exacerbate client's hallucinatory experiences, e.g., stressors that may trigger sensory-perceptual disturbances. *Although hallucinations may have a biochemical etiology, they may be exacerbated by outside stressors in a vulnerable client, and identifying such stressors may help to prevent severity of the hallucinatory experience.*

7. Praise client for reality-based perceptions, reduction/cessation in aggressive/acting-out behaviors, and appropriate social interaction and group participation. *Warranted praise reinforces repetition of functional behaviors when given at appropriate times during the treatment regimen, such as when medication has begun to take effect.*

8. Educate client and family/significant others about client's symptoms, the importance of medication compliance, and continued use of therapeutic support services after discharge *to facilitate client and family/significant other's knowledge base, ensure client's continued therapeutic support, and possibly prevent relapse after discharge from the hospital.*

9. Distract client from delusions that tend to exacerbate aggressive or potentially violent episodes. *Engaging client in more functional, less anxiety-provoking activities increases the reality base and decreases the risk for violent episodes that may be provoked by troubling delusions.*

10. Focus on the meaning or feeling engendered by client's delusional system rather than focus on the delusional content itself *to help meet client's needs, reinforce reality, and discourage the false belief without challenging or threatening the client.*

11. Accompany client to group activities, beginning with the more structured, less threatening ones first, and gradually incorporating more informal, spontaneous activities *to increase client's socialization skills and expand the reality base in a nonthreatening way.*

12. Assist with personal hygiene, appropriate dress, and grooming until client can function independently *to prevent physical complications and preserve self-esteem.*

13. Establish routine times and goals for self-care, and add more complex tasks as the client's condition improves. *Routine and structure tend to organize and promote reality in the client's world.*

14. Spend intervals of time with the client each day, engaging in nonchallenging interactions *to ease the client out into the community by first developing trust, rapport, and respect.*

15. Assess the client's self-concept. *A low self-concept may result from or perpetuate social isolation.*

16. Act as a role model for social behaviors in interactions by maintaining good eye contact, appropriate social distance, and a calm demeanor *to help the client identify appropriate social behaviors.*

17. Keep all appointments for interactions with the client *to promote client trust and self-esteem.*

18. Listen actively to client's family/significant others, allowing them to express fears and anxieties about mental illness, giving them support and empathy, and emphasizing client's strengths *to provide ventilation of pent-up emotions and calm irrational fears while acknowledging realistic concerns; to promote hope and bonding between family/significant other and client.*

Additional Treatment Modalities

It is very important to have health practitioners work together in mental health treatment. Consequently, team meetings are common on the psychiatric units, where psychiatric nurses, psychiatrists, psychologists, social workers, occupational and recreational therapists, pharmacologists, special education teachers (for children and adolescents), and other support workers all communicate regarding the clients' conditions and treatment plans.

Briefly described below are the activities and goals of these collaborative professionals in their respective fields.

Psychopharmacology

Psychopharmacology is the somatic treatment of choice today. The psychopharmacist dispenses medications for psychiatric clients according to the physician's prescription. He or she keeps informed on new developments in psychotropic drugs and educates the staff regarding the actions and side effects of the newer neuroleptic drugs. The psychopharmacist also consults with the psychiatrist regarding chemical properties of the medications and their interactions with food and other drugs. In many institutions, the psychopharmacist also has the responsibility of client education.

For an extensive discussion of the psychotrophic drugs used for the treatment of schizophrenia, refer to Chapter 23.

Psychotrophic drugs often have serious side effects. Two of the most serious are akathisia and neuroleptic malignant syndrome (NMS).

When a client is discharged to the family and community, one important criterion is that he or she accept responsibility for self-care, particularly with respect to medication. This has important implications for health teaching by nurses (see Client and Family Teaching Guidelines on page 310).

Somatic Therapy

Somatic therapy had its origin in the concept of the sanitarium, a place where persons with mental illness could go for rest and healthy physical treatment. The idea of the sanitarium was to offer the clients fresh air, vitamins, a healthy diet, and rest and relaxation. This is still a good idea, although more than palliative treatment is available today.

Somatic therapies are infrequently used today, except for electroconvulsive therapy (ECT), which is used most often for severe depression and for some schizophrenic syndromes that are short-term and have affective symptoms (Valente, 1991). ECT is also useful for the client with catatonic schizophrenia. A course of treatment usually consists of 6 to 12 episodes. Nursing implications for the client receiving therapy are explanation, renegotiation of client's consent, nurturance, monitoring, orientation, support, family teaching, and analgesics for headache following treatment. ECT is discussed in detail in Chapter 23.

Other somatic therapies that have fallen into disuse are psychosurgery (lobotomy), insulin coma therapy, hydrotherapy, and narcotherapy. Therapeutic use of seclusion, restraints, and jackets is discussed later in this section.

Milieu Therapy

Milieu therapy is a 24-hour environment that shelters, protects, supports, and enhances the client with mental illness. This is the model currently in use on psychiatric units today (see Figure 13-4). It is characterized by indi-

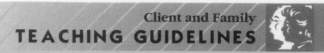

Client and Family
TEACHING GUIDELINES

Medications

Teach the Client and Family	Strategies	Rationale
Right to informed consent and disclosure regarding benefits, side effects, anticipated prognosis with and without medication, alternatives	Initially, and any time the medication or dosage is changed, written permission is obtained from the client. Items in the left column are discussed with the client. Nurse consults with physician regarding disclosure beneficial to client versus disclosure that may be harmful.	Client has the right to choose the extent to which society may intervene. Client experiences autonomy, self-esteem, and self-control. Client develops trust because of the regard for his or her concerns.
Correct storage and administration of medications	Explain, demonstrate, and request return demonstration on handling, administration. Work with client to prepare a check chart on medication, dosage, and times. Gain control of the environment: reduce distractions, simplify instructions, teach in small segments, reinforce often.	Safety of client and others is assured. Client who is involved develops ownership of process; compliance. Client will be able to focus better, minimize frustration, feel successful.
Symptoms that may be reduced or eliminated by the use of medication; action of medication	Encourage client's own desire to prevent relapse; explain in a matter-of-fact way that many people have various illnesses and take medication for them.	Offers client hope and reinforcement. Shares rationale for treatment.
Side effects that may be experienced	Show client how to use a journal to record feelings, thoughts, and behaviors over time.	Helps client to assume responsibility for self-care; documents treatment effect.
Food and drug interactions to be avoided	Inform client about symptoms and events that must be reported, and to whom.	Keeps side effects from getting out of control and causing complications.
How to use the support of family and friends	Include significant others in teaching sessions. Offer complete education, answer questions, engage in discussion.	Elicits the support of significant others, decreases family anxiety, allows nurse to be a client advocate.

From Collins-Colon T: Do it yourself: medication management for community-based clients, *J. of Psychosocial Nursing* 28(6):25–29, 1990 and Weiss F: The right to refuse: informed consent and the psychosocial nurse, *J of Psychosocial Nursing* 28(8):25–30, 1990.

vidualized treatment programs, self-governance, humanistic attitudes, enhancing environment, and links to the family and community. The purpose of milieu therapy is to assist the client in learning to manage and cope with stress, as well as to correct maladaptive behaviors.

Psychosocial Rehabilitation

As the clients move toward community living, a similar model, the psychosocial rehabilitation model, helps them readjust to community living (Boyd, 1994; Olfson et al, 1993). This model, with assistance of community services, encourages clients to participate with others in the community. This enables clients to develop skills and talents that have lain dormant during their illnesses. The model differs from the hospital-based program in that there is more emphasis on autonomy, and fewer constraints (Harris, 1990). Psychosocial rehabilitation is coordinated by psychiatric nurses who assess physical

problems, oversee the functioning of the client in the environment, dispense medications, meet with families, and refer clients to job training and to appropriate service providers in the community. With the loss of hospital beds, future trends point toward case management and psychosocial rehabilitation (Mann et al, 1993; Maurin, 1990; Thompson and Strand, 1994).

Individual Psychotherapy

Individual psychotherapy may be given by a psychiatrist, a psychologist, a psychiatric social worker, a psychiatric clinical nurse specialist, or a specialist in family and child counseling, all of whom are educationally prepared at the master's or doctorate level, and work autonomously with their clients. The purpose of psychotherapy is to effect a positive change in the client by helping him or her develop effective coping patterns and overcome the feeling of helplessness most clients experience. There are

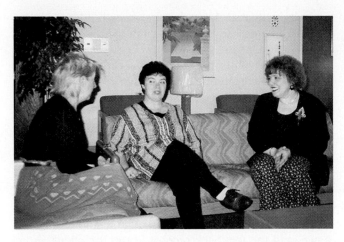
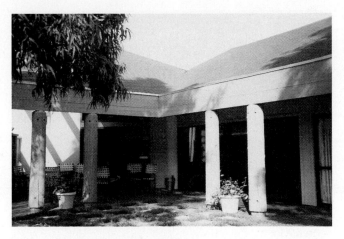

Figure 13-4 Therapeutic milieu. These scenes show a particularly enhancing and restful physical environment. Indoor and outdoor photographs are of Grossmont Behavioral Health Unit, La Mesa, California. (Courtesy Grossmont Hospital/Sharp Health Care, San Diego, California.)

many types of therapy, as described in Chapter 22. The choice of therapy depends on the client's condition and symptoms, as well as the therapist's area of expertise. The levels of therapy are as follows:

Supportive therapy allows the person to express feelings and reinforces effective coping mechanisms. It is particularly effective for clients with schizophrenia (Olfson et al, 1993).

Re-educative therapy is useful for the higher-functioning client. It is a cognitive technique that uses role-playing to explore new ways of perceiving and behaving.

Reconstructive therapy is not considered helpful for clients with schizophrenia (Olfson et al, 1993). It consists of psychoanalysis or intensive therapy groups and delves into all aspects of the client's life (Weiden and Havens, 1944).

Group Therapy

Group therapy is discussed in detail in Chapter 22. However, the type of group therapy suitable for clients with schizophrenia varies according to their level of functioning. Nurses generally use the Rogerian model, which helps clients to express and clarify feelings and promotes feelings of acceptance. This therapy uses the technique of reflection, is evocative, is not confrontative, and may allow behavioral try-outs.

Family Therapy

For a detailed discussion on family therapy, refer to Chapter 22. For the client with schizophrenia, especially one with paranoia, it may be necessary to begin with individual family therapy in which each family member has a therapist. This type of family therapy is also recommended as a first step for extremely disturbed families. Later, the family may progress to conjoint (nuclear) family therapy, in which communication patterns are emphasized among family members and the integrity of each family member is supported. According to Bellack and Mueser (1993), intervention programs that include

educating families through family therapy have helped them cope with the client's illness and show positive effects on the course of the schizophrenia.

Behavior Modification

Behavior modification is a precise approach to bringing about behavioral change. Those types that are used for schizophrenia are listed below.

Operant conditioning is widely used in child and adolescent units and is useful for anyone needing to control the behavior of other individuals. It operates on the principle of reinforcing desirable behaviors, so that they will reoccur, and ignoring negative behaviors. The techniques used include relaxation and self-control procedures. Results from using this form of therapy indicate that intolerable behaviors such as withdrawal, screaming, incontinence, and incoherence lessened. In some cases, it was then possible to prepare chronically ill, hospitalized persons to live in the community, as both positive and negative symptoms of schizophrenia had improved (Liberman et al, 1994).

Cognitive therapy explores the connection between distorted thinking and negative behavior. For example, the client who engages in all-or-nothing thinking may not be participating in a craft session because "I can never do anything right." For high-functioning patients, "homework" is assigned to separate out negative thoughts from negative feelings. Intensive cognitive-behavior therapy has been used in connection with reduction of neuroleptic dosages, in clients who have negative symptoms, suffer medication side effects, and are minimally responsive to medication.

Imagery is often combined with relaxation therapy. The client pictures past pleasant memories. Imagery is sometimes combined with role-playing.

Assertiveness training deconditions the anxiety arising from interpersonal relationships, which are usually a problem for the client with schizophrenia. This training

ADDITIONAL TREATMENT MODALITIES

Psychopharmacology
Somatic Therapy
Milieu Therapy
Psychosocial Rehabilitation
Individual Psychotherapy

- Supportive Therapy
- Re-educative Therapy
- Reconstructive Therapy

Group Therapy
Family Therapy
Behavior Modification

- Operant Conditioning
- Cognitive Therapy
- Imagery
- Assertiveness Training
- Exercise, Movement Therapy, and Dance Therapy

Occupational and Recreational Therapy
Therapies to Prevent Acting Out or Assault

promotes expressive, spontaneous, goal-directed, self-enhancing behavior.

Exercise, movement therapy, and dance therapy promote identification of the body image through kinesthetic stimulation, as well as providing a form of coping for stress. (See Chapter 24.)

Occupational and Recreational Therapy
Occupational therapy is a diagnostic tool that assesses the functional level and progress of the client with schizophrenia. The occupational therapist uses crafts as a tool to check hand-eye coordination, perception, and fine muscle tone. Some visit the clients' homes to provide special equipment or needed therapy. In fact, today's psychosocial rehabilitation programs depend on active-directive learning principles designed to help the client regain or improve skills, or to develop alternate, compensatory skills useful for community living (Boyd, 1994).

The recreational therapist's emphasis is on body kinesics, movement therapy, and resocialization through recreation. The emphasis is on cooperation rather than competition, especially for the client with schizophrenia. The therapist works on client motivation, planning trips and outings. For a more detailed description of occupational and recreational therapy, see Chapter 24.

Special Therapies to Prevent Acting Out or Assault
Given that there is a possibility for violent behaviors in seriously ill clients with schizophrenia, clinicians take steps to avoid impending assault. There are two ideas to be considered. The first idea is to predict when violence

may occur due to the emotional stress, attitude, or behavior of others toward the client with schizophrenia (Vincent and White, 1994). The second idea is to employ de-escalation skills to reduce the threat of violence, and/or physical methods to contain it (Turnbull et al, 1990).

De-escalation skills are useful techniques that can be used for interpersonal relationships in any context but are especially important for the psychiatric nurse. The skills range from using nonthreatening verbal and nonverbal messages to safely disengaging and controlling the aggressor physically. The choice to use the techniques set forth in Table 13-6 will depend on the stage of the threat, the speed of escalation of the impending violence, and the feedback received from the client, representing the effectiveness of the technique.

Physical methods to contain violence include placing clients in restraints or seclusion. The Understanding and Applying Research box on page 314 describes research on the seclusion experience of the client and the nursing responsibilities toward the client in seclusion.

Violence in interpersonal relationships frequently arises due to differing expectations regarding therapeutic or social rules and their enforcement; it also may be triggered by substance abuse. Negative reinforcement may play a part, in that violent behavior intimidates people and drives them away from the aggressor, who experiences self-gain in control (Morrison, 1994). Although the expression of aggressive behavior may be influenced by defective functioning of the central nervous system (Harper-Jaques and Reimer, 1992), mental health practitioners need to be aware of the ways anger, aggression, and violence are reinforced, whatever the inciting event. (See Chapters 25 and 26.)

■ ■ ■ ■ ■ ■ EVALUATION

At its most basic level, evaluation follows specific intervention statements and behavioral objectives incorporating the concepts of quality, quantity, and time. For example, if a goal is to resocialize a client who has been isolating herself while on the unit, an intervention might consist of having the client join the current affairs discussion group along with other clients on the unit. To evaluate the effectiveness of this intervention, specific behavioral client outcomes to be accomplished are stated in measurable terms. For example, a beginning behavioral objective might be: "On her second day on the unit, Mary will accompany the nurse to the current affairs discussion group and remain with the group for 15 minutes."

Note that the outcome is criteria-specific as to time (on the second day), quality of experience (going to discussion group with the nurse), and quantity (for 15 minutes). These criteria can be seen and measured. If all criteria are met, the minimal acceptable level of performance will progress, so that by the third day, the client outcome might read: "Mary will go to the discussion

TABLE 13-6 De-escalation of aggressive behavior

Concept	Behavior	Rationale
1. Managing the environment	Persuade the client to move to another area. Enlist help from colleagues to remove other clients, but have one colleague near you.	Prevents anxiety contagion; protects others.
2. Showing confidence and leadership	(Hold regular drills with staff to practice strategies.) Give clear instructions. Be brief. Be assertive. Negotiate options. If the client has a weapon, instruct him/her to put it on the floor.	Prevents panic when crises occur. Avoids misunderstandings, not knowing what to do. Allows client to feel he or she has some room to exercise options.
3. Encouraging verbalization	Ask questions that are open-ended and nonthreatening. Use "How?", "What?", "When?", to get details, but *not* "Why?" Keep voice calm and modulated.	Refocuses on the client's problem and not on his or her intent to act out the anger. Stops anger from escalating.
4. Using nonverbal expression	Allow the client body space; do not stand closer than about 8 feet. Keep body at a 45-degree angle. Assume an open posture; hands at sides, palms outward.	Conveys nonthreatening message, willingness to listen and accommodate client.
5. Personalizing yourself and showing concern	Remind the client who *you* are; the world may be nasty, but *you* haven't done any harm to him or her. Use words such as "we" or "us." Show that you are listening; use encouragers such as "go on . . ." to show empathy.	Encourages and reflects cooperation.
6. Using disengagement breakaways	Manage hair pulls, strangle holds, grabs, and hugs according to safety instructions, videos, and return demonstrations.	Prevents injury to self, client, and others.
7. Using removal, seclusion, and restraints	Rehearse these procedures regularly.	Allows client to regain self-control.
8. Accurately documenting the event. Holding a debriefing session with staff	Keep a detailed record: time, place, circumstances. Review and discuss the event.	Keeps an accurate account, e.g., for legal aspects. Helps staff to de-escalate and learn.

Adapted from Turnbull J et al: Turn it around: short-term management for aggression and anger. *J of Psychosocial Nursing* 28(6):6–10 and 13, 1990.

Understanding and Applying
RESEARCH

Kennedy BR, Williams CA, Pesut DJ: Hallucinatory experiences of psychiatric patients in seclusion, *Arch of Psychiatric Nursing* 8(3):169–176, 1994.

The purposes of this study were to describe seclusion experiences (especially hallucinations) of clients with psychiatric disorders, and to examine the relationships between frequency of hallucinations and the sensory stimulation provided by staff contact. According to relevant theories, there are two models to account for hallucinatory experiences: Model A proposes that people with schizophrenia who are secluded experience sensory deprivation and generate their own stimuli through hallucinating. Model B proposes that people with schizophrenia have reduced ability to erect sensory-perceptual barriers and thus are vulnerable to any stimuli, which may induce hallucinations. Seclusion, therefore, would be soothing for them.

Twenty-five clients with schizophrenia and schizoaffective disorder were interviewed within five days of their seclusion experience, and the prevalence of hallucinations was measured by standard interview questionnaires. Clients were also asked why they thought they had been placed in seclusion, what problems they had during the experience, and who they thought might help them.

Results indicated that the clients were able to verbalize that their self-destructive impulses, agitation, and combativeness were the reasons they had been placed in seclusion. Fifty-two percent reported hallucinations, but 70% of those had experienced hallucinations before being placed in seclusion. The direction of the findings was consistent with Model A, although results did not reach statistical significance. All types of hallucinations were reported, but those in seclusion were not significantly greater in number than hallucinations before seclusion. There were no significant relationships between hallucinating and interactions with staff while in seclusion.

However, there were several important implications for nursing. When asked who might help them, 88% of the clients indicated that nurses were the most helpful. Yet, documentation did not indicate this. Documentation on clients in seclusion needs to be more precise and done more frequently. Also, both clients and staff need debriefing from the emotional experience of seclusion. In addition, many clients complained that the seclusion room was cold, an environmental condition over which nursing has control. Standards of care for clients in seclusion would seem essential to avoid unnecessary discomfort.

---

group on her own, remain for a half hour, and make at least one comment."

Nursing process is not a static concept. It is an ongoing design for interaction with the environment and is evaluated as such. If the criteria were evaluated and found to be not met on the second day, for instance, the client outcomes and nursing interventions would have to

be reconsidered and perhaps rewritten at a level closer to the client's ability to perform. If outcomes are revised and are still not met, the rest of the nursing process will need to be examined in total. Thus, eventual success with the nursing process demands patience and persistence, as gains are made in small increments, especially in clients with chronic schizophrenia.

Summary of Key Concepts

1. The schizophrenias are the largest group of mental disorders.

2. Biologic factors are foremost in the research and interest in the etiology of schizophrenia. Five biologic models currently considered are heredity/genetic, neuroanatomic/neurochemical, neurotransmitter function, immunologic, and stress/disease/trauma/drug abuse.

3. The five major subtypes of schizophrenia are paranoid, disorganized, catatonic, undifferentiated, and residual.

4. Diagnostic criteria for schizophrenia include two or

more symptoms of hallucinations, delusions, disorganized or catatonic behavior, or disorganized speech that are evident for at least one month.

5. Involving the client with schizophrenia and the client's family or significant others in the treatment plan is very important and contributes to more effective treatment.

6. Psychopharmacology is a widely used intervention for symptoms of schizophrenia.

7. Milieu therapy, psychosocial rehabilitation, psychotherapy, and behavior modification techniques are some treatments used with clients with schizophrenia.

REFERENCES

American Psychiatric Association: *Diagnostic and statistical manual of mental disorders,* ed 4, Washington, D.C., 1994, APA.

Andreasen N, Carpenter W: Diagnosis and classification of schizophrenia, *Schizophrenia Bulletin* 19(2):199–214, 1993.

Arieti S: *Interpretation of schizophrenia,* ed 2, New York, 1974, Basic Books.

Arieti S: Schizophrenia: The manifest symptomatology, the psychodynamic and formal mechanisms. In Arieti S, editor: *American handbook of psychiatry,* vol I, New York, 1959, Basic Books.

Bawden E: Reaching out to the mentally ill homeless, *J of Psychosocial Nursing* 28(3):6–13, 1990.

Bellack A, Mueser K: Psychosocial treatment for schizophrenia, *Schizophrenia Bulletin* 19(2):317–336, 1993.

Bendik M: Reaching the breaking point: Dangers of mistreatment in elder caregiving situations, *J of Elder Abuse & Neglect* 4(3):39–59, 1992.

Benes F: Neurobiological investigations in cingulate cortex of schizophrenic brain, *Schizophrenia Bulletin* 19(3):537–549, 1993.

Betemps E, Ragiel C: Psychiatric epidemiology: facts and myths on mental health and illness, *J of Psychosocial Nursing* 32(5):23–28, 1994.

Bogerts B: Recent advances in the neuropathology of schizophrenia, *Schizophrenia Bulletin* 19(2):431–445, 1993.

Boyd M: Integration of psychosocial rehabilitation into psychiatric nursing practice, *Issues in Mental Health Nursing* 15:13–26, 1994.

Breier A et al: Effects of clozapine on positive and negative symptoms in outpatients with schizophrenia, *Am J Psychiatry* 151(1):20–26, 1994.

Brown J: Role of selenium and other trace elements in the geography of schizophrenia, *Schizophrenia Bulletin* 20(2):387–398, 1994.

Calev A, Edelist S: Affect and memory in schizophrenia: negative emotion words are forgotten less rapidly than other words by long-hospitalized schizophrenics, *Psychopathology* 26:229–235, 1993.

Cannon J, Marco E: Structural brain abnormalities as indicators of vulnerability to schizophrenia, *Schizophrenia Bulletin* 20(1):89–102, 1994.

Castle D, Murray R: The epidemiology of late-onset schizophrenia, *Schizophrenia Bulletin* 19(4):691–700, 1993.

Clementz B, McDowell J, Zisook S: Saccadic system fixing among schizophrenic patients and their first-degree biological relatives, *J of Abnormal Psychology* 130(2):277–287, 1994.

Cohen C: Poverty and the course of schizophrenia: implications for research and policy, *Hospital and Community Psychiatry* 44(10):951–956, 1993.

Collins-Colon T: Do it yourself: medication management for community-based clients, *J of Psychosocial Nursing* 28(6): 25–29, 1990.

Crow T: Molecular pathology of schizophrenia: more than one disease process? *British Medical Journal* 12:66–68, January 1980.

D'Angelo E: Conceptual disorganization in children at risk for schizophrenia, *Psychopathology* 26:195–202, 1993.

Dauner A, Blair D: Akathisia: When treatment creates a problem, *J of Psychosocial Nursing* 28(10):13–18, 1990.

DeMann J: First person account: the evolution of a person with schizophrenia, *Schizophrenia Bulletin* 20(3):579–582, 1994.

Draine J et al: Predictors of reincarceration among patients who received psychiatric services in jail, *Hospital and Community Psychiatry* 45(2):163–167, 1994.

Dworkin R et al: Childhood precursors of affective vs. social deficits in adolescents at risk for schizophrenia, *Schizophrenia Bulletin* 19(3):563–577, 1993.

Dworkin R et al: Social competence deficits in adolescents at risk for schizophrenia, *J of Nervous and Mental Disease* 182(2):103–108, 1994.

Dzurec L: How do they see themselves? Self-perception and functioning for people with chronic schizophrenia, *J of Psychosocial Nursing* 28(8):10–14, 1990.

Elkashef A et al: Basal ganglia pathology in schizophrenia and tardive dyskinesia: an MRI quantitative study, *Am J Psychiatry* 151(5):752–755, 1994.

Evans D et al: Self-perception and adolescent psychopathology: a clinical-developmental perspective, *Amer J Orthopsychiatry* 64(2):293–300, 1994.

Fields J et al: Assessing positive and negative symptoms in children and adolescents, *Am J Psychiatry* 151(2):249–253, 1994.

Fortinash K, Holoday-Worret P: *Psychiatric nursing care plans,* ed 2, St. Louis, 1995, Mosby.

Fortinash K: Assessment of mental status. In Malasanos L et al, editors: *Health Assessment,* St. Louis, 1990, Mosby.

Fuentes I et al: Relationships between electrodermal activity and symptomatology in schizophrenia, *Psychopathology* 26: 47–52, 1993.

Goldman R et al: Neuropsychological prediction of treatment efficacy and one-year outcome in schizophrenia, *Psychopathology* 26:122–126, 1993.

Green M et al: Dichotic listening during auditory hallucinations in patients with schizophrenia, *Am J Psychiatry* 151(3): 357–362, 1994.

Gundel H, Rudolf G: Schizophrenic autism: proposal for a nomothetic definition, *Psychopathology* 26:304–312, 1993.

Gur R et al: Clinical subtypes of schizophrenia: Differences in brain and CSF volume, *Am J Psychiatry* 151(3):343–350, 1994.

Gur R, Pearlson G: Neuroimaging in schizophrenia research, *Schizophrenia Bulletin* 19(2):337–353, 1993.

Gureje O et al: Early brain trauma and schizophrenia in Nigerian patients, *Am J Psychiatry* 151(3):368–371, 1994.

Harper-Jaques S, Reimer M: Aggressive behavior and the brain: a different perspective for the mental health nurse, *Arch of Psychiatric Nursing* 6(5):312–320, 1992.

Harris J: Self-care actions of chronic schizophrenics associated with meeting solitude and social interaction requisites, *Arch of Psychiatric Nursing* 4(5):298–307, 1990.

Hemsley D et al: The neuropsychology of schizophrenia: act 3, *BBS* 16(1):209–215, 1993.

Hietala J et al: Striatal D_2 dopamine receptor characteristics in neuroleptic-naive schizophrenic patients studied with positron emission tomography, *Arch Gen Psychiatry* 51:116–123, 1994.

Hoffman R: Commentary: dissecting psychotic speech, *J of Nervous and Mental Disease* 182(4):212–215, 1994.

Janicak P et al: *Principles and practice of psychopharmacotherapy,* Baltimore, 1993, Williams and Wilkins.

Joseph M: The neuropsychology of schizophrenia: beyond the dopamine hypothesis to behavioral function, *BBS* 16(1):203–205, 1993.

Kaplan HI, Sadock BJ: *Synopsis of psychiatry: behavioral sciences, clinical psychiatry,* ed 7, Baltimore, 1994, Williams and Wilkins.

Keltner N, Folks D: *Psychotropic drugs,* St Louis, 1993, Mosby.

Kendler K, Diehl S: The genetics of schizophrenia: a current, genetic-epidemiologic perspective, *Schizophrenia Bulletin* 19(2):261–285, 1993.

Kennedy B et al: Hallucinatory experiences of psychiatric patients in seclusion, *Arch of Psychiatric Nursing* 8(3):169–176, 1994.

Kennedy M: Relationship between psychiatric diagnosis and patient aggression, *Issues in Mental Health Nursing* 14:263–273, 1993.

Lenzenweger M: Psychometric high-risk paradigm, perceptual aberrations, and schizotypy: an update, *Schizophrenia Bulletin* 20(1):121–135, 1994.

Lewandowski L: Brain-behavior relationships. In L Hartlage et al, *Essentials of Neuropsychological Assessment,* New York, 1991, Springer Publishing Co.

Liberman R et al: Optimal drug and behavior therapy for treatment-refractory schizophrenic patients, *Am J Psychiatry* 151(5):756–759, 1994.

Lieberman J and Koreen: Neurochemistry and neuroendocrinology of schizophrenia: a selective review, *Schizophrenia Bulletin* 19(2), 371–429, 1993.

Linszen D et al: Cannabis abuse and the course of recent-onset schizophrenic disorders, *Arch of General Psychiatry* 51(4):273–279, 1994.

Macciardi F et al: Analysis of the D_4 dopamine receptor gene in an Italian schizophrenia kindred, *Arch of General Psychiatry* 51(4):288–293, 1994.

Malone J: Schizophrenia research update: implications for nursing, *Journal of Psychosocial Nursing* 28(8), 4–9, 1990.

Mann N et al: Psychosocial rehabilitation in schizophrenia: beginnings in acute hospitalization, *Arch of Psychiatric Nursing* 7(3):154–162, 1993.

Mannion E et al: Designing psychoeducational services for spouses of persons with serious mental illness, *Comm Mental Health J* 30(2):177–190, 1994.

McCain N, Smith J: Stress and coping in the context of psychoneuroimmunology: a holistic framework for nursing practice and research, *Arch of Psychiatric Nursing* 8(4):221–227, 1994.

McEnvoy J et al: Insight about psychosis among outpatients with schizophrenia, *Hosp and Comm Psychiatry* 44(9):883–884, 1993.

Meador K, Nichols F: The neurological examination as it relates to neuropsychological issues. In L Hartlage et al, editors: *Essentials of neuropsychological assessment,* New York, 1991, Springer Publishing.

Morrison E: The evolution of a concept: aggression and violence in psychiatric settings, *Arch of Psychiatric Nursing* 8(4):245–253, 1994.

Mulvey E: Assessing the evidence of a link between mental illness and violence, *Hosp and Comm Psychiatry* 45(7):663–668, 1994.

Natale A, Barron C: Mothers' causal explanations for their son's schizophrenia: relationship to depression and guilt, *Arch of Psychiatric Nursing* 8(4):228–237, 1994.

Oke S et al: The contingent negative variation in positive and negative types of schizophrenia, *Am J Psychiatry* 151(3):432–433, 1994.

Olfson M et al: Inpatient treatment of schizophrenia in general hospitals, *Hosp and Comm Psychiatry* 44(1):40–43, 1993.

Orrison W et al: *Functional Brain Imaging,* St. Louis, 1995, Mosby.

Osmon D: The neuropsychological examination. In L Hartlage et al, editors: *Essentials of neuropsychological assessment* New York, 1991, Springer Publishing.

Peplau H: Future directions in psychiatric nursing from the perspective of history, *J of Psychosocial Nursing* 18–28, 1989.

Peplau H: Principles of psychiatric nursing. In Arieti S, editor: *American handbook of psychiatry,* vol. II, New York, 1959, Basic Books.

Perry W, Braff D: Information-processing deficits and thought disorder in schizophrenia, *Am J Psychiatry* 151(3):363–367, 1994.

Plum F: Prospects for research on schizophrenia: 3. Neuropsychology: Neuropathological findings, *Neuroscience Research Progress Bulletin* 10:348–388, 1972.

Previc F: A neuropsychology of schizophrenia without vision, *BBS* 16(1):207–208, 1993.

Sabate O et al: Failure to find evidence of linkage or association between dopamine D_3 receptor gene and schizophrenia, *Amer J Psychiatry* 151(1):107–111, 1994.

Scherling D: Prenatal cocaine exposure and childhood psychopathology, *Amer J Orthopsychiatry* 64(1):9–19, 1994.

Shore D: *Recent developments in schizophrenia research: Relevance for psychiatric nurses.* Plenary session address to American Psychiatric Nurses' Association Convention, Denver, 1989.

Smothergill D, Kraut A: Toward the more direct study of attention in schizophrenia: alertness decrement and encoding facilitation, *BBS* 16(1):208–209, 1993.

Stirling J et al: Expressed emotion and schizophrenia: the ontogeny of EE during an 18-month follow-up, *Capsules and Comments in Psychiatric Nursing* 1(1):40–41, 1994.

Takei N et al: Prenatal exposure to influenza and the development of schizophrenia: Is the effect confined to females? *Am J Psychiatry* 151(1):117–119, 1994.

Thompson J, Strand K: Psychiatric nursing in a psychosocial setting, *J of Psychosocial Nursing* 32(2):25–29, 1994.

Trygstad L: The need to know: biological learning needs identified by practicing psychiatric nurses, *J of Psychosocial Nursing* 32(2):13–18, 1994.

Tsuang M: Genetics, epidemiology, and the search for causes of schizophrenia, *Am J Psychiatry* 151(1):3–6, 1994.

Turnbull J et al: Turn it around: short-term management for aggression and anger, *J of Psychosocial Nursing* 28(6):6–10 and 13, 1990.

Turner B: First person account: the children of madness, *Schizophrenia Bulletin* 19(3):649–650, 1993.

Valente S: Electroconvulsive therapy, *Arch of Psychiatric Nursing* 5(4):223–228, 1991.

vonKarmen D et al: CSF dopamine B-hydroxylase in schizophrenia: associations with premorbid functioning and brain computerized tomography scan measures, *Am J Psychiatry* 151(3):372–378, 1994.

Vincent M, White K: Patient violence toward a nurse: predictable and preventable? *J of Psychosocial Nursing* 32(2):30–32, 1994.

Weiden P, Havens L: Psychotherapeutic management techniques in the treatment of outpatients with schizophrenia, *Hosp and Comm Psychiatry* 45(6):549–555, 1994.

Weiss, F: The right to refuse: informed consent and the psychosocial nurse, *J of Psychosocial Nursing* 28(8):25–30, 1990.

CHAPTER 14

Personality Disorders

Pamela E. Marcus

Comorbid More than one psychiatric diagnosis occurring at the same time in the same individual.

Devaluation Dealing with emotional conflict or stressors by attributing exaggerated negative qualities to self or others.

Forensic psychiatry A branch of psychiatry that studies individuals who commit crimes and enter the court system, some of whom are incarcerated.

Idealization The tendency of a person with borderline personality disorder to idealize persons or groups beyond their capabilities when they are meeting that person's needs.

Ideas of reference Incorrect interpretations of incidents and external events as having a particular or special meaning that is specific to the person.

Milieu therapy Re-creates a community atmosphere on an inpatient hospital unit, a partial hospitalization unit, and a day treatment setting, in order to facilitate interaction between client peers to identify and problem-solve issues that occur while relating to others.

Nuclear family A family made up of the parental diad and the individual's siblings.

Object constancy The ability to maintain a relationship regardless of frustration and changes in the relationship. Also a stage in growth and development when the toddler can maintain the image of the mother even when she is not within the toddler's sight.

Object relations The stability and depth of an individual's relations with significant others as manifested by warmth, dedication, concern, and tactfulness.

Personality traits Behaviors and enduring patterns of perceiving, relating to, and thinking about the environment and oneself that are exhibited in a wide range of social and personal contexts.

Projective identification Projecting one's emotional conflicts and stressors to another who does not fully disavow what is projected. The individual remains aware of his or her own affects or impulses but misattributes them as justifiable reactions to the other person.

Splitting Keeping the positive and negative aspects of self and others separate from each other. An individual who uses the unconscious defense mechanism of splitting cannot tolerate ambiguity. Therefore, people, events, or ideas are either good or bad, right or wrong, black or white, but not gray.

State disorders The diagnoses made on Axis I are considered state disorders. These diagnoses constitute behavior patterns that are not as pervasive or long-lasting as trait disorders.

Trait disorders The diagnoses made on Axis II are considered trait disorders. The Axis II is used exclusively for the description of personality disorders and mental retardation, which are considered trait diagnoses. The symptoms of a personality disorder or mental retardation are not time-limited and do not occur only in a time of crisis.

Transitional objects Objects that remind one of a significant person. For example, the boss keeps a picture of his wife on his desk, which reminds him of her during work hours.

- Discuss three elements of personality development as described by Freud in the psychosexual stages of development.

- Describe two contributions made by Margaret Mahler and Otto Kernberg to object relations theory.

- Identify two biologic indices that are often abnormal in clients with a personality disorder.

- Describe one behavior, in one or two words, that differentiates between Clusters A, B, and C of Axis II in the DSM-IV.

- Discuss two nursing diagnoses for each cluster of the personality disorders.

- Identify a plan of care for two different personality disorders, including two treatment modalities that are collaborative and two outcome criteria relevant to the client's DSM-IV diagnosis.

DEFINITION OF PERSONALITY DISORDERS

The definition of personality disorders, as classified by the DSM-IV, are long-standing, pervasive, maladaptive patterns of behavior and relating to others that are not caused by Axis I disorders (Kaplan and Sadock, 1990). According to the DSM-IV, a personality disorder is an "enduring pattern of inner experience and behavior that deviates markedly from the expectations of the individual's culture, is pervasive and inflexible, has an onset in adolescence or early adulthood, is stable over time, and leads to distress or impairment" (APA, 1994). All human beings have a personality made up of one's definition of self, skills used to relate to others, and a defense structure. When studying personality disorders, one has to determine to what degree these qualities are compromised. One can determine these behaviors by observing how individuals relate to others, their perception of surroundings, and their ability to problem-solve. Mansfield, when describing someone with a personality disorder, states that "the term personality disorder, also called a 'disorder of the self,' refers to a lack of a genuine sense of 'self' and a consequent impairment of self-regulating abilities. Instead of looking within themselves to locate feelings or to make decisions, persons with personality disorders look outside themselves for evaluations, directions, rules, or opinions to guide them" (Manfield, 1992).

Definition of Axis II in DSM-IV

When reviewing the diagnostic criteria for the various personality disorders (Axis II), it is important to differentiate personality traits from personality disorders. DSM-IV has defined six general diagnostic criteria for a personality disorder as listed in the box below.

Personality traits are those behaviors, patterns of perceiving, relating to others, and thinking about the environment and oneself that are exhibited in a wide range of social and personal contexts (APA, 1994). These traits may be adaptive or maladaptive, depending on whether the trait is inflexible or causes significant functional impairment or subjective distress. When this occurs, one is

---

DSM-IV CRITERIA

Personality Disorder

A. An enduring pattern of inner experience and behavior that deviates markedly from the expectations of the individual's culture. This pattern is manifested in two (or more) of the following areas:

   (1) cognition (i.e., ways of perceiving and interpreting self, other people, and events)

   (2) affectivity (i.e., the range, intensity, lability, and appropriateness of emotional response)

   (3) interpersonal functioning

   (4) impulse control

B. The enduring pattern is inflexible and pervasive across a broad range of personal and social situations.

C. The enduring pattern leads to clinically significant distress or impairment in social, occupational, or other important areas of functioning.

D. The pattern is stable and of long duration and its onset can be traced back at least to adolescence or early adulthood.

E. The enduring pattern is not better accounted for as a manifestation or consequence of another mental disorder.

F. The enduring pattern is not due to the direct physiologic effects of a substance (e.g., a drug of abuse, a medication) or a general medical condition (e.g., head trauma).

Reprinted with permission from *Diagnostic and statistical manual of mental disorders*, ed 4, Washington, D.C., 1994, American Psychiatric Association.

---

said to have a personality disorder. The symptoms of a personality disorder are not time-limited nor do they occur only in a time of crisis (APA, 1994; Kaplan and Sadock, 1990; Kreisman and Straus, 1989). Behaviors are long-standing, enduring, and are not responsive to short-term psychotherapy or pharmacological measures.

Diagnoses made on Axis I are considered **state disorders.** These diagnoses constitute behavior patterns that are not as long in duration (Kreisman and Straus, 1989). Often the symptoms of these disorders can be alleviated through the use of medication, psychotherapy, and milieu therapy for severe symptoms. Personality disorder diagnoses are classified on Axis II of the DSM-IV in a cluster format as follows:

Cluster A:

- Paranoid, schizoid, and schizotypal are described as the odd and/or eccentric cluster.

- These diagnoses are more likely to be **comorbid,** that is, both diagnoses may be present in the same individual with psychotic disorders.

Cluster B:

- Antisocial, borderline, histrionic, and narcissistic are described as the dramatic and emotional cluster.

- The Cluster B group is often comorbid with affective disorders.

Cluster C:

- Avoidant, dependent, and obsessive-compulsive compose the anxious and fearful cluster.

- These diagnoses are often affiliated with anxiety disorders (APA, 1994; Oldham and Skodol, 1992; Widiger and Rogers, 1989).

Individuals with personality disorder diagnoses in each cluster may be predisposed to developing a comorbidity with specific Axis I diagnoses. However, this is not a hard-and-fast rule, and there are no consistent research findings that bear this out (APA, 1994; Oldham and Skodol, 1992; Widiger and Rogers, 1989).

THEORIES OF PERSONALITY DEVELOPMENT
Freudian Theories

To understand personality disorders, it is important to understand the theories of personality development. Sigmund Freud was one of the early published students of human development and inner psychological conflict. Chapter 8 provides a thorough discussion of Freud's theories.

If individuals have difficulty during the genital stage, their sense of self and ability to relate to others will be compromised. They will therefore be unable to attain their identified goals or form values. They will also experience difficulty in identifying their strengths and weaknesses, likes and dislikes, and which types of skills they want to acquire. Individuals who have difficulty resolving the genital stage can manifest symptoms and behaviors that are described within the whole range of personality disorders.

Object Relations

As theorists studied human behavior further, particularly observing development of personality structure and relatedness, the theory of object relations began to be developed. This theory has many contributors and is being reevaluated and expanded as the study of human relations and personality development and disorders is more clearly understood. Tyson and Tyson clarify the difference between interpersonal relations and object relations in the following manner: "The first (interpersonal relations) has to do with the actual interactions between people. **Object relations** (or 'internalized' object relations) refers to the intrapsychic dimensions of experiences with others—that is, to the mental representations of the self and of the other and of the role of each in their interactions" (Tyson and Tyson, 1990). Object relations, then, is the stability and depth of an individual's relations with significant others as manifested by warmth, dedication, concern, and tactfulness.

SEPARATION-INDIVIDUATION PHASE

When studying object relations from a developmental standpoint, Margaret Mahler identified and studied the separation-individuation phase of development occurring between 3 and 25 months. Mahler's Theory of Separation and Individuation evolved from a longitudinal study where she observed normal mothers and their babies during the child's first three years of life. The term *separation* in this context refers to the child's gradually developing an intrapsychic self-representation that is distinct and separate from the representation of the mother. The term *individuation* is used in this context to recognize the infant's attempts to form a distinctive identity and to develop characteristics that are unique to that individual (Mahler, 1963; Tyson and Tyson, 1990).

Mahler described four stages of the process of separation-individuation: differentiation, practicing, rapprochement, and object constancy. These stages are explained in Box 14-1 (Mahler, 1963; 1972a).

KERNBERG'S THEORIES

Otto Kernberg studied individuals with severe personality disorders and formulated some ideas about these disorders and their development, primarily with borderline and narcissistic personality disorders. Kernberg (1984) believes that a person who is emotionally healthy has an integrated working structure of the id, superego, and ego. This means that the ego is intact, with sufficient ability to determine reality from fantasy and to separate self from another object. The superego is functional, not too

rigid or punishing, but a filter for the ego. The id is integrated and not in conflict with the other two structures.

Kernberg identified two essential tasks that the early ego must accomplish for the internalization of object relations. The first task involves the ability of the child to distinguish between self and other people in order to formulate healthy feelings about self and identification with the other person. This is similar to Mahler's differentiation stage. The second task that Kernberg discussed in relation to the internalization of object relations is that there is an integration of "good" and "bad" self-images, as well as an integration of "good" and "bad" object (the other person's) images. This consolidation of images leads to total self and object representations that are dif-

---

Box 14-1   Mahler's Stages of Separation-Individuation

1. **Differentiation.** Occurs when the child is between 3 and 8 months old. During this stage, the child begins to differentiate his or her own image from that of the mother or significant nurturer.

2. **Practicing.** Occurs when the child is between 8 and 15 months old. The task of this stage is for the child to actively explore his or her world in a manner in which the child seems oblivious to the mother. This occurs when the child begins to walk and is able to explore the environment around him or her, as locomotion becomes more stabilized.

3. **Rapprochement.** Occurs when the child is between 15 and 22 months old. The child begins to return to mother for emotional needs when the exploration of the surroundings (which is done during the practicing phase) is completed. During this time the toddler becomes moody and in distress with temper tantrums, even when the mother is with the child. The child wishes to have things his or her way, which may not be what the mother had planned. The task is for the child to deal with the conflict between his or her wish for independence and individuation, and with wanting to be loved and comforted by the mother.

4. **The Beginning of Object Constancy.** Occurs around 25 months. Object constancy involves the ability to maintain a relationship regardless of frustration and changes in the relationship. The toddler at 25 months can think about mother even when mother is not close to the child and can therefore comfort himself or herself by the mother's representation. This comfort may include a blanket or stuffed toy that may remind the child of mother.

From Mahler MS: Thoughts about development and individuation, *Psychoanalytic Study Child* 18:307–324, 1963, and Mahler MS: On the first three subphases of the separation-individuation process, *International J of Psychoanalysis*, 53:333–338, 1972a.

ferentiated from one another and realistic in that both structures have good and bad, satisfaction and frustration in their systems.

In the borderline personality disorder, or what Kernberg calls the "borderline personality organization," this is a particularly important aspect. He identifies splitting as a primary defense of the individual with borderline personality disorder. **Splitting** is the inability to synthesize the positive and negative aspects of self and others. The person with a borderline personality disorder exhibits splitting by his or her difficulty in perceiving that self and other people have both good and bad aspects. There is a tendency to idealize persons or groups when those persons meet the needs of the individual with borderline personality disorder. This process is called **idealization.** At the other extreme, a person with a borderline personality can devalue persons or groups when needs are not perceived to be met. This process is called **devaluation.** The person with borderline personality disorder views self and others as either all good or all bad and is unable to reach a state of **object constancy,** which means that one is unable to hold the memory of significant others in mind. This individual is unable to use **transitional objects** that represent the significant other person and which help the individual remember the other person. For example, an individual with object constancy can think of his or her loved one when experiencing something that may remind him or her of the other person, such as a favorite song or a tangible object. An individual who is unable to obtain object constancy cannot picture his or her loved one when that individual is away from him or her. Therefore, the person views the absence of the significant other as an abandonment.

Masterson identified four defenses that block the client's developmental growth from the stages of individuation-separation to autonomy: projection, clinging, denial, and avoidance. Masterson believes that the client with borderline personality disorder becomes stuck in the subphases of the individuation-separation stage. This leads to the client's failure in achieving object constancy.

A client with borderline personality disorder does not relate to people as wholes but as parts. He or she is unable to sustain a relationship through the frustration of everyday living and tends to experience anger and rage when feeling rejected or ignored. This individual is unable to evoke the image of the other when the other is not present. If a significant person in the client's life dies, the client with borderline personality disorder cannot mourn but may exhibit one or more of the six constituent states: depression, anger and rage, fear, guilt, passivity and helplessness, emptiness and void.

Another defense against the client's anxiety that is important in understanding the individual with a Cluster B personality disorder is **projective identification.** This defense is a primitive type of projection. Kernberg (1984) describes this defense as having the following characteristics:

- the tendency to continue to experience the impulse that is simultaneously being projected onto the other person
- fear of the other person under influence of that projected impulse
- the need to control the other person under the influence of this mechanism

BIOLOGIC CONTRIBUTIONS TO PERSONALITY DISORDERS

As researchers in the biologic aspects of behaviors began to study some of the physiologic markers consistent with the Axis I diagnoses, some of the same studies were used with individuals with personality disorders, with consistent results. There have been family studies, including twin studies, that demonstrate a strong genetic influence, thus suggesting there are some ties between biologic factors and personality organization (Coryell and Zimmerman, 1989; Kavoussi and Siever, 1991; Marin et al, 1989; Siever, 1992; Siever and Davis, 1991).

One interesting aspect of this research is noted in the studies done on individuals with schizotypal personality disorder who demonstrate impaired eye tracking behavior. (See Understanding and Applying Research on page 322.) Impaired eye tracking behavior is described as "the ability to track a smoothly moving target" (Siever, 1992). This is important for cognitive interpretation of information in the environment. Individuals with schizophrenia demonstrate difficulty with smooth-pursuit eye movements, and this is thought to reflect disrupted neurointegrative functioning of the frontal lobes (Siever, 1992). The impaired eye tracking studies are associated with the "deficit" traits of schizophrenia, namely the social isolation, detachment, and inability to relate to others.

Another biologic test indicative of cognitive-perceptual difficulties that is often seen in clients who have schizotypal personality disorder is *backward masking.* This test of neurointegrative functioning involves a "process in which a visual stimulus is rapidly followed by another visual stimulus and the subject is asked to identify the original stimulus" (Kavoussi and Siever, 1991). Siever noted that individuals with this personality disorder have results that are similar to those noted in individuals with schizophrenia, but not as severe (Siever, 1985).

There are some neurochemical measures that are important indicators of biologic manifestations of the schizotypal personality disorder. Siever (1992) reported that cerebrospinal fluid homovanillic acid is increased in preliminary studies of schizotypal clients and correlates with positive psychotic-like criteria for schizotypal personality but without the negative or deficit symptoms. He also reported that plasma homovanillic acid is increased in clients with schizotypal personality disorder as compared with client controls (Kavoussi and Siever, 1991). In 1988 Schultz et al found that clients with borderline

Understanding and Applying
RESEARCH

Lencz et al: Impaired eye tracking in undergraduates with schizotypal personality disorder, *Amer J Psychiatry* 150:152–153, 1993.

This study was conducted to test the hypothesis that non-client study subjects who fit the diagnostic criteria for schizotypal personality disorder demonstrate an impairment in eye tracking movements. The sample studied consisted of 32 individuals. The following tests were given to all subjects: Schizotypal Personality Questionnaire and the Structured Clinical Interview for DSM-III-R Personality Disorders (SCID-II). The researchers used an oculogram to measure the smooth-pursuit eye movements. In addition, IQ and other tests were taken, on digit span, arithmetic, block design, and digit symbol.

The results of this study demonstrated that there was a statistically significant difference in the mean eye movement rating of the group with schizotypal personality disorder as compared to the group with no symptoms of schizotypal personality disorder. These results support previous findings of a relationship between impairments in smooth-pursuit eye movements and schizotypal personality disorder.

The clinician treating a person with a schizotypal personality disorder needs to recognize that the client has difficulties with social interaction as part of the impairments in the smooth-pursuit eye movements. Problem solving and exploration of the client's issues must include nonverbal tools, such as art, music, or movement therapy to enhance the therapy experience.

---

personality disorder who also have schizotypal personality disorder demonstrate evidence of a worsening of psychotic-like symptoms in response to an infusion of amphetamines.

In clients who have difficulty with affective regulation, some biologic indices are important to consider. The dexamethasone suppression test (DST), the thyrotropin-releasing hormone test (TRH), and EEG sleep studies have been used in research as biologic markers of affective disorders. Abnormal DST and TRH results were found in clients with borderline personality disorder, prompting researchers to question whether these clients have a variant of mood disorders. However, in studies that separated clients with borderline personality disorder into groups with and without depression, it was reported that the nondepressed subjects had a higher percentage of normal DST and TRH results. Marin et al (1989) suggest that these results may be related to depression rather than to the personality disorder.

Several studies demonstrate disturbances in central serotonergic neurotransmission indicating that aggressive and suicidal behaviors in individuals with a personality disorder correlate with reduced levels of the cerebrospinal fluid 5-hydroxyindoleacetic acid, a major metabolite of serotonin, which indicates a reduction in serotonin activity (Brown et al, 1982). Mann (1986) found increased postsynaptic serotonergic receptors in suicide victims. Stanley and Stanley (1990) demonstrated information on both presynaptic and postsynaptic serotonergic "markers" which suggests that a reduction in serotonin neurotransmission is an underlying biochemical "risk factor" for suicide. Marin et al (1989) and Kavoussi and Siever (1991) surveyed several studies that involve serotonin and its metabolites and found that there seems to be serotonergic reduction in behaviors such as impulsiveness, motor aggression, and suicidal tendencies. Brown and Linnoila (1990) studied the cerebrospinal fluid metabolites of serotonin (5-HIAA) which demonstrated that there is a relationship between reduced serotonergic activity and aggressive and impulsive behavior.

There may also be a dysfunction of the brain system's ability to modulate and inhibit aggressive responses to environmental stimuli (Siever and Davis, 1991). There is some data that EEG slow-wave activity and a low threshold for sedation discriminate individuals with antisocial personality disorder from individuals with a long-term depression (Siever and Davis, 1991).

That individuals with personality disorders manifest some biologic markers is exciting for researchers and clinicians, as this information provides some suggestions that may be useful when treating this population. There is a need for future research in this area as the functions of the brain and the neurotransmitters become better known and understood.

CLINICAL DESCRIPTION AND EPIDEMIOLOGY

The following section describes each personality disorder, the epidemiology, and common behaviors of each disorder. These descriptions are organized by cluster.

Cluster A Personality Disorders

Cluster A, often described as the "odd" or "eccentric" cluster, consists of the following personality disorders: paranoid, schizoid, and schizotypal. The clients in this cluster all have difficulty relating to others, isolate them-

CLINICAL SYMPTOMS

Cluster A Personality Disorders

Paranoid personality disorder

- Distrust, suspicion
- Difficulty adjusting to change
- Sensitivity, argumentation
- Feelings of irreversible injury by others—often without evidence
- Anxiety, difficulty relaxing
- Short temper
- Difficulty with problem solving
- Lack of tender feelings toward others
- Unwillingness to forgive even minor events
- Jealousy of spouse or significant other—often without evidence

Schizoid personality disorder

- Lack of desire to socialize; enjoys solitude
- Lacks strong emotions
- Detached, self-absorbed affect
- Lacks trust in others
- Brief psychotic episodes in response to stressful events
- Difficulty expressing anger
- Passive reactions to crises

Schizotypal personality disorder

- Incorrect interpretation of external events/belief that all events refer to self
- Superstition, preoccupation with paranormal phenomena
- Belief in possession of magical control over others
- Constricted or inappropriate affect
- Anxiety in social situations

Box 14-2   Epidemiology of Cluster A Personality Disorders

Paranoid personality disorder

- Diagnosed in 0.5%–2.5% of the general population
- 10%–30% of the paranoid population are in inpatient psychiatric settings
- 2%–10% are in outpatient mental health clinics
- Increased risk in families who have one or more members already diagnosed with paranoid personality disorder
- Males are diagnosed more often than females
- Substance abuse is common

Schizoid personality disorder

- Males are diagnosed slightly more often than females
- Increased prevalence in families with members who have schizophrenia or schizotypal personality disorder

Schizotypal personality disorder

- Diagnosed in 3% of the general population
- 30%–50% also have major depression
- Individuals with schizotypal personality disorder seek treatment for anxiety and/or depression, not for the personality disorder features
- First-degree relatives of individuals with schizophrenia are at increased risk
- Males are diagnosed slightly more often than females

selves, and are unable to socialize comfortably. The boxes above provide summaries of the key clinical symptoms and epidemiology of each disorder.

Cluster B Personality Disorders

Cluster B personality disorders have components of dramatic behavior, a description widely used when describing individuals with a Cluster B personality disorder. The four diagnostic categories that make up this cluster are antisocial, borderline, histrionic, and narcissistic. Each personality disorder has unique features; each shares a dramatic quality in the way the individual lives his or her life. The boxes on page 324 summarize the key clinical symptoms and epidemiology of each of these disorders.

Cluster C Personality Disorders

Cluster C personality disorders are described as the anxious or fearful cluster. They include avoidant personality disorder, dependent personality disorder, and obsessive-compulsive personality disorder. The boxes on page 325 summarize the key clinical symptoms and epidemiology of these disorders.

Unspecified Personality Disorders

This category describes individuals whose personality pattern meets the general criteria for a personality disorder, but not the criteria for any specific personality disorder. It is also used for an individual whose personality

CLINICAL SYMPTOMS

Cluster B Personality Disorders

Antisocial personality disorder

- Irresponsibility
- Failure to honor financial obligations, plan ahead, provide children with basic needs
- Involvement in illegal activities
- Lack of guilt
- Difficulty learning from mistakes
- Initial charm dissolves to coldness, manipulation, blaming others
- Lacks empathy
- Irritability
- Abuse of substances

Borderline personality disorder

- Intense, stormy relationships
- Sees people as "all good" or "all bad"
- Impulsivity
- Self-mutilation
- Difficulty identifying self
- Negative or angry affect
- Feelings of emptiness and boredom
- Difficulty being alone, feeling of abandonment
- Engages in impulsive acts (e.g., binging, spending money, reckless driving, unsafe sex)
- Suicidal ideations

Histrionic personality disorder

- Fluctuation in emotions
- Attention-seeking, self-centered attitude
- Sexual seduction and flamboyance
- Attentiveness to own physical appearance
- Dramatic, impressionistic speech style
- Vague logic—lack of conviction in arguments, often switching sides
- Shallow emotional expression
- Craving for immediate satisfaction
- Complaints of physical illness, somatization
- Use of suicidal gestures and threats to get attention

Narcissistic personality disorder

- Grandiose view of self
- Lacks empathy toward others
- Need for admiration
- Preoccupation with fantasies of success, brilliance, beauty, ideal love

Box 14-3   Epidemiology of Cluster B Personality Disorders

Antisocial personality disorder

- Usually diagnosed by age 18
- Have a history of conduct disorders before age 15
- Males are diagnosed more often than females
- Characteristics are evident by early childhood in males and by puberty in females
- High percentage of diagnosed individuals are in substance abuse treatment settings and prisons
- Incidence is more common in the lower socioeconomic classes
- Substance abuse is common
- Impulsive behavior is common

Borderline personality disorder

- Diagnosed in 2% of the general population
- 10% of this population is in outpatient mental health clinics
- 20% are in inpatient psychiatric settings
- 75% of diagnosed individuals are female
- 60% of the diagnosed disorder population has borderline personality disorder
- Diagnosed individuals have a history of physical and sexual abuse, neglect, hostile conflict, and early parental losses or separation

Histrionic personality disorder

- Females are diagnosed more often than males
- Diagnosed in 2%–3% of the general population
- 10%–15% of the individuals who seek treatment have this disorder

Narcissistic personality disorder

- Diagnosed in less than 1% of the general population
- Diagnosed in 2%–16% of the clinical population
- 50%–75% of those diagnosed are male

pattern meets the general criteria for a personality disorder, but the person is considered to have a personality disorder that is not included in the current classification, such as passive-aggressive personality disorder.

PROGNOSIS

When providing nursing care to clients with personality disorders, it is important to consider the prognosis for improvement. This is especially important during the planning and evaluating portions of the nursing care

CLINICAL SYMPTOMS

Cluster C Personality Disorders

Avoidant personality disorder

- Fearful of criticism, disapproval, or rejection
- Avoid social interactions
- Withhold thoughts or feelings
- Negative sense of self, low self-esteem

Dependent personality disorder

- Submissive, clinging
- Unable to make decisions by themselves
- Cannot express negative emotions
- Difficulty following through on tasks

Obsessive-compulsive personality disorder

- Preoccupation with perfection, organization, structure, control
- Procrastination
- Abandonment of projects due to dissatisfaction
- Excessive devotion to work
- Difficulty relaxing
- Rule-conscious behavior
- Self-criticism and inability to forgive own errors
- Reluctance to delegate
- Inability to discard anything
- Insistence on others' conforming to own methods
- Rejection of praise
- Reluctance to spend money
- Background of stiff and formal relationships
- Preoccupation with logic and intellect

Box 14-4   Epidemiology of Cluster C Personality Disorders

Avoidant personality disorder

- Diagnosis is equal for males and females
- Diagnosed in 0.5%–1% of the general population
- 10% are diagnosed in outpatient settings

Dependent personality disorder

- Most frequently diagnosed personality disorder
- More females are diagnosed than males
- Symptoms are demonstrated early in life
- Children or adolescents with chronic physical illness or separation anxiety disorder may be predisposed

Obsessive-compulsive personality disorder

- Diagnosed in 1% of the general population
- Diagnosed in 3%–10% of the population who seek treatment
- Males are diagnosed twice as often as females

---

plan. By definition, individuals with personality disorders have demonstrated pervasive and inflexible behaviors and thoughts that deviate from their cultural expectations (APA, 1994). These patterns first begin in adolescence or early adulthood and are stable over time. The symptoms lead to distress and functional and relationship impairment in the individual. With this definition in mind, the prognosis for individuals with personality disorders is guarded.

Realistic expectations for improvement include a commitment by the client to explore and evaluate his or her thoughts and behaviors, especially when under stress. The nurse plays a powerful role by providing support, tools for this exploration, and client teaching. If the client can use the knowledge of his or her dysfunctional patterns to predict how he or she will respond when faced with a stressor, innovative options for problem

solving can be planned. In this way, the individual learns new responses and can improve functioning. This process often needs to be repeated over time before behavioral and thought patterns change. Therefore, long-term treatment aimed at problem solving and cognitive reframing is indicated for this client.

DISCHARGE CRITERIA

Clients with personality disorders are treated in both inpatient and outpatient settings, such as day treatment facilities, partial hospital units, clinics, and private office practices. To determine when to discharge a client from an inpatient hospital setting, it is important to consider the risk factor of safety for the client and others. Some clients with personality disorders have suicidal ideas that are part of their day-to-day thought process. When evaluating clients with this ongoing theme, it is important to ascertain whether the client has a suicidal plan and if he or she intends to implement that plan. Refer to the Assessment section of Chapter 26, Suicide, for assessment of suicide risk.

Individuals with a personality disorder who are hospitalized often have more than one psychiatric diagnosis. Their lives can be complex and chaotic. Psychiatric follow-up, whether in a partial hospitalization program, a day treatment center, or with an outpatient psychotherapist, is important in order to assist the client in working through some of the issues that contributed to the crisis that culminated in the hospital stay. Prior to discharge from the hospital, it is important for the client to have a plan for outpatient follow-up and the first post-hospital appointment established.

Client teaching is a powerful tool to help the client understand the psychiatric problems that he or she is experiencing as well as to help prevent a relapse of symptoms. Prior to discharge from the hospital, each client should receive education in the following areas:

- the need for follow-up in an outpatient setting
- the psychiatric symptoms that indicate a need for emergent treatment
- an understanding of any medications that the client may be receiving

This client teaching can take place in a group setting or on an individual basis. If one of the milieu activities is a relapse prevention group and/or a medication group, it is helpful for the primary nurse to review the material specific to each client prior to his or her discharge.

If the client is being treated in an outpatient setting, the following issues must be considered prior to discharge from treatment:

- The client no longer has thoughts of wanting to harm self or others.
- The client controls self-destructive impulses, such as substance abuse when feeling upset or shoplifting when feeling empty.
- The client has an understanding of the symptoms that precipitated the need for psychotherapy.
- The client understands the types of symptoms that indicate a need for further treatment in the future.
- The client can use community 12-step groups if this is relevant to his or her problems, such as Alcoholics Anonymous, Narcotics Anonymous, Co-Dependents Anonymous, Incest Survivors Anonymous, and Overeaters Anonymous.

THE NURSING PROCESS ■ ■ ■ ■ ■ ■ ■ ■ ■ ■ ■ ■ ■ ■ ■ ■ ■ ■

■ ASSESSMENT

When assessing an individual with a personality disorder, interview the client in a comfortable, quiet, private, safe environment. There should be no interruptions during the assessment. Individuals with these disorders may be withdrawn, defensive, guarded, and impulsive, or they may be charming and friendly.

The nurse should not be judgmental or confrontational during the interview. If the client demonstrates an escalation of anger or makes hostile, threatening comments to the assessment questions, suggest that a break may help the client regain composure. Do not threaten the client with seclusion or restraints, because this may provoke him or her to impulsively lose control. See Nursing Care in the Community on page 327.

Box 14-5 represents a comprehensive evaluation that can be used with clients who have a personality disorder. Five domains of human behavior are examined: physical, emotional, cognitive, social, and spiritual.

■ ■ NURSING DIAGNOSES

The nursing diagnosis is developed based on the in-depth assessment of the client's health status. The nursing diagnosis is a statement that defines the problem, its characteristics and contributing factors, and guides the development of the nursing care plan (Carpenito, 1992). The following are nursing diagnoses that are most common when caring for clients with a personality disorder.

NANDA Diagnoses for Paranoid, Schizoid, and Schizotypal Personality Disorders (Cluster A)

Altered thought processes
Ineffective individual coping
Anxiety
Social isolation

NANDA Diagnoses for Antisocial, Borderline, Histrionic, and Narcissistic Personality Disorders (Cluster B)

Risk for violence: directed at others
Ineffective individual coping
Risk for violence: self-directed
Risk for self-mutilation
Personal identity disturbance
Chronic low self-esteem
Ineffective individual coping
Impaired social interaction

NANDA Diagnoses for Avoidant, Dependent, and Obsessive-Compulsive Personality Disorders (Cluster C)

Anxiety
Chronic low self-esteem
Ineffective individual coping
Impaired social interaction

Nursing Care in the Community

Personality Disorders

The community health nurse often encounters many dilemmas when working with clients who have Axis II diagnoses. The extent of client's illness may not be immediately apparent. Interactions require constant vigilance, as suggestions may be distorted into criticism or blame, and professional attention may be perceived as interest in personal involvement. Any attempt by the nurse to be helpful may be negated by a help-rejecting attitude, and the client's distressed complaints will continue. Other mental health professionals may be disparaged, in a less than subtle attempt to gain an alliance with the current provider. It is a signal to be cautious when the client says that every other person misunderstands him or her.

The client may also attempt to manipulate the nurse emotionally by expressing thoughts of self-harm, such as continued drinking, drug abuse, or self-mutilation, to justify prolonged attention and subsequent hospitalization. The nurse must always remain calm and impassive, no matter how much the client acts out self-threatening behaviors. Clients must be encouraged to consider the outcomes of their behaviors and think about other options they could pursue. Control of the interaction and self-awareness are especially important for the mental health nurse in the community, because there will not be a team of nurses to provide a reality check.

Clients with Axis II disorders are often charming and have insightful humor, although they seem unable to use their intellectual gifts to help themselves break the cycles of substance abuse and/or self-mutilation. They are engaging and often pit those who would help them against each other. A cohesive team approach is essential, as the demands of this group of clients tend to "burn out" individual case workers. All decisions concerning their care should be made in consensus with the psychiatrist, psychologist, social worker, and any other professional involved in the case.

Nursing Assessment Questions

Personality Disorders

These questions involve *the nurse's observation of the client's appearance, general nutritional status, and level of observable anxiety manifestations.*

1. Does the client appear appropriately dressed, is eye contact maintained, does he or she appear properly nourished? Does the client exhibit signs of anxiety, such as pacing, foot tapping, sighing, facial tension? Does the client appear hypervigilant? Does the client appear withdrawn?

The following questions are suggestions for the nurse to ask the client *to determine if there are disturbances in the client's relationships, thought processes, and behavior.*

2. How would you describe yourself? What do you like about yourself? What would you like to change about yourself?

3. Describe your relationship with your spouse or significant other, your children, your parents, and other family members. Describe your relationship with your friends. What do you talk about? What types of activities do you do together?

4. How do you feel about your job? Do you get along with your boss and coworkers?

5. If you have a personal problem, who do you trust to help you with it?

6. What are your main worries? How often do you think about them? Do you talk to anyone about these worries? Does that help?

7. Do you ever feel like hurting yourself or anyone else? Have you ever been suicidal? Have you ever hurt yourself by cutting your skin or burning yourself? How often does this occur?

8. Have you ever felt hopeless, helpless, worthless, and a burden? Do you feel this now? Are you getting any support from friends or family?

9. Do you ever use alcohol and/or illegal drugs? Have you ever gone to the doctor to get tranquilizers to reduce your nervousness? What did the doctor give you? What are you taking now?

10. What are your religious beliefs and practices?

Box 14-5 Assessment of Individuals with Personality Disorders

Physical domain

- Is there evidence of appropriate ADLs?
- Is the client neatly groomed?
- Is the client dressed appropriately?
- Does the client appear adequately nourished?
- Is there evidence of a regular exercise program in his or her life?
- Is there evidence of any physical illnesses?
- Does the client concentrate on somatic concerns?
- Is the client able to maintain eye contact?
- Is the client experiencing tension?
- Does the client demonstrate sympathetic stimulation, cardiovascular excitation, superficial vasoconstriction, and/or pupil dilation?
- Does the client report trouble sleeping?
- Is the client glancing about?
- Is the client demonstrating extraneous movements, such as foot shuffling, hand or arm movements?
- Does the client show facial tension?
- Is his or her voice quivering?
- Does the client report increased wariness?
- Is the client having an increase in perspiration?
- Does the client have a history of any of the following physical conditions?
    - temporal lobe epilepsy
    - progressive central nervous system disorder
    - head trauma
    - hormonal imbalance
    - mental retardation
    - abuse of alcohol and/or drugs
    - mania
- Is the client dressed inappropriately or in a seductive manner?
- Does the client have a high incidence of accidents?
- Is the client overly concerned with physical attractiveness?

Emotional domain

- Does the client demonstrate demanding, hostile behavior?
- Does the client have a history of aggressive actions?
- Is the client emotionally volatile?
- Does the client have poor impulse control?
- Does the client indicate having thoughts of harming self or others?

- Is the client suspicious of others?
- Is the client fearful or highly anxious?
- Does the client express feelings of helplessness?
- Does the client appear apprehensive?
- Does the client's thought pattern include feelings of uncertainty?
- Does the client discuss concerns about unspecified consequences?
- Does the client have persistent worries?
- Does the client demonstrate critical behavior toward self and others?
- Does the client have low self-esteem?
- Is the client concerned about how others will evaluate him or her?
- Does the client inflate his or her importance?
- Does the client describe feelings of guilt or regret?
- Does the client lack remorse and justify hurting another with excuses?
- Does the client lack empathy?
- Is the client vindictive?
- Does the client demonstrate a low frustration tolerance?
- Does the client show a lack of motivation?
- Is the client dependent on others to meet his or her needs?
- Is the client's behavior passive?
- Does the client discuss feelings of inadequacy?
- Does the client deny strong emotions, such as anger and joy?
- Is the client describing feelings of hopelessness?
- Does the client demonstrate inappropriate sexually seductive behavior?
- Does the client manifest a constricted affect?
- Does the client exhibit an inappropriate affect, such as silly or aloof facial expressions?
- Does the client display lability of his or her mood?

Cognitive domain

- Does the client demonstrate inaccurate interpretation of stimuli, both internal and/or external?
- Does the client have difficulty understanding abstract ideas?
- Is the client able to identify problem areas?
- Is the client able to identify options to solve the problems?
- Does the client's identification of the problem area involve blaming others or self?

Box 14-5   Assessment of Individuals with Personality Disorders—cont'd

- Is the client vindictive in his or her problem solving?
- Does the client lie?
- Is the client able to identify both good and bad traits in others?
- Is the client able to distinguish positive and negative options to problem solving?
- Does the client ruminate over issues of concern?
- Is the client's thought pattern redundant?
- Is the client able to tolerate a delay in gratification?
- Is the client able to identify his or her value system?
- Does the client have difficulty learning from his or her mistakes?
- Is the client impulsive?
- Does the client manifest any memory deficits in long-term or short-term memory?
- Is the client preoccupied?
- Does the client have a lack of consensual validation?
- Does the client describe any delusions?
- Does the client experience any hallucinations? What type: auditory, visual, tactile, gustatory, smell? What is the content of the hallucinations?
- Does the client reveal any perceptual experiences?
- Does the client confirm having any ideas of reference?
- Does the client discuss any odd beliefs or magical thinking that influence his or her behavior?
- Is the client's speech impoverished, digressive, vague, or inappropriately abstract?

Social domain

- Does the client prefer to be alone?
- Does the client express a desire to socialize but have concerns that he or she will not be accepted by others?
- Is the client dependent on others for meeting his or her needs?
- Does the client participate in family activities?
- Does the client have any friends?
- Does the client have unstable relationships that consist of conflict and concerns about abandonment?
- Is the client able to identify the dynamics of relationship problems?
- Is the client using manipulative behavior as a means of getting needs met?
- Does the client show evidence of splitting: Does the client place great value on relating with one person while becoming critical and angry with the other? Does the client devalue and complain about one individual to another person with whom the client has a positive relationship?

- Does the client identify his or her sense of self by indicating membership in a relationship?
- Is the client attention-seeking, wanting to be the center of attention?
- Is the client preoccupied with how others view him or her?
- Is this client extremely sensitive to praise and criticism of others?
- Is the client reluctant to give time, gifts, and support to his or her friends unless the client can profit?
- Does the client choose solitary activities?
- Does the client engage in any social activities?
- Does the client feel increasingly anxious when in a social situation?
- Does the client express no desire to have a sexual experience with another person?
- Does the client have multiple sexual partners?
- Is this client indifferent to praise and criticism of others?
- Does the client expect others to exploit him or her?
- Does the client exploit others to get his or her needs met?
- Does the client question the loyalty or trustworthiness of friends or associates? Does the client question the fidelity of his or her spouse or sexual partner?
- Does the client read hidden meanings into benign remarks of others?
- Does the client bear grudges toward others?
- Is the client reluctant to confide in others?
- Is the client preoccupied with self to the exclusion of others?
- Does the client fail to honor financial obligations?
- Does the client fail to plan ahead, such as traveling without a clear plan or quitting work without plans to begin another job?
- Does the client provide his or her children with the basic needs for health?
- Does the client engage in illegal activities?
- Does the client abuse drugs or alcohol?
- Does the client demonstrate a belief that he or she is owed a sense of entitlement?

Spiritual domain

- Does the client have a belief in a higher power?
- Is the client able to state a meaning and purpose to his or her life?

CASE 📁 STUDY

James, a 32-year-old single man, was evaluated by a nurse in an outpatient clinic at the recommendation of his father, due to an increase in his isolative behavior. James did not want to come in for the interview, since he did not consider "being alone" a problem. He was oriented three times, but was not spontaneous with answers to the nurse's assessment questions. His affect was flat, he kept his eyes averted with no eye contact, and his leg was shaking. He was unkempt, with a disheveled appearance and mismatched clothing. He had a vague, wandering, nonspecific way of discussing his problem and his lifestyle.

His mother had been recently hospitalized with pneumonia—however, he did not see that as part of his problem. He perceived his boss as "disliking" him, because the boss thought he was "weird." He has no friends, finds socializing difficult, and tends to withdraw further when forced to interact with others. He is suspicious of the interviewer and of his father's motives for asking him to seek psychiatric intervention.

The problem he identified was that he felt he had to "do more around the house" in his mother's absence. That seemed "unfair and like a burden" to James. "She just got sick so she wouldn't have to cook supper or do the laundry," James stated. "The doctors put her in the hospital so they can make more money off of her. Dad is in on it; he sent me here so you could make money." James has not visited his mother in the hospital, because he is afraid he will get "germs" there. Although he saw no reason for this interview, he consented to return to the clinic to "help" his father.

Critical Thinking and Assessment

1. What questions should the nurse ask James to determine symptoms in the physical domain?

2. How can the nurse assess the emotional domain?

3. How could James's problems in the cognitive domain be assessed?

4. What information about James helps to determine his functioning in the social domain?

5. What questions could the nurse ask James to assess how he functions in the spiritual domain?

COLLABORATIVE DIAGNOSES

DSM-IV Diagnoses*	NANDA Diagnoses**
Cluster A	
Paranoid Personality Disorder	Altered thought process
Schizoid Personality Disorder	Ineffective individual coping
Schizotypal Personality Disorder	Anxiety
	Social isolation
Cluster B	
Antisocial Personality Disorder	Risk for violence: directed at others
	Ineffective individual coping
Borderline Personality Disorder	Risk for violence: self-directed
Histrionic Personality Disorder	Risk for self-mutilation
	Personal identity disturbance
Narcissistic Personality Disorder	Chronic low self-esteem
	Ineffective individual coping
	Impaired social interaction
Cluster C	
Avoidant Personality Disorder	Anxiety
	Chronic low self-esteem
Dependent Personality Disorder	Ineffective individual coping
Obsessive-Compulsive Personality Disorder	Impaired social interaction

*Reprinted with permission from *Diagnostic and statistical manual of mental disorders,* ed 4, Washington, D.C., 1994, American Psychiatric Association.

**Reprinted with permission from *NANDA nursing diagnoses: definitions and classifications, 1995–1996,* Philadelphia, 1994, North American Nursing Diagnosis Association.

options to change these maladaptive patterns to more effective coping strategies.

The outcome criteria are derived from the nursing diagnosis and are the expected client responses or behaviors that occur as a result of the plan of care. Outcomes are written in clear, measurable terms.

Outcome Identification for Personality Disorders

Client will:

1. Demonstrate absence of suicidal ideation

2. No longer have any thoughts of harming others

3. Refrain from self-mutilation

■ ■ ■ OUTCOME IDENTIFICATION

An individual with a personality disorder has disturbances in self-image and relationships throughout life. Identifying outcomes includes the client's ability to demonstrate understanding of problem areas and to display healthy and effective adaptive behaviors. The focus is on helping the individual find patterns of maladaptive behavior, thoughts, and emotions that produce distress. The nurse and the client can work together to explore

4. Reach and maintain the highest functioning possible, as demonstrated by the ability to function at home, work, and in the community

5. Identify two impulsive behavior patterns that take place during times of stress

6. Recognize when he or she is experiencing cognitive distortions during a stressful period of time

7. Be able to identify a cognitive distortion used most often during times of stress

8. Identify one new method of problem solving

9. Reward self, both with an item (such as some flowers) and a positive thought when able to successfully identify and change a cognitive distortion

10. Identify some patterns of isolative behavior

11. Tolerate short interactive periods with the nurse, family members, and peers

12. Identify with positive role models

13. Contribute one statement in a group setting directed toward facilitating increased socialization

■ ■ ■ ■ PLANNING

When planning interventions with a client with a personality disorder, it is important for the nurse to recognize that changes in behavior or thoughts often occur slowly. These changes are a result of the client's perception of the need for that change. Individuals with a personality disorder have disturbed interpersonal relationships and values that do not reflect the views held by the general population. Due to these disturbances, the nurse must collaborate with the client on the goals identified during treatment.

■ ■ ■ ■ IMPLEMENTATION

The implementation of the plan of care for clients with personality disorders includes interventions focused toward modifying life-long disruptive and dysfunctional behaviors and thoughts, with the promotion of safety.

Nursing Interventions

1. Assess the client for suicidal ideation and determine the level of lethality *to prevent harm or injury.*

2. If warranted, place the client on suicidal precaution, depending on his or her level of lethality (for example, a client who has verbalized plans to hang self while on the unit should be placed on close individual observation as long as those plans are still viable, with no means or provisions to carry out the intent) *to prevent suicide.*

3. Establish a contract for safety with the client by asking client to write a statement indicating that he or she will not harm himself or herself. If the suicidal impulse becomes too strong, encourage the client to seek out a staff member to discuss the increase in in-

> ## CASE 📖 STUDY
>
> Jean has been working with a nurse for the past three years in outpatient psychotherapy. She was recently arrested for stealing some candy and lipstick at a local department store following an argument with her boyfriend. During the session following the arrest, the nurse suggested that Jean explore the dynamics of the incident and how this was related to the argument with her boyfriend. Jean became angry, then scared, expressing concern that she may lose the respect and the therapeutic relationship with the nurse. She ran out of the room, yelling that the nurse did not understand her pain, and slammed the door. Several minutes later, Jean returned, apologized, and asked the nurse to forgive her.
>
> **Critical Thinking and Outcome Identification**
>
> 1. Why would the nurse suggest to Jean that her behavior of stealing requires further discussion and understanding of the dynamics that lead to this impulsive behavior?
>
> 2. What changes in behavior are anticipated as a result of Jean's gaining understanding into her impulsive behavior?
>
> 3. Describe two outcomes that would be realistic for Jean.

tensity of suicidal ideation *to protect the client from acting on suicidal impulses.*

4. Encourage the client to attend all unit group sessions *to receive support from peers and to provide opportunities for problem solving.*

5. Assess the client for an escalation of anger-to-rage and possible impulsive actions against others (obtain a history of violence if possible) *to prevent harm or injury to others.*

6. Contract with the client that he or she will no longer threaten staff or peers during hospitalization *to ensure the safety of others.*

7. Teach the client other options to manage the angry, impulsive feelings and behavior (such as leaving the room where the conflict is occurring) or using a quiet area (such as an unlocked seclusion room) until the impulse to do harm passes. *Removing the client from a stimulating, provocative environment may decrease angry impulses.*

8. Discuss angry feelings in a group setting that is focused on exploring alternative options for problem solving. *Alternative actions may distract client from angry feelings and help to focus his or her energy on constructive activities.*

NURSING CARE PLAN

Sam was admitted to the psychiatric unit directly from the E.R. because he was involved in a fight with another man at a bar. He was under the influence of PCP as well as alcohol while at the bar. The E.R. staff assessed him as medically stable, but suggested admission due to his potential for violence.

When Sam arrived on the unit, he was angry, loudly stating that he had been treated unfairly in the E.R. and that he did not need admission to the psychiatric unit "with all those nuts!" He demanded a TV in his room and a cigarette. When the staff denied his requests, he became louder and threatening. He told the charge nurse that he would get his way, that he has friends on the hospital board, and that there would be an investigation into the hospital treatment of his case if he is not allowed to smoke or to watch TV in private. He reminded the nurse that he was admitted for fighting in a bar, and he "knows how to get his way."

DSM-IV Diagnosis

Axis I: Substance abuse (alcohol and PCP)

Axis II: Antisocial personality disorder

Axis III: Medically stable, R/O withdrawal symptoms

Axis IV: Psychosocial stressors severe, 5: substance abuse, history of negative self-appraisal

Axis V: GAF: current 40
           past year 60

Nursing Diagnosis: Risk for violence: directed at others. Risk Factors: a perception that others are denying him his rights and control over his environment; a history of violence against others; an increase in verbal demands, a loud voice, and verbally threatening behavior.

Client Outcomes	Nursing Interventions	Evaluation
• Sam will be able to maintain control of his anger so that he will not threaten or harm others.	• Monitor the client for escalation of the anger to rage or impulsive action *to predict any increase in impulsivity and prevent injury to self or others.* • Contract with the client that he will no longer threaten staff or client peers during the hospitalization *to assist Sam in impulse control.*	• Sam was able to discuss his feelings about entering the hospital without threatening or aggressive behavior.
• Sam will use the interactions with the nurse, members of the interdisciplinary team, and groups in the milieu to discuss alternative options to deal with situations that provoke angry, potentially violent responses.	• Teach the client other options to manage the angry feelings, such as leaving the area where the conflict is occurring and using a quiet area such as an unlocked seclusion room until the impulse to do harm passes *to provide other ways to handle angry feelings, rather than violence.* • Discuss angry feelings in the group setting, how the anger can escalate out of control, and what to do to control violent impulses *to use group input to provide alternative solutions to deal with angry feelings rather than resorting to violence.*	• Sam was able to control angry outbursts and ask for his needs in a calm manner during his hospital stay and shared his feelings with the group.

Nursing Diagnosis: Ineffective individual coping related to intoxication from alcohol and PCP, as evidenced by the client's loud and threatening behavior.

Client Outcomes	Nursing Interventions	Evaluation
• Sam will be able to determine his basic needs and make requests in a calm, thoughtful manner, and make some choices about his treatment and care.	• The nurse will observe for symptoms of intoxication and withdrawal from alcohol and PCP, which may require medication and administer medications as needed. *Symptoms of intoxication and withdrawal of both substances may include irritability and loss of impulse control.* • The nurse will assist Sam to become adjusted to the unit by providing a tour, giving statements of support, and telling Sam how the hospitalization will help him. Provide Sam with choices in his care when appropriate. *The client will feel in control with an understanding of the environment and expectations as well as being able to make some decisions regarding his care.*	• Sam was able to decrease his loud and threatening behavior after medication was given to decrease withdrawal symptoms, and he was able to make some decisions regarding his care.

NURSING CARE PLAN ■ ■ ■ ■ ■ ■ ■ ■   ■ ■ ■ ■ ■ ■

Nursing Diagnosis: Chronic low self-esteem related to long-term negative feedback toward self, and the belief that he is unable to deal with problems, as evidenced by self-destructive behavior (drinking and physical fighting in the bar), inability to accept constructive limit-setting from the nursing staff, and the degradation of others to increase own feelings of self-worth.

Client Outcomes	*Nursing Interventions*	*Evaluation*
• Sam will be able to discuss during a one-to-one session with his primary nurse or in a problem-solving milieu group that his threatening behavior and degradation of others reveal his own feelings of low self-esteem.	• Encourage Sam to attend all verbal milieu groups for problem solving, particularly those that discuss behavior and feelings. *Sam will obtain feedback from other group members about his threatening and degrading behavior toward others, therefore hearing the same feedback from several sources.* • Discuss how threatening behavior and derogatory remarks toward others distance people. *This discussion will help Sam determine his part in the process of others not attending to his needs, therefore reinforcing his low self-esteem.*	• Sam asked for an identified need without threatening another person. He determined other options to meet the identified need if the other person elected not to assist Sam.
• Sam will be able to identify a positive attribute to his personality.	• Assist Sam to list the strengths and areas needing adjustment as he views self. *Sam only identifies negative parts of self. Listing both strengths and weaknesses helps Sam have a more balanced view of self.* • Provide positive feedback to Sam when he accomplishes something within the unit milieu or in discussion with others. *Positive feedback reinforces functional behavior.*	• Sam was able to identify two strengths in his character that he values, and agrees to recognize these strengths in the future.

9. Assess the client for evidence of self-mutilation. *Clients who are self-destructive are likely to repeat such acts and may require further interventions.*

10. Obtain a contract from the client that he or she will approach a staff member when the urge to self-mutilate is present *to ensure the safety of the client.*

11. Place the client on an individual, close watch until the urge to harm self passes or until the client is able to identify another way to obtain emotional relief (for example, wrapping in a sheet or participating in a movement therapy group) *to protect the client from harmful impulses and redirect the impulses toward alternative, constructive methods.*

12. If self-mutilation occurs, attend to the wounds in a matter-of-fact manner *to provide safe care to the client in a nonjudgmental way.*

13. Encourage the client to keep a journal of thoughts and feelings experienced prior to the urge to self-mutilate *to help the client acknowledge feelings and thoughts and helps decrease impulsivity.*

14. Medicate the client with an anxiolytic or antipsychotic medication, prn as ordered *to assist the client to control his or her intense anxiety or rage rather than to self-mutilate.*

15. Use physical restraints if all attempts of least restrictive measures have been unsuccessful *to protect the client.*

16. Assist the client to recognize thought patterns that contribute to impulsive behavior. This can be done by helping the client understand the role intense feelings (for example, abandonment, anger, rage, or anxiety) play in precipitating impulsive behavior or distorted thinking. Using a journal to document such feelings and thoughts and receiving feedback during group sessions are helpful, instructive methods. *Clients can be taught to manage impulsive behavior and distorted beliefs through a variety of methods within the milieu.*

17. Suggest alternative behaviors that can be learned to deal with the intense feelings, such as:

Recognizing the intense emotional state, and writing in a journal or thinking about an action that may help to relieve the intensity of the feeling without resorting to impulsive or self-destructive acts.

Talking about the intense feeling while looking into a mirror, telling the mirror what the client wished to express to the object of anger.

NURSING CARE PLAN ■ ■ ■ ■ ■   ■ ■ ■ ■ ■ ■

Angela is a 29-year-old single female who became suicidal after her boyfriend, Al, told her their relationship was over. She started to drink and use Valium to calm down after Al told her they were through. The relationship had become stormy, with frequent threats from Al that he would stop seeing her. Angela became vengeful, went to Al's parent's house where he was staying, and threw a rock into their living room window, shouting that she loves Al and cannot live without him. She shouted, "I don't want to hurt anyone. I just want to die!" and ran into the street in front of an oncoming car. The driver slammed on the brakes and hit Angela hard enough to knock her down and cause a pelvic fracture. She was admitted to the local hospital, still vowing to harm herself if Al did not return to her.

DSM-IV Diagnoses

Axis I: Substance abuse (alcohol and Valium)

Axis II: Borderline personality disorder

Axis III: Pelvic fracture

Axis IV: Psychosocial stressors, 5: Breakup of intense personal relationship, substance abuse, suicide attempt

Axis V: GAF: current, 30
           past year, 60

Nursing Diagnosis: Risk for violence, self-directed. Risk Factors: intense feelings of abandonment, increased anxiety level, and a history of suicidal attempts.

Client Outcomes	Nursing Interventions	Evaluation
• Angela will not act on her suicidal thoughts.	• Place the client on suicide watch and assess her level of depressed thoughts *to prevent any further suicide attempts through early intervention.*	• Angela decreased her suicidal ideation within two days of hospitalization.
• Angela will honor the terms of her contract for safety.	• Present Angela with a contract for safety which states that she will inform the staff if her suicidal ideation increases *because early preventive measures can be taken to prevent a suicidal gesture.*	• She was able to use the contract for safety to assist with impulse control.
• Angela will contact the staff when she experiences suicidal thoughts.	• Teach Angela to inform the staff if there is an increase in her suicidal ideation *to help her become an active participant in her suicide prevention and more aware of how her thoughts and feelings influence her behavior.*	• Angela contacted staff when she had suicidal thoughts, feelings of abandonment, and other troubling feelings.

Nursing Diagnosis: Ineffective individual coping related to ending a significant relationship, as evidenced by client's vengeful behavior, her impulsive behavior to do self-harm, and her use of drugs and alcohol.

Client Outcomes	Nursing Interventions	Evaluation
• Angela will identify impulsive behavior patterns that take place during times of stress, record these feelings in a journal and share them in appropriate groups.	• Teach Angela to link her feelings and behavior to her response to the events in her relationship with the use of a journal about her thoughts and feelings, one-to-one discussions with her assigned nurse, and the use of the groups in the inpatient milieu. *A journal will help Angela acknowledge her feelings and thoughts, determine her impulsive behavioral patterns, and decrease her reaction to those thoughts and feelings.*	• Angela was able to talk about her intense feelings of loss and emptiness with her assigned nurse and in the verbal groups on the unit. She was able to use her journal as a coping mechanism when the emotions became overwhelming.

NURSING CARE PLAN

Client Outcomes	Nursing Interventions	Evaluation
• Angela will be able to identify at least one new method of problem solving to manage negative thoughts and impulses.	• Teach the client healthy ways of dealing with intense feelings of anger and sadness, such as expressing these feelings to supportive friends and family members. Teach her to employ a behavior to help cope with the intense emotion, such as listening to music, taking a hot bath, going to an exercise class, buying flowers, or writing in the journal. *These activities will help Angela learn new coping patterns to deal with intense, painful emotions.*	• Angela was able to use her journal by writing poetry to problem-solve and calm herself when feelings became intense during the hospitalization.

Nursing Diagnosis: Dysfunctional grieving related to ending a significant relationship with Al, as evidenced by the client's use of drugs and alcohol, vengeful behavior, suicidal ideation, and impulsive behavior to do self-harm.

Client Outcomes	Nursing Interventions	Evaluation
• Angela will identify feelings generated by the ending of the relationship with Al, such as anger, fear of being alone, and sadness.	• Discuss Angela's feelings about the end of the relationship with Al in an open manner *to encourage her to be able to discuss her hurt feelings, fear of loneliness, and abandonment issues to facilitate healthy mourning of the loss of the relationship.*	• At the end of the hospitalization, Angela was able to talk about the end of her relationship with Al without suicidal thoughts or cravings for alcohol or Valium.
• Angela will share her loss with group members who also experienced losses.	• Encourage Angela to attend group problem-solving sessions on the unit to discuss her loss with other peers in the unit *to give Angela a better perspective on how others have dealt with losses.*	• Angela shared her loss with appropriate group members.
• Angela will use healthy methods to deal with her loss and not use alcohol or Valium to mask her feelings.	• Encourage Angela to write her thoughts and feelings about the end of the relationship in her journal, *because recognizing the thoughts and feelings about the loss of the relationship may help her come to terms with the unresolved issues associated with the loss.*	• Angela developed journal writing as a healthy method of dealing with her loss and working through painful issues.

Identifying healthy options to deal with the anger, such as discussing the issue with the person who is involved in the interaction.

Role-playing with the nursing staff different ways to approach the problem that precipitated the intense feelings.

Introducing the issue in the problem-solving milieu group meeting to receive feedback from peers.

Rewarding self with something that is pleasant and healthful, such as buying flowers or reading a novel.

Learning alternative ways to cope with intense feelings can reduce anger/anxiety and provide constructive ways of managing life stressors.

18. Help the client explore behavior that relates to the community, such as safe driving and responsibilities

for the environment *to help the client focus on changes that he or she can do to live in a more healthy and responsible way.*

19. Evaluate the client's family system by observing the family dynamics and determining the client's role within the family. *How the client interacts within the family system and the role the client takes (for example, victim, placator, etc.) offers the nurse insight into how the client views self.*

20. Engage the client in frequent short interactions several times during the shift *to illustrate the value of interacting with others.*

21. Use milieu groups, such as problem-solving groups and groups that concentrate on self-care and community responsibilities *to help the client understand the value of interacting with others.*

22. Teach the client assertiveness techniques *to improve the client's ability to relate to others.*

Client and Family
TEACHING GUIDELINES

SET Method

Clients with personality disorders often have difficulties recognizing problem areas and identifying options that could be solutions. The nurse could incorporate teaching clients and family members to problem-solve more effectively as part of the care plan. One area of difficulty is communication. Kreisman and Straus (1989) suggest using the "SET" method of communication. This was originally developed for clients with borderline personality disorder who were in crisis and were unable to communicate effectively. Kreisman and Straus's "SET" is a three-part system of communication. This is a particularly useful tool when the client is impulsive, is having outbursts of rage, is harmful to self or others, or is making unreasonable demands on others for caregiving. In the SET method:

- the **S** stands for **Support,** the nurse states a personal statement of concern for the client

- the **E** is for **Empathy,** in which the nurse acknowledges the individual's chaotic feelings in a neutral way, with the emphasis on the client's painful experience, not the staff member's feelings

- the **T** is a **Truth** statement used to highlight the client's responsibility for his or her behavior and life (Kreisman and Straus, 1989)

For example, Charles had become enraged when his wife, Margaret, did not go shopping and cook some meals for him before she went away for a business trip. His anger mounted, and he drank to deal with his intense feelings.

He came to his partial hospitalization program, reporting a hangover.

His primary nurse began the discussion about Charles's response to Margaret's travel on business with the following statement:

Nurse:	"I know it is hard for you when Margaret has to go away." **(E)**
Charles:	"You got that right. It makes me so angry that she can't complete all her work here."
Nurse:	"Okay, I hear you **(S),** but in her job, travel is a big part of how business is conducted." **(T)**
Charles:	"Yeah, I know, and I think she's good at what she does. I just get so lonely, so empty, I then get angry and scared."
Nurse:	"Can you look at what type of things you can do when she is away that may help your feelings of emptiness?" **(T)**
Charles:	"Like what?"
Nurse:	"Like going to the movies on the night Margaret is out of town, and see something she wasn't interested in. Treat yourself to carry-out Chinese or fast-food, so that you can have dinner without a lot of fuss. Does that sound like something that may help?" **(T)**
Charles:	"I'll try."

23. Provide direct feedback to the client about his or her interaction with others in a nonjudgmental fashion *to facilitate learning new social skills.*

Additional Treatment Modalities

A team approach, involving nursing staff, the psychiatrist, psychologist, social worker, occupational therapist, art therapist, music therapist, movement therapist, and recreational therapist provides the most comprehensive interventions for a client with a personality disorder in an inpatient, partial hospitalization, or day treatment setting.

Occupational therapy

The occupational therapist assesses a client's abilities and disabilities and helps the client increase functioning and independent living skills in areas such as self-care, work, or leisure activity. The occupational therapist teaches adaptive skills for home, school, or job functioning. Groups such as stress management, enhancing par-

enting skills, conflict resolution, time management, money management, budgeting, feeling, and self-awareness are often planned and co-led by the occupational therapist.

Art therapy

The art therapist uses art as a means of helping the client express thoughts and feelings he or she may not be able to verbalize. This intervention helps the client to understand problem areas from a symbolic standpoint. The art therapist also teaches the client an alternative means of expression and self-soothing. For example, a client who is feeling intense rage and has feelings of wanting to self-mutilate may use art to draw these feelings rather than act on them.

Music therapy

The music therapist uses music to help the client express feelings and thoughts that may not be easily verbalized. Music is used to help the client relax and learn alternative self-soothing strategies.

ADDITIONAL TREATMENT MODALITIES

- Occupational Therapy
- Art Therapy
- Music Therapy
- Movement Therapy
- Recreational Therapy
- Medication Therapy
- Individual Therapy
- Group Therapy
- Family Therapy
- Milieu Therapy

Movement therapy

Movement therapy teaches clients how they move their bodies when stressed and helps them learn methods of relaxation. Movement therapy is helpful for clients who become "numb" when feeling intense feelings, such as abandonment or anger, to use methods of self-touching to reestablish a feeling state rather than self-mutilate.

Recreational therapy

Recreational therapy helps clients with personality disorders explore ways to enjoy themselves without the use of self-destructive behaviors, such as abusing alcohol or drugs. This modality is helpful for clients who have difficulty socializing, because recreation strengthens social skills.

Medication therapy

Medications can play a major role in helping the client with a personality disorder. Clients who are demonstrating violence against others may require medications to gain emotional and behavioral control over their impulses. Keltner and Folks (1993) suggest that clients who are able to take an oral anxiolytic or the sedative-hypnotic class may respond well to the use of a benzodiazepine. Clients who are very agitated or psychotic may respond to the use of a neuroleptic or antipsychotic class medication. Clients with extreme violence who are unable to control this impulse may be given intravenous or intermuscular sedative-hypnotics such as barbiturates, benzodiazepines such as diazepam, or antipsychotics such as haloperidol.

Clients who demonstrate depression along with the symptoms of a personality disorder may benefit from antidepressants. Tricyclic antidepressants (TCA) are helpful in decreasing depression and the neurovegetative signs in clients with both depression and personality disorders. The selective serotonin reuptake inhibitors (SSRIs) demonstrate a reduction in depressed symptoms in clients with both depression and a personality disorder. The SSRIs have some advantages over the TCAs. There is a reduced probability of completed suicide with an overdose, and there are fewer side effects with the SSRIs than the TCAs. SSRIs are more expensive than TCAs, which may be limiting to clients who are unable to afford the cost. Some physicians are prescribing an SSRI with a TCA for clients who have severe depression. Monitoring side effects is an important nursing function.

Soloff et al (1991) studied the impact of medications on individuals with borderline personality disorder and schizotypal personality disorder. They reported that haloperidol helped the client increase global functioning, decrease schizotypal symptoms, decrease hostility, and increase impulse control. They also reported that amitriptyline (a TCA medication) decreased hostility and increased impulse control for clients with borderline personality disorder who were evaluated as being unstable.

Individual therapy

Individual therapy helps the client explore problem areas, define new options, and discuss how the new behavior may help solve the original problem. With the emphasis in the health care system on short-term therapy, individual therapy is now problem-solving oriented as opposed to explorative based on early trauma.

Group therapy

Group therapy is also problem-solving oriented. The work in group therapy is done based on the repeated dynamics of the individuals in the group. This is especially beneficial for clients with a Cluster B personality disorder, who are dramatic and require a lot of attention. The group members will help the client to understand the effect his or her behavior has on each of them so that the client can use this information when relating to significant people in his or her everyday life.

Family therapy

Family therapy is helpful for clients with a personality disorder, as the dynamics of the family system are often repeated in other relationships in the client's life, such as with his or her boss or spouse. The family sessions consist of an assessment of the family system and an exploration of how the family dynamics are affected by the current problems that caused the client to seek care. Due to the current philosophy of short-term therapy, exploration of earlier dynamics and/or trauma is focused on the current issue.

Milieu therapy

When a client is hospitalized in an inpatient psychiatric setting or participates in a partial hospitalization program or a day treatment facility, the client becomes part of that milieu (environment). The purpose of **milieu therapy** is to re-create a community setting on these units so that the client can interact with other client peers in order to identify and problem-solve issues that occur while relating to others. Such relationship issues may be discussed in community meetings or other problem-solving groups, such as coping skills group.

The community meetings may be used to delegate tasks of the unit, such as cleaning off the tables at the end of the meal. This meeting can be used to ask each member to think through a daily goal for therapy and discuss how he or she plans to meet that goal. If something happens on the unit (for example, if someone becomes aggressive or brings drugs or alcohol on the unit), these concerns are discussed in the community meeting.

Problem-solving groups, such as coping skills group, may pick a common area of concern; the group works together to explore the issues and options necessary to solve the dilemma.

As in any other community, socializing is an important part of the interaction. In an inpatient, partial hospital-ization program or day treatment milieu, socialization groups discuss problems with socializing. The socialization group may use a discussion of a movie the group has just seen or current events read from a magazine or a newspaper as a means of enriching the discussion.

■ ■ ■ ■ ■ ■ EVALUATION

The evaluation stage of the nursing process is ongoing and takes place to ensure accountable nursing practice. There are two steps to the evaluation stage:

1. The nurse compares the client's current functioning with the outcome criteria.

2. The nurse asks questions to determine possible reasons if the outcome criteria were not met (Fortinash and Holoday-Worret, 1995).

Summary of Key Concepts

1. A personality disorder is a long-standing, pervasive, maladaptive pattern of behavior and relating to others that is not caused by an Axis I disorder.

2. There are several theories for the development of a personality disorder. In psychodynamic theory, there is a belief that an individual who develops a personality disorder has deficits in his or her psychosexual development or a failure to achieve object constancy. There is recent research that has hypothesized biologic considerations as possible causal factors for individuals developing personality disorders.

3. The DSM-IV Axis II is set up in a three-cluster format.

4. Clients with personality disorders have difficulty relating to others at home, at work, and in the community.

5. When working with individuals with personality disorders, it is important to assess each client for the risk of violence toward self and/or others.

6. Clients with personality disorders often exhibit self-destructive behavior, such as self-mutilation, eating disorders, alcohol or substance abuse, and shoplifting.

7. Realistic expectations for improvement include a commitment by the client to explore and evaluate his or her thoughts, relationships, and behaviors, especially when under stress.

REFERENCES

Akhtar S: *Broken structures: severe personality disorders and their treatments,* Northvale, N. J., 1992, Jason Aronson.

American Psychiatric Association: *Diagnostic and statistical manual of mental disorders,* ed 3, revised, Washington, D.C., 1987, American Psychiatric Association.

American Psychiatric Association: *Diagnostic and statistical manual of mental disorders,* ed 4, Washington, D.C., 1994, American Psychiatric Association.

American Psychiatric Association: *The American Psychiatric Association's psychiatric glossary,* Washington, D.C., 1984, American Psychiatric Press.

Brown GL et al: Aggression, suicide and serotonin relationships to CSF amine metabolites, *Am J Psychiatry* 139:741–745, 1982.

Brown GL, Linnoila MI: CSF serotonin metabolite (5-HIAA) studies in depression, impulsivity, and violence, *J of Clin Psych* 51: 31–43, April 1990.

Carpenito LJ: *Nursing diagnosis: application to clinical practice,* Philadelphia, 1992, JB Lippincott.

Coryell WH, Zimmerman MBA: Personality disorder in the families of depressed, schizophrenic, and never-ill probands, *Am J Psychiatry* 146: 496–502, April 1989.

Erikson EH: *Childhood and society,* New York, 1950, WW Norton.

Fortinash KM, Holoday-Worret PA: *Psychiatric nursing care plans* ed 2, St. Louis, 1991, Mosby.

Freud S: The development of the libido and the sexual organizations, *Standard Edition* 16:320–338, 1917.

Freud S: The ego and the id. *In standard edition* 19:3–66, 1923.

Freud S: The dissolution of the Oedipus Complex. *In standard edition* 19:72–79, 1924.

Gunderson JG: *Borderline personality disorder,* Washington, D.C., 1984, American Psychiatric Press.

Horner AJ: *The primacy of structure: psychotherapy of underlying character pathology,* Northvale, N.J., 1990, Jason Aronson.

Houseman C: The paranoid person: a biopsychosocial perspective, *Arch of Psychiatric Nurs* 5(6):176–181, 1990.

Kaplan HI, Sadock BJ: *Pocket handbook of clinical psychiatry,* Baltimore, 1990, Williams and Wilkins.

Kavoussi R, Siever L: Biologic validators of personality disorders. In Olham JM, editor: *Personality disorders: new perspectives on diagnostic validity,* Washington, D.C., 1991, American Psychiatric Association.

Keltner NL, Folks DG: *Psychotropic drugs,* St. Louis, 1993, Mosby.

Kernberg OF: *Severe personality disorders: psychotherapeutic strategies,* New Haven, Conn., 1984, Yale University Press.

Kernberg OF: *Borderline conditions and pathological narcissism,* Northvale, N.J., 1985, Jason Aronson.

Kreisman JJ, Straus H: *I hate you—don't leave me: understanding the borderline personality,* Los Angeles, 1989, The Body Press.

Lencz T et al: Impaired eye tracking in undergraduates with schizotypal personality disorder, *Am J Psychiatry* 150(1):152–153, 1993.

Mahler MS: Thoughts about development and individuation, *Psychoanalytic Study Child* 18:307–324, 1963.

Mahler MS: A study of the separation-individuation process and its possible application to borderline phenomena in the psychoanalytic situation, *Psychoanalytic Study Child* 26:403–424, 1971.

Mahler MS: On the first three subphases of the separation-individuation process, *International J of Psychoanalysis* 53:333–338, 1972a.

Mahler MS: Rapprochement subphase of the separation-individuation process, *Psychoanalytic Quarterly* 41:487–506, 1972b.

Manfield P: *Split self split object: understanding and treating borderline, narcissistic, and schizoid disorders,* Northvale, N.J., 1992, Jason Aronson.

Mann JJ et al: Increased serotonin-2 and beta-adrenergic receptor binding in the frontal cortices of suicide victims, *Arch of Gen Psych* 43:954–959, 1986.

Marin D et al: Biological models and treatments for personality disorders, *Psych Annals* 19:143–146, March 1989.

Masterson JF: *Psychotherapy of the borderline adult: a developmental approach,* New York, 1976, Brunner/Mazel.

Oldham JM, Skodol AE: Personality disorders and mood disorders. In Tasman A, Riba MB, editors: *American Psychiatric Press review of psychiatry,* vol 11, Washington, D.C., 1992, American Psychiatric Press.

Siever LJ: Biologic markers in schizotypal personality disorder, *Schizophrenic Bull* 11:564–575, 1985.

Siever LJ: Schizophrenia spectrum personality disorders. In Tasman A and Riba MB, editors: *American Psychiatric Press review of psychiatry,* vol 11, Washington, D.C., 1992, American Psychiatric Press.

Siever LJ, Davis KL: A psychobiological perspective on the personality disorders, *Amer J of Psych* 148(12):1647–1658, 1991.

Soloff PH et al: Pharmacotherapy and borderline subtypes. In Oldham JM, editor: *Personality disorders: new perspectives on diagnostic validity,* Washington, D.C., 1991, American Psychiatric Press.

Stanley M, Stanley B: Postmortem evidence for serotonin's role in suicide, *J of Clin Psych* 51:22–27, April 1990.

Steele, RL: Staff attitudes toward seclusion and restraint: anything new? *Perspectives in Psychiatric Care* 29:23–28, July–September 1993.

Townsend MC: *Nursing diagnoses in psychiatric nursing: a pocket guide for care plan construction,* ed 3, Philadelphia, 1994, FA Davis Co.

Tyson P, Tyson R: *Psychoanalytic theories of development: and integration,* New Haven, Conn., 1990, Yale University Press.

Widiger TA, Rogers JH: Prevalence and comorbidity of personality disorders, *Psych Annals* 19:132–136, March 1989.

CHAPTER 15

Substance-Related Disorders

Ona Z. Riggin
Barbara A. Redding

Abuse A maladaptive pattern of substance use leading to problems in psychosocial, biologic, cognitive/perceptual, or spiritual/belief dimensions of life.

Alcoholism A chronic, progressive, and potentially fatal biogenic and psychosocial disease characterized by impaired control over drinking, tolerance and physical dependence that lead to loss of control, distorted thinking, and other social consequences.

Blackout Acute anterograde amnesia without recognition formation of long-term memory, e.g., a period of memory loss during which there is no recall for activities, resulting from the ingestion of alcohol and/or other drugs.

Codependency An emotional, psychologic, and behavioral pattern of coping that an individual develops as a result of prolonged exposure to a dysfunctional pattern of behavior within the family of origin. The individual experiences difficulty with identity development and setting functional boundaries, which lead to taking care of others rather than self.

Cross-tolerance A condition in which tolerance to one drug often results in a tolerance to chemically similar drugs. Tolerance is originally produced by long-term administration of one drug, which is manifested toward a second drug that has not been administered previously (for example, tolerance to alcohol is accompanied by cross-tolerance to volatile anesthetics or barbiturates).

Dependence, physical A physiological state of adaptation to a drug or alcohol, usually characterized by the development of tolerance to drug effects and the emergence of a withdrawal syndrome during prolonged abstinence.

Dependence, psychologic The compulsive use of substances leading to a state of craving a drug or alcohol for its positive effect or to avoid negative effects associated with its absence or the ability to exercise behavioral restraint.

Detoxification Treatment that assists the individual to withdraw from the physical effects of alcohol and/or other addictive substances and helps eliminate severe withdrawal symptoms that can occur with abrupt withdrawal. It can be provided in a hospital, day treatment, or outpatient setting.

Dual diagnosis The simultaneous occurrence of a substance-related disorder and a medical or psychiatric disorder in an individual.

Enmeshed An individual's inability to differentiate or establish a personal identity. Enmeshed individuals have diffuse boundaries within the family and live solely for each other. Member roles are permeable with a tendency to cut off outside interactions.

Half-life Time required for the serum concentration of a drug to decrease by 50%. Drugs dosed at intervals less than their half-life will accumulate in the body, often to toxic levels.

Relapse/Relapse prevention Resumption of a pattern of substance use or dependency after a period of sobriety, and/or the process in which indicators or warning signs appear prior to the individual's actual resumption of the substance. Relapse prevention is a means of helping the chemically dependent individual maintain behavioral changes over a prolonged period of time.

Sobriety The state of complete abstinence from alcohol and/or other drugs of abuse in conjunction with a satisfactory quality of life.

Teratogens Substances that cause developmental malformations in the fetus.

Tolerance Physiological adaptation to the effect of drugs that diminishes effects with constant dosages or maintains the intensity and duration of effects through increased dosage.

- Trace the historical evolution of substance abuse.

- Identify the major concepts relative to substance abuse.

- Compare and contrast the etiological factors relative to substance abuse.

- Describe the effects of alcohol and other drugs on biologic, psychosocial, cultural, cognitive, and spiritual dimensions of clients across the life span.

- Apply the nursing process for clients with substance-related disorders.

- Identify community resources used in rehabilitating clients with substance-related disorders.

- Discuss disease concepts specific to substance abuse and addiction.

- Describe the current treatment modalities in managing the care of clients with substance-related disorders.

Substance-related disorders are a significant health problem in today's society. Problems associated with **abuse** of alcohol, tobacco, and other drugs continue to consume a major proportion of the health care dollar. In addition to treating problems related to substance abuse, secondary complications of drug use account for a large percentage of admissions to emergency rooms and inpatient facilities.

Individuals of all age groups, cultures, and ethnic populations are affected by substance abuse. Health care providers are in a unique position to provide preventive, screening, diagnostic, treatment, and rehabilitation services. Since the age of onset for developing problems with alcohol or drugs is occurring more frequently during the elementary school years, prevention must begin in the preschool years. The nurse is in an ideal position to provide preventive education services about substance use to individuals, families, and the community at large.

HISTORICAL AND THEORETICAL PERSPECTIVES

The use and abuse of alcohol and other substances have been reported for centuries. References to the use of alcohol are reported in the Old Testament. Greek and Roman mythology had gods of wine (Dionysus and Bacchus, respectively). Alcohol was a part of the meal as well as a staple in many early cultures' diets. In addition, it was used in celebrations of births, death, coronations, and religious ceremonies. Cannabis was used as a minor pain reliever, an additive to beer to produce hallucinogenic effects, and as a component of ritualistic ceremonies.

Medical Use

In early times, alcohol was used to cleanse wounds, as an anesthetic, and as an ingredient in salves and tonics. Many drugs, specifically elixirs, were alcohol-based. In the late 1800s and early 1900s, patent medicines and remedies were sold by traveling medicine men, physicians, and pseudophysicians. A large number of these medicines and remedies contained drugs such as opium, heroin, and alcohol. Since the production of these substances was not governed by law, poisonings (especially of infants), deaths, and addiction occurred in large numbers. In the nineteenth century, morphine and codeine were extracted from opium. The production of synthetic narcotics followed. Today, the production and use of medications subject to abuse are regulated by federal laws.

ETIOLOGY

The literature on substance abuse indicates that no one theory adequately explains the etiology for substance abuse. Historically, **alcoholism** and abuse of other substances have been viewed from a psychological or moral perspective, with the indication that those who abuse substances are weak and have the capacity to refrain from use if they desire. More recently it has become accepted that alcoholism is a disease with a hereditary predisposition. Major etiological factors of substance abuse are summarized in Box 15-1.

Biologic Theories

One of the earliest observations that some people have a predisposition to alcoholism was proposed by Jellinek (1946). Jellinek conjectured that the addictive process and the "loss of control" over the use of alcohol may have a biochemical basis. The most widely accepted classification for alcoholism was proposed by Jellinek (1977) when he noted that alcoholics pass through various stages, including the prealcoholic symptomatic phase, the prodromal phase, the crucial phase, and the chronic phase.

Jellinek's work was reinforced in the late 1950s by research reports based on Scandinavian twin studies. The longitudinal research focused on twins of alcoholic parents who were reared in three different environments, i.e., their own parents, foster parents who were alco-

---

Box 15-1   Etiological Theories Related to Substance-Related Disorders

Biologic theories

- genetic predisposition to alcoholism
- low response to ethanol

Psychological theories

- regression and fixation at the pregenital, oral level of psychosexual development
- dependent personality
- low self-esteem
- basic depressive personality organization
- intolerance for frustration and pain
- lack of success
- lack of meaningful relationships
- difficulty with intimacy

Family theories

- enmeshment
- emotional compensation
- underlying familial problems
- separation/individuation issues

Learning theories

- positive effect of mood alterations
- media reinforcement
- peer pressures

---

holics, and foster parents who did not consume alcohol. After 25 years, the incidence of alcoholism in all three groups was almost identical. The research strongly suggested that a genetic factor predisposed the twins to alcoholism.

In 1973 and 1974 Goodwin et al studied identical twins of alcoholic and nonalcoholic fathers. All twins in the study were adopted at birth. Fifty percent of the twins were placed in alcoholic homes, and 50% were placed in nonalcoholic homes. The twins of alcoholic fathers developed alcoholism at a significantly higher rate than twins of nonalcoholic fathers, even when they were raised in nonalcoholic homes. Twins of nonalcoholic fathers who were raised in alcoholic homes did not develop alcoholism at a greater rate than that of the general population.

Schuckit (1985) reports that children of alcoholics are four times more likely to become alcoholic, even if they are adopted by nonalcoholic families at birth. Identical twins have a 60% or greater chance of becoming alcoholic, while fraternal twins have a 30% chance or less. The research further substantiated the finding that when children of nonalcoholic parents are reared by parents who are alcoholics, they are not at increased risk for becoming alcoholic.

In 1994, Schuckit reported on research in which young adults who had a low response to ethanol were followed for approximately a decade. The data revealed that a strong relation existed between a less intense response to ethanol and the later development of dependence on alcohol and/or alcohol abuse.

At the present time, research based on computerized laboratory tests, radiologic examinations, and genetic linkage have revealed differences between alcoholics and nonalcoholics. Further replication of studies is necessary before conclusive results can be postulated.

Psychologic Theories

Various psychologic theories have been proposed to explain substance abuse. The earliest theories focus on a psychoanalytic perspective and view the substance abuser as regressed and fixated at the pregenital, oral levels of psychosexual development. The individual seeks need satisfaction through oral behaviors that include smoking and ingestion of substances or food.

Interpersonal theories focus on the individual with a dependent personality who is unable to fulfill gratification needs, or the individual with an inadequate personality or low self-esteem who uses substances to feel a sense of control, reduce anxiety, and thereby feel more competent.

Knott (1987) stated that there is no addictive personality for alcoholism. He identified several psychodynamic factors that are associated with alcoholism, including a basic depressive personality organization, an intolerance for frustration and pain, a lack of success, a lack of affectionate and meaningful relationships in life, low self-esteem, lack of self-regard, and risk behaviors.

Problems with sexual identity, difficulty with intimacy, marked narcissistic trends, and personal insecurity have also been implicated. Generally speaking, theories of psychologic causation are less well-accepted at the present time and are considered to be insufficient to adequately explain the need for excessive substance use.

Family Theories

Family systems theory (Bowen, 1978) can be used as a conceptual model to describe the interrelated and interdependent concepts that provide an understanding of emotional family functioning. Several of Bowen's concepts exemplify what happens in the family with an individual who abuses substances.

Children from these families have a tendency to be "nondifferentiated" and **enmeshed** in the family system. Enmeshed individuals have an inability to differentiate or establish a personal identity. They have diffuse boundaries within the family and live solely for each other. Family secrets and myths are used as survival measures by family members, with a tendency to cut off outside interactions. The "multi-generational transmission process" can be used to trace existence of the disease in the extended family.

Scheitlin (1990) states that alcoholism in the family reaches far beyond the alcoholic and has adverse effects on the spouse, children, and others in the immediate and work environments. It is estimated that approximately 28 million Americans are children of alcoholics. The development of a systems perspective that includes alcoholism and substance abuse as a family disease emphasizes the need to treat the family as well as the substance abuser.

Stanton and Todd et al (1982) propose that adolescents who are reared in enmeshed families have a higher tendency to turn to substances to compensate for feelings of dependency, inadequacy, and fear of separation. They state that the adolescent uses substances to keep the family in crisis in an effort to avert the emergence of underlying familial problems.

Learning Theories

Learning theory based on operant conditioning models and modeling theory provides additional explanations for substance use. In accordance with operant conditioning theories, drug use develops and is reinforced through the positive effect of mood alterations that occur as a result of chemical alterations in the body.

Differential reinforcement of the effects of drugs occurs at many levels. Media portrayals of "good times" with alcohol and drugs serve as powerful reinforcing mechanisms for adolescents and young adults. Peer group pressures and the need to belong to the group also have positive reinforcing powers. Children and adolescents reared in homes where substances are readily available frequently model the behavior of adults and role models who use substances to feel good.

Initially, the effect of substances produces pleasant physical and emotional sensations. The individual experiences increased feelings of self-confidence; relief from tension, anxiety, and fear; and a general feeling of well-being. Unfortunately, drugs serve as their own reinforcers and become a necessary way of life for the drug user. When negative consequences occur due to excessive use, the initial learned or conditioned response remains, and the negative response is insufficient to stop use of the substance. At this time, other interventions, including conditioning with less dangerous drugs, for example, methadone or antabuse, may be required.

EPIDEMIOLOGY

Substance abuse is the number one health problem in the United States. As such, it places an undue burden on the health care system and increases the cost of health care. Substance abuse affects every facet of society and places an enormous strain on the quality of life, not only for the abuser but also for the family.

There are more deaths, illnesses, accidents, and disabilities from substance abuse than from any other preventable health problem. The cost of substance abuse has been estimated to be a staggering $238 billion per year. Of this cost, $99 billion is attributed to alcohol, $67 billion to illicit drugs, and $72 billion to smoking (Rice, 1990).

The impact on individuals who abuse substances, as well as the impact on their families and on society, varies for each substance. Productivity losses, illness, accidents, and premature deaths account for the major cost for alcohol, while crime and juvenile detention play a major role for illicit drug-related costs. With regard to smoking, more than 63% of the cost is attributed to premature deaths due to lung cancer; coronary heart disease; and chronic bronchitis, emphysema, and other smoke-related chronic lung disease (Horgan, 1993).

Many elementary schoolchildren begin to experiment with alcohol, tobacco, and illicit drugs in the fifth and sixth grades (Figure 15-1). Since alcohol and cigarettes usually precede the use of illicit drugs, they are referred to as "gateway drugs." It is estimated that by the eighth grade, 70% of youth report having tried alcohol, 44% have smoked cigarettes, 10% have tried marijuana, and 2% have used cocaine. By the twelfth grade, these percentages have increased as follows: 80% alcohol, 63% tobacco, 37% marijuana, and 8% cocaine (Horgan, 1993). The age at which an individual first uses drugs is a strong predictor of heavy use throughout his or her lifetime. Use at an early age also subjects the individual to the probability of early dependence and addiction. The incidence and prevalence of substance abuse are summarized in Box 15-2.

Demographic Differences

Demographic variables, including ethnicity, race, gender, education, and place of residence, affect the use of drugs. Caucasian high school seniors are at highest risk for alcohol and cigarette use, African-American high school seniors are at lowest risk, and Hispanic high school seniors fall somewhere in the middle.

Statistics from the NIDA High School Senior Survey (1992) indicate that about 48% of male Native Americans and Caucasian high school seniors drink heavily. Comparable statistics placed Hispanics at 45%, African-Americans at 24%, and Asian-Americans at 18%. Similar results were revealed for nicotine use. Statistics for high school students who smoked one-half pack of cigarettes or more per day were as follows: 18% Native Americans, 12% Caucasians, 5% Hispanics, and 4% Asian-Americans (Horgan, 1993).

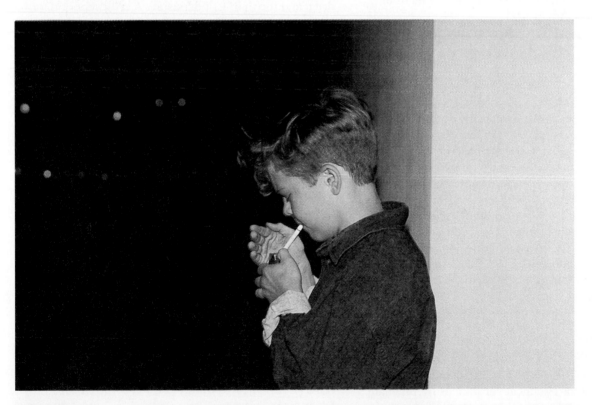

Figure 15-1 Many children have experimented with alcohol or cigarettes by the time they are age 11 or 12. Cigarettes and alcohol are considered "gateway drugs" because they usually lead to the use of other drugs.

(Copyright © Cathy Lander-Goldberg, Lander Photographics.)

> ### Box 15-2   Epidemiology
> ### for Substance-Related Disorders
>
> **Alcohol**
>
> - 18 million people in the United States drink alcohol heavily
> - 10 million people in the United States are alcoholics
> - High school seniors and young adults ages 18–25 are at highest risk for heavy alcohol use, followed by people ages 26–34
> - By the eighth grade, 70% of youth report having tried alcohol, 44% have smoked cigarettes, 10% have tried marijuana, and 2% have used cocaine
> - By the twelfth grade, the percentages are 80% alcohol, 63% tobacco, 37% marijuana, and 8% cocaine
>
> **Illicit drug use**
>
> - Use of illicit drugs by high school seniors has decreased from 40% in 1970 to 14% in 1992
> - Marijuana use has decreased from 35% in 1979 to 13% in 1991
> - Cocaine use has decreased from 9% in 1979 to 2% in 1991
>
> **Nicotine use**
>
> - The number of adult smokers has decreased from 42% in 1965 to 26% in 1991
> - 15% of the population (or 56% of smokers) smoked a pack or more a day in 1991

Patterns of substance use by gender are in flux. Generally, more high school males than females consume alcohol and use marijuana and cocaine. The gap in use, however, is narrowing. A reversal is noted in cigarette use from previous trends where females were more likely to smoke cigarettes than males. Recent findings reveal that high school males also smoke more than females. Individuals' educational level, coupled with the area in which they live, has an additional influence on alcohol, tobacco, and drug use. Individuals with less formal education who live in highly metropolitan areas are most likely to use substances.

SUBSTANCE ABUSE IN SPECIAL POPULATIONS
Perinatal Concerns

The use and abuse of chemical substances by pregnant women are on the increase. Tobacco (in the form of cigarettes) continues to be the most common drug pregnant women use. Approximately 25%–30% of women

expose their children to nicotine in utero. While some mothers stop smoking during the first three or four months of pregnancy, 75% resume tobacco use following pregnancy.

According to the National Household Survey on Drug Abuse conducted in 1988 by NIDA, estimates indicate that three out of every five women of childbearing age drink alcohol (NIDA, 1988). One in every 10 American women consumes 2 or more drinks daily, 14 or more drinks weekly, or up to 60 drinks monthly, and is classified as a moderate drinker. Approximately 6%–8% of pregnant women have serious alcohol problems (Ewing, 1992). Ten percent of women of childbearing age acknowledged using an illicit drug within 30 days prior to the 1988 NIDA Household Survey (Cook et al, 1990). In particular, cocaine use has risen among young women. Many of these women are polydrug users who may use cocaine, tobacco, alcohol, marijuana, and/or other drugs. An estimated 375,000 infants born each year in the United States have been exposed to illicit substances in utero (Kelly et al, 1991).

Many of the substances abused by pregnant women are **teratogens** to the offspring, causing developmental malformations in the fetus. However, since many pregnant women are polydrug users, it is difficult in most instances to predict the outcome in their offspring. The effect of substances on fetuses is dependent on a number of factors, including the amount and pattern of maternal consumption, the properties of the chemical substance/drug, and the timing of exposure. A critical period for vital organ development occurs during the embryonic phase, from the second through the eighth week after conception. Drug exposure after this period is more likely to result in intrauterine growth retardation and more subtle mental and behavioral deficits (Cook et al, 1990).

Generally, intrauterine drug exposure has been associated with

- low birth weight (small for gestational age), decreased length, and small head circumference
- specific congenital physical malformations
- mild to severe withdrawal effects that include irritability, tremors, seizures, and hypertonia, abdominal distention, increased respiratory rate, and vomiting
- central nervous system damage that may delay or impair neurobehavioral development

These neurobehavioral effects may include subtle behavioral abnormalities or latent developmental deficits and/or delays that are frequently not obvious at birth (Cook et al, 1990).

FETAL ALCOHOL SYNDROME/FETAL ALCOHOL EFFECTS

Many infants who have been exposed to alcohol during the prenatal period demonstrate a) low birth weight; b) certain facial characteristics; and c) neurological abnormalities, including developmental and/or intellectual delays. The facial characteristics include microcephaly (head circumference below the third percentile), microthalmia (small eyes) and/or short palpebral fissures, poorly developed philtrum (median groove between upper lip and nose), thin upper lip, short nose, small chin, and flattening of the maxillary area (see Figure 15-2).

Infants and children who have all three of these characteristics (a, b, and c) are identified as having *fetal alco-* *hol syndrome* (FAS). Those with at least one of the characteristics (a, b, or c) are identified as having *fetal alcohol effects* (FAE). In addition, these children may also have a variety of defects affecting other organ systems, including cardiac defects, visual problems, hearing defects, dental malalignments, and minor genital anomalies. As children with FAS and FAE become older, they may exhibit such behaviors as hyperactivity, which evolves into problems of easy distractibility, inability to attend to

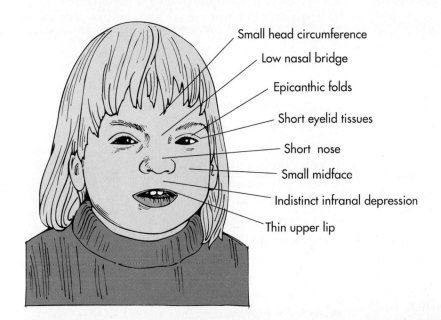

Small head circumference
Low nasal bridge
Epicanthic folds
Short eyelid tissues
Short nose
Small midface
Indistinct infranal depression
Thin upper lip

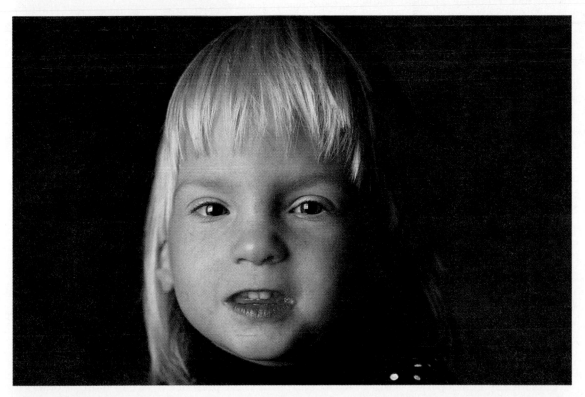

Figure 15-2 Fetal alcohol syndrome. Milder forms of alcohol-induced changes on the fetus and the infant are known as fetal alcohol effects.

relevant data, and the inability to ignore irrelevant information. In addition, these individuals show poor coordination and short attention spans, dependency, stubbornness or sullenness, social withdrawal, teasing or bullying, crying or laughing too easily, impulsivity, and periods of high anxiety.

Whether working with an adolescent or an adult client, one must recognize that some of these individuals may have or develop other medical or psychological problems; therefore, it is important to consider the existence of comorbidity, the presence of two or more disorders in the same person.

Those with FAS/FAE who have awareness of the etiology of the syndrome manifest a high incidence of depression, anger, suicidal ideation, antisocial behavior, and drug and alcohol use. Many of these men and women are unable to lead normal, independent lives. Their family or caregivers must make plans for long-term community support and care.

COCAINE USE

Cocaine use by the pregnant mother and the effect on her child show great variability. Some of the infants have severe effects (for example, missing digits, cerebral stroke, and malformations of major body systems), while other children appear to compensate for or show no effects of cocaine exposure. As more of these children enter the school system, an increase in learning and behavioral problems may be documented. When a child experiences such problems, the exposure during fetal life to alcohol and other drugs, including cocaine, should be explored.

Adolescent Substance Abuse

Adolescent substance abuse is a major health and social problem. Rates of substance use and abuse among American high school students and college students remain the highest in the industrialized world (Johnson et al, 1988). The true measure of the problem is further complicated by the fact that substance abuse in adolescence is an illicit behavior with potential legal complications. Adolescent peers are reluctant to volunteer information about drinking behaviors or other drug use (Kozel and Adams, 1986).

Another problem related to adolescent drug use concerns the DSM-IV classification for substance abuse. The labels of dependence and abuse do not adequately describe the problem in adolescence, nor are they helpful in treating adolescents. It is more appropriate to use the term "problematic use," because adolescents drink in response to specific events, emotional crisis, or peer group pressure (Flynn, 1992). They do not develop the usual signs of psychologic or physical dependence because they have not used alcohol for a sufficient period of time. **Psychologic dependence** is the compulsive use of substances leading to a state of craving a drug or alcohol for

its positive effect or to avoid negative effects associated with its absence or the ability to exercise behavioral restraint. **Physical dependence** is a physiological state of adaptation to a drug or alcohol, usually characterized by the development of tolerance to drug effects and the emergence of a withdrawal syndrome during prolonged abstinence. Adolescents who have continuing problems with drinking alcohol and using other drugs manifest a pervasive, recurrent pattern that has serious consequences in several areas of their lives, including family, school, social relationships, and job performance. Legal consequences frequently occur as a result of drug use in adolescence.

The following are significant factors that place the adolescent at risk for substance use/abuse:

- school drop-out
- emotionally disadvantaged background
- children of drug abusers
- victims of abuse—child/parental, sexual
- experienced trouble with law
- history of mental problems
- suicide attempts
- long-term physical pain
- dysfunctional families; divorce
- feelings of inferiority—emotional, physical, academic

The Client and Family Teaching Guidelines on page 349 lists signs of substance use for parents to be aware of and strategies to prevent substance abuse.

Impaired Professionals

The issue of substance dependence in health care professionals has received increasing attention from professional groups. Statistics concerning substance dependency in nurses vary greatly from one study to another. Statistics reported by the American Nurses Association (ANA) indicated that 5% of 2.4 million nurses were chemical abusers and 8%–10% were chemically dependent (ANA, 1984).

Sullivan and Handley (1992) concluded that the prevalence of alcohol and drug problems in nurses and student nurses does not exceed that of others in society. The authors also identified that published research is limited in scope because results are based on small nonrandomly selected samples. Few studies have been replicated, and long-term research is lacking. Additional research is needed to obtain more accurate information on the problem of impairment in nurses and other health care professionals.

Persons with Dual Diagnosis

Comorbidity is the presence of two or more disorders in the same person. They may be medical or psychological conditions as well as substance-related disorders, and

Client and Family
TEACHING GUIDELINES

Signs of adolescent drug use/abuse

- Sudden behavioral changes
- Sweating, especially at night
- Needle marks
- Inebriation
- Change in nutritional intake
- Nasal congestion
- Rhinorrhea with cocaine use
- School problems

Prevention of adolescent substance use/abuse

- Provide positive role modeling by parents and adults in the adolescent's world
- Reinforce positive behaviors and the dangers of substance use
- Support adolescent in coping with the social pressure exerted by peers
- Establish normative expectations for adolescent behaviors
- Help adolescent anticipate pressures and reinforce behaviors to cope with realities
- Encourage involvement in life skills training programs where the emphasis is on positive skills training, resistance training, and group support
- Monitor the adolescent's television viewing since media may portray legal and illegal substance use as a part of daily life

may occur simultaneously or sequentially. If occurring simultaneously, it is also known as **dual diagnosis.** Dual diagnosis indicates that an individual has two initial unrelated disorders that interact and cause increased manifestations of the other disorder (Lehman et al, 1987). Individuals may be labeled with a dual diagnosis on the basis of self-reports because the assessment tools available to identify the characteristics related to the dually diagnosed are of questionable reliability and validity (Drake et al, 1990).

The literature shows that there is a relationship between substance-use disorders and individuals who experience depression or anxiety (Landry et al, 1991). Many individuals who are experiencing depression will self-medicate with psychoactive substances to feel better. Likewise, individuals who abuse substances develop depressive symptoms due to the losses they experience and actual biochemical changes that may result. Treatment is difficult because treating either disorder without attention to the other may exacerbate the coexisting problem.

The literature also indicates that individuals with personality disorders have a higher incidence of dual diagnosis. Many of them are discharged from the hospital earlier than usual or leave against medical advice. Ross et al (1988) reported that 47% of individuals admitted to a drug and alcohol treatment unit had a lifetime diagnosis of antisocial personality disorders. Dulit et al (1990) found that borderline personality and substance abuse disorders were interrelated in two-thirds of the population that they studied.

Another type of dual diagnosis is related to clients with schizophrenia who use alcohol and drugs. Most research findings support prevalence rates of substance abuse in people with schizophrenia that are similar to the prevalence rate in the general population. However, Mueser et al (1990) found the use of stimulants and hallucinogens appreciably greater among persons with schizophrenia, ranging from 4.5%–15% above the norm. Cuffel (1992) states that alcohol abuse and stimulant abuse among clients with schizophrenia have steadily increased since the 1960s. Findings of the research indicate prevalence rates for alcohol abuse of approximately 40% and stimulant abuse of approximately 19%.

Persons with HIV Disease

The transmission of human immunodeficiency virus (HIV) occurs through infected blood or blood products and through sexual contact. Sexual contact is considered the major route of transmission. In the United States, the incidence of heterosexual transmission continues to rise. The use of alcohol and other drugs is certainly one of the causes that contributes to "sexual risk-taking behavior" such as failure to use a condom, multiple partners, or engagement in alternative sexual acts. The second major factor that often puts the individual at risk is injectable–drug abuse that includes intravenous (IV), intradermal (skin-popping), and intramuscular (steroid abuse route). Intravenous drug use is the second most common risk factor among cases of AIDS in the United States and continues to increase.

Alcohol is known to have immunosuppressive effects that may increase an individual's susceptibility to the HIV virus or, if the individual has been exposed, increase the onset of symptoms of HIV disease. It is also believed that the effects of alcohol on the immune system and on the HIV infection may be influenced by the individual's drinking habits. Persons with chronic alcoholism who have a history of liver disease may be at greater risk for HIV infection.

CLINICAL DESCRIPTION

The DSM-IV (APA, 1994) includes the diagnostic classification Substance-Related Disorders. Subcategories exist in each of these classes. Most of the categories include dependence, abuse, intoxication, withdrawal, delirium, psychotic disorders with delusions, psychotic disorders with hallucinations, mood disorders, anxiety disorders, sexual dysfunction, sleep disorders, and disorder NOS (Not Otherwise Specified). The DSM-IV criteria for Substance Abuse and Substance Dependence are found on pages 350 and 351.

Although alcohol is the most frequently abused drug, a variety of other psychoactive drugs are abused, including barbiturates, benzodiazepines, opioids, cocaine, stimulants, and nicotine. A brief description of each type of drug follows. Refer to Chapter 22, Psychopharmacology and Other Biologic Therapies, for additional information.

Alcohol Abuse

Alcohol abuse and dependence have many physiologic complications affecting several body systems. These complications will be discussed in the following section along with signs and symptoms of alcohol withdrawal.

DSM-IV CRITERIA

Substance Abuse

A. A maladaptive pattern of substance use leading to clinically significant impairment or distress, as manifested by one (or more) of the following, occurring within a 12-month period:

  (1) recurrent substance use resulting in a failure to fulfill major role obligations at work, school, or home (e.g., repeated absences or poor job performance related to substance use; substance-related absences, suspensions, or expulsions from school; neglect of children or household)

  (2) recurrent substance use in situations in which it is physically hazardous (e.g., driving an automobile or operating a machine when impaired by substance use)

  (3) recurrent substance-related legal problems (e.g., arrests for substance-related disorderly conduct)

  (4) continued substance use despite having persistent or recurrent social or interpersonal problems caused or exacerbated by the effects of the substance (e.g., arguments with spouse about consequences of intoxication; physical fights)

B. The symptoms have never met the criteria for Substance Dependence for this class of substance.

Reprinted with permission from *Diagnostic and statistical manual of mental disorders,* ed 4, Washington, D.C., 1994, American Psychiatric Association.

NEUROLOGIC SYSTEM

Excessive use of alcohol produces several changes in the neurologic system that result from damage to brain cells. The following discussion describes common resulting syndromes.

Blackouts occur most frequently with excessive use of alcohol and present as an early sign of alcoholism. Individuals who experience blackouts enter a fugue-like amnestic state during which recollection of activities are lost from conscious recall. These individuals remain conscious and appear to function normally to those in their environment. Blackouts may last for a relatively short period of time, 24–48 hours, or they may last for a week or longer.

Pathologic intoxication usually has a sudden onset manifested by agitation, altered consciousness, aggressiveness, fear, and anxiety. It may be accompanied by mental confusion, disorientation, delusions, and hallucinations. Suicide attempts may occur due to hallucinations or the heightened state of anxiety and agitation. The attacks last from a few moments to a day or more and usually end with a long period of sleep. The next day a "hangover" occurs, which is commonly characterized by headache, gastrointestinal upsets, and general malaise. Most often, the individual has very little if any recollection of what transpired during the time of pathologic intoxication.

Substance withdrawal delirium (delirium tremens or DTs) is the most severe form of alcohol withdrawal. It occurs approximately 24–72 hours after the individual has had the last drink. Delirium tremens occur in heavy drinkers and are manifested by an acute psychotic state. Approximately 5% of all alcoholics hospitalized for alcohol withdrawal develop DTs. Confusion and disorientation regarding time and place are common. Other symptoms include vivid visual and auditory hallucinations that are accusatory and threatening to the patient, illusions (light cords appearing as snakes), severe agitation, profuse sweating, tachycardia, tachypnea, and possible grand mal seizure activity (Box 15-3). The condition may be life-threatening if immediate medical intervention does not occur.

Acute alcoholic hallucinosis occurs after a prolonged period of drinking. The syndrome is characterized by threatening auditory hallucinations. This condition is differentiated from DTs in that the individual remains oriented to time and place; during lucid periods, the person usually can recall occurrences after recovery. Some individuals incorporate the auditory hallucinations into an elaborate delusional system that may be threatening to those in the immediate environment.

Wernicke's syndrome and *Korsakoff's syndrome* occur after many years of excessive alcohol intake. The syndromes affect the entire neurologic system. Korsakoff's syndrome is an amnestic syndrome caused by deficiency in the B vitamins, including thiamin, riboflavin, and folic

DSM-IV CRITERIA

Substance Dependence

A maladaptive pattern of substance use, leading to clinically significant impairment or distress, as manifested by three (or more) of the following, occurring at any time in the same 12-month period:

(1) tolerance, as defined by either of the following:

    (a) a need for markedly increased amounts of the substance to achieve intoxication or desired effect

    (b) markedly diminished effect with continued use of the same amount of the substance

(2) withdrawal, as manifested by either of the following:

    (a) the characteristic withdrawal syndrome for the substance (refer to Criteria A and B of the criteria sets for Withdrawal from the specific substances)

    (b) the same (or a closely related) substance is taken to relieve or avoid withdrawal symptoms

(3) the substance is often taken in larger amounts or over a longer period than was intended

(4) there is a persistent desire or unsuccessful efforts to cut down or control substance use

(5) a great deal of time is spent in activities necessary to obtain the substance (e.g., visiting multiple doctors or driving long distances), use the substance (e.g., chain-smoking), or recover from its effects

(6) important social, occupational, or recreational activities are given up or reduced because of substance use

(7) the substance use is continued despite knowledge of having a persistent or recurrent physical or psychologic problem that is likely to have been caused or exacerbated by the substance (e.g., current cocaine use despite recognition of cocaine-induced depression, or continued drinking despite recognition that an ulcer was made worse by alcohol consumption)

Specify if:

With Physiological Dependence: evidence of tolerance or withdrawal (i.e., either Item 1 or 2 is present)

Without Physiological Dependence: no evidence of tolerance or withdrawal (i.e., neither Item 1 nor 2 is present)

Course specifiers (see text for definitions):

Early Full Remission

Early Partial Remission

Sustained Full Remission

Sustained Partial Remission

On Agonist Therapy

In a Controlled Environment

Reprinted with permission from *Diagnostic and statistical manual of mental disorders,* ed 4, Washington, D.C., 1994, American Psychiatric Association.

---

acid. It is characterized by amnesia, disorientation to time and place, falsification of memory, and severe peripheral neuropathy, i.e., tingling, muscle weakness, sore burning muscles, parathesias, and extreme pain on movement. Extremities, especially lower extremities, are affected. Precaution must be taken in moving clients because of the severe pain they experience. An important nursing care requirement is to prevent footdrop.

Wernicke's syndrome, also referred to as *alcoholic encephalopathy,* most frequently occurs simultaneously with Korsakoff's syndrome but may occur as an isolated condition. It is a neurologic disease characterized by ataxia, ophthalmoplegia (particularly involving the sixth cranial nerve), nystagmus, and confusion. It is caused by severe deficiency in Vitamin B_1 due to the lack of adequate food intake. The early stage responds rapidly to large doses of parenteral thiamin. If the condition is not adequately treated at an early point, it progresses to a chronic, severe lifetime condition that requires custodial care. The chronic condition is becoming more rare in re-

cent years due to the rapid use of thiamine as a treatment modality (Kaplan and Sadock, 1994).

EFFECTS ON THE LIVER

The liver is characteristically the body organ most affected by excessive use of alcohol. Alcohol passes directly into the bloodstream through the stomach and intestinal walls. It is processed by the liver where enzymes change alcohol into acetaldehyde, which is further metabolized into acetate, carbon dioxide, and water. Alcohol metabolism releases excessive amounts of hydrogen into the liver; this inhibits certain metabolic processes, including metabolism of fats. As a result, the unburned fat becomes deposited into the liver and causes hepatic steatosis, or "fatty liver" (Lieber and Leo, 1982).

Alcoholic hepatitis occurs after a prolonged period (usually several years) of alcohol abuse. It is an inflammatory condition of the liver characterized by fever, chills, nausea, pain in the upper abdomen, and jaundice. Treatment consists of abstinence with nutritional support.

Box 15-3   Alcohol Withdrawal Symptoms and Treatment

Withdrawal symptoms

- Tremulousness ("the shakes"); onset 3–36 hours after the last drink
- Increased psychomotor hyperactivity with tremors
- Insomnia
- Acute anxiety and hyperalertness
- Tachycardia (120–140 beats/min)
- Hypertension
- Anorexia
- Agitation
- Possible nausea, abdominal cramps, vomiting
- Weakness
- Craving for alcohol or sedative drug
- Acute hallucinosis
  - Auditory or visual hallucinations assume prominence; this may indicate that alcohol withdrawal delirium is impending
- Alcohol withdrawal delirium (the horrors, delirium tremens, DTs); onset 24–72 hours after last drink; most serious of withdrawal phases (5%–36% mortality)
  - Disorientation
  - Hallucinations
  - Delusions
  - Delirium
  - Severe agitation

Treatment of withdrawal

Impending withdrawal

- Monitor vital signs every 3 hours; notify physician of any abnormal readings
- Provide a quiet, nonstimulating environment, yet keep a light on in room
- Administer sedating medications promptly as ordered (do not undersedate); ensure medications are taken
- Frequently orient client to place, person, time; quietly and simply explain all procedures, routines, expected components of treatment process
- Accurately record intake and output (including emesis, diarrhea, estimated loss from diaphoresis)
- Do not force fluids until it has been established that client is dehydrated; however, ensure that client takes estimated minimum of fluids per 24-hour period
- Allow ambulation ad lib if ordered and *if client is stable,* since this channels excess agitation
- Allow client to express fears regarding withdrawal; provide nonjudgmental, caring concern
- Institute seizure precautions (oral airway, upright siderails, remove potentially harmful objects)
- Assist client with activities of daily living (bathing, eating, mouthcare) without overstimulating client (e.g., no shaving, nail care)
- Provide small, frequent, high-carbohydrate feedings that are easily digested; administer antiemetic PRN before meals (offer patient flavored fluids, gelatins); administer vitamins as ordered, such as multivitamin, B-complex including thiamine, vitamin C
- Test urine for specific gravity and stools for guaiac to detect GI dysfunction
- Be there; spend time with client and family

Alcohol withdrawal delirium

- Monitor vital signs qh
- Assess neurologic status qh
- Stimulate patient to cough and deep breathe q2h
- Carefully evaluate bladder and bowel functions
- Inspect skin for signs of breakdown or traumatic injury
- IVs, tube feedings, catheter if ordered
- Restrain client to prevent injury if needed
- Check client at least every 15 minutes
- Administer anticonvulsant medications as ordered

From Beare P, Myers JL: *Principles and practice of adult health nursing,* ed 2, St. Louis, 1994, Mosby.

Approximately 50% of clients who continue to drink progress to cirrhosis of the liver (Galamos, 1985).

Cirrhosis of the liver due to alcohol abuse occurs in fewer than one-third of alcoholics. However, alcohol abuse continues to be the leading cause of cirrhosis. Alcohol abuse causes scarring of the small veins in the liver and the resultant impaired circulation that causes the liver to become hypertrophied. Ascites, hypertension, and esophageal varices often result, and hepatic failure may lead to death (Francis and Miller, 1991).

EFFECTS ON THE GASTROINTESTINAL TRACT

Gastritis is a frequent complication that results from alcohol intake. The amount of alcohol and the length of time required to produce this effect vary from individual to individual. Alcohol stimulates acid production in the stomach, which damages the stomach lining and results in gastritis and gastric ulcers. Malabsorption of vitamins, especially thiamine, folic acid, and B_{12}, may occur in the small intestine. Since alcohol supplies calories and displaces the need for food, malnutrition is common. Heavy alcohol use over a prolonged period may affect the pancreas, resulting in pancreatitis and pancreatic insufficiency.

EFFECTS ON THE CARDIOVASCULAR SYSTEM

Alcohol abuse over a long period may affect the cardiovascular system. Alcoholic cardiomyopathy with congestive failure and atrial fibrillation may occur. Other manifestations include narrow pulse pressure, tachycardia, elevated diastolic pressure, hypertension, and peripheral edema. According to Donahue et al (1986), the risk of hemorrhagic stroke is doubled for light consumers of alcohol and tripled for heavy drinkers. It is not common to delay elective surgery for individuals who consume excessive amounts of alcohol because of the negative effects of alcohol on the cardiovascular system.

EFFECTS ON OTHER SYSTEMS

Excessive alcohol intake may affect any system in the body. Male alcoholics may experience impotence due to erection problems. Effects on the reproductive system are substantiated for mothers and their unborn infants, as discussed under fetal alcohol syndrome. Female alcoholics frequently experience infertility and decreased menstruation, a process called "telescoping" that occurs as a result of more rapid development of dependence.

Acute myopathy is another common sequelae of long-term alcohol abuse, characterized by sudden leg cramps. If alcohol abuse continues, chronic myopathy may occur, resulting in weakness and atrophy of the leg muscles. Alcoholics are also at risk for metabolic bone disease (Bikle, 1980).

Effects of alcohol on the endocrine system are less well-documented. It is believed that alcohol affects the hypothalamic-pituitary adrenal system, causing hypoglycemia which, in turn, causes the alcoholic to drink.

Abuse of Other Drugs
BARBITURATES

First introduced in 1903, barbiturates are used as hypnotics, sedatives, and anticonvulsants. Phenobarbital and barbital are long-acting drugs with a **half-life** (the time required for the serum concentration of a drug to decrease by 50%) of 12–24 hours. Amobarbital (Amytal) has an intermediate active half-life of 6–12 hours; pentobarbital (Nembutal) and secobarbital (Seconal) are short-acting drugs with a half-life of 3–6 hours (Kaplan and Sadock, 1994).

Barbiturates are frequently abused drugs because they are legitimately manufactured in large quantities and available in many forms. Secobarbital, pentobarbital, and amobarbital are the three most frequently abused barbiturates. When they are available through the black mar-

ket, the strength of the drug is unknown because most of it has been replaced with sugar and other substances (Kaplan and Sadock, 1994). Abuse of barbiturates, as well as prescriptions for barbiturates, have been reduced since they have been classified as controlled substances and are under federal legal control with the implementation of the Harrison Narcotic Act in 1914.

Barbiturate abuse occurs most frequently among young users or among middle-aged individuals who abuse prescription drugs. Consumption is through oral or intravenous routes. Young abusers may substitute barbiturates for heroin or morphine because they are cheaper and more readily available. Barbiturates have a **cross-tolerance** to other chemically similar drugs including alcohol, benzodiazepines, and heroin. Intravenous users experience a sudden warm "rush" followed by a prolonged drowsy feeling.

Individuals who present with mild barbiturate intoxication experience the following symptoms: sluggishness in coordination, emotional lability, aggressive impulses, slowness of speech, thought disorders, and faulty judgment. Neurologic signs include nystagmus (involuntary eye oscillations), diplopia (double vision), strabismus (deviation of the eye), ataxic gait, positive Romberg's sign (swaying of the body when standing with the feet close together and eyes closed), hypotonia, dysmetria (disturbance to control range of movement in muscular acts), and decreased superficial reflexes. The diagnosis of barbiturate intoxication is confirmed by blood tests (Kaplan and Sadock, 1994).

Barbiturates are especially dangerous because all patterns of overuse have potentially deleterious effects on the individual's health. They are a common cause of lethal accidents and are frequently used in suicide attempts. Barbiturates found in home medicine cabinets may be consumed by children and may result in fatal drug overdoses. Death occurs as a result of deep coma, which progresses to respiratory arrest and cardiovascular failure. Lethal doses vary widely from individual to individual. There is a narrow therapeutic index for sedative effects with the therapeutic dose being very close to the lethal dose (Kaplan and Sadock, 1994).

BENZODIAZEPINES

Benzodiazepines, introduced in the early 1960s, have largely displaced therapeutic uses of barbiturates. Prior to barbiturates, alcohol was the most frequently sought after substance for anxiety and insomnia. Benzodiazepines potentiate the sedative and central nervous system (CNS) depression effects of alcohol and barbiturates. The benzodiazepines rarely produce unconsciousness or death when taken alone (Paul, 1988).

Benzodiazepines have a wide range of pharmacologic differences, including rapidity of onset of action, half-life, and ways in which they are metabolized in the body (Scharf et al, 1988).

Benzodiazepines that have a rapid onset of action are more likely to have abuse potential. Diazepam (Valium) is the most rapidly absorbed of the group and produces an affective euphoria. It is the most widely abused benzodiazepine and one of the most widely abused prescription drugs. The scientific community lacks agreement on the abuse potential of diazepam when prescribed for medical reasons.

The benzodiazepines, including diazepam, are not likely to produce abuse in clients who do not have a history of chemical dependence. Although the specific mechanisms are unknown, individuals with a chemical dependency react differently to diazepam than do individuals with no chemical dependency. **Tolerance** (physiological adaptation to the effect of drugs that diminishes effects with constant dosages or maintains the intensity and duration of effects through increased dosage) in individuals with a chemical dependency is rapid for sedative and euphoric effects and negligible for anti-anxiety effects (Francis and Miller, 1991).

OPIOIDS

Included in this classification of drugs are opium alkaloids derived from opium (juice of the opium poppy *Pavaver somniferum*) of which morphine is the best known. Other opiate alkaloids are heroin, codeine, and hydromorphine (Dilaudid). Synthetic opioids made in the laboratory include meperidine (Demerol), methadone, and propoxyphene (Darvon).

The most widely abused opiate is heroin. There are an estimated 400,000–600,000 heroin addicts in the United States. Male heroin addicts outnumber female addicts, three to one. Most heroin addicts have a long history of chemical dependence, starting with substance abuse at an early age and progressing to heroin in their late twenties and early thirties. Most heroin addicts spend more than $200 a day to support their habit. Many obtain money through engaging in criminal activity or pushing and selling drugs (Kaplan and Sadock, 1994).

Tolerance to opiates develops rapidly; however, tolerance to the respiratory depressant effect of opiates does not. Most deaths occur as a result of respiratory arrest. An overdose of morphine is life-threatening. In addition to marked analgesic effects, the triad of coma, pinpoint pupils, and respiratory depression signal opiate overdose.

Emergency medical intervention with an opiate antagonist is necessary in the case of an overdose. Naloxone (Narcan) is administered intravenously, beginning with an initial dose of 0.4 mg. The dose may be repeated up to 4 or 5 times in the initial 30–45 minutes, depending on vital signs and the client's level of responsiveness. It is imperative to insure an open airway and provide continuous monitoring of vital signs until the client is fully responsive and out of danger. Naloxone has a short duration of action (4–5 hours); therefore, continuous monitoring is imperative to prevent recurrence of toxic symptoms from the opiate effects (Kaplan and Sadock, 1994).

WITHDRAWAL FROM OPIATES

Morphine and heroin addicts consume huge amounts (up to 5000 mg) of the drug. Withdrawal symptoms begin 6–8 hours after the last dose and reach their peak intensity within 48–72 hours. Withdrawal symptoms include severe muscle cramps, abdominal cramps, bone aches, vomiting with severe diarrhea, diaphoresis, rhinorrhea, lacrimation, pupillary dilation, hypertension, tachycardia, and temperature irregularities including fever. The term *cold turkey,* which denotes the abstinence syndrome, comes from another common symptom, the appearance of gooseflesh. A single dose of morphine can alleviate all symptoms.

METHADONE TREATMENT

Methadone treatment is the treatment of choice for morphine and heroin addicts. Methadone is a synthetic opioid given to addicts to suppress withdrawal symptoms. A methadone dose of 20–80 mg/day is usually sufficient to stabilize a client. Methadone maintenance is continued until the client can be withdrawn from methadone. Methadone itself is addicting, but clients can be withdrawn by gradually decreasing the total daily dose until the client is methadone-free. Special precautions need to be exercised in maintaining and withdrawing pregnant clients from opiates. Usually smaller doses of methadone are indicated (10–40 mg/day) (Kaplan and Sadock, 1994).

COCAINE

Cocaine (snow, coke, girl, lady) is a highly addictive alkaloid derived from *Erythroxylon coca,* a plant indigenous to Bolivia and Peru. The addictive properties of cocaine were not fully recognized until the 1980s when both the general public and physicians became aware of the problem. Cocaine use peaked in 1985 when 12 million used the drug and decreased significantly to 8 million users in 1988 (Adams et al, 1989).

Pharmacologic effects of cocaine that block reuptake of serotonin and the catecholamine neurotransmitters, particularly dopamine, produce an intense feeling of euphoria. This makes cocaine a highly addictive drug. A single dose of cocaine, especially in the form of "crack," may cause psychologic dependence. The main effect of cocaine is relatively brief (30–60 minutes) when used intravenously or sniffed. However, cocaine remains in the brain for approximately 10 days. After the acute drug effect, there is usually a period of depression that may be sufficiently severe to precipitate suicidal ideation (Kaplan and Sadock, 1994).

Individuals who inhale while they smoke cocaine may experience swelling and inflammation of the nasal passages and ulceration of the nose. Those who are sensitive to crack may experience sudden cardiac arrest. As with all intravenous use, the risk of sharing needles may cause infection and emboli at the injection site and predispose the individual to the risk of contracting HIV disease.

Cocaine intoxication is characterized by extreme irritability, agitation, aggressiveness, impulsive sexual activity, and manic excitement. The course of intoxication is usually self-limiting to approximately 24 hours, after which time withdrawal symptoms occur. These withdrawal symptoms are often referred to as the "crash."

Abrupt withdrawal creates an intense craving for the drug. Clients experience severe depression with suicidal ideation. They become hypersomnolent and complain of fatigue, anhedonia, and general malaise. Symptoms usually subside in a number of weeks. An inherent danger is that clients will seek other mood-altering substances, including alcohol and benzodiazepines, to fill the void they experience from giving up cocaine.

The treatment for cocaine users is varied and requires cooperation by the family, employer, and health professionals. Many individuals require hospitalization to assure separation from the drug and other substances. Urine testing for toxicologic analysis should be a part of the continuing treatment program. Psychotherapy is helpful in addressing underlying psychologic problems, and family support for the individual should be sought. Support groups such as Cocaine Anonymous (CA) are critical in helping the individual remain abstinent. The underlying depression and possible psychosis require medical treatment with antidepressant and antipsychotic medications.

STIMULANTS

Stimulant drugs include caffeine, ephidrine, propanolamine (PPA), and amphetamine. Amphetamines have the greatest abuse potential. Amphetamine was first synthesized in 1887; however, it was not marketed until 1932 under the name Benzedrine. The Benzedrine inhaler is available as a nonprescription drug for nasal congestion and asthma. Amphetamines and amphetamine congeners (drugs that have a similar action on muscle groups) compose a large group of central nervous system stimulant drugs. Among the best known are dextroamphetamine (Dexedrine), methamphetamine (Methedrine), and methylphenidine (Ritalin) (Kaplan and Sadock, 1994).

Amphetamine is a highly addictive drug. Although it is not as addictive as cocaine, occasional users soon begin to abuse the drug and use it intravenously, which leads to physical and psychosocial morbidity. In the United States, amphetamine abuse reached epidemic proportions in the 1970s.

The therapeutic use of the drug according to the Food and Drug Administration (FDA) is restricted to attention deficit/hyperactivity disorder in children and adults, narcolepsy, and obesity. Black market use of the drug continues. It is particularly popular with students, athletes, entertainers, and truck drivers because it produces a sense of well-being and reduces fatigue. The amphetamine that has been called the drug of the '90s is "ice," a pure form of methamphetamine. "Ice" is inhaled or used intravenously. Of greatest concern is the fact that "ice" is a synthetic drug that can be easily synthesized in illicit domestic laboratories (Kaplan and Sadock, 1994).

Since tolerance develops rapidly for amphetamines, some abusers may consume up to one gram per day. Death may occur with doses of 120 mg in nonusers. Life-threatening, adverse effects include cardiac arrest, stroke, and neurologic involvement, including twitching, tetany, convulsions, coma, and death.

Amphetamines also have severe psychologic effects that include restlessness, dysphoria, insomnia, irritability, confusion, and panic. Intoxication of high doses of amphetamines may lead to induced paranoia and ideas of reference. Homicidal behavior also has been reported. Diagnosis of amphetamine intoxication is made on the basis of symptoms and history. Specific laboratory tests to detect amphetamine in the urine are the most reliable to diagnose "intoxication"; however, urine testing is ineffective if more than 48 hours have elapsed since the last dose. Withdrawal symptoms usually peak in 48–72 hours after the drug is discontinued; symptoms may last for several weeks. The most frequent and dangerous symptom is depression with suicidal ideation (Kaplan and Sadock, 1994).

NICOTINE

Nicotine dependence is classified under Nicotine Use Disorder, and nicotine withdrawal is classified under Nicotine Induced Disorder in the DSM-IV. More than one-third of the world population uses nicotine. The most frequent form of ingestion is through cigarette smoking. Although nicotine use in the United States has declined in recent years, it continues to be heavily used by certain groups and populations, including women, adolescents, African-Americans, the elderly, and psychiatric clients. Nicotine use has increased in other countries, especially Japan and some European countries. Individuals with other substance-abuse problems, especially alcohol abuse, are generally heavy smokers. Many, in fact, "chain-smoke"—that is, they light their next cigarette from the one they are currently smoking.

Dependence on nicotine occurs in a relatively short period of time. The average smoker uses 20–30 cigarettes a day. Individuals who chain-smoke may use several packs a day. Withdrawal of nicotine causes marked withdrawal symptoms, including irritability, restlessness, difficulty concentrating, insomnia, and depression. Many individuals gain weight due to increased appetite. Without medical assistance, 80% of smokers who quit will relapse within the first two years. In recent years nicotine gum, nicotine nasal sprays, and nicotine patches have been used to decrease withdrawal symptoms and craving. Medical supervision is advised when these methods are used to monitor the amount of nicotine that the client is receiving.

Prognosis

Sobriety, abstinence from use of alcohol or drugs together with a satisfactory quality of life, is the goal for complete recovery from substance abuse or dependence. Many clients relapse several times before achieving sobriety. The course of the disorders vary with the class of substance, route of administration, and other factors (APA, 1994). A diagnosis of substance abuse is more likely in persons who have begun using substances only recently. For many, substance abuse with particular substances can evolve into substance dependence for the same substances, particularly for substances that have a high potential for development of tolerance, withdrawal, and patterns of compulsive use (APA, 1994).

The course of substance dependence is variable. The course is usually chronic, lasting years, with periods of heavy intake and partial or full remission. During the first 10 months after the onset of remission, one is particularly vulnerable to relapse.

Discharge Criteria

Client will

- Maintain abstinence
- Admit to lifelong dependence on psychoactive substances
- Express knowledge of continual process of recovery ("one day at a time")
- Verbalize realistic goals

- Maintain attendance in support group (Alcoholics Anonymous, Narcotics Anonymous)
- Express increased self-esteem
- Verbalize decreased guilt, loneliness, shame, despair, anger
- Demonstrate methods and strategies for managing anxiety, frustration, and anger
- List tangible substitutes to replace drug-seeking, drug-taking behaviors (hobbies, school, employment, volunteer work, social functions)
- State feeling in control of own life
- Express hope for future
- Attend self-help group (client and family)
- Abandon people and situations that influence and contribute to drug-taking behaviors
- State consequences of psychoactive substances on biopsychosocial/cultural/spiritual well-being
- State names and phone numbers of resources to contact when unable to cope or feel need to revert to substance-taking behaviors
- Investigate substance abuse assistance programs such as the Employee Assistance Program (EAP)
- Continue with Alcoholics Anonymous (AA) if warranted
- Support family and/or significant others to attend Alanon/Alateen

THE NURSING PROCESS ■ ■ ■ ■ ■ ■ ■ ■ ■ ■ ■ ■ ■ ■

■ ASSESSMENT

In gathering information about drug use, the nurse uses a systematic approach by integrating questions into the general history regarding legal substances, including over-the-counter drugs, inhalants, and prescription drugs. Specific questions are asked about the use of nicotine, caffeine, and alcohol, including first use, patterns of use, frequency, and quantity. In addition, information should be asked about other drug categories listed in Box 15-4.

A client's positive response regarding the use of any of these drugs should alert the interviewer to obtain further information about the specific drug, including age of first use, the period of heaviest lifetime use, patterns of use, presence or absence of binges, and any occurrence of blackouts. It is important to ascertain use during the immediate past to determine the possibility of withdrawal symptoms and/or toxicity. In many instances, such as when the client is a poor historian due to the effects of drug use/abuse, it is important to corroborate the history with a family member, significant others, and previous treatment facilities. If the client is on methadone, it is essential for the nurse to ascertain when the last dose was administered.

The other components of a complete health history include a psychosocial history, family history, risk for suicide or violence (toward self or others), and a mental status examination. See Understanding and Applying Research on page 357 for a discussion of recommendations for assessment of elderly clients with alcoholism.

Box 15-4   Drug Categories Considered in an Assessment

- nicotine: cigarettes, chewing tobacco, pipe smoking, snuff, etc.
- alcohol: beer, wine, whiskey, gin, etc.
- cannabis: marijuana, "pot," "hashish"
- cocaine: "crack," etc.
- central nervous system depressants: barbiturates, benzodiazepines, methaqualone, (quaaludes, sopers)
- central nervous system stimulants: caffeine, amphetamines, diet pills
- opioids: heroin, codeine, methadone
- hallucinogens: lysergic acid diethylamide (LSD), mescaline, phencyclidine (PCP), mushrooms, peyote
- inhalants: glue, paint, aromatic hydrocarbons
- anabolic steroids
- synthetics: meperidine hydrochloride (Demerol), propoxyphene hydrochloride (Darvon)
- over-the-counter (OTC) drugs: antihistamines, cough syrups, sleeping pills, etc.
- designer drugs: mcthylcncdioxylmethamphetamine (Ecstasy), fentanyl analogues (China white, synthetic heroin), painkillers, mood elevators

Physical Examination

Physical assessment of the client may alert the nurse to the physical indicators of substance abuse. Particular attention is given to the areas of assessment listed in Table 15-1. During the assessment process, the nurse observes for and questions the client regarding the incidence of accidents and injuries. Clients who have a history of trauma and repeat hospital admissions may abuse substances, ruling out other possible causes for accidents or injury incidents. The nurse should also assess the client for alterations or disturbances in cognition, sensory perception, emotion, or behavior.

Screening Instruments

In addition to a complete history and physical examination, screening instruments are useful in identifying potential drug use. The instrument most frequently incorporated into the interview is the CAGE test (see Box 15-5). A positive response to two out of the four items of the CAGE indicates a potential problem for alcoholism.

Other frequently used instruments are:

- Short Michigan Alcohol Screening Test (SMAST) (Seltzer, 1975)
- Alcohol Use Disorders Identification Test (AUDIT) (Babor et al, 1989)
- Brief Trauma Scale (Skinner et al, 1984)

Understanding and Applying
RESEARCH

Krach P: Discovering the secret: nursing assessment of elderly alcoholics in the home, *Journal of Gerontological Nursing* 16(11):32–38, 1992.

Nurses, more than any other professionals, have the ability to conduct assessments covering many facets due to their educational backgrounds and the quantity and quality of time that they spend with the elderly. This study conducted functional assessments on older alcoholics in a home setting to provide data that would assist nurses to better assess and intervene with them.

Fifteen individuals participated in the study, all of whom were 55 years of age or older. All of the participants were surveyed in the home to assess their levels of functioning in five areas: physical, mental, social, economic, and self-care capacity.

The data from this study suggest that a comprehensive functional assessment of the older alcoholic is much more appropriate than a symptom-oriented approach. Symptoms of alcohol abuse, such as confusion, self-neglect, or repeated falls, can sometimes be attributed to the effects of aging, rather than suspected as signs of alcoholism. A functional assessment in the home setting allows the nurse to make an accurate evaluation of the older alcoholic and to develop an effective treatment plan.

The following interventions were suggested to be effective when working with an older alcoholic in a home setting:

- Confront less aggressively
- Avoid use of terminology such as *alcoholic* or *alcoholism*
- Use whatever is important in the person's life as a possible motivating force for change
- Include significant others in treatment plan
- Build on strengths; remember that you are working with survivors

Nurses must successfully work with elderly alcoholics by exploring personal attitudes toward aging and alcoholism and by developing an understanding of the aging process and alcoholism to differentiate alcohol-related changes from those related to normal aging.

TABLE 15-1   Significant areas for physical assessment of the client with substance abuse

Area of assessment	Observable signs
Temperature	elevated
Pulse	rapid; regular; irregular
Respirations	rapid; shallow; depressed
Height	
Weight	weight loss; malnourished appearance
Eyes	conjunctivitis; red/bloodshot; pupils, dilated or pinpoint; teariness; nystagmus
Nose	congested; red; rhinorrhea
Skin	cool; clammy; bruises; abrasions; sweating; petechiae (small hemorrhagic spots on the skin); telangiectasis (vascular lesions formed by dilation of a group of small blood vessels); erythematous palms; gooseflesh; needle marks
Oral cavity	mucosa red, irritated; edematous, coated tongue
Abdomen	epigastric tenderness; distended abdomen; vomiting; diarrhea; hepatomegaly (enlargement of the liver)
Speech	slurred; incoherent; deviations in volume and sound
Cognition	impaired; memory disturbance; thought blockage
Neuromuscular coordination	motor incoordination; fine muscle tremor; unsteady, weaving, shuffling gait; clumsiness
Sensorium	distortion in orientation, time, place, and person

Box 15-5   CAGE Screening Test for Alcoholism

1. Have you ever felt you ought to **C**ut down on your drinking?

2. Have people **A**nnoyed you by criticizing your drinking?

3. Have you ever felt **G**uilty about your drinking?

4. Have you ever had a drink first thing in the morning to steady your nerves or get rid of a hangover (**E**ye-opener)?

From Ewing JA: Detecting alcoholism: the CAGE questionnaire. *JAMA*, 252:1905–1907, 1984.

Laboratory Tests

In addition to the history and physical examination, part of the assessment process includes laboratory testing for drug use. Ethical issues continue to be a concern with drug testing, such as potential infringement of civil rights and the issue of obtaining the client's informed consent. (Refer to Chapter 3, Legal and Ethical Issues, for a discussion on informed consent.)

A comprehensive urine screen is an important part of early detection, treatment, and follow-up. A significant number of false positives and false negatives are reported, so it is important to be familiar with the values reported by a specific laboratory.

The use of laboratory tests for diagnosing substance abuse continues to become more complex and sophisticated. A large number of variables may affect the results,

including the uniqueness of the drug, the dosage taken, frequency of use, the type of body fluid tested (urine, blood, stool), differences in drug metabolism, half-life of the drug, sample collection time and its relationship to time of use, and sensitivity of the test itself.

Several laboratory tests may be ordered while the diagnosis of alcohol or other drug use is being considered. The most commonly used laboratory tests are the blood alcohol level (BAL), the gamma-glutamyl transferase (GGT), and the mean corpuscle value (MCV). In most states, the BAL is used to determine legal intoxication. The serum GGT levels rise in response to ingestion of alcohol. About 60%–80% of individuals with chronic alcohol abuse will have an increased GGT, whether or not other signs of liver damage are present. The MCV is elevated in 35% of individuals who are heavy or chronic alcohol abusers. An additional test that may be performed is the Aspartate aminotransferase (AST). An elevation of the AST level indicates liver damage in 35% of heavy alcohol users.

■ ■ NURSING DIAGNOSIS

Nursing diagnoses are made from the information obtained during the assessment phase. The accuracy of diagnoses depends on a careful, in-depth assessment.

Nursing Diagnoses for Substance-Related Disorders

Priority diagnoses (dependent on substance abused)

Alcoholism
Thought processes, altered
Individual coping, ineffective

CASE 📁 STUDY

Acute Alcoholism

Nancy Smith is a 28-year-old, married female who, when out to dinner with her husband, had four margaritas and became intoxicated. When she left the restaurant, she experienced difficulty walking and fell. She became verbally abusive with her husband. As he attempted to put her into the car, she became combative. He transported her to the Emergency Room where she told the admitting nurse, "I am going home. There's nothing wrong with me."

Critical Thinking and Assessment

1. What is Nancy's most immediate problem?
2. Is Nancy a danger to herself or others? Why or why not?
3. What symptoms displayed by Nancy are typical of an individual with a suspected diagnosis of alcoholism?
4. Given Nancy's behavior, how would you assess her for alcoholism?
5. What laboratory tests could be used to assess her involvement with alcohol?

Nutrition, altered
Trauma, risk for
Denial, ineffective
Violence, risk for
Family processes, altered
Family processes: alcoholism, altered

Other possible nursing diagnoses

Adjustment, impaired
Body image disturbance
Family coping: disabling, ineffective
Decisional conflict (specify)
Altered family processes
Fear
Injury, risk for
Oral mucous membrane, altered
Powerlessness
Protection, altered
Rape trauma
Role performance, altered
Self-esteem disturbance
Sleep pattern disturbance
Social interaction, impaired
Aspiration, risk for
Breathing pattern, ineffective
Decreased cardiac output
Diarrhea

COLLABORATIVE DIAGNOSES

DSM-IV Diagnoses*	NANDA Diagnoses**
Alcohol Use Disorders	Adjustment, impaired
Alcohol-Induced Disorders	Body image disturbance
Amphetamine Use Disorders	Family coping, ineffective Disabling
Amphetamine-Induced Disorders	Individual coping, ineffective
Caffeine Use Disorders	Decisional conflict (specify)
Caffeine-Induced Disorders	Denial, ineffective
Cannabis Use Disorders	Family processes, altered
Cannabis-Induced Disorders	Fear
Cocaine Use Disorders	Injury, risk for
Cocaine-Induced Disorders	Oral mucous membrane, altered
Hallucinogen Use Disorders	Powerlessness
Hallucinogen-Induced Disorders	Protection, altered
Inhalant Use Disorders	Rape trauma
Inhalant-Induced Disorders	Role performance, altered
Nicotine Use Disorders	Self-esteem disturbance
Nicotine-Induced Disorders	Sleep pattern disturbance
Opioid Use Disorders	Social interaction, impaired
Opioid-Induced Disorders	Thought processes, altered
Phencyclidine Use Disorders	Trauma, risk for
Phencyclidine-Induced Disorders	Violence: risk for, self-directed or directed at others
Sedative, Hypnotic, or Anxiolytic-Use Disorders	Aspiration, risk for
Sedative, Hypnotic, or Anxiolytic-Induced Disorders	Breathing pattern, ineffective
Other (or Unknown) Substance Use Disorders	Decreased cardiac output Diarrhea
Other (or Unknown) Substance-Induced Disorders	Fluid volume deficit
	Gas exchange, impaired
	Health maintenance, altered
	Hypothermia
	Infection, risk for
	Noncompliance (specify)
	Nutrition: altered, less than body requirements
	Parenting, altered
	Role performance, altered
	Self-mutilation, risk for
	Sexual dysfunction

*Reprinted with permission from *Diagnostic and statistical manual of mental disorders,* ed 4, Washington, D.C., 1994, American Psychiatric Association.

**Reprinted with permission from *NANDA nursing diagnoses: definitions and classifications, 1995–1996,* Philadelphia, 1994, North American Nursing Diagnosis Association.

Fluid volume deficit

Gas exchange, impaired

Health maintenance, altered

Hypothermia

Infection, risk for

Noncompliance (specify)

Parenting, altered

Role performance, altered

Self-mutilation, risk for

Sexual dysfunction

■ ■ ■ OUTCOME IDENTIFICATION

Outcome criteria are derived from nursing diagnoses and are the expected client responses to be achieved.

Client will:

1. Maintain vital signs within normal range.

2. Verbalize a reduction in delusional thinking, absence of hallucinations, absence of suicidal or homicidal ideation.

3. Maintain normal fluid hydration.

4. Remain free of seizure activity.

5. Verbalize "I feel safe in my environment."

6. Verbalize a desire to stop drinking/drug use.

7. State that there is a reduction in the symptoms of withdrawal (which may occur weeks after last use).

8. Participate in the therapeutic activities of the treatment plan (individual/group).

9. Ingest well-balanced diet of sufficient calories to meet prescribed nutritional needs.

10. Express need to contact family members/significant others regarding support.

11. Explore factors that may interfere with treatment plan, for example, lack of social or family support, lack of financial resources, seeking old "drinking buddies."

12. Develop realistic goals for rehabilitation, for example, continue with 12-step program.

13. Verbalize "recovery is a lifelong process" that occurs one day at a time.

14. Verbalize the ability to sleep without sedation.

15. Express the desire to establish relationships with nondrinking friends and avoid situations that previously invoked alcohol intake.

■ ■ ■ PLANNING

Because the client frequently has a long history of alcohol and other drug abuse, the nurse must develop a plan of care that meets the individual's ongoing needs. Client care is based on the data gathered during the assessment process and the immediate needs, as well as the long-range goals of treatment and aftercare.

Collaboration among the nurse, the client, the family, and the treatment team is essential in the development and revision of the plan of care. For the client who abuses substances, the road to abstinence and recovery requires realistic outcome criteria and a consistent plan of care.

■ ■ ■ ■ ■ IMPLEMENTATION

The nurse providing care for a client who abuses alcohol and other drugs will consider a plan of care that meets the client's needs in relation to an identified stage in the recovery process. Recovery from a substance abuse problem is a long-term process often interrupted by periods of relapse. The nurse realistically recognizes this problem and develops a plan that meets the client's individual needs.

The plan includes helping the client with withdrawal symptoms/complications of substance use, providing nutritional support as needed, helping the client resolve anger/potential violence toward self or others, providing support to increase the client's self-worth, helping the client set realistic short-term/long-term goals, reintegrating the client with the family/significant others, providing resources for vocational rehabilitation, and monitoring the client's progress post-discharge. A clinical pathway for treating clients with alcoholic dependency is included in Appendix D.

Nursing Interventions

1. Monitor the client's vital signs, while observing for signs and symptoms of substance overdose, withdrawal, and drug-to-drug interactions *to establish baseline information about the client's condition.*

2. Assess the physiologic and psychologic symptoms of withdrawal and the effects of medications prescribed during the withdrawal process *to provide safe, effective treatment during withdrawal.*

3. Initiate therapeutic interventions to treat withdrawal symptoms, including anxiety and other complications, *to help the client safely withdraw from the addictive substance.*

4. Provide psychologic support to the client/family/significant others *to include the family in the client's treatment process.*

5. Provide a safe, calm, nonthreatening environment for the client who is in withdrawal *because of possible illusions, delusions, or hallucinations experienced during withdrawal, the potential danger to self or others, and grand mal seizures.*

6. Support the client in meeting nutritional/metabolic needs either orally or intravenously, dependent on the client's ability to take and retain fluids, *to provide adequate hydration as needed.*

7. Refer to a nutritionist as needed, considering the client's personal, cultural, or spiritual preferences, *to offer holistic and interdisciplinary care.*

NURSING CARE PLAN ■ ■ ■ ■ ■ ■ ■ ■ ■ ■ ■ ■ ■ ■ ■ ■

Mr. Jamison is a 36-year-old African-American veteran who has been homeless for the last six months. He is admitted to the psychiatric acute care unit of the Veteran's Hospital with a diagnosis of polysubstance abuse that includes heavy use of alcohol and nicotine and occasional use of cocaine. He has no other illnesses, but he appears malnourished. He has been separated from his wife of 10 years for the last eight months. He is the father of two boys, ages 4 and 6. Mrs. Jamison has returned to work as a computer technician at a local data processing company.

Previous to his drug use, Mr. Jamison owned a small electrical shop. On admission he indicated a desire to get his life together so he can be rehabilitated and reunited with his wife and children. The wife states that she loves her husband and will do whatever she can to assist with treatment and rehabilitation.

Since admission to the unit, Mr. Jamison has reported that he has not been able to sleep at night. He has been visited by his minister and his wife who report that the children "are eager to have Daddy well and home."

DSM-IV Diagnoses

AXIS I	Alcohol Dependence
	Nicotine Dependence
	Cocaine Dependence
AXIS II	No Diagnosis
AXIS III	Medical Diagnoses: Malnourished; Sleep Disturbance
AXIS IV	Severity of Psychosocial Stressors (Extreme = 5)
	Homeless; Financial: Loss of Job; Interpersonal: Loss of Family
AXIS V	Global Assessment of Functioning: Current GAF = 40; Highest GAF in last year = 70

Nursing Diagnosis: Ineffective individual coping related to personal vulnerability and inadequate coping methods, as evidenced by dependence on alcohol and nicotine, being separated from wife and family, and homelessness.

Client Outcomes	*Nursing Interventions*	*Evaluation*
• Mr. J will verbalize that he is "powerless" over alcohol.	• Support Mr. J's statement that he is powerless over alcohol *to begin breaking through denial. Additional support by the nurse can help him to replace his dependence on alcohol.*	• Mr. J verbalizes that he is powerless over alcohol.
• Mr. J will use effective coping skills that were previously successful, and newly acquired skills to manage problems related to substance abuse.	• Assess Mr. J's usual coping style through interview/counseling techniques and help him explore strengths and weaknesses *because, to build new coping skills, previous effective coping methods must be explored.*	• Mr. J is effectively integrating existing coping skills with newly acquired coping methods at the time of discharge.

Nursing Diagnosis: Self-esteem disturbance related to negative thoughts and feelings about self, as evidenced by failure of marriage, failure as a father and in business, and alcohol use/abuse.

Client Outcomes	*Nursing Interventions*	*Evaluation*
• Mr. J will begin to verbalize positive comments about self to nursing staff.	• Reinforce Mr. J's statements of self-worth *to build self-esteem with continuing support from the nurse and others.*	• Mr. J shares his feelings of self-worth with his wife and children at the time of discharge.
• Mr. J will express hope for a drug-free future.	• Support Mr. J's expressed plan for the future *because clients need the opportunity to discuss future plans while in a therapeutic environment.*	• Mr. J has a concrete plan for action, including a new job and continuation in a 12-step treatment plan.

NURSING CARE PLAN ■ ■ ■ ■ ■ ■ ■ ■ ■ ■ ■ ■ ■ ■ ■ ■ ■

Nursing Diagnosis: Altered family processes, related to the effects of chronic use of alcohol and cocaine as evidenced by separation from wife and children for eight months.

Client Outcomes	Nursing Interventions	Evaluation
• Mr. J will initiate contact with family through phone call and request for family visits.	• Provide Mr. J with encouragement to initiate contact with wife and children *to provide a solid family support system to help reintegrate him back into the family and stop substance use/abuse.*	• Mr. J returned home with his family at the time of discharge.
• Mr. J will attend family counseling sessions with Mrs. J.	• Teach Mr. and Mrs. J about the benefits of family therapy *because both adult family members need support with resolution of disabling effects of substance-abuse problems.*	• Mr. and Mrs. J are attending family therapy sessions at discharge.
• Mrs. J will attend weekly Al-Anon meetings.	• Support Mrs. J in her decision to attend Al-Anon meetings *to help her learn new ways to effectively deal with partner.*	• Mrs. J is attending Al-Anon at the time of Mr. J's discharge.

Nursing Diagnosis: Altered nutrition: less than body requirements related to lack of interest in food and/or substitution of alcohol or drug for nutrients, as evidenced by malnourishment and vitamin and mineral deficiencies.

Client Outcomes	Nursing Interventions	Evaluation
• Mr. J will eat a minimum of 50% of provided nutrients at each meal.	• Provide preferred foods high in proteins, carbohydrates, and vitamins, especially the B vitamins *so Mr. J will eat more of favored foods and become better nourished in accordance with metabolic needs.*	• Mr. J ate 100% of well-balanced meals at the time of discharge.
• Mr. J will select a diet including "desired" foods.	• Offer encouragement with dietary choices until Mr. J feels secure *to help him realize he is able to make appropriate choices for himself.*	• Mr. J selected a balanced diet based on the food pyramid at the time of discharge.

Nursing Diagnosis: Sleep pattern disturbances related to the effects of psychological stress as evidenced by irritability, restlessness, depression, and the inability to fall asleep and stay asleep during the night without a sedative.

Client Outcomes	Nursing Interventions	Evaluation
• Mr. J will sleep soundly through the entire night without sedation for one week.	• Provide information regarding supportive measures to induce sleep, such as the use of relaxation techniques, white noise, and a soothing back rub *to help him relax and use these techniques as a substitute for alcohol use.*	• Mr. J was sleeping throughout the night without sedation at the time of discharge.

8. Increase carbohydrate intake as needed *to decrease some of the client's cravings for illicit substances and satisfy the client's oral needs (for example, hard candies and other such snacks).*

9. Initiate the necessary vitamin and mineral replacement therapeutic regimen. *Low levels of vitamin B can occur even in the absence of dietary deficiencies and malabsorption. Other vitamins affected are A, C, D, E, and K. Iron, magnesium, and zinc levels may also be affected by the ingestion of alco-* hol. (See Box 15-3 on page 352 for treatment of alcohol withdrawal symptoms.)

10. Provide support to the client in working through denial. Establish a therapeutic, caring relationship when working with the client who denies that a substance abuse problem exists. A variety of techniques may be used with the client, including psychotherapeutic techniques, confrontation, and behavioral approaches as described below in this chapter. Family therapy may also be indicated. *Providing support*

TABLE 15-2   Disorders related to excessive alcohol intake and abuse of other substances

Problem	Suspected cause
Hypoglycemia	Limited food intake, depletion of glycogen stores, inhibition of gluconeogenesis
Lactic acidosis	Excessive production of lactic acid by hepatocytes
Hyperuricemia	Reduced renal clearance of uric acid associated with lactic acid accumulation in the body and the need to eliminate it
Esophagitis	Direct toxic effect, vomiting
Gastritis	Direct toxic effect, increased secretin and histamine production
Duodenal ulceration	Increased secretin and histamine production
Malabsorption	Pancreatic insufficiency, mucosal damage associated with reduced transport activity and disaccharidase production, hyperperistalsis
Fatty liver	Triglyceride accumulation in hepatocytes
Hyperlipidemia	Increased lipoprotein production, increased lipoprotein clearance, mobilization of nonhepatic fat stores
Hyperketonemia	Excessive fat metabolism
Alcoholic hepatitis	Hepatocyte inflammation and necrosis related to alcohol and its metabolism
Cirrhosis	Scarification of liver tissue associated with long-term fatty infiltration or hepatitis
Pancreatitis	Alcohol-induced inflammation of the pancreas leading to increased secretin production
Anemias	Direct toxic effect, malabsorption of nutrients, malnutrition, decreased transferrin synthesis
Beriberi heart disease	Thiamine deficiency
Cardiomyopathy	Direct toxic effect, malnutrition
Skeletal myopathies	Direct toxic effect
Reduced bone density with increased fracture risk	Excessive excretion of calcium in the urine, poor diet, malabsorption of vitamin D, reduced liver hydroxylation of vitamin D
Impaired immune response	Malnutrition, direct toxic effect
Hemorrhagic displays	Impaired production of blood-clotting proteins
Wernicke-Korsakoff syndrome	Thiamine deficiency
Tuberculosis/pneumonia	Reduced resistance to infection, atelectasis
Cancer of the gastrointestinal system (neck, throat, stomach, pancreas)	Indirect toxic effects
Impotency	Neuropathy and CNS depressant
Peripheral neuritis	Malnutrition, especially vitamin deficiencies (B complex)
Malnutrition	Alcohol is high in calories and acts as appetite suppressant

From Beare P, Myers JL: *Principles and practice of adult health nursing*, ed 2, St. Louis, 1994, Mosby.

and empathy, yet not enabling the client, assists the client in working through the denial process and helps develop awareness that many of his or her life problems are related to substance-abuse. (See Chapter 22, Interactive Therapies and Methods of Implementation.)

11. Intervene with secondary complications exhibited by the client as a result of substance abuse. (Table 15-1 on page 358 shows the areas for assessment of problems that the clients may demonstrate.) *The prolonged use/abuse of alcohol or other drugs may cause a variety of complications or damage to all major body systems* (see Table 15-2 above).

12. Establish a caring, empathetic relationship through individual and group interactions *to help the client improve self-esteem and deal with thoughts of guilt*

and remorse. Clients who abuse substances have a tendency to feel inadequate and unwanted.

13. Encourage client's efforts to establish/reestablish/strengthen family and significant other supports through a variety of measures such as role-playing; providing a quiet, congenial environment for the client to meet with family; and possibly remaining with the client and family during the first visit. Inform the family of the client's needs prior to their meeting. *Clients who abuse substances frequently have lost meaningful contact with their family/significant others.*

14. Teach the client, family, and significant others about substance abuse, symptoms, management, and treatment outcomes individually, as a group, or with written material. *Client, family, and significant others*

need opportunities to learn about substance abuse. Information about substance abuse, especially taught in a group, provides a common base for understanding and provides opportunities for client and family to interact with and learn from others.

15. Support the client and family members in maintaining active involvement with 12-step support groups, such as AA, Al-Anon, Al-a-Teen, ACoA, NA, and CA. *Past experience in working with substance abuse clients indicates that lifelong membership in a 12-step program is essential to remain drug-free.*

16. Encourage the family to be flexible and patient regarding the client's participation in support groups. *Establishing a new lifestyle, such as engaging in a support group network, takes time, effort, and motivation.*

17. Teach the client, family/significant others about substance abuse and the preventive aspects by providing factual information and suggestions for preventing the use of alcohol and other drugs. *The nurse should be available as an advocate and a resource regarding the dangers of substance abuse and the need for a healthy lifestyle.*

18. Support client in establishing a social support system by putting him or her in touch with community organizations where the client may find alternative housing, make new friends, and build inner strength that will assist in the recovery process. *The client is faced with the enormous task of establishing new social support systems and cannot do it without support and guidance.*

Additional Treatment Modalities

Collaborative interventions include the entire team involved with the client's treatment and rehabilitation. These interventions include, but are not limited to, medications for the treatment of withdrawal symptoms and vitamin and mineral deficiencies, conditioning therapy, psychotherapy, vocational rehabilitation counseling, and relapse prevention. Additional modalities used in the treatment of substance-related disorders include behavioral therapy and techniques, group therapy, and family therapy. The various other modalities and collaborative interventions are summarized in the Additional Treatment Modalities box on this page.

Withdrawal/Detoxification

Sudden withdrawal of a drug in a physically dependent individual requires immediate medical intervention. If severe withdrawal symptoms occur, the client must be **detoxified.** Gradual weaning from the drug or the use of an alternative drug that blocks the occurrence or minimizes withdrawal symptoms is required. Early symptoms of withdrawal include tremors, diaphoresis, rapid pulse (120–140 beats per minute), elevated blood pressure (150/90 or above), and insomnia. In addition, clients experience hyperalertness and a feeling of internal jitters.

ADDITIONAL TREATMENT MODALITIES

Withdrawal/Detoxification

- Medical interventions
- Vitamin therapy

Psychotherapy

- Individual therapy
- Group therapy
- Family therapy

Behavior therapy

- Aversive conditioning with Disulfiram (Antabuse)

12-Step Support Groups

- Alcoholics Anonymous (AA)
- Narcotics Anonymous (NA)
- Al-Anon
- Al-a-Teen
- Adult Children of Alcoholics (ACoA)

Halfway Houses
Day or Night Hospitalization

Auditory and visual hallucinations and grand mal seizures may occur when and if treatment strategies are unsuccessful. Adequate and rapid medical intervention in clients who are withdrawing from alcohol should eliminate more severe symptoms, including delirium tremens.

Most detoxification units have an established drug protocol managed and monitored by the nurse. A typical protocol provides for 25–50 mg of chlordiazepoxide every 2–4 hours. The client's vital signs are monitored every 15 minutes until vital signs are stable. Close monitoring of vital signs is indicated for 48–72 hours or longer. If the client does not respond to the medication, larger doses of the medication are indicated. It is not unusual to give 50–100 mg of chlordiazepoxide at 2–4 hour interims. As much as 10–20 times the normal dose may be needed to prevent withdrawal symptoms. Higher doses of medication require close monitoring by the nurse and physician to guard against drug overdose. Adequate treatment and careful monitoring prevent grand mal seizures and possible cardiovascular collapse and death.

Clients experiencing severe withdrawal symptoms from alcohol usually require B vitamins, including thiamin (vitamin B_1), folic acid, and B_{12} due to inadequate dietary intake and malabsorption. Thiamine replacement helps in preventing Wernicke's syndrome (Francis and Franklin, 1988).

It is necessary to monitor the client's fluid and electrolytes. Replacement therapy may be indicated due to vomiting, diarrhea, and diaphoresis. Caution should be taken not to overhydrate the client. Alcohol intake with elevated blood alcohol levels causes diureses. But as the blood alcohol level drops, fluid retention occurs and the individual becomes overhydrated. The sequence may result in congestive heart failure. Monitoring the client for signs of overhydration is essential. Other medications indicated include anticonvulsants to prevent seizures and magnesium sulfate to raise the seizure threshold. If indicated, potassium replacement is used to restore electrolyte balance and vitamin B replacement therapy.

Detoxification from other drugs requires similar precautions to those mentioned above. Individuals addicted to heroin and on methadone therapy require careful monitoring of methadone levels in addition to vital signs. Overdose of methadone may lead to cardiovascular collapse and death.

Individuals who are heavy users of hallucinogens may present with toxic psychosis. It is important to ascertain the specific drug, because nursing care approaches differ. Individuals experiencing psychosis due to PCP are belligerent and strike out. They do not respond well to interpersonal approaches. Conversely, individuals experiencing a "bad trip" from LSD respond to verbal reassurance and reorientation (Vourakis and Bennett, 1979).

Psychotherapy

Psychotherapy with clients who abuse alcohol or other drugs may take many forms including individual, group, and family therapy.

Individual Therapy   Individual psychotherapy is indicated for alcoholics who have a high level of anxiety, inadequate coping mechanisms, and low tolerance for frustration.

Communication during the initial contact with the therapist is crucial. The therapist must be empathetic, supportive, and assume an active role in therapy. Alcoholics are conditioned to experience rejection. Reticence in overtly addressing the problem of alcoholism and the client's psychologic defenses may be interpreted by the client as rejection. Removal of intellectual and emotional barriers between the client and the therapist should be an early goal.

Psychotherapy with clients who are alcoholic has many attendant problems. Clients continue to test the therapeutic bond between client and therapist throughout the period of therapy. Therapists must be aware of several occurrences during the process of therapy, in-

cluding the possibility of **relapse** (resumption of a pattern of substance abuse or dependency), the onset of depression, and the refusal to continue in therapy. Many clients with alcoholism become depressed when they give up alcohol and are forced to learn new ways of coping because previous coping patterns and defenses are no longer adequate. Spouse and family understanding of the problem is essential. Involving the spouse in conjoint couples therapy and the family in family therapy can aid the psychotherapeutic process. Referral of the spouse and teens to 12-step support groups provides support for them and helps family members gain a better understanding of the disease process, the client's defense patterns, and the client's need for support.

Group Therapy   Group therapy has certain advantages for clients with alcoholism that are difficult to achieve in individual therapy. In a group setting, clients with similar experiences and problems can confront and support each other in a relatively safe environment (see Figure 15-3). The therapist's role is to facilitate group members' participation and to assist in clarifying interpersonal interactions within the group. Clients in recovery who have maintained sobriety can share experiences and serve as role models for newly admitted clients.

Group discussions are best facilitated when ground rules and goals are established with clients early in the group therapy experience. Sobriety, regular attendance, willingness to share experiences and confront defenses, and confidentiality are common ground rules. Goals include sobriety; a desire to change and learn new ways of coping with problems; and a willingness to recognize and identity feelings and thoughts, such as guilt, depression, inadequacy, anxiety, and fear.

Family Therapy   In recent years family therapy has gained credibility with clients with alcoholism. Family therapy is a treatment modality based on family systems theory. The recognition and acceptance of alcoholism as an illness that affects all members of the family indicates the need for family therapy. Often when the family member who abuses alcohol suddenly attains sobriety, the dynamics of the entire family change. It is a well-known fact that some clients relapse because the family does not know how to relate to the person when he or she is sober. For instance, the spouse of a client with alcoholism experiences difficulty giving up the power position in the family that was assumed while the client was abusing alcohol.

Family members in alcoholic families have a tendency to lack trust for one another, feel unloved and unwanted, and carry a heavy burden of guilt. Family myths and family secrets are coveted. Family therapy provides opportunities to learn healthy ways of interacting with one another and of solving problems. Hope and trust can be instilled, and children can be relieved of the heavy burdens that they carry, not the least of which is the guilt they experience related to the belief that they are responsible for the parent's drinking problem.

CLINICAL ALERT   !

When a client who is addicted to heroin is admitted to a detoxification unit, the nurse should contact the methadone clinic to ascertain when the last dose was administered to prevent overdosage of methadone, which can be life-threatening.

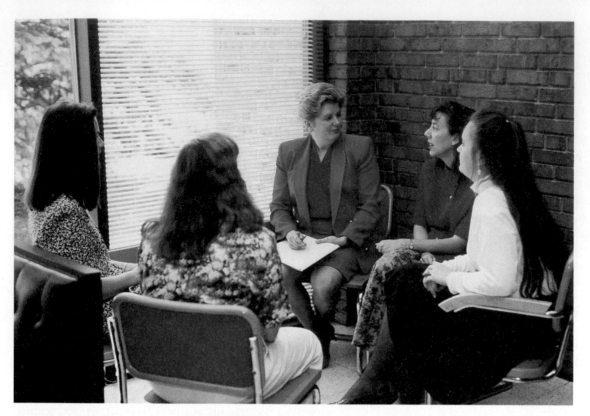

Figure 15-3 Group therapy can be effective for clients with substance abuse.

Family therapy provides a structure in which the entire family can be educated about alcoholism as a disease. Children who are at high risk for developing problems with alcohol due to genetic predisposition and environmental circumstances can be helped to understand the importance of refraining from alcohol use. Family members can be enlisted to support the client's attendance at AA meetings, even if attendance conflicts with planned family activities.

Behavioral Therapy *Aversive Conditioning with Disulfiram (Antabuse)* Aversive conditioning is the most frequently used technique of behavior therapy. The client is conditioned by pairing the sight, smell, and taste of alcohol with an emetic. Induced nausea and vomiting act as aversions to alcohol. Following the conditioning experience the client is placed on disulfiram (Antabuse). Antabuse inhibits the enzyme aldehyde dehydrogenase; even a small amount of alcohol can cause a toxic reaction because of acetaldehyde accumulation in the blood.

Clients must be in good health, highly motivated, and cooperative. They are warned about the consequences of using the drug disulfiram, if and when even small amounts of alcohol are ingested. Clients experience flushing and feelings of heat in the face, chest, and upper limbs. Other symptoms include pallor, hypotension, nausea, general malaise, dizziness, blurred vision, palpitations, air hunger, and numbness of upper extremities. The most serious consequence is severe hypotension.

CLINICAL ALERT !

All clients on Antabuse therapy should carry a card similar to that carried by diabetics stating they are on Antabuse therapy and should be taken to an emergency room if found in a debilitated state, which may include nausea, vomiting, headache, difficulty breathing, and rapid or irregular heartbeat.

Most clients receive 250 mg disulfiram daily. If larger doses are prescribed, toxic psychoses may occur with memory impairment and confusion (Kaplan and Sadock, 1994). Clients on Antabuse therapy should carry a card similar to that given to diabetic clients. The card states that they are on Antabuse therapy and require medical treatment instead of incarceration if found in a debilitated state.

Other Behavioral Techniques Other behavioral therapy techniques employed with alcoholic clients include skills training to assist them in refusing drinks, assertiveness training, relaxation training, and **relapse prevention** therapy (a means of helping the chemically dependent individual maintain behavioral changes over a prolonged period of time). Most clients relapse a minimum of 3–4 times before they attain sobriety (complete abstinence from alcohol or other drugs of abuse in conjunction with a satisfactory quality of life).

12-Step Support Groups

Alcoholics Anonymous (AA) is the original self-help group for recovering alcoholics. AA was founded in 1935 by two alcoholics, a stockbroker and a surgeon. It is built on the premise that support and encouragement from other alcoholics can aid them on the road to recovery. New members are assigned a sponsor (a recovering alcoholic who provides 24-hour assistance as needed). AA meetings are built on a 12-step program that allows individuals with alcoholism to restructure their lives and make the necessary changes. The 12 steps of Alcoholics Anonymous are listed in Box 15-6.

A variety of AA groups are available in each community. Meetings may be open or closed. During open meetings, spouses, friends, and significant others are invited to attend; they are also open to observers such as nursing and other health professional students. Closed meetings are restricted to individuals in the recovery process. Some groups are identified for special populations such as women, nonsmokers, identified business interests, and specialized professional groups.

Narcotics Anonymous (NA) embraces a similar philosophy to AA. It is a support group for individuals addicted to narcotics, especially opiates. Since many substance abusers are polysubstance abusers, attendees may have problems with one or more substances.

Al-Anon and *Al-a-Teen* self-help groups operate independent of AA groups. They are formed to help family members of people with alcoholism cope with common problems.

Al-Anon is a support group for spouses and friends of alcoholics. Opportunities are provided to learn about alcohol as a disease and to share common problems and solutions with other spouses. Behaviors and issues common to the disease process are dealt with, such as avoidance, enabling, self-inflicted guilt, and shame.

Al-a-Teen is a nationwide support group for teens (children over 10 years of age) who have alcoholic parents. Similar to Al-Anon, the group helps remove self-guilt as the cause of the parent's drinking and restore feelings of self-worth. The group meetings are beneficial and therapeutic.

Adult Children of Alcoholics (ACoA) is a support group for adults that were reared in alcoholic homes. Children of alcoholics are frequently deprived of nurturing and loving parents. They enter adulthood with poor self-concepts and experience interpersonal difficulties. The support groups provide opportunities to discuss problems and feel acceptance from others who have had similar experiences.

Adult children of alcoholics may manifest **codependent** behaviors that focus on control, enabling, making excuses for others' behaviors (especially the behavior of alcoholics), inability to trust self, and feelings of inadequacy and insecurity. Codependent individuals have a constant need to assume responsibility and take care of others' needs.

Many codependent behaviors—for example, caring, nurturing, assisting and supporting others, and self-denial—are often associated with women and especially nurses. Individuals who were reared in alcoholic homes may experience a higher degree of codependency; however, recent findings indicate that individuals from nonalcoholic homes may have similar behaviors. The overresponsible behaviors, especially of codependent spouses, may be more easily explained on the basis of stress rather than on inadequate or disturbed personalities (Montgomery and Johnson, 1992).

Halfway houses   Clients who are discharged from acute treatment settings often need additional time to begin the rehabilitation process. Halfway houses provide shelter as well as support, group therapy, and direct access to AA

Box 15-6   The Twelve Steps of Alcoholics Anonymous

1. We admitted we were powerless over alcohol, that our lives had become unmanageable.

2. Came to believe that a Power greater than ourselves could restore us to sanity.

3. Made a decision to turn our will and our lives over to the care of God as we understood Him.

4. Made a searching and fearless moral inventory of ourselves.

5. Admitted to God, to ourselves, and to another human being the exact nature of our wrongs.

6. Were entirely ready to have God remove all these defects of character.

7. Humbly asked him to remove our shortcomings.

8. Made a list of all persons we had harmed, and became willing to make amends to them all.

9. Made direct amends to such people wherever possible, except when to do so would injure them or others.

10. Continued to take personal inventory, and when we were wrong promptly admitted it.

11. Sought through prayer and meditation to improve our conscious contact with God as we understood Him, praying only for knowledge of His will for us and the power to carry that out.

12. Having had a spiritual awakening as the result of these steps, we tried to carry this message to alcoholics and to practice these principles in all our affairs.

The Twelve Steps are reprinted with permission of Alcoholics Anonymous World Services, Inc. Permission to reprint this material does not mean that AA has reviewed or approved the contents of this publication. AA is a program of recovery from alcoholism *only*—use of the Twelve Steps in connection with programs and activities which are patterned after AA, but which address other problems, does not imply otherwise.

meetings. An opportunity is provided for gradual reen-trance into the family and progressive re-entry into the work world and society. Halfway house placement is highly recommended for clients who have been alien-ated from their families or have no place to live.

Day or night hospitalization   Partial hospitalization is recommended for clients who need additional thera-peutic support from professionals. Some clients resume employment and spend the night in the hospital, while others spend the day at the treatment center and go home at night. As with the halfway house, partial hospi-talization provides additional therapeutic support during early or difficult phases of rehabilitation.

■ ■ ■ ■ ■ ■ EVALUATION

The purpose of evaluation is to ascertain changes that oc-cur as a result of nursing and other interdisciplinary in-terventions. The nurse observes for changes in the client's behaviors and responses to treatment and inter-ventions using the outcome criteria. It is important to recognize that resolution of the acute phase is merely the first step in treatment. Success for the recovery process and rehabilitation are dependent on many factors, in-cluding access to 12-step support groups, continuing health care, support of family/significant others, voca-tional rehabilitation and community support. (See Nurs-ing Care in the Community below.)

It is recognized that many clients relapse several times during the rehabilitation process. For this reason, it is dif-ficult to predict the time when clients finally achieve ac-ceptance of the fact that they are powerless over alcohol and/or drugs. As they attain sobriety, they develop a commitment to change their lifestyle, which often af-fects their relationships with family, significant others, and coworkers. Many clients develop a lifetime commit-ment to their 12-step program.

Nursing Care in the Community

Substance-Related Disorders

The nurse working with clients with chemical dependen-cies in the community often experiences judgmental feel-ings toward chronic relapse. Relapse is a common occur-rence that causes frustration not only for the client but also the nurse, who may feel hopeless in the face of the client's self-destructive behavior. Allowance must be made for the state of impairment in the thought processes as a result of chronic alcohol or drug use. It is crucial to un-derstand that, in some cases, relapse is a part of the treat-ment process and that continual reinforcement of positive interactive and coping skills will ultimately make a differ-ence in the client's behavior.

Stamina is perhaps the most essential quality the nurse must cultivate. Repeatedly offering help and support when nothing seems to work requires almost superhuman endurance. A knowledge of the predictable stages the al-coholic or drug abuser will go through can help the nurse accept the client and encourage behavioral change. It is important to evaluate the client's acceptance of his or her dependence on alcohol/drugs and the detrimental impact it has had on the client's lifestyle. The client, who is in de-nial of a problem, needs a stern reality check, not referrals to community programs. The developmental level of the client must be considered in getting the client to admit to a substance use/abuse problem. Teenagers, for example, will listen and talk to a peer counselor more readily than an adult. The client's level of prior functioning also must be included, because many clients present with dual diag-noses and may be impaired in their ability to function well even when sober. Depression is a consistent comorbid finding, and monitoring for suicidal thoughts is crucial for the mental health nurse, especially with the client who would rather be dead than drunk.

The nurse must continually recommend contact with AA or other support groups, give encouragement and coun-seling to family members, enlist the help of other profes-sionals such as social workers, and investigate the oppor-tunity to enroll the client in a community service group to increase his or her sense of involvement and self-worth. In-teraction between nurse and client in the community set-ting is based on the client's choice and not involuntary de-tainment, so the cultivation of the relationship is essential. The relationship requires a rigorous and nonaccusatory honesty, suggesting that both parties aspire to high stan-dards of behavior and responsibility.

Another problem that may occur in the community is blatant drug use, visible paraphernalia, and/or groups of drug abusers obviously "under the influence" of some sub-stance, whether controlled or not. This may feel threaten-ing or at least distinctly uncomfortable for the visiting nurse. The best way to handle this problem is a profes-sional, "matter-of-fact" attitude, including identifying one-self clearly to everyone and stating the purpose of the visit.

Summary of Key Concepts

1. Assessment for substance abuse should be a part of every client history and physical examination.

2. Alcohol is the number one drug of abuse in American society today at all age levels.

3. Nicotine use is a major health problem and, along with alcohol, serves as a "gateway" to illicit drug use.

4. Fetal alcohol syndrome is 100% preventable if the pregnant woman abstains from alcohol throughout her pregnancy.

5. A positive family history of alcoholism is the number one risk factor for developing alcoholism.

6. The incidence of substance abuse varies with cultural groups. Native Americans have the highest incidence of alcohol abuse.

7. Dual diagnosis/comorbidity requires in-depth assessment followed by treatment of both the substance abuse and the psychiatric diagnosis.

8. Current DSM-IV diagnoses of abuse and dependency do not adequately describe substance use in the adolescent population. It is preferable to use such terms as "problematic" drinking or excessive substance use.

9. An individual who uses drugs indiscriminately is identified as a polydrug user.

10. Secondary complications of alcoholism may be causative factors for disease conditions in any of the major organs or body systems.

11. Commitment to long-term treatment and rehabilitation programs, including 12-step groups, is essential for recovery from substance abuse.

REFERENCES

Adams EH et al: *Overview of selected drug trends* (NIDA Publication No. RP0731), Rockville, Md., 1989, National Institute on Drug Abuse.

American Nurses Association: *Addictions and psychological dysfunction in nursing,* New York, 1984, American Nurses Association.

American Psychiatric Association: *Diagnostic and statistical manual of mental disorders,* ed 4, Washington, D.C., 1994, American Psychiatric Association.

Babor TF et al: *AUDIT: the alcohol use disorders identification test, guidelines for use in primary care,* Geneva, 1989, World Health Organization.

Beare P, Myers JL: *Principles and practice of adult health nursing,* ed 2, St. Louis, 1994, Mosby.

Bikle D: Effects of alcohol disease on bone, *Comprehensive Therapy* 14(2):16–20, 1980.

Bowen M: *Family therapy in clinical practice,* New York, 1978, Jason Aronson.

Cigarette smoking among adults, *MMWR* 41(20), 1990.

Cook P et al: *Alcohol, tobacco, and other drugs may harm the unborn,* Rockville, Md., 1990, U.S. Department of Health and Human Services, Office for Substance Abuse Prevention.

Cooper ML: Alcohol and increased behavioral risks for AIDS, *Alcohol Health & Research World* 16: 64–72, 1990.

Cuffel BJ: Prevalence estimates of substance abuse in schizophrenia and their correlates, *The J of Nervous Disease* 180(9): 589–592, 1992.

Donahue RP et al: Alcohol and hemorrhagic stroke, *JAMA* 255:2311–2314, 1986.

Drake RE et al: Diagnosis of alcohol use disorders in schizophrenia, *Schizophrenia Bull* 16(1):57–67, 1990.

Dupont RL, Saylor KE: Sedatives/hypnotics and benzodiazepines. In Francis RJ, Miller SI: *Clinical textbook of addictive disorders,* New York, 1991, Guilford Press.

Dulit RA et al: Substance use in borderline personality disorder, *AJP* 147(8):1002 1007, 1990.

Ewing H: Care of women and children in the prenatal period. In Fleming MF, Barry KL, editors: *Addictive disorders,* St. Louis, 1992, Mosby.

Ewing JA: Detecting alcoholism: the CAGE questionnaire, *JAMA,* 252:1905–1907, 1984.

Fleming MF, Barry, KL: *Addictive disorders,* St. Louis, 1992, Mosby.

Flynn S: Adolescent substance abuse. In Fleming MF, Barry KL, editors: *Addictive disorders,* St. Louis, 1992, Mosby.

Francis RI, Franklin IE: Alcohol and other psychoactive substance use disorders. In Talbott IA et al, editors: *Textbook of psychiatry,* Washington, D.C., 1988, American Psychiatric Association.

Francis RJ, Miller SI: Addiction treatment: the widening scope. In Francis RJ, Miller SI, editors: *Clinical textbook of addictive disorders,* New York, 1991, Guilford Press.

Galamos JT: Alcoholic liver disease: fatty liver, hepatitis and cirrhosis. In Berk JE, editor: *Gastroenterology,* Philadelphia, 1985, W.B. Saunders.

Goodwin DW et al: Alcohol problems in 4 adoptees raised apart from biological parents, *Arch of Gen Psychiatry* 28:228, 1973.

Goodwin DW et al: Drinking problems in adopted and nonadopted sons of alcoholics, *Arch of Gen Psychiatry* 31:164, 1974.

High school senior survey. Unpublished data, Institute for Health and Aging, University

of California at San Francisco (1990). In Horgan et al: *Substance abuse: the nation's number one health problem,* Princeton, N.J., 1990, Institute for Health Policy, Brandeis University, The Robert Wood Johnson Foundation.

Jellinek EM: *The disease concept of alcoholism,* New Haven, Conn., 1960, Hillhouse Press.

Jellinek EM: Phases of alcohol addiction, *Quarterly J of Studies on Alcohol* 38:114–130, 1977.

Jellinek EM: *Phases in drinking history of alcoholics,* New Haven, Conn., 1946, Hillhouse Press.

Johnson L et al: *Details of annual survey,* Ann Arbor, 1988, University of Michigan News and Information Services.

Kaplan HI, Sadock BJ: *Synopsis of psychiatry: behavioral sciences, clinic psychiatry* ed 7, Baltimore, Md., 1994, Williams and Wilkins.

Kelly SJ et al: Birth outcomes, health problems, and neglect with prenatal exposure to cocaine, *J of Ped Nursing* 17:130–136, 1991.

Knott DH: The addictive process. Lecture presented June 1987 at the University of Utah Summer School on Alcoholism and Other Drug Dependencies, Salt Lake City. In Varcarolis EM: *Foundations of psychiatric mental health nursing,* ed 2, Philadelphia, 1994, W.B. Saunders.

Kozel NJ, Adams EH: Epidemiology of drug abuse: an overview, *Science* 234:970–974, 1986.

Krach P: Discovering the secret: nursing assessment of elderly alcoholics in the home, *J of Geron Nursing,* 16(11):32–38, 1992.

Landry MJ et al: Anxiety, depression and substance use disorder: diagnosis, treatment and prescribing practices, *J of Psychoactive Drugs* 23(4):397–416, 1991.

Lehman A et al: Assessment and classification of patients with psychiatric and substance abuse syndromes, *Hosp and Comm Psychiatry* 40(10):1019–1024, 1987.

Lieber CS, Leo MA: Alcohol and the liver. In Lieber CS, editor: *Medical disorders of alcoholism: pathogenesis and treatment,* Philadelphia, 1982, W.B. Saunders.

McDonald DI: *Drugs, drinking and adolescents,* Chicago, 1989, Year Book.

Mendelson JH, Mello NK: Diagnostic criteria for alcoholism and alcohol abuse. In Mendelson JH, Mello NK, editors: *The diagnosis and treatment of alcoholism,* New York, 1985, McGraw-Hill.

Montgomery P, Johnson B: The stress of marriage to an alcoholic, *J of Psychosocial Nursing* 30(10):12, 1992.

Mueser PR et al: Prevalence of substance abuse in schizophrenics: demographic and clinical correlates, *Schizophrenia Bull* 16(1):31–56, 1990.

National Institute of Drug Abuse. *National household survey on drug abuse: Population estimates 1988,* Washington, D.C., 1988, U.S. Department of Health and Human Services.

Nurses: help your patients stop smoking, Washington, D.C., 1992, U.S. Department of Health and Human Services.

Office of National Drug Control Policy: *National drug control strategy, part 1 (September 1989),* Washington, D.C., 1989, U.S. Government Printing Office.

Office of National Drug Control Policy: *National drug control strategy: reclaiming our community from drugs and violence (February 1994),* Washington, D.C., 1994, U.S. Government Printing Office.

Paul SM: Anxiety and depression: a common neurobiological substrate? *J of Clin Psychiatry* 49:13–16, 1988.

Rice DP: Unpublished data, Institute for Health and Aging, University of California at San Francisco (1990). In Horgan C et al: *Substance abuse: the nation's number one health problem,* Princeton, N.J., 1990, Institute for Health Policy, Brandeis University, The Robert Wood Johnson Foundation.

Robins LN et al: Lifetime prevalence of specific psychiatric disorders in three sites, *Arch of Gen Psychiatry* 41:949–958, 1984.

Ross HE et al: The prevalence of psychiatric disorders in patients with alcohol and other drug problems, *Arch Gen Psychiatry* 17(3):321–336, 1988.

Scharf MB et al: Therapeutic substitution: clinical differences among benzodiazepine compounds, *US Pharmacist* H1–H13, December 1988.

Scheitlin K: Identifying and helping children of alcoholics, *Nurse Practitioner* 15(2):34–36, 1990.

Schuckit MA: Low level response to alcohol as a predictor of future alcoholism, *Amer J of Psychiatry* 15:184–189, 1994.

Schuckit M: Genetics and the risk of alcoholism, *JAMA* 254:2614–2617, 1985.

Seltzer MS et al: A self administered Short Michigan Alcoholism Screening Test (SMAST), *J of Studies on Alcohol* 36(1):117–126, 1975.

Skinner HA et al: Identification of alcohol abuse using laboratory tests and a history of trauma, *Annals of Internal Medicine* 101:847–851, 1984.

Stanton MD, Todd TC et al: *The family therapy of drug abuse and addiction,* New York, 1982, Guilford Press.

Sullivan EJ: Comparison of chemically dependent and nondependent nurses on familial, personal and professional characteristics, *J of Studies on Alcohol* 48:563–568, 1987.

Sullivan EJ, Handley SM: Alcohol and drug abuse in nurses, *Annual Review of Nursing Research* 10:113–125, 1992.

Vourakis C, Bennett G: Angel dust: not heaven sent, *Amer J of Nursing* 79:649–653, 1979.

CHAPTER 16

Delirium, Dementia, and Amnestic and Other Cognitive Disorders

Geraldine I. Strachan
George G. Glenner

Agnosia The loss of comprehension of auditory, visual, or other sensations, although the senses are intact.

Agraphia The loss of the ability to write.

Alexia The loss of the ability to understand and interpret the written word.

Alzheimer's disease A neurodegenerative disease characterized by progressive, irreversible, and lethal structural damage to the brain due to the presence of β-amyloid proteins and leading to loss of cognitive functions and symptoms of progressive dementia.

Aphasia Expressive—the inability to speak or write (also known as Broca's aphasia).

Global—complete loss of all motor and sensory uses of oral and written speech; expression and comprehension are severely impaired.

Receptive—the inability to comprehend what is being said or written (also known as Wernicke's aphasia).

Apraxia The loss of the ability to carry out purposeful, complex movements and to use objects properly.

Catastrophic reaction A sudden or gradual negative change in the behavior of clients with dementia, caused by their inability to understand and cope with stimuli in the environment.

Delirium A disturbance of consciousness and change in cognition that develops over a short period of time and tends to fluctuate during the course of the day, characterized by disorientation to time and place; reduced ability to focus, sustain, or shift attention; incoherent speech; continual aimless physical activity.

Dementia A global impairment of intellectual (cognitive) functions (e.g., thinking, remembering, reasoning) that usually is progressive and of sufficient severity to interfere with a person's normal social and occupational functioning.

Dysarthria Difficulty in articulating words; this is especially frustrating, because the client knows what words to use but has trouble forming them (more commonly found in vascular dementias and strokes).

Neuritic plaques Maltese-cross–appearing clumps composed of amyloid fibers found in the brains of persons with Alzheimer's disease.

Neurofibrillary tangle The accumulation of twisted filaments inside brain cells, which is one of the characteristic structural abnormalities found upon autopsy that confirms the diagnosis of Alzheimer's disease.

Sundowner's syndrome The confusion and irritation common in clients with dementia at the end of the day, probably resulting from general tiredness and an inability to process any more information after a long day of struggling to interpret their environment correctly.

- Identify and differentiate between primary and secondary dementias.

- Discuss the various theories of the nature and development of Alzheimer's disease and rationale of the most currently accepted theories.

- Classify the progressive symptoms of Alzheimer's disease into three stages (onset/mild, middle/moderate, terminal/severe).

- Identify the neurological deficits, particularly of Alzheimer's disease, and list the resulting behavioral problems.

- Differentiate behavioral problems in Alzheimer's disease from other mental disorders.

- Assess cognition, functional levels, and stress of client and family to plan appropriate nursing interventions and use positive behavior interactions to affect outcomes.

- Describe and plan therapeutic activities for clients experiencing dementia.

- Refer clients' families to appropriate community resources for support and current information about Alzheimer's disease.

- Teach appropriate information about dementia and Alzheimer's disease to families/caregivers and evaluate results.

Dementia is a global impairment of intellectual (cognitive) functions, which is usually progressive and of sufficient severity to interfere with a person's normal social and occupational functioning. Many diseases and pathological processes are categorized under this medical syndrome, of which Alzheimer's disease is the most prevalent. Dementia is often confused with the lay term *senility,* which refers to the deterioration of both cognitive abilities and body function with advancing age. This confusion has obscured the significance and incidence of Alzheimer's disease until the past decade.

Alzheimer's disease (AD) affects short-term memory first and then a whole range of intellectual abilities, such as speech, reading, writing, and comprehension. These clients grow confused and unaware of their surroundings and later become progressively incapable of caring for their basic activities of daily living (ADL) such as feeding, grooming, and toileting. Morbidity increases and death follows.

Alzheimer's disease was first reported in 1907 by Dr. Alois Alzheimer, a neurologist, in his paper about a 51-year-old woman diagnosed with what was then called presenile dementia. Since then, progress has been made in understanding and treating this disease, which is still described as progressive, irreversible, incurable, and lethal.

As grim as this may seem, there is hope. Scientists are currently on the verge of new frontiers in technology and research in Alzheimer's disease and have refined the techniques of differential diagnosis. More important to the nursing profession is the development of new and better methods of assessing, diagnosing, determining positive outcomes, planning, implementing, and evaluating clients and their care.

The family also deserves special attention, because without support the burdens of caring for someone with Alzheimer's disease can be overwhelming. Placement in a long-term care facility is usually the final step in the family caregiver's commitment. Many years of concern precede this decision for out-of-home care. Emotional stresses as well as financial expenses become significant. Health care and in-home services, special equipment and foods, and loss of income for the client and the caregiver are only a few of the cost factors encountered. More than 50% of nursing home care cost is paid from the private funds of clients and their families.

HISTORICAL AND THEORETICAL PERSPECTIVES

Dementia in individuals over 65 years of age (late onset type) has been well known since the time of Hippocrates, the father of medicine (460–375 B.C.), and Galen, the father of experimental physiology (130–200 A.D.). Early onset dementia was first described by Griesinger in his textbook on psychiatric pathology. He differentiated this condition from arterial disease and neurosyphilis, stressing gross brain atrophy, which was found at autopsy.

Alois Alzheimer (1864–1915), a German-trained neurologist, was inspired by the neurologist Franz Nissl (1860–1919) to study neuropathology. In 1895 Nissl moved to Germany to work with the psychiatrist Emil Kraepelin (1856–1926) on the structural basis of psychiatric disease. Kraepelin transferred his operations to Munich in 1903, taking Nissl and Alzheimer with him. At about the same time, a revolution in histological techniques was taking place, in both microscope technology and the advent of metallic stains for nervous tissue. In 1899 Ramón y Cajal demonstrated the usefulness of this new staining technique in studying the structure and form of nervous tissue. Nissl produced his stain for neuronal cell bodies in 1892, and in 1902 Max Bielschowsky, a German neuropathologist (1869–1940), produced the silver-based stain that allowed Alzheimer to demonstrate

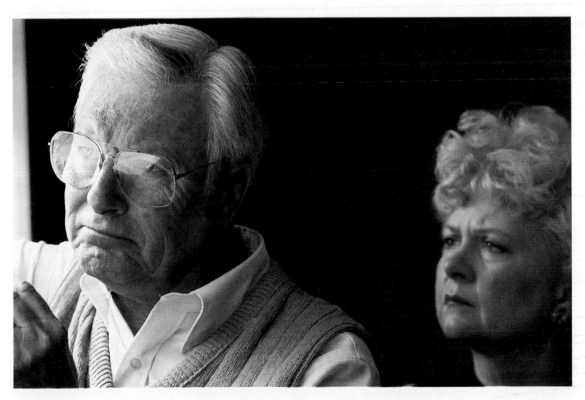

A wife feels sorrow over her husband's loss of faculties due to Alzheimer's disease.

(Copyright © Cathy Lander-Goldberg, Lander Photographics.)

the now-familiar neuritic (senile) plaques and neurofibrillary tangles in the brain. In 1906 Alzheimer announced his findings of these lesions in the brain of a 51-year-old woman suffering from dementia and paranoia, and he published them in 1907.

In 1910 Kraepelin referred to cases similar to that of Dr. Alzheimer's as Alzheimer's disease or "presenile" dementia (now called early onset dementia in DSM-IV), the frequency of which we now know to be much less than that of "senile" dementia (or late onset dementia in DSM-IV). The incorporation of Alzheimer's disease in Kraepelin's classic text categorized Alzheimer's disease as a psychiatric process rather than a neurological one, and thus for many decades designated it as the responsibility of specialists in psychiatry.

Early descriptions of Alzheimer's lesions affecting individuals with Down's syndrome over the age of 40 were described initially by Jervis in 1948 and tended to relate Alzheimer's disease to an accelerated aging process (which at that time Down's syndrome was thought to be).

It was not until the publication in 1968 to 1970 of an important series of papers by the team of British clinical pathologists, Tomlinson, Blessed, and Roth, that Alzheimer's disease moved into its modern era. These authors compared the brains of individuals over age 65 without dementia to an age-matched group with dementia. Much to their surprise they found that 62% of cases with dementia had the tangles and plaques described by Alzheimer. Using a neuropsychological test, they showed that the severity of dementia correlated with the number of cerebral plaques. Only 22% of these cases had evidence of arteriosclerosis and brain softening, indicative of cerebrovascular disease.

The application of the electron microscope magnified images up to 400,000 diameters, which further defined the lesions of Alzheimer's disease. The tangles revealed by the microscope were composed of parts of two twisted ribbon-like structures, termed *paired helical filaments.* The senile plaques and vascular lesions were made of bundles of twisted, nonbranching structures—the fibers of amyloid.

The major recent advance in the knowledge of the development of Alzheimer's disease is derived from the discovery of the chemical nature of the amyloid deposits making up the plaques and vascular lesions. Glenner and Wong (1984) defined these as being composed of a unique protein, the β-protein. This discovery has led to other studies and implications of the nature and treatment of Alzheimer's disease.

ETIOLOGY
Alzheimer's Disease

The cause of Alzheimer's disease is unknown, but several theories have been suggested and are currently being investigated. Among these are the following:

- infectious agents
- neurotoxic agents
- angiopathy and blood-brain barrier incompetence
- neurotransmitter and receptor deficiencies
- abnormal proteins and their products

INFECTIOUS AGENTS

A fibrillar protein, termed the *prion,* is associated with the infectious process in Creutzfeldt-Jakob disease. The prion has the characteristics of amyloid fibrils and is found in the gray matter of the brain (the cortex). This finding suggested a relationship with Alzheimer's disease (Prusiner, 1991; Prusiner, 1984). However, the order in which the amino acids occur in the amyloid fibrils of Alzheimer's disease deposits was found to be distinctly different from that of the prion. This negated a chemical identity between these two types of dementia.

NEUROTOXIC AGENTS

Aluminum toxicity has been the most frequently hypothesized causative toxic factor in the development of Alzheimer's disease. This resulted from the following (Perl and Brody, 1980):

- evidence of increased aluminum levels in the brain, correlated with aging
- chemical evidence of aluminum silicates in plaques
- electron probe evidence of aluminum concentration in tangles

It has been suggested that the development occurs by way of ingestion (aluminum utensils and antacids containing aluminum), inhalation and olfactory nerve involvement, or cutaneous absorption (deodorants). Against the etiologic significance of these findings is the lack of Alzheimer-type lesions in clients suffering from aluminum intoxication ("dialysis dementia"), the absence of an increased incidence of Alzheimer's disease in aluminum factory workers, and the invariable presence of Alzheimer lesions in clients with Down's syndrome. The localization of aluminum to tangles and plaques may be the result of aluminum binding to preformed amyloid fibrils and thus is a purely secondary phenomenon.

ANGIOPATHY AND BLOOD-BRAIN BARRIER INCOMPETENCE

Physical alterations of capillary walls have been noted in studies of the brains of persons with Alzheimer's disease. These changes include lumpy thickening and nodular vessels and loss of the fine network of nerve fibers normally investing the blood-contacting surfaces. It has been suggested that these lesions, and the resulting devastation of nerves, destroy the barrier that prevents many blood serum components from entering the brain (the blood-brain barrier). The fact that amyloid deposition in the walls of blood vessels and in capillaries in the cerebral cortex almost always accompanies Alzheimer's disease was recently demonstrated. This has reaffirmed that these vascular lesions result in blood-brain barrier incompetence (Glenner, 1983; Scheibel et al, 1987). Thus serum proteins leak into the grey matter (cortex) of the brain. Evidence that a serum protein, SAP, can be identified and isolated from the amyloid core of neuritic plaques (Scheibel, Duong, and Tomiyasu, 1987) strongly suggests that blood-brain barrier incompetence exists in Alzheimer's disease.

NEUROTRANSMITTER AND RECEPTOR DEFICIENCIES

The consistent finding of depleted activity of the neurotransmitter, choline acetyltransferase (an enzyme involved in the synthesis of the neurotransmitter acetylcholine), in the brains of clients with Alzheimer's disease led to many studies based on several theories. These theories suggested that this depletion was the result of one of the following:

- an enzyme (neurotransmitter synthesizing) deficiency
- a depletion or absence of a neurotransmitter
- the destruction of a group of cells at the base of the brain that is believed to innervate the cortical cells. Loss of this innervation is thought to result in cortical cell death.

Based on these "cholinergic theories," therapeutic attempts to increase the level of acetylcholine were made. This was accomplished by administering the precursors to acetylcholine, lecithin and choline, by directly infusing acetylcholine, and by introducing cholinesterase inhibitors, such as physostigmine and tetrahydroaminoacridine (Cognex). Thus far these approaches have been highly controversial and have led to uncertain results.

In Alzheimer's disease, dysfunction in a variety of neuronal systems is associated with neurotransmitter receptors. These are proteins incorporated in nerve cell membranes that bind specific neurotransmitter molecules. Reduction in many types of receptors (e.g., of serotonin, glutamate, and somatostatin) occurs in the cortex in Alzheimer's disease, but a consistent receptor abnormality occurring in Alzheimer's disease has not been found (Bowen et al, 1987; Whitehouse, 1987). There is a growing consensus that the neuroreceptor and neurotransmitter defects in Alzheimer's disease are the result of prior cell damage and death, not the cause.

ABNORMAL PROTEINS AND THEIR PRODUCTS

The consistent evidence of amyloid fibrillar deposits in plaques, cerebral vessels, and tangles demonstrates that these are twisted, β-pleated sheet fibrils (Glenner et al, 1971) and that Alzheimer's disease is a form of cerebral amyloidosis (Prusiner, 1984). This signifies that these lesions may be directly or indirectly responsible for neuronal cell death and are the final stage of the pathogenetic process leading to Alzheimer's disease.

The discovery of the major protein that makes up the amyloid fibrillar deposits, the β-protein, in both Alzheimer's disease and Down's syndrome has initiated biochemical and molecular biological studies. This protein was first isolated and purified, and its amino acid sequence determined from amyloid-laden cerebral vessels of clients with Alzheimer's disease and Down's syndrome (Wong et al, 1985). Based on its presence as amyloid fibrils in 100% of individuals with Down's syndrome, it was suggested that the β-protein was a chemical marker for Down's syndrome and that the gene encoding for its precursor would be found on chromosome 21, the abnormally tripled chromosome found in Down's syndrome (Glenner and Wong, 1984).

Current knowledge suggests that there are complex genetic sequences of events leading to cerebrovascular amyloidosis, plaques, and tangles.

The identification of abnormal enzyme(s) responsible for amyloid formation in the brain could result in the development of specific inhibitors and thus a treatment for Alzheimer's disease. Such findings could also lead to a *true diagnostic test* for Alzheimer's disease.

Nature of Alzheimer's Disease

Alzheimer's disease is a neurodegenerative disorder in which, predominantly, the cortex of the brain containing nerve cells involved in memory and cognition is destroyed. The loss of gray matter causes a separation of the brain from the skull, widening of crevices that produce its convoluted appearance (sulci), and dilatation of the cisterns that collect waste fluid and substances from the brain (ventricles).

The degradation of the gray matter is caused by the accumulation of destructive lesions, which are the hallmarks of the disease. These are the senile **neuritic plaques** which are composed of amyloid fibers and **neurofibrillary tangles** which are composed of paired helical filaments that destroy nerve cells and amyloid deposits in the walls of cerebral blood vessels. Although the exact process of gray matter destruction by these lesions is not completely known, certain assumptions can be made. In Alzheimer's disease an abnormal βPP circulates in the blood and forms amyloid fibrils in blood vessel walls. The amyloid fibrils disrupt the vessel, causing it to leak. This abnormal βPP then enters the brain tissue, where it blocks receptors necessary for proper metabolism of nerve cells. This leads to an interference in nerve function and the formation of tangles that destroy the nerve cells. The precursor also seeps into brain areas, where digestive enzymes cleave it to release the β-protein that accumulates to form senile plaques (Prelli et al, 1988) (Fig. 16-1). These plaques, where they contact nerve fibers, envelop the nerve fibers and cause their destruction.

Primary and Secondary Dementias

Because there is no definitive diagnostic test other than at autopsy (and the rare familial cases with known genetic

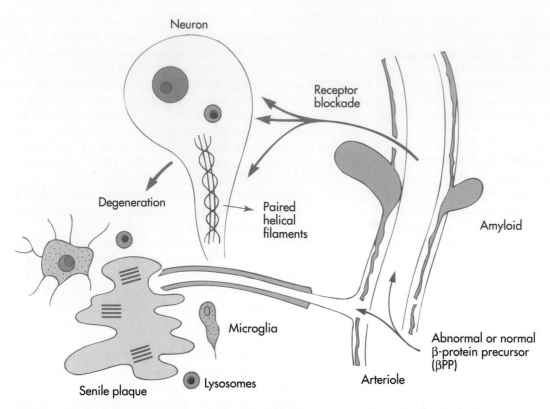

Figure 16-1 Diagram of the theory of brain damage in Alzheimer's disease. An abnormal β protein precursor (βPP) circulates in the blood, forming amyloid fibrils. These fibrils break the blood-brain barrier, causing leakage into brain tissue. There it blocks receptors necessary for proper metabolism of nerve cells and leads to the formation of paired helical filaments (tangles), which destroy the nerve cell. The βPP also seeps into other brain areas where it accumulates to form senile plaques.

(Courtesy George G. Glenner.)

mutations), the diagnosis of Alzheimer's disease must be specified by ruling out all other causes of dementia.

The vast majority of dementias (80%) are designated as primary dementias and are caused by degenerative diseases that are either untreatable or rarely treatable. They progress to irreparably destroy nervous tissue. The possible exception to this is multi-infarct dementia caused by hypertension or diabetes, whereby control of the hypertension or diabetes with medication may eliminate the progression of the disease. Diseases that cause primary dementia and the frequency of their occurrence are illustrated in Table 16-1.

Secondary dementias are a group of processes that represent about 20% of dementia cases. The vast majority of these are treatable and/or curable. For example, the metabolic disease, vitamin B_{12} deficiency, mimics most of the Alzheimer's disease symptoms. When the client is treated by a physician with injections of vitamin B_{12}, before irreversible damage occurs, the dementia symptoms can be eliminated and the well-being of the client readily restored. This is also the case with certain superficial benign tumors (meningiomas), which, when completely re-

TABLE 16-1 Etiological factors of primary dementia

Diseases that cause primary dementia	Incidence at autopsy (%)
Alzheimer's disease (AD)	62.6
Vascular dementia (formerly called multi-infarct dementia [MID])	21.4
Mixed Alzheimer's disease and vascular dementia (MIX)	6.3
Parkinson's disease	5.7
Pick's disease	3.0
Creutzfeldt-Jakob (including Gerstmann-Sträussler-Sheinker) disease	0.5
Other cases: Diffuse Lewy body disease Progressive supranuclear palsy Binswanger's disease Down's syndrome	0.5

From Glenner GG: Alzheimer's disease, *Encyclopedia of human biology* 1:103–111, 1994.

TABLE 16-2 Etiological factors in secondary dementia

Toxic causes	Other electrolyte disturbances	Infective causes	Cerebral disease
Barbiturate intoxication	Hepatic disease	Chronic respiratory infection with cardiac decompensation	Slow-growing cerebral tumor, e.g., frontal meningioma
Alcoholism	Porphyria	Pulmonary tuberculosis	
Polypharmacy	Nutritional	Bacterial endocarditis	Multiple cerebral emboli
Metabolic disorders	Undernutrition by prolonged neglect or self-isolation	Endocrine disease	
Potassium loss from self-purgation	Chronic malabsorption syndrome	Myxedema	Normal pressure hydrocephalus*
	Vitamin B_{12} deficiency	Pituitary insufficiency	
	Nicotinic acid encephalopathy	Addison's disease	

*Normal pressure hydrocephalus is a disorder characterized by dementia, gait disorder, and urinary incontinence. Dilatation of the ventricles in the absence of increased cerebrospinal fluid is a prominent manifestation. A shunt is usually effective treatment.

moved by a surgeon, will eliminate the dementia symptoms. Etiological factors in secondary dementia are discussed in Table 16-2.

EPIDEMIOLOGY

It is estimated that 4 million people in the United States have Alzheimer's disease, of which 120,000 die each year (Box 16-1). One out of three families with a member age 65 or older will include a person with Alzheimer's disease. More than 50% of nursing home clients have been diagnosed with probable or possible Alzheimer's disease. The age of the youngest autopsy-diagnosed case was 38, whereas the average age of clients with Alzheimer's disease is about 75. The percentage of cases under age 60 is only 0.1%. The life span of a client with Alzheimer's disease is halved, with death ranging from 5 to 15 years after symptoms are first noted. A few cases of 20 to 30 years duration are on record. Generally the younger the client, the more rapidly the disease progresses and the more likely it is to be familial.

Death resulting from Alzheimer's disease can be caused by many factors, the most common being aspiration pneumonia, because the client's inability to swallow properly causes regurgitation of food into the lungs. Other causes may be thrombophlebitis and emboli, urinary tract infection, and infected decubitus ulcers.

CLINICAL DESCRIPTION

Alzheimer's disease is described as a "global" disease affecting all regions of the gray matter (cortex) of the brain. This is the outer surface in which the intellectual processes arise. However, two characteristics make diagnosis difficult in its earliest stage. Initially the hippocampus is attacked by neurofibrillary tangles, producing recent memory loss. This is usually followed by nonsymmetrical, or uneven, deterioration of the temporoparietal regions, producing cognitive deficits in learning, atten-

tion, judgment, orientation, and/or speech and language use. To further complicate matters, occasionally other regions of the brain may be affected. Thus a panorama of symptoms results. The situation is compounded by the insidious onset of the disease, which to the untrained observer may be perceived as inattention, restlessness, mild forgetfulness, and depression.

Therefore, a client with Alzheimer's disease does not present a uniform or coherent history, nor can the time of onset be clearly defined. This can present a serious problem in differential diagnosis. Frequently, family members who have not seen the person for a while fail to notice the subtle changes that have occurred. Rash judgments based on a short visit often lead to conflict between the family caregiver and relatives of the client, particularly when institutionalization comes into question. The loss of a job or a serious auto accident may, unfortunately, be the most convincing evidence of serious cognitive loss and usually motivates the family members to act on behalf of their loved one.

Box 16-1   Epidemiology of Alzheimer's Disease

- 4 million people are affected
- 120,000 people die each year
- one out of six people over age 65 are affected
- fourth most common cause of death
- accounts for 50% of skilled nursing facility admissions
- $90 billion are spent per year on medical bills, nursing home costs, and lost productivity

From *Progress report on Alzheimer's disease 1993*, NIH Pub No 93-3409, National Institute on Aging.

Frequently the first symptoms of dementia are noted following a surgical procedure in which general anesthesia is used. Since the reserve of neurons is markedly depleted by the Alzheimer's disease process, a transient loss of oxygen during anesthesia further depletes the number of functioning nerve cells, thus making the initial symptoms of Alzheimer's disease apparent for the first time.

Caregivers may seek medical care for a loved one when specific behavioral difficulties have been observed, such as the following:

- trouble with shopping, which requires performing tasks sequentially, correlating lists, planning, remembering, and calculating money
- problems in the areas of driving, involving accidents or episodes of getting lost
- missing social engagements and appointments
- difficulty with financial tasks, particularly balancing a checkbook, getting bills paid, or understanding financial statements
- aimless pacing or wandering away from home
- inability to recognize people they should know or misidentifying friends and family members
- inability to do common household tasks, e.g., cooking and cleaning

Although clients themselves may notice early signs of cognitive impairment, many will employ one or more of the defense mechanisms of denial, repression, projection, aggression, regression, or rationalization. Some will succeed in deceiving family, friends, and employers for a time. Distinguishing these behaviors from cognitive deficits further complicates the diagnostic process.

A careful history may reveal many or all of the following symptoms:

Altered thought processes (paranoia)

Confused or disoriented state

Impaired intellect and memory (especially short-term memory in the early stage)

Sensory/perceptual alterations (hallucinations)

Decreased sensorium

Loss of body functions

Self-care deficit

Fear, anxiety, depression

Panic/rage reactions (catastrophic reactions)

Self-concept disturbance/powerlessness

Compromised physical ability

Social isolation, apathy

Impaired verbal communication

Emotional lability

Sleep disturbances

Dementia of the Alzheimer Type

Dementia, as stated before, is a global impairment of intellectual functions that usually is progressive and of sufficient severity to interfere with a person's normal social and occupational functioning. The dementia associated with Alzheimer's disease is classified as dementia of the Alzheimer's type (DAT). The diagnostic criteria for dementia of the Alzheimer's type are listed in the box on page 379.

Delirium

Delirium is a state of mental confusion and excitement characterized by disorientation for time and place, usually with illusions and hallucinations. The mind wanders, speech is incoherent, and the client is often in a state of continual, aimless physical activity.

Delirium is characterized by a clouding of consciousness with a reduced capacity to shift, focus, and sustain attention. The client may or may not be agitated or sleepy and may or may not display hallucinations. The duration of onset ranges from hours to days, and symptoms fluctuate over the course of a day (Rockwell, 1991). There may be periods of lucidity or a change in cognition such as memory deficit, language disturbance, or perceptual impairment. Clients may be agitated or withdrawn, tearful, and even sad. As such, they can appear depressed. Delirium always has an organic basis that needs to be carefully assessed.

Delirium is usually seen in clients with Alzheimer's disease when a severe infection or other medical condition is superimposed on the preexisting conditions. At least 22% of elderly clients become delirious at some point during hospitalization (Lyness, 1990). Delirium can also be the first or only indicator of illnesses ranging from pneumonia to myocardial infarction to drug toxicity. Failure to recognize delirium can lead to significant morbidity and mortality, both from the underlying illness and from inadvertently self-inflicted injuries. When delirium overlies dementia of the Alzheimer's type, differentiating becomes more difficult yet more vital to positive client outcomes. The DSM-IV criteria for delirium are listed in the box on page 379. A comparison of delirium, depression, and dementia is found in Table 16-3.

Amnestic Disorders

Amnestic disorders are characterized by a disturbance in memory that is due to either the direct physiological effects of a general medical condition or the persisting effects of a substance use/abuse or toxin exposure. The main focus is memory disturbance and can be specified as transient (duration of hours or days but less than one month) or chronic (duration of more than one month). The DSM-IV criteria for amnestic disorders are listed in the box on page 381.

DSM-IV CRITERIA

Dementia of the Alzheimer's Type

A. The development of multiple cognitive deficits manifested by both:

   1) memory impairment (inability to learn new information and to recall previously learned information)

   2) one (or more) of the following cognitive disturbances:

      a) **aphasia** (language disturbance)

      b) **apraxia** (inability to carry out motor activities despite intact motor function)

      c) **agnosia** (failure to recognize or identify objects despite intact sensory function)

      d) disturbance in executive functioning (e.g., planning, organizing, sequencing, abstracting)

B. The cognitive deficits in criteria A1 and A2 each cause significant impairment in social or occupational functioning and represent a significant decline from a previous level of functioning.

C. The course is characterized by gradual onset and continuing cognitive decline.

D. The cognitive deficits in criteria A1 and A2 are not due to any of the following:

   1) other central nervous system conditions that cause progressive deficits in memory and cognition (e.g., cerebrovascular disease, Parkinson's disease, Huntington's disease, subdural hematoma, normal pressure hydrocephalus, or tumor)

   2) systemic conditions that are known to cause dementia (e.g., hypothyroidism, vitamin B_{12} or folic acid deficiency, niacin deficiency, hypercalcemia, neurosyphilis, HIV infection)

   3) Substance-induced conditions

E. The deficits do not occur exclusively during the course of delirium.

F. The deficits are not better accounted for by another Axis I disorder (e.g., Major Depressive Disorder or Schizophrenia).

Reprinted with permission from *Diagnostic and statistical manual of mental disorders*, ed 4, Washington, D.C., 1994, American Psychiatric Association.

Other Dementias

VASCULAR DEMENTIA (MULTI-INFARCT DEMENTIA)

Vascular dementia, formerly called multi-infarct dementia, results from the occlusion or obstruction of small arteries or arterioles in the cortex of the brain by the increased number of the cells of the vessel, so nutrients cannot enter the brain. Occasionally, rupture of these vessels may occur, producing hemorrhage into the brain substance or vessel blockage, causing "softening" (strokes) and open spaces (lacunae). Paralysis rarely occurs, since the damage tends to be limited to the gray matter. Computerized tomography (CT), magnetic resonance imaging (MRI), or positron emission tomography (PET) scans often reveal otherwise undetectable strokes. The DSM-IV criteria for vascular dementia are listed in the box on page 381.

PARKINSON'S DEMENTIA

Parkinson's dementia is associated with *Parkinson's disease,* which was first described in 1817 by Parkinson in his *Essay on the Shaking Palsy* as "involuntary tremulous motion, with lessened muscular power, in parts not in action and even when supported; with a propensity to bend the trunk forwards, and to pass from a walking to a running pace; the senses and intellects being uninjured."

DSM-IV CRITERIA

Delirium

A. Disturbances of consciousness (i.e., reduced clarity of awareness of the environment) with reduced ability to focus, sustain, or shift attention.

B. Change in cognition (such as memory deficit, disorientation, language disturbance, perceptual disturbance) that is not better accounted for by a pre-existing, established, or evolving dementia.

C. The disturbance develops over a short period (usually hours to days) and tends to fluctuate during the course of the day.

D. There is evidence from the history, physical examination, or laboratory findings that the disturbance is caused by the direct physiological consequences of a general medical condition or intoxication or withdrawal from substance abuse.

Reprinted with permission from *Diagnostic and statistical manual of mental disorders*, ed 4, Washington, D.C., 1994, American Psychiatric Association.

TABLE 16-3 Delirium, depression, and dementia comparison

	Delirium	Depression	Dementia
Onset	Rapid (hours to days)	Rapid (weeks to months)	Gradual (years)
Course	Wide fluctuations; may continue for weeks if cause not found	May be self-limited or may become chronic without treatment	Chronic; slow but continuous decline
Level of consciousness	Fluctuates from hyperalert to difficult to arouse	Normal	Normal
Orientation	Client is disoriented, confused	Client may seem disoriented	Client is disoriented, confused
Affect	Fluctuating	Sad, depressed, worried, guilty	Labile; apathy in later stages
Attention	Always impaired	Difficulty concentrating; client may check and recheck all actions	May be intact; client may focus on one thing for long periods
Sleep	Always disturbed	Disturbed; excess sleeping or insomnia, especially early-morning waking	Usually normal
Behavior	Agitated, restless	Client may be fatigued, apathetic; may occasionally be agitated	Client may be agitated or apathetic; may wander
Speech	Sparse or rapid; client may be incoherent	Flat, sparse, may have outbursts; understandable	Sparse or rapid; repetitive; client may be incoherent
Memory	Impaired, especially for recent events	Varies day to day; slow recall; often short-term deficit	Impaired, especially for recent events
Cognition	Disordered reasoning	May seem impaired	Disordered reasoning and calculation
Thought content	Incoherent, confused, delusions, stereotyped	Negative, hypochondriac, thoughts of death, paranoid	Disorganized, rich content, delusional, paranoid
Perception	Misinterpretations, illusions, hallucinations	Distorted; client may have auditory hallucinations; negative interpretation of people and events	No change
Judgment	Poor	Poor	Poor; socially inappropriate behavior
Insight	May be present in lucid moments	May be impaired	Absent
Performance on mental status exams	Poor but variable; improves during lucid moments and with recovery	Memory impaired; calculation, drawing, following directions usually not impaired; frequent "I don't know" answers	Consistently poor; progressively worsens; client attempts to answer all questions

From Holt J: How to help confused patients, *Am J Nurs* 93:32–36, 1993.

The muscular stiffness, the immobile face, and the mumbling speech were later emphasized clinically. These characteristic motor signs are still diagnostic criteria. Nerve cells in the substantia nigra (brain stem), where dopamine is produced, develop pigmented lesions within them that are a sign of the disease. These were first described by Lewy in 1913 and are called *Lewy bodies.* In about 30% of cases of Parkinson's disease the amyloid lesions of Alzheimer's disease can be seen whereas, conversely, about 50% of clients with Alzheimer's disease demonstrate typical parkinsonian symptoms.

PICK'S DISEASE

Pick's disease, named after the Czechoslovakian physician Arnold Pick (1851–1924), is a degenerative process of nerve cells, usually localized to the frontal and temporal lobe of the brain. It is distinguished clinically by changes in personality early in the course of the disease, deterioration of social skills, emotional blunting, behavioral disinhibition, and prominent language abnormalities.

CREUTZFELDT-JAKOB DISEASE

Creutzfeldt-Jakob (CJ) disease, first described by Jakob in 1921, is an infectious (but not contagious) process that can be transmitted by corneal grafts, infected electrodes, and injected crude growth hormone derived from human pituitaries. It is believed to be caused by an infectious agent, called a prion, and produces a spongy appearance to the brain (spongioform encephalopathy) with vacuolization of nerve cells (the creation of a clear space in cell protoplasm filled with fluid or air). Its course is more rapid than that of Alzheimer's disease. Creutzfeldt-Jakob disease begins with the insidious onset

DSM-IV CRITERIA

Amnestic Disorders

A. The development of memory impairment as manifested by impairment in the ability to learn new information or the inability to recall previously learned information.

B. The memory disturbance causes significant impairment in social or occupational functioning and represents a significant decline from a previous level of functioning.

C. The memory disturbance does not occur exclusively during the course of a delirium or a dementia.

D. There is evidence from the history, physical examination, or laboratory findings that the disturbance is the direct physiological consequence of a general medical condition (including physical trauma).

Reprinted with permission from *Diagnostic and statistical manual of mental disorders,* ed 4, Washington, D.C., 1994, American Psychiatric Association.

DSM-IV CRITERIA

Vascular Dementia

A. The development of multiple cognitive deficits manifested by both:

1) memory impairment (impaired ability to learn new information or to recall previously learned information)

2) one (or more) of the following cognitive disturbances:

a) aphasia

b) apraxia

c) agnosia

d) disturbance in executive functioning

B. The cognitive deficits in criteria A1 and A2 each cause significant impairment of occupational functioning and represent a significant decline from a previous level of functioning.

C. Focal neurological signs and symptoms (e.g., exaggeration of deep tendon reflexes, extensor plantar response, pseudobulbar palsy, gait abnormalities, weakness of an extremity) or laboratory (MRI) evidence indicative of cerebrovascular disease (e.g., multiple infarctions involving cortex and underlying white matter) that are judged to be etiologically related to the disturbance.

D. The deficits do not occur exclusively during the course of delirium.

Reprinted with permission from *Diagnostic and statistical manual of mental disorders,* ed 4, Washington, D.C., 1994, American Psychiatric Association.

of confusion, depression, and altered sensation, progressing in weeks or months to dementia, ataxia, palsy, and sometimes cortical blindness. Even though Creutzfeldt-Jakob disease constitutes only 0.5% of primary dementia cases, it is advisable to remove a client with chronic dementia from any donor list, because there is a risk of transmitting the disease.

GERSTMANN-STRÄUSSLER-SHEINKER DISEASE

Gerstmann-Sträussler-Sheinker (GSS) disease is, like Creutzfeld-Jakob disease, an infectious process but has a genetic component, a mutation in the prion protein, that results in a familial disease.

DIFFUSE LEWY BODY DISEASE

Diffuse Lewy Body disease is a late-life primary degenerative dementia noted predominantly in men in which Lewy bodies, as seen in Parkinson's disease, are present in neurons in the gray matter. Early ataxic gait, psychiatric symptoms (hallucinations, delusions, and violent or aggressive behavior) are not uncommon. It is associated with Alzheimer's disease lesions as well as those of Parkinson's disease.

PROGRESSIVE SUPRANUCLEAR PALSY

Progressive supranuclear palsy is a degenerative disease that particularly affects the nucleus of the neuron and presents clinically with dementia, progressive paralysis of downward (vertical) gaze, difficulty in articulation of joints **(dysarthria),** muscular rigidity (most marked in

the neck), and ataxic gait. Males are affected more than twice as often as females.

BINSWANGER'S DISEASE

Binswanger's disease affects small arteries and arterioles in the brain, producing moderate to severe narrowing defects such as those seen in multi-infarct dementia. Lesions appear in the white and gray matter. Dementia is a common but not constant symptom, with dizziness, ataxic gait, and hemiparesis occurring.

DOWN'S SYNDROME DEMENTIA

Down's syndrome dementia is difficult to diagnose, despite the extensive Alzheimer's disease-type lesions seen in the cortex of the brain upon autopsy. Only about 50% of individuals with Down's syndrome over age 40 can be determined as having dementia, which is usually first manifested as memory loss. This is probably due to the difficulty in ascertaining dementia in the face of mental deficiency.

CEREBRAL VASCULAR ACCIDENTS

Cerebral vascular accidents (CVA) are stroke-like episodes that occur in approximately 20% of clients with Alzheimer's disease and are due to the effects of cerebrovascular amyloid deposits either blocking the vessel or causing it to rupture to produce a cerebral hemorrhage. This lesion occurs predominantly in the gray matter and therefore does not result in paralysis. However, if the vessel ruptures in the leptomeninges, i.e., on the brain surface, severe hemorrhage can result in paralysis and death.

Stages of Alzheimer's Disease

Although up to 15 different stages in the progression of Alzheimer's disease have been proposed by various sources, it is both effective and practical to reduce these to three major categories. These three categories are detailed below and summarized in Table 16-4.

STAGE 1: ONSET OR MILD

- Recent memory loss: Without this symptom the diagnosis of Alzheimer's disease cannot be made. The magnitude of this loss is best depicted in the following example: If an automobile accident occurred 2 days ago with a woman driver being injured, the failure to remember the injured person's gender is not serious, but failure to remember the accident is suggestive of severe recent memory loss.

- Cognitive loss is always present but to varying degrees. There is progressive loss of intellectual abilities, e.g., communicating verbally or in writing, calculating, and recognizing of persons, places, or things that should be known to the client are impaired.

- Anxiety and confusion may or may not be caused by the memory loss but are believed in most cases to be independent of it. Depression may complicate diagnosis and should be identified and treated. Personality change is often seen. This will be addressed in detail later in this chapter.

- Behavioral problems begin to manifest themselves in the inability to begin and complete tasks without assistance.

STAGE 2: MIDDLE OR MODERATE

- All the symptoms of Stage 1 increase.

- Behavior problems increase, which may include restless pacing and agitation, wandering, and getting lost. Catastrophic reactions (see Box 16-3 on page 394), Sundowner's syndrome (see Box 16-5 on page 397), and perseveration (involuntary persistence of same verbal or motor activity) may occur.

- Confusion increases, leading to incidence of incontinence first of bladder and later of bowel.

- Abnormal tension of muscles (hypertonia) with resulting unsteady gait may appear.

STAGE 3: TERMINAL OR SEVERE

- All the symptoms of Stage 2 increase.

- Urinary and fecal incontinence are prominent.

- Ineffective swallowing leads to choking while eating and aspiration pneumonia (a frequent immediate cause of death).

- Emaciation is a frequent occurrence even in the case of adequate nutrition.

- Constant supervision and assistance are necessary and total bedridden state occurs.

PROGNOSIS

There is no known medical treatment that can prevent, arrest, or modify the course of Alzheimer's disease, but means to modify and lessen some of its symptoms exist. As noted, family education and counseling can ease the demands of caring for a client with Alzheimer's disease

TABLE 16-4   Stages of Alzheimer's disease

Stage 1: onset or mild	Stage 2: middle or moderate	Stage 3: terminal or severe
Recent memory loss	Stage 1 symptoms increase	Stage 2 symptoms increase
Cognitive loss in	Behavior problems increase, which	Incontinence, total
• communicating	may include the following:	Choking
• calculating	• catastrophic reactions	Emaciation
• recognition	• Sundowner's syndrome	Total care needed
Anxiety and confusion	• perseveration	Progressive gait disturbances leading
Mild behavior problems such as the	• aimless pacing	to nonambulatory status
inability to initiate and complete a task	• wandering	
	Confusion	
	Incontinence, mild	
	Hypertonia	

and can avoid family caregiver conflicts. Positive interventions by the caregiver can result in behavioral modification and reduce anxiety, avoid incontinence, and eliminate sleep disturbances and depression. (See the Understanding and Applying Research box below.) A planned therapeutic activity program can increase the client's awareness, verbal and physical response, and level of function. Drug intervention may be necessary (specifics will be addressed later).

DISCHARGE CRITERIA

The characteristics of Alzheimer's disease and other primary dementias do not fall into categories of final discharge. The client and the caregivers will be flowing from one level of need to another. Before adjustments in care are made, the following indications of success in specific areas should be considered.

The client is

- absent from risk of self-harm or caregiver abuse

- accomplishing activities of daily living (ADL) and independent activities of daily living (IADL) with minimal possible assistance
- free from catastrophic reactions and is able to communicate needs and wants
- is participating in a therapeutic activity program tailored to assessed needs

The primary caregiver(s) has

- integrated correct knowledge of Alzheimer's disease or the related disease into daily routines of caregiving
- used positive behavior interactions at all times
- instituted plans and developed resources for self-care
- appropriate legal and financial plans for the client and self in place
- appropriate back-up systems in place in case of emergencies (e.g., sudden illness or death of the client or of the caregiver[s])

Understanding and Applying
RESEARCH

Woods P, Ashley J: Simulated presence therapy: Using selected memories to manage problem behaviors in Alzheimer's disease patients. *Geriatr Nurs* 16:9–14, 1995.

A 1000-client survey in 42 skilled nursing facilities reported that 64% of clients with Alzheimer's disease demonstrated significant behavioral problems. The three most common problems were social isolation (93%), agitation (67%), and verbal or physical aggression (7%). Eighty-eight percent displayed more than one type of problem behavior. As an alternative intervention for behavioral disruptions, researchers have found that reminiscence by a special family member provides a calming effect. The authors conducted two studies based on the hypothesis that maladaptive behaviors would decrease when an environment of fond memories and pleasant experiences was created. The intervention used, called simulated presence therapy (SPT), was designed to replicate a caregiver's presence through the use of an audio tape of a family member reminiscing about the client's cherished memories, loved ones, and family anecdotes. The client listened to the tape through a portable cassette player and headphones.

The first study involved 27 cognitively impaired residents from four nursing homes whose ages ranged from 76 to 94 years of age. Family members of these clients made a 15-minute-long tape which conveyed affection and positive emotion through reminiscence. For one month, the tapes were played for the clients when they displayed disruptive behavior, and nursing staff recorded the clients' behavioral responses as either improved, unchanged, or worsened behavior. Results showed that 22 of the 27 subjects (81.5%) showed positive responses to SPT. The behavior of the 18% whose response was not positive did not worsen, but remained unchanged.

The second, and more controlled, study included 9 residents ranging from 71 to 97 years of age from 2 units in a 120-bed nursing home. Subjects were selected based on their positive Diagnosis of Alzheimer's Type confirmed behavioral problems, retained capacity for verbal interaction, and willingness of their families to participate. All subjects were considered to have moderate cognitive impairment. For 2 months, clients listened to the tapes once each morning, and once each afternoon or early evening. Observations of behavior were made before and after SPT. An average of 47 episodes of problem behaviors were recorded per patient. Results showed that problem behaviors improved with SPT 91% of the time. Seven percent of the time, behavior remained unchanged or worsened with SPT. SPT was refused 2% of the time. All 9 residents exhibited positive responses to SPT for at least some of their episodes of problem behavior, ranging from 100% to 68%.

Although these studies were preliminary, SPT proved successful in interrupting problem behaviors among clients with DAT. One reason for its success is that it relies on remote memory which is more likely to be retained by these clients than is recent memory. Because of the deficit in their recent memory, clients perceive each time the tape is played as the first time. Managing behavioral problems is one of the most difficult tasks for families and caregivers. SPT shows promise as an alternative intervention to medications and restraints. Nurses are encouraged to use interventions similar to SPT, which evoke positive memories, in an attempt to decrease maladaptive behaviors in clients with cognitive disorders.

■ ASSESSMENT

Assessment of clients with dementia is difficult and must rely, to a great degree, on information from sources other than the client (usually the family caregiver). This is especially true of clients with Alzheimer's disease, since often the first symptom reported is recent memory loss, and even remote memory may be adversely affected by the concurrent symptoms of disorientation, depression, delusions, or hallucinations.

Assessment Environment

When interviewing the client or administering an assessment test, a positive physical and emotional environment is critical. The room should be free from distractions, quiet, and away from the noise of any activity. Visual and auditory deficits may be present in the client, and the evaluator must establish eye contact, speak directly to the client in a low-frequency range (since high tones are usually less discernible), and enunciate clearly. Hearing aids or glasses, if usually worn by the client, should be in clean, working condition. Any printed material from which a client response is expected should be presented in large, heavy type that is easily read. If English is a second language, someone who speaks the client's primary language should administer the test and/or translate for the client and interviewer to yield valid results. Paraphrasing questions is permissible to clarify an item. Sufficient time needs to be allotted, since the client may take longer to process the information and form a correct response. In general, the attitude of the evaluator must be friendly, nonthreatening, and nonjudgmental. Giving positive feedback to the client by saying "You're doing fine," "That was good," or "This is a really hard one," can help relieve the stress of testing. Avoid indications that a response is correct or incorrect.

Administering a test in sections is permissible if the client has become too fatigued, has too short an attention span, or shows signs of anxiety. It is best to test the client alone, without an informant/caregiver so that responses are entirely the client's own and not colored by hints or responses from someone else.

Interviews with the caregiver also should include the same courtesies as used with the client and should be conducted separately and in private. This will ensure honest responses and avoid the danger of talking about the client in front of him or her.

Cognitive Assessment Tools

A variety of tools can lend insight into a person's cognitive status. Among the most common are

- Mini-Mental Status Examination (MMSE)
- NIMH Dementia Mood Assessment Scale (DMAS)
- Blessed Dementia Rating Scale (Blessed DRS)

Mini-Mental Status Examination (MMSE)

This tool, developed by Folstein, appears to be the most useful and popular. It can be administered in as short a time as 5–10 minutes and provides standardized methods of data collection, scoring, and interpretation in specific areas of cognitive impairment (see Fig. 10-1 in Chap-

---

Nursing Care in the Community

Cognitive Disorders

With the increased population of elderly persons, more community attention has been focused on the support of families whose aging members are acting in unusual and troubling ways. The community mental health nurse may be asked to evaluate a person who no longer seems able to provide self-care and is resistant to help from caregivers. The nurse will need to assess the reports of caregivers, observe the behavior of the client, evaluate medication regimen/compliance, and attempt an individual interaction including an assessment of mental status.

The nurse should attempt to determine if the behavior change is a result of a cognitive disorder or if it has another explanation. Sometimes the identified behavior is merely an "acting-out" demand for more attention, which might be rectified by a brief intervention, such as providing a more comfortable environment in terms of temperature or stimulation level. Apparent confusion may be due to a malfunctioning hearing aid or the need for one. The elderly person may have a urinary tract infection without showing signs of it. This infection can lead to restlessness and agitation. Some medications may have the effect of stimulation rather than sedation, which might induce the untrained caregiver to increase the dosage, thereby compounding the problem. Taking multiple medications concurrently also can have adverse effects.

The caregiver's need for support should also be carefully appraised by the nurse, and consideration should be given to establishing a pattern of respite care, which would give the family members needed time for themselves. The community nurse must be aware of options for caregiver respite, such as day treatment facilities or visiting care assistants.

ter 10 for this tool). When repeated it may indicate any change in the disease process. It can also be used in the differential diagnosis of dementias (e.g., in Huntington's disease the ability to recall three items will remain significantly higher than in Alzheimer's disease).

NIMH Dementia Mood Assessment Scale (DMAS)

Increased precision is possible with this tool but the test itself is quite lengthy. Data is collected through a clinical interview. Objective information from the family or professional caregiver is also obtained. Scoring is more complicated than with the MMSE; however, it can give a detailed baseline for future comparison and differential diagnosis.

Blessed Dementia Rating Scale (Blessed DRS)

The Blessed scale is short, practical, and easy to use and has been used as a standardized assessment scale. It begins to determine loss of function ability as it measures loss of ability to perform ADLs. Scoring is easy yet informative.

Neurological Deficits

The previously discussed pathological changes in the brain (neuritic plaques, neurofibrillary tangles, and fibrillar deposits in cerebral vessels) result in neurological deficits with ensuing behavioral changes. Determining the status of a client with Alzheimer's disease or another related dementia must involve assessment of neurological deficits such as the following (Zgola, 1987): (The memory aid "PALMER" may help to remember these areas.)

Perception and Organization

How well does the client interpret

- sensory cues?
- relationships between objects and between self and environment?

How well does the client organize

- movement such as sitting, standing, transferring?
- tasks such as dressing in proper sequence?
- solutions to simple puzzles?

Attention Span

How well does the client

- initiate an activity?
- sustain an activity (shortened attention span or loss of interest)?
- terminate an activity when completed or in an established pattern (perseveration)?

Language

How well does the client

- express thoughts verbally (expressive **aphasia**)?
- comprehend the spoken word (receptive aphasia)?
- read and comprehend the written word (**alexia**)?
- express thoughts in writing (agraphia)?

Nursing Assessment Questions

Cognitive Disorders

The following questions may be helpful in assessment and can be asked of the caregiver.

1. Has onset been rapid or slow? Hours, days, weeks? (Time of onset determines type of disorder.)

2. Is disorientation to person, place, and/or time present? Is it consistent or transient? Is it consistent with previous symptoms of Alzheimer's disease or other underlying dementia? (Sensorium can establish type of disorder.)

3. Is there any known underlying medical condition or indication of substance use/abuse? What substance is suspected? (These conditions may adversely affect the primary condition.)

4. Is cognitive impairment present? Is it consistent or fluctuating? (This is a primary symptom of Alzheimer's disease.)

5. Is psychomotor agitation present or absent? Is it consistent or transient? (Agitation may lead to diagnosis of other dementias.)

6. Is the client's mood consistent or unstable?

7. What is the client's level of consciousness? Does it fluctuate?

8. Has the sleep/wake cycle been altered?

9. Is the client able to maintain attention and focus? (Questions 6–9 help to determine diagnosis of delirium, dementia, or depression.)

Memory

How well does the client remember

- recent events immediately following their occurrence (immediate recall)?
- recent events within a matter of minutes (recent memory)?
- events from past events of months or years ago (remote or long-term memory)?

Emotional Control

Is the client's emotional control

- consistent with and appropriate to the situation?
- sustained for an appropriate length of time?
- changed from previous behavior?

Reasoning and Judgment

How well has the client

- made appropriate decisions based on good advice or facts?
- conformed to social conventions?
- reacted appropriately in an emergency situation?

CASE STUDY

Henry has been brought to the emergency room by his wife, Ann, for treatment of a large skin tear on his right forearm, which is bleeding and wrapped in a large gauze roller bandage. While the wound is being treated, the nurse interviews Ann and notes that her appearance is disheveled, grooming is poor, and there are dark circles under her eyes. Henry is 68 and has been retired for 7 years, and Ann is 64 and still trying to work part-time as a clerk to supplement their income. Ann relates that Henry has been "acting crazy," "never sits still," "has accidents in the bathroom," and that he has kept her up for the last three nights. She states that she is exhausted and says, "If I don't get some sleep, I'm going to hit him or something." Further questioning reveals that Henry lost his job as a clerk because of low production and errors in mathematics. Henry's affect is flat and he states, "I can't remember how I hurt myself." His hygiene and grooming are poor, which is evidenced by his untidy appearance, soiled clothing, and offensive body odor. Ann confirms that neither has seen a physician "in a long time," since Henry decided that doctors "are all useless."

Critical Thinking and Assessment

1. What are the primary immediate and long-term needs of Henry and Ann?

2. What approach should be used to gain their confidence?

3. Which assessment tools might be used to determine their psychosocial status?

4. What questions might elicit information about Ann's knowledge regarding Henry's behavior?

5. What approaches might be successful in getting this couple to seek future help?

Emotional Status

Mood and State of Mind

Each time a nurse approaches a client, an informal assessment of mood and state of mind is done. The Omnibus Budget Reconciliation Act (OBRA) of 1987 requires a more formal psychiatric assessment of a client prior to admission to a Skilled Nursing Facility (SNF) and before the administration of any psychotropic medications or physical restraints. Consistent use of the following guidelines to assess clients' symptoms and behaviors will ensure a reliable data assessment tool. Significant quoted statements from the client should be noted to increase the objectivity and usefulness of the report. Regular documented Mental Status Examinations (MSE) further assist the professional staff in communicating information in a systematic way.

Depression

Secondary depression can be a concomitant condition with the client with dementia or Alzheimer's disease, and signs and symptoms should be thoroughly assessed and treatment plans developed. (See Chapter 12, and also Table 16-3.) Tools such as the Zung or Beck depression scales can be used in most stages of Alzheimer's disease as long as some language ability is still present enough to communicate such feelings as sadness, guilt, and suicidal ideation. Occurrences of adverse fatigue, weight loss, loss of appetite, insomnia or social withdrawal needs consultation and follow-up.

Functional Ability

Determination of a client's functional ability is essential as nursing diagnoses are formulated. Excess disability can occur when the caregiver responds verbally or physically with more assistance than is necessary and diminishes the client's speaking or activity skills. Maintaining independence in ADLs and IADLs is vital if clients with Alzheimer's disease are to retain their self-esteem and engage in worthwhile activities.

Behavior

Behaviors often found in clients with Alzheimer's disease and other cognitive disorders can be grouped in the following manner.

Behaviors that are related to mood:

- pacing, wandering, and rummaging may indicate anxiety
- decreased or inappropriate socialization may signify apathy
- refusal to eat, bathe, or groom may mean depression
- hoarding or accusations of thievery may manifest paranoia

Behaviors that result from perceptual/cognitive deficits:

- day/night reversal
- inappropriate eating (eating too rapidly or too much, eating nonfood items)

CLINICAL ALERT !

Signs of Silent Aspiration (choking):

Watering eyes

Reddening of the face

Gurgly or "wet" sounding respirations

Change in rate or ease of respiration

Grimacing

Coughing

Gagging

Throat clearing

- falls/accidents (walking into walls or furniture, not being aware of hazards)

- delusions, hallucinations, paranoia

Behaviors that result from the destruction of impulse control:

- inappropriate toilet activities

- inappropriate sexual behavior (masturbating in public, display of penis or breasts, sexually explicit comments or language, inordinate sexual drive)

- inappropriate social behavior (undressing in public, being offensive, rude, or aggressive)

When any change in behavior from previous observations occurs, the client should be immediately assessed. The client often cannot evaluate or communicate to others about distressing signs or symptoms of an illness. Determining how a client feels involves use of honed observation skills, especially in the area of assessing body language.

Physical Manifestations

Weight changes of three to five pounds or more should be noted and an assessment made for treatable problems unrelated to the dementing illness. Frequently, a change in eating patterns occurs, which may lead to weight gain or loss. If no other clinical signs or symptoms are noted, the client's immediate environment must be examined next. The nurse should observe and correct distracting lighting, seating arrangement (groups should be homogenous and compatible), noise level, and physical comfort of table and chairs. Emaciation during Stage 3 of Alzheimer's disease is often seen and appears to be the result of the body's inability to process foods rather than poor intake.

Choking is a risk during Stage 3 of Alzheimer's disease and the resulting aspiration pneumonia is frequently the immediate cause of death.

The caregiver monitoring feeding should watch for a swallow after each bite, indicated by the larynx rising and returning to the resting position.

Clients with dementia often suffer from *dehydration,* because they cannot recognize the discomfort of thirst or remember when they last had a drink. It is a nursing responsibility to ensure adequate hydration. Diluted juices are a good resource, since they are palatable and also provide some much-needed calories. If choking problems are present, thickening agents may need to be added to facilitate swallowing.

Changes in *gait* are often noted and again nurses must be alert to other disease processes, such as vision problems, inner ear disturbances, pain from osteoarthritis or an injury, which the client may not be able to identify, and neuropathy resulting from vascular or diabetic problems and general decrease of the "righting reflex" (the reflexes that enable any animal to maintain the body in a definite relationship to the head and thus maintain its body right side up). Treating underlying problems usually will result in better gait in the client in the early stages of Alzheimer's disease, but as the disease progresses, decrease in sensory interpretation, neurologic deficits, and hypertonia will require increased awareness and interventions by the caregiver to prevent falls.

Clients may complain of *feeling cold* even on the warmest summer days. The level of activity and the amount of body fat present are among several factors that influence body comfort with regard to heat or cold. The best way to judge a client's response to environmental temperature is to actually feel the skin, and if perspiration is present, the amount of clothing should be reduced. Conversely, if the skin feels cold to the touch, the client needs the additional layers of clothing even though it might appear to be excessive.

Incontinence, first of urine and then of feces, may begin in the second stage of Alzheimer's disease and become permanent during the third stage. Other possible causes of incontinence should be identified before attributing the problems to Alzheimer's disease. Many medications can affect bladder continence as well as a client's levels of awareness and consciousness.

Fecal incontinence may have many of the same causes as those attributed to bladder incontinence (e.g., drug side effects, cognitive deficits, and memory loss). It may also be related to a decrease in muscle control, chronic laxative abuse, long-term poor bowel habits, lack of exercise, or a diet low in fiber and fluids.

Physical and Laboratory Examination

Other tests are done to rule out other causes. Physical examination must be careful and thorough to rule out neoplasia (i.e., growths or tumors in the brain), metabolic disorders (i.e., hormone or vitamin imbalances), systemic illnesses (i.e., hypertension, inflammatory signs indicative of infection processes), and side effects of med-

---

CLINICAL ALERT   !

Types of urinary incontinence

Stress—involuntary loss of small amounts of urine associated with coughing, sneezing, laughing, etc.

Urge—loss of larger amounts of urine due to inability to delay voiding after feeling the sensation of a full bladder.

Overflow—loss of small amounts of urine due to stresses on an overly full bladder.

Functional—loss of large amounts of urine due to cognitive deficits that lead to not recognizing cues from the bladder, inability to find the bathroom, or increasing apraxia.

ication. Vision, hearing, pupillary changes and eye movements, motor and sensory function, and reflexes are areas to be specifically examined to determine deficits and assist in the differential diagnosis.

Blood studies including a complete blood count (CBC), sedimentation rate (ESR), glucose, urea nitrogen (BUN), electrolytes, calcium and phosphorus, bilirubin, vitamin B_{12}, folate, and a complete thyroid panel will further enable an accurate diagnosis and rule out treatable diseases. Specific screening related to toxic metals and fluids should be performed on those clients known to have been exposed to these agents.

Radiologic studies may include a chest x-ray, CT, MRI, or PET. These imaging studies will not reveal Alzheimer's disease in the early stage but are used to rule out other pathological factors such as brain tumors or strokes.

Some studies that may be indicated to rule out other disease processes are electrocardiogram, routine urinalysis, and (when indicated) electroencephalogram, lumbar puncture, urine for heavy metals, and arterial blood gases.

■ ■ ■ NURSING DIAGNOSIS

Nursing diagnoses are made from the information obtained during the assessment phase of the nursing process. The accuracy of diagnosis depends on a careful, in-depth assessment.

NANDA Diagnoses for Delirium, Dementia, and Amnestic and Other Cognitive Disorders

Safety and/or health risks:

Aspiration, risk for
Body temperature, risk for altered
Constipation
Diarrhea
Health maintenance, altered
Home maintenance management, impaired
Injury, risk for
Nutrition, altered
Pain
Physical mobility, impaired
Poisoning, risk for
Protection, altered
Self-care deficits (bathing/hygiene, dressing/grooming, feeding, toileting)
Suffocation, risk for
Swallowing, impaired
Trauma, risk for
Urinary elimination, altered
Urinary retention

Perceptual/cognitive disturbances

Anxiety
Body image disturbance

Confusion (acute, chronic)
Diversional activity deficit
Environmental interpretation syndrome, impaired
Hopelessness
Incontinence (bowel, stress, reflex, urge, functional, total)
Memory, impaired
Relocation syndrome
Sensory/perceptual alterations (visual, kinesthetic, gustatory, tactile, olfactory)
Powerlessness
Sleep pattern disturbances
Thought processes, altered

Problems in communicating and relating to others

Communication, impaired verbal
Decisional conflict
Fatigue
Self-esteem, disturbance in
Sexual dysfunction
Sexuality patterns, altered

Disruption in coping abilities (client and/or family)

Adjustment, impaired
Caregiver role strain
Caregiver role strain, risk for
Coping, ineffective individual
Coping, ineffective family (disabling or compromised)
Denial, ineffective
Family processes, altered
Fear
Grieving, anticipatory
Social isolation (client and family)
Therapeutic regime, ineffective management of

Client and family teaching needs

Caregiver role, potential for growth

■ ■ ■ OUTCOME IDENTIFICATION

Outcome criteria are derived from nursing diagnoses and are the expected client responses to be achieved.

Outcome Identification for Delirium, Dementia, and Amnestic and Other Cognitive Disorders

Client will:

1. reach and maintain the highest functional level possible within capacity.

2. maintain optimal physical status.

3. participate in a therapeutic activity program for cognitive stimulation and socialization and to meet other psychosocial needs.

4. participate in planning for care as able, especially making legal/financial decisions while capacity for decision making is still intact.

COLLABORATIVE DIAGNOSES

DSM-IV Diagnoses*

Dementia

Dementia of the Alzheimer's type (early or late onset)

Vascular dementia (formerly called multi-infarct dementia [MID])

Dementia due to HIV disease

Dementia due to head trauma

Dementia due to Parkinson's disease

Dementia due to Huntington's disease

Dementia due to Creutzfeldt-Jakob disease

Dementia due to other general medical conditions (e.g., normal pressure hydrocephalus, hypothyroidism, brain tumor, vitamin B_{12} deficiency)

Dementia not otherwise specified

Substance-induced persisting dementia (not separately coded)

Dementia due to multiple etiologies (not separately coded)

Delirium Disorders

Delirium due to a general medical condition (e.g., hepatic encephalopathy, electrolyte imbalance, etc. General medical conditions may also be coded on Axis III)

Delirium not otherwise specified

Substance-induced delirium (not separately coded)

Delirium due to multiple etiologies (not separately coded)

Amnestic Disorders

Amnestic disorder due to a general medical condition (e.g., physical trauma or vitamin deficiency)

Amnestic disorder not otherwise specified

Substance-induced persisting amnestic disorder (not separately coded; includes medication side effects)

Other Cognitive Disorders

Cognitive disorders not otherwise specified (e.g., mild neurocognitive disorder or postconcussional disorder following head trauma)

NANDA Diagnoses**

Thought processes, altered
Verbal communication, impaired
Anxiety
Powerlessness
Hopelessness
Health maintenance, altered
Risk for violence
Self-esteem disturbance
Impaired adjustment
Coping, ineffective (individual, family, community)
Grieving, anticipatory (family and individual)
Knowledge deficit (pathology, neurology, therapy, medication)
Denial, ineffective (individual-family)
Social isolation (individual-family)
Caregiver role strain
Family processes, altered
Sensory/perceptual alterations
Sleep pattern disturbance
Injury, risk for
Self-care deficit
Physical mobility, impaired
Nutrition, altered
Sexual dysfunction
Sexual patterns, altered
Home maintenance, impaired
Aspiration, risk for
Constipation
Fatigue
Environmental interpretation syndrome, impaired
Memory, impaired
Confusion (acute, chronic)

*Reprinted with permission from *Diagnostic and statistical manual of mental disorders*, ed 4, Washington, D.C., 1994, American Psychiatric Association.

**Reprinted with permission from *NANDA nursing diagnoses: definitions and classifications, 1995–1996*, Philadelphia, 1994, North American Nursing Diagnosis Association.

Caregiver will:

1. maintain optimum personal physical and mental health status.

2. initiate contacts with support services for legal and financial planning, support groups or individual counseling, case management, and respite services.

3. increase knowledge base regarding the disease process, positive behavior interactions, and therapeutic activities.

■ ■ ■ ▫ **PLANNING**

A few common issues need to be specifically addressed to achieve appropriate planning for the client with a cognitive disorder:

Short-Term and Long-Term Goals

Nurses in diverse roles will have contact with a client and the family for varying lengths of time. Acute care nurses may have only hours or days to formulate and im-

NURSING CARE PLAN ■ ■ ■ ■ ■ ■ ■ ■ ■ ■

Gail, a 63-year-old female, has been referred to a home health nurse by her primary physician for evaluation for home care. The diagnosis given is probable Alzheimer's disease with a secondary diagnosis of controlled hypertension. After an interview with Hal, Gail's husband, who is 64 and still working as a sales representative, the following is determined:

- 2-year history of recent memory loss
- history of being well groomed but now refuses to bathe and change clothes and dresses inappropriately, putting on clothes in the wrong sequence
- appears to understand spoken language, if thoughts are stated slowly and simply
- expressive language lacks correct grammar with evidence of word searching and parroting words used by the interviewer
- Gail's widowed sister, Ann, comes to stay with her during the day and stays overnight if the husband has to be out of town

- recent episodes of crying, negativity, and angry verbal outbursts have caused the sister concern and fear
- Hal is staying away more often and leaving care to the sister, who is losing weight and dropping out of her personal social activities

DSM-IV Diagnoses

Axis I	Dementia of the Alzheimer's Type with Perceptual Disturbances
	Dementia of the Alzheimer's Type with Behavioral Disturbances
Axis II	R/O Dependent Personality Disorder
Axis III	Hypertension
Axis IV	Problems with Access to Health Care Services
	Other Psychosocial Problems
Axis V	GAF rating 35

Nursing Diagnosis: Self-care deficit related to perceptual and cognitive alterations secondary to neurological damage in the brain as evidenced by inability to recognize the need for self-care (bathing, changing), inability to sequence properly (dressing in the right order), and inability to reason and judge (inappropriate choice of clothing).

Client Outcomes	*Nursing Interventions*	*Evaluation*
• Gail will bathe 3 times a week.	• Determine habitual time and manner of bathing. *Establishing a pattern based on Gail's previous habits will use her retained remote memory.*	• Gail was successfully bathed by the Home Health Aide twice in the first week with the help of Ann. The second week Ann was successful on two occasions with HHA assisting. Extend HHA for 1 more week and reevaluate.
	• Ensure privacy *to preserve dignity and self-esteem.*	
	• Determine room and water temperature. *Comfort and safety will encourage positive client response.*	
	• Reduce sensory stimulation (e.g., noise from TV, radio, other people) to enable client to attend to the task at hand). Mirrors may need to be covered if the reflection is incorrectly interpreted by the client to be an observer. *Limiting the number of responses required by Gail will facilitate her cooperation and independence.*	
	• Provide a Home Health Aide (HHA) three times a week for 2 weeks. *Caregivers, Ann and Hal, will increase their knowledge and skills and thus enhance their confidence and ease in assisting Gail. The HHA will teach the caregivers ways in which to maintain skin integrity and general health. The supervising nurse will check on general health status and hypertension.*	

NURSING CARE PLAN

Client Outcomes	Nursing Interventions	Evaluation
• Gail will be well groomed.	• Determine areas of dysfunction in grooming. • Set adequate routines of visual and verbal cues to assist in grooming routines. • Assist directly only as necessary to complete task. • Employ positive reinforcement. • Refer for dental prophylaxis and assist the family to preplan with dentist and hygienist for a successful visit. • Assist Hal and Ann in formulating follow-up plan for daily oral hygiene. *These interventions will reduce stress for client and caregivers, avoid excess disability, provide a positive environment, and avoid unnecessary physical disabilities.*	• Ann and Hal have been successful on 5 out of 7 successive days in cuing Gail to complete her dental hygiene and in helping with combing her hair. An appointment has been made with the dentist who previously cared for her, and Hal has informed the dentist of the present situation. Evaluate success of visit later.

• Gail will dress herself appropriately.	• Assess clothing supply.
	• Simplify dressing choices for Gail by the following:
	  • remove clothes not currently being worn
	  • assemble coordinated outfits on one hanger and limit these to six to eight choices
	  • stack clothes in the order in which they are to be put on
	• Assess clothes and assist family to choose those that are appropriate yet easy for Gail to put on, e.g., eliminate buttons, buckles, pantyhose, etc., and replace with elastic waists, snaps, velcro fasteners, knee- or thigh-high hose. *The client will retain control and independence by making some simple decisions and will be socially acceptable, thus increasing self-esteem and reducing stress for all.*
		• Family/nurse/HHA see the improvement in Gail's appearance and Gail is responding with smiles at the compliments about her appearance. Hal is having some adjustment problems in changing her dress style (not putting on hose and heels as she had) and in moving some of his favorite outfits out of the closet. Ann comments favorably on the ease of dressing Gail now and on Gail's increased comfort evidenced by her willingness to participate in activities and calmer interactions.

Nursing Diagnosis: Altered thought processes related to inability to process and synthesize information as evidenced by recent memory loss, decreased ability to analyze, reason, and form judgments, and interruption in logical stream of thought.

Client Outcomes	Nursing Interventions	Evaluation
• Gail will use her intellect and judgment to the best of her ability.	• Develop a stimulating therapeutic activities program. *Cognitive stimulation in deficit areas and positive reinforcement will promote self-esteem and encourage Gail to attain the highest functional level possible.*	• Hal and Ann have found that Gail enjoys walks and they have established routines. Gail has recognized some previously familiar birds and indicated she wanted bird seed to feed them. She also enjoys simple puzzles and assisting Ann in laundry tasks.

NURSING CARE PLAN

Client Outcomes	Nursing Interventions	Evaluation

• Gail will retain some control in her life by exercising her right to choose.	• Assess environment and activities and collaborate with all caregivers to
	  • simplify choices in food, clothes, colors, and activities
	  • use multiple sensory cues, especially auditory, visual, and tactile senses, to indicate choices. *Choices, even simple ones, give control back to Gail and improve her self-esteem, making her more willing to try to participate in daily activities.*
		• Gail is responding to the use of multiple cues by increasingly exercising her right to choose. (During the first week Gail made an independent choice five times. During the second week she made seven choices.)

• Gail will be oriented to place, time of day, scheduled activities, and family members.	• Develop simple calendars with daily routines and easy-to-read clocks. • Encourage family members to repeat their names and relationships often in conversations. *These actions will assist in overcoming recent memory loss. Establishing routine decreases the stress of making decisions; verbal cues reinforce recognition and eliminate the need to chat.*	• After 2 weeks, Gail knows the time for her walks with Hal and indicates that she wants her supply of bird seed. She is less frequently confused regarding the identification of persons and never fails to recognize Hal and Ann.
• Gail will use remote memory.	• Formulate daily periods of reminiscence using old photos, specially designed picture books, and rummage boxes. *The use of multiple sensory cues to stimulate remote memory is building on the retained strength of habitual skills to stimulate use of remote memory.*	• Gail looked at old photographs with Hal and Ann and indicated her recognition with short phrases or smiles. She independently sought out the box of various colored and textured yarns and handle them with satisfaction, indicating that she remembers knitting when she was well.
• Gail will have decreased **catastrophic reactions** (see Box 16-3).	• Analyze with all caregivers what the previous causative factors may have been. • Simplify the environment (evaluate furniture and objects, colors, noise level). *Through analyzing and simplifying the environment, the client's safety is maintained and the stressors causing the catastrophic incidents are reduced. Collaborative planning will ensure consistent successful approaches to tasks, and client and caregiver stress will be reduced.*	• Gail had two catastrophic reactions during the last 2 weeks. Hal and Ann analyzed each incident and discovered that the underlying causes were (1) increased ambient noise from street repairs in front of the house and (2) being rushed to leave for a dental appointment.

NURSING CARE PLAN

Nursing Diagnosis: Ineffective family coping—compromised related to inadequate understanding of the process of Alzheimer's disease by the caregivers, inability of spouse to adequately manage the emotional conflicts, role changes, temporary abandonment, weak support systems, ineffective communication/relationship with secondary caregiver, as evidenced by Hal being away from home more and Ann's loss of weight and social withdrawal.

Family Outcomes	*Nursing Interventions*	*Evaluation*
• Hal and Ann will verbalize realistic perception of their roles and responsibilities in caring for Gail.	• Facilitate meeting with all family members. *Sharing knowledge of status and prognosis will establish the core of a support system based on mutual respect and understanding.* • Address knowledge deficits and obtain feedback from participants. *Understanding allays fears and promotes rational planning; each person retains knowledge in unique ways and common understandings are vital to successful planning and implementation.* • Collaborate in developing roles for each caregiver. *Understanding each one's role, including expectations and limitations, will reduce behaviors that might lead to abuse or abandonment and elicit positive care outcomes for the client.*	• Hal and Ann have met with other family members who live in the area, and these family members expressed gratitude for being included and enlightened: they offered assistance with outings and evening care. On two consecutive nursing visits Hal and Ann have successfully reviewed information on the pathologic and neurologic deficits of Alzheimer's disease and are coping with Gail's behavior manifestations. Interventions have been successful on four occasions. They have congratulated each other.
• Hal and Ann will express their feeling in a mutually supportive manner.	• Facilitate sessions directly or provide referrals to appropriate health professionals. *Caregivers need permission to express themselves in a nonjudgmental, supportive environment.*	• Hal and Ann join each other for breakfast on most weekdays to plan for the day and critique the previous day's activities. Revisions of plans have been accepted in most cases.
• Hal and Ann will demonstrate cooperation of all family/support persons in planning, problem solving, and decision making regarding Gail's care and Hal's and Ann's personal needs.	• Inform family of support services in the community. • Encourage attendance at support groups or individual counseling sessions. *Support services and groups provide external assistance and concern for the caregiver's needs.* • Facilitate positive methods, e.g., calendars, defining responsibilities and problem-solving tasks. *Sharing and preplanning will avoid conflict and pursue positive outcomes.*	• Hal and Ann attended an Alzheimer's disease support group together while a grandchild stayed with Gail. Hal was late one evening but later apologized to Ann.

NURSING CARE PLAN ■ ■ ■ ■ ■ ■ ■   ■ ■ ■ ■ ■ ■

Family Outcomes

- Hal and Ann will exhibit effective coping strategies.

Nursing Interventions

- Promote healthful methods of caregiver self-care, i.e., socialization, exercise, adequate diet, and time for personal renewal. *Developing positive coping strategies will restore positive physical and mental health and revive a functional family unit.*

Evaluation

- Ann has only regained two pounds but admits to eating better and feeling more energetic. She attended a sewing class, resuming a previous social activity. Hal is having dinner with an old friend before attending Lions Club meetings, while Ann stays with Gail for the evening.

Box 16-3   Catastrophic Reactions

Often clients with dementia are unjustly labeled as noncompliant, disruptive, uncooperative, or threatening/violent. Usually a client with dementia is only reacting to being overwhelmed by the inability to interpret the environment because of cognitive deficits. Clients are not trying to annoy, get attention, or hurt the caregiver but are trying their best to understand a world they can no longer comprehend. A *catastrophic reaction* can be a display of verbal or physical aggression, verbal outbursts, worry, anger, tension expressed in body language or facade, rapid changes in mood, stubborn resistance, pacing or wandering, paranoia, crying, or hysterical laughter.

Analysis of a Catastrophic Reaction

Was the person

- Trying unsuccessfully to comprehend more than one or two sensory messages at once?
- Feeling insecure (e.g., being in new surroundings or surrounded by unfamiliar staff)?
- Having a minor mishap (e.g., spilling a drink or dropping something) or failing at a task?
- Asked to reason, make a judgment, or make too complex a choice?
- Experiencing negative interactions such as scolding, arguing, anger, frustration, or irritation?
- Experiencing a hallucination, delusion, or illusion?

Interventions for a Catastrophic Reaction

- Reassure the client that the environment is safe, and that nothing is threatening or harmful.

- Use positive behavior interactions.
- Be careful of invading the person's "personal space" without permission. Step back several feet and remove your hands from the person.
- Eliminate or reduce all outside stimulation.
- Identify and remove the source of the problem or remove the person.
- Give a reassuring touch, a hug, or holding a hand if the person is not extremely angry or after the person has calmed down somewhat.
- Redirect the client to a less demanding and stressful activity and environment.
- Be patient and allow sufficient time for the client to calm down. This may take only a few minutes or hours, varying with each client and situation.

If the nurse can't stop or minimize the reaction:

- Leave the client alone for a while in a quiet, safe place within view of staff or at least "back off" a few feet and provide some personal space.
- When the nurse returns or readdresses the client, act as if nothing has happened.
- Have another person intervene (change of face) and leave the area. Two people gesturing and talking will only add to the client's confusion and will reinforce negative behaviors.

Box 16-4   Types and Levels of Care for Cognitive Disorders

Acute Care

The client's or caregiver's first attempt to seek help may be associated with a routine physical checkup, emergency situations, or an acute illness requiring hospitalization. Therefore, nurses in clinics, physicians' offices, emergency room/urgent care units, or acute care facilities must be alert to the signs and symptoms of dementia. The care given to the client depends, in part, on the caregiver's mental and physical health; therefore, stress-related problems experienced by caregivers need to be addressed.

Day Care

With the increasing cost of long-term care, the option of using daycare services instead of long-term care facilities becomes even more viable. Not only is day care cost effective, but it also offers support for families who opt to care for the person with Alzheimer's disease in the home.

Social day care centers for the elderly offer many opportunities for interaction in terms of recreation, education, and other meaningful activities. Caregivers in these settings often are the first to notice decreasing mental and physical abilities in the client with Alzheimer's disease, and are in the position to offer counseling and referral for appropriate care.

Adult day health care licensing regulations throughout the country vary, but in general the focus of these centers is on education, rehabilitation, training, and maintenance of physical functions as well as mental status.

Dementia day care began in the early 1980s when the need was recognized for specialized respite, education, and support for the caregivers of clients with dementia and for therapeutic activity programs and appropriate behavior management approaches for the client with dementia.

In-Home Care

As the disease progresses, an increasing amount of support and care will be necessary in the home. The role of case management agencies, to coordinate and provide direct care for the client and the caregiver, will increase. Often home care and day care, provided together, will enable the client to stay at home longer, thus increasing the quality of life, conserving financial and emotional resources, and postponing institutionalization.

Residential Care Facility (RCF)

There are many residential care options, and state regulations vary. The services offered may include housekeeping and communal meals, which could be sufficient in the early stages of Alzheimer's disease, but as deficits in memory and decision making increase, more supervision will be necessary in areas of ADL and IADL. A Residential Care Facility (RCF) is often a more appropriate placement than a Skilled Nursing Facility (SNF) in the moderate stage of the dementia, since physically, the client may be very active and otherwise well. For effective care, all staff involved in residential care should be dementia-competent, i.e., keenly aware of the effects of Alzheimer's disease and trained to interact positively for the successful outcome achievement.

Skilled Nursing Facility (SNF)

As the disease progresses and behavior problems increase (especially night wandering and incontinence) and other disease entities develop, the need for more professional assistance becomes evident, and a skilled nursing facility (nursing home) may be the best option. Financing this phase of the long-term care continuum is becoming increasingly problematic. The financial resources of the client, family, and state and federal government all become involved.

---

plement a treatment plan and their opportunities to assess, diagnose, identify outcomes, plan, implement, and evaluate will therefore be focused on resolution of immediate problems (e.g., trauma crisis, pre- or postoperative care, and stabilization of medical, health, and safety needs).

Goals for long-term care nurses, whether in the home, residential care setting, or a skilled nursing facility, are more focused on maintaining the client's highest functional level, educating the caregiver about effective and realistic outcomes and interventions, and referring to available options for care in the home and in the community.

Flexibility and Change

Care plans are not cast in concrete and must be changed as often as assessment indicates. Acute care nurses may need to adapt the care plan to fit the client's needs as each shift changes, whereas nurses in long-term care need to set routine times (e.g., every 3 months) to closely examine the client's needs and adjust care accordingly.

Collaboration

Cooperation by both acute and long-term care nurses and other members of the health care team is critical, as the collective knowledge and experience at all levels assure more effective, realistic client outcomes and caregiver gratification. A clinical pathway for dementia is included in Appendix D.

■ ■ ■ ■ ■ IMPLEMENTATION

The care and treatment of clients with cognitive disorders present the nurse/caregivers with a variety of situations that can be both challenging and gratifying. Each plan of care should reflect the unique qualities of the individual with special consideration given to the family as well as the client. It is the nurse who keeps the health care team focused on both short-term and long-term goals that address the problems arising from dementia and delirium.

Caregiver and support system integrity must be maintained by involving the family and significant others in planning, intervention, and evaluation. Client and Family Teaching Guidelines below list issues that need to be addressed in their involvement. Treatment options for acute, chronic, and terminal care need to be addressed early. The client and the caregivers need a realistic knowledge base regarding diagnosis, treatment, and prognosis. As the therapeutic relationship between the nurse, client, and family/caregivers develops, the nurse will be able to introduce these delicate and often painful topics while preserving hopefulness and family integrity. Types and levels of care are detailed in Box 16-4.

Nursing Interventions

1. Keep all interactions with the client pleasant, calm, and reassuring *to decrease anxiety, because clients with cognitive disorders mirror the emotional climate around them.*

2. Attempt to understand the client's feelings *to decrease frustration and meet clients' needs.*

3. Respond to the client's feelings and validate them with words, body language, and actions *to make client feel understood and increase feelings of self-worth.*

4. Help the client maintain self-esteem by avoiding or simplifying difficult activities and always keeping interactions on an adult level without infantilizing or patronizing. Use proper names versus "pet" terms, e.g., "granny" and "honey." If errors or failures occur, assure the client that no harm has been done and

avoid any criticism. Avoid negative responses and commands. Avoid "why" questions. *Clients with dementia are often aware that there is something wrong with their performance, and they do not totally comprehend their environment. They are sensitive to criticism and may not be able to respond to "why" questions, which may provoke a sense of failure.*

5. Provide the client the opportunity to make simple choices. *Choosing offers some control to the client and aids in maintaining a sense of independence.*

6. Set up fairly structured routines. *This helps overcome short-term memory losses, promotes independence, and reduces anxiety.*

7. Praise successes and facilitate the use of remaining strengths *to increase self-esteem and reduce a sense of failure.*

8. Simplify the verbal message using no more than five or six words at a time. Accompany words with touch and visual clues *to decrease confusion and increase clarity of the message.*

9. Repeat the message if needed, allowing time for responses. Use the same words. Don't go on to another message until you are sure the first one has been grasped, or leave and return to explain in a different way. *Using these techniques may avoid or lessen such common behavior problems as* **catastrophic reactions** *(Box 16-3) and* **Sundowner's syndrome** *(Box 16-5) and deter the development of excess disability.*

Additional Treatment Modalities

Interdisciplinary Team

The nurse can most effectively provide care to a client with a cognitive disorder by collaborating with other health care professionals in developing and implementing a plan of care. A gerontologic assessment team might be composed of a nurse practitioner or home health nurse; a physician with expertise in the care of the older adult with cognitive disorders; a psychiatrist, psychologist, or social worker; a nutritionist; a pharmacist; and rehabilitation specialists (e.g., speech, physical, occupational), each with a special knowledge of gerontology or geriatrics. A Clinical Pathway for dementia is presented in Appendix D. It details the collaborative treatment interventions for this condition.

A number of practical considerations, especially in regard to the client's safety, nutrition, polypharmacy, and potential for falls, may only be discernible as a result of a home visit by a geriatric or geropsychiatric nurse specialist, social worker, or other home health specialist.

Pharmacological Interventions

Pharmacological intervention with cognitive disorders can be successful in two areas:

Client and Family
TEACHING GUIDELINES

Cognitive Disorders

1. A strong professional and family support network is important for the caregiver who must carry out exhausting tasks.

2. Psychiatric intervention for the caregiver may aid in adjusting and coping with difficulties that arise.

3. The caregiver must be allowed the time and opportunity to mourn and complete the grieving process.

4. Verbalizing concerns and feelings is important for coping.

5. Action regarding finances must be taken while the client still retains the capacity to make decisions.

Box 16-5 Sundowner's Syndrome

A phase of confusion and irritation may be seen in clients at the close of the day. It probably is due to general mental and physical tiredness, which interferes with the ability to process further information. It may be evidenced by increased confusion, irritation, and signs of anxiety.

ADDITIONAL TREATMENT MODALITIES

Interdisciplinary team

Pharmacological interventions

　　Drugs used to modify behavior and increase function

　　Drugs used in the therapy of Alzheimer's disease

Experimental biologic interventions

Therapeutic activity program

• those that aim at modifying behavior to enhance the client's functional level

• experimental and FDA-approved drugs used for therapy of Alzheimer's disease

Multiple drug administration can cause secondary dementia, and therefore drugs to combat symptoms such as anxiety are used singly and are given in a dosage to produce optimal functioning while eliminating adverse symptoms. Frequently the drug is administered in a high dose and then reduced to obtain the best functioning level for the client. This process of determining the optimal drug dose is termed *titration* and usually requires frequent observation by the physician, nurse, and/or family caregiver. Many drugs may have adverse side effects. Unless otherwise indicated, no drug should be stopped abruptly, since this may result in the client's confusion or disorientation.

Drugs Used to Modify Behavior and Increase Function

Antidepressants such as the tricyclics, monoamine oxidase inhibitors (MAOIs), and selective serotonin reuptake inhibitors (SSRIs), may be used for clients exhibiting persistent depressive symptoms. Of these, tricyclics such as amitriptyline (Elavil), amoxapine (Ascendin), doxepine (Adapin), and related drugs, e.g., desyrel (Trazodone), can produce severe side effects, particularly on the cholinergic system. The MAOIs have less of these effects but react with other drugs and certain foods. The more frequently used is phenelzine (Nardil). The SSRIs are rapidly becoming the most frequently prescribed antidepressant drugs and include fluoxetine (Prozac), paroxetine (Paxil), fluvoxamine (Fluvox), and sertraline (Zoloft).

Antianxiety medication or the sedative-hypnotics may relieve anxiety as well as treat insomnia. They are the benzodiazepines such as diazepam (Valium), chlordiazepoxide (Librium), triazolam (Halcion), and other mild tranquilizers. Buspirone HCl (BuSpar) is an antianxiety agent that is not chemically or pharmacologically related to benzodiazepines, barbiturates, or other sedative/anxiolytic drugs.

Antipsychotic drugs that are used to treat hallucinations and combative behavior may have severe anticholinergic effects. The most commonly used one is haloperidol (Haldol).

The drugs used to modify behavior and increase function are discussed in detail in Chapter 23.

Experimental Drugs in the Therapy of Alzheimer's Disease

Most of the experimental drugs presently undergoing trials have been developed based on the "cholinergic hypothesis." This now-outmoded theory assumed that Alzheimer's disease was caused by a depletion or lack of the neurotransmitter acetylcholine, and drugs were developed to prevent its depletion or loss. It is now known that loss of the neurons in the gray matter causes the depletion of acetylcholine and that this neuron loss cannot be reversed. However, such drugs as tetrahydroaminoacridine (THA, Tacrine, Cognex), based on the cholinergic hypothesis, may, in the early stages of the disease before neuronal damage is complete, act to modify some of the effects of an acetylcholine neurotransmitter depletion. Other experimental drugs of this type are physostigmine (Synapton), velnacrine (Mentane), and E2020. Several other drugs based on other theories are acetyl-1-carnitive, phosphatidylserine, and nimodipine.

Experimental Biological Interventions

The failure to develop, to date, an experimental animal model with all the features of Alzheimer's disease, has markedly retarded rapid advances in therapy. However, experimental techniques are being attempted in animals, such as the replacement of damaged neurons by cerebral injections of fetal cells, and cells genetically modified to secrete nerve growth factor, a compound that in experimental systems increases the activity of nerve cells (Gage, 1990). Application of these methods to human disease has not yet been attempted.

Therapeutic Activity Program

An activity is described as any project a person enjoys and that produces a positive feeling. A *therapeutic activity program* is a total plan of care, based on assessment of the client's needs and a history of previous endeavors. It is specifically designed to meet the identified needs and to keep the person functioning at the highest possible level (Stehman et al, 1991).

Building on retained strengths (e.g., retained remote memory, use of habitual skills, preserved large and fine motor skills, and intact emotional responses) is the basis of success. It is exceedingly difficult, if not impossible, for the person with Alzheimer's disease to learn new skills. "Use it or lose it!" is a truism, especially when working with clients with dementia. Once a skill is lost, it is virtually gone forever and not able to be learned.

For persons with dementia a therapeutic program is considered a primary treatment, since often the first neurological losses result in the inability to plan, initiate, carry out in ordered steps (sequence), or remember activities by themselves. It is therefore the role of the caregiver to assist the client throughout the activity, from beginning to end. Positive reinforcement should be used at each step of the way.

Success of a therapeutic activity program can be measured on some objective terms by addressing the following questions:

- Has the number of times per day or week that the client is actively involved increased or decreased?

- Have incidents of catastrophic reactions or Sundowner's syndrome decreased?

- Have incidents of the client aimlessly pacing or wandering and getting lost decreased?

- Has the level of functioning in ADL and IADL remained stable, or is it decreasing at a slower pace than before the program was initiated?

- Are caregivers feeling less stress, which might be indicated by fewer incidents of anger or crying, improved sleep patterns, or enhanced feelings of physical and mental well-being?

Summary of Key Concepts

1. Only 20% of clients over the age of 65 who suffer from a cognitive disorder are thought to have a reversible, treatable disease. Most cognitive disorders are thought to be incurable, irreversible, and ultimately fatal, although this process may last as long as 20 years.

2. Alzheimer's disease is the most prevalent cognitive disorder.

3. The five current theories regarding the cause of Alzheimer's disease state that it is the result of infectious agents, neurotoxic agents, angiopathy and blood-brain incompetency, neurotransmitter and receptor deficiencies, and abnormal proteins and their products.

4. Regardless of the biologic cause, the effect of these diseases is altered neurochemistry or neurophysiology that disrupts metabolism in the brain.

5. The pathological process of cognitive disorders results in neurological deficits, such as reduced ability to perceive the environment and organize appropriate responses, decreased attention span, language

■ ■ ■ ■ ■ ■ EVALUATION

Evaluating the client's progress and the degree to which nurses have achieved satisfactory client and caregiver outcomes is especially challenging when Alzheimer's disease and other dementias are involved. Factors that may influence success vary greatly with each situation and must be carefully considered in this process. Below are some questions that need to be clearly answered and understood before specific topics are addressed.

- Is the dementia reversible or irreversible?

- What is the setting, i.e., acute care or long-term care?

- What is the caregiving situation?

- What other medical/psychiatric problems need to be addressed?

- What is the current drug profile and degree of compliance?

- What are the resulting behavior problems to be addressed?

- What is the highest functional level that can be achieved?

- Have the medical and nursing diagnoses been made using all available resources of the interdisciplinary team?

When the answers to the above questions have been agreed upon, then the nurse, in conjunction with other health and social service professionals, will be better able to focus the degree to which specifics in the Client/Family Outcomes have been realized.

deficits, memory loss, changes in emotional responses, and a decline in the ability to reason and form judgments.

6. Alzheimer's disease is considered to have three stages: mild, moderate, and severe.

7. A variety of cognitive assessment tools can be used to determine medical and nursing diagnoses.

8. The nurse should plan and supervise therapeutic activity programs to achieve the highest possible functional status for the client and prevent excess disability.

9. Caring for a person with a cognitive disorder is a significant physical and emotional burden for the caregivers.

10. All nursing care for clients with cognitive disorders should be done in collaboration with the client's caregivers.

11. Care plans should be formulated that are based on assessment of both the client's needs and the caregiver's needs.

12. The success of care plans should be based on successful functional status and not on a curative basis.

REFERENCES

AD Center, University of Kentucky: *Caring for the cognitively impaired patient,* Silver Springs, Ky., 1990, ADEAR.

Alzheimer A: Über eine eigenartige Erkrankung der Kirnrinde, *Allgemeine Zeitschrift für Psychiatrie* 64:146–148, 1907.

Bowen DM, Francis PT, Palmer AM: The biochemistry of cortical and subcortical neurons in Alzheimer's disease. In Glenner GG, Wurtman RJ, editors: *Advancing frontiers in Alzheimer's disease research,* Austin, Tex, 1987, University of Texas Press.

Corder EH et al: Gene dose of apolipoprotein E type e4 allele and the risk of Alzheimer's disease in late-onset families, *Science* 261:921–923, 1993.

Engels GL: Grief and grieving, *Amer J Nurs,* 64:93–98, 1964.

Gage FH et al: Gene therapy in the CNS: intracerebral grafting of genetically modified cells, *Prog Brain Res* 86:205–217, 1990.

Glenner, GG: Alzheimer's disease, *Encyclopedia of Human Biology* 1:108–111, 1994.

Glenner GG: Alzheimer's disease: multiple cerebral amyloidosis, *Banbury Report 15: Biological Aspects of Alzheimer's Disease,* Cold Spring Harbor Symposium, 137–144, 1983.

Glenner GG: Amyloid deposits and amyloidosis (medical progress), *N Eng J Med* 302:1333–1343, 1980.

Glenner GG: Amyloid deposits and amyloidosis: the β-fibrilloses (Medical Progress Report), *N Engl J Med* 302:1283–1292, 1333–1343, 1980.

Glenner GG et al: The creation of "amyloid" fibrils from Bence Jones proteins *in vitro,* *Science* 174:712–714, 1971.

Glenner GG, Wong CW: Alzheimer's disease and Down's syndrome: sharing of a unique cerebrovascular amyloid fibril protein, *Biochem Biophys Res Commun* 122:1131–1135, 1984.

Glenner GG, Wong CW: Alzheimer's disease: initial report of the purification and characterization of a novel cerebrovascular amyloid protein, *Biochem Biophys Res Commun* 120:885–890, 1984.

Goate A et al: Segregation of a missense mutation in the amyloid precursor protein gene with familial Alzheimer's disease, *Nature* 349:704–706, 1991.

Holt J: How to help confused patients, *Am J Nurs* 93:32–36, 1993.

Ikeda S et al: Gerstmann-Sträussler-Scheinker disease showing β-protein amyloid deposits in the peripheral regions of PrP-Immunoreactive amyloid plaques, *Neurodegeneration* 1:281–288, 1992.

Jervis GA: Early senile dementia in mongoloid idiocy, *Am J Psychiatry* 105:102–106, 1948.

Kidd M: Paired helical filaments in electron microscopy of Alzheimer's disease, *Nature* 197:192–194, 1963.

Kraepelin E: *Klinische Psychiatric in Psychiatrie,* ed 8, 2(1), Leipzig, 1910, Barth.

Kübler-Ross E: *On death and dying,* New York, 1969, Macmillan.

Lyness JM: Delirium: Masquerades and misdiagnosis in elderly patients, *Journal of the American Geriatrics Society* 38(11):1235–1238, 1990.

Moore K: Stroke: the long road back, *RN,* 3:50–54, 1994.

Perl DP, Brody AR: Alzheimer's disease: x-ray spectrometric evidence of aluminum accumulation in neurofibrillary tangle-bearing neurons, *Science* 208:297–299, 1980.

Prelli F et al: Differences between vascular and plaque core amyloid in Alzheimer's disease, *J Neurochem* 51:648–651, 1988.

Prusiner SB: Molecular biology of prion diseases, *Science* 252:1515, 1991.

Prusiner SB: Some speculations about prions, amyloid, and Alzheimer's disease, *N Engl J Med* 310:661–663, 1984.

Ramsdell JW: Geriatric assessment in the home, *Geriatric Home Care* 7(4):677–693, 1991.

Rockwell E: *Behavior problems in Alzheimer's disease* (accompanies the video "Speaking for Them"), Silver Springs, Md., 1991, Alzheimer's Disease Education and Referral Center (ADEAR).

Scheibel AB et al: Denervation microangiopathy in senile dementia, Alzheimer type, *Alzheimer Dis Assoc Disord* 1:19–37, 1987.

Stehman J et al: *Training Manual for Alzheimer's Care Specialists,* Manuscript submitted for publication, 1991.

Task Force on DSM-IV, American Psychiatric Association: *DSM-IV Criteria,* Washington, D.C., 1994, American Psychiatric Association.

Thomas M, Isaac M: Alois Alzheimer: a memoir, *Top Neurol Sci* 10:306–307, 1987.

Tomlinson BE et al: Observations on the brains of demented old people, *J Neurol Sci* 11:205–242, 1972.

Torack RM: *The pathologic physiology of dementia,* Berlin-Heidelberg, 1978, Springer-Verlag.

van Duinen SG et al: Hereditary cerebral hemorrhage with amyloidosis of Dutch origin is related to Alzheimer's disease, *Proc Nat Acad Sci U S A* 84:5991, 1987.

Whitehouse PJ: Neurotransmitter receptor alterations in Alzheimer disease: a review, *Alzheimer Dis Assoc Disord* 1:9–18, 1987.

Wong CW et al: Neuritic plaques and cerebrovascular amyloid in Alzheimer's Disease are antigenically related, *Proc Nat Acad Sci USA* 82:8729–8732, 1985.

Woods P, Ashley J: Simulated presence therapy: using selected memories to manage problem behaviors in Alzheimer's disease patients, *Geriatr Nurs* 16:9–14, 1995.

Zgola J: *Doing things: a guide to programming activities for persons with Alzheimer's disease and related disorders,* Baltimore, 1987, The Johns Hopkins University Press.

CHAPTER 17

Disorders of Childhood and Adolescence

Vincent R. Pieranunzi
Richard Lucas

Acting out The expression of internal affective states through external activities and behaviors that are often destructive and/or maladaptive.

Autism A pervasive developmental disorder characterized by marked impairment of social and cognitive abilities.

Encopresis The repeated involuntary or intentional passage of feces into inappropriate places.

Enuresis Repeated involuntary or intentional voiding of urine into bed or clothes.

Pervasive developmental disorders A collection of disorders in which the child experiences deficits in a broad range of developmental areas.

Therapeutic play Age-appropriate play activities used purposefully by the nurse for assessment, intervention, and promotion of normal growth and development in children.

Tic A sudden, rapid, recurrent, nonrhythmic, stereotyped movement or vocalization considered irresistible but often suppressible for short periods of time.

- Distinguish between developmental disorders, attention-deficit disorders, and mental retardation.

- Distinguish between conduct disorder, oppositional defiant disorder, and the effects of abuse and depression.

- Examine the behavioral characteristics of the major childhood and adolescent mental disorders.

- Understand the implications of child and adolescent disorders on later functioning and the development of adult mental disorders.

- Apply the nursing process in a developmentally appropriate manner with children and adolescents.

T he nurse encounters children and adolescents in a wide variety of health care settings. Often, these encounters will initially be for other health problems. The astute nurse, however, will be alert to the possible presence of mental health problems. Depression, for example, can often present as vague somatic complaints.

In addition, children and adolescents are members of families. As nurses work with adults with mental health problems, they must be aware of the often concurrent mental health needs of their children. Stress and the presence of major mental disorders in adults can often predispose their children for abuse and neglect. It is important for the nurse to understand the mental health issues facing children and adolescents. This chapter will familiarize the reader with the major mental disorders affecting children and adolescents and offer direction for applying the nursing process to this population.

HISTORICAL AND THEORETICAL PERSPECTIVES

History tells a story of a lack of concern for and little attention paid to understanding or treating children. Despert documented indifference and even cruelty to children through time. DeMause found that the further back one goes, the lower the level of child care and the less effective parenting were present. Children tended to be seen as miniature adults with no understanding of development.

Around the turn of the century, children and adolescents began to have more individual attention. Laws established separate Juvenile Courts in 1889. In the early 1900s, William Healy started the Juvenile Psychopathic Institute in Chicago. Ernest Southard became the director of an outpatient clinic specifically for children in Boston (Hirschberg, 1980).

Historically, psychopathology in childhood and adolescence resulted from multiple biopsychosocial factors. The rapid rate of development in childhood and adolescence distinguishes these periods from adulthood. Two theories broadly classify development: reactive and structural.

Reactive theories maintain that the child's mind starts as a blank slate, and environmental influences promote healthy or pathological development. The major reactive theories include stimulus-response, learning, classical conditioning, and operant conditioning. These theories imply that symptoms are learned behavior, and improvement comes through relearning and environmental change.

Structural theories start with the belief that the child has a genetically determined ability for developing behavior and acts on the environment. Major structural theorists include Bowlby, (attachment), Freud (psychosexual developmental lines), Erickson (psychosocial development), and Piaget (cognitive development). Treatment under a structural theory involves a reorganization within the child or adolescent (e.g., resolution of intrapsychic conflicts, alternation of family patterns of interaction, or acquiring a new schema) (Lewis, 1980).

MENTAL RETARDATION
Etiology and Epidemiology

Despite extensive evaluations, no clear etiology can be found in 30%–40% of individuals with mental retardation. When found, etiology may be primarily biologic or primarily psychosocial, or a combination of the two. Major factors include the following:

- Heredity accounts for approximately 5% and includes the following examples: Tay-Sachs disease, tuberous sclerosis, Down's syndrome, and fragile X syndrome.

- Early problems in embryonic development account for approximately 30% and include chromosomal changes such as trisomy 21 or prenatal exposure to toxins (for example, maternal alcohol consumption, infections).

- Pregnancy and perinatal problems make up about 10% and include fetal malnutrition, prematurity, hypoxia, viral and other infections, and trauma.

- General medical conditions acquired during infancy or childhood contribute to approximately 5% and include infections, traumas, and poisoning (for example, lead).

- Environmental influences and other mental disorders contribute to about 15%–20%. Factors include deprivation of nurturance and social, linguistic, and other stimulation, and severe mental disorders (for example, autistic disorder) (APA, 1994).

Although studies vary, the prevalence of mental retardation is estimated at 1% (APA, 1994).

Clinical Description and Prognosis
GENERAL

Individuals typically present with problems in adaptive functioning defined as "how effectively individuals cope with common life demands and how well they meet the standards of personal independence expected of someone in their particular age group, sociocultural background, and community setting." Several factors may influence adaptive functioning: education, motivation, personality characteristics, social and vocational opportunities, and other coexisting mental and physical conditions (APA, 1994).

SUBTYPES

Mild mental retardation constitutes 85% of individuals with mental retardation. These children typically develop social and communication skills during the preschool years, suffer only minimal sensorimotor problems, and often do not get identified until a later age. They can generally acquire academic skills up to approximately the sixth-grade level. In adulthood they generally achieve social and vocational skills adequate for minimum self-support. They usually require supervision, guidance, and assistance. But, in most cases, they live successfully in the community—some independently, some in supervised settings.

DSM-IV CRITERIA

Mental Retardation

A. Significant subaverage intellectual functioning: an IQ of approximately 70 or below on an individual administered IQ test (severity determined as follows: mild-IQ 50–55 to approximately 70; moderate-IQ 35–40 to 50–55; severe-IQ 20–25 to 50–55; profound-IQ below 20–25).

B. Concurrent deficits or impairments in present adaptive function (i.e., the person's effectiveness in meeting the standards expected for his or her age by his or her cultural group) in at least two of the following areas: communication, self-care, home living, social/interpersonal skills, use of community resources, self-direction, functional academic skills, work, leisure, health, and safety.

C. Onset before age 18.

Reprinted with permission from *Diagnostic and statistical manual of mental disorders,* ed 4, Washington, D.C., 1994, American Psychiatric Association.

Moderate mental retardation makes up about 10% of the entire population with mental retardation. Most individuals with mental retardation acquire some communication skills during early childhood and may benefit from vocational training, but they seldom advance academically beyond the second-grade level. With moderate supervision, they can usually provide for their own personal care and learn to travel in familiar areas. Peer relationships often deteriorate in adolescence because of problems in recognizing socially correct interactions. During adulthood they generally can perform unskilled or semiskilled work and live in the community in supervised setting.

Severe retardation constitutes 3%–4% of individuals with mental retardation. They typically acquire little if any communicative speech during early childhood but may learn to talk and develop elementary self-care skills in the school-age period. They may profit from learning to sight read some "survival" words. As adults they may be able to perform simple skills in tightly supervised settings. They can generally live in the community in group homes or with their families unless some other handicap requires specialized nursing or other care.

Only 1%–2% of mentally retarded individuals suffer from profound retardation. Most also have an identified neurological condition causing their retardation. They have considerable sensorimotor problems recognized in early childhood and require a highly structured setting with constant monitoring and aid in an individualized relationship for optimal development. Under this sort of care, they may develop enough motor skills, self-care skills, and communication to perform simple tasks in a closely supervised and sheltered setting (APA, 1994).

ASSOCIATED FEATURES

Individuals with mental retardation demonstrate no consistent or specific personality or behavioral features. Individual traits range from passive, placid, and dependent styles to aggressive and impulsive styles. Individuals with more severe retardation and associated communication deficits demonstrate more aggression and impulsivity due to frustration and lack of ability to interact with their environment adequately. Some medical conditions that cause mental retardation have specific problems associated with them, such as the self-injurious behavior found in Lesch-Nyhan syndrome. Individuals with mental retardation frequently suffer further because of their vulnerability to exploitation. They may have rights and opportunities denied or suffer outright physical or sexual abuse.

Individuals with mental retardation have a comorbid mental disorder an estimated three to four times more often than the general population. Any mental disorder may present in retarded individuals, and no evidence indicates any difference in the nature of the mental disorder. However, problems occur frequently in diagnosing mental disorders due to communication skills deficits and other handicaps. The most commonly diagnosed

mental disorders include attention-deficit/hyperactivity disorder, mood disorder, pervasive developmental disorder, stereotypic movement disorder, and mental disorders due to a general medical condition (for example, dementia due to head trauma) (APA, 1994).

PERVASIVE DEVELOPMENTAL DISORDER: AUTISTIC DISORDER

Pervasive developmental disorders are a collection of disorders in which the child experiences deficits in a broad range of developmental areas. **Autism,** characterized by marked impairment of social and cognitive abilities, is the most common of these disorders.

Epidemiology

Studies suggest the rate of autistic disorder is 2–5 cases per 10,000. Rates are four to five times higher in males than in females. Females, however, tend to have more severe mental retardation. Siblings of individuals with the disorder have an increased risk of developing autistic disorder (APA, 1994).

Clinical Description
BEHAVIORAL MANIFESTATIONS

A variety of behavioral symptoms may present including any of the following: hyperactivity, short attention span, impulsivity, aggressiveness, self-injurious behaviors, and temper tantrums. Abnormalities of eating (for example, limiting intake to a few foods or eating nonnutritious objects) or sleeping (for example, recurrent awakenings with rocking) may be found. Individuals often have restricted, repetitive, and stereotyped patterns of behavior, interest, and activity. They become preoccupied in a way that is abnormal, either in intensity or focus, with an inflexible adherence to specific, nonfunctional routines or rituals; or they use stereotypical and repetitive mannerisms or become persistently preoccupied with parts of objects.

They may demonstrate an obsessive need to maintain sameness and orderliness by insisting on lining up objects over and over again. They may be unable to tolerate even minor changes in the environment and have a catastrophic reaction to minor changes such as a new chair or seating arrangement at dinner. They may demand maintaining nonfunctional and unreasonable adherence to rituals and routines.

They often demonstrate stereotypic motor activities (for example, clapping hands, spinning, rocking, swaying) and posture (for example, walking on tiptoes, odd postures, or strange hand movements). Play cannot be disrupted from preoccupation with objects such as buttons. They frequently show a fascination with movement of such things as fans, revolving objects, or the opening and closing of doors or drawers. They may become highly attached to some unusually inanimate object such

DSM-IV CRITERIA

Autistic Disorder

A. A total of six (or more) items from the following three areas:

(1) qualitative impairment in social interaction, as manifested by at least two of the following:

(a) marked impairment in the use of multiple nonverbal behaviors such as eye-to-eye gaze, facial expression, body postures, and gestures to regulate social interaction.

(b) failure to develop peer relationships appropriate to developmental level.

(c) a lack of spontaneous seeking to share enjoyment, interests, or achievements with other people (e.g., by a lack of showing, bringing, or pointing out objects of interests)

(d) lack of social or emotional reciprocity.

(2) qualitative impairments in communication as manifested by at least one of the following:

(a) delay in, or total lack of, the development of spoken language (not accompanied by an attempt to compensate through alternative modes of communication such as gesture or mime).

(b) in individuals with adequate speech, marked impairment in the ability to initiate or sustain a conversation with others.

(c) stereotyped and repetitive use of language or idiosyncratic language.

(d) lack of varied, spontaneous make-believe play or social imitative play appropriate to developmental level.

(3) Restricted repetitive and stereotyped patterns of behavior, interests, and activities, as manifested by at least one of the following:

(a) encompassing preoccupation with one or more stereotyped and restricted patterns of interest that is abnormal either in intensity or focus.

(b) apparently inflexible adherence to specific, nonfunctional routines or rituals.

(c) stereotyped and repetitive motor mannerisms (e.g., hand or finger flapping or twisting, or complex whole-body movements).

(d) persistent preoccupation with parts of objects.

B. Delays or abnormal functioning in at least one of the following areas with onset before 3 years: (1) social interaction, (2) language as used in social communication, (3) symbolic or imaginative play.

C. The disturbance not better accounted for by Rett's Disorder or Childhood Disintegrative Disorder

Reprinted with permission from *Diagnostic and statistical manual of mental disorders*, ed 4, Washington, D.C., 1994, American Psychiatric Association.

---

as a piece of string or rubber band and ignore typical items like a blanket or teddy bear.

EMOTIONAL MANIFESTATIONS

Individuals with autistic disorder typically lack emotional reciprocity (for example, not actively participating in simple social play or games, instead preferring solitary activities or only attempting to involve others as tools or "mechanical" aids). Mood or affect abnormalities such as giggling or weeping for no apparent reason or no emotional reaction when a reaction is expected can be present. There may be inappropriate reaction to danger, with no fear exhibited to real danger or excessive fear exhibited to harmless objects. Self-injurious behavior can include head banging or biting of various body parts. If sufficient cognitive ability develops during development, depression may appear secondarily to a realization of these individuals' serious impairment.

COGNITIVE MANIFESTATIONS

Approximately 75% of individuals with autistic disorder have some degree of mental retardation, most commonly in the moderate range (IQ 35–50). Other cognitive skills may also be impaired. Communication problems usually present so severely in both verbal and nonverbal areas that spoken language may be absent. Individuals who do speak may not be able to begin or sustain a conversation with others, or they use such stereotyped and repetitive or idiosyncratic language that others find it difficult to continue a conversation with them. Speech may often contain abnormalities of pitch, intonation, rate, and rhythm (for example, monotonous or inappropriate sing-song pitch and rhythm or questionlike raises of tone at the end of declarative sentences). Grammar is often immature, stereotyped, and repetitive (for example, inappropriate repetition of jingles or commercials, regardless of meaning) or metaphorical (for example, the grammar can only be understood by those familiar with the individual's idiosyncratic use of language). Individuals may not be able to understand simple questions, directions, or jokes. Other children may develop excellent long-term memory of insignificant items such as train schedules, baseball statistics, or songs.

PERCEPTUAL MANIFESTATIONS

Individuals may respond oddly to sensory stimuli (for example, they have a high pain threshold, oversensitivity to sound or touch, exaggerated response to light or color, or a fascination with a particular sensory stimulation).

SOCIAL MANIFESTATIONS

Autistic disorder presentation depends on the developmental level and chronological age, but autism at any age represents an extremely severe and disabling disorder. Markedly abnormal or impaired development in social interaction and communication and markedly restricted range of activity and interests severely impair the individual's ability to function in society without a significant amount of active intervention and treatment.

Social interaction problems are major and sustained. Individuals typically cannot recognize and use nonverbal social clues and behaviors to regular social interaction and communication. Peer relationships produce varied difficulties, depending on developmental level. Young individuals may have little or no interest in friendship, while older individuals may have an interest but experience serious problems understanding and dealing with expected and accepted social conventions. They often lack the ability to demonstrate spontaneous efforts to seek shared enjoyments in interests or achievements (for example, they may not show or discuss with others the things or ideas they find interesting). Individuals with autistic disorder often appear oblivious to others, have no concept of their needs, and do not notice their distress or joy.

They often lack the developmental skill to use a varied, spontaneous, make-believe play activity or to use social imitation appropriate to their age. Play becomes mechanical, out of context with others, and lacks the imagination generally expected.

The nature of impairments in social interaction may change over time, depending on developmental levels. Infants may refuse to cuddle, may show an indifference or aversion for affection or physical contact, may fail to demonstrate eye contact or facial responsiveness, or may not smile socially or respond to parents' voices. Young children may treat adults as interchangeable or cling mechanically to one specific person. Even if the child becomes willing to engage in social interactions, the interactions demonstrate unusual behavior (for example, expecting others to answer ritualized questions in specific ways, showing little sense of personal space boundaries, and being inappropriate in social interactions) (APA, 1994).

Prognosis

Language skills and overall intellectual level are the strongest factors related to ultimate prognosis. Available studies that have followed the course of this disorder suggest that only a small percentage of individuals with

the disorder go on to live and work independently as adults. In about on-third of cases, some degree of partial independence is possible. The highest functioning adults with autistic disorder typically continue to exhibit problems in social interaction and communication together with restricted interests and activities.

OTHER PERVASIVE DEVELOPMENTAL DISORDERS

Rett's Disorder

The essential feature of Rett's disorder is development of multiple specific deficits following normal prenatal and perinatal periods and apparent normal development for the first five months of life. Between 5–48 months, head growth decelerates with a loss of prior purposeful hand skills and subsequent characteristic stereotyped hand movements resembling hand-wringing or hand washing. Interest diminishes in social activities, and problems in coordination of gait and trunk movement develop. An associated impairment in language develops with severe psychomotor retardation. Rett's disorder appears much less frequently than autistic disorder and has been seen only in females. The duration of the disorder is lifelong, and the loss of skills is generally persistent and progressive. Recovery is usually limited. Communication and behavioral difficulties usually remain constant throughout life (APA, 1994).

Childhood Disintegrative Disorder

This very rare disorder, apparently slightly more common in males, is distinguished by a marked regression in multiple areas of functioning following at least two years of apparently normal development. Before ten years of age, clinically significant loss of previously acquired skills appears in at least two of the following areas: expressive or receptive language, social skills or adaptive behavior, bowel or bladder control, play, or motor skills. Individuals show social, communicative, and behavioral problems generally seen in autistic disorder. Qualitative problems in social and communicative skills and restricted, repetitive, and stereotyped patterns of behavior, interests, and interests develop. Usually the loss of skills reaches a plateau with limited improvement, but in some instances loss of skills is progressive. The disorder follows a continuous course and usually duration is lifelong (APA, 1994).

Asperger's Disorder

This disorder contains many similar features of autistic disorder: severe and sustained impairment in social interaction, and restricted, repetitive patterns of behavior, interests, and activities that produce significant impairment in social, occupational, or other important areas of functioning. However, in contrast to autistic disorder, no

DSM-IV CRITERIA

Attention-Deficit/Hyperactivity Disorder

A. Either (1) or (2):

(1) Six or more of the following symptoms of inattention have persisted for at least six months to a degree that is maladaptive and inconsistent with developmental level:

Inattention

(a) often fails to give close attention to details or makes careless mistakes in schoolwork, work, or other activities.

(b) often has difficulty sustaining attention in tasks or play activities.

(c) often does not seem to listen when spoken to directly.

(d) often does not follow through on instructions and fails to finish schoolwork, chores, or duties in the workplace (not due to opposition behavior or failure to understand instructions).

(e) often has difficulty organizing tasks and activities.

(f) often avoids, dislikes, or is reluctant to engage in tasks that require sustained mental effort (such as schoolwork or homework).

(g) often loses things necessary for tasks or activities (e.g., toys, school assignments, pencils, books, or tools).

(h) is often easily distracted by extraneous stimuli.

(i) is often forgetful in daily activities.

(2) Six or more of the following symptoms of hyperactivity-impulsivity have persisted for at least six months to a degree that is maladaptive and inconsistent with developmental level:

Hyperactivity

(a) often fidgets with hands or feet or squirms in seat.

(b) often leaves seat in classroom or in other situations in which remaining seated is expected.

(c) often runs about or climbs excessively in situations in which it is inappropriate (in adolescents or adults, may be limited to subjective feelings or restlessness).

(d) often has difficulty playing or engaging in leisure activities quietly.

(e) is often "on the go" or often acts as if "driven by a motor."

(f) often talks excessively.

Impulsivity

(g) often blurts out answers before questions have been completed.

(h) often has difficulty awaiting turn.

(i) often interrupts or intrudes on others (e.g., butts into conversations or games).

B. Some hyperactive-impulsive or inattentive symptoms that caused impairment were present before age 7 years.

C. Some impairment from the symptoms is present in two or more settings (e.g., at school [or work] and at home).

D. There must be clear evidence of clinically significant impairment in social, academic, or occupational functioning.

E. The symptoms do not occur exclusively during the course of a pervasive developmental disorder, schizophrenia, or other psychotic disorder and are not better accounted for by another mental disorder (e.g., mood disorder, anxiety disorder, dissociative disorder, or personality disorder).

Reprinted with permission from *Diagnostic and statistical manual of mental disorders*, ed 4, Washington, D.C., 1994, American Psychiatric Association.

---

clinically significant delays in language, cognitive development, age-appropriate self-help skills, adaptive behavior, or curiosity about the environment occur (APA, 1994). This disorder follows a continuous course, and usually duration is lifelong.

ATTENTION-DEFICIT/HYPERACTIVITY DISORDER

Epidemiology

Attention-deficit/hyperactivity disorder (ADHD) has been reported in various cultures. Western countries report variations in prevalence that likely arise from varying diagnostic practices rather than from differences in actual clinical presentation. DSM-IV reports the prevalence at an estimated 3%–5% of all school-age children. Data appear too limited to estimate the rate in adolescents and adults. Males receive the diagnosis more frequently with the range varying from 4:1 to 9:1, depending on whether the diagnosis is made in the general population or in clinic settings. Family members of individuals with ADHD have a higher rate of mood and anxiety disorders, learning disorders, substance-related disorders, and antisocial personality disorder. By the time these individuals reach treatment, they often also meet the criteria for a diagnosis of oppositional defiant disorder or conduct disorder. A higher prevalence also exists for the following disorders: mood disorders, anxiety disorders, learning disorders, and communication disorders. ADHD often coexists with and typically precedes Tourette's disorder (APA, 1994).

Etiology

Although not necessarily a cause, the following histories have been noted when the diagnosis has been made: child abuse or neglect, multiple foster placements, neurotoxin exposure (for example, lead poisoning), infections (for example, encephalitis), drug exposure in utero, low birth weight, and mental retardation. ADHD also has been found more often in the first-degree relatives of children with ADHD (APA, 1994).

Clinical Description
BEHAVIORAL MANIFESTATIONS

Behavioral manifestations typically occur in several places and must take place in at least two settings in order to make the diagnosis. The level of problems typically varies from time to time in the same or different settings. Symptoms generally worsen in situations that require sustained attention and lack appeal or variety to the child or adolescent, such as listening to teachers, performing monotonous tasks, or reading lengthy materials. Symptoms may actually disappear or become minimal when under strict control, such as during a diagnostic interview or when receiving frequent rewards for appropriate behavior. Symptoms tend to worsen in unstructured, group situations such as the typical classroom and playground.

Hyperactivity presents in many forms: fidgeting or squirming in one's seat, getting up when expected to remain seated, excessive running or climbing when dangerous or inappropriate, or loud and disruptive play during quiet activities, demonstrating a driven verbal or motor quality. Even though toddlers developmentally present with a lot of activity and inquisitiveness, toddlers with ADHD present different qualitatively; they are always on the go, darting back and forth, unable to remain still for completion of simple tasks such as putting on a coat or listening to a simple story, or running, jumping, and climbing on furniture.

School-age children may settle down somewhat but still display excessive overactivity; they demonstrate difficulty remaining seated by hanging onto the edge of their seats, squirming as if the need to shed their skin, playing with objects, or tapping their hands and feet. At home they frequently do not finish meals or even finish watching a television show. They make excessive noise, interrupting others during quiet times and talking constantly, such as giving a running commentary on a televi-

sion show. Adolescents often can express a subjective feeling of restlessness and report a preference to engage in active rather than sedentary activities.

Impulsivity manifests itself in the following ways: impatience, failing to delay responses, blurting out answers before the question has been finished, difficulty waiting for one's turn or problems waiting in line without pushing and shoving, and frequently interrupting others to the point of social, academic, or occupational problems. In addition, they may also make comments out of turn; fail to listen to directions; initiate inappropriate contact with others by interrupting conversations; grab others by their clothing, limbs, or belongings; touch things that are off limits to them; and clown around at times of expected quiet. Accidents may result by knocking over objects, running into people, grabbing dangerous objects such as a hot pan, or taking dangerous risks without consideration of the consequences, such as riding a bicycle at night without reflective lights. They often exhibit temper outbursts, bossiness, stubbornness, and excessive and frequent insistence that their requests be met.

EMOTIONAL MANIFESTATIONS

Individuals with this disorder may develop a number of other problems as a result of the underlying attention and hyperactive-impulsive problems, including any of the following: low frustration tolerance, mood lability, demoralization, dysphoria, and poor self-esteem.

COGNITIVE MANIFESTATIONS

Inattention can take place in one or several settings. Schoolwork or other activities may contain careless errors showing lack of close attention to details. Work may be messy, with evidence of not thinking through the project or schoolwork, or of not persisting to adequate completion. Often it appears the child is daydreaming and not listening to what is being said or asked. Shifts may occur from one unfinished task to another, with a growing clutter surrounding the child's path. Although chores or schoolwork often do not get completed, care must be taken in attributing this symptom to ADHD, because other problems such as oppositional behavior often occur and would be considered a normal developmental task during early childhood. These individuals often have problems with organization skills, find tasks that require sustained mental effort unpleasant, and become aversive to such tasks (especially homework). Materials needed for such tasks typically become scattered, lost, or carelessly handled and damaged. Trivial stimuli such as household noises often distract these individuals, who then leave their assigned task to attend to the interrupting stimuli. They often forget and miss appointments, fail to meet schoolwork deadlines, or forget lunch money. As a result, academic achievement is often impaired.

PERCEPTUAL MANIFESTATIONS

Perceptual problems are not usually a problem in ADHD.

Understanding and Applying
RESEARCH

Kelly SJ: Child maltreatment, stressful life events, and behavior problems in school-aged children in residential treatment. *Journal of Child and Adolescent Psychiatric Nursing* 5:2, 1992.

This study examined children in residential treatment to determine the prevalence of maltreatment, stressful life events, and behavior problems. A sample of 44 children, ages 5–13, were included: 61% male and 39% female. At the time of the study, the mean time in residential treatment was 8.6 months.

The Child Behavior Checklist was used to determine social competence and behavior problems in the subjects. A modified use of the Coddington Life Events Record was used to examine stressful life events. The child's social worker was used to determine the presence of maltreatment in the child's history.

The study hypothesis was supported. Every child in the study has experienced at least one episode of maltreatment, mainly physical and emotional abuse, and seeing his or her mother abused. Over 55% percent of the subjects' parents abused drugs or alcohol. Stressful life events were noted in the majority of the subjects and included separation from their mother, death of a sibling, foster care, and serious illness of a parent.

The study has important ramifications for nursing care. Children who experience major life traumas and stress are much more likely to go on to develop long-term mental illness. Seeing and experiencing abuse and neglect predispose them to becoming abusers themselves. Nurses working with children need to be aware of the impact of these factors on a child's current and long-term mental health.

SOCIAL MANIFESTATIONS

Social problems may occur due to losing the train of conversation and changing topics inappropriately, not following expected rules of games or activities, and appearing uninterested in others. Family members frequently develop resentment and antagonism, particularly when the variability of symptoms leads parents to believe that their children's troublesome behavior is willful. ADHD can cause rejection by peers, and conflict with family and school authorities. Others often interpret inadequate self-application as laziness, irresponsibility, and oppositional behavior (APA, 1994).

Prognosis

In most cases, the disorder is relatively stable through early adolescence. In most persons, symptoms are reduced in late adolescence and adulthood, although a few experience the full range of symptoms into mid-adulthood. Other adults retain only some of the symptoms.

CONDUCT DISORDER
Etiology

The following factors have been identified as predisposing to conduct disorder: parental rejection and neglect, difficult infant temperament, inconsistent child-rearing practices with harsh discipline, physical or sexual abuse, lack of supervision, early institutional living, frequent changes of caregivers, large family size, association with a delinquent peer group, and certain family psychopathology. See Understanding and Applying Research above. Conduct disorder occurs more frequently when a

biological or adoptive parent has antisocial personality disorder; a biological parent has alcohol dependence, a mood disorder, schizophrenia, or a history of ADHD or conduct disorder; or a sibling has conduct disorder (APA, 1994).

Rogeness reviewed biological issues in conduct disorder. Findings indicate that clients with decreased noradrenergic activity and conduct disorder respond poorly to signs of impending punishment and therefore tend to have trouble internalizing societal rules. Studies tend to show that serotonin inhibits aggression, which leads to theories that low serotonin plays a role in aggressive **acting-out** behaviors (the expression of internal affective states through external activities and behaviors that are often destructive and/or maladaptive). The source of these neurotransmitter changes remains unclear, although some studies support psychosocial stress, such as parental neglect, as well as genetic factors (Rogeness, 1994).

Epidemiology

According to DSM-IV, rates appear higher in urban than in rural settings and vary depending on the nature of the population sampled and methods of ascertainment used; for males under 18, rates vary from 6%–16%; for females, rates vary from 2%–9% (APA, 1994). Bauermeister reports that a pattern of conduct disorder is highest in 13- to 16-year-olds with a sharp decline thereafter. In boys the prevalence reached a high point from 10–13 years of age with a gradual decline from ages 10–20. In girls a gradual increase occurs in late childhood and early adolescence, peaking at age 16 followed by a sharp decline (Bauermeister, 1994).

DSM-IV CRITERIA

Conduct Disorder

A. A repetitive and persistent pattern of behavior in which the basic rights of others or major age-appropriate norms or rules are violated, as manifested by the presence of three or more of the following criteria in the past 12 months, with at least one criterion present in the past 6 months:

Aggression to people or animals

(1) often bullies, threatens, or intimidates others

(2) often initiates physical fights

(3) has used a weapon that can cause serious physical harm to others (e.g., a bat, brick, broken bottle, knife, gun)

(4) has been physically cruel to people

(5) has been physically cruel to animals

(6) has stolen while confronting a victim (e.g., mugging, purse snatching, extortion, armed robbery)

(7) has forced someone into sexual activity

Destruction of property

(8) has deliberately engaged in fire-setting with the intention of causing serious damage

(9) has deliberately destroyed others' property (other than by fire-setting)

Deceitfulness or theft

(10) has broken into someone else's house, building, or car

(11) often lies to obtain goods or favors or to avoid obligations (i.e., "cons" others)

(12) has stolen items of nontrivial value without confronting a victim (e.g., shoplifting, but without breaking and entering; forgery)

Serious violations of rules

(13) often stays out at night despite parental prohibitions, beginning before age 13 years

(14) has run away from home overnight at least twice while living in parental or parental surrogate home (or once without returning for a lengthy period)

(15) is often truant from school, beginning before age 13 years

B. The disturbance in behavior causes clinically significant impairment in social, academic, or occupational functioning.

C. If the individual is age 18 years or older, criteria are not met for antisocial personality disorder (APA, 1994).

Reprinted with permission from *Diagnostic and statistical manual of mental disorders.* ed 4, Washington, D.C., 1994, American Psychiatric Association.

Clinical Description

BEHAVIORAL MANIFESTATIONS

Conduct disorder presents mainly with a repetitive and persistent pattern of behavior that violates the basic rights of others or major age-appropriate societal norms or rules. The behavior typically presents in a variety of settings, including home, school, and the community. But it can be difficult to detect because the child or adolescent tends to minimize the problems, and adults may not have full knowledge due to their inability to adequately supervise the child or adolescent.

Clients with conduct disorder often initiate aggressive behavior and react aggressively toward others. They bully, threaten, and intimidate; initiate physical fights; use weapons in ways that could easily lead to injury; act cruelly to people or animals; steal with confrontation; and force sexual activity. The severity of these behaviors may involve rape, assault, or (though rarely) may result in homicide. Deliberate destruction of property may result in fire damage, vandalism, and destruction of others' property for simple vengeance. In addition to theft or robbery, deceitfulness may include frequent lying or breaking of promises to obtain goods or favors, or to

avoid obligations or responsibility. Running away for safety in order to avoid physical or sexual abuse does not meet the criteria; the running away typically occurs in conjunction with violation of other norms and rules.

They also frequently attempt to avoid consequences by attempting to blame others. Early onset of behavior usually associated with adults may occur and includes sexual activity, drinking, smoking, use of illegal substances, and other high-risk–taking acts. These behaviors frequently lead to school suspensions, unplanned pregnancy, physical injury, sexually transmitted diseases, legal problems, dismissals from work or other activities, and the inability to attend regular schools. They generally exhibit callous behavior but may express guilt or remorse because they have learned it may reduce or prevent punishment. Although they may project an image of "toughness," they often experience low self-esteem with resulting poor frustration tolerance, irritability, temper outbursts, and reckless behavior.

EMOTIONAL MANIFESTATIONS

Individuals with conduct disorders usually have little empathy or concern for the feelings, wishes, and well-being of others. Suicide ideation, attempts, and completions occur at a higher rate than expected.

PERCEPTUAL MANIFESTATIONS

Clients with conduct disorder often misperceive the intentions of others, especially in ambiguous situations. They typically perceive others as more threatening and hostile and therefore feel justified in responding aggressively.

COGNITIVE MANIFESTATIONS

Individuals with conduct disorder may have various learning disorders or impairments in cognitive functioning, such as borderline intelligence, but none appears specific to conduct disorder.

SOCIAL MANIFESTATIONS

Accidents rates appear higher. Peer relationships often are impaired due to the behaviors associated with conduct disorder (APA, 1994).

Prognosis

Less severe symptoms tend to emerge initially. Males dominate in the childhood-onset group and tend to exhibit more fighting, stealing, vandalism, and school discipline problems. Females tend to have symptoms of lying, running away, substance use, and prostitution. Males tend to use more confrontational aggression; females more nonconfrontational behaviors. An onset of conduct disorder before age 10 (childhood-onset type) generally indicates a more severe and persistent type that often develops into adult antisocial personality disorder. These individuals typically are male, display more physical aggression, more likely have oppositional defiant disorder during childhood, and meet full criteria for conduct disorder prior to puberty. Adolescent-onset type individuals (no symptoms of conduct disorder prior to age 10) display less aggression, are likely to have better peer relationships and display conduct problems in groups (APA, 1994).

OPPOSITIONAL DEFIANT DISORDER
Etiology

Oppositional defiant disorder occurs more often in families where child care has been disrupted by a succession of different caregivers, or where harsh, inconsistent, or neglectful child-bearing practices occur. The disorder occurs more commonly when serious martial problems are present (APA, 1994).

Epidemiology

Rates vary considerably from 2%–16% based on the nature of the population sample and method of assessment. Oppositional defiant disorder occurs more frequently in

---

DSM-IV CRITERIA

Oppositional Defiant Disorder

A. A pattern of negativistic, hostile, and defiant behavior lasting at least 6 months, during which four or more of the following are present:

(1) often loses temper

(2) often argues with adults

(3) often actively defies or refuses to comply with adults' requests or rules

(4) often deliberately annoys people

(5) often blames others for his or her mistakes or misbehavior

(6) is often touchy or easily annoyed by others

(7) is often angry and resentful

(8) is often spiteful or vindictive

Note: Consider a criterion met only if the behavior occurs more frequently than is typically observed in individuals of comparable age and developmental level.

B. The disturbance in behavior causes clinically significant impairment in social, academic, or occupational functioning.

C. The behaviors do not occur exclusively during the course of a psychotic or mood disorder.

D. Criteria are not met for conduct disorder, and, if the individual is age 18 years or older, criteria are not met for antisocial personality disorder, (APA, 1994).

Reprinted with permission from *Diagnostic and statistical manual of mental disorders*, ed 4, Washington, D.C., 1994, American Psychiatric Association.

---

males prior to puberty and with approximately equal frequency after puberty. The disorder also occurs more commonly when at least one parent has a history of one of the following: mood disorder, oppositional defiant disorder, conduct disorder, ADHD, antisocial personality disorder, or a substance-related disorder. ADHD commonly occurs, and learning disorders and communication disorders tend to be associated with oppositional defiant disorder (APA, 1994).

Clinical Description
BEHAVIORAL MANIFESTATIONS

The essential features of negativism, defiance, disobedience, and hostile toward authority figures typically present with persistent stubbornness, resistance to directions, and unwillingness to compromise, give in, or negotiate with adults. Evidence of defiance can also present as deliberate or persistent testing of limits, typically by ignoring directions, arguing, and refusal to accept blame for misbehavior. Hostility may be directed at adults or peers and includes deliberately annoying others verbally or through nonserious aggression. Symptoms invariably present at home but may be absent or minimal at school and are generally directed toward those the child knows best. Individuals with oppositional defiant disorder do not tend to regard themselves as troublesome but blame others for making unreasonable demands or blame the circumstances.

EMOTIONAL MANIFESTATIONS

During school years the following problems may be seen: low self-esteem, mood lability, and low frustration tolerance.

COGNITIVE AND PERCEPTUAL MANIFESTATIONS

Cognitive and perceptual symptoms do not usually present as significant symptoms in oppositional defiant disorder.

SOCIAL MANIFESTATIONS

During early childhood, evidence of difficult temperament (for example, high reactivity, difficulty in being soothed) or high motor activity has been noted. There may be swearing and precocious use of alcohol, tobacco, or illicit drugs. A cycle of parent and child bringing out the worst in each other frequently appears (APA, 1994).

Prognosis

Onset is typically gradual, usually occurring over the course of months or years. In a significant number of cases, oppositional defiant disorder develops into conduct disorder.

TIC DISORDER: TOURETTE'S DISORDER
Etiology and Epidemiology

Although genetically transmitted in an autosomal dominant pattern, penetrance of Tourette's disorder in females is only about 70% but in males reaches 99% (APA, 1994).

Tourette's disorder occurs in approximately 4–5 persons per 10,000. It is approximately 1.5–3 times more common in males than females. Other disorders associated with Tourette's disorder include ADHD, obsessive-compulsive disorder, and learning disorders (APA, 1994).

Clinical Description
BEHAVIORAL MANIFESTATIONS

Tics present as a physical symptom seen as behavior. A **tic** is defined as "a sudden, rapid, recurrent, nonrhythmic, stereotyped motor movement or vocalization." Although experienced as irresistible, it can often be suppressed for a varying length of time. Stress typically exacerbates tics,

and absorbing activities such as reading or sewing may reduce them. Sleep markedly decreases tics.

Simple motor tics include eye blinking, neck jerking, shoulder shrugging, facial grimacing, and coughing. Simple vocal tics include throat clearing, grunting, sniffing, snorting, and barking. Complex motor tics include facial gestures, grooming behaviors, jumping, touching, stamping, smelling an object, and echokinesis (imitation of another's movements). Complex vocal tics include repeating words or phrases out of context, coprolalia (repeating socially unacceptable words, typically obscene or swear words), palilalia (repeating one's own sounds or words), and echolalia (repeating the last heard word, sound, or phrase).

In Tourette's disorder the number, type, frequency, complexity, and severity of the tics vary over time. Most common tics in Tourette's disorder involve the head and parts of the body such as the torso and limbs. Common vocal tics include clicks, grunts, barks, sniffs, snorts, and coughs. Coprolalia occurs in less than 10% of the cases. Complex motor tics reported in Tourette's disorder include touching, squatting, deep knee bends, retracing steps, and twirling during walking. The most frequent initial tic is blinking. Other initial tics reported include tongue protrusion, squatting, sniffing, hopping, skipping, throat clearing, stuttering, uttering sounds or words, and coprolalia. Other relatively common issues include hyperactivity, distractibility, and impulsivity. Reti-

---

DSM-IV CRITERIA

Tourette's Disorder

A. Both multiple motor and one or more vocal tics have been present at some time during the illness, although not necessarily concurrently.

B. The tics occur many times a day (usually in bouts) nearly every day or intermittently throughout a period of more than one year, and during this period there was never a tic-free period of more than three consecutive months.

C. The disturbance causes marked distress or significant impairment in social, occupational, or other important areas of functioning.

D. The onset is before age 18.

E. The disturbance is not due to the direct physiological effects of a substance (e.g., stimulants) or a general medical condition (e.g., Huntington's disease or postviral encephalitis.)

Reprinted with permission from *Diagnostic and statistical manual of mental disorders,* ed 4, Washington, D.C., 1994, American Psychiatric Association.

nal detachment can occur from head banging; orthopedic problems from knee bending, neck jerking, or head turning; and skin problems from picking.

EMOTIONAL MANIFESTATIONS

Shame, self-consciousness, and depressed mood may occur as a secondary result of problems stemming from Tourette's disorder.

COGNITIVE MANIFESTATIONS

Obsessions and compulsions make up the most common cognitive features seen in a client with Tourette's disorder.

PERCEPTUAL MANIFESTATIONS

Perceptual problems are not a typical problem area in Tourette's disorder.

SOCIAL MANIFESTATIONS

Frequently reported associated symptoms include social discomfort and rejection by others that interfere with social, academic, and occupational functioning. In severe cases tics may interfere with activities of daily living, such as reading or eating, or cause medical complications (APA, 1994).

Prognosis

Tourette's disorder may begin as early as two years of age but typically presents during childhood or early adolescence. Although it is almost always a lifelong disorder, in most cases symptoms diminish during adolescence and adulthood (APA, 1994).

OTHER TIC DISORDERS
Chronic Motor or Vocal Tic Disorder

This disorder resembles Tourette's disorder, except the tics may be either motor or vocal and need not be multiple. It also tends to be less severe (APA, 1994).

Transient Tic Disorder

This diagnosis is made if the tics last more than one year. Otherwise, the criteria are the same as for Tourette's but typically with less severity (APA, 1994).

Tic Disorder Not Otherwise Specified

This diagnosis is used when other more specific diagnoses cannot be made. Examples include tics lasting less the 4 weeks or tics with an onset after 18 years of age (APA, 1994).

SEPARATION ANXIETY DISORDER
Etiology and Epidemiology

Separation anxiety disorder appears to be more common in first-degree relatives and may be more common in children whose mothers have panic disorder. It may develop after some life stress (for example, death of relative or pet, illness in the child or parent, or a change in the environment) (APA, 1994).

This disorder occurs in approximately 4% of children and adolescents and is more common in females. It typically presents before late adolescence (APA, 1994).

Clinical Description
BEHAVIORAL MANIFESTATIONS

With a need to know the whereabouts of their parents or others, individuals with separation anxiety often display attempts to stay in touch with frequent telephone calls. Because of significant discomfort in being away from home, they may become resistant to traveling alone and reluctant to attend activities that other peers enjoy and look forward to such as camp, school, and sleepovers at friends' houses. They may not stay in a room alone. Clients with separation anxiety disorder may demonstrate clinging behavior and attempt to shadow their parents around home and even more so outside the home. Bedtime can be quite difficult, with the child or adolescent insisting the parent remain with them until they fall asleep. During the night these individuals may attempt to get in bed with the parents or another significant figure; if their way is obstructed, they may sleep outside the parents' or other's door.

Physical complaints often appear during actual or anticipated separation and frequently include stomachaches, headaches, nausea, and vomiting. Older children and adolescents may experience a racing or pounding heart, dizziness, and faintness. The somatic complaints often lead to numerous trips to physicians and subsequent medical procedures.

EMOTIONAL MANIFESTATIONS

Individuals with this disorder may experience recurrent excessive distress away from home or major attachment figures. Some become extremely distraught and miserable away from home and become preoccupied with reunion fantasies. They may become extremely fearful that some imagined harm will happen to the significant other(s). Fears about danger to themselves or their families may present as fear of animals, monsters, the dark, muggers, burglars, kidnappers, accidents, or plane or train travel. Fears may also present as concerns about death and dying. They may show various moods, such as excessive worry that no one loves them and they therefore want to die, or unusual anger when someone tries to separate them from their parent or significant other. The depressed mood may at times justify a diagnosis of depression. As adulthood is reached, some of these individuals may develop panic disorder with agoraphobia.

COGNITIVE MANIFESTATIONS

Nightmares often contain elements of the individual's fears, such as family death through fire, murder, or other

DSM-IV CRITERIA

Separation Anxiety

A. Developmentally inappropriate and excessive anxiety concerning separation from home or from those to whom the individual is attached, as evidenced by three or more of the following:

1. recurrent excessive distress when separation from home or major attachment figures occurs or is anticipated.

2. persistent and excessive worry about losing or possible harm befalling major attachment figures.

3. persistent and excessive worry that an untoward event will lead to separation from a major attachment figure (e.g., getting lost or being kidnapped).

4. persistent reluctance or refusal to go to school or elsewhere because of fear of separation.

5. persistent and excessive fear or reluctance to be alone or without major attachment figures at home, or without significant adults in other settings.

6. persistent reluctance or refusal to go to sleep without being near a major attachment figure or to sleep away from home.

7. repeated nightmares with the theme of separation.

8. repeated complaints of physical symptoms (such as headaches, stomachaches, nausea, or vomiting) when separation from major attachment figures occurs or is anticipated.

B. The duration of the disturbance is at least 4 weeks.

C. The onset is before age 18.

D. The disturbance causes clinically significant distress or impairment in social, academic (occupational), or other important areas of functioning.

E. The disturbance does not occur exclusively during the course of a pervasive developmental disorder, schizophrenia, or other psychotic disorder and, in adolescents and adults, is not better accounted for by panic disorder with agoraphobia (APA, 1994).

Reprinted with permission from *Diagnostic and statistical manual of mental disorders,* ed 4, Washington, D.C., 1994, American Psychiatric Association.

---

catastrophe. Academic difficulties may result from refusal to attend school and thus increase the problem with social avoidance.

PERCEPTUAL MANIFESTATIONS

When alone, young children may experience perceptual problems such as seeing people peering into their room, scary creatures reaching for them, and eyes staring at them.

SOCIAL MANIFESTATIONS

With a typically close-knit family, clients with separation anxiety disorder may exhibit social withdrawal, apathy, sadness, or concentration difficulties at work or play when away from the parents or significant others. Families frequently experience in significant conflict, with parental resentment and frustration. At times, however, these children may also become unusually conscientious, compliant, and eager to please. Parents often describe these children as demanding, intrusive, and in need of constant attention; the children may physically strike out (APA, 1994).

Prognosis

Typically these are periods of severity and reduction of symptoms. Both the anxiety about possible separation and the avoidance of situations involving separation may persist for many years.

ELIMINATION DISORDERS: ENCOPRESIS

Etiology and Epidemiology

Certain conditions such as inadequate, inconsistent toilet training and psychosocial stress (for example, entering school or the birth of a sibling) may predispose to **encopresis** (APA, 1994), which is the repeated passage of feces into inappropriate places, whether involuntary or intentional.

Approximately 1% of 5-year-olds have encopresis. It is more common in males (APA, 1994).

Clinical Description

Most often the fecal soiling is involuntary, but at times it may be intentional. It must not be due to the direct physiological effects of a substance such as laxatives or a medical condition except through a mechanism involving constipation. Involuntary soiling often involves constipation, impaction, and retention with subsequent overflow. The underlying reason for constipation typically involves a psychological reason such as anxiety specific to a place or a more general pattern of oppositional or anxious behavior.

DSM-IV CRITERIA

Encopresis

A. Repeated passage of feces into inappropriate places (e.g., clothing or floor) whether involuntary or intentional.

B. At least one such event a month for at least three months.

C. Chronological age is at least four years (or equivalent developmental level).

D. The behavior is not due exclusively to the direct physiological effects of a substance (e.g., laxatives) or a general medical condition except through a mechanism involving constipation (APA, 1994).

Reprinted with permission from *Diagnostic and statistical manual of mental disorders,* ed 4, Washington, D.C., 1994, American Psychiatric Association.

DSM-IV CRITERIA

Enuresis

A. Repeated voiding of urine into bed or clothes (whether involuntary or intentional).

B. The behavior is clinically significant as manifested by either a frequency of twice a week for at least three consecutive months or the presence of clinically significant distress or impairment in social, academic (occupational), or other important areas of functioning.

C. Chronological age is at least five years (or equivalent developmental level).

D. The behavior is not due exclusively to the direct physiological effect of a substance (e.g., a diuretic) or a general medical condition (e.g., diabetes, spina bifida, or a seizure disorder) (APA, 1994).

Reprinted with permission from *Diagnostic and statistical manual of mental disorders,* ed 4, Washington, D.C., 1994, American Psychiatric Association.

Associated Features

Individuals with encopresis often feel ashamed about the condition and attempt to avoid situations that would lead to further embarrassment, such as camp, school, and sleepovers. Impairment generally relates to the ability of the child's self-esteem to withstand social ostracism, anger, punishment, and rejection by caregivers. Smearing as an associated feature may be due to an attempt to clean or hide feces or may be more clearly deliberate. When deliberate, the individual often exhibits features of oppositional defiant disorder or conduct disorder (APA, 1994).

Prognosis

Encopresis can persist for years with remissions and exacerbations but rarely becomes chronic (APA, 1994).

ELIMINATION DISORDERS: ENURESIS
Etiology and Epidemiology

Enuresis is the repeated voiding of urine into bed or clothes, whether involuntary or intentional. Some possible predisposing factors include delayed or lax toilet training, psychosocial stress, a dysfunction in the ability to concentrate urine, and a lower bladder volume threshold for involuntary voiding (APA, 1994).

At 5 years of age, 7% of boys and 3% of girls experience enuresis. At 10 years of age, 3% of boys and 2% of girls experience it (APA, 1994).

Clinical Description and Associated Features

The diagnostic criteria for enuresis present the typical problem of voiding in inappropriate places during the day or night when control is expected. The actual amount of impairment usually comes from interference with social activities or its effect on self-esteem, along with the degree of social ostracism and degree of caregiver acceptance or rejection and punishment. Other disorders sometimes seen with enuresis include encopresis, sleepwalking disorder, and sleep terror disorder (APA, 1994).

Prognosis

Enuresis persists at age 18 in only 1% of boys and less for girls. Only about 1% of cases continue into adulthood. About 75% of all children with enuresis have a first-degree relative who had the disorder (APA, 1994).

DEVELOPMENTAL DISORDERS: LEARNING DISORDER, COORDINATION DISORDER, COMMUNICATION DISORDER
Etiology

Learning disorders are associated with a number of factors, such as genetic predisposition, perinatal injury, and various neurological or medical conditions. However, these conditions do not inevitably predict learning disorders. Certain medical conditions have a strong association to learning disorders: lead poisoning, fetal alcohol syndrome, and fragile X syndrome. A number of factors must be ruled out when evaluating for a learning disorder: normal variations in academic attainment, lack of opportunity, poor teaching, cultural factors, and impaired hearing or vision (APA, 1994).

Epidemiology

Learning disorders are found in about 2%–10% of children depending on the nature of assessment and the definitions applied. Approximately 5% of public school students have an identified learning disorder. Reading disorder is estimated at 4% of school-age children in the United States, and approximately 1% of school-age children have mathematics disorder. Prevalence has not been clearly established for disorder of written expression, but it is rare when not associated with other learning disorders. Motor coordination disorder may reach as high as 6% in 5- to 11-year-old children. Developmental expressive language disorder occurs in approximately 3%–5% of children and is acquired in fewer children. The developmental type of mixed receptive-expressive language disorder is estimated at up to 3% of school-age children. About 2%–3% of 6- and 7-year-olds show phonological disorder, which falls to 0.5% by age 17. Stuttering occurs in 1% of prepubertal children and drops to 0.8% in adolescence. Males dominate with a three-to-one ratio (APA, 1994).

Clinical Description
LEARNING DISORDERS

Learning disorders encompass problems with reading, writing, math, and a not otherwise specified category. They are diagnosed by individually administered, standardized tests when performance is substantially below expected (generally defined as 1-2 standard deviations below the average) and when there is significant interference with academic achievement or activities of daily living. Many problems can result from learning disorders, including demoralization, low self-esteem, and deficits in social skills. Children and adolescents with learning disorders drop out of school at a rate of nearly 40% (approximately 1.5 the average rate). Ten to 25% of individuals with conduct disorder, oppositional defiant disorder, ADHD, major depression, or dysthymic disorders have learning disorders as well. Language delay may occur in learning disorders, and learning disorders may be associated with a higher rate of developmental coordination disorder. Underlying abnormalities in cognitive abilities may exist (e.g., deficits in visual perception, linguistic processes, attention, memory, or a combination) that often precede or are associated with learning disorders.

COORDINATION DISORDERS

Developmental coordination disorder is only diagnosed if motor coordination significantly interferes with academic achievement or activities of daily living and not due to a medical condition (for example, cerebral palsy or muscular dystrophy). Specific activities or tasks that may be impaired or altered include walking, crawling, sitting, tying shoelaces, buttoning shirts, or zipping pants. Communication disorders also may be associated (APA, 1994).

COMMUNICATION DISORDERS

Expressive language disorder features vary but may include a limited amount of speech, limited range of vocabulary, difficulty acquiring new words, word-finding or vocabulary errors, shortened sentences, simplified grammar use, omissions of critical parts of a sentence, use of unusual word order, and slow rate of language development. Intelligence measured by performance tests is usually normal. Expressive language disorder may be acquired as a result of a neurological or medical condition (for example, encephalitis, head trauma, or irradiation) or developmental (i.e., no known neurological condition). Mixed receptive-expressive language disorder symptoms include receptive difficulties (e.g., markedly limited vocabulary, errors in tense, difficulty recalling words or producing developmentally appropriate sentences, and general difficulty expressing ideas) and language development problems (e.g., difficulty understanding words, sentences, or specific types of words). As with expressive language disorder, mixed receptive-expressive language disorder may be developmental or acquired. A child may initially appear confused or inattentive, follow commands incorrectly, and give inappropriate responses to questions. The child may appear quiet or unusually talkative. Other communication disorders include phonological disorder (problems using expected speech sounds) and stuttering (a disturbance in normal fluency and time patterns of speech) (APA, 1994).

Prognosis

Reading disorder prognosis is good with early identification and intervention but may persist into adult life. The degree of impairment usually depends on the overall intelligence level in mathematics disorder. Brighter children may be able to function at or near grade level in early grades but by the fifth grade the reading disorders almost always become apparent. The course of disorder of written expression has not been clearly defined. Motor coordination disorder has a variable course and may last into adolescence or adulthood. Approximately one-half of children with developmental expressive language disorder outgrow it, while the other half have long-lasting difficulties. In the acquired type, recovery depends on the severity and location of the injury as well as age at time of occurrence. Recovery may be rapid and complete or the injury may get progressively worse. The prognosis for mixed receptive-expressive language disorder of the acquired type is worse than for expressive language disorder. The acquired type has a variable prognosis like expressive language disorder. Phonological disorder prognosis varies according to cause and severity. In severe cases speech may not be recognizable and the disorder may persist, while mild cases may remit spontaneously. Stuttering typically occurs insidiously and, when noticed, has a waxing and waning course. Recovery occurs in up to 80%, of cases; spontaneously in 60%. Recovery typically occurs at age 16 (APA, 1994).

DISCHARGE CRITERIA

Client will:

- Engage in self-care within level of capability
- Demonstrate emotional control within capacity
- Attend to tasks, schoolwork, and performance without undue anger or frustration
- Exhibit healthy self-concept and self-estem
- Demonstrate functional eating habits and behaviors appropriate for age and stature
- Use cognitive, communication, and language skills to make self understood and to get needs met
- Demonstrate interactive skills appropriate for level of development
- Verbalize satisfaction with gender identity and sexual preference
- Interact meaningfully with staff, peers, and family within capability
- Seek attention and assistance appropriately from significant persons and refrains from undue or unnecessary interactions with strangers
- Adhere to treatment regimen, including medication as needed
- Play appropriately with peers
- Engage in educational and vocational programs within capacity
- Use adaptive coping techniques and stress-reducing strategies
- Respond satisfactorily to others' attentions and requests
- Use community resources to enhance quality of life
- Engage in ongoing individual and family therapy

CHILD ABUSE

Child abuse, which may include physical or sexual abuse, neglect, or being a witness to violence, produces many problems that need to be addressed in childhood and adolescence. There is a significant increase in rates of physical aggression and antisocial acts by victims of child abuse. Aggressive behavior and inappropriate sexual behavior make up the single most common symptom in sexually abused children. Other problems include delinquency, violence, running away, substance abuse, and teen pregnancy (Bellis and Putnam, 1994).

In 1993 the National Research Council reported that 9.4–107 cases of child abuse occurred per 1000 children per year (Bellis and Putnam, 1994). In 1990 the U.S. Advisory Board on Child Abuse reported 1.5 million cases of child abuse and 3.3 million cases of children being exposed to violence. It gave rates of 5.7 cases of physical abuse per 1000 children per year and 2.5 cases of sexual abuse per 1000 children per year (Lewis, 1994). See Chapter 25, Survivors of Violence, for a more detailed discussion of this issue.

ADOLESCENT SUICIDE

Adolescent suicide does not neatly fall under any diagnostic category. Depression and self-destructive behaviors, including substance abuse, recklessness, delinquency, impulsive behaviors, and sexual promiscuity, have been strongly associated with adolescents at risk for suicide. Suicide accounts for 12% of adolescent deaths and ranks second only to accidents as a leading cause of death in adolescents. The adolescent suicide rate tripled between 1950 and 1980, increasing from 2.7 per 100,000 to 8.5 per 100,000. The yearly prevalence of self-destructive behavior ranges stand out at a much higher rate of 4% to as high as 20%. Firearms use is the most common method to commit suicide, and adolescents have been able to obtain the weapons no matter how securely they are stored at home.

Identified risk factors include the following:

1. Psychiatric Diagnosis: affective (depression and anxiety) and antisocial disorders, borderline personality disorder, alcohol and drug abuse, and disruptive disorders (conduct disorder, oppositional defiant order, attention-deficit hyperactivity disorder)

2. Psychosocial Factors: long-term stressors, especially involving a loss (particularly of a family member through suicide), history of physical or sexual abuse, school failure, alcohol and drug abuse, and a chaotic and nonsupportive family

3. Biologic Factors: dysfunction of the hypothalamic-pituitary-adrenal axis and dysregulation of serotonin and noradrenergic metabolism

No matter what the etiology, a pattern of self-destructive behavior typically presents before suicide behaviors. Generally these behaviors present as disruptive, hostile, or isolating in nature. Many adolescents also seek medical attention within one to three months before an attempt, providing an opportunity for early evaluation (Sulik and Garfinkel, 1992).

Working with children and adolescents is a challenge for the nurse in any context. However, when these clients are experiencing problems related to a major mental disorder, the nurse's skills and expertise are even more greatly challenged. The steps of the nursing process are followed, just as they are with any other client. However, a greater challenge exists in the areas of assessment and intervention.

A thorough knowledge of growth and development is essential to fully understand any deviations from the norm. This understanding will greatly impact nursing care. In addition, the child and adolescent usually present with family members. Thus, the nurse has a unique opportunity to assess and care for the whole family. This is a benefit in terms of acquiring a wider range of assessment data; however, it does present problems of its own. Often, the child or adolescent may be the "symptom-bearer" for the family. In other words, the mental health problems that the child or adolescent is experiencing may be, in fact, a reflection of a broader family psychopathology. The child or adolescent may be the "identified client" but may be scapegoated by the family. Any attempt the nurse makes to broaden the approach to include other family members in the assessment and planning process may be met with stiff resistance. Overcoming this resistance is a major component of working with children and adolescents in the context of the family.

Lastly, applying the nursing process to the child or adolescent with mental illness can be frustrating. Seeing the outcomes of nursing care successfully met in the identified client can be rewarding, and children and adolescents are often motivated, amazingly resilient clients. However, discharging them to family systems that may not be willing or able to continue the treatment gains made can lead to frustration for the nurse. All these factors suggest that nursing care of children and adolescents is very challenging! Nevertheless, it is a very rewarding population to work with because these children and adolescents often present as motivated clients quite open to the support offered in the nurse-client relationship.

■ ASSESSMENT

When nurses approach children and adolescents in order to assess them, they must be aware of normal growth and development. Many expressions of normal child or adolescent behavior can mimic symptoms of major mental disorders. Separation anxiety, temper tantrums, night fears, testing of limits in adolescents, sexual experimentation, moodiness, and a host of other symptoms are all normal in children and adolescents as they move along the developmental continuum. In addition, anxiety often presents differently in younger children, perhaps in the form of aggressiveness. Thus, nurses must understand what is "normal" in a client before they can accurately assess any potentially abnormal symptomatology.

Developmental Stage

The nurse begins with an assessment of normal aspects of growth and development to establish a baseline assessment. Developmental milestones, language skills, school performance, level of abstract thinking, and other factors provide the nurse with a comparison to begin examining specific symptoms. Nurses must be aware of the normal course of development. Many children experience developmental delays as a result of abuse, neglect, or the complication of a major mental disorder. Box 17-1 below lists key developmental tasks accomplished in childhood and adolescence.

Physical Assessment

A thorough physical assessment is important in ruling out any complicating factors that may be affecting the child. For example, in a child with encopresis, determining if there is any physical trauma from sexual abuse is an important differentiating factor in assessment. Children often use physical problems such as asthma to gain attention from parents and to manipulate their home and school environments. In addition, a physical assessment allows the nurse to note any evidence of child abuse. Many behavioral problems in children can be linked to abusive and neglectful home environments and must be assessed before an adequate diagnoses of mental disorders can be made.

Box 17-1 Developmental Tasks of Childhood and Adolescence

1. Evolution of self-identity (including gender).
2. Separation and individuation from parents.
3. Clarification and prioritization of values, beliefs, and interests.
4. Establishment of meaningful relationships with the same and opposite sex.
5. Achievement of intimacy.
6. Understanding and appropriate expression of emotion.
7. Development of meaningful purpose in life.
8. Building of competence and the honing of skills.
9. Determination of career goals and lifestyles.

CLINICAL ALERT !

Many children engage in sexual experimentation as a normal part of their development. The nurse must be able to differentiate between what may be normal activity and what may in fact be evidence of sexual abuse. In young children, mimicking sexual activity can suggest that the child has been exposed to such sexual activity, or may have been involved in the activity—both of these constitute sexual abuse. The nurse must assess the sexualized play of the child, first from the basis of what is normal for other children that age—e.g., what sexual play would be considered normal for children of that age in any context. Then the nurse must carefully observe and interview the child to determine if the sexualized play has come about as a result of exposure or involvement in sexual activity. The nurse then proceeds accordingly in the intervention process.

Family Life

The child's or adolescent's home environment must be carefully assessed to fully understand the context of the symptoms. How does the child get along with brothers and sisters? What typical methods do the parents use for disciplining children? What marital problems potentially exist in the parents that may be significantly impacting the children in the home? What economic factors may be increasing stress in the home? The nurse must gain a clear picture of what occurs within the family to understand what is actually happening with the child or adolescent. It is important to determine what each family member perceives as the key problem issue.

Activities of Daily Living

On inpatient settings in particular, the nurse has a unique opportunity to observe and assess the child's or adolescent's activities of daily living. Often passed over as routine or unimportant, these activities reveal much about the child's or adolescent's developmental state and can deepen the nurse's understanding of underlying affective issues. All children participate in ADLs. However, the level of independent self-care should be consistent with the child's age. An underdeveloped self-care ability may indicate neglect, developmental delays (often found in developmental disorders), or even depression. An over-developed self-care may indicate a child who has been left to fend for himself or herself. It may indicate a child conditioned to please adults. The nurse must assess the child's or adolescent's self-care level and make a determination as to whether it is developmentally appropriate and the implications inherent in any deviations from the norm.

CASE ⬢ STUDY

Billy, an eight-year-old male, was admitted to the Child Inpatient Mental Health Unit for disruptive behavior at school and aggressiveness toward his four-year-old sister. Billy had been on the unit for six days and consistently refused to comb his hair, brush his teeth, make his bed, or wear appropriate clothing. Every morning was like a "war" as staff attempted to get Billy to do his ADLs. He would frequently end up in "time-out" for his resistance and would need to be "one-to-one'd" by a staff member. Occasionally, his behavior would escalate, and he would need to be restrained.

Critical Thinking and Assessment

1. What would be considered "normal" in terms of growth and development for self-care in a child Billy's age?

2. What gains might Billy be acquiring by battling with the staff around ADL issues?

3. What possible acting-out behaviors are noted in his interactions with the staff?

4. How would time-outs and even seclusion and restraint reinforce Billy's negative behavior?

In addition, activities of daily living may become areas for acting out. Children and adolescents are sensitive to power issues in interpersonal relationships. In an attempt to introduce some level of control into their environment, these clients may use simple activities as ways to exert independence or to defy authority. This can be especially acute on inpatient units where children or adolescents are admitted against their wishes by their parents and do not perceive a need to be in the hospital. Sensitive and consistent intervention by the nurse can do much to alleviate the child's or adolescent's need to act-out and involve staff in power plays. However, the assessment potential for these simple activities should not be overlooked by the nurse.

■ ■ NURSING DIAGNOSIS

The nursing diagnosis process for children and adolescents is similar to that for other clients. Accurate diagnosis always follows a thorough and astute assessment. As has been stated, the key to working effectively with children and adolescents is the accurate assessment of growth and development issues. This allows for an accurate, realistic diagnostic process. The family must be taken into consideration in this process as well.

All currently used NANDA nursing diagnoses are applicable to children and adolescents. However, due to the tendency for children and adolescents to act-out the many issues they struggle with, some diagnoses may be more important. Safety issues are significant with any client in the mental health setting. It is even more crucial for children and adolescents, because even children who are developing normally may have little impulse control. Thus, diagnoses such as Risk for Violence: Self or Other Directed and Risk for Injury are important for the nurse to consider. This is especially true in some of the pervasive developmental disorders where autistic behaviors can lead to self-mutilating activities and, in the case of attention-deficit/hyperactivity disorder, where extreme impulsivity and hyperactive behavior can result in injury.

Communication and relationship issues present a challenge for the diagnostic process. Children, especially young children, often do not have adequate verbal skills with which to communicate needs and feelings to the nurse. In some developmental disorders this may be even more of a complicating factor. For adolescents, mistrust of authority and power may cause difficulty in the development of the nurse-client relationship and hinder care. Thus, diagnoses related to difficulties in communication may be indicated. In addition, the diagnosis of altered growth and development should be considered when there is a series of deficits that impact nursing care and discharge planning.

Finally, family issues may be more pertinent for the nurse to consider than in other client care situations. Alterations in Role Performance and/or Parenting and Family Coping are all important diagnoses for the nurse to consider. The needs of the family should always be considered in the process of assigning a nursing diagnosis.

■ ■ ■ OUTCOME IDENTIFICATION

Outcome criteria flow from the nursing diagnoses and, as in all nursing care situations, must be realistic, clear,

and stated in measurable terms. Outcome criteria for children and adolescents should focus on supporting normal growth and development and the movement toward gains in developmental deficits. Safety issues, as previously noted, are always important with any psychiatric population, particularly children and adolescents. Some examples of outcome criteria for children and adolescents are as follows:

1. Expresses thoughts and feelings through appropriate play activities.
2. Absence of aggressive acting-out behaviors.
3. Expresses appropriate attention-seeking/help-seeking behaviors.
4. Participates in age-appropriate play/milieu activities.
5. Demonstrates age-appropriate peer relationships.
6. Demonstrates age-appropriate relationships with adults.
7. Participates in developmentally appropriate self-care activities.

■ ■ ■ ■ PLANNING

Planning and delivering nursing care to children and adolescents require nurses' understanding of the developmental issues and limitations of their clients. The plan of care must be realistic and must include an understanding of family issues and dynamics. It must also take into account the issue of vulnerability. Mental health problems encountered in childhood and adolescence often predispose the client to future problems. Reducing vulnerability and enhancing developmentally appropriate coping strategies are crucial parts of the plan of care. Supporting the family so that client gains can be maintained is also crucial. This necessitates careful and realistic discharge planning.

■ ■ ■ ■ ■ IMPLEMENTATION

For the child or adolescent client, nursing interventions must allow for the developmental stage of the client relative to communication issues and care outcomes. For example, young children are not primarily verbal in their communication. They may have difficulty articulating feelings and thoughts in a manner that aptly reveals their true thoughts. For these younger children, nursing intervention must take place in expressive **therapeutic play** activities (age-appropriate play activities used purposefully by the nurse for assessment, intervention, and promotion of normal growth and development in children). Play is the language of the child. Working with the child client in this way will decrease anxiety and enable a greater therapeutic alliance to be forged. It also provides the context for ongoing assessment as the child will continue self-expression through play activity. Play is also developmentally appropriate for the child. It enables him or her to begin to make gains in developmental deficits.

COLLABORATIVE DIAGNOSES

DSM-IV Diagnoses*	NANDA Diagnoses**
Autistic Disorder	Social Isolation
	Self-Care Deficit
	High Risk for Self-Mutilation
Conduct Disorder	High Risk for Violence:
	Directed at Self or Others
	Impaired Social Interaction
Separation Anxiety	Anxiety
Disorder	Ineffective Individual Coping

*Reprinted with permission from *Diagnostic and statistical manual of mental disorders,* ed 4, Washington, D.C., 1994, American Psychiatric Association.

**Reprinted with permission from *NANDA Nursing diagnoses: definitions and classifications, 1995–1996,* Philadelphia, 1994, North American Nursing Diagnosis Association.

NURSING CARE PLAN

Kelly is an 11-year-old male admitted with a diagnosis of conduct disorder. He has had many problems in school and was recently suspended for fighting. He frequently threatens other children and at home is noted to physically abuse his younger sister and brother. He has a history of cruelty to animals to the point that the family has had to get rid of a dog. He has stolen from both parents on numerous occasions. Kelly has run away from home on two occasions, once staying away all night. His parents were feeling overwhelmed and brought Kelly into the Young Adolescent Inpatient Mental Health Unit for treatment.

Nursing assessment reveals a defiant young man who refuses to talk and stares at the wall. Family history is significant for depression in the mother and alcohol abuse in the father. Kelly's 9-year-old sister is described as quiet and doing well in school. His 5-year-old brother is considered "hyper" and is the object of frequent beatings by Kelly. There has been some spousal abuse between the parents. As the parents described Kelly's home and school functioning, he would frequently burst out with protestations and blame others for his actions.

After the family interview, the nurse engaged Kelly in an age-appropriate play activity to continue assessment. Kelly reveals a very low self-esteem and a great deal of anxiety about the future of his parents' marriage and, thus, the home. He sees himself as a failure and feels that he is in the hospital because he is "bad."

DSM-IV Diagnoses

AXIS I	Conduct Disorder
AXIS II	Learning Disorder
AXIS III	Medical Diagnosis: Asthma
AXIS IV	Severity of Psychosocial Stressors: 3 (Moderate)
	• Family Conflict
	• School Performance Problems
	• Recent School Change
AXIS V	GAF: 45

Nursing Diagnoses: Risk for violence: directed at others. Risk factors: history of aggressive acting-out behavior and poor impulse control as evidenced by: acting-out behaviors in school, suspended for fighting recently, threatening other children and physically abusing his siblings and family pets.

Client Outcomes	*Nursing Interventions*	*Evaluation*
• Kelly will refrain from any aggressive acting-out behavior while on the unit.	• Set firm but realistic limits on Kelly's behavior with clear consequences for his actions *to provide structure and expectations to help Kelly gain control.*	• Kelly had only two episodes of acting out while on unit.
• Kelly will verbalize awareness of factors/situations that precipitate violent behaviors	• Discuss with Kelly factors that precipitate violent behaviors *to help Kelly connect anger-provoking events with acting-out behaviors.*	• Kelly verbalizes awareness of enviornmental triggers that cause him to act out.

• Kelly will express anger in appropriate ways. Examples:
  • Physical activities/ exercise
  • Sports/hobbies
  • Talking to staff members
	• Engage Kelly in unit activities and groups *to allow Kelly to express anger in a therapeutic safe milieu.*
	• Encourage verbal and nonverbal expression of feelings in socially acceptable ways *to help Kelly vent feelings rather than act on them.*
		• Kelly has expressed his anger in appropriate ways, such as playing volleyball with the group and talking to staff and peers.

• Kelly will follow through with behavioral contract established by staff.	• Develop a behavioral contract for Kelly *to provide structure and expectation of behaviors.*	• Kelly has complied with goals of the behavioral contract.

NURSING CARE PLAN

Nursing Diagnosis: Impaired social interaction, related to lack of consistent positive peer relationships, and poor parental role modeling as evidenced by threatening and bullying behaviors.

Client Outcomes	Nursing Interventions	Evaluation
• Kelly will interact in age-appropriate milieu activities with peers in a positive manner.	• Engage Kelly in specific age-appropriate activities *to increase self-esteem and facilitate development of the nurse-client relationship.* • Offer praise and support for Kelly's appropriate peer interactions. Set limits on any negative interactions *to encourage repetition of functional behaviors.*	• Kelly regularly engaged in peer activities on the unit without bullying or threatening peers.
• Kelly will engage in a therapeutic alliance with his primary nurse.	• Meet with Kelly during an age-appropriate play activity at specified periods of time throughout the shift *so that Kelly can have something to look forward to and begin to learn positive attention and help-seeking behaviors.*	• Kelly consistently met with his primary nurse and shared his thoughts and feelings in an appropriate manner.
• Kelly will identify and use support systems while on the unit.	• Teach Kelly the importance of peer and staff support throughout the treatment process *to provide Kelly with security that others are there to support him.*	• Kelly was seen approaching select peers and staff for problem solving.

These activities enable the child to gain a mastery of his or her environment, which can be important in building self-confidence. By teaching parents about the importance of play, nurses can facilitate the child's play activities at home, thus further consolidating treatment gains.

Group play activities are also important for the same reasons. Childhood is an important time of developing peer skills and positive interpersonal relationships. The nature and quality of these skills will dramatically impact future development. The nurse can use group activities in the milieu to assess as well as intervene in these areas. Group activities allow the nurse to teach and model appropriate behaviors, reinforce positive gains, and promote reality testing.

Intervening with adolescents is often more difficult than with children. Adolescents often present as unwilling clients brought by parents or at the request of school authorities. In addition, it is a normal developmental stage for adolescents to mistrust authority and test limits. In the presence of a major mental disorder, these behaviors can be intensified. Thus, the key nursing intervention with the adolescent client is the establishment of a therapeutic alliance.

Adolescents are primarily verbal; expressive activities tend to diminish in effectiveness with this age group. Nursing interventions that support the development of the nurse-client relationship become foundational to care. The nurse must communicate empathy to the adolescent. Power plays and automatic siding with parents will effectively block the establishment of a therapeutic alliance. The nurse must communicate understanding of the difficult contexts that the adolescent exists in and the difficult growth and development issues at this stage in his or her life. The nurse should avoid acting like an adolescent in order to appear acceptable to the client. This is seen as contrived by most adolescents and will diminish respect for the nurse. Adolescents are primarily looking for effective role models. When parents cannot provide this due to a wide variety of factors, adolescents will look to gangs and others. The nurse has an excellent opportunity to be a surrogate role model and model effective, appropriate, productive adult behavior. Nurses who are successful with adolescents can be themselves with their clients and convey a warmth and empathy that tear down defensive walls. In addition, successful nurses will model consistent, caring, adult relationships with other staff and clients. In this way, the full therapeutic effects of the milieu can be brought to play for the adolescent client.

Group activities provide an important opportunity for the nurse to interact with adolescent clients. Because adolescents are at a stage developmentally where they are testing adult behaviors and forming increasingly adult-like relationships, group activities allow them the opportunity to develop interpersonal skills, enact modeled behavior, communicate with peers and staff, and learn about appropriate ways to function in an adult world. Milieu-related groups as well as formal therapy groups all provide the nurse with a powerful means to intervene and develop relationships with adolescent clients.

Following is a list of key nursing interventions used in the care of children and adolescents.

Nursing Interventions

1. Maintain a safe environment by assessing it for potential dangers, for the presence of suicidal ideation or plans, and for cues and signals indicating frustration, anger, or behavioral changes *to provide safety and prevent violence.*

2. Demonstrate acceptance of painful feelings and issues that underly acting-out behavior without condoning the behavior itself *to help the child or adolescent develop patterns of positive attention-seeking and help-seeking behaviors.*

3. Maintain a therapeutic environment *to maximize the opportunities in the milieu for the mastery of social-emotional skills, and the acquisition of confidence and increasing self-esteem.*

4. Use developmentally appropriate language and activities *to develop a therapeutic alliance with the child or adolescent.*

5. Work effectively with the family *to facilitate treatment gains and to prepare the child or adolescent and other family members for discharge.*

Additional Treatment Modalities

Numerous collaborative interventions are used with children and adolescents. Medication usage is increasing in this population, and the nurse is often called on to administer these medications to clients. Most of the medications used are the same ones used for adults; thus, the same issues related to side effects, informed consent, and safety apply. In addition, younger children may not be able to clearly articulate side effects of medications. The nurse must therefore use even more astute observational skills to determine if medication side effects are present.

Recreational and occupational therapies are important treatment modalities in this population because of the emphasis on developmentally appropriate play activities and the need for continued development of gross and fine motor skills. The nurse should be involved in these activities whenever possible, because they provide further opportunities for ongoing assessment as well as nonthreatening avenues for the development of the therapeutic alliance.

■ ■ ■ ■ ■ ■ EVALUATION

The evaluation phase is incorporated into the discharge planning process. The discharge planning process with children and adolescents focuses on preparing the client for return to the home or to an out-of-home placement. Many youngsters may spend time in group homes or foster care, or long-term treatment facilities called 24-hour schools. When the discharge plan calls for out-of-home placement, the nurse has a tremendous challenge. He or she must help the client and the client's family deal with a sense of failure or inadequacy, as well as the grief associated with separation and loss. Discharge planning should include helping the child or adolescent prepare for the out-of-home placement, decreasing anxiety, and understanding what the new routines and activities will be. In addition, the nurse should help the client understand why the out-of-home placement has been chosen as a continuing treatment option over a return home. Many times, the child or adolescent may have a distorted view of this treatment choice and see it as failure on his or her part to make treatment gains. Parents may share these feelings of guilt. Working with the family and the client can help prepare them for the separation and set up positive expectations for the outcome of treatment.

When the child or adolescent is to return home, many similar issues must be addressed. The family must be included in the discharge plan. Treatment approaches and gains must be clearly explained so that parents will have the greatest opportunity to continue these activities post-discharge. A great deal of teaching is needed to ensure that parents understand normal growth and development so they can properly interact with and evaluate their child's behavior. Aftercare plans should be clearly explained and realistic for the family to attain. The nurse must be especially aware of the potential for abuse and neglect in the family and act accordingly. Consulting with social workers and other discharge planning resources may be crucial to insuring the child's or adolescent's safety after discharge.

Ethical discharge planning with this population also involves the timely and sensitive termination of the nurse-client relationship. While difficult for most clients, children and adolescents (especially younger ones) may have a difficult time understanding the termination of the relationship. Acting-out behaviors prior to discharge are quite common and should not be seen as the loss of treatment gains. The nurse must handle these behaviors with sensitivity and consistency and proceed with the discharge planning process.

Summary of Key Concepts

1. Of mentally retarded individuals, 85% are only mildly retarded; 10% are moderately retarded; 3%–4% are severely retarded; and 1%–2% are profoundly retarded.

2. The most commonly diagnosed mental disorders are attention-deficit/hyperactivity disorder, mood disorder, pervasive development disorder, stereotype movement disorder, and mental disorders due to a general medical condition.

3. Children with autistic disorder present with repetitive movements, no emotional reciprocity, impaired communication (both verbal and nonverbal), and an indifference to affection. Seventy-five percent have some degree of mental retardation.

4. Children with attention-deficit/hyperactivity disorder may have the following histories: child abuse or neglect, multiple foster placements, neurotoxin exposure, infections, drug exposure in utero, low birth weight, and mental retardation.

5. AHDH causes problems in academics, social relationships, self-esteem, and occupation due to its demanding, impulsive, and seemingly lazy manifestations.

6. One of the main characteristics of conduct disorder is the client's violent and/or aggressive behavior with little concern for those his or her actions affect.

7. Like autistic disorder, Tourette's disorder involves repetitive movements, sounds, and actions; however, unlike autistic disorder, these symptoms diminish during adolescence and adulthood.

8. Separation anxiety is a disruptive disorder that prevents children from engaging in normal activities due to incessant fear that their loved ones will be harmed in their absence.

9. Encopresis and enuresis are often caused by anxiety.

10. Children with learning disorders (including reading disorder, mathematics disorder, and disorder of written expression) compose 5% of public school children.

11. Aggressive behavior and inappropriate sexual behavior make up the single most common symptom in sexually abused children.

12. Treated early, many of the problems that affect children and adolescents can be resolved. Treatment may help the client acquire skills and abilities for a more healthy adult life. However, if these disorders are not treated early, the client may be predisposed to long-term mental health problems.

13. Working with a young population challenges the nurse to include the family more intensely than with other populations.

REFERENCES

American Psychiatric Association: *Diagnostic and statistical manual of mental disorders,* ed 4, Washington, D.C., 1994, American Psychiatric Association.

Bauermeister J et al: Epidemiology of disruptive behavior disorders. In Lewis M, editor: *Child and adolescent psychiatric clinics of North America: disruptive behaviors,* vol 3, no 2, Philadelphia, April 1994, W. B. Saunders.

Bellis, Putnam: The psychobiology of childhood maltreatment. In Lewis M, editor: *Child and adolescent psychiatric clinics of North America: child abuse,* vol 3, no 4, Philadelphia, October 1994, W. B. Saunders.

Fortinash K, Holoday-Worret P: *Psychiatric nursing care plans,* ed 2, St. Louis, 1995, Mosby.

Hirshberg JC: Child psychiatry: introduction. In Kaplan et al., editors: *Comprehensive textbook of psychiatry/III,* ed 3, vol 3, Baltimore, 1980, Williams and Wilkins.

Kelly SJ: Child maltreatment, stressful life events, and behavior problems in school-aged children in residential treatment. *Journal of Child and Adolescent Psychiatric Nursing* 5:2, 1992.

Lewis M: A structural overview of psychopathology in childhood and adolescence. In Kaplan et al, editors: *Comprehensive textbook of psychiatry/III,* ed 3, vol 3, Baltimore, 1980, Williams and Wilkins.

Otnow Lewis D: Etiology of aggressive conduct disorders: neuropsychiatric and family contributions. In Lewis M, editor: *Child and adolescent psychiatric clinics of North America: disruptive behaviors,* vol 3, no 2, Philadelphia, April 1994, W. B. Saunders.

Rogeness G: Biologic findings in conduct disorder. In Lewis M, editor: *Child and adolescent psychiatric clinics of North America: disruptive behaviors,* vol 3, no 2, Philadelphia, April 1994, W. B. Saunders.

Sulik LR, Garfinkel BD: Adolescent suicidal behavior: understanding the breadth of the problem. In Lewis M, editor: *Child and adolescent psychiatric clinics of North America: mood disorders,* vol 1, no 1, Philadelphia, July 1992, W. B. Saunders.

CHAPTER 18

Eating Disorders

Anne Clarkin-Watts

Affective instability Rapidly fluctuating moods in which the individual is emotionally reactive to external events and lacks coping skills to manage feeling states.

Anorexia nervosa An eating disorder classified in DSM-IV, characterized by self-starvation, weight loss below minimum normal weight, intense fear of being fat even when emaciated, distorted body image, and amenorrhea in females.

Binge eating disorder (BED) (proposed) A pattern of binge eating without the purging characteristic of bulimia nervosa. BED is commonly known as compulsive overeating. Is included in DSM-IV as a proposed diagnosis for further study.

Body image disturbance A perceptual disturbance in the way an individual's body shape, size, weight, and proportions are subjectively perceived and experienced by him or her. Typically, persons with anorexia complain of feeling "fat" or see their stomach, hips, and thighs as fat when they are clearly underweight.

Bulimarexia An obsession with thinness and dieting and a compulsive cycle of binging and purging. This syndrome is now labeled *bulimia nervosa*.

Bulimia nervosa An eating disorder classified in DSM-IV, characterized by recurrent episodes of binge eating subjectively experienced as out of control, followed by inappropriate compensatory behavior to prevent weight gain, such as self-induced vomiting, overuse of laxatives, diuretics, diet pills, fasting, or excessive exercise. Also present is excessive preoccupation with body shape and weight.

Comorbidity The co-occurrence of two or more psychiatric or other disorders. The simultaneous appearance of the disorders may be due to a causal relationship between the two, an underlying predisposition to both, or the disorders may be completely unrelated. Depression is a common comorbid disorder in clients with eating disorders. There are different theories about the association between eating disorders and mood disorders.

Dichotomous thinking A cognitive distortion common to people with eating disorders, in which an individual views a situation as all or nothing, black or white, all good or all bad. If a situation is less than perfect, it is perceived as a failure.

Enmeshed families A pattern of family relationships in which children are pressured to conform to parental expectations rather than express their individuality. Overinvolvement among family members, discouragement of outside relationships, and blurring of boundaries occur; i.e., a mother will "feel" her daughter's emotions.

Interoceptive deficits Inability to correctly identify and respond to bodily sensations. Individuals with eating disorders are often out of touch with their bodies and either fail to recognize or else mistrust physical sensations such as hunger, satiety, fatigue, or pain, as well as emotional states.

Purging The use of self-induced vomiting, the abuse of laxatives, diuretics, syrup of ipecac, diet pills, or enemas to avoid weight gain following a binge. One or more of these behaviors as well as periods of fasting and excessive exercise during an episode of bulimia nervosa may be used.

Secondary gain Any benefit, such as personal attention or sympathy from others, or escape from unwanted responsibilities, as a result of illness. Individuals with eating disorders may experience secondary gain when family or friends pay a great deal of attention to their eating behavior; i.e., preparing special meals or making special arrangements in an attempt to encourage them to eat.

- Identify the behavioral and psychological symptoms of anorexia nervosa and bulimia nervosa.

- Compare and contrast the medical complications of anorexic and bulimic behavior.

- Analyze the complex interplay of biologic, sociocultural, familial, and psychologic factors that contribute to the etiology of eating disorders.

- Explain the "vicious cycle" of eating disorder behavior.

- Discuss the psychological issues that underlie eating disorder behavior.

- Describe the type of therapeutic relationship that is most effective with clients with eating disorders, including the approach and attitude the nurse should demonstrate to achieve this relationship.

- Apply the nursing process—assessment, diagnosis, outcome identification, planning, implementation, and evaluation—for clients with eating disorders.

E ating disorders have many facets and many causes. Although they have become quite common and are seen in a wide variety of clinical settings, eating disorders are considered to be a relatively new phenomenon. Self-starvation, gorging, and purging behaviors have existed for centuries but, historically, have been rare and poorly understood conditions. The incidence of **anorexia nervosa,** characterized primarily by self-starvation and distorted body image, and **bulimia nervosa,** characterized primarily by binge eating and purging behavior, has increased dramatically in the past quarter-century. With this increase has come a rapidly growing body of literature, including medical research, psychiatric research, psychological literature, and popular press, as well as enormous media attention. This information has helped educate us about eating disorders, but many controversies and conflicts have ensued.

Throughout history, it appears that women have used food as a symbol to express a variety of issues in a variety of contexts. Because food has always been a compelling cultural symbol (of wealth, of nurturing, and of survival), the rejection of food and denial of appetite are always attention-getters.

The increase in eating disorders in the late twentieth century has coincided with three major cultural trends: the fashion industry, the diet and fitness industry, and the women's movement. A trend toward thinness in fashion, the creation of the diet and fitness industry, and the changes in the women's movement have all contributed to the current epidemic of eating disorders. Box 18-1 summarizes these cultural trends.

HISTORICAL AND THEORETICAL PERSPECTIVES

Eating disorders are not just a late twentieth-century fad of young, fashion-conscious American women; they have existed in various forms for hundreds of years. The explosion of written material on eating disorders includes some careful and thorough research into the history of both anorexia nervosa and bulimia nervosa (Bell, 1987; Brumberg, 1989).

Box 18-1   Cultural Trends and Eating Disorders

Fashion Industry

Cultural ideals of beauty have always been reflected in the fashion of the day. The trend in fashion since the 1960s has been more and more toward thinness. In the late twentieth century, fashion has become a huge industry, fueled by advertising dollars, exerting great influence on women. With the media as the vehicle, women are bombarded with images of the thin, fit, "perfect" woman, an ideal unattainable for most women (Fig.18-1). Epidemiological studies show that 0.1% of women have a natural body type that matches the ideal, leading most to believe that their normal, healthy shape is too fat.

Diet and Fitness Industry

The second trend is the birth of the diet and fitness industry. Since the 1950s, weight management has moved out of the doctor's office into multibillion-dollar businesses, which are run by opportunistic entrepreneurs who are not part of the health professions. Again, with the media's help, women are deluged with an array of products, including pills, powders, packaged food, diet books, videos, and a variety of health club and diet program memberships designed to help them attain the perfect body.

Women's Movement

A third trend is the ongoing women's movement. Although women's struggles for equality are not new, women's roles have changed dramatically during the past 20 to 25 years. Pressure to be "superwoman"—to balance motherhood, marriage, and career—is new and has influenced women of all generations. The need for women to achieve academically and professionally while still fulfilling their traditional female roles creates conflicts, even as it affords women greater societal rights and freedom.

Professional women need to be assertive and even aggressive to successfully compete in the business world, yet women are still socialized to be passive and accommodating. Some feminist writers such as Susie Orbach and Susan Wooley view the drive for thinness as possibly symbolizing a woman's attempt to destroy her femininity in order to compete in a man's world or as male society's backlash against the women's movement. Pressuring women to strive for an impossible ideal of thinness may promote feelings of inadequacy that drive women to constantly diet and exercise to please men (Orbach, 1978; Wooley and Wooley, 1985).

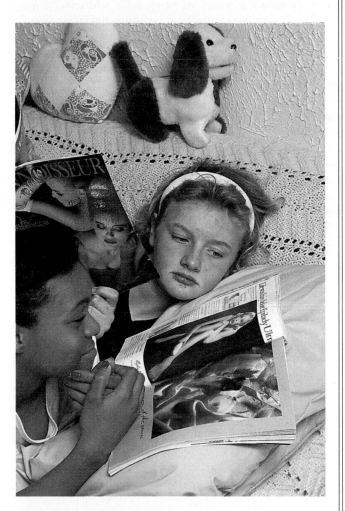

Figure 18-1   Fashion magazines are one example of the media's influence on women's perceptions of themselves.

(Copyright © Cathy Lander-Goldberg, Lander Photographics)

Incidence in History

Brumberg, in *Fasting Girls*, and Bell, in *Holy Anorexia*, note that medieval women commonly starved themselves in devotion to Christ. These women were canonized as miracles of female holiness for their refusal of food, sustaining themselves only on the Christian Eucharist and prayer. Both authors detail the case of Saint Catherine of Siena, Italy (1347–1380), who kept an extensive diary of her fasting and self-induced vomiting. Her piety also included self-flagellation and other self-punishing behavior, not very different from the self-destructive behavior common today among clients with anorexia and bulimia. Medieval physicians called this phenomenon "anorexia mirabilis" (miraculously inspired loss of appetite). Like Catherine, many "holy anorectics" occasionally binged and purged. This demonstrates the intertwining of anorexic and bulimic behaviors from the beginning of their known existence.

Fasting continued in the ensuing centuries in Europe as a demonstration of piety but also of mysticism and magic. Skeptics accused persons with anorexia of Satanism, of witchcraft, and of malingering (Brumberg, 1989).

Many persons with anorexia nervosa binged and purged, but few clinical accounts of normal weight bulimia nervosa existed until the twentieth century when case histories began to appear in psychoanalytical literature. In "The Case of Ellen West," American psychoanalyst Binswanger described a woman he treated in approximately 1915. She dieted from 165 lbs to 92 lbs, but she also binged and purged with excessive exercise, laxative abuse, and self-induced vomiting. She was obsessed with food and clinically depressed, and she committed suicide 13 years later (Binswanger, 1958). In *The Fifty Minute Hour*, psychiatrist Robert Lindner described the case of "Laura," a client with bulimia nervosa.

Since these were psychoanalytical case studies, the writings did not include any discussion of sociocultural or biologic influences but instead focused on the bulimic symptom complex as a manifestation of oral impregnation fears, oral eroticism, rejection of femininity, and unconscious hatred of the mother. A few less well-known case studies noted bulimic behavior among young girls in boarding schools and refugee children (Johnson and Connors, 1987). These cases are clearly related to separation issues, which are a primary factor in the development of bulimia nervosa among college women today.

In the 1950s, binge eating among the overweight and obese population was described as another form of an eating disorder (Hamburger, 1951; Stunkard, 1959). This common condition was compared with alcoholism with similar cravings and secret binges, followed by shame and guilt. The term *compulsive overeating* has been used most commonly to describe this disorder.

In the mid-1970s, psychologist Marlene Boskind-Lodahl coined the term **bulimarexia** to describe a group of women of normal and low-normal weight she saw at Cornell University's mental health clinic, who share the anorectic's fear of fat and drive for thinness but are not emaciated and who regularly binge and purge. In her 1983 book, she describes her extensive clinical experience and groundbreaking research with this group, who represented the first wave of the current outbreak of eating disorders. Bulimarexia has never been formally used as a diagnosis. The DSM-III-R and DSM-IV chose *Bulimia Nervosa* rather than *bulimarexia* for its formal nomenclature (Boskind-Lodahl, 1976; Boskind-Lodahl and White, 1983).

ETIOLOGY

A wide variety of etiological theories regarding eating disorders have been explored. Except for a few extremists, there has been a convergence among many disparate etiological views from biology, sociology, psychoanalysis, and other models to form a new model of eating disorders as multifaceted, multidetermined syndromes. Most of the current literature describes eating disorders as complex, with biological, sociocultural, and psychodynamic variables (Box 18-2).

Box 18-2 Etiological Factors Related to Eating Disorders

Biologic Factors

- Family history of depression
- Tendency to be overweight

Sociocultural Factors

- Diet and fitness industry
- Fashion industry
- Women's movement
- Developmental peer pressure

Psychologic Factors

- Low self-esteem
- Perfectionism
- Affective instability
- Interoceptive deficits
- Ineffectiveness
- Compliance—a "people pleaser"

Familial Factors

- Enmeshment
- Poor conflict resolution
- Separation/individuation issues
- Some incidence of alcoholism or physical or sexual abuse

Biologic Factors

There is a connection between eating disorders and depression. It is generally believed that biogenetic factors predispose individuals to affective illness. Additionally, a biological tendency to be overweight may increase the likelihood of body dissatisfaction and dieting behavior, which, along with other factors, may trigger an eating disorder to develop.

Many researchers have failed in their attempts to find consistent neurological and/or endocrinological markers in clients with eating disorders (Braun and Chouinard, 1992).

Sociocultural Factors

By adolescence the pre-anorexic or pre-bulimic woman has been exposed to countless advertisements, fueled by the diet and fashion industries, that encourage her to eat, dress, and exercise to look beautiful. She has equated food with pleasure, comfort, and love and may have been nurtured, punished, or rewarded with food within her family.

Frequently the person with anorexia nervosa or bulimia nervosa may also have been observing her grandmother's and mother's often unsuccessful struggles to balance all of society's expectations. These include the need to maintain a feminine image and still achieve the superwoman role. Food plays a significant role in this dichotomy. Such conflicting dynamics influence the woman's eating patterns.

Psychologic Factors

Although the same sociocultural pressures challenge all adolescents, only a few, approximately 8%, develop eating disorders. Some teens seem to cope more effectively than others, based on their personalities and support systems. Personality traits common among those with eating disorders include the following:

- perfectionism
- social insecurity
- **affective instability:** rapidly fluctuating moods
- **interoceptive deficits:** inability to correctly identify and respond to bodily sensations
- immaturity
- compliance
- a sense of ineffectiveness in dealing with the world

These traits increase vulnerability to eating disorders. Self-esteem is another important factor. Studies show that individuals diagnosed with eating disorders have lower self-esteem than other diagnostic groups.

Cognitive therapy literature describes certain distorted thinking patterns as characteristic of eating disorders (Bauer and Anderson, 1989). They include **dichotomous thinking** (individuals view situations as either all good or all bad), erroneous control issues (individuals

feel solely responsible for the happiness and failure of others), and personalization (individuals compare themselves endlessly with others and believe everything other people do is a reaction to them).

Familial Factors

Personality characteristics can be partially influenced by family environment. Despite early stereotypes of "eating disorder families" described by family therapist Salvador Minuchin (1978), a clear picture of a "type" of family that has a member with an eating disorder is difficult to portray. They come from all socioeconomic levels, races, and cultures. Some common characteristics do exist in their interactional patterns. The family environments of persons with eating disorders are often tense, rigid, and enmeshed. **Enmeshed families** have poor boundaries, overinvolvement among members, and a pattern of relating in which individuality is discouraged and conformity is expected. These families discourage the direct expression of feeling. They tend to demonstrate poor conflict-resolution skills, in which disagreement may be displayed as denial of conflicts, conflict avoidance, repetitive and unproductive arguments, or escalation to violence. The result is ongoing tension, fear of conflict, and a belief that conflict is bad and dangerous. These families often put a great deal of importance on outward appearance, social acceptance, and achievement. Many family environments include substance abuse, severe mood disorders, and even sexual abuse.

In extremely dysfunctional families, the damage can be severe. Sexual abuse has devastating effects. But even in the families without physical or sexual abuse, the child may not feel encouraged to be independent, to trust herself, or to have confidence in her own individual abilities. She may learn to avoid conflict, to please others, and to fear adult responsibilities. Because she did not learn to be autonomous or independent, adolescence is a crisis. The sense of self never fully developed and the pressures to separate and be an individual in adolescence can be terrifying, not only to the child but also to the parents.

Confronted with this crisis, it is not surprising that a young woman feels overwhelmed. She experiences her life as out of control and desperately wants to feel in control. The myth of thinness as the key to confidence and success portrayed in the diet program advertisement may be very compelling and be perceived as a good way to "get control of my life." The young woman, then, begins dieting, loses weight, and begins to feel better about herself. Consequently, she continues dieting and losing weight, focusing on this as an accomplishment and feels more in control. Unfortunately, this behavior is often reinforced by **secondary gains** such as attention and envy from her peers. Later, when people tell her she is getting too thin and should eat more, she feels a sense of power and control she has never felt before. By losing weight, she not only has gotten attention but also has been able to cause envy and frustrate those who try to make her eat normally. These secondary gains can be very rewarding, especially to an individual with low self-esteem. The diet has thus distracted her from her actual conflicts and given her a sense of mastery, albeit false, which she does not want to give up.

Sometimes a young woman in this situation cannot stick to the diet. Binging often begins as a reaction to the deprivation of dieting. Binge eating not only relieves hunger but also numbs pain and distracts from actual conflicts. It may also represent an angry rebellion against the pressure to be thin. The binge is temporary, however, and the problems soon come back. With them comes guilt about eating, and panic about loss of control and weight gain. So, the young woman purges to undo the binge—and the guilt. Figure 18-2 illustrates the interrelationship of all the etiological factors in the cycle of eating disorders.

EPIDEMIOLOGY

Studies report wide discrepancies in estimates of prevalence of bulimia nervosa. Methodological problems, particularly the criteria used to define bulimia, the low re-

sponse rate of samples, and the use of self-report questionnaires are probably responsible for the discrepancies. Studies using strict DSM-IV criteria estimate that 5%–8% of high-school–age and college-age women and 1% of all males are bulimic. The rate drops to 2% and less than 1% among the general population. Binge eating without purging at least once a week occurs in approximately 5%–20% of all women and slightly fewer men.

The studies of prevalence of anorexia nervosa are less methodologically flawed. A rate of 0.5%–1% in high-school–age and college-age women is more consistently reported. Anorexia nervosa is much less common in males. The incidence and prevalence of eating disorders are summarized in Box 18-3.

Sex Ratio

Eating disorders are predominantly female disorders. Some researchers believe eating disorders are underreported in men, and that men are not encouraged to seek help for what is labeled a "female" problem. Most samples report that 95%–99% of clients with eating disorders are female.

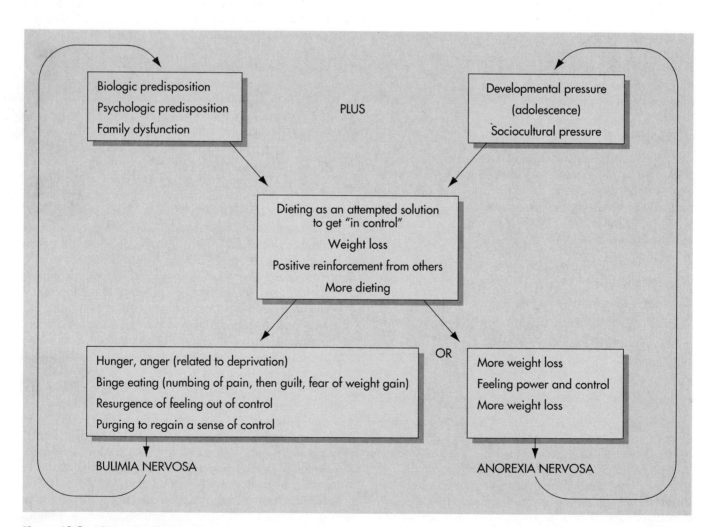

Figure 18-2 The cycle of eating disorders.

Age of Onset

The average age of onset of bulimia nervosa is age 18 with 80% of cases reported with an onset between the ages 15 to 30. In anorexia nervosa, the peak ages of onset are ages 14 and 18. The range of onset ages for both disorders is 9 to 50 years of age.

Cross-Cultural Studies

Incidence and prevalence of eating disorders around the world show similar rates among European countries, United States, Canada, Mexico, Japan, and other westernized countries with plentiful food supplies.

Underdeveloped countries do not show any cases of eating disorders, and it is generally believed that abundance of food is necessary for an outbreak of eating disorders.

In the United States, there is no evidence of any significant differences among racial, ethnic, or socioeconomic groups. There was a gap in past decades, with clients with eating disorders being predominantly white, upper-middle-class women, but this gap has disappeared in more recent studies.

Mortality

In anorexia nervosa, the mortality rate after 10 years is 6% to 7%. After 20 to 30 years it rises to somewhere between 18%–20%. In bulimia nervosa, estimates of mortality range from 0% to 19%. This discrepancy is likely due to the fact that many deaths from purging are recorded as cardiac arrest or cardiomyopathy and never connected directly to bulimia nervosa.

Suicide is frequently the cause of death in persons with eating disorders, occurring in 2% of cases.

Comorbidity

Comorbidity is the concurrent existence of two or more disorders. Eating disorders are often accompanied by other Axis I disorders and by Axis II disorders. The previous section on etiology mentioned the high incidence of depression in eating disorders (50%–80%). Depression seems to occur more frequently with bulimia nervosa than with anorexia nervosa. Less common than depression but also frequently seen in clients with bulimia are generalized anxiety disorders, panic, or substance abuse disorders.

In anorexia nervosa, depressive disorders are also the most frequent Axis I diagnosis, followed by anxiety disorders, especially panic, agoraphobia, social phobia, and obsessive-compulsive disorder (Halmi et al, 1991). Recent studies have begun to look at the incidence of dissociative disorders in clients with eating disorders (Vanderlinden et al, 1993). This is discussed later in this chapter.

Box 18-3   Epidemiology for Eating Disorders

- Average age(s) of onset is 14–18 for anorexia nervosa; 18 for bulimia nervosa.
- 5%–8% of high-school–age and college-age women and 1% of all men have bulimia nervosa.
- 2% of women and less than 1% of men in the general population have bulimia nervosa.
- 5%–20% of the general population (male and female) binge regularly (but do not purge).
- 1% of high-school–age and college-age women have anorexia nervosa. Anorexia nervosa is much less common in males.
- 95%–99% of clients with eating disorders are female.
- Mortality rates for bulimia nervosa are from 0%–19%, for anorexia nervosa, from 6%–20%.
- Similar incidence and prevalence rates are found among western countries; eating disorders are not found in underdeveloped countries.
- Comorbidity:

  Axis I   Mood Disorders

  Anxiety Disorders

  Dissociative Disorders

  Substance-Related Disorders

  Axis II   Borderline Personality Disorder

  Avoidant Personality Disorder

  Obsessive-Compulsive Personality Disorder

Numerous studies have investigated the phenomenon of *comorbid personality,* which is well known to eating disorder clinicians. Varying rates of prevalence of comorbid personality disorders are reported, from one-third to three-fourths of clients with eating disorders having an Axis II diagnosis (Gartner, Marcus, and Halmi, 1989; Herzog et al, 1992.

Borderline Personality Disorder is the Axis II diagnosis most commonly associated with eating disorders, with avoidant and obsessive-compulsive personality disorders also prevalent (Herzog et al, 1992).

In the discussion of eating disorders, borderline personality disorder, and dissociative disorders, the issue of sexual abuse must be raised. Many researchers have investigated a possible link between a history of sexual abuse and the development of eating disorders, borderline personality disorder, and dissociative identity disorder. The media have also focused attention on a possible connection. Well-controlled research studies report a high incidence (25%–30%) of childhood sexual abuse among clients with eating disorders. However, this is not

Understanding and Applying RESEARCH

Levin A et al: Multiple personality in eating disorder patients, *Int J Eat Disord* 13(2):235–239, 1993.

The researchers describe two cases of individuals who presented for inpatient treatment for eating disorders and were subsequently found to have Dissociative Identity Disorder, formerly known as Multiple Personality Disorder in DSM-III-R. The intertwining of the eating disorder symptoms and the dissociative phenomena resulted in an atypical clinical picture for an eating disorder. The authors describe how the diagnosis of Dissociative Identity Disorder (which was the primary Axis I diagnosis) was crucial for the successful treatment of these clients. They also propose that undiagnosed comorbid Dissociative Identity Disorder may be responsible for the refractory course seen in some clients with eating disorders. The authors encourage clinicians to assess for Dissociative Identity Disorder in clients with eating disorders who are resistant to treatment.

a significantly higher incidence than is reported in females in the general psychiatric population. Thus childhood sexual abuse is a risk factor for the development of a psychiatric disorder but not specifically for an eating disorder. However, those clients with eating disorders who had been sexually abused had a higher incidence of comorbid dissociative disorders, obsessive-compulsive disorders, and phobias (Connors and Morse, 1993; Folsom et al, 1993; Waller, 1993).

The phenomenon of dissociative disorders, especially dissociative identity disorder (formerly multiple personality disorder), in clients with eating disorders is a new, quite compelling area of research. Studies are beginning to investigate how a history of sexual (and physical) abuse contributes to the development of an eating disorder, and the ramifications of this phenomenon on treatment. (See Understanding and Applying Research above.)

CLINICAL DESCRIPTION

Eating disorders are an easily recognizable group of psychiatric diagnoses. Refusal to eat, severe weight loss, and self-induced vomiting are unmistakable indicators of an eating disorder. However, making a precise DSM-IV diagnosis and determining specific nursing diagnoses to reflect a particular client's case can be confusing and complicated tasks.

Eating disorders is a relatively new diagnostic category in DSM. This reflects the recent rapid increase in

prevalence from obscurity to a common phenomenon seen by most clinicians in most health care settings. Although there is extensive literature on eating disorders, clinicians and researchers are still learning about the phenomenon. Evolving knowledge is reflected in each revision of DSM criteria. DSM-IV has brought new refinements in eating disorder diagnoses.

Anorexia Nervosa and Bulimia Nervosa are the two specific eating disorder diagnoses in DSM-IV. The Eating Disorder Not Otherwise Specified category (NOS) is provided to diagnose those individuals with eating disorder symptoms that do not meet the criteria for Anorexia Nervosa or Bulimia Nervosa. The box on page 433 details the DSM-IV criteria for these three diagnoses. The clinical symptoms of Anorexia Nervosa and Bulimia Nervosa are listed in the boxes on pages 434 and 435.

Obesity is not included as an eating disorder in DSM-IV because it has not been established that all cases of obesity involve underlying psychiatric illness. In cases where psychologic factors are directly affecting an individual's obesity, this can be classified within DSM-IV as Psychological Factors Affecting Medical Condition. Obesity itself is classified in the International Classification of Diseases (ICD-10) as a general medical condition (APA, 1994).

Inclusion or exclusion of **Binge Eating Disorder** (BED) in DSM-IV has been a controversial issue. Although it was not included in DSM-IV as a separate diagnosis, it is cited as an example of an Eating Disorder Not Otherwise Specified and is included in the DSM-IV classification (Appendix B) as a proposed diagnosis for further study. Further research may lead to its inclusion as a separate eating disorder diagnosis in the next revision of the DSM. BED is described specifically as recurrent episodes of binge eating, in which the individual eats more than most people would during a similar period of time and feels out of control while eating. Specific behavioral indicators for loss of control are included, such as eating when not hungry, eating until uncomfortably full, eating alone due to embarrassment, etc. Other criteria include distress, guilt, and disgust regarding the behavior. A frequency of two binge episodes a week for 6 months is required (APA, 1994; Spitzer et al, 1992, 1993).

Anorexia Nervosa and Bulimia Nervosa are classified as distinct diagnoses but have many overlapping features. In clinical practice, many low-weight persons with anorexia binge and purge occasionally, and many purge small amounts of food but never binge. The subtypes assist the clinician in making the most precise diagnosis. For example, if an individual meets the criteria for both Bulimia Nervosa and Anorexia Nervosa, the diagnosis of Anorexia Nervosa, Binge Eating/Purging Type would be made, because it is the only category that includes ALL of the symptoms (neither subtype of Bulimia Nervosa deals with weight loss).

In clinical practice, the author has counseled several clients with anorexia in their late 30s and 40s who con-

DSM-IV CRITERIA

Eating Disorders

Anorexia Nervosa

A. Refusal to maintain body weight at or above a minimally normal weight for age and height (e.g., weight loss leading to maintenance of body weight less than 85% of that expected; or failure to make expected weight gain during period of growth, leading to body weight less than 85% of that expected).

B. Intense fear of gaining weight or becoming fat, even though underweight.

C. Disturbance in the way in which one's body weight or shape is experienced, undue influence of body weight or shape on self-evaluation, or denial of the seriousness of the current low body weight.

D. In postmenarcheal females, amenorrhea, i.e., the absence of at least three consecutive menstrual cycles. (A woman is considered to have amenorrhea if her periods occur only following hormone, e.g., estrogen, administration.)

Specify type:

Restricting Type: during the current episode of Anorexia Nervosa the person has not regularly engaged in binge-eating or purging behavior (i.e., self-induced vomiting or the misuse of laxatives, diuretics, or enemas)

Binge-Eating/Purging Type: during the current episode of Anorexia Nervosa, the person has regularly engaged in binge-eating or purging behavior (i.e., self-induced vomiting or the misuse of laxatives, diuretics, or enemas)

Bulimia Nervosa

A. Recurrent episodes of binge eating. An episode of binge eating is characterized by both of the following:

1. eating, in a discrete period of time (e.g., within any 2-hour period), an amount of food that is definitely larger than most people would eat during a similar period of time and under similar circumstances

2. a sense of lack of control over eating during the episode (e.g., a feeling that one cannot stop eating or control what or how much one is eating)

B. Recurrent inappropriate compensatory behavior in order to prevent weight gain, such as self-induced vomiting; misuse of laxatives, diuretics, enemas, or other medications; fasting; or excessive exercise.

C. The binge eating and inappropriate compensatory behaviors both occur, on average, at least twice a week for 3 months.

D. Self-evaluation is unduly influenced by body shape and weight.

E. The disturbance does not occur exclusively during episodes of Anorexia Nervosa.

Specify type:

Purging Type: during the current episode of Bulimia Nervosa, the person has regularly engaged in self-induced vomiting or the misuse of laxatives, diuretics, or enemas.

Nonpurging Type: during the current episode of Bulimia Nervosa, the person has used other inappropriate compensatory behaviors, such as fasting or excessive exercise, but has not regularly engaged in self-induced vomiting or the misuse of laxatives, diuretics, or enemas.

Eating Disorder Not Otherwise Specified (NOS)

Disorders of eating that do not meet the criteria for a specific eating disorder. Examples include the following:

1. For females, all of the criteria for Anorexia Nervosa are met except amenorrhea.

2. All of the criteria for Anorexia Nervosa are met except that, despite significant weight loss, the individual's current weight is in the normal range.

3. All the criteria for Bulimia Nervosa are met except that the frequency of binge eating is less than twice a week or the duration has been less than 3 months.

4. Average weight individual who regularly uses inappropriate compensatory behavior but does not binge eat.

5. Repeatedly chewing and spitting out but not swallowing large amounts of food.

6. Binge eating disorder: recurrent episodes of binge eating in the absence of the regular use of inappropriate compensatory behaviors characteristic of Bulimia Nervosa.

From American Psychiatric Association: *Diagnostic and statistical manual of mental disorders,* ed 4, Washington, D.C., 1994.

tinued to menstruate at 70% to 75% of ideal body weight. These cases presented as "classic" cases of Anorexia Nervosa but had to be diagnosed as Eating Disorder Not Otherwise Specified, because the criterion for amenorrhea in Anorexia Nervosa was not met.

PROGNOSIS

The prognosis for eating disorders is considered to be poor as compared to other diagnostic groups. The course of the illness is variable. A few individuals recover fully from a single, time-limited (usually less than a year)

CLINICAL SYMPTOMS

Anorexia Nervosa

Behavioral Symptoms

- Self-starvation—reported intake restriction and refusal to eat
- Rituals or compulsive behaviors regarding food, eating, and/or weight loss
- May engage in self-induced vomiting, laxatives, diuretics, or excessive exercise to lose weight

Physical Symptoms

- Weight loss 15% below ideal weight
- Amenorrhea—absence of three or more menstrual cycles when expected to occur (primary or secondary)
- Slow pulse, decreased body temperature
- Cachexia, sunken eyes, protruding bones, dry skin
- Growth of lanugo on face
- Constipation

Psychological Symptoms

- Denial of the seriousness of current low weight
- Body image disturbance, claiming to see self as fat when emaciated or to experience parts of the body (such as stomach, buttocks, hips, and thighs) as unrealistically large, as depicted in Figure 18-3.
- Intense and irrational fear of weight gain that does not diminish as weight is lost
- Constant striving for "perfect" body
- Self-concept unduly influenced by shape and weight
- Preoccupation with food, cooking, nutritional information, and feeding others
- May exhibit delayed psychosexual development or lack age-appropriate interest in sex and relationships

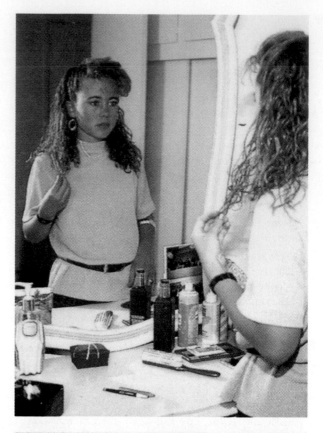

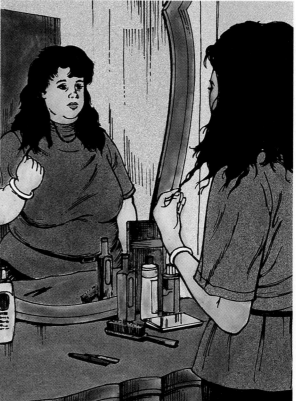

Figure 18-3   Clients with eating disorders have a distorted view of their physical appearance, perceiving themselves as unrealistically large. A) A girl views herself in the mirror. B) The unrealistically large image the girl sees of herself in the mirror.

episode of anorexia nervosa or bulimia nervosa. Some teenagers who become anorexic recover their normal weight within a year but later develop bulimia nervosa. Others with anorexia nervosa follow a chronic course over many years, either remaining at a consistent low weight or slowly deteriorating to lower and lower weights. Others demonstrate an episodic pattern of weight restoration followed by relapse. Bulimia nervosa is commonly episodic, with periods of remission free of binging and purging followed by relapse. A chronic, unremitting course of bulimia nervosa is possible as well.

Since long-term, methodologically sound outcome studies with large samples and good control groups are

CLINICAL SYMPTOMS

Bulimia Nervosa

Behavioral Symptoms

- Recurrent episodes of binge eating (rapid consumption of a large amount of food in a discrete period of time) (Fig. 18-4)
- Engages in purging behavior such as self-induced vomiting, use of laxatives, diuretics, diet pills, ipecac, enemas, excessive exercise, or periods of fasting to compensate for the binge

Physical Symptoms

- May experience fluid and electrolyte imbalances from purging:

    hypokalemia

    alkalosis

    dehydration

- Cardiovascular:

    hypotension

    cardiac arrhythmia/dysrhythmia

    cardiomyopathy

- Endocrine:

    may experience menstrual dysfunction

- Gastrointestinal:

    constipation, diarrhea

    gastroparesis (delayed gastric emptying)

    esophageal reflux, esophagitis

    Mallory-Weiss tears (in esophagus)

- Dental:

    enamel erosion

- Parotid gland enlargement

Psychological Symptoms

- Body image disturbance, seeing self as unrealistically fat when at or near ideal weight or experiencing parts of the body as unrealistically fat or out of proportion
- Persistent overconcern with weight, shape, and proportions
- Constant striving for "perfect" body
- Self-concept unduly influenced by body weight and shape

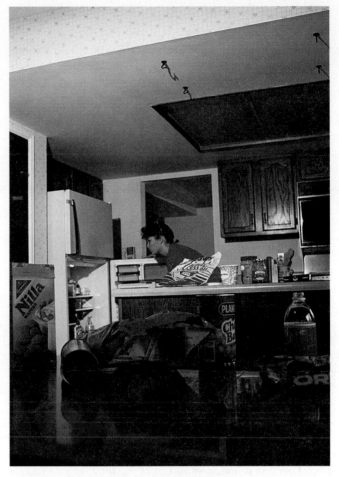

Figure 18-4   Binge eating is a significant symptom of bulimia nervosa.

(Copyright © Cathy Lander-Goldberg, Lander Photographics)

nonexistent, it is difficult to accurately assess prognosis. The existing outcome studies, few and flawed as they are, suggest that multidisciplinary treatment, using cognitive techniques, behavioral techniques, pharmacology, and individual and group therapy, seems to most effectively reduce binge/purge episodes and restore normal weight for the long term (Halmi, 1992; Wilson and Fairburn, 1993).

The discussion of comorbidity indicates that the presence of personality disorders and/or dissociative disorders suggests a much poorer prognosis (Glassman et al, 1990; Levin et al, 1993). Severe depression increases the risk of suicide. Lower weight in both anorexia nervosa and bulimia nervosa and later onset have been associated with poorer prognosis (Glassman et al, 1990).

DISCHARGE CRITERIA

Client will

- Be free from self-harm
- Achieve minimal (within 15%) normal weight as determined by the treatment team

- Consume adequate calories to maintain minimal normal weight

- Demonstrate ability to comply with the treatment regimen recommended for postdischarge (i.e., compliance with medication, food plan, control over binge/purge behavior, plan for follow-up care)

- Verbalize awareness and understanding of the psychological issues related to the eating disorder behavior and the maladaptive use of food and weight control to try to cope with these issues

- Demonstrate the use of improved coping abilities to respond to stress and to manage emotional issues

- Exhibit more functional behaviors within the family system

- Demonstrate decreased enmeshment with family members

- Attend group therapy sessions that encourage healthy eating patterns and positive self-image and self-concept

- Interact with peers who assist client to maintain healthy coping patterns

- Keep appointments to monitor behaviors and medications

Comorbid Disorders Commonly Found in Eating Disorders

Mood disorders

Dysthymic disorder

Major depressive disorder

Anxiety disorders

Generalized anxiety disorder

Agoraphobia

Panic disorder

Social phobia

Obsessive-compulsive disorder

Post-traumatic stress disorder

Dissociative disorders

Dissociative identity disorder

Substance-related disorders

Personality disorders

Borderline personality disorder

Obsessive-compulsive personality disorder

Avoidant personality disorder

THE NURSING PROCESS ■ ■ ■ ■ ■ ■ ■ ■ ■ ■ ■ ■ ■ ■ ■ ■ ■

■ ASSESSMENT

Nursing assessment of clients with eating disorders involves sensitivity, thoroughness, and keen observation skills (Fig. 18-5). The first few minutes of the interview are crucial, since first impressions set the tone for the entire treatment experience. Clients with eating disorders are very sensitive to others and are quick to judge them as trustworthy or not. If a therapeutic alliance can be forged immediately, much of the power struggles can be avoided.

Because many clients with eating disorders have one or more coexisting disorders, it is critical for the nurse to assess for the disorders listed in the box on page 437.

■ ■ NURSING DIAGNOSIS

Nursing diagnoses are made from the information obtained during the assessment phase of the nursing process. The accuracy of diagnosis depends on a careful, in-depth assessment.

NANDA Diagnoses for Anorexia Nervosa

Safety and/or health risks

Risk for self-mutilation

Altered nutrition: less than body requirements

Fluid volume deficit

Perceived constipation or actual constipation

Risk for altered body temperature

Altered growth and development

Perceptual/cognitive/emotional disturbances

Anxiety

Body image disturbance

Self-esteem disturbance

Powerlessness

Hopelessness

Problems in communicating and relating to others

Social isolation

Impaired social interaction

Sexual dysfunction

Disruptions in coping abilities

    Ineffective individual coping
    Ineffective family coping
    Ineffective denial

Client and family teaching needs

    Knowledge deficit regarding nutrition and medical
       side effects of anorexic behavior
    Noncompliance with refeeding process

NANDA Diagnoses for Bulimia Nervosa

Safety and/or health risks

    Risk for self-mutilation
    Altered nutrition: less than body requirements
    Fluid volume deficit
    Perceived constipation or constipation

Perceptual/cognitive/emotional disturbances

    Anxiety
    Body image disturbance
    Self-esteem disturbance
    Powerlessness
    Hopelessness

Problems in communicating and relating to others

    Social isolation
    Impaired social interaction
    Sexual dysfunction

CASE STUDY

Sarah is a 20-year-old college student who was brought to the emergency room by her boyfriend after she fainted in the shower. The boyfriend took the nurse aside and confided that Sarah was bulimic and that he was concerned that her eating disorder was related to the fainting episode. He went on to say that Sarah was very secretive and somewhat defensive about the bulimia. The initial physical exam of Sarah showed no injuries from the fall and her vital signs were normal. Her parotid glands appeared enlarged. Her weight appeared within a normal range. Her affect was tense and anxious. She avoided eye contact with the nurse and mumbled that she had been up late recently studying and had not been getting enough sleep.

Critical Thinking and Assessment

1. How should the nurse approach Sarah? How can the subject of bulimia nervosa be brought up?

2. If Sarah responds defensively or with denial, how should the nurse respond?

3. What further physical assessments should be done?

4. What other information is needed to complete the nursing assessment?

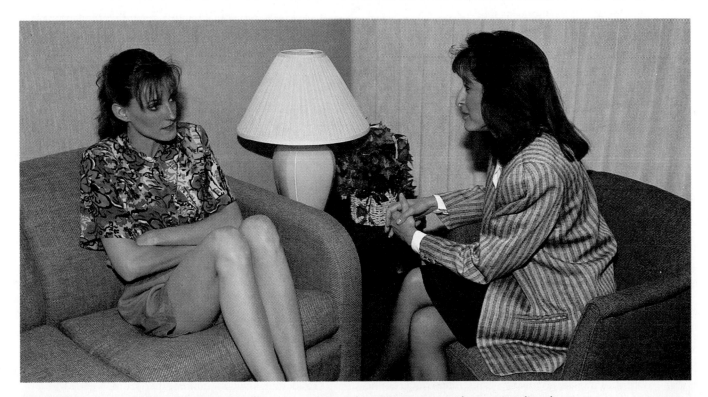

Figure 18-5 An initial assessment interview between a nurse and a young woman with an eating disorder.

(Copyright © Cathy Lander-Goldberg, Lander Photographics)

Nursing Assessment Questions

Eating Disorders

1. "How do you feel about being here today?"
   (To determine if self-referred or forced into treatment and to assess willingness to engage in treatment)

2. "Have you ever talked with anyone before about your eating disorder?"
   (To assess level of self-disclosure and to reduce anxiety and feelings of shame)

3. "Have you been in therapy before?"
   (To assess treatment history and get details of previous treatment, including the name of clinician, dates of treatment, outcomes, and client's experience of the treatment)

4. "Describe your weight throughout your life."
   (To determine patterns and perceptions regarding weight)

   Include the following:

   Current weight—including fluctuations during past 6 months

   Desired weight

   Lowest and highest adult weight (excluding pregnancy)

   Lowest and highest adolescent weight

   Perception of childhood weight

   Perception of adolescent weight

   Perception of present weight

   Childhood experiences related to weight

5. "How do you feel about the way your body looks?"
   (To assess body dissatisfaction and body image distortion)

6. Assess dieting history:

   "When did you first diet?"

   "What started it?"

   "What happened?"

   "Did you lose/gain?"

   "Has anyone encouraged you to lose weight?"

   "What dieting behaviors have you used?"
   (To determine use of fasting, structured diet, restriction, diet products/programs)

7. Assess binge eating:

   "Do you binge eat?"

   "When was the first time?"
   (Get details about typical binge eating, including when, where, duration, frequency, type and amount of food, any rituals or patterns involved)

   Ask if secrecy, hiding, stealing, or lying is involved.
   (To determine use of fasting, structured diet, restriction, diet products/programs)

8. Help client identify feeling states associated with the binge: before binging, in the planning stages, and during and after the binge
   (Ask client to focus on past binge episodes to answer this question, help client to identify feelings "Did you feel angry? Anxious?", etc.)
   (To determine client's feelings regarding binge behaviors)

9. Assess food cravings:
   Time of day, weekends, where in menstrual cycle, associated with places (car, work, home, store)
   (To determine if client can associate dysfunctions with specific times/situations)

10. Assess purging behavior:
    (To identify client's usual methods of purging)

Type:	Frequency: (Times/week)	Amount:	First used: (Age)	Last used: (Date)
Vomiting				
Diuretics				
Laxatives				
Diet pills				
Ipecac				
Thyroid pills				
Amphetamines				
Cocaine				
Exercise				

11. Assess menstrual history:
    (Onset of menses, regularity, PMS, menstrual dysfunction, any hormone therapy)
    (To determine effect of dysfunctional behaviors on menses)

12. Assess medical side effects of eating disorder
    (To identify any concomitant medical problems)

13. Assess comorbidity

Disruptions in coping abilities

Ineffective individual coping
Ineffective family coping

Client and family teaching

Knowledge deficit regarding nutrition, side effects of bulimic behavior
Noncompliance with treatment program

■ ■ ■ OUTCOME IDENTIFICATION

Outcome criteria are derived from nursing diagnoses and are the expected client responses to be achieved.

Outcome Identification for Anorexia Nervosa

Client will

1. Participate in therapeutic contact with staff
2. Consume adequate calories for age, height, and metabolic need
3. Achieve minimum normal weight
4. Maintain normal fluid and electrolyte levels
5. Resume normal menstrual cycle
6. Demonstrate improvement in body image with more realistic view of body shape and size
7. Demonstrate more effective coping skills to deal with conflicts
8. Manage family dysfunction more effectively
9. Verbalize awareness of underlying psychological issues
10. Achieve ideal body weight for age, height, and metabolic need
11. Perceive body weight and shape as normal and acceptable
12. Resume sexual interest and age-appropriate sexual behavior

13. Demonstrate absence of food rituals, preoccupation with food, or fears of food
14. Resolve family issues

Outcome Identification for Bulimia Nervosa

Client will

1. Participate in therapeutic contact with staff
2. Maintain normal fluid and electrolyte levels
3. Consume adequate calories for age, height, and metabolic need
4. Cease binge/purge episodes while in inpatient setting
5. Demonstrate more effective coping skills to deal with conflicts
6. Manage family dysfunction more effectively
7. Verbalize awareness of underlying psychological issues
8. Cease binge/purge episodes completely, cease dieting behavior
9. Perceive body shape and weight as normal and acceptable
10. Resolve family and other underlying issues

COLLABORATIVE DIAGNOSES

DSM-IV Diagnoses*	NANDA Diagnoses**
Anorexia Nervosa	Altered nutrition: less than body requirements
	Body image disturbance
	Anxiety
	Social isolation
Bulimia Nervosa	Fluid volume deficit
	Self-esteem disturbance
	Ineffective individual coping

*From American Psychiatric Association: *Diagnostic and statistical manual of mental disorders,* ed 4, Washington, D.C., 1994, APA.

**From North American Nursing Diagnosis Association: *NANDA nursing diagnoses: definitions and classifications 1995-1996,* Philadelphia, 1994.

CASE 📓 STUDY

Laura is a 27-year-old married mother of a 3-year-old child. Laura is hospitalized following a suicide attempt, in which she overdosed on a combination of 100 laxatives and a full bottle of her antidepressant medication. She is currently seeing a psychiatrist for depression and bulimia nervosa. The nursing assessment reveals that Laura currently binges and purges up to three times per day. Purging consists of self-induced vomiting as well as the use of laxatives (usually 5 or 6 pills every day). She is within normal weight range at 140 lb at 5'9". Laura is participating in milieu activities willingly, although her affect is depressed. She is eating very little at meals and has agreed not to purge while in the hospital.

Critical Thinking and Outcome Identification

1. How will the nurse determine Laura's therapeutic involvement with staff and peers?
2. What are realistic expectations of Laura for eating regular meals? What data should be monitored to track her improvement in nutritional status?
3. How will the nurse recognize improvements in eating behavior and cessation of purging?
4. How will Laura demonstrate awareness of the psychologic issues underlying her bulimia?

■ ■ ■ ■ PLANNING

The nurse's attitude toward the client with an eating disorder is as critical in the plan of care as any specific therapeutic intervention. Clients with eating disorders appear fragile, and although they are vulnerable, they can also be quite rigid and frustrating. If a good working alliance is not formed, with the nurse taking a firm, yet compassionate approach, client care quickly turns into a series of power struggles and the treatment is doomed to fail. Therefore the plan of care will include consistent, collaborative efforts by client, family, and interdisciplinary staff.

■ ■ ■ ■ ■ IMPLEMENTATION

For the client with an eating disorder, the nurse needs to implement a balanced plan of action that includes behavioral interventions to interrupt the cycle of eating disorder behavior. Psychological interventions are used to improve coping skills, communication skills, and insight into underlying issues. Implementation of the plan will provide a safe, structured environment to prevent self-harm; promote weight gain and/or nutritional restoration; help the client express in words what she is acting out with the behavior; teach more effective coping skills, monitor the use of medications, and coordinate the multidisciplinary efforts of the treatment team. Specific issues faced by a community nurse working with a client with eating disorders are discussed in Nursing Care in the Community below.

Nursing Interventions

1. Provide safety and prevent violence by providing a safe environment.

   Assess any risk of suicide (suicide ideation, gesture, plan) *to prevent self-harm* (see care plan on suicide in Chapter 24).

2. Engage the client in a therapeutic alliance *to encourage expression of thoughts and feelings, especially any self-destructive urges.*

3. Restore minimal weight and nutritional balance through a behavioral program *to promote health and wellness.*

   Anorexia includes refeeding with food, food supplements, and tube feeding when necessary.

   Bulimia includes eating meals prescribed by dietitian and avoidance of purging by nurse remaining with the client for at least one hour after each meal.

4. Create a structured, supportive environment with clear, consistent, firm limits *to help establish a predictable routine and promote internal locus of control that the client now lacks.*

Nursing Care in the Community

Persons with Eating Disorders

The most overt problems encountered in community nursing with a client with an eating disorder involve the potential for a power struggle over the client's participation in a treatment regimen. It is not possible for the community mental health nurse to continually observe the client's eating patterns, including starvation and self-induced vomiting. The client may have learned to be somewhat evasive about his or her real intent or emotions. He or she may say the "right" thing, what the nurse wants him or her to say, which confuses the issue. Only if the client's physical state deteriorates does the nurse obtain a clear picture of what is actually occurring.

The nurse must use the observations of family, friends, and other professionals to validate the reports of the client. This may be achieved by offering support groups not only for the clients themselves but also for their families and significant others. The nurse can suggest to these persons how to support the client in reality testing and offer encouragement rather than criticism. They must be educated about the signs of the disorder, potential problems, and suggestions for positive changes in communication dynamics.

The community nurse plans interventions to empower the client to participate effectively in treatment. A written contract may be an effective tool to give the client a feeling of involvement. Clients may be taught to identify situations that have been problematic for them in the past. They must know that help is readily available and be able to stop their habitual patterns to ask for help. The nurse can teach coping skills to an individual or to groups. Bonding techniques can be taught to further the support group of the client, especially those clients in their teens or early twenties, who are most in need of a comforting peer group.

The nurse must be aware of community support groups for clients with anorexia nervosa and bulimia nervosa. Overeaters Anonymous (OA) often has affiliated groups for persons with other eating disorders. OA is an effective resource for those suffering from all types of eating disorders. Clients may concurrently be experiencing depression, requiring antidepressant medication that must be monitored for effectiveness and side effects. As in any prolonged illness, hospitalization must always be an option if the client's eating disorder behaviors become life-threatening.

5. Construct a behavioral plan that includes weight-gain goals, specific eating goals (eating 75% of all meals), and consequences for compliance (preferably increased privileges for compliance rather than punishment for noncompliance. *Structure helps the client gain self-control and reduces the anxiety generated by noncompliance and unpredictable routine.*

6. Encourage the client to express thoughts, feelings, and concerns about body and body image. *Verbalization helps to solidify concerns and helps the client to transform a pervasive sense of shame, guilt, and fear into specific areas of conflict, and clarifies the underlying issues (intimacy, sex, adult responsibility).*

7. Continue to help the client increase understanding of body image distortion. *The goal is for the client to recognize that preoccupation with breasts, hips, stomach, legs, etc., actually symbolizes underlying issues that will not resolve by changing her body.*

8. Assist the client to recall positive eating experiences, such as a time when client was able to eat a small portion of sweets and stop without binging *to emphasize the fact that the client is capable of engaging in successful episodes of eating, and to promote hope.*

9. Assume a caring yet matter-of-fact approach without being overly sympathetic or overly confrontive and authoritarian *to assist the client to maintain clear boundaries and to avoid power struggles.*

10. Intervene with the client's anxiety by helping the client associate feelings of anxiety with unmet needs and expectations that may represent threats to the self-system. *The client's recognition that anxiety can be the result of unconscious conflicts can in itself bring relief and start the process of problem solving.*

11. Offer positive feedback and praise when the client adheres to the treatment plan and strives to maintain the goals of the individual contract. *Praise increases self-esteem, promotes compliance, and encourages repetition of positive behaviors.*

    Examples:

    "You have maintained your weight for 3 days."

    "You listen attentively in group."

12. Engage the client in therapeutic interactions and groups:

    Individual Therapy

    Group Therapy

    Family Therapy

    Occupational/Recreational Therapy

    to express feelings and conflicts engendered by eating disorder behaviors in a supportive environ-

ment, and reduce/rechannel anxiety in a more structured and meaningful way.

13. Assist the client to identify issues of low self-esteem, separation, family dysfunction, and fear of maturity *to uncover and process the psychologic conflicts that underlie the eating disorder.*

14. Discuss with the client how obsession with food and weight helps the client avoid more difficult life problems and challenges *to assist the client to increase awareness and gain insight about the dynamics of the disorder.*

15. Collaborate with the dietitian to provide information to the client about adequate nutrition for the client's height and body type *to counter erroneous information about ideal weight and size and provide education regarding cultural pressures to be unrealistically thin.*

16. Collaborate with the social worker, family therapist, physician, and other members of the interdisciplinary team *to promote consistency in implementing the treatment plan.*

17. Teach adaptive therapeutic strategies (cognitive, behavioral, assertive) *to promote realistic thoughts, feelings, and behaviors and help the client to realize that it is irrational to believe that losing weight will solve his or her problems.*

18. Teach the client, family, and significant others about the disorder, symptom management, and prevention. *Knowledge promotes power and control and reduces fear and anxiety.*

19. Educate the family about healthy boundaries and normal separation and individuation vs. overprotectiveness and family enmeshment *to help the family relinquish unnecessary controls and promote mutually satisfying interpersonal relationships among family members.* (See Client and Family Teaching Guidelines on page 442.)

CLINICAL ALERT !

Purging

If the client is compliant with his or her contract but does not make expected weight gain, the nurse may suspect the client is purging and report this to the treatment team, who may recommend that the nurse confront the client with his or her purging behaviors. Increased supervision after meals and during administration of supplements to prevent purging will follow. The nurse remains in the room with the client for an hour following eating or has the client sit at the nursing station for that time period. The contract may be amended to include these changes. If weight gain does not occur in a few days, tube feeding may be initiated.

Eating Disorders

Teach the client's family members:

To not focus exclusively on the client's weight and food intake as indicators of progress. Help them to understand that eating disorder behaviors are symptomatic of underlying psychologic issues. Specify and explain common underlying issues such as low self-esteem, separation/individuation conflicts, fear of maturity, and conflict avoidance.

To encourage the client to share what she has learned in group and individual therapy regarding the particular psychologic issues underlying the eating disorder.

To encourage the client to verbalize thoughts and feelings about family interactions that she may previously have been fearful or reluctant to disclose directly.

To relinquish control over the client's behavior; to stop monitoring what, when, and/or how much she eats and what she weighs.

To understand how their monitoring and controlling behaviors serve to reinforce the eating disorder behavior by setting up a power struggle in which the client feels controlled and rebels against this indirectly by worsening her behavior.

Teach the client:

To stop acting out conflicts and feelings with the eating disorder behavior. To stop trying to get needs met indirectly through behaviors, but rather to identify and verbalize conflicts, needs, and feelings.

To express thoughts and feelings verbally in group and one-to-one interactions. To transform diffuse feelings of guilt, anxiety, fear, emptiness, and sadness into concrete concerns. These feelings are expressed as experiences related to the body, and about being fat. Ask the client to be very specific about the feeling: "What specifically are you afraid will happen?" or "When you say 'I'm freaking out' what thoughts are going through your head?"

Additional Treatment Modalities

Biologic

Clients with anorexia who are more than 15% below ideal body weight should be closely monitored medically. After the initial assessment and treatment for effects of starvation such as amenorrhea, osteoporosis, and vitamin and mineral deficiencies, the client should be closely monitored while refeeding takes place.

Clients with bulimia need to be initially assessed for acute fluid and electrolyte imbalance and for any of the

ADDITIONAL TREATMENT MODALITIES

Biologic
Pharmacological
Psychotherapeutic

- Individual psychotherapy
- Behavioral therapy
- Cognitive therapy
- Family therapy
- Group therapy
- Expressive therapies

Adjunctive therapy

- Occupational therapy
- Nutrition education and counseling

Social Work

- Interdisciplinary treatment team
- Community support groups

dangerous side effects related to their individual purging behaviors. If purging is not completely stopped during treatment, the electrolytes need to be continually monitored.

There are many other accepted modalities of treatment for eating disorders. These are listed in the box above and are discussed in the following section.

Pharmacologic

Tricyclic antidepressants and, more recently, selective serotonin reuptake inhibitors (SSRIs) such as fluoxetine (Prozac), sertraline (Zoloft), and paroxetine (Paxil) have been effective in treating the comorbid eating disorder/affective disorder (Pope and Hudson, 1984). The dosage of SSRIs needed to obtain decreased binge urges, known as the "anti-bulimic" effect, is usually 60 mg or more (Devlin and Walsh, 1989). Buproprion (Wellbutrin) is contraindicated with bulimia nervosa because of high incidence of seizures during clinical trials.

Antipsychotics may be used for extreme agitation or in clients exhibiting psychotic symptoms. Antianxiety medications are avoided due to their addictive qualities and also because clients with eating disorders need to learn to tolerate and cope with their anxiety rather than avoid it.

Often the medical side effects of eating disorders require the use of medication. Hypokalemia may be treated with potassium supplements, either orally or intravenously. Nutritional anemia may be treated with iron supplements. Gastroparesis, or delayed gastric emptying, may be treated with metoclopramide (Reglan). Infected parotid glands may be treated with antibiotics. Laxative dependence is often treated with a combination of stool softeners, bran, fiber, fluids, and decreasing doses of laxatives

NURSING CARE PLAN ■ ■ ■ ■ ■ ■ ■   ■ ■ ■ ■ ■ ■

Melissa is a 19-year-old college freshman who is hospitalized for severe cachexia (95 lb at 5'7") with hypokalemia, nutritional anemia, and cardiac disrhythmia. She had arrived home after flunking out of her first semester at college, and her parents, who had not seen her in several months, immediately took her to the family doctor who hospitalized her. Melissa's doctor reports that she has been dieting and excessively exercising for the past 2 years but that she had always kept her weight within 10% of ideal body weight and that she had been in individual psychotherapy for a year before going to college. Melissa now states that she did not continue with therapy in college, as she had promised. Melissa minimizes her weight loss, complains of feeling fat, is sullen and angry, and wants to be discharged.

DSM-IV Diagnoses

AXIS I   Anorexia Nervosa, Binge-Eating/Purging Type

AXIS II   R/O Borderline Personality Disorder

AXIS III   Deferred

AXIS IV   3 Moderate: move away from home to college

AXIS V   GAF = 50 on admission, 65 within past year

Nursing Diagnosis: Altered nutrition, less than body requirements, related to self-starvation, possible purging behavior, as evidenced by severe weight loss, hypokalemia, and cardiac disrhythmia.

Client Outcomes	Nursing Interventions	Evaluation
• Melissa will consume adequate calories for age, height, and metabolic need (e.g., 75% of each meal will be consumed by the end of the hospital stay).	• Initiate refeeding, in collaboration with treatment team (Box 18-4). *Starving behavior is out of control and Melissa cannot begin eating again on her own.*	• Melissa ate only 25% of meals on Day 1, but on Day 2, she ate 50% and drank all three dietary supplements. After 7 days, she was eating 75% of all meals and the supplements were discontinued.
	• Encourage Melissa to choose her own menu. *Melissa may be more cooperative if she feels she has some control over the refeeding process.*	• Melissa selected her own meals on Day 3.
• Melissa will achieve minimal normal weight (less than 15% below ideal weight: for 5'7", approximately 115 lb).	• Weigh daily with back facing the scale. *Melissa's obsession with weight may be reinforced by her knowledge of daily weight changes. Not knowing may help her tolerate weight gain and help her to let go of her overcontrol of her body.*	• Melissa achieved her goal weight by discharge.
• Melissa will gain an average of 4 lb per week.	• Continue to implement the refeeding plan and contract as needed *to maintain client's expected weight.*	

Nursing Diagnosis: Body image disturbance, related to underlying psychological conflicts (fear of growing up, fear of sexuality) as evidenced by complaints of body dissatisfaction, fear of weight gain, and minimizing weight loss when more than 15% below minimal normal weight (e.g., 95 lb at 5'7").

Client Outcomes	Nursing Interventions	Evaluation
• Melissa will demonstrate realistic perceptions of body shape and size.	• Encourage expression of thoughts and feelings regarding body. *Verbalizing specific concerns may help Melissa uncover psychologic issues related to her body image.*	• Client verbalized awareness that she is underweight and that her dissatisfaction with her body has to do more with psychologic issues than with her weight.
• Melissa will demonstrate increased insight into body image distortion.	• Collaborate with dietitian to give fact-based information to counter irrational beliefs about body size and shape, e.g., "You are 20 lb below minimum healthy weight for your age and height," *to provide reality orientation of discrepancy between ideal weight and current weight.*	• Melissa verbalized that she perceives herself as heavier than her actual weight.

NURSING CARE PLAN

Client Outcomes	Nursing Interventions	Evaluation
• Melissa will demonstrate an enhanced self-concept based on positive attributes, rather than totally based on her body shape.	• Give Melissa feedback regarding positive qualities that she demonstrates in the milieu. *Melissa's self-concept is overly defined by her body, and she needs to view herself more realistically.*	• Melissa verbalized positive qualities about herself that were unrelated to her body.

Nursing Diagnosis: Noncompliance with the treatment plan, related to underlying psychologic conflicts (control issues or separation issues), as evidenced by anger, refusal to self-disclose to the staff, and requests to be discharged.

Client Outcomes	Nursing Interventions	Evaluation
• Melissa will participate in therapeutic contacts with staff.	• Engage Melissa in therapeutic alliance. Example: using Melissa's input to develop a collaborative treatment plan. *Including Melissa as a part of the treatment team increases her power base and decreases power struggles, strengthening the therapeutic alliance.*	• Melissa participated as part of the treatment team.
• Melissa will comply with the interdisciplinary treatment plan.	• Use interdisciplinary-designed contracts, with clear expectations and consequences, *to increase client compliance and further reduce power struggles.*	• Melissa complied with the expectations of her behavioral contract.
• Melissa will acknowledge her condition and the need for treatment.	• Use reality orientation to challenge Melissa's minimization of the seriousness of her condition. Give information about lab results, medical status, etc. *Melissa's denial will decrease when challenged with concrete information.*	• Melissa verbalized awareness of the need for hospitalization and treatment.

Box 18-4   Refeeding Procedure

If Melissa does not eat 75% of her meals on Day 1, she will receive three dietary supplements on Day 2. Supplements will continue daily until she eats 75% of her meals. If she does not finish her supplements on Day 2, she will be tube fed on Day 3. Tube feeding will continue until she eats 75% of all meals for 1 day.

(if taking very high doses, such as 50 to 100 laxatives at a time, abrupt withdrawal is quite dangerous and gradual withdrawal is done under close supervision.)

Psychotherapeutic

Individual Psychotherapy   Some type of individual psychotherapy is generally recommended as the preferred treatment for eating disorders. Psychodynamically oriented therapists recommend long-term, insight-oriented therapy to repair early developmental failures or traumas, which are seen as primary etiological factors. All but the most conservative psychoanalytical therapists, however, do recommend an active therapeutic stance and encourage the use of behavioral techniques for symptom management and cognitive restructuring to alter distorted thinking patterns.

Cognitive therapists are more likely to recommend structured, short-term individual therapy with less insight orientation and more focus on thought patterns.

Most therapists, whatever their orientation, use hospitalization as a means to manage acute exacerbations of either the eating disorder symptoms or concomitant affective disorder symptoms.

Behavioral Therapy   Either within the context of individual outpatient therapy or in a hospital setting, behavioral therapy is used for symptom management. Behavioral contracts for weight gain, for regulating eating behavior, and for diminishing binge/purge behaviors are commonly used tools in inpatient and outpatient treatment. Exposure plus response prevention, in which clients eat "scary" or binge foods and are then prevented from purging, is an effective intervention for bulimia nervosa.

Cognitive Therapy   Most treatment programs and therapists mention the use of cognitive therapy in the treatment of eating disorders. Most clients demonstrate distorted thoughts and beliefs related to food and weight as well as to self-concept. Techniques such as reframing, cognitive restructuring, and rational-emotive therapy are commonly used to alter these cognitive distortions.

Family Therapy Adolescents with eating disorders almost always participate in family therapy as part of their treatment. Educating the family about eating disorders is very important, as the eating disorder behavior often becomes the focal point of the family, leading to overinvolvement and constant power struggles that inadvertently reinforce the behavior. Families may cater to individuals with eating disorders by buying and preparing separate meals for them, by not expecting them to adhere to family rules regarding meals, and even by not setting age-appropriate limits for them. This may represent a well-intentioned attempt to decrease their stress levels in hopes that they will then stop the eating disorder behavior. Unfortunately, individuals may welcome this extra nurturing and escape from responsibility, experiencing this as a benefit of the eating disorder behavior. Decreasing these secondary gains and uncovering any underlying family dysfunction are the initial goals of family therapy. Improving family interactions and interrelationships are goals for the longer term.

Group Therapy Group psychotherapy is widely used in both inpatient and outpatient settings for the treatment of eating disorders. The rationale is twofold. Clients with anorexia and bulimia often set themselves apart from others with their unusual stance toward food and eating, resulting in secretiveness, feeling misunderstood, and secondary gains related to feeling "special." Being in a group with others with eating disorders allows them a safe place to self-disclose and be accepted/understood, while preventing manipulation and secondary gains related to being "different."

Expressive Therapies Art therapy, music therapy, dance/movement therapy, journal writing, and poetry are often used as part of a multidisciplinary approach to eating disorders. Because the eating disorder symptoms are an indirect expression, on a physical level, of emotional pain, many clients have great difficulty translating their pain into the words needed for "talking" therapy. The use of nonverbal techniques may allow for greater self-disclosure and exploration of underlying issues.

Adjunctive Therapy

Occupational Therapy Many clients with eating disorders need assistance in learning how to plan meals, shop, and cook for themselves, especially if they have not eaten properly for many years. Although the dietitian will do the actual meal planning, occupational therapy can help the client carry out the plan.

Nutrition Education and Counseling Although clients with eating disorders are obsessed with food, most have inaccurate, outdated, or distorted information about nutrition. Consultation with a registered dietitian in both inpatient and outpatient settings is an important part of treatment. The dietitian should be the one to calculate the client's ideal weight range, plan a refeeding program, and supervise meal planning. The dietitian can provide nutritional counseling and assist the client with meal planning on an ongoing basis.

Social Work

Clients with chronic eating disorders often do not function well in society. Hospital social workers can be helpful in finding community resources for those clients needing help with day treatment services, alternative living situations such as Board and Care homes, group homes, residential treatment facilities, or vocational rehabilitation. Social workers are also often used to provide family therapy.

Interdisciplinary Treatment Team

An interdisciplinary approach to treatment is recommended for eating disorders. In both inpatient and outpatient settings, a successful treatment outcome depends on the collaboration of nursing, medical, psychiatric, psychological, dietary, social work, counseling, and occupational therapy professionals. Different clinical settings employ varying combinations of disciplines (some use psychiatric nurses, psychologists, and occupational

---

CASE STUDY

Eileen is a 16-year-old young woman admitted to the hospital for increasingly out-of-control bulimic symptoms, including binging and purging up to 10 times a day and abuse of laxatives.

During her first week of hospitalization, the primary focus was correcting Eileen's fluid and electrolyte balance and monitoring her to prevent purging. Eileen slept a great deal her first week. She participated superficially in group sessions, complaining mainly of physical discomfort related to stopping purging and laxatives. During the second week of treatment, the team set goals to help Eileen become "more involved" in the psychologic issues related to her bulimia. The interventions included encouraging Eileen to work on underlying issues of self-esteem and family dysfunction.

Critical Thinking and Evaluation

1. How will the nurse evaluate Eileen's progress in working on underlying issues? What are three specific client outcomes that would indicate such progress?

2. What specific observations should the nurse make during group sessions to evaluate Eileen's progress?

3. What verbalizations made by Eileen would indicate progress in her work on "underlying issues"?

therapists but no social workers, etc.), so the exact composition of the treatment team may vary. Nurses are often called on to provide services of other disciplines that are not represented in a particular setting, such as doing discharge planning or family education if no social workers are available. Clinical specialists often co-facilitate group therapy with mental health workers or with other nurses. Nurses are usually the coordinators of the multidisciplinary team as well.

Interdisciplinary treatment team meetings are the recommended forum for sharing assessment information and developing the multidisciplinary treatment plan. Nurses are usually the ones who coordinate this plan and see that it is implemented. As the health care system changes and managed care takes over more of the mental health care industry, hospital stays become shorter and specialty units such as eating disorder units may disappear. Clients with eating disorders are more likely to be admitted to general psychiatric units or even medical units. Nursing is thus taking more of a leadership role in the coordination of the treatment team.

Community Support Groups

Community-based support and self-help groups are available in some areas. Overeaters Anonymous, a 12-step program, can be very useful for individuals with binge

eating disorder. National nonprofit organizations such as Anorexia Nervosa and Associated Disorders (ANAD) and Anorexia Bulimia Care (ABC) provide support groups for people with anorexia nervosa and bulimia nervosa. Names and addresses of other organizations providing help for eating disorders can be found in Appendix C.

■ ■ ■ ■ ■ ■ EVALUATION

The nurse will evaluate the progress of the client with an eating disorder in an organized, timely manner in accordance with the outcomes delineated in the care plan. For the client with an eating disorder, the evaluation will include physiologic, behavioral, psychologic, and social spheres. Monitoring lab values, vital signs, weight, and food/fluid intake will provide the data to evaluate physiological responses to treatment. Observing and recording the client's affect, level of program participation, specific eating behaviors, peer interactions, and responses to staff provide evaluative data to track behavioral responses to treatment. Listening to and interacting with the client in group therapy, milieu activities, and during individual interactions regarding specific issues, the treatment plan, or contract provides more data to evaluate the client's psychologic and behavioral responses to treatment.

Summary of Key Concepts

1. Eating disorders are syndromes with physiological, behavioral, and psychological features.

2. Self-starvation, binge eating, and purging behaviors have existed for many centuries, having various psychological meanings in different cultural eras. Until recently, eating disorders were a rare occurrence.

3. The recent outbreak of eating disorders is related to current cultural trends in the fashion industry, the diet industry, and the women's movement.

4. Eating disorders have a multidetermined etiology, including biologic, sociocultural, psychologic, and familial factors.

5. There is a high incidence of depression among clients with eating disorders and their families. It is believed that some biological link may exist between the two disorders.

6. Personality traits common among those with eating disorders include low self-esteem, perfectionism, affective instability, interoceptive deficits, ineffectiveness, and people pleasing.

7. Common dynamics of families of origin of persons with eating disorders include enmeshment, poor conflict resolution, and incomplete separation and may include alcoholism and physical or sexual abuse.

8. Ninety-five to 99% of individuals with eating disorders are female. Bulimia nervosa is more common

than anorexia nervosa. Eating disorders are most common among high-school and college students.

9. Clients with eating disorders often have other psychiatric diagnoses. Common Axis I diagnoses are depressive, anxiety, and dissociative disorders. Common Axis II diagnoses are borderline, avoidant, and obsessive-compulsive personality disorders.

10. Anorexia Nervosa and Bulimia Nervosa are distinct diagnoses in DSM-IV but have many overlapping features.

11. Prognosis for eating disorders is considered poor. The course of the illness may be chronic or episodic, requiring long-term or repeated treatment episodes.

12. Interdisciplinary treatment is indicated to deal with the multifaceted nature of eating disorders.

13. Medical complications from eating disorders can be life threatening. Self-induced vomiting and abuse of laxatives and diuretics can cause serious electrolyte imbalances that may lead to cardiac disrhythmias and cardiac arrest.

14. The nurse must take a firm, professional, yet compassionate approach to avoid the power struggles that commonly undermine treatment of individuals with eating disorders.

15. The plan of care must balance behavioral interventions that interrupt the cycle of behavior with psychologic interventions that deal with underlying issues.

16. A safe, structured environment must be provided to prevent self-harm, promote nutritional restoration, help the client understand the meaning of his or her behavior, and learn more effective coping skills.

17. Refeeding must be done in a structured manner with clear expectations and consequences. Positive reinforcement is more effective than punishment. Consistency is crucial.

18. The client must understand how he or she is using the eating disorder to avoid psychological issues.

The nurse assists the client to refocus attention from gaining weight to underlying issues and conflicts.

19. Antidepressants are used to treat the comorbid depression in clients with eating disorders and may help decrease binge urges in clients with bulimia. The mechanism is unknown.

20. Long-term individual psychotherapy of various modalities is generally recommended for all clients with eating disorders. Group and family psychotherapies are also widely used.

REFERENCES

American Psychiatric Association: *Diagnostic and statistical manual of mental disorders,* ed 4, Washington, D.C., 1994, APA.

Bauer B, Anderson W: Bulimic beliefs: food for thought, *J Coun Dev* 67:416–419, 1989.

Bell R: *Holy anorexia,* Chicago, 1987, University of Chicago Press.

Binswanger L: The case of Ellen West. In May R, Angel E, Ellenburger H, editors: *Existence,* New York, 1958, Basic Books.

Boskind-Lodahl M: Cinderella's stepsisters: a feminist perspective on anorexia nervosa and bulimia, *Signs* 343–356, 1976.

Boskind-Lodahl M, White W: *Bulimarexia: the binge/purge cycle,* New York, 1983, Norton.

Braun C, Chouinard M: Is anorexia nervosa a neuropsychological disease? *Neuropsych Rev* 3:171–212, 1992.

Brumberg J: *Fasting girls,* New York, 1989, New American Library.

Connors M, Morse W: Sexual abuse and eating disorders: a review, *Int J Eat Disord* 13(1):1–11, 1993.

Devlin M, Walsh B: Eating disorders and depression, *Psych Annals* 19(9):473–476, 1989.

Folsom V et al: The impact of sexual and physical abuse on eating disordered and psychiatric symptoms, *Int J Eat Disord* 13:249–257, 1993.

Gartner A, Marcus R, Halmi K: DSM-IIIR personality disorders in patients with eating disorders, *Am J Psychiatry* 146:1585–1591, 1989.

Glassman JN et al: Some correlates of treatment response to a multicomponent psychotherapy program in outpatients with eating disorders, *Ann Clin Psychiatry* 2:33–38, 1990.

Halmi K: A clinical overview of anorexia nervosa, Presentation at conference: Eating Disorders: A practical clinical update, San Francisco, 1992.

Halmi K et al: Comorbidity of psychiatric diagnoses in anorexia nervosa, *Arch Gen Psychiatry* 48:712–718, 1991.

Hamburger W: Emotional aspects of obesity, *Med Clin North Am* 35:483–499, 1951.

Herzog D et al: The prevalence of personality disorders in 210 women with eating disorders, *J Clin Psychiatry* 53:147–152, 1992.

Johnson C, Connors M: *The etiology and treatment of bulimia nervosa,* New York, 1987, Basic Books.

Levin A et al: Multiple personality in eating disorder patients, *Int J Eat Disord* 13(2):235–239, 1993.

Lindner R: The case of Laura. In *The fifty minute hour,* New York, 1955, Holt, Rinehart & Winston.

Minuchin S, Rosman B, Baker L: *Psychosomatic families: anorexia nervosa in context,* Cambridge, Mass., 1978, Harvard University Press.

Orbach S: *Fat is a feminist issue,* New York, 1978, Berkeley Books.

Pope H, Hudson J: *New hope for binge eaters,* New York, 1984, Harper & Row.

Spitzer R et al: Binge eating disorder: a multisite field trial of the diagnostic criteria, *Int J Eat Disord* 11:191–203, 1992.

Spitzer R et al: Binge eating disorder: its further validation in a multisite study, *Int J Eat Disord* 13:137–153, 1993.

Stunkard A: Eating patterns and obesity, *Psychiatr Q* 33:284–292, 1959.

Vanderlinden J et al: Dissociative experiences and trauma in eating disorders, *Int J Eat Disord* 13:187, 1993.

Waller G: Association of sexual abuse and borderline personality disorder in eating disordered women, *Int J Eat Disord* 13:259–263, 1993.

Walsh B, Devlin M: The pharmacologic treatment of eating disorders, *Psychiatr Clin North Am* 15:149–160, 1992.

Wilson G, Fairburn C: Cognitive treatments for eating disorders, *J Consult Clin Psychol* 61:261–269, 1993.

Wooley S, Wooley O: Intensive outpatient and residential treatment for bulimia. In Garner D, Garfinkel P, editors: *Handbook of psychotherapy for anorexia nervosa and bulimia,* New York, 1985, Guilford Press.

CHAPTER 19

Sexual Disorders

Kathryn Thomas
Shelly F. Lurie

Depo-Lupron (Leuprolide) A synthetic analog of naturally occurring gonadotropin-releasing hormone. It inhibits gonadotropin secretion, thus suppressing testicular testosterone.

Depo-Provera (Medroxyprogesterone Acetate) A medication used in the adjunctive treatment of sexual disorders; a sexual appetite suppressant; lowers testosterone level to a prepubescent level.

Ego dystonic pedophile A person who is cognitively aware that his or her behavior is inappropriate and is affected by this. This person might voluntarily seek treatment to deal with his or her disorder.

Ego syntonic pedophile A person who is cognitively aware that his or her behavior is inappropriate but is not troubled by this. This person will not voluntarily seek treatment because he or she sees no need to do so.

Estradiol Endocrine testing for the female that determines level of estradiol in the bloodstream. Estradiol levels may reflect level of sexual desire.

External vacuum pump A cylindrical vacuum pump applied to the penis. When operated it brings blood into the penis and traps it there, thus improving erection.

Intracorporal injections Injections of various medications into the right and left corpus cavernosum to improve erection.

Lovemap Term coined by Money. Refers to an idiosyncratic image in the mind-brain that depicts the idealized lover and love-making activities.

Nocturnal penile tumescence A test that uses a strain gauge around the penis to depict the pattern of arousal while the client sleeps.

Paraphilias Sexual deviations/disorders presenting with inappropriate sexual fantasies involving deviant sexual acts, inappropriate sexual urges, and acting out of these fantasies and urges.

Penile-brachial index (PBI) A test that determines the difference between the penile and the brachial blood pressure in order to assess vascularization to the penis.

Penile plethysmography A diagnostic test that may help determine a person's arousal pattern and level of arousal. This test may reveal what arouses a client and how significant the arousal is.

Psychoeducation A type of therapy that educates the client with a paraphilic disorder to identify situations/objects that may trigger inappropriate sexual activity, and develop awareness of relapse prevention strategies and the importance of treatment compliance.

Recidivisim Chronic, repetitive acting out of sexual behaviors considered to be unacceptable which have or have not resulted in criminal conviction.

Sensate focus A learned exercise developed by Masters and Johnson that involves concentrating on the sensations produced by touching.

Triggers Stimuli that heighten unacceptable sexual cravings.

Vaginal dilators A graduated series of cylindrical dilators introduced into the vagina to decrease involuntary spasm.

Vaginal plethysmography A test that uses a vaginal probe to assess blood flow to the vagina. Blood flow is an indicator of arousal.

Victimizer Another term used to define a sex offender; may be used when discussing familial transmissions of the paraphilia.

Yohimbine An alpha adrenoreceptor blocker that may facilitate blood flow to the genitalia (especially in men) and therefore improve arousal.

LEARNING OBJECTIVES

- Discuss possible etiologies for the origins of sexual dysfunctions.
- Describe various sexual dysfunction diagnoses.
- Examine techniques used in diagnosing various sexual dysfunctions.
- Compare and contrast various treatment modalities.
- Apply the nursing process in caring for clients with sexual dysfunctions.
- Describe the different diagnoses of the sex offender (paraphilic) population.
- Discuss the focus of treatment for paraphilic disorders.
- Explain at least two types of treatment and effects on illness symptomatology.
- Analyze the relationship between treatment and recidivism.
- Apply the nursing process in caring for clients with sexual (paraphilic) disorders.

This chapter discusses the two categories of sexual disorders: sexual dysfunctions and paraphilias. Sexual dysfunctions will be covered in the first part of the chapter, paraphilias in the second.

SEXUAL DYSFUNCTIONS: HISTORICAL AND THEORETICAL PERSPECTIVES

In 1966 William Masters and Virginia Johnson published their classic work, *Human Sexual Response*. As a result they became famous, practically overnight. Their work was based on the direct laboratory observation of more than 10,000 male and female volunteers (Masters and Johnson, 1966). From this research, they were able to determine exactly what happens to the body during erotic stimulation, from excitement to plateau to orgasm and, finally, to resolution. In 1970, they published a second text, *Human Sexual Inadequacy,* in which they discussed their work in helping others overcome sexual dysfunction. In this book, Masters and Johnson outlined the probable causes for dysfunction and gave detailed prescriptions for treatment.

Masters and Johnson were not the first people to explore the area of sexual dysfunction. Many prominent sexologists—Henry Havelock Ellis, Sigmund Freud, Niles Newton, and Theodoor van de Velde—addressed these issues in earlier eras (Brecher, 1971). However, these works were more theoretical and were not based on scientific data.

For the early pioneers, the treatment focus for sexual dysfunction was psychoanalytical. Childhood experiences were believed to exert a subconscious influence on sexual behavior as an adult. Such infantile feelings as fear of castration and penis envy, coupled with fantasies, fears, and experiences, combined to create sexual dysfunctions. The treatment was aimed at uncovering these old traumas.

Masters and Johnson radically moved the theoretical perspective to the behavioral sphere. They postulated that sex therapy should be a series of specifically directed exercises guided by a therapist. Their original treatment program consisted of couples therapy in which the clients worked with a male/female treatment team. Couples came to St. Louis and lived in a hotel for 13 days. Day one and day two were devoted to assessment. By day three the couple came together with the treatment team to discuss the issues uncovered and to begin the specific exercises. The remaining days were spent practicing the homework assignments and having roundtable discussions regarding their progress and feelings with the therapists. Masters and Johnson additionally developed many specific techniques such as sensate focus and the squeeze technique (discussed later in the chapter).

Since the late 1960s, much has been learned about sexual dysfunctions and about sexuality in general. Though they have their benefits, structured treatment programs such as Masters and Johnsons' have not proved to be a panacea. Sexuality is too complex to be reduced to a sex manual solution. In recent years, approaches that combine behavioral, cognitive, and communication methods as well as psychodynamic techniques have been readily employed. Helen Singer Kaplan (1974) identified the need for behavioral techniques to be reintegrated with psychoanalysis in treatment. She also is responsible for separating the desire phase from the excitement (arousal) stage.

Many others have researched other approaches. Hartman and Fithian (1972) outlined a treatment approach based on careful observational research. Others such as Anon (1976), Leiblum and Rosen (1989), and LoPiccolo and Friedman (1988) have developed other strategies and therapeutic perspectives. The latest treatments involve biologic techniques such as injection, prosthesis, and surgical interventions.

ETIOLOGY

Etiological possibilities for sexual dysfunctions fall in several different categories: biologic, psychologic, and couple oriented (Box 19-1).

Biological Factors

Biologic factors that may contribute to sexual dysfunction include vascular, neurologic, and endocrine, as well as a range of diseases such as cancer, degenerative diseases, and genital infections (Kaplan, 1974; Wagner and Kaplan, 1993). Vascular factors include cardiac disease and disease of the blood vessels. Neurologic factors may be stroke, head injuries, spinal cord disorders, epilepsy, or peripheral nerve disorders. Endocrine factors include diabetes and altered hormonal levels. The effects of medications can be considered here. It is well known that antipsychotics, antidepressants, and antihypertensives, as well as sedatives, tranquilizers, narcotics, and alcohol can all adversely affect sexual functioning.

Psychologic Factors

As previously noted, early childhood experiences formed the hallmark of beliefs about causation. Indeed, many still believe that psychosocial factors are more important in the etiology of sexual dysfunctions than other reasons. There is currently much literature and discussion about the impact of childhood sexual trauma on later sexual functioning (Beitchman et al, 1992). Repressive childhood

---

Box 19-1   Etiologic Factors for Sexual Dysfunctions

Biologic factors

Vascular	Cardiac disease
	Diseases of the blood vessels
Neurologic	Stroke
	Head injuries
	Spinal cord disorders
	Epilepsy
	Peripheral nerve disorders
Endocrine	Diabetes
	Altered hormonal levels, especially testosterone

Psychologic factors

Childhood experiences
Anxiety and stress
Misinformation and lack of sex education

Couple-oriented factors

Differences in sexual desire or interests
Lack of communication
Lack of trust

Understanding and Applying
RESEARCH

LeMone P: Human sexuality in adults with insulin dependent diabetes mellitus, *Image: J of Nursing Scholarship* 25(2):101–105, 1993.

This was a qualitative study involving 11 men and women designed to explore human sexuality in adults with insulin-dependent diabetes mellitus (IDDM). The author contends that human sexuality may be affected by the process of chronic disease such as IDDM. In this study she attempted to formulate a theory of the process of change in sexuality experienced by adults with chronic illness.

Seven subjects were selected from a physician-provided list; four subjects heard about the study and volunteered for it. This was a purposive sampling strategy. Subjects ranged in age from 27–70 and had been diagnosed with IDDM after the age of 21. There were six men and five women, all Caucasians.

Data collection involved audiotaped 30- to 60-minute interviews in a private location, often the subject's home. Open-ended questions about sexuality were asked, such as, "Tell me about your experiences with sexual functioning since you were diagnosed with diabetes." Data collected was organized according to open coding; codes were then grouped into categories.

Subjects reported changes in interrelated components of sexuality that occurred as the result of the illness or treatment of the illness. Men reported changes in function with hyperglycemia. Hypoglycemia in both males and females was reported to cause a decrease in the ability to be sexually aroused. All female subjects reported monilial infections with hyperglycemia and thus avoided intercourse due to pain. Four men reported inability to achieve an adequate erection. Subjects also reported that IDDM has negatively affected their relationships.

The investigator used grounded theory concerning the impact of IDDM on sexuality. She discusses the impact of the findings and the outcomes of transforming experiences. She suggests the need to value self by accepting self as a diabetic, accepting feeling different, and of maintaining control.

The study helps further understanding of the effects of chronic disease on human sexuality. However, it engaged a small sample size, nonrandom sampling, and a descriptive design. Thus, it cannot be generalized, and further study is necessary. Nurses should consider the impact of chronic disease on clients' sexual functioning and provide interventions that address client's self-acceptance.

---

environments that include religious, familial, or cultural restrictions have also been implicated (Money, 1986).

Other issues such as anxiety and stress may also contribute to changes in sexual functioning. Partially, these relate to anxiety about sexual performance. Masters and Johnson (1970) coined the term *spectatoring*. This psychologic factor refers to the tendency to monitor one's own sexual activity, thus detracting from the actual experience. Stress from any source has been noted to lower sexual drive and to decrease both testosterone and luteinizing hormone levels (Morokoff and Gilliland, 1993). Stress may be the result of many nonsexual causes, such as worry about money, job, or job security.

Misinformation and a lack of sex education may account for some degree of sexual dysfunction. One example is ignorance about the placement and function of the clitoris, which may severely affect obtaining sexual pleasure. Myths, such as those that assert that men are always ready for sex and women are never interested, have also influenced attitudes toward sex.

Couple-Oriented Factors

Couple-oriented factors involve differences in sexual drives and interests. Money (1986) used the term **lovemap** to describe one's idealized picture of who and what make up one's sexual arousal pattern. Lovemaps vary from individual to individual. Thus, a couple may not be well matched in the types of behaviors that interest them. Communication is another couple-oriented factor that may impact sexual functioning. Couples often do not discuss what they do or don't enjoy sexually, or share their feelings about the experience. Trust between partners is also a crucial factor.

EPIDEMIOLOGY

The prevalence of sexual dysfunction disorders is difficult to determine. This is partially due to a lack of research, but also to a lack of such problems being reported. Masters and Johnson (1970) suggested that 50% of all couples have a sexual dysfunction. Spector and Carey (1990) believe that sexual problems are quite common in our society.

Forty-six percent of couples presenting for sex therapy at one treatment center complained of low sexual desire (LoPiccolo and Friedman, 1988). Kaplan (1974) estimates that 50% of all males will experience erectile problems sometime in their lives. Spector and Carey (1990) say that erectile dysfunction is the most common cause of why males seek therapy.

In relationship to orgasmic disorder, Renshaw (1988) found that females with primary orgasmic dysfunction

DSM-IV CRITERIA

Sexual Dysfunctions

Sexual desire disorders

Hypoactive sexual desire disorder

A deficiency or absence of sexual fantasy or drive for sexual activity

Sexual aversion disorder

Aversion to or avoidance of genital sexual contact with a partner

Sexual arousal disorders

Female sexual arousal disorder

Inability to attain or maintain an adequate lubrication/ swelling response of sexual excitement

Male erectile disorder

Inability to attain or maintain an adequate erection

Orgasmic disorders

Female orgasmic disorder

Delay in or absence of orgasm after sexual excitement phase (must be persistent or recurrent)

Male orgasmic disorder

Delay in or absence of orgasm following sexual excitement phase (must be persistent or recurrent)

Premature ejaculation

Onset of orgasm and ejaculation with minimal sexual stimulation (must be persistent or recurrent)

Sexual pain disorders

Dyspareunia

Genital pain associated with sexual intercourse (not due to a general medical condition)

Vaginismus

Involuntary contractions of the perineal muscles with penetration (not due to a general medical condition)

Sexual dysfunction due to a general medication condition

Use same subtypes as above, but indicate which medical condition it is due to

Substance-induced sexual dysfunction

Use same subtypes and above and indicate specific substance

Sexual dysfunction not otherwise specified

Does not meet criteria for the category of sexual dysfunction

Adapted from *Diagnostic and statistical manual of mental disorders,* ed 4, Washington, D.C., American Psychiatric Association, 1994.

---

constituted 32% and females with secondary orgasmic dysfunction constituted 37% of all clients seen at a sex clinic. Kinsey et al (1953) noted that 10% of women interviewed reported lifelong anorgasmia. By contrast, Masters and Johnson (1970) found inhibited male orgasm rare. They reported only 17 cases in an 11-year period.

Kaplan (1974) cites premature ejaculation as the most common of all sexual dysfunctions. For pain disorders, Renshaw (1988) reported 8% for dyspareunia and 5% for vaginismus, but other investigators cited higher averages. There appears to be a relatively high incidence of sexual dissatisfaction in the population yet a serious lack of research and understanding of the issues.

CLINICAL DESCRIPTION

The DSM-IV (1994) divides the sexual dysfunctions into sexual desire disorders, sexual arousal disorders, orgasmic disorders, sexual pain disorders, sexual dysfunction due to a general medical condition, substance-induced sexual dysfunction, and sexual dysfunction not other-

wise specified (see the DSM-IV box above). The first three categories are based on Kaplan's (1974) stages of the sexual response cycle.

PROGNOSIS

In order to guide and properly educate their clients, nurses must understand how successful therapy can be for the individual or for the couple. There are some prognostic data available for sexual dysfunctions in general. However, this data cannot be used specifically for each dysfunction. For example, sexual desire disorders tend to have a more negative prognosis that do orgasmic disorders.

Masters and Johnson (1970) found that primary impotence treatment had a 40.6% failure rate, while the failure rate for secondary impotence treatment was 26.2%. Premature ejaculation treatment failed only 2.2% of the time. Concerning intervention rates for orgasmic dysfunction in males, the failure rate was 19.7% and for females 19.3%. When Masters and Johnson did follow-up five years later, they found that only 5.1% had relapsed. More recently sex therapists have suggested that approximately two-thirds of all treatment is successful. Zilbergeld and Evans (1980) noted a relapse rate of 54%. This may not be due to a lessening of therapeutic effectiveness but rather to different criteria for data collection. Many professionals believe that desire phase disorders are the least easily treated. This is perhaps due to the variety of origins of desire.

DISCHARGE CRITERIA

Client will:

1. express satisfaction with one's sexuality.

2. develop insight into the disorder, etiology of the disorder, and the symptoms.

3. develop appropriate strategies to impact on the specific disorder.

4. communicate effectively with significant other regarding sexuality.

5. demonstrate ability to communicate needs and desires sexually.

6. develop appropriate coping strategies.

Sexuality is an essential and sensitive part of every human being. All nurses should have the goal of helping their clients achieve positive sexual expressions. Facilitating this goal is a rewarding albeit difficult task.

For any given client or couple, it is difficult to predict how long interventions and treatment need to last. Some disorders are more difficult to treat (for example, sexual desire disorders); some are relatively simple (for example, orgasmic disorders and premature ejaculation). However, the assumption that this will be true in any given case is short-sighted. Individual factors will speed or complicate the recovery period; thus, flexibility must be built in. The astute nurse is consistently aware of this. Additionally, it is not up to the nurse alone to know when goals are met. Individuals vary in the outcomes they expect. Sexual expression and satisfaction are for the individual alone to decide. As long as the expression and satisfaction are not harmful to another, they should not be determined by anyone else except the client.

THE NURSING PROCESS ■ ■ ■ ■ ■ ■ ■ ■ ■ ■ ■ ■ ■ ■ ■ ■ ■

■ ASSESSMENT

For many reasons, sexuality is a sensitive topic for most people. When discussing sexuality with clients, consider these sensitivities. Nurses are not immune to the feelings, beliefs, values, and attitudes that affect others. Therefore, when the nurse is dealing with client-related sexual dysfunction issues, it may be uncomfortable for both parties. Yet, a holistic nursing assessment must consider sexuality as important as other functions. An important step in decreasing discomfort is to have the nurse examine his or her own feelings and comfort with the topic.

The nurse will be better equipped to deal with others in the important area of human sexuality by combining self-understanding, a firm knowledge base, expert use of the nursing process, and nonjudgment.

Assessment is a crucial phase in working with clients with sexual dysfunction. A clear understanding of the complexity of the symptoms and what areas of functioning are affected is needed. Sexual dysfunctions may arise throughout various phases of the sexual response cycle. Dysfunctions may reflect individual functioning or be couple-related. Sexual assessment must be seen in the context of overall assessment factors such as background, physical health, religious and cultural beliefs, education, occupation, significant relationships, and social relationships. In addition to the assessment of the specific complaint, the nurse must also consider the individual's or couples' perspective of the problem and desire to change.

Box 19-2 presents a sample sexual history form. The following guidelines should apply when doing a sexual assessment:

1. Before beginning a sexual assessment, examine one's own feelings, attitudes, values, and level of comfort.

2. Ensure a private, quiet space for assessment, ample time, and an unhurried attitude.

3. Questions on sexuality should not be the first asked. Begin with background information and fit the sexual assessment into the context of the overall assessment.

4. Questions asked about sexuality should begin with the least sensitive areas and move to areas of greater sensitivity. For example, begin by asking when client(s) first learned about sex.

5. Maintain appropriate eye contact and a relaxed, interested manner.

Box 19-2   Sample Sexual History Form

- Identifying Information
    - Age
    - Gender
    - Other pertinent information
- What brings the person for treatment?
- Informants for the history
- Family history
    - Parents
    - Siblings
    - Extended family
    - Family health history
    - Social history
- Personal history
    - Date, place, and circumstances of birth
    - Childhood health history
    - Social history
    - Educational history
    - Occupational history

    Habits (tobacco, alcohol, and drugs)
    Religious/spiritual history
    Adult health history
    Psychiatric history
    Legal history
- Sexual history
    - Early childhood sexual history (doctor play, sexual experiences with adults)
    - Masturbation history
    - Teenage experiences
    - Same sex and opposite sex experiences
    - History of significant relationships
    - Current sexual partner/activities
    - Fantasies
    - Use of erotica
    - Contraception/STD protection
    - Satisfaction
    - Questions and concerns

---

6. Be professional and matter-of-fact about information asked or obtained. Avoid extreme reactions.

7. Use language that is professional but understood by the client(s) being interviewed.

8. Remember, the nurse's tone of voice and manner reflect trust. If clients feel they can trust the nurse, they will be more open.

■ ■ NURSING DIAGNOSIS

After a thorough gathering of assessment data, the nurse is in a position to analyze the findings and arrive at diagnoses. Diagnoses of sexual dysfunctions should be viewed in relation to the psychiatric diagnoses, DSM-IV, as well as nursing diagnoses that reflect the specific problems. A combination of both help to ensure that adequate plans for intervention will be developed. Determination of diagnoses is done on an individual basis and carefully selected from all that is known.

NANDA Diagnoses for Sexual Dysfunctions

Sexual dysfunction
Knowledge deficit, human sexuality
Fear
Anxiety
Role performance, altered
Self-esteem disturbance
Communication, impaired, verbal
Social isolation
Pain

CASE ◆ STUDY

Kelly is a 28-year-old, never-married female who tells the nurse that she has never had an orgasm. On assessment the nurse learns that Kelly has had a total of three male sexual partners. Her first intercourse experience was at age 19. She said she has never masturbated but sometimes fantasizes about sex and can get aroused by reading a sexually explicit story or seeing a movie with sex scenes. She has been in a three-year monogamous, committed relationship to a man she is considering marrying. She said that they have sex 2–3 times per week. She generally enjoys it but is unable to achieve orgasm. Lately this has become a problem for her and her partner. He fears that he is unable to please her.

Critical Thinking and Assessment

1. What are the symptoms that Kelly exhibits that pertain to sexual dysfunctioning?

2. What about Kelly's background leads the nurse to believe that she has sexual problems?

3. How could Kelly's sexual problem affect other areas of her relationship?

■ ■ ■ OUTCOME IDENTIFICATION

In this phase the nurse determines clear outcome criteria or expected client outcomes from the nursing diagnosis. Client will:

1. Verbalize specific problem in the sexual area by time of the second visit with nurse.

2. Write a list of feelings associated with sexual problem by time of the second visit with nurse.

3. Seek a physical examination (if appropriate) by time of the third visit with nurse.

4. Participate in sex therapy sessions (if appropriate) by time of the fourth visit with nurse.

5. Practice strategies learned in sex therapy as recommended by the sixth week in therapy.

6. Describe two strategies learned to enhance sexual functioning after the sixth week in therapy.

7. Incorporate strategies learned in sex therapy into routine sexual activity by the time of discharge.

■ ■ ■ ■ PLANNING

Planning for client care comes about as the result of thorough assessment and analysis. Following formulation of DSM-IV diagnoses and nursing diagnoses that reflect

COLLABORATIVE DIAGNOSES

DSM-IV Diagnoses*	NANDA Diagnoses**
Sexual desire disorder	Sexual dysfunction
Hypoactive sexual desire	Fear
Sexual aversion disorder	Anxiety
	Role performance
	Self-esteem disturbance
Sexual arousal disorders	Communication
Female sexual arousal	impaired
disorder	
Male erectile disorder	
Orgasmic disorders	Knowledge deficit
Female orgasmic disorder	Social isolation
Male orgasmic disorder	
Premature ejaculation	
Sexual pain disorder	Pain
Dyspareunia	
Vaginismus	
Sexual dysfunction due to general medical condition	
Substance-induced sexual dysfunction	
Sexual dysfunction not otherwise specified	

*Reprinted with permission from *Diagnostic and statistical manual of mental disorders*, ed 4, Washington, D.C., 1994, American Psychiatric Association.

**Reprinted with permission from *NANDA nursing diagnoses: definitions and classifications, 1995–1996*, Philadelphia, 1994, North American Nursing Diagnosis Association.

client status, the nurse is ready to begin an individualized plan of care that will address all the issues. Client care will be based on realistic, mutually arrived upon goals.

In working with clients and couples with sexual dysfunction, the nurse needs to carefully consider the long-term goals and what each participant is willing to do to work toward those goals. These may differ in each situation, based on each person's values and attitudes and how each perceives the problem. For example, the client with a primary orgasmic dysfunction may have difficulty with masturbatory exercises that form one basis for treatment because he or she believes that touching one's own genitals is unacceptable and that orgasmic release must come only from partnered sexuality. Obviously, such individually held beliefs will influence implementation of a care plan.

■ ■ ■ ■ ■ IMPLEMENTATION

Development of an individualized plan of care is crucial. To do so, one must be aware of the specific nature of the problem and possible etiologies. Implementation includes education, counseling, and assistance in identifying specific strategies and support. The nurse must be aware of various treatment modalities and prognosis of recovery with treatment. The importance of following through on a plan of care, including physical exam and treatments, and on specific sex therapy needs for the individual or the couple must be stressed. The nurse will help the client(s) express concerns about sexual functioning; express feelings about the impact of this; and help enhance client knowledge base, self-esteem, and communication skills. The nurse will also recommend physical exam and/or treatment, sex therapy, monitor client compliance and success in treatment, and help develop appropriate discharge planning.

Sexuality is a sensitive area of intervention. Having a trusting, open, and comfortable relationship with clients is essential. Without this, many sexual problems will go unrecognized and untreated.

The nature of sexuality is partially one of relationships with others. Therefore, the nurse must be aware of significant others and the impact on them as well. Implementation of any plan of care often involves a couple relationship and must be seen in this context. Thus, it is often helpful to view the problem as couple-oriented instead of placing the blame on either partner. Interventions aimed at the couple, in these instances, are most effective.

Nursing Interventions

1. Help client(s) understand human sexual functioning. Teach them about the human sexual response cycle. Recommend appropriate reading materials, such as Masters and Johnson's *Human Sexual Response. This knowledge forms a foundation for understanding other issues related to sexual disorders.*

NURSING CARE PLAN

Lisa and Victor are a married couple who talk with the nurse about problems in their sexual relationship. Lisa is 34 years old; Victor is 35. Both say they are in good physical health and neither takes any medication routinely. They have two children: Amanda, age 4, and Brandon, age 2. The couple met 6½ years ago and become sexually involved shortly afterward. They lived together for approximately 8 months and married 5½ years ago.

They say that their sexual relationship was good prior to marriage and to the birth of their children. They had sexual intercourse about 2–4 times per week and both enjoyed it. Lisa says she occasionally has masturbated and continues to do so. Victor says that as an adolescent he masturbated once a day but this has gradually decreased. He says he is not masturbating currently and has no interest in doing so.

Lisa says that Victor's interest in sex has gradually declined and that now he rarely wants to be sexual. She feels he sometimes will have sex just to please her. Victor agrees

that his interest in sex has declined. He says he is currently busy and preoccupied with fears and worries. According to Victor, he and a partner started their own business three years ago, and it has been a constant struggle. He admits that his sexual drive is down but says he can get an erection with adequate stimulation. Lisa complains that they have not been able to talk about the problem; she says they fight whenever sex is mentioned.

DSM-IV Diagnosis (Victor)

AXIS I	Hypoactive sexual desire disorder
AXIS II	Deferred
AXIS III	None known
AXIS IV	Severity of psychosexual stressors (moderate = 3) job stress and anxiety
AXIS V	GAF = 70 within past year

Nursing Diagnosis: Sexual dysfunction, related to fear, anxiety, and lack of communication, as evidenced by the couple's lack of sexual intimacy, and decrease in sexual interest and in masturbation in the husband.

Client Outcomes	Nursing Interventions	Evaluation
• Both Lisa and Victor will discuss how they perceive the problem with each other, in the presence of the nurse at the first visit.	• Assess for perception of problem through taking sexual and couple history *to clearly delineate problem in sexual functioning and how couple perceives it.* • Ask each client to discuss how he or she perceives the problem. Allow each an equal amount of time *to help understand the problem thoroughly and to open communication between the partners.*	• Lisa and Victor both identified problem as decrease in sexual interest on Victor's part.
• Lisa and Victor will identify one way to be intimate with each other after the first visit.	• Discuss with couple alternative methods of intimacy they may practice, such as massage or partnered bath taking. *Couple will experience decreased pressure for genital sex that will help with relaxation.* • Give couple suggestions for readings on sexuality. *Sexual books in the market outline alternative ways to be sexual.*	• Lisa and Victor agreed to give each other a half-hour massage this week.
• Victor will have exam done by primary care physician by end of second week.	• Discuss with clients need to rule out any physical disorder that may have relationship to sexual change. *Sexual dysfunction may be the result of a medical disorder. Before other forms of treatment are planned, this should be determined.* • Refer client to primary care physician if necessary *to rule out physical problems.*	• Victor sought out physical exam and was given clean bill of health.
• Lisa and Victor will agree to enter sex therapy with a qualified therapist after results of physical exam.	• Encourage client to receive treatment for sexual problems. *Sex therapy may be helpful in overcoming sexual difficulty and anxiety. Educate couple about techniques of sexual therapy. They may be better informed to make appropriate choices.* • Refer couple to qualified sex therapist *for continued professional help.*	• Lisa and Victor see a sex therapist and work with him or her.

NURSING CARE PLAN

Nursing Diagnosis: Anxiety related to job stress, performance anxiety, and lack of communication, as evidenced by Victor's statements that he is anxious and distracted from sexual interaction.

Client Outcomes	Nursing Interventions	Evaluation
• Victor will describe nature of anxiety by the second visit.	• Encourage Victor to be aware of anxiety and how it affects his sexuality. *Knowing what anxieties are will help alleviate need to worry when involved in other activities.* • Ask Victor to discuss what type of issues create anxiety. *Members of the couple are aware of them and create a strategy to overcome them.*	• Victor able to discuss worries, success of business, and financial security.
• Victor will practice sensate focus exercises with wife during intimacy after the first visit.	• Educate Victor on sensate focus exercises. *This will train Victor to focus on body feeling and not on anxiety during intimacy with wife.* • Recommend reading materials for couple that describe sensate focus exercises as part of education *to enhance learned skills.*	• Victor reports he is able to focus on body sensations during intimacy.

Nursing Diagnosis: Communication, impaired verbal related to anxiety, self-esteem disturbance, embarrassment as evidenced by Lisa's statement that they could not discuss sexual issues without fighting.

Client Outcomes	Nursing Interventions	Evaluation
• Lisa and Victor will discuss sexual concerns in first session with nurse.	• Encourage couple to be more open verbally about sexual needs and concerns. *Open discussion facilitates mutual understanding and decreases blame.* • Ask direct questions about sexuality and keep focused on this during sessions. *Help decrease anxiety and open up couple communication around sex.*	• Both Lisa and Victor able to discuss sexual concerns at first session.
• Lisa and Victor will discuss sex with each other one hour each week after first session.	• Encourage couple to set aside time to discuss sexual needs *to be able to express needs and thus facilitate sexuality.*	• Lisa and Victor say they are able to discuss needs with each other. Lisa says she would like more time together, and Victor says he would like Lisa to initiate.

2. Educate client(s) about sexual dysfunctions, including possible etiologies, symptoms, and treatment options. Various methods of assessment should be included: physical, urological, gynecological, and laboratory examinations, as well as a psychosocial sexual assessment. *Education helps to ensure that client(s) understand why changes in sexuality are happening to them and symptoms that may signal a problem.*

3. Help client(s) enhance communication skills around intimacy/sexuality. Teach and reinforce positive communication skills. *The inability to communicate is often the root of a sexual dysfunction problem.*

4. Support client(s) in exploring fears/anxieties related to anxiety in a private, trusting, open atmosphere. Encourage client's recall of early learning about sexuality, possibly through journal writing. *An open forum for discussing sexuality will help the client(s) overcome some of the repressions they have felt and be more open to satisfying sexual experiences.*

5. Help client(s) enhance self-esteem related to sexuality. Encourage positive self-talk and body image exercises. Discuss variations of sexual expression techniques. *Lack of self-esteem is often a contributing factor in sexual dysfunction.*

6. Refer client(s) to physical treatment modalities or sex therapy as applicable, *to maximize the client's(s') success in dealing with sexual dysfunction.*

Client and Family
TEACHING GUIDELINES

Sexual Dysfunctions

Teach the client and significant other:

How to bring more intimacy, caressing, and spontaneity into the relationship without demand only for orgasmic release. Ask the couple what they can develop sexually that is unique to them. Have them find something they can do to create more pleasure in their relationship, for example, full-body or specific-area massage, sexual play at spontaneous moments, or variation in times or locations to be sexual.

To enhance communication, interest in one another, and caring in the relationship.

To assist in creating a more sexual atmosphere in the couple relationship without demand for intercourse alone. This demand can lead to anxiety.

Additional Treatment Modalities

Once careful assessment is done to determine the specific diagnosis of sexual dysfunction, a range of treatment modalities can be instituted.

Psychophysiologic

Physiologic causation must be ruled out in advance of deciding on one or more forms of treatment. Various medical specialties have produced new diagnostic and therapeutic procedures that have quickly changed the practice of sex therapy/clinical sexology.

For men, various psychophysiologic methods are employed in both diagnosis and treatment. **Nocturnal Penile Tumescence** involves the determination of erectile response during the sleep cycle. The client is generally seen in a sleep lab where penile plethysmography is used to monitor erection. **Penile plethysmography** involves the use of a strain gauge that fits around the penis and detects erection. This information, processed through mechanical and computerized equipment, provides a graphic portrayal of the erectile pattern. This testing is time-consuming and relatively expensive, but it clearly detects whether erection is possible without competing psychologic stimuli. Determination of erectile potential can also be done by daytime evaluation using visual erotic stimuli and the plethysmograph. Wineze et al (1988) found that laboratory exposure to erotic pictures produced erection in dysfunctional men.

Medical testing for males may include endocrine measures, particularly testosterone and prolactin. Testosterone is the predominantly male sex hormone produced in the testes which is responsible for the male sex drive. In general, a higher level of testosterone in males is associated with greater sexual desire; a higher level of prolactin is associated with decreased sexual interest. The

ADDITIONAL TREATMENT MODALITIES

Psychophysiological Modalities

- Yohimbine
- Aphrodisiacs
- Hormonal replacement (testosterone and estrogen)
- Intracavernosal injections
- Vascular surgery
- Penile prosthesis
- External vacuum devices
- Vibrators

Psychosocial Modalities

- Sensate focus
- Body therapies (massage, chakra balancing, tantric yoga)
- Communication therapy
- Education
- Masturbation training
- Erotic stimuli training
- Seman's stop-start technique
- Gradual dilatation of the vagina

penile-brachial index (PBI) is also a useful measure. This monitors the difference between penile and brachial blood pressures. There are other invasive and noninvasive tests for evaluation of arterial and venous blood flow to the penis, including pulse wave assessments, intracorporal pharmacological testing, ultrasound (the use of sound waves to evaluate structures and functions within the male genitalia), and cavernosography. Neurological assessments that carefully evaluate various minute components of neural control of erection are also available.

In women, there is a noticeable lack of assessment and treatment in the psychophysiologic realm. **Vaginal plethysmography** is used to determine blood flow to the vagina, which is an indicator of arousal. However, this procedure is inconsistent and invasive. Endocrine studies can be used, but the hormonal control of female sexuality is more complex and affected by the menstrual cycle. Thus, the findings may not be very useful in diagnosis. **Estradiol** measurement is sometimes done, which determines the level of estradiol in the bloodstream, possibly reflecting levels of desire.

Today practitioners have several methods of treatment. Drug and hormonal therapies often are used as adjuncts. The use of the drug **yohimbine,** an alpha adrenoreceptor blocker, is believed to facilitate blood flow to the genitalia, especially in men. Hormonal replacement may also prove useful. This may involve testosterone in males, low levels of testosterone in females, or estrogen replacement in females.

Intracorporal injections of vasodilators have gained popularity. An injection of prostaglandins, papaverine, or combinations of these and other drugs is made directly into the corpus cavernosa and produces erection. Wagner and Kaplan (1993) have detailed this extensively, along with client satisfaction, complaints, and follow-up considerations. In males, surgery can be done to alter penile arterial blood flow or to implant prosthetic devices. Prosthetic devices come in two different general forms and have been developed over time with more satisfactory results. There is a semirigid rod that can be made of silicone or metal, and there are inflatable pumps of varying degrees of sophistication.

External vacuum pumps improve erection and orgasmic function in males. The vacuum draws blood into the corpus cavernosa of the penis and traps it there. In China a sophisticated system has been developed that uses herbal tonics, an electronic pumping device, and a vagina-like container filled with warm fluid, and a self-control apparatus for the client. Although it has proved useful in China, the system has not yet been used in the United States.

Elaborate physiological methods of treatment are not available for women but clearly need to be developed. Currently, various types of vibrators are available that can be useful therapeutically for females. However, they are marketed as toys or relaxation devices instead of biomedical instruments and therefore do not have the sanction or the quality of medical instruments.

Psychosocial

There are effective sex therapy techniques for both males and females as well as couples. These techniques were first developed by Masters and Johnson and have become more effective and comprehensive over the years. Masters and Johnson (1970) developed the **sensate focus** technique that involves focusing on body sensations, especially those in the breasts and genitals, while shutting out other stimuli.

Body therapies have been used in the field for several decades, including hands-on healing, massage, spiritual energizing techniques, chakra balancing, and the adaptation of Eastern principles of sexuality such as Tantric yoga. Couples massage is often utilized to enhance pleasure and provide nonverbal communication. Often couples are instructed to give one another weekly hour-long massages that are nondemand; in other words, the partner being massaged must only receive the sensations without feeling the need to reciprocate. Nondemand also implies that there is no demand for sexual arousal or sexual desire completion. Massage has proved effective for individuals who may have reactions to touch and need to develop the ability prior to being able to improve their sexual response.

Sex therapy practitioners and clinical sexologists have a wide range of other psychosocial techniques. In general, homework assignments and supportive counseling form the basis of therapy. Often sex therapy involves weekly or bimonthly visits to the therapists where the client(s) have the opportunity to discuss symptoms, progress, feelings, and observations, as well as other aspects of the psychological/cultural or couple states that may impact treatment.

Education provides a first-line technique for sex therapy. Cognitive restructuring, involving replacing negative thoughts about sexuality with positive thoughts, can be helpful as well. Communication training is also beneficial. For desire phase disorders, erotic materials may be used to help train the individual to be more sexually focused. Clients are often asked to include sexual thinking and feelings into their daily schedule. Masturbation training can be done for males and females to help them be more sensitive to sexual stimulation. It may then train males and females to become orgasmic or improve orgasmic potential. Becoming orgasmic may also entail the use of cognitive restructuring of beliefs about sexuality and techniques to reduce the fear of losing control.

For males, the stop-start technique helps overcome premature ejaculation. This technique, developed in 1956 by Semans, has the couple practice foreplay and stimulation until the point of ejaculation. Then, direct stimulation is stopped until the feeling subsides. The couple resumes the procedure a total of three times. This technique trains the male to be more aware of the sensation of impending ejaculation and to better control the timing.

Once medical causations for the sexual pain disorders of dyspareunia and vaginismus have been ruled out, appropriate strategies can be used. Insertions of a finger or **vaginal dilator** in the vagina are begun slowly. The gradual introduction of ever larger inserters, coupled with relaxation techniques, will help the woman overcome her fear and pain and help decrease involuntary spasm. Sets of dilators may be purchased from medical supply firms for this purpose.

The tools and methods of sex therapy have been important developments in the field. But without the sensitivity and attention to other factors in the client's sexual realm, they may not provide satisfactory results. Some other factors include cultural and religious values, other psychologic disorders, poor sexual learning, and body image issues.

Anon (1976) created what is known as the PLISSIT model of sexual intervention. This is an excellent model for the collaborative care of clients with sexual dysfunctions. The P stands for giving *permission*, i.e., giving permission for people to be sexual and to have sexual feelings. If the problem persists, go to LI, giving *limited information*, i.e., information and education concerning specific sexual problem(s). If the problem persists, go to SS, making *specific suggestions*, i.e., calling on the specific treatments for various dysfunctions. If the problem persists, refer to a sex therapist/clinical sexologist for IT, *intensive therapy*.

■ ■ ■ ■ ■ ■ **EVALUATION**

Evaluation of the effectiveness of intervention is an ongoing process and involves many levels. If the outcome criteria are thorough and carefully defined, evaluation is a relatively simple process of determining whether these outcomes were met. The nursing process is cyclical, thus, if the nurse determines that outcome criteria were not met, he or she must go back to the assessment phase to determine if some key underlying factors were overlooked.

To better understand this cyclical nature in the area of sexual dysfunction, refer to the nursing care plan on page 457 concerning Lisa and Victor. During assessment the nurse learned that Victor had a decreased sexual desire over the past few years. One of the nursing diagnoses identified was anxiety that may be due to job stress, performance anxiety, and lack of communication. One outcome criteria the nurse determined with Victor was that he would practice sensate focus exercises during intimacy with his wife. The nurse then taught Victor how to do sensate focus. If, on evaluation, Victor says he still cannot focus on his body and is easily distracted, what should the nurse do next?

The answer here is for the nurse to go back to assessment. Was something missed? Perhaps something was overlooked in Victor's history, perhaps he put on weight that has affected his body image, or perhaps he has a fear of being touched. Couple issue may have been missed. Lisa may have rejected Victor in the past, and he is still angry. If any of these or additional issues are found in assessment, the nurse must revamp the care plan to include them. Nursing diagnosis, outcome criteria, and interventions will then change. If nothing is missed in assessment, perhaps the outcome criteria were unrealistic. The issue of Victor's anxiety may be complex and deep, and it may be unrealistic to assume that he will develop insight by the second visit. The need for ongoing evaluation can be seen in this example.

Nursing Care in the Community

Sexual Dysfunction

Many people find sexual dysfunctions difficult to discuss because of the traditional reluctance about such matters. The sources of clients' problems may be found in a variety of factors, including natural changes of the aging process, side effects of various medications, rape, or a history of abuse. Some clients may have kept their problems secret for extended periods of time, or may not have been aware of the original cause.

Some individuals may experience gender-related conflict or desire for types of sexual experience not condoned by society. Any of these problems may be presented to the community mental health nurse with, "You are a nurse and have probably seen it all." The nurse must respond with calmness and poise to such an opening, as someone who will neither be judgmental nor condone hurtful behavior. The nurse must have patience as the client attempts to express feelings that may have never been shared. The nurse also needs to acknowledge that there are no easy answers to the client's questions but emphasize readiness to explore individualized options. The nurse may want to remind the client that thoughts are not harmful to others, that there is individual or group support available, and that the client has a choice about putting ideas into action.

Sexual problems associated with the maturing process are increasingly common as the population which came of age with the Pill now must cope with the complexities of AIDS, menopause, and viripause (as some have dubbed the male version of hormonal change). Women may experience depression and lack of sexual desire due to diminished hormone levels and related painful intercourse. Men may feel stuck in their careers or in relationships. Sexually active adults who are not in secure monogamous relationships must always have concerns about sexually transmitted diseases (STDs), which may be somewhat eased with specific instructions about risk factors and protected intimacy.

Clients in the community may also include those who have already contracted STDs such as HIV, genital herpes, or full-blown AIDS. These individuals can be helped individually and in support groups to reduce their guilt and evaluate their situations in order to decide what sort of relationships are possible for them. They must be encouraged to be scrupulously honest with prospective partners and to explore safer forms of intimacy in their relationships.

The community mental health nurse must have current information about medications, especially anti-depressants, which have side effects that impact on a client's sexual activity such as impaired desire, delayed orgasm, and impotency. Many people tolerate such side effects in silence, feeling that they are still suffering from depression or that they have developed some other abnormality to add to their problems. They will need assurance that their problems are physiological, not emotional.

The difference that the mental health nurse will find working in the community setting is that relationships with clients are more sustained, holistic, and balanced. A nurse-client partnership is easier to establish, and there may be more interaction and fewer power struggles than in the hospital. For sensitive topics such as sexual disorders, this collaboration can lead to effective consensual treatment strategies.

PARAPHILIAS: HISTORICAL AND THEORETICAL PERSPECTIVES

The **paraphilias** are a group of behaviors commonly accepted by the clinical description of sexual deviations. Paraphilias present inappropriate sexual fantasies involving deviant sexual acts, inappropriate sexual urges, and acting out of these fantasies and urges.

Once a psychiatric syndrome is described clinically, several steps, including laboratory studies, delimitation from other disorders, follow-up studies, and family studies are necessary to establish diagnostic validity. It is generally acknowledged that no psychiatric syndrome has yet to be fully validated by the complete series of these steps. However, many syndromes have had a substantial body of data published in most phases of the validation.

Little is known, however, about the data in the other areas establishing clinical validity. For instance, there are some laboratory tests and follow-up studies of sexual deviance; however, there are few family studies of paraphilias.

ETIOLOGY

It is also unclear as to what may predispose an individual to developing a paraphilic disorder. Several studies have attempted to suggest etiological factors and the prevalence of sexual deviancies. Research has not concluded cause-and-effect etiology of the paraphilias.

Biological Factors

It is important to acknowledge that people do not voluntarily decide what types of sexual arousal patterns they will have. Researchers suggest possible etiologies (Box 19-3). In the biologic domain, two areas will be addressed: chromosomal functioning and hormonal levels.

In 1942, Klinefelter and his colleagues described Klinefelter's syndrome as a condition characterized by 1) the development of gynecomastia (enlarged breasts) at the time of puberty, 2) aspermatogenesis (low sperm production), and 3) an increased secretion of follicle stimulating hormone (FSH) by the pituitary gland in the brain.

In this particular syndrome, the client presents with 47 chromosomes instead of the normal 46. There is an extra X chromosome present. The client may be thought of as a male (XY) with an extra X chromosome or as a female (XX) with an extra Y chromosome. Clients with this syndrome look like a male at birth. Hence, parents will naturally raise them as males and assign them a male sex role. Money (1957) described a Klinefelter's case of an otherwise normal 8-year-old boy who insisted he felt more comfortable dressed in girl's clothing. Klinefelter's clients have very small testes and produce little testosterone and virtually no sperm. They also experience problems with sexual orientation and the nature of their erotic desires.

Stoller (1968) hypothesized that biological factors such as hormonal and chromosomal abnormalities may be etiological factors in considering the development of sexual disorders (Stoller's "biological force" hypothesis). However, he also suggested that environmental factors, such as early life experiences, may contribute to the development of a paraphilic disorder.

Hereditary/Environmental Factors

Gaffney et al (1984) found evidence that suggests familial transmission of paraphilic disorders. Groth (1979) has identified children who were sexually active with adults during childhood as being environmentally influenced and therefore potentially predisposed for developing a pedophilic disorder. This is an example of victim turned **victimizer,** or sex offender.

EPIDEMIOLOGY

According to the DSM-IV, although paraphilias are not generally diagnosed in clinical facilities, the sizeable commercial market in paraphiliac pornography and paraphernalia suggests that its prevalence in the community is "likely to be higher" (APA, 1994). The paraphilias most common as presenting problems are pedophilia, voyeurism, and exhibitionism. About one-half of the clients with paraphilias seen clinically are married (APA, 1994).

CLINICAL DESCRIPTION

The essential diagnostic features of a paraphilia are "recurrent, intense sexually arousing fantasies, sexual urges, or behaviors generally involving 1) nonhuman objects, 2) the suffering or humiliation of oneself or one's partner, or 3) children or other nonconsenting persons, that occur over a period of at least 6 months" (APA, 1994). Another criterion is that "the behavior, sexual urges, or fantasies cause clinically significant distress in social,

---

Box 19-3 Etiologic Factors for Paraphilias

Biologic Factors

- Chromosomal Functioning
- Hormonal Levels

Hereditary Predisposition

Experiential Factors

- History of Sexual Abuse

Environmental Factors

occupational, or other important areas of functioning" (APA, 1994). The DSM-IV box below summarizes the criteria and description of the paraphilias.

PROGNOSIS

Nurses should be cautioned in attempting to predict **recidivism** (the chronic, repetitive inappropriate acting out of sexual behaviors considered to be unacceptable which have or have not resulted in criminal conviction).

Clients currently undergoing treatment for a sexual disorder may have a lower level of sexual recidivism (Berlin, 1991). Berlin's 1991 study revealed a higher re-offense rate for those clients not receiving (or who have never received) treatment than those engaged in treatment. Hence, treatment compliance is a therapeutic issue that nurses treating this population must address.

It is important for nurses to also acknowledge that treatment efficacy cannot be proven at this time. Further studies are warranted in this area.

DSM-IV CRITERIA

Description of Paraphilias

Exhibitionism

The exposure of one's genitals to an unsuspecting person(s), followed by sexual arousal.

Fetishism

Utilization of objects, e.g. panties, rubber sheeting, for purposes of sexual arousal.

Frotteurism

Rubbing up against a nonconsenting person to heighten sexual arousal.

Pedophilia

Fondling and/or other types of sexual activities with a pre-pubescent child (usually under the age of 13 having not yet developed secondary sex characteristics). Heterosexual pedophiles are sexually attracted to female children under the age of 13. Homosexual pedophiles are sexually attracted to male children under the age of 13. **Ego syntonic pedophiles** do not view this type of behavior as troublesome and will not voluntarily seek treatment for it. **Ego dystonic pedophiles** are concerned and troubled with this type of behavior and might voluntarily seek treatment to deal with it.

Should specify if:

- homosexual pedophilia
- heterosexual pedophilia
- bisexual pedophilia (sexual attraction to both males and females)
- limited to incest (sexual attraction to a child in one's immediate family)
- exclusive type (sexually attracted to children only)
- nonexclusive type (may also be sexually attracted to adults of either sex)

Sexual masochism

Sexual arousal is achieved by being the receiver of pain (either physical or emotional), humiliation, or being made to suffer.

Sexual sadism

Sexual arousal is achieved by the infliction of pain (either physical or emotional) or humiliation onto another person.

Transvestic fetishism

The act of cross-dressing (heterosexual males wearing female clothing) to achieve sexual arousal.

Voyeurism

Sexual arousal is achieved by observing unsuspecting persons who are naked, in the act of disrobing, or engaging in sexual activity ("peeping tom").

Paraphilia NOS (not otherwise specified)

These disorders do not meet the criteria for the aforementioned categories:

- Telephone scatologia: obscene phone calling; "900" sex lines
- Necrophilia: sexual activity with corpses
- Partialism: exclusive focus on a particular body part for sexual arousal
- Zoophilia: sexual activity involving participation with animals (bestiality)
- Coprophilia: sexual arousal by contact with feces
- Klismaphilia: sexual arousal generated by use of enemas
- Urophilia: sexual arousal by contact with urine
- Ephebophilia: fondling and/or other types of sexual activities with pubescent children who are developing secondary sex characteristics, e.g., pubic hair, breasts; these children are usually between the ages of 13–18
- Paraphilic coercive disorder: rape; aggressive sexual assault involving an act of sexual intercourse against one's will and without consent

Adapted from *Diagnostic and statistical manual of mental disorders,* ed 4, Washington, D.C., 1994, American Psychiatric Association.

DISCHARGE CRITERIA

Client will:

1. State nature of specific paraphilic disorder and its impact on self and others (breakdown/absence of cognitive distortions).

2. Identify **triggers**—stimuli that heighten unacceptable sexual cravings and provoke inappropriate sexual behaviors.

3. Develop appropriate relapse prevention strategies.

4. Communicate and problem-solve effectively.

5. Practice appropriate coping strategies.

6. Identify support systems.

THE NURSING PROCESS ■ ■ ■ ■ ■ ■ ■ ■ ■ ■ ■ ■ ■ ■ ■ ■ ■

■ ASSESSMENT

The client with a sexual disorder may exhibit a variety of behavioral symptoms depending on the nature of the disorder. Some symptoms are more difficult to assess than others. The pedophile may exhibit perceptual disturbances. It is not uncommon to hear a pedophile state, for example, "The child looked older than he was." This may also be perceived as a cognitive distortion (an unconscious defense mechanism).

Cognitive distortions may be present in the client with a sexual disorder. Two cognitive distortions most often present in this client population are denial and rationalization. Denial is a defense mechanism used to avoid dealing with problems and responsibilities related to one's behaviors. Rationalization justifies upsetting behaviors by creating reasons (rationale) that would allow the individual to believe the behaviors were warranted or appropriate. These are the most critical issues that the nurse needs to address early in the therapeutic process. A client making a statement such as, "Well, the child didn't fight me and agreed to have sex with me" is a good indication that such cognitive distortions are present.

Another symptom requiring assessment is a disturbance in feeling. Clients with a paraphilic disorder commonly lack remorse for their victims. If they do experience remorse, they may be unable to acknowledge it secondary to the presence of cognitive distortions. Occasionally, pedophiles may claim to experience feelings of "being loved" by the child with whom they have had inappropriate sexual activity.

Clients with a paraphilic disorder should also be assessed for the presence of behavioral and relating disturbances. These are assessed in the client's inability to develop age-appropriate relationships, altered relationships with others, and social withdrawal that may occur secondary to embarrassment or media attention.

■ ■ NURSING DIAGNOSIS

After collecting client assessment data, the nurse is ready to begin formulating diagnoses. In doing so, the nurse may find the client to have symptoms indicative of more than one diagnosis, such as a paraphilic disorder, a psychoactive substance disorder, and/or a personality disorder. Multiple diagnoses will not be addressed in this chapter. However, it is important for the nurse to be aware of this possibility.

When addressing nursing diagnoses for the client with a paraphilic dirsoder, the nurse has many diagnoses from which to choose and will select those that are specific and appropriate to each individual, based on an analysis of comprehensive data collected during the assessment phase.

Nursing Assessment Questions

Paraphilias

1. What brings you here for treatment?
   (To assess client's level of insight)

2. Do you think you have a sexual disorder?
   (To determine if cognitive distortions are present)

3. Do you think you've caused any harm, either physically or emotionally to your victims?
   (To determine if there are disturbances of feelings present)

4. What impact has this problem created on your lifestyle? Relationships?
   (To determine the presence of disturbances in relationships)

NANDA Diagnoses for Paraphilias

Sexuality patterns, altered
Denial, ineffective
Knowledge deficit (of illness and aspects of treatment)
Noncompliance (therapeutic regimen)
Individual coping, ineffective
Social interaction, impaired

■ ■ ■ OUTCOME IDENTIFICATION

Client-centered outcomes should relate to the client's nursing diagnoses and be the opposite of the defining characteristics. Outcomes should be stated in clear, measurable, behavioral terms and include a time frame when feasible in which the client is expected to achieve them. Outcomes may be described as expected or anticipated and are viewed as specific goals to be achieved through the implementation of the plan of care. Examples of behavioral terms the nurse may want to use in developing client-centered outcomes include such words and "Client will . . . state, list, perform, participate, etc."

Outcome Identification for Paraphilias

Client will:

1. State two sexually inappropriate behaviors within three days of admission.
2. Write a list of triggers that provoke inappropriate sexual acting out within the first week of admission.
3. List several relapse prevention strategies appropriate to the client's disorder within the second week of admission.
4. Actively participate in weekly sexual disorders group psychotherapy sessions.
5. Describe two appropriate coping strategies within one week of admission.
6. Verbalize two appropriate methods to meet sexual needs by the time of discharge.
7. Explain the importance of medication compliance and follow-up with outpatient group psychotherapy by time of discharge.

■ ■ ■ ▣ PLANNING

Once diagnoses have been established and client problem identification has occurred, the nurse is ready to begin developing a plan of care specific to the individual client. Client care should be based on mutually agreed upon, realistic, client-centered outcomes. The nurse needs to involve the client in the development of an individualized plan of care, with the expectation that the client will participate in the planning process.

In the population of clients with paraphilic disorders, it is not uncommon to find the presence of cognitive distortions. Nurses must be aware of this as they obtain client input into the development of the plan of care. For example, a client who is in denial of a paraphilic disorder may not be able to fully cooperate with the planning of care or view client-centered outcomes as realistic.

■ ■ ■ ▣ ▣ IMPLEMENTATION

The nurse should work with the client to develop an individualized plan of care that will help the client identify the presence of cognitive distortions (if appropriate), prevent reoffending by identifying triggers that provoke inappropriate sexual activity, and develop effective relapse prevention strategies. The nurse should also explain the significance of treatment on recidivism, and stress the importance of medication compliance and follow-up with outpatient group psychotherapy.

Providing nursing care to such a client may be difficult because of the sensitive nature of this disorder. Nurses must recognize this and be aware of their own comfort

---

COLLABORATIVE DIAGNOSES

DSM-IV Diagnoses*	NANDA Diagnoses**
Exhibitionism	Altered sexuality patterns
Fetishism	Ineffective denial
Frotteurism	Knowledge deficit
Voyeurism	Ineffective individual coping
	Altered family process
	Impaired social interaction
	Anxiety
Pedophilia	High risk for injury to others
	Disturbances in self-concept: personal identity, self-esteem
Sexual masochism	High risk for self-mutilation
	Disturbances in self-concept: personal identity, self-esteem
Sexual sadism	High risk for self-mutilation
	Disturbances in self-concept: personal identity, self-esteem
Transvestic fetishism	Altered role performance
	Disturbances in self-concept: personal identity, self-esteem

(These nursing diagnoses may be applied to all medical diagnoses for the client with a paraphilic disorder.)

*Reprinted with permission form *Diagnostic and statistic manual of mental disorders,* ed 4, Washington, D.C., 1994, American Psychiatric Association.

**Reprinted with permission from *NANDA nursing diagnoses: definitions and classifications, 1995–1996,* Philadelphia, 1994, North American Nursing Diagnosis Association.

NURSING CARE PLAN ■ ■ ■ ■ ■ ■ ■ ■ ■   ■ ■ ■ ■ ■

Robert is a 50-year-old vice president of a major corporation who has been diagnosed as having voyeurism. He intermittently acted-out by engaging in voyeuristic activities at his country club in the ladies locker room. He would secretly masturbate while "peeping." His wife is currently unaware of his behavior but suspects something is wrong. When she confronted Robert regarding her suspicions, he denied any problems.

Robert voluntarily came for treatment primarily out of concern that his wife would discover his disorder. He also began to recognize that he spends a great deal of time on the job fantasizing and/or engaging in voyeuristic and masturbatory activities. Robert has been lying to his wife about his whereabouts for approximately 10 years.

The treatment team focused on assisting Robert in developing appropriate coping strategies. Treatment also included psychoeducation regarding trigger identification and appropriate relapse prevention strategies. The need for couples counseling to disclose the "secret" of Robert's behavior was also addressed. Robert was given Depo-Provera 500 mg IM q wk to help him control his inappropriate sexual acting-out.

DSM-IV Diagnoses

AXIS I	Voyeurism
AXIS II	Deferred-compulsive traits noted
AXIS III	Medical Diagnoses (None)
ACIS IV	Severity of psychosocial stressors (moderate = 3), marital conflict, job stress, anxiety
AXIS V	GAF = 61 within past year and currently

Nursing Diagnosis: Altered sexuality patterns, related to use of cognitive distortions (denial) and sexual behaviors in a socially unacceptable manner, as evidenced by engaging in sexual behavior without regard for others, and public masturbation.

Client Outcomes	Nursing Interventions	Evaluation
• Robert will identify two sexual behaviors that are socially unacceptable within first week of admission.	• Assess for presence of cognitive distortions via a thorough sexual history. *If cognitive distortions are present, Robert may not be able to identify socially unacceptable behaviors, and further treatment is warranted.* • Discuss with Robert what are socially unacceptable sexual behaviors and why *to educate the client about problematic sexual behaviors and their implications on society.* • Encourage client's participation in a sexual disorders group. *These clients frequently believe they are the only ones experiencing inappropriate sexual behaviors, which may lead to feelings of hopelessness, embarrassment, and isolation. Group therapy provides confrontation, support, and hope.*	• Robert readily identified his voyeuristic and public masturbatory behaviors as inappropriate, after one week of admission.

Nursing Diagnosis: Ineffective individual coping, related to inability to trust wife with his secret and inadequate problem-solving skills, as evidenced by use of maladaptive coping methods such as lying, ineffective communication with wife (unable to discuss thoughts and feelings regarding disorder), anxiety, and fear of discovery by wife.

Client Outcomes	Nursing Interventions	Evaluation
• Robert will effectively communicate his thoughts and feelings about his disorder and behaviors with wife and selected staff, within one week of admission.	• Encourage Robert to verbalize his thoughts and feelings concerning his current coping methods (lying, nondisclosure) *to illustrate to Robert the impact of his present coping strategies on him and his wife.*	• Robert verbalized many thoughts and feelings about the impact this could have on his marriage.

NURSING CARE PLAN

Client Outcomes	Nursing Interventions	Evaluation
• Robert will identify two concerns he has about disclosing his disorder and behaviors to his wife, by the time of discharge.	• Educate Robert and his wife about his disorder, its implications and treatment. *Educating Robert and his wife about his disorder and aspects of treatment will alleviate their fears and anxiety, develop trust, and establish an effective, supportive relationship.*	• At the time of discharge, Robert was able to share his "secret" with his wife who was very supportive and eager to learn more about how she could help her husband cope with his disorder.
• Robert will formulate two relapse prevention strategies by the time of discharge, such as calling wife before leaving work so that she will expect him at a certain time, to avoid reoffending.		• Robert discussed two relapse prevention strategies with staff. He will call his wife before leaving work and he will discuss inappropriate thoughts with his wife or therapist.

Nursing Diagnosis: Knowledge deficit of illness and aspects of treatment, related to cognitive distortions, anxiety, and uncertainty, as evidenced by failure to seek prior treatment for his disorder and behaviors.

Client Outcomes	Nursing Interventions	Evaluation
• Robert will verbalize an understanding of his illness within one week of admission.	• Assess Robert's current level of knowledge regarding his illness and readiness to learn by asking direct questions. *A client must exhibit readiness to learn for learning to occur.* • Create a climate conducive to learning, such as a quiet, private, safe environment. *Learning may occur when the nurse has the client's complete attention and distractions are avoided.*	• Robert has successfully identified triggers that provoke sexual thoughts/feelings, and has developed appropriate relapse prevention strategies at the time of discharge.
• Robert will identify triggers, such as unstructured time, that provoke inappropriate thoughts and feelings, within one week of admission.	• Teach the importance of trigger identification and development of relapse prevention strategies as critical steps in treatment *to help Robert gain more effective control of inappropriate behaviors.* • Suggest that Robert write a list of triggers that provoke sexually inappropriate activity and review this list with him *to assess Robert's insight into his disorder and symptom occurrence.*	
• Robert will formulate two relapse prevention strategies, such as opened lines of communication with wife, to avoid reoffending, by the time of discharge.	• Help Robert develop appropriate relapse prevention strategies for his identified triggers *to construct a realistic plan to avoid reoffending.* • Encourage Robert's participation in a sexual disorders group *to receive feedback from peers regarding realistic qualities of trigger identification and relapse prevention strategies.*	

level when discussing sexual issues with these clients. Identifying the presence of a paraphilic disorder may have devastating effects on clients and their significant others. It is important for nurses to include significant others in the interventions to the extent that they can participate.

Nursing Interventions

1. Help the client confront cognitive distortions through direct questioning methods that promote reality orientation as to the client's offending behavior. Open confrontation by the nurse may be needed, including an explanation of the impact of these distortions on treatment outcomes. Journaling may assist in the breakdown of cognitive distortions and help the client track inappropriate sexual fantasies. *Client needs to be aware of the problem and acknowledge it before treatment can begin.*

2. Educate the client and significant others about paraphilic disorders and aspects of treatment, such as identifying triggers that provoke inappropriate sexual activity and methods that help avoid relapse. Encourage active participation in the education process by compiling lists in a journal for review by the client and the nurse. Copies of these lists should be placed in the client's medical record to inform other team members about the client's progress. *This knowledge forms a foundation for treatment.*

3. Enhance the client's compliance with treatment by openly discussing with him or her the effect of inappropriate sexual behaviors on others. Provide research studies regarding the effects of treatment on recidivism rates and handouts about the scope of treatment and how compliance can assist in regaining control of sexual behaviors. *Compliance with treatment reduces the risk of relapse.*

4. Teach the client appropriate coping strategies, assertiveness skills, and problem-solving techniques *to promote follow-through of the treatment plan and facilitate appropriate sexual behaviors.*

5. Promote the client's development of appropriate social skills and provide support and encouragement to the client for efforts at control of the disorder. Peer-to-peer mentorship may be appropriate to enhance appropriate social skills and feelings of acceptance. *The client may feel guilty over his or her behavior and become socially isolated. Support and encouragement of the client will signify that there are healthy, functional, acceptable aspects of his or her personality.*

Additional Treatment Modalities
Pharmacologic

The need for medications is based on the collaborative efforts of the multidisciplinary team to assess the intensity and impulsivity of the client's disorder and symptoms.

CLINICAL ALERT !

The nurse should be alert to signs of noncompliance with treatment or signs indicative of potential relapse, as evidenced by such things as the client's refusal to take medications and/or attend therapy sessions. Client statements such as "I don't know why I need this, I'm just here because the courts sent me", social withdrawal, presence of cognitive distortions, and lack of candidness may all be viewed as risk factors for noncompliance.

ADDITIONAL TREATMENT MODALITIES

Pharmacologic

- Depo-Provera
- Depo-Lupron

Psychotherapy/Psychoeducation Groups

- Individual and group

    Insight-oriented

    Goal-directed

- Occupational/Recreational Therapy
- Family/Couples Therapy

Depo-Provera (Medroxyprogesterone Acetate) 500 MG IM q wk has been prescribed with some success for clients with a paraphilic disorder (Berlin, 1981). This form of external control helps clients develop their own internal controls to avoid relapse. Clients have reported that this medication lowers the frequency and intensity of inappropriate sexual thoughts and fantasies.

There are several side effects the nurse needs to be aware of. Since this type of medication decreases testosterone levels and sperm production, the client receiving Depo-Provera may not be able to father a child. Common side effects include weight gain, increased blood pressure, and fatigue. The nurse may suggest a dietary consultation to help the client maintain weight and decrease the possibility of weight gain. Blood pressures need to be taken prior to each dose. In general, if the diastolic is 100 mmhg or greater, the medication should be withheld. The nurse must communicate with the physician regarding blood pressure readings and whether to administer the medication.

The medication is viscous and should be given in no more than 250 mg (2½ ccs) in each deltoid. The gluteal muscle may also be used in administering Depo-Provera. It is not necessary to administer this medication via "Z" track because there is no conclusive evidence that this method of injection increases absorption. Clients may complain of pain in the injection sites and need to be reassured that the pain will subside within a day. If given in the deltoid, the nurse may want to instruct the client to engage in range-of-motion exercises (moving shoulder and arm in a circular motion).

Depo-Provera should not be administered without informed consent and the client's signature on a consent form that explains about the medication and its therapeutic and nontherapeutic effects. The nurse may review this with the client after a decision has been made by the physician to include this as part of the client's individualized plan of care.

Depo-Lupron (Leuprolide) is a relatively new form of treatment, and there is not much experience with its use in the paraphilic population. This medication may be a more powerful antiandrogenic drug. It acts similarly to Depo-Provera by lowering testosterone levels in the client with a paraphilic disorder. This medication is usually prescribed as 7.5 mg IM once a month. It is also available in a nondepo form; the usual prescribed dosage is 1 mg subcutaneous daily.

Side effects include a decrease in libido (the desired result), bone pain, gynecomastia, hair growth, weight gain, high blood pressure, dizziness, headaches, mood swings, and phlebitis. The nurse must have the knowledge to assess for the presence of any and all nontherapeutic effects.

In the beginning of treatment with Lupron, clients should be prescribed Fludimide 250 mg p.o. TID to enhance the testosterone-suppressing aspects of Lupron by blocking testosterone receptors. This should be prescribed secondary to the increase in testosterone production within the first 2–4 weeks after having started treatment with Lupron.

Again, it is important for the nurse to monitor the client's blood pressure prior to administering Lupron. The same criteria for Depo-Provera apply here.

CASE STUDY

Martin is a 24-year-old college student who attends the local university and lives at home with his parents and two older sisters. He was referred for treatment after conviction for raping a 22-year-old female. Martin has been an active participant in an 8-member outpatient sex offender group for the last 5 years. The Department of Parole and Probation is about to release him back into the community without any further legal requirements. The nurse group leader finds herself feeling uncomfortable with Martin's desire to be discharged outright from group. Her discomfort is related to the seriousness of the disorder, not to the amount of progress he has made. Martin has been compliant with treatment within the last 5 years. His treatment consisted of weekly group attendance with participation, compliance with medications when prescribed, development and implementation of appropriate relapse prevention strategies, and sound understanding of the nature of his disorder.

Critical Thinking and Evaluation

1. What criteria does the nurse use to effectively evaluate Martin's readiness for discharge from therapy?
2. What concerns might the nurse have regarding Martin's prognosis after discharge?
3. With whom might the nurse consult in rendering her decision regarding Martin's discharge from the therapy group?
4. Would family therapy be indicated upon discharge from the group therapy session? Discuss the rationale for this intervention.
5. How could the nurse be responsible if Martin relapses after discharge from the group?

Psychotherapy/Psychoeducation Groups

Nurses may lead or co-lead psychotherapy/psychoeducation groups with the physician or another member of the treatment team if they have the appropriate group psychotherapy credentials.

The purpose of group psychotherapy/**psychoeducation** are 1) to address cognitive distortions; and 2) to provide education to this client population regarding identification of triggers, relapse prevention strategies, importance of treatment compliance, self-esteem issues, appropriate coping strategies, and problem-solving skills.

Recreational and occupational therapy may also be provided to assist the client in time structuring, which may be viewed as a relapse prevention strategy. (See Chapter 24 for further information.)

Family/couples therapy may also be recommended, depending on the individual client care needs. This form of therapy is usually provided by the social worker and may also be provided by a masters-prepared nurse or physician.

■ ■ ■ ■ ■ ■ EVALUATION

Nurses must continually evaluate the effectiveness of their interventions on the behavior to successfully treat this population. If identified nursing interventions are not helping the client achieve his or her outcomes, revisions must be made in the nursing care plan. The nurse may want to discuss the plan with the client and obtain his or her assistance in revising it. The areas in which client outcomes have been successfully achieved should be identified as "resolved." If newly identified problems arise, these should also be addressed in the client's plan of care.

In treating the client with a paraphilic disorder, it is not unrealistic to expect the client to acknowledge the presence of the paraphilic disorder, identify triggers, develop relapse prevention strategies, and state the importance of treatment compliance post discharge. If these outcomes are not met by the time of discharge, the client would be at a greater risk for reoffending. The need to protect both the client and society from possible relapse or recidivism is critical.

The minimal expected period for outpatient treatment is two years, although actual time for treatment may be considerably longer. These clients need to be carefully monitored for any changes in their status that could lead to relapse. Monitoring may occur through weekly outpatient group therapy or, if group is not indicated, by periodic visits with the client's therapist.

A client is formally discharged from outpatient treatment based on the level of progress and current status regarding the paraphilic behaviors.

Summary of Key Concepts

1. The nurse must have an understanding of human sexuality, be aware of his or her feelings and values regarding sexuality, and be committed to incorporating sexuality into client care in a nonjudgmental manner.

2. Sexual dysfunctions are the most common of all sexual problems that come to the attention of health care practitioners. Estimates of the prevalence of sexual dysfunctions are as high as 50%.

3. The lack of sex education and the high rate of sexual repression may contribute to the high incidence of sexual dysfunctions.

4. Establishment of a plan of care should include the significant other. In a couple situation, blame should not be placed on either person.

5. Specific, realistic outcome criteria developed by the client (or client and significant other) are necessary for implementing the plan of care.

6. Nursing interventions include education about human sexual functioning, sexual response, and sexual dysfunctions; helping clients improve their communication; support for the clients' fears and anxieties; support for enhancement of self-esteem; and referral for professional help.

7. Many complex diagnostic and treatment modalities have been developed for sexual dysfunctions in the past few decades. These include psychophysiologic methods and psychosocial methods. They include neurologic, endocrine, and vascular treatments, as well as specific sex therapy techniques. Therapeutic modalities are currently more developed for males than for females.

8. Permission-giving for sexual feelings and behaviors may be the single most important intervention.

9. Paraphilia is defined as sexual deviations/disorders presenting with inappropriate sexual fantasies involving deviant sexual acts, inappropriate sexual urges, and acting out of these fantasies and urges.

10. Family history positive for the presence of a paraphilic disorder and/or history of victimization may predispose other family members to developing a similar or different paraphilic disorder.

11. Establishing a plan of care should include the client to the extent that he or she is able to participate, and goals should reflect mutual agreement between the nurse and the client.

12. Interventions should be based on the client's individual needs. Included in the plan of care are confrontation of cognitive distortions, exploring the effects of inappropriate sexual behaviors on others, psychoeducational group therapy to teach the client how to identify triggers that provoke inappropriate sexual thoughts, development of relapse prevention strategies and the effects of treatment on illness symptomatology, the importance of treatment compliance during hospital stay and postdischarge, and development of appropriate coping strategies and problem-solving skills.

13. The client with a paraphilic disorder who is compliant with treatment has a lesser risk of recidivism.

REFERENCES

Abel GG et al: Sexually aggressive behavior. In Curran, WJ et al, editors: *Forensic psychiatry and psychology*, Philadelphia, 1986, F.A. Davis.

Abel GG et al: Self-reported sex crimes of non-incarcerated paraphiliacs, *J Interpersonal Violence* 2(1):3–25, 1987.

Abel GG, Osborn C: Stopping sexual violence, *Psychiatric Annals* 22(6):301–306, 1992.

American Psychiatric Association: *Diagnostic and statistical manual of mental disorders*, ed 4, Washington, D.C., 1994, APA.

Anon J: The PLISSIT model, *J Sex Education and Therapy* 2(1):1–15, 1976.

Arndt WB Jr: *Gender disorders and the paraphilias*, Madison, Conn., 1991, International Universities Press.

Baker HJ, Stoller J: Can a biological force contribute to gender identity? *Amer J Psychiatry* 124(12):1653–1658, 1968.

Beitchman J et al: A review of the long-term effects of child sexual abuse, *Child Abuse and Neglect* 16:101–118, 1992.

Bergner RM: Money's "lovemap" account of the paraphilias: a critique and reformulation, *Amer J Psychotherapy* 42(2): 254–259, 1988.

Berlin FS: Special considerations in the psychiatric evaluation of sexual offenders against minors. In Rosner R, Schwartz H, editors: *Juvenile psychiatry and the law: critical issues in American psychiatry and the law*, vol 4, New York, 1989, Plenum Press.

Berlin FS: The paraphilias and Depo-Provera: Some medical, ethical and legal considerations. *Bull Amer Ac of Psychiatry and the Law* 17(3):233–239, 1989.

Berlin FS et al: A five-year plus follow-up survey of criminal recidivism within a treated cohort of 406 pedophiles, 111 exhibitionists and 109 sexual aggressives: issues and outcomes, *Amer J Forensic Psychiatry* 12(3):5–28, 1991.

Berlin FS, Malin HM: Media distortion of the public's perception of recidivism and psychiatric rehabilitation, *Amer J Psychiatry* 148 (11):1572–1576, 1991.

Berlin FS, Meineke CF: Treatment of sex offenders with antiandrogen medication: conceptualization, review of treatment modalities and preliminary findings, *Amer J Psychiatry* 138:601–608, 1981.

Brecher E: *The sex researchers*, New York, 1971, New American Library.

Gaffney GS et al: Is there familial transmission of pedophilia? *J Nervous and Mental Disease* 172:546–548, 1984.

Groth AN: *Men who rape*, New York, 1979, Plenum Press.

Hartman W, Fithian M: *Treatment of sexual dysfunction: a bio-psycho-social approach*, Long Beach, Calif., 1972, Center for Marital and Sexual Studies.

Kaplan H: *The new sex therapy*, New York, 1974, Brunner/Mazel.

Kaplan HI, Sadock BJ: Paraphilias. In Kaplan HI, Sadock, BJ, editors: *Synopsis of psychiatry, behavioral sciences, clinical psychiatry*, ed 6, Baltimore, 1991, Williams and Wilkins.

Kiersch TA: Treatment of sex offenders with Depo-Provera, *Bull Amer Ac of Psychiatry and the Law* 18(2):179–187, 1990.

Kim MJ et al: *Pocket guide to nursing diagnoses*, ed 5, St. Louis, 1993, Mosby.

Kinsey A et al: *Sexual behavior in the human female*, Philadelphia, 1953, W.B. Saunders.

Klinefelter HF et al: Syndrome characterized by gynecomastia, aspermatogenesis without A-Leydigism, and increased excretion of FSH, *J Clin Endocrinology* 2(2):615–627, 1994.

Leiblum S, Rosen R: *Principles and practice of sex therapy*, New York, 1989, Guilford Press.

LeMone P: Human sexuality in adults with insulin-dependent diabetes mellitus, *Image: J of Nursing Scholarship* 25(2):101–105, 1993.

LoPiccolo J, Friedman J: Broad spectrum treatment of low sexual desire: integration of cognitive, behavioral and systematic therapy. In Leiblum S, Rosen R, editors: *Sexual desire disorders*, New York, 1988, Guilford Press.

Masters W, Johnson V: *Human sexual inadequacy*, Boston, 1970, Little Brown.

Masters W, Johnson V: *Human sexual response*, Boston, 1966, Little Brown.

Meyer WJ et al: Depo-Provera treatment for sex offending behavior: an evaluation of outcome, *Bull Amer Ac Psychiatry and the Law* 20(3):249–259, 1992.

Money J et al: Imprinting and the establishment of gender role, *Arch Neurology and Psychiatry* 77:333–336, 1957.

Money J: *Lovemaps*, Buffalo, N.Y., 1986, Prometheus Books.

Money J: *Lovemaps: clinical concepts of sexual/erotic health and pathology, paraphilia, and gender transposition in childhood, adolescence, and maturity*, New York, 1986, Irvington Publishers.

Money J: *Venuses penuses: sexology, sexosophy and exigency theory*, Buffalo, N.Y., 1986, Prometheus Books.

Money J: Treatment guidelines: antiandrogen and counseling of paraphilic sex offenders, *J Sex and Marital Therapy* 13(3):219–223, 1987.

Morokoff P, Gillilland R: Stress, sexual functioning and marital satisfaction, *J Sex Research* 30:43–53, 1993.

Renshaw D: Profile of 2376 patients treated at Loyola Sex Clinic between 1972 and 1978, *Sexual and Marital Therapy* 3: 111–117, 1988.

Schiavi R et al: Erectile function and penile blood pressure in diabetes mellitus, *J Sex and Marital Therapy* 20(2):119–124, 1994.

Semans R: Premature ejaculation: a new approach, *Southern Med J* 49:353–358, 1956.

Simon WT, Schouten PG: Plethysmography in the assessment of sexual deviance: an overview, *Arch Sexual Behavior* 20(1):75–91, 1991.

Spector I, Carey M: Incidence and prevalence of the sexual dysfunctions: a critical review of the literature, *Arch Sexual Behavior* 19:389–408, 1990.

Wagner G, Kaplan, HS: *The new injection treatment for impotence*, New York, 1993, Brunner/Mazel.

Wilson GD: An ethological approach to sexual deviation. In Wilson GD, editor: *Variant sexuality: research and theory*, Baltimore, 1987, The Johns Hopkins University Press.

Wincze J et al: Comparison of nocturnal penile tumescence response and penile response to erotic stimulation during waking states in comprehensively diagnosed groups of males experiencing erectile difficulties, *Arch Sexual Behavior*, 17:333–348, 1988.

Zilbergeld B, Evans M: The inadequacy of Masters and Johnson, *Psych Today* 14:29–43, 1980.

CHAPTER 20

Adjustment Disorders

Merry A. Armstrong

Adjustment disorders Short-term disturbances in mood or behavior with nonpsychotic manifestations resulting from identifiable stressors. The severity of the reaction is not predictable by the severity of the stressor.

Adult developmental theory A theory that suggests that although persons may complete developmental tasks of childhood, they continue to evolve as maturity progresses. Adulthood is divided into four age categories, and central themes of adult experience and development are articulated.

Holism A term with various interpretations and meanings. In the broadest sense, holism refers to a belief system in which persons are unified, complex, interdependent systems with interrelated physical, mental, emotional, spiritual, and social dimensions.

Loss A process characterized by a series of overlapping stages that include common psychological and behavioral manifestations of recognition, adjustment, and resolution.

- Describe five major criteria for an adjustment disorder.

- Analyze the relationship of life events to adjustment disorders.

- Discuss the implications of the diagnosis of adjustment disorder with depressed mood for the nonpsychiatric hospitalized client.

- Apply the nursing process to clients who exhibit symptoms of adjustment disorders.

- Explain the major therapeutic goals for clients who have a diagnosis of adjustment disorder.

T his chapter discusses the diagnostic category of **adjustment disorders,** or problematic responses to life events. Problematic responses are behaviors, feelings, or thoughts that interfere with an individual's functioning or sense of well-being. Some of the symptoms of adjustment disorders are similar to those in other diagnostic groups, such as affective mood disorders or anxiety disorders. However, adjustment disorders are considered less serious and often represent transient episodes in the lives of otherwise mentally healthy individuals.

For example, clients treated for a physical illness are sometimes referred to a mental health practitioner because of complaints of depression, dysphoria, or anxiety resulting from difficulty adjusting to their diagnosis. Depending on the nature of the symptoms and their temporal relationship to life events, many of these clients are diagnosed as having an adjustment disorder.

In this situation the diagnosis implies that the mental health practitioner has reason to believe that the client's problematic symptoms will abate when the physical illness is resolved as a central issue. Like all clients, the client diagnosed with an adjustment disorder would be continually assessed for new or intensifying symptoms that might indicate a developing major depressive disorder or other mental illness.

Additionally, individuals seeking outpatient therapy for assistance in dealing with responses to such things as specific problematic life events may also be diagnosed as having an adjustment disorder. After obtaining an appropriate developmental history, completing a mental status assessment, and systematically eliminating other potential diagnoses, the mental health practitioner may decide that the client has an adjustment disorder. The term *mental health practitioner* is used because in some states advanced practice nurses (APN), licensed clinical social workers (LCSW), or other licensed, qualified personnel determine DSM-IV pathology. The diagnosis of adjustment disorder suggests the probability that the client possesses or can rally sufficient resources to resolve his or her problematic response within an appropriate time, in this case by responding to therapeutic intervention as a primary treatment modality.

HISTORICAL AND THEORETICAL PERSPECTIVES

Problematic responses to either developmental or situational stressors have been discussed in psychiatric literature for many years. However, adjustment disorders were first professionally categorized and described in 1968 in the second edition of the *Diagnostic and Statistical Manual of Mental Disorders* (DSM-II) as "transient situational disturbance" (APA, 1968). The DSM-III (1980) grouped adjustment disorders by clinical presentation. If the client described symptoms of depression without symptoms of major depression, he or she was diagnosed as having an adjustment disorder with depressed mood.

The DSM-III-Revised (1987) used adjustment disorders as a classification for conditions that did not fulfill criteria for a major psychiatric disorder. Nine types of adjustment disorder were identified.

The DSM-IV (1994) considers adjustment disorders transient episodes of dysfunction in response to specific stressors. To be diagnosed as having an adjustment disorder, the client must demonstrate criteria for one of six classifications: adjustment disorder with depressed mood, with anxiety, with mixed anxiety and depressed mood, with disturbance of conduct, with mixed disturbance of emotions and conduct, and unspecified. Adjustment disorders may be acute (symptoms last six months or less), or chronic (symptoms persist for more than six months), or when the precipitating stressor had long-lasting effects. Examples of these disorders will be presented later in the chapter.

As a part of their role, many mental health practitioners are required to arrive at conclusions (diagnoses) about the mental condition of their clients. Without the immediacy or specificity of laboratory tests such as blood values or radiologic studies to rely on, the practitioner initiates a relationship with the client. The developing therapeutic relationship is the forum in which dialogue, discussion, observation, and professional assessment converge to provide material supporting a mental health diagnosis. As the therapeutic relationship continues, diagnoses (medical or nursing) may change depending on the client's symptoms, behaviors, or as other new information becomes known to the professional staff. The diagnosis of adjustment disorder suggests that troublesome symptoms may abate with time and therapeutic intervention. Conversely, adjustment disorders may be precursors to more serious mental health problems. In either case, continual reassessment of client symptoms, condition, and situation is required.

ETIOLOGY

The interaction of personality, crisis, stress, developmental factors, and cultural influences must be considered when investigating the formation of adjustment disorders.

Crisis and Stress Models

Situational events requiring major physical and/or psychologic adjustment occur normally during a person's lifetime. Most people develop a repertoire of skills to manage difficult situations. However, because of the intensity, timing, or repetition of the stressor or situation, prior methods are sometimes not sufficient to mitigate the problem. Using the model suggested by the crisis theory one might say that an adjustment disorder results from an individual's inability to use existing coping methods or create new methods in response to a situation. This inability to use former methods or formulate new strategies results in a situation in which the client feels overwhelmed, confused, and helpless, further depleting his or her ability to rally resources. These feelings may be manifested as depression, anxiety, or other combinations of emotional experience.

Stress-adaptation theory, originally formulated by Selye, (1956, 1978) suggested a biological response to stress called the *general adaptation syndrome* (GAS). *Stress* was defined as a situation that required a physiologic response or change. It was noted that people may respond to the same stressful situation in different ways. For example, one individual might experience a headache in response to an argument, while another might experience physical or psychologic sensations of relief. An experience might be labeled pleasant or unpleasant, but if a biologic adjustment is required, the GAS is activated and the stress response is present. The stress-adaptation and crisis models are similar in that the client feels overwhelmed and without resources to respond to a situation.

PRECIPITATING FACTORS

Adjustment disorders can be triggered by a stressor or series of stressors that may be developmental (adolescence, menopause), situational (job change, divorce, hospitalization), or adventitious (earthquake, war, flood).

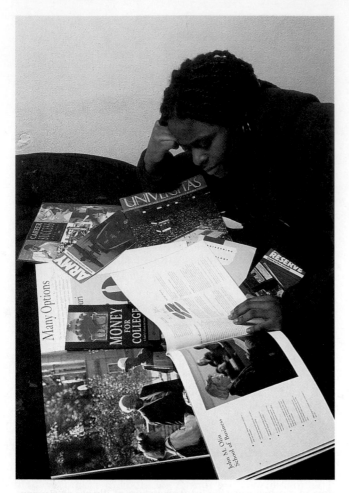

Figure 20-1 Adolescents face developmental and situational challenges as they contemplate decisions for their future, such as options for employment or college.

Life events requiring major adjustments can be either developmental, situational, adventitious, or a combination of all three.

For example, serious developmental and situational challenges occur in early adulthood when adolescents graduate from high school and must decide their direction. Accomplishing the developmental tasks of establishing personal identity as well as negotiating situational stressors (decisions after graduation from high school to explore career, school, surfing, peace corps, military, etc.) that determine one's life course are complex endeavors.

Likewise, people in their middle and older years have significant developmental challenges that may result in transient situational adjustment problems. For example, retirement is often referred to as a benefit and goal of late adulthood, yet it is sometimes experienced as a loss of identity and purpose. Other life events related to individual physical or psychologic development may include the loss of a significant other or the diagnosis of a major disease process. Changes in employment, marital status,

child bearing, and other life occurrences may also present individuals with significant responsibilities to manage. Illness, major family changes, and/or developmental crises are not uncommon occurrences, and often occur simultaneously.

LOSS

A key process underlying life change is that of **loss,** described by Kubler-Ross (1969) and since explored and refined by others (Levine, 1987 Walsh and McGoldrick, 1991). Loss is a process characterized by a series of overlapping stages that include common psychologic and behavioral manifestations of recognition, adjustment, and resolution. Numerous examples of loss have been articulated in this chapter, and all change includes loss. To manage a desired change such as retirement, marriage, or establishing a family requires loss of previous status, freedom, or identity. Walsh and McGoldrick (1991) stated that losses require movement through a process of mourning in order to get what is needed from the experience or relationship to continue on with one's life. How persons get what they need from the experience is often contextually determined and influenced by culture and socialization. The nurse plays an instrumental role in educating the client about the loss process and in helping the client mourn loss.

Grief, mourning, and bereavement are other expressions of loss and are discussed in Chapter 27, Grief and Loss. According to DSM-IV criteria, persons experiencing severe or prolonged difficulties with grief and bereavement would not be diagnosed with adjustment disorders.

Developmental Influences

Erikson (1963) proposed a developmental theory of the personality through achievement of specific tasks at different stages of the life cycle. Erikson postulated that difficulties in adjustment occurred when age-appropriate behaviors or tasks were not completed, resulting in an inability to move forward with developmental tasks. The **adult developmental theory** suggests that individuals continue to evolve as maturity progresses.

Colarusso and Nemiroff (1981) contended that individuals continue to refine their sense of identity and self and that adulthood was characterized by normative crises based on adult developmental tasks. According to these authors, themes of adult developmental tasks are intimacy, love, and sex; issues related to the body; time and death; relationship to children; relationship to parents; mentor relationships; relationship to society; work; play; and finances. As people mature, themes of adult development are continuous and important sources of information for the therapist in the process of identifying the dynamics of the client problem or symptoms.

Colarusso and Nemiroff (1981) used the developmental concept of Erikson's (1963) model and suggested that adulthood is divided into rough age groupings: early adulthood (ages 20–40), middle adulthood (ages 40–60), late adulthood (ages 60–80), and late-late adulthood (ages 80 and beyond). These authors further suggested that adult developmental strands existed on a continuum and were experienced differently, depending on issues active in each age category.

For example, the strand, or theme, of adult development, "time and death," might likely be applied as an active developmental task for a person in middle adulthood rather than for someone in early adulthood. So a person in middle adulthood may, at the same time, experience being diagnosed with a chronic health problem, responsible for substantial financial and work responsibilities, involved in parenting teenagers, and experiencing the death of a parent.

If adults experience developmental challenges unique to their age and situation, as Colarusso and Nemiroff (1981, 1987) contended, how can mental health professionals help clients identify, attain, and utilize new skills? A common precipitating event that stimulates adult development is the personal experience of an illness, or the illness of a loved one. Clients at risk for, or who have adjustment disorders, are commonly cared for by nurses in general hospitals, long-term care facilities, rehabilitation centers, or in the home. Nurses have unique opportunities for long-term assessment and subsequent intervention regarding clients' emotional and psychologic difficulties. For example, one of the activities in a mental health assessment is the determination of the meaning of the situation for the client. Being briefly hospitalized for a hernia repair probably does not have the same meaning for a client of the same age who is hospitalized for stabilization of newly diagnosed diabetes.

Cultural, Social, and Psychologic Influences

Growth and development must be examined with consideration of contextual aspects of sociocultural influences. This chapter would not be complete without mentioning the scope and volume of currently debated issues of psychologic and personality development. Extending beyond historic disputes of nature versus nurture theories, scholars question classification systems of mental illness (Kirk and Kutchins, 1992) and traditional scientific research methods (Blier, 1986).

In addition, debate continues in the human sciences regarding differences in development and experience according to one's gender and socialization (Gilligan, 1982; Jordan et al, 1991; Lerner, 1988; Lewis, 1986; Meth and Pasick, 1990; Napier, 1991; Pittman, 1991). Gender, culture, and social factors influence the results of measurements such as the intelligence quotient (IQ). If gender, culture, and social factors partially determine a person's reality, how do we give nursing care using standard nursing diagnoses that may not reflect the reality of our clients?

For example, a nurse caring for a client identifies that the client has problems related to the death of a spouse and applies the nursing diagnosis of dysfunctional grieving. However, behaviors that the nurse perceives as problems may be appropriate in the client's culture. If that is the case, whose problems is the nurse stating? Instead of identifying the client's problems, the nurse might have demonstrated cultural bias in expecting all people to resolve issues in the same way. The nurse must be aware that clients must resolve their grief in a culturally and socially appropriate manner and include assessment activities that reveal this information. This sounds like a simple solution, but different cultures also proscribe speaking to persons outside the family about intimate details. Therefore, the nurse must also be aware of communication patterns of the culture and other social customs.

Lowenberg (1989), a nurse researcher, explored the practices of consumers and practitioners of American health care and uses the framework of an evolving paradigm of health care, **holism.** Historically, illness was thought to represent social deviance (Davis, 1972; Parsons, 1951), and that stigma and labeling were applied to a variety of problems culturally interpreted as illness. The author observed that emerging concepts of holism and health suggested that people's physical, mental, emotional, spiritual, and social aspects were interrelated and interdependent. Using this concept, some people have redefined the illness experience from biologic deterioration to a more positive interpretation of illness as a warning sign that adjustments in living are needed. Lowenberg (1989) observed that the emerging health paradigm (holism) considered illness as an opportunity for growth and development.

Contributions of Nursing Research

Nursing research has contributed information leading to a greater understanding of individual experience. Although nursing research has not addressed the diagnosis of adjustment disorders specifically, it has explored meanings of many life events for individual clients and caregivers, using qualitative research techniques (Armstrong, 1992; Beck, 1992; Bergum, 1989; Heifner, 1993; Lowenberg, 1989; Main et al, 1993; Mickley et al, 1992; Murphy, 1993; Tanner et al, 1993). Understanding the process of an illness experience can help nurses and other professionals develop effective assessment techniques, methods for intervention, and models for evaluation of treatment. See Understanding and Applying Research on page 478.

EPIDEMIOLOGY

Adult adjustment disorders are thought to be common, although data to support this opinion are scarce (Popkin,

Coward D: The lived experience of self-transcendence in women with advanced breast cancer, *Nurs Sci Quarterly*, 3(4):162–169, 1990.

Understanding and Applying RESEARCH

The purpose of this study was to describe the experience of self-transcendence in women with advanced breast cancer. Five women who had lived with metastatic disease from 2 to 7 years described experiences from which they derived an increased sense of self-worth, purpose in life, and interconnectedness with others. Self-transcendence involved reaching out beyond self to help other women, to permit others to help them, or to just accept unchangeable situations. Nurses may be able to establish and maintain conditions in which self-transcendence occurs.

Reading about their experiences, one imagines that at several points during their illness these women may have been candidates for a diagnosis of adjustment disorder. This study describes unique ways that a person with a diagnosis of adjustment disorder experiences the continuum of a disease process. As a result of understanding this process, nurses may consider additional options for including the client in supportive nursing therapies and mutual and creative care planning.

DSM-IV CRITERIA

Adjustment Disorders

A. A reaction to an identifiable psychosocial stressor (or multiple stressors) that occurs within three months of onset of the stressor(s).

B. Symptoms of distress are marked and in excess of a normal and expectable reaction to the stressor(s), OR the client experiences significant social or occupational impairment.

C. The disturbance does not meet criteria for Axis I or II disorder. A diagnosis of adjustment disorder may be made in the presence of an Axis I or II disorder if the pattern of symptoms is not attributable to these disorders, and an identified stressor exists.

D. This diagnosis is not used when symptoms represent bereavement.

E. Symptoms of the disorder must resolve within 6 months of the cessation of the stressor.

However, symptoms persisting longer than 6 months because of the chronicity of the stressor (a chronic physical disease) or as the result of enduring consequences of a stressor (divorce, loss of employment) may be considered chronic adjustment disorders.

Reprinted with permission from *Diagnostic and statistical manual of mental disorders*, ed 4, Washington, D.C., 1994, American Psychiatric Association.

1989). A factor contributing to difficulty in gathering statistics regarding adjustment disorder treatment is that the clinical or symptomatic findings in adjustment disorder vary widely, thus making the diagnosis difficult. The DSM-IV (1994) cites prevalence rates in outpatient populations between 5% and 20%.

Studies were conducted on the findings of psychiatric consultation/liaison personnel who assessed clients in acute care hospitals. Adjustment disorders in medically ill inpatient clients (Popkin et al, 1990; Razavi et al, 1990; Snyder et al, 1990) were commonly identified. Many clients with terminal diagnoses or severe chronic illness displayed symptoms of either major depression or adjustment disorder.

CLINICAL DESCRIPTION

Six subtypes of adjustment disorder are noted in the DSM-IV. They are coded on Axis IV according to symptom type and with stressor(s) noted. Because adjustment disorder can present with various combinations of symptomatology, it is difficult to categorize discrete symp-

toms. General clusters of symptoms are provided in Box 20-1.

PROGNOSIS

Data are not currently available related to specific prognoses for adjustment disorders. Most practitioners believe that because the diagnosis of adjustment disorder ordinarily precludes a major psychiatric problem, there is hope that the client can resolve problems by developing coping methods and mobilizing resources.

DISCHARGE CRITERIA

At the time of discharge, the client will:

• Verbalize absence of thoughts of self-harm.

• Identify goals for continuing care after discharge, if indicated.

• Identify and analyze coping resources and plans for using resources.

• Describe stressors and effective ways of managing stressful situations in the past.

Box 20-1   Types of Adjustment Disorders

Adjustment Disorder with Depressed Mood

Used when the predominant symptomatology are depressed mood, tearfulness, and feelings of hopelessness.

Adjustment Disorder with Anxious Mood

Used when the predominant symptomatology are nervousness, worry, and jitteriness.

Adjustment Disorder with Mixed Anxiety and Depressed Mood

Used when predominant manifestation is a combination of depression and anxiety.

Adjustment Disorder with Disturbance of Conduct

Used when the client's conduct violates the rights of others or major age-appropriate societal norms and rules (for example, vandalism, fighting, defaulting on legal responsibilities).

Adjustment Disorder with Mixed Disturbance of Emotions and Conduct

Used when predominant symptomatology are combinations of emotions (for example, depression or anxiety) and a disturbance of conduct.

Unspecified

Used for maladaptive reactions (such as physical complaints, social withdrawal, or work or academic inhibition) to psychosocial stressors not classifiable in other specific subtypes.

Reprinted with permission from *Diagnostic and statistical manual of mental disorders*, ed 4, Washington, D.C., 1994, American Psychiatric Association.

THE NURSING PROCESS ■ ■ ■ ■ ■ ■ ■ ■ ■ ■ ■ ■ ■ ■ ■ ■ ■

■ ASSESSMENT

Because clients are not often hospitalized for treatment of adjustment disorder, nurses are more likely to assess clients with an adjustment disorder in an outpatient or home setting. See Nursing Care in the Community on page 480. Outpatient clients may request treatment based on the symptoms of one or more adjustment disorders. Adjustment disorder subtypes with anxious or depressed mood are the most frequently diagnosed in adult clients (Popkin, 1989).

Nurses need to assess for precipitating stressors that preceded the onset of symptoms of adjustment disorder. Assessment of behavioral symptoms and mood and affect congruity are key to initial nursing assessment. Symptoms depend on the type of adjustment disorder and might include the following:

- **Sensory-Perceptual:** Nervousness, worry, and jitteriness; other symptoms congruent with feeling anxious and/or depressed, such as headache, backache, lethargy.

- **Thinking Disturbances:** Preoccupation with thoughts of death (not suicidal thoughts), inability to attend to tasks, decreased concentration, inattention to external environment, inability to attend to detail, inability to concentrate, and short attention span leading to learning impairment. Feelings of ambivalence and inability to make decisions. Denial of physical illness and noncompliance with treatment recommendations.

- **Feeling Disturbances:** Feelings of sadness and sorrow, feelings of emptiness and worthlessness, decreased self-esteem, inability to articulate feelings, excessive worry about life events.

- **Behavioral and Relating Disturbances:** Lack of interest in external events, disruption in relationships, social withdrawal, loss of interest in hobbies, withdrawal from work or academic endeavors, spiritual distress, increased or decreased psychomotor activity, hyperverbal patterns, difficulty continuing conversations, becoming easily distracted, insomnia, violation of age-appropriate norms or rules, violation of rights of others.

■ ■ NURSING DIAGNOSES

In adjustment disorders, nursing diagnoses are prioritized based on symptoms. Data gathered in the assessment phase of the nursing process provide information about the client's history, symptoms, and (especially in the case of adjustment disorder) behavior and responses to life stressors. The collaborative and multidisciplinary

Nursing Care in the Community

Adjustment Disorders

Adjustment disorders are commonly found in the community mental health field. Some are the long-term results of predictable crises of maturation and development, such as death of a loved one, employment problems, and financial issues. In such cases, therapeutic strategies have been fairly well-established, and the nurse can follow up the initial crisis intervention to reassure the client that the situation should improve with time. Clients with these problems can be introduced to support groups focused on similar issues and, if necessary, be prescribed medication to help mitigate the process until the individual has established balanced coping patterns. These clients usually respond well to education and exposure to peers who have experienced similar problems. However, prolonged adjustment difficulties may require more intensive interventions. The nurse may consider longer-term work with the client, focusing on changes in living situation and perhaps even in lifestyle, to reduce stress, occupy free time, and increase coping abilities.

Unpredictable and at times catastrophic crises are much more difficult to manage, requiring active and decisive action on the part of the community mental health nurse. Rape or mugging would be examples of such overwhelming trauma, initially managed by crisis intervention, and then requiring extremely careful supervision to avoid excessive emotional reactions, such as homicidal or suicidal feelings. Nonjudgmental debriefing must be continued to put the situation in perspective and allow clients to both ventilate and distance themselves from the trauma.

Prolonged difficulties, such as marital problems, chronic ill health, or financial problems, require a new level of coping ability. Adjustment should be achieved within 3–6 months without attendant anxiety, depression, or changes in typical behavior. The community mental health nurse is in a good position to monitor how well the client has reconciled to the current situation and how positive he or she is about the future.

Finally, if the symptoms of adjustment difficulties continue for longer than approximately 6 months, the long-term needs of the client are addressed by giving referrals to an appropriate therapist and a support group, for ongoing treatment. Adjustment disorders often require long-term psychosocial and practical interventions designed to promote the client's future safety and well-being through the development of healthy, effective coping skills.

Nursing Assessment Questions

Adjustment Disorders

1. What has happened in your life in the recent past?
   (To determine if the client can identify a stressor or stressors preceding an adjustment disorder)

2. In the overall picture of your life, in what way did that event affect you?
   (To determine the meaning of the event to the person)

3. What have you done in the past when such events occurred?
   (To determine whether the client has adequate coping skills and potential resources)

4. Tell me about your family and friends and their roles in this event.
   (To determine current support networks and obtain information about family/significant others)

NANDA Diagnoses for Adjustment Disorders

Risk for violence, self-directed or directed at others
Anxiety
Ineffective individual coping
Spiritual distress
Impaired adjustment
Dysfunctional grieving
Self-esteem disturbance
Impaired social interaction

■ ■ ■ OUTCOME IDENTIFICATION

Based on symptoms related to the specific adjustment disorder, outcome criteria may vary. However, regardless of the symptoms, client safety is a prime concern. Client outcomes, which are derived from nursing diagnoses, are the expected and anticipated client behaviors or responses to be achieved.

Outcome Identification for Adjustment Disorders

Client will:

1. Verbalize absence of thoughts of self-harm.

2. Identify goals for continuing care after discharge.

3. Discuss plans for goal achievement.

effort in adjustment disorders is appropriately directed toward helping the client rally resources to achieve a functional level of daily living.

CASE 📁 STUDY

C. F., An 18-year-old unemployed Caucasian, single female presented to the community clinic with complaints of lack of energy. After completion of a thorough medical assessment, the nurse talked with the client about recent events in her life. Living at home with her parents and two younger siblings, C. F. shared with the nurse that she graduated from high school two months earlier and was uncertain what direction to take with her life. Her boyfriend wanted them to get married. She wanted to continue on to junior college. Her parents were noncommittal, except that they were urging her to do something and start paying rent. She visited a favorite aunt who recommended she seek counseling.

For approximately three weeks, C. F. had noticed symptoms of increased irritability, occasional crying spells, withdrawal from friends, and impulses to run away. Before coming to the clinic, she had been home watching a movie on television and began feeling increasingly depressed and confused about what to do with her life.

Critical Thinking and Assessment

1. C. F. is experiencing two types of problematic life events. What are they?
2. What is C. F.'s risk for suicide?
3. Which behaviors has C. F. demonstrated, indicating her ability to identify or mobilize resources?
4. Apply concepts of the loss process to C. F.'s situation.

COLLABORATIVE DIAGNOSES

DSM-IV Diagnoses*	NANDA Diagnoses**
Adjustment Disorder with Depressed Mood	Ineffective Individual Coping Social Isolation Spiritual Distress Ineffective Denial
Adjustment Disorder with Anxious Mood	Anxiety Ineffective Individual Coping Sleep Pattern Disturbance
Adjustment Disorder with Disturbance of Conduct	Ineffective Individual Coping Anxiety Impaired Adjustment Altered Role Performance Defensive Coping
Adjustment Disorder with Mixed Disturbance of Emotions and Conduct	Ineffective Individual Coping Defensive Coping Sleep Pattern Disturbance Anxiety Impaired Adjustment Social Isolation Spiritual Distress Ineffective Denial

*Reprinted with permission from *Diagnostic and statistical manual of mental disorders,* ed 4, Washington, D.C., 1994, American Psychiatric Association.

**Reprinted with permission from *NANDA nursing diagnoses: definitions and classifications, 1995-1996,* Philadelphia, 1994, North American Nursing Diagnosis Association.

4. Analyze coping resources and plans for using resources.
5. Describe stressors and effective ways of managing stressful situations in the past.
6. Evaluate any planned life changes in advance for potential sources of distress.

■ ■ ■ ■ PLANNING

Data from nursing assessment and collaboration with the health care team provide direction for treatment of clients with adjustment disorder. Because clients have different needs, depending on the symptoms of adjustment disorder, nursing care will be (as always) individualized. Symptoms of adjustment disorder are presumed to be short-term, so continuing care may be planned once the client is discharged from an inpatient unit. Continuing care is appropriate if the client's symptoms are active at the time of discharge and provide the opportunity to monitor the client's progress after discharge. The nurse must be alert to detect differences in symptoms or their intensity while caring for the client. For example, a client with adjustment disorder with depressed mood may begin to express thoughts of suicide.

■ ■ ■ ■ ■ IMPLEMENTATION

For the client diagnosed with an adjustment disorder, nursing interventions will be individualized, depending on the symptoms the client exhibits. Any plan of care should include ongoing assessment of symptoms.

Nursing Interventions

1. Assess any risk of suicidal ideation, gesture, or plan to *provide for client's safety and prevent violence to self.*
2. Help the client identify coping strategies *to encourage use of internal resources.*
3. Support activities that increase socialization *to decrease isolation and foster growth of social support networks.*

NURSING CARE PLAN

Mr. Y, a 57-year-old client in a general medical unit, is well-known to the nursing staff. He has been hospitalized many times during the past few years for stabilization of diabetes mellitus, which is difficult to control. During his most recent admission, his involvement with plans for his care has not been typical, because his interest is minimal. Also, he has eaten foods high in sugar content that belong to his roommate. He denies this behavior, is difficult to engage in client education, and is increasingly withdrawn. He says he does his blood glucose testing at home and administers his insulin appropriately.

Mr. Y has recently retired from his job at a manufacturing plant because of his diabetes, and his retirement benefits are adequate to support his lifestyle. When asked if he feels sad or depressed about his retirement, he denies it in an angry tone of voice. His wife of 10 years died about 8 months ago. He says he has grieved for his wife, acknowledges feeling less sad about her death, and states that he is more at peace with his situation as time goes by. He is able to talk about the good times they had together. At the same time, he acknowledges disappointment at spending his retirement alone and says he feels depressed that his retirement is not as he hoped it would be.

He denies suicidal ideation. Visiting friends told the nurses that he has been reluctant to attend social activities. They say he has told them that he prefers to spend his time alone and just doesn't feel like being with people. Mr. Y's inpatient nurse knows that he will be discharged soon and initiates home health follow-up.

DSM-IV Diagnoses

AXIS I	Adjustment Disorder with Depressed Mood
AXIS II	None
AXIS III	Diabetes Mellitus
AXIS IV	Extreme = 4 (diabetes, death of spouse)
AXIS V	GAF: = 80 within the last year, GAF, current = 60 at time of evaluation

Nursing Diagnosis: Risk for violence, self-directed. Risk factors: chronic illness, retirement, change in marital status.

Client Outcomes	Nursing Intervention	Evaluation
• Mr. Y will not harm self while in hospital.	• Observe Mr. Y's behavior frequently during routine client care. *Close observation is necessary to protect client from self-harm.*	• Mr. Y remained safe, unharmed.
• Mr. Y will refrain from verbal suicidal threats or behavioral gestures.	• Listen closely for suicidal statements and observe nonverbal indications of suicidal intent, such as giving away possessions. *Such behaviors are critical clues regarding risk for self-harm. Clues regarding potential behavior are verbal and nonverbal.*	• Absence of verbalized or behavioral indications of suicidal intent by Mr. Y.
• Mr. Y will deny any plans for suicide.	• Ask direct questions to determine suicidal intent, plans for suicide, and means to commit suicide. *Suicide risk increases if plans and means exist.*	• Mr. Y denies active suicidal plan.
• Mr. Y will agree to terms of a no-harm contract, and will seek staff when feeling suicidal.	• Obtain verbal or written agreement from Mr. Y not to harm self and to seek staff if suicidal feelings and impulses emerge *to confirm that help is available if client loses control.*	• Mr. Y agrees to term of contract, and sought staff to help maintain control.

Nursing Diagnosis: Ineffective individual coping, related to response to situational crisis (retirement), as evidenced by isolative behavior, changes in mood, and decreased sense of well-being.

Client Outcomes	Nursing Interventions	Evaluation
• Mr. Y will identify positive coping strategies, such as structuring leisure time.	• Develop trusting relationship with Mr. Y. *to demonstrate caring and encourage Mr. Y to practice new coping skills in a safe therapeutic setting.*	• Mr. Y voices trust in nurse-client relationship.
• Mr. Y will combine past effective coping methods with newly acquired coping strategies.	• Praise Mr. Y for adaptive coping. *Positive feedback encourages repetition of effective coping by Mr. Y.*	• Mr. Y discusses plans for use of past and newly learned coping methods.

NURSING CARE PLAN

Client Outcomes	Nursing Interventions	Evaluation
• Mr. Y will cope adaptively by putting anger into words versus actions.	• Assist Mr. Y to express anger and to explore angry feelings. *Verbalization of feelings in a nonthreatening relationship may help client resolve conflicts and provide opportunity to vent feelings.*	• Mr. Y verbalizes feelings of anger and loneliness appropriately.
• Mr. Y will verbalize understanding of loss as a process that needs to be worked through over time.	• Determine stage of loss. *Interventions vary with stage of loss process. Identification of stage is necessary for effective interventions.*	• Mr. Y verbalizes knowledge that loss is a natural process and will resolve in time.
	• Explain to Mr. Y the feelings and behaviors associated with each stage of loss to *help Mr. Y understand that feelings such as anger are appropriate and acceptable to resolve loss at this stage.*	• He verbalizes his understanding of loss stages and identifies his own loss process.

Nursing Diagnosis: Impaired social interaction, related to alteration in role (Mr. Y is now retired), as evidenced by disruption in usual social activities and isolating behaviors.

Client Outcomes	Nursing Intervention	Evaluation
• Mr. Y will increase socialization and involvement in activities according to capabilities.	• Review Mr. Y's resources possesses and identify positive activities that he enjoys and can resume to *encourage Mr. Y to focus on positive aspects of self and situation.*	• Mr. Y spends more time socializing with client peers than being alone
• Mr. Y will effectively use social support systems inside and outside the hospital.	• Explore Mr. Y's social support system and his desire to seek help. Identify role changes now that he lives alone. *Opportunity to discuss socialization and preferences for activities helps Mr. Y identify his own socialization patterns and demonstrates therapeutic alliance.*	• Mr. Y socilaizes with select client peers and identifies aftercare social network and acitivities.

4. Help the client name thoughts, feelings, and concerns *to help the client identify patterns of thought and provide opportunities for validation of feeling, reflection, and problem solving.*

5. Teach the client, family, and significant others about the disorder including symptom management *to provide control and reduce fear and anxiety.* (See Client and Family Teaching Guidelines on page 484.)

6. Engage client in a therapeutic alliance *to encourage discussion of thoughts and feelings, particularly noting any suicidal ideation or increase in symptoms of depression.*

7. Support client's progress toward goals *to foster self-esteem and encourage repetition of positive behaviors.*

8. Collaborate with multidisciplinary treatment team *to promote consistency in implementing the treatment plan. Consistency provides structure and communicates involvement of the entire team in the treatment of the client; expectations of the client are agreed on and articulated.*

9. Help the client identify symptoms of anxiety and predisposing situational stressors *to promote problem solving and increased feelings of control.*

10. Help the client recall prior instances of success *to foster self-esteem, support creative problem solving, and instill hope for the future.*

Additional Treatment Modalities

The nurse is an integral part of the multidisciplinary team that identifies key (or target) symptoms or behaviors, designs interventions to address key symptoms, and decides on evaluative methods to measure client movement toward or away from desired outcomes. Before the team meeting, representatives from each discipline

---

Client and Family
TEACHING GUIDELINES

Adjustment Disorders

Teach the client, family, and/or significant other:

To identify the symptoms of adjustment disorders and that:

Symptoms usually resolve completely

Symptoms can be managed using a variety of techniques (for example, relaxation exercises can be taught to mitigate anxiety)

Symptoms should be reported to their care provider

Thoughts of self-harm or suicide need to be reported immediately to their care provider

Their response to a life event is normal because individual people have unique responses to life events.

They have dealt with difficult life situations in the past using particular coping methods. Reinforce prior successes.

Dosage, frequency, and effects of medication. Include information about common side effects of medication and when to call the physician with questions or concerns regarding medication management.

---

should complete their own assessment activities and bring pertinent information to the planning session. In this way, primary functions of the individual disciplines within the team are identified, clarified, and maximized toward resolving the client's problems. Because each discipline has a unique perspective on the treatment issues of each client and focuses collective energy on resolving problems, the resulting team plan is greater than the sum of its parts. For example, the nonverbal client may respond to therapies designed by occupational or art therapists while being relatively nonresponsive to verbal interventional techniques.

Medications

Medications are used sparingly for clients with adjustment disorders because the disorders are expected to resolve after their immediate causes are identified and processed. Also because symptoms of adjustment disorder may in some cases progress to include symptoms of major mental disorders, mental health nurses may prefer to observe the client without the effects of medication. Benzodiazepines are often prescribed for brief periods of time to treat symptoms of anxiety. Antidepressants may

be prescribed if symptoms are problematic and interfere with the client's ability to mobilize resources.

Adjunctive therapies

Collaborative approaches to client care frequently include the use of adjunctive therapies. For example, recreational therapies may be used with the client diagnosed with an adjustment disorder. Discovering the client's preference in leisure activities and providing appropriate resource materials may help the client become more comfortable socially and inspire him or her to become self-directed in pursuing recreational activities. If the client is able to exercise, physical exercise and/or movement can be a constructive outlet for tension and anxiety while enhancing self-esteem.

Supportive therapies

Clinical nurse specialists, physicians, social workers, and psychologists are prepared to provide therapeutic support for clients diagnosed with an adjustment disorder. Since clients with adjustment disorders are typically treated on an outpatient basis, they have a variety of treatment options and referral sources. Depending on professional preference, assessment of the client's problems, and identification of desired outcomes, therapists may employ a variety of interventional methods. Cognitive behavior therapy, interpersonal or psychodynamic psychotherapy, and brief strategic therapeutic techniques may all be effectively used. Family therapy may be indicated when the stressor triggering the adjustment disorder occurs within a family system and the client and family require assistance in resolving the problem. Other therapeutic intervention techniques include biofeedback, relaxation exercises, hypnosis, meditation, journaling, and visual imaging activities.

■ ■ ■ ■ ■ ■ EVALUATION

Evaluation of outcomes for adjustment disorders depends on the original features of the particular disorder. For the client with depressed or anxious mood, the absence of original problematic symptoms signifies resolution. For most clients, resolution of symptoms signifies a successful outcome to the treatment.

If the client is hospitalized, the nurse is expected to evaluate the client's plan of care and response to interventions at least once every 24 hours. Thoughtful discharge planning with attention to follow-up home health care or a visit to the primary physician's office can allay potential problems once the client is discharged. If the client is not completely free of symptoms before discharge, the treatment team should examine options for placement following the need for acute hospitalization.

Summary of Key Concepts

1. Adjustment disorders are transient episodes of clinically significant emotional or behavioral nonpsychotic symptoms in response to identifiable psychosocial stress or stressors. Symptoms have developed within three months after the stressful event.

2. The diagnosis of adjustment disorder is considered if the client's behaviors or symptoms are different from usual patterns of response and if the symptoms have persisted for less than six months (acute) or unless symptoms are in response to an ongoing stressor or stressors (chronic).

3. The severity of the reaction to the stressor is not predictable from the stressor and is unique to the individual.

4. In an adult population, the most commonly diagnosed adjustment disorders are adjustment disorder with depressed mood and adjustment disorder with anxious mood.

5. Clients with adjustment disorder are often treated as outpatients because the severity of their symptoms or subjective distress does not warrant inpatient hospitalization.

6. Supportive psychotherapy is the most frequently used treatment modality with clients with adjustment disorders.

7. Clients diagnosed with adjustment disorder may experience a resolution of symptoms or an exacerbation and increase of symptoms, supporting the diagnosis of a major psychiatric disorder such as major depression.

8. Research is needed to establish the frequency and incidence of adjustment disorders and to measure outcomes of specific therapeutic interventions.

9. Attempting to understand the client's experience from his or her point of view fosters the therapeutic process. Application of clinical models are of little value unless anticipated outcomes of care are meaningful to the client.

10. Clients know more than anyone else about their lives and must be considered the resident experts in determining meaning of life events, mobilizing inner strengths, and determining preferences for care.

REFERENCES

American Nurses Association *Statement on psychiatric-mental health clinical nursing practice and standards of psychiatric-mental health clinical nursing practice,* Washington, D.C., 1994, American Nurses Publishing.

American Psychiatric Association: *Diagnostic and statistical manual of mental disorders,* ed 2, Washington, D.C., 1968, American Psychiatric Association.

American Psychiatric Association: *Diagnostic and statistical manual of mental disorders,* ed 3, Washington, D.C., 1980, American Psychiatric Association.

American Psychiatric Association: *Diagnostic and statistical manual of mental disorders,* ed 3 revised, Washington, D.C., 1987, American Psychiatric Association.

American Psychiatric Association: *Diagnostic and statistical manual of mental disorders,* ed 4, Washington D.C., 1994, American Psychiatric Association.

Armstrong M: Being pregnant and using drugs: a retrospective phenomenological inquiry. Unpublished doctoral dissertation. San Diego, Calif., 1992, University of San Diego.

Beck C: The lived experience of postpartum depression: a phenomenological study, *Nurs Research* 41(3):166–170, 1992.

Bergum V: *Woman to mother: a transformation,* Boston, 1989, Bergin & Garvey.

Blier R: *Science and gender,* New York, 1986, Pergamon Press.

Colarusso C, Nemiroff R: *Adult development: a new dimension in psychodynamic theory and practice,* New York, 1981, Plenum Press.

Colarusso C, Nemiroff R: Clinical implications of adult development, *Amer J Psychiatry* 144(10):1263–1269, 1987.

Coward D: The lived experience of self-transcendence in women with advanced breast cancer, *Nurs Sci Quarterly* 3(4):162–169, 1990.

Davis F: Deviance disavowal: the management of strained interaction by the visibly handicapped. In Davis F, editor: *Illness, interaction and the self,* Belmont, Calif., 1972, Wadsworth.

Erikson, EH: *Childhood and society,* ed 2, New York, 1963, W.W. Norton.

Gilligan C: *In a different voice: psychological theory and women's development,* Cambridge, Mass., 1982, Harvard University Press.

Heifner C: Positive connectedness in the psychiatric nurse-patient relationship, *Arch Psychiatric Nursing* 7(1):11–15, 1993.

Jordan J et al: *Women's growth in connection: writings from the stone center,* New York, 1991, Guilford Press.

Kirk S, Kutchins H: *The selling of DSM: the rhetoric of science in psychiatry,* New York, 1992, Aldine de Gruyter.

Kubler-Ross E: *On death and dying,* New York, 1969, Macmillan.

Lerner H: *Women in therapy,* Northvale, N.J., 1988, Jason Aronson Press.

Levine S: *Healing into life and death,* New York, 1987, Doubleday.

Lewis H: Is Freud an enemy of women's liberation? Some historical considerations. In Bernay T, Cantor D, editors: *The psychology of today's woman: new psychoanalytic visions,* Cambridge, Mass., 1986, Harvard University Press.

Lowenberg J: *Caring and responsibility: the crossroads between holistic practice and traditional medicine,* Pittsburgh, 1989, University of Pennsylvania Press.

Main M et al: Information sharing concerning schizophrenia in a family member: adult siblings' perspectives, *Arch Psychiatric Nursing* 7(3):147–153, 1993.

Meth R, Pasick R: *Men in therapy: the challenge of change,* New York, 1990, Guilford Press.

Mickley J et al: Spiritual well-being, religiousness and hope among women with breast cancer, *Image: J Nursing Scholarship* 24(4):267–272, 1992.

Murphy S: Coping strategies of abstainers from alcohol up to three years post-treatment, *Image: J Nursing Scholarship* 25(1):29–35, 1993.

Napier A: Heroism, men, and marriage, *J Marital and Family Therapy* 17(1):9–16, 1991.

Nemiroff R, Colarusso C: *Psychotherapy and psychoanalysis in the second half of life,* New York, 1985, Plenum Press.

Parsons T: *The social system,* New York, 1951, The Free Press.

Pittman F: The secret passions of men, *J Marital and Family Therapy,* 17(1):17–23, 1991.

Popkin M: Adjustment disorder and impulse control. In Kaplan H, Saddock B, editors: *Comprehensive textbook of psychiatry/V,* Baltimore, 1989, Williams and Wilkins.

Popkin M: Adjustment disorders in medically ill inpatients referred for consultation in a university hospital, *Psychosomatics* 31(4): 410–414, 1990.

Razavi D et al: Screening for adjustment disorders and major depressive disorders in cancer inpatients. *British J Psychiatry* 156:79–83, 1990.

Selye H: *Stress without distress,* New York, 1956, New American Library.

Selye H: *The stress of life,* New York, 1978, McGraw-Hill.

Spector R: *Cultural diversity in health and illness,* ed 3, Norwalk, Conn., 1991, Appleton & Lange.

Tanner C et al: The phenomenology of knowing the patient, *Image: J Nursing Scholarship* 25(4):273–280, 1993.

Walsh F, McGoldrick M: *Living beyond loss,* New York, 1991, W.W. Norton.

Therapeutic Modalities

Safe Camp
HOBO

Communication symbols are used by modern "knights of the road," the hobos and by the homeless. This "safe camp" sym-bol portrays relief from worldly stressors for individuals in crisis and in need of respite. The chapters in Part Five discuss the various modalities of treatment used to relieve stressors and treat mental disorders.

CHAPTER 21

Crisis Intervention

Donna C. Aguilera

Appraisal As related to crisis, the ongoing perceptual process by which a potentially harmful event is distinguished from a potentially beneficial or irrelevant event.

Cognition Awareness and subjective meaning of an event.

Coping Various strategies, conscious or unconscious, to deal with stress and tensions arising from perceived threats to psychological integrity. It is the process of attempting to solve life problems.

Ego dissonance Inconsistency between attitudes and behaviors.

Equilibrium A state of emotional balance.

Generic approach A method of crisis intervention that focuses on the characteristic course of the particular kind of crisis rather than on the personal aspects of each individual in crisis.

Individual approach A method of crisis intervention emphasizing professional assessment of the interpersonal and intrapsychic processes of the person in crisis.

Paradigm A side-by-side example to show a clear pattern.

- Describe the historical development of crisis intervention.
- Identify and define the phases of crisis.
- Discuss the balancing factors that affect emotional equilibrium.
- Compare and contrast maturational crises, situational crises, and adventitious crises.
- Compare and contrast the generic and individual approaches of crisis intervention.
- Define and describe the steps of crisis intervention and apply them to the problem-solving process.

HISTORICAL DEVELOPMENT

The origin of modern crisis intervention dates back to the work of Eric Lindemann and his colleagues following the Coconut Grove fire in Boston on November 28, 1942. In what was at that time the worst single-building fire in the country's history, 493 people perished when flames swept through the crowded nightclub. Lindemann and others from Massachusetts General Hospital played an active role in helping survivors who had lost loved ones in the disaster.

Lindemann's clinical report (Lindemann, 1944) on the psychological symptoms of the survivors became the cornerstone for subsequent theorizing on the grief process, a series of stages through which a mourner progresses toward accepting and resolving loss. Lindemann came to believe that the clergy and other community caregivers could play a critical role in helping bereaved people through the mourning process and thereby head off later psychological difficulties. This concept was further developed with the establishment of the Wellesley Human Relations Service in Boston in 1948, one of the first community mental health services noted for its focus on short-term therapy in the context of preventive psychiatry.

From his experience working with grief reactions, Lindemann concluded that a conceptual frame of reference built around the concept of an emotional crisis, as shown by bereavement reactions, would be worthy of investigation and useful for the development of preventive efforts. Certain inevitable events in life can be described as hazardous situations, for example, bereavement, the birth of a child, and marriage. He proposed that in each of these situations emotional strain would be generated, stress would be experienced, and a series of adaptive mechanisms would occur that could lead to mastery of the new situation or to failure with more or less lasting impairment to function. Although such situations create stress for all people exposed to them, they become crises for those who are especially vulnerable to this stress and who do not have the emotional resources to adapt.

Lindemann's theoretical frame of reference led to the development of crisis intervention techniques. In 1948 he and Gerald Caplan established the Wellesley Project, a community-wide mental health program in Boston.

According to Caplan (1961), the most important aspects of mental health are the state of the ego, the stage of its maturity, and the quality of its structure. Assessment of the ego's state is based on three main areas: 1) the capacity of the person to withstand stress and anxiety and to maintain ego equilibrium, 2) the degree of reality recognized and faced in solving problems, and 3) the repertoire of effective coping mechanisms the individual can employ in maintaining a balance in the biopsychosocial field.

Caplan believes that all the elements that compose a person's total emotional milieu or environment must be assessed in an approach to preventive mental health. The material, physical, and social demands of reality, as well as the individual's needs, instincts, and impulses, must all be considered important behavioral determinants.

CRISIS
Definition and Description

A psychological crisis refers to an individual's inability to solve a problem. All individuals exist in a state of emotional **equilibrium,** or balance. When something different occurs (either positive or negative), such as a change or a loss that creates a state of disequilibrium, the individual strives to regain and maintain the previous level of equilibrium. A person in crisis is at a turning point. Often the problem cannot be readily solved by using coping mechanisms that have worked before. As a result, tension and anxiety make it more difficult to find a solution. A person in this situation feels helpless, caught in a state of emotional upset, and unable to take action to solve the problem.

Caplan defines crisis as occurring "when a person faces an obstacle to important life goals that is, for a time, insurmountable through the utilization of customary methods of problem-solving. A period of disorganization ensues, a period of upset, during which many abortive attempts at solution are made" (Caplan, 1961). In essence, the individual is viewed as living in a state of emotional equilibrium—with the goal always to return to or maintain that state. The individual must either solve the problem or adapt to nonsolution. In either case, a new state of equilibrium develops, sometimes better and sometimes worse in terms of positive mental health. There is a rise in inner tension, there are signs of anxiety, and there is disorganization of function, resulting in a prolonged period of emotional upset. This Caplan refers to as "crisis." The outcome is governed by the kind of interaction that takes place during the crisis period between the individual and the key figures in his or her emotional milieu.

Crisis is characteristically self-limiting and lasts from four to six weeks. This transitional period represents both the danger of increased psychological vulnerability and an opportunity for personality growth. In any particular situation, the outcome may depend to a significant degree on the availability of appropriate help. On this basis, the length of time for intervention is from four to six weeks, with the average being four weeks (Jacobson, 1965). Because time is so important, the therapeutic intervention commands the concentrated attention of both therapist and client. A goal-oriented sense of commitment develops, in sharp contrast to the more modest pace of traditional treatment modes.

Phases of Crisis

According to Caplan (1974), a crisis has four developmental phases:

1. An initial rise in tension as the stimulus continues and more discomfort is felt.

2. A lack of success in coping as the stimulus continues and more discomfort is felt.

3. A further increase in tension acts as a powerful internal stimulus that mobilizes internal and external resources. In this stage, emergency problem-solving mechanisms are tried. The problem may be redefined, or there may be resignation and the giving up of certain aspects of the goal as unattainable.

4. If the problem continues and can be neither solved nor avoided, tension increases and a major disorganization occurs.

A stressful event is seldom so clearly defined that its source can be determined immediately. Internalized changes occur at the same time as the externally provoked stress. As a result, some events may cause a strong emotional response in one person, yet leave another person apparently unaffected. Much is determined by the presence or absence of factors that can effect a return to equilibrium.

Whenever a stressful event occurs, certain recognized balancing factors can bring about a return to equilibrium; these factors are perception of the event, available situational supports, and coping mechanisms, as shown in the paradigm in Figure 21-1. A **paradigm** is a side-by-side example to show a clear pattern. The upper portion of the paradigm illustrates the "normal" initial reaction of an individual to a stressful event.

In column *A* of Figure 21-1, the balancing factors are operating and crisis is avoided. However, in column *B* the absence of one or more of these balancing factors may block resolution of the problem and thus increase disequilibrium and precipitate crisis.

Balancing Factors Affecting Equilibrium

Between the perceived effects of a stressful situation and the resolution of the problem are three recognized balancing factors that may determine the state of equilibrium: perception of the event, situational supports, and coping mechanisms. Strengths or weaknesses in any one of the factors can be directly related to the onset of crisis or to its resolution.

PERCEPTION OF THE EVENT

Cognition, or the awareness and subjective meaning of a stressful event, plays a major role in determining both the nature and degree of coping behaviors. Differences in cognition, in terms of the event's threat to an important life goal or value, account for large differences in coping behaviors. The concept of *cognitive style* (Cropley and Field, 1969) suggests uniqueness in the way people take in, process, and use information from the environment.

Cognitive styles, or the characteristic modes for organizing perceptual and intellectual activities, play an important role in determining an individual's coping responses to daily life stresses. According to Inkeles (1966), cognitive style helps to set limits on information-seeking in stress situations. It also strongly influences perceptions of others, interpersonal relationships, and responses to various types of psychiatric treatment.

For example, in stressful situations a person whose cognitive style is identified as "field-dependent" is very dependent on external objects in the environment for orientation to reality. This type of individual tends to use such coping mechanisms as repression and denial. In contrast, the "field-independent" person tends to prefer intellectualization as a defense mode.

If the event is perceived realistically, the relationship between the event and feelings of stress is recognized. Problem solving can be appropriately oriented toward reduction of tension, and successful solution of the stressful situation is more probable.

Lazarus (1966) and colleagues (1974) focused on the importance of the mediating cognitive process, *appraisal*, to determine the various coping methods individuals use. **Appraisal,** in this context, is an ongoing perceptual process by which a potentially harmful event is distinguished from a potentially beneficial or irrelevant event. It has been found that an individual's Sense of Coherence (SOC) significantly affects cognitive appraisal, specifically secondary appraisal (McSherry and Holm, 1994). SOC is a global orientation that expresses the extent to which one has a pervasive, enduring though dynamic feeling of confidence to comprehend, manage, and learn from a crisis (Antonovsky, 1987).

When a threatening situation exists, a *primary* appraisal is made to judge the perceived outcome of the event in relation to one's future goals and values. This is followed by a *secondary* appraisal, whereby one perceives the range of coping alternatives available either to master the threat or to achieve a beneficial outcome. As coping activities are selected and initiated, feedback cues from changing internal and external environments lead to ongoing *reappraisals* or to changes in the original perception.

As a result of the appraisal process, coping behaviors are never static. They change constantly in both quality and degree as new information and cues are received during reappraisal activities. New coping responses may occur whenever new significance is attached to a situation. One's SOC level appears associated with the way in which one appraises and copes with stressful situations (McSherry and Holm, 1994).

If, in the appraisal process, the outcome is judged to be too overwhelming or too difficult to be dealt with by using available coping skills, an individual is more likely to use defense mechanisms to repress or distort the reality of the situation. An appraisal of a potentially successful outcome, however, more likely leads to the use of direct action modes of coping, such as attack, flight, or compromise. It has been recognized that high SOC persons report significantly higher levels of perceived coping resources than low SOC persons (McSherry and Holm, 1994).

If the perception of the event is distorted, a relationship between the event and feelings of stress may not be recognized. Thus, attempts to solve the problem are ineffective, and tension is not reduced. In other words, what does the event mean to the individual? How is it going to affect his or her future? Can the person look at it realistically, or does the person distort its meaning?

SITUATIONAL SUPPORTS

Situational supports are those persons who are available in the environment and who can be depended on to help solve the problem. By nature, human beings are dependent on others to supply them with reflected appraisals of their own intrinsic and extrinsic values. In establishing life patterns, certain appraisals are more significant to the individual than others because they tend to reinforce the individual's self-perception. Dependency relationships may be more readily established with those whose appraisals tend to support the individual against feelings of insecurity and with those who reinforce feelings of ego integrity.

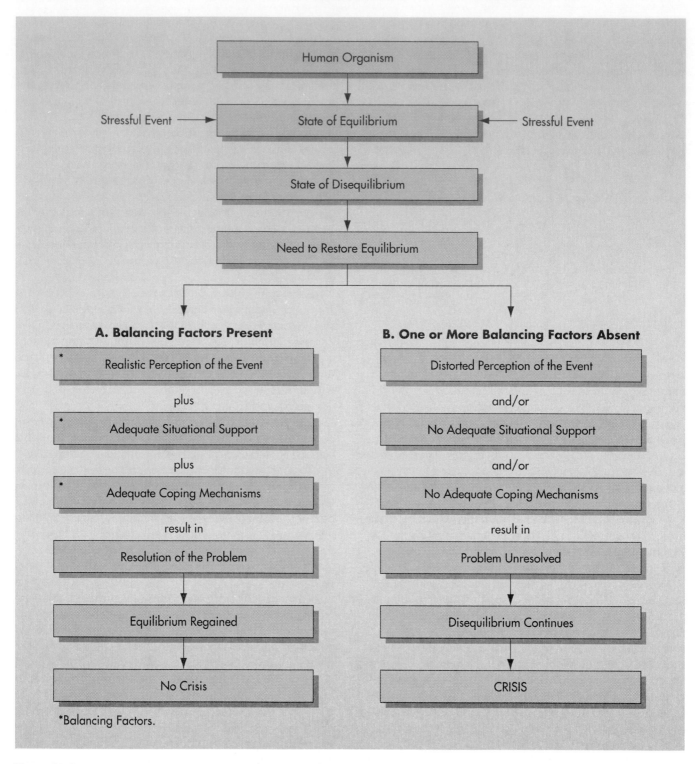

Figure 21-1 A paradigm illustrating the effect of balancing factors in a stressful event.

(From Aguliera DC: *Crisis intervention: theory and methodology,* ed 7, St. Louis, 1994, Mosby.)

These meaningful relationships with others provide a person with nurturance and support, resources vital for coping with stressors. Social isolation denies a person availability of social interactions and opportunities to develop meaningful relationships. Sudden or unexpected social isolation results in the loss of usual resource supports. Lacking these, a person is much more vulnerable to daily living stressors.

Loss, threatened loss, or feelings of inadequacy in a supportive relationship may also leave a person in a vulnerable position. Confrontation with a stressful situation, combined with a lack of situational support, may lead to a state of disequilibrium and possible crisis.

Appraisal of self varies across ages, sexes, and roles. The belief system that forms the basis of the self-concept and self-esteem develops out of experiences with significant others in a person's life. Although self-esteem is fairly stable within a certain range, it does fluctuate according to internal and external environmental variables. In order to achieve and maintain a sense of value and self-worth, a person must feel loved by others and capable of achieving an ideal self, one that is strong, capable, good, and loving of others.

When self-esteem is low or when a situation is perceived as particularly threatening, the person is strongly in need of and seeks out others from whom positive reflective appraisals of self-worth and ability to achieve can be obtained. The lower the self-esteem or the greater the threat, the greater the need to seek situational supports. Conversely, a person avoids or withdraws from contacts with those perceived as threatening to self-esteem, whether the threat is real or imagined. Any potentially stressful situation can set off questions of self-doubt about how one is perceived by others, the kind of impression being made, and the real or imagined inadequacies that might be disclosed (Mechanic, 1974). However, not everyone who faces a threat to self-image will suffer a decrease in self-esteem (Jalajas, 1994). Whether self-esteem decreases will depend upon whether the threat to the self-image can be reaffirmed (Jalajas, 1994).

Success or failure of a coping behavior is always strongly influenced by the social context in which it occurs. The environmental variable most centrally identified is the person's significant others. From them, a person learns to seek advice and support in solving daily problems in living. Confidence in being liked and respected by these peers is based on past testing and reaffirmation of the expected supportive responses.

Self-esteem has an important influence on how threats to the self-concept result in a loss of well-being (Jalajas, 1994). Any perceived failure to obtain adequate support to meet psychosocial needs may provoke, or compound, a stressful situation. The receipt of negative support could be equally detrimental to a person's self-esteem.

COPING MECHANISMS

People use many methods to cope with anxiety and reduce tension. Lifestyles are developed around patterns of response which, in turn, are established to cope with stressful situations. These lifestyles are highly individual and quite necessary to protect and maintain equilibrium.

Over the years, it has been unusual to find the term *coping* used interchangeably with such similar concepts as adaptation, defense, mastery, and adjustive reactions. Coping activities take a wide variety of forms, including all the diverse behaviors that people engage in to meet actual or anticipated challenges. In psychological stress

theory, the term **coping** emphasizes various strategies used, consciously or unconsciously, to deal with stress and tensions arising from perceived threats to psychologic integrity. It is not synonymous with mastery over life problems. Rather, it is the *process* of attempting to solve them (Lazarus, 1966).

Coleman (1950) defined *coping* as an adjustive reaction made in response to actual or imagined stress in order to maintain psychological integrity. Within this concept, human beings are perceived as responding to stress by attack, flight, or compromise reactions. These reactions become complicated by various ego-defense mechanisms whenever the stress becomes ego-involved.

Attack reactions usually attempt to remove or overcome the obstacles seen as causing stress in life situations. They may be primarily constructive or destructive in nature. Flight, withdrawal, or fear reactions may be as simple as physically removing the threat from the environment (such as putting out a fire) or removing oneself from the threatening situation (such as running away from the fire area). They might also involve much more complex psychological maneuvering, depending on the perceived extent of the threat and the possibilities for escape.

Compromise or substitution reactions occur when attack or flight from the threatening situation is thought to be impossible. This method is most commonly used to deal with problem solving and includes accepting substitute goals or changing internalized values and standards.

Masserman (1948) demonstrated that, in situations of extended frustration, individuals find it increasingly possible to compromise for substitute goals. This often involves use of *rationalization,* a defense mechanism whereby "half a loaf" does indeed soon appear to be "better than none."

Tension-reducing mechanisms can be overt or covert and can be consciously or unconsciously activated. They have been generally classified into such behavioral responses as aggression, regression, withdrawal, and repression. The selection of a response is based on tension-reducing actions that successfully relieved anxiety and reduced tension in similar situations in the past. Through repetition, the response may pass from conscious awareness during its learning phase to a habitual level of reaction as a learned behavior. In many instances, the individual may not be aware of *how*, let alone *why*, he or she reacts to stress in given situations. Except for having vague feelings of discomfort, the individual may not notice the rise and consequent reduction in tension. When a new stress-producing event arises and learned coping mechanisms are ineffectual, discomfort is felt on a conscious level. The need to "do something" becomes the focus of activity, narrowing perception of all other life activities.

Normally, defense mechanisms are used constructively in the process of coping. This is particularly evident whenever there is danger of becoming psychologically overwhelmed. Almost all defense mechanisms are seen as important for survival. None is equated with a pathological condition unless it interferes with the process of coping, such as being used to deny, to falsify, or to distort perceptions of reality.

According to Bandura et al (1977), the strength of the individual's conviction in his or her own effectiveness in overcoming or mastering a problematical situation determines whether coping behavior is even attempted in the first place. People fear and avoid stressful, threatening situations they believe exceed their ability to cope. They behave with assurance in those situations in which they judge themselves able to manage and in which they expect eventual success. It is the perceived ability to master that can influence the choice of coping behaviors as well as the persistence used once a coping behavior is chosen.

Available coping mechanisms are what people *usually* do when they have a problem. They may sit down and try to think it out or talk it out with a friend. Some cry it out or try to get rid of their feelings of anger and hostility by swearing, kicking a chair, or slamming doors. Others may get into verbal battles with friends. Some may react by temporarily withdrawing from the situation in order to reassess the problem. These are just a few of the many coping methods people use to relieve their tension and anxiety when faced with a problem. Each coping mechanism has been used at some time in the developmental past of the individual, has been found effective in maintaining emotional stability, and has become part of the lifestyle in meeting and dealing with the stresses of daily living.

Types of Crises

MATURATIONAL CRISES

A maturational crisis involves the normal life transition that creates changes with individuals and how they perceive themselves, their role, and their status. Transitional periods throughout the life cycle are key times for maturational growth to occur. Examples of these crucial times are adolescence, parenthood, midlife, and retirement. How an individual has accomplished developmental tasks throughout the life span significantly determines whether the new transitional period will be viewed as a crisis or an opportunity for maturation.

A young adult who has had difficulty with the task of middle childhood (i.e., industry versus inferiority) and learning the necessary socialization skills for that age group is also likely to experience difficulty leaving the parental home, establishing a new family, and obtaining employment and social competence. A transitional crisis can be an out-of-sequence life transition, such as a normal occurrence happening unexpectedly (for example, premature death of a parent or a young child). Out-of-sequence events tend to be more difficult to experience, because the individual is unprepared for such traumatic occurrences; thus, they can have negative maturational effects.

SITUATIONAL CRISES

A situational crisis occurs when a specific, external event disturbs an individual's psychological equilibrium. This can be an event that affects the person individually or within that person's peer group. Situational crises usually center around losses that impact the individual and result in **ego dissonance** (inconsistency between attitudes and behaviors). Examples of situational crises are loss of employment, loss of a loved one or valued object, loss of health, and loss of status.

The loss of an important person in one's life may result in confusion and ambivalent, unresolved feelings surrounding the loss. The loss may be compounded by a change in one's status, finances, and support systems. The loss of employment can result in financial stress, resulting in a deeper sense of loss of one's role and a possible sense of failure, as well as decreased self-worth and self-esteem.

It is normal to mourn the loss of a loved one and to experience grief, but it is also common to mourn the loss of an idea, an idealized object, or changes within oneself. The changes that occur in one's body over time and in loved ones help define and redefine the self. In periods of stability, one defines one's life by attempting to understand its meaning and finiteness. Each transition from one developmental stage to another leads to termination of a previous life structure; each transition is an ending, a process involving separation or loss. Levinson described transition as an opportunity to review and evaluate one's past, to take what was best from one's life and separate it from the difficult and traumatic events. A transition is a time of bridging the past with the hopes and promises of the future. During transitions, changes can be attempted in both the self and the individual's world. It involves a letting go of unfinished or painful experiences and incorporating the best of one's development and experience (Levinson et al, 1978).

ADVENTITIOUS CRISES

Adventitious crises are precipitated by acts of God, providence, or fate. They are the unpredictable tragedies that occur without warning. Examples are earthquakes, tidal waves, floods, famine, and other natural disasters. Civil uprising, riots, and war are also included in this category. Often, it is the unpredictability of such disasters that leaves such fear, confusion, and ego dissonance in their victims. Only a minority of those who experience a natural disaster develop psychologic disorders, suggesting that there are individual differences in responses to such stressors (Phifer, 1990).

CRISIS INTERVENTION

Crisis intervention can offer the immediate help that a person in crisis needs to reestablish equilibrium. It is an inexpensive, short-term therapy that focuses on solving the immediate problem. The minimum therapeutic goal of crisis intervention is resolution of the individual's immediate crisis and restoration to at least the precrisis level of functioning. A maximum goal is improvement of functioning above the precrisis level. For specific interventions a nurse may encounter in the community, see Nursing Care in the Community below.

Methods of Crisis Intervention

Jacobson et al (1968, 1980) state that crisis intervention may be divided into two major complementary categories: generic and individual.

GENERIC APPROACH

The **generic approach** proposes that there are certain recognized patterns of behavior in most crises. Many studies have substantiated this, for example, Lindemann's (1944) studies of bereavement of a relative. He refers to these sequential phases as "grief work" and found that failure of a person to grieve appropriately or to complete the process of bereavement could potentially lead to future emotional illness. Kaplan and Mason (1960) and Caplan (1974) studied the effect on the mother of the birth of a premature baby and identified four phases or tasks that she must work through to ensure healthy adap-

tation to the experience. Janis (1958) suggests several hypotheses concerning the psychologic stress of impending surgery and the patterns of emotional responses that follow a diagnosis of chronic illness. Rappoport (1963) defines three subphases of marriage during which unusual stress could precipitate crises.

The generic approach focuses on the characteristic course of the *particular kind of crisis* rather than on the psychodynamics of each individual in crisis. A treatment plan is directed toward an adaptive resolution of the crisis. Specific intervention measures are designed to be effective for all members of a given group rather than for the unique differences of one individual. Recognition of these behavioral patterns is an important aspect of preventive mental health.

Jacobson et al (1968) state that generic approaches to crisis intervention include

direct encouragement of adaptive behavior, general support, environmental manipulation and anticipatory guidance. . . . In brief, the generic approach emphasizes 1) specific situational and maturational events occurring to significant population groups, 2) intervention oriented to crisis related to these specific events, and 3) intervention carried out by non-mental health professionals.

Nursing Care in the Community

Crisis Intervention

Crisis intervention is a lifeline to the public. A skilled crisis nurse acts as the gatekeeper for the entire mental health system and activates the legal network in emergency situations. The nurse must often make decisions that directly impact the lives of clients in the community, when assessing an individual's danger to himself or herself, or to others. In a way, the entire community could be considered as the client.

Psychiatric nurses working in the community are especially necessary in catastrophic situations such as fires, floods, or earthquakes, both to those who have been traumatized by the event itself and those who have lost friends or relatives. Victims of the event may have a psychiatric diagnosis, and the disease may intensify as a result of the stress of the event. They may even feel responsible for the disaster and will not respond to reassurance. Immediate psychiatric assessment and intervention are needed to help the person manage the disease behaviors through personal comfort and possibly medication.

Friends and relatives of trauma victims may also experience overwhelming emotional response that requires psychiatric intervention. They should be referred to a community contact, given reassurance, and provided with information about how long such upsetting feelings may last, including referrals if they continue to feel disrupted.

The nurse must be able to intervene in the needs of the individual as well as the community.

The crisis nurse may also offer support to individual clients who are lonely and stressed. Some clients check in daily with familiar workers and become well-known to crisis service personnel. Strategies focus on identifying an immediate precipitating event, evaluating the client's personal safety, and working with him or her to reestablish emotional equilibrium. Interventions range from giving referrals to programs such as AA and suggesting private therapists, to commonsense advice about daily problems. It is routine to counsel a heartbroken lover, a recently discharged client with adjustment difficulties, or a parent whose child has become estranged through drug abuse. Some people call as proxies for friends or family members who are too upset or disorganized to be coherent.

The crisis nurse must be familiar with the most recent diagnostic manual and capable of making assessments based on sparse information. He or she must be aware of personal limitations yet be able to take responsibility for rapid independent action, such as calling paramedics or the police. As in other community situations, it is better to err on the side of caution than to hesitate due to fear of intruding on individual clients.

This approach has been found feasible as a mode of intervention that can be learned and implemented by nonpsychiatric physicians, nurses, social workers, and others. It does not require a mastery of knowledge of the intrapsychic and interpersonal processes of an individual in crisis.

INDIVIDUAL APPROACH

The **individual approach** differs from the generic in its emphasis on assessment by a professional of the interpersonal and intrapsychic processes of the person in crisis. It is used in selected cases, usually with those who are not responding to the generic approach. Intervention is planned to meet the unique needs of the individual in crisis and to reach a solution for the particular situation and circumstances that precipitated the crisis. It differs from the generic approach, which focuses on the characteristic course of a particular kind of crisis.

Unlike extended psychotherapy, the individual approach deals relatively little with the developmental past of the individual. Information from this source is seen as relevant only for the clues that may result in a better understanding of the present crisis situation. Emphasis is placed on the immediate causes for disturbed equilibrium and on the processes necessary for regaining a precrisis or higher level of functioning.

Jacobson (1968) cites the inclusion of family members or other important persons in the process of the individual's crisis resolution as another area of differentiation from most individual psychotherapy. In comparison with the generic approach, the individual approach is viewed by Jacobson as emphasizing the need for greater depth of understanding of the biopsychosocial process, intervention oriented to the individual's unique situation, and intervention carried out only by mental health professionals.

Morley et al (1967) recommend several attitudes that are important adjuncts to the specific techniques, which are listed in Box 21-1.

Steps in Crisis Intervention

There are certain specific steps involved in crisis intervention (Morley et al, 1967). Although each cannot be placed in a clearly defined category, crisis intervention involves the following sequence of phases.

ASSESSMENT

Assessment requires the nurse to use active focusing techniques to obtain an accurate assessment of the precipitating event and the resulting crisis that brought the individual to seek professional help. The nurse may have to judge whether the help-seeking person presents a high suicidal or homicidal lethality and whether hospitalization is necessary. If hospitalization is not deemed necessary, the intervention proceeds.

> ### Box 21-1 Attitudes Important in the Individual Approach of Crisis Intervention
>
> 1. View the work being done as the treatment of choice.
> 2. Assess the presenting problem(s) only.
> 3. Recognize that the treatment is time-limited.
> 4. Eliminate unrelated problems.
> 5. Be active and directive.
> 6. Act as a resource person or information giver, and take an active role as a liaison with other helping resources.
> 7. Assist in problem solving.
>
> From Morley et al: Crisis: paradigms of intervention, *J Psychiatr Nurs* 5:538, 1967.

PLANNING THERAPEUTIC INTERVENTION

Intervention is aimed at restoring the person to at least the precrisis level of equilibrium. In this phase, determination is made of the length of time since onset of the crisis. It is important to know how much the crisis has disrupted the person's life and the effects of this disruption on others. Information is also sought to determine the individual's strengths, what coping skills have been successfully used in the past, what coping skills are being used presently, and what people might be used as supports. Search is made for alternative methods of coping that for some reason are not presently being used.

INTERVENTION

The nature of intervention techniques is highly dependent on the preexisting skills, creativity, and flexibility of the nurse. Morley suggests some of the following, which have been found useful:

A. *Helping the individual to gain an intellectual understanding of the crisis.* Often the individual sees no relationship between a hazardous situation occurring in life and the extreme discomfort of disequilibrium it causes. The nurse could use a direct approach, describing to the client the relationship between crisis and the event.

B. *Helping the individual bring into the open present feelings not previously accessible.* Frequently the person may have suppressed some very real feelings such as anger or other inadmissible emotions toward someone that "should be loved or honored." It may also be denial of grief, feelings of guilt, or failure to complete the mourning process following bereavement. An immediate goal of intervention is the reduction of tension by providing means for the individual to recognize these feelings and bring them into the open. It is sometimes necessary to produce emotional catharsis and reduce immobilizing tension.

C. *Exploration of coping mechanisms.* This requires helping the person examine alternate ways of coping. If behaviors used in the past for successfully reducing anxiety have not been tried, the possibility of their use in the present situation is explored. New coping methods are sought, and frequently the person devises some highly original methods that have not been tried.

D. *Reopening the social world.* If the crisis has been precipitated by loss of someone significant to the person's life, the possibility of introducing new people to fill the void can be highly effective. It is particularly effective if supports and gratifications provided by the "lost" person in the past can be achieved to a similar degree from new relationships.

RESOLUTION OF THE CRISIS AND ANTICIPATORY PLANNING

During this phase, the nurse reinforces those adaptive coping mechanisms that the individual has used successfully to reduce tension and anxiety. As coping abilities increase and positive changes occur, they may be summarized to allow the person to reexperience and reconfirm the progress made. Assistance is given as needed in making realistic plans for the future. There is discussion of ways in which the present experience may help in coping with future crises.

Problem Solving in Crisis Intervention: Application of Crisis Theory

John Dewey (1910) proposed the classical steps of problem solving:

1. A difficulty is felt.
2. The difficulty is located and defined.
3. Possible solutions are suggested.
4. Consequences are considered.
5. A solution is accepted.

With minor changes, this approach to the steps in problem solving has persisted over the years. Johnson (1955) simplified problem solving by reducing the number of steps to three: preparation, production, and judgment.

According to Guilford (1967), the general problem-solving model involves the following processes:

1. *Input* (from environment and soma).
2. *Filtering* (attention aroused and directed).
3. *Cognition* (problem sensed and structured).
4. *Production* (answers generated).
5. *Cognition* (new information obtained).
6. *Production* (new answers generated).

7. *Evaluation* (input and cognition tested, answers tested; new tests of problem structure, new answers tested).

When professional help is sought because a person is in crisis, the nurse must use logic and background knowledge to define the problem and plan intervention. The *crisis approach to problem solving* involves an assessment of the individual and the problem, planning of therapeutic intervention, intervention, and resolution of the crisis and anticipatory planning (Morley et al, 1967).

ASSESSMENT OF THE INDIVIDUAL AND THE PROBLEM

The first therapy session is directed toward determining the crisis-precipitating event and what factors are affecting the individual's ability to solve problems. It is important that both nurse and client define a situation clearly before taking any action to change it. Questions such as "What do I need to know?" and "What must be done?" are asked. The more specifically the problem can be defined, the more likely it is that the "correct" answer will be sought.

Clues are investigated to point out and explore the problem or what is happening. The nurse obtains factual knowledge about the problem area by asking questions and through observation. It is important to know what has happened within the immediate situation. How the individual has coped in past situations may affect present behavior. Observations are made to determine the level of anxiety, expressive movements, emotional tone, verbal responses, and attitudinal changes.

It is important to remember that the nurse's task is to focus on the immediate problem. There is not enough time and *no need* to go into the client's past history in depth.

One of the nurse's first questions usually is "Why did you come for help today?" The word *today* should be emphasized. Sometimes the individual will try to avoid stating the reason by saying, "I've been planning to come for some time." The usual reply is, "Yes, but what happened that made you come in *today?*" Other questions to ask are "What happened in your life that is *different? When* did it happen?"

The next area on which to focus is the individual's perception of the event: What does it mean to the person? How does it affect the future? Is the event perceived realistically, or is the meaning distorted?

The client is then questioned about available situational supports: Who in the environment can the nurse find to support the person? With whom does the client live? Who is the client's best friend? Who does the client trust? Is there a member of the family to whom the client feels particularly close? Crisis intervention is sharply time-limited, and the more people involved in helping the person, the better. Also, if others are involved and familiar with the problem, they can continue to give support when therapy is terminated.

The next area of focus is ascertaining what the person usually does with a problem that is difficult to solve. What coping skills are used? Has anything like this ever happened before? How does the person reduce tension, anxiety, or depression? Has this method been used before? If not, why not, if it usually works? What does the person think would reduce symptoms of stress? The client usually thinks of something; coping skills are so very individual. Methods of coping with anxiety that have not been used in years may be remembered.

One of the most important parts of the assessment is to find out whether the person is suicidal or homicidal. The question must be *very direct and specific:* Is the person planning to commit suicide or homicide? How? When? The nurse must determine and assess the lethality of the threat. Is the person merely thinking about it, or has a method already been selected? Is it a lethal method—a loaded gun? Has the person picked out a tall building or bridge? Can the person tell you when it will happen, for example, after the children are asleep?

If the threat does not seem imminent, the person is accepted for crisis therapy. If the intent is carefully planned and details are specific, hospitalization and psychiatric evaluation are arranged in order to protect the person or others in the community.

PLANNING THERAPEUTIC INTERVENTION

After identifying the precipitating event and the factors that are influencing the individual's state of disequilibrium, the nurse plans the method of intervention. Determination must be made as to how much the crisis has disrupted the individual's life. Is the person able to work? go to school? keep the house? care for the family? Are these activities being affected? This is the first area to examine for the degree of disruption. How is this state of disequilibrium affecting others in the person's life? How does the person's spouse, roommate, or family feel about this problem? What do they think the client should do? Are they upset?

This is basically a search process in which data are collected. It requires the use of cognitive abilities and recollection of past events for information relative to the present situation. The last phase of this step is essentially a thinking process in which alternatives are considered and evaluated against past experience and knowledge, as well as in the context of the present situation.

Tentative solutions are advanced about *why* the problem exists. This step requires familiarity with theoretical knowledge and anticipation of more than one answer. In the study of behavior, it is important to seek causal relationships. Clues observed in the environmental conditions are examined and related to theories of psychosocial behavior to suggest reasons for the individual's disturbed equilibrium.

INTERVENTION

In the third step, intervention is initiated. Action is taken with the expectation that if the *planned action* is taken, the *expected result* will occur.

After the necessary information is collected, the problem-solving process is continued to initiate intervention. The nurse defines the problem from the information that has been given and reflects it back to the individual. This process clarifies the problem and encourages focusing on the immediate situation. The nurse then explores possible alternative solutions to the problem to reduce the symptoms produced by the crisis. At this time, specific directions may be given as to tentative solutions. Then the individual can leave the first session with some positive guidelines for going out and testing alternative solutions. At the next session, the individual and nurse evaluate the results. If none of these solutions has been effective, they work toward finding others.

The nurse may validate observations and tentative conclusions by reviewing the case with a colleague when he or she thinks it may be helpful or necessary. Briefly, the nurse identifies the crisis-precipitating event, symptoms that the crisis has produced in the individual, degree of disruption evident in the individual's life, and plan for intervention. Planned intervention may include one technique or a combination of several techniques. It may be helping the individual to gain an intellectual understanding of the crisis or helping the person explore and ventilate feelings. Other techniques may be helping the individual find new and more effective coping mechanisms or using other people as situational supports. Finally, a plan is presented for helping the person establish realistic goals for the future.

ANTICIPATORY PLANNING

An evaluation determines whether the planned action has produced the expected results. Appraisal must be objective and impartial to be valid. Has the individual returned to a normal level or a higher level of equilibrium in functioning? The problem-solving process is continued as the nurse and the individual work toward resolution of the crisis.

Summary of Key Concepts

1. The most important aspects of mental health are the state of the ego, the stage of its maturity, and the quality of its structure.

2. Caplan refers to a crisis as showing a rise in inner tension, signs of anxiety, and disorganization of function, all of which result in a prolonged period of emotional upset.

3. If adaptive mechanisms are used and a state of equilibrium is regained, a crisis can result in personal growth.

4. Differences in coping mechanisms are caused by the way each individual perceives the threat.

5. The more realistically an individual views the stressful event, the more success the individual has in solving the problem quickly.

6. Because appraisal of the event is an ongoing process, coping behaviors are never static as new significance is attached to the event.

7. Lack of situational support may compound a stressful situation into a crisis.

8. Coping is the process of attempting to solve problems—not the mastery over life problems.

9. There are three basic reactions to stress: attack, flight, or compromise.

10. Tension-reducing responses—aggression, regression, withdrawal, and repression—are based on past successful responses.

11. Success in handling maturational, or transitional, crises depends on how the individual accomplished developmental tasks.

12. There are two approaches to crisis intervention. The generic approach focuses on the characteristic course of a particular kind of crisis. The individual approach focuses on meeting the unique needs of an individual.

13. There are four typical phases in crisis intervention: assessment, planning therapeutic interventions, intervention, and resolution of the crisis and anticipatory planning.

REFERENCES

Aguiler DC: *Crisis intervention: theory and methodolgy,* ed 7, St Louis, 1994, Mosby.

Antonovsky A: *Unraveling the mystery of health: how people manage stress and stay well,* 1987, San Francisco, Jossey-Bass.

Bandura A et al: Cognitive processes mediating behavioral change, *J Pers Soc Psychol* 35:125, 1977.

Caplan G: *Support systems and community mental health: lectures in concept development,* New York, 1974, Behavioral Publications.

Caplan G: *An approach to community mental health,* New York, 1961, Grune & Stratton.

Coleman JC: *Abnormal psychology and modern life,* Chicago, 1950, Scott Foresman.

Cropley A, Field T: Achievement in science and intellectual style, *J Appl Psychol* 53:132, 1969.

Dewey J: *How we think,* Boston, 1910, Health.

Guilford JP: *The nature of human intelligence,* New York, 1967, McGraw-Hill.

Inkeles A: Social structure and the socialization of competence, *Harv Ed Rev* 36:265–283, 1966.

Jacobson G: Crisis theory, *New Dir Ment Health Serv* 6:1, 1980.

Jacobson G: Crisis theory and treatment strategy: some sociocultural and psychodynamic considerations, *J Nerv Ment Dis* 141:209, 1965.

Jacobson G et al: Generic and individual approaches to crisis intervention, *Am J Public Health* 58:339, 1968.

Jalajas DS: The role of self-esteem in the stress process: empirical results from job hunting, *Journal of Applied Social Psychology* 24, 22:1984–2001, 1994.

Janis IL: *Psychological stress, psychoanalytical and behavioral studies of surgical patients,* New York, 1958, John Wiley.

Johnson DM: *The psychology of thought and judgment,* New York, 1955, Harper & Row.

Kaplan DM, Mason EA: Maternal reactions to premature birth viewed as an acute emotional disorder, *Am J Orthopsychiatry,* 30:539, 1960.

Lazarus RS: *Psychological stress and the coping process,* New York, 1966, McGraw-Hill.

Lazarus RS et al: The psychology of coping: issues in research and assessment. In

Coehlo GV et al, editors: *Coping and adaptation.* New York, 1974, Basic Books.

Levinson DJ et al: *The seasons of a man's life,* New York, 1978, Alfred A. Knopf.

Lindemann E: Symptomatology and management of acute grief, *Am J Psychiatry* 101:101–148, 1944.

Masserman JH: *Principles of dynamic psychology,* Philadelphia, 1946, W.B. Saunders.

McSherry WC, Holm JE: Sense of coherence: Its effects on psychological and physiological processes prior to, during, and after a stressful situation, *Journal of Clinical Psychology,* 50(4):476–487, 1994.

Mechanic D: Social structure and personal adaptation: some neglected dimensions. In Coehlo GV et al, editors: *Coping and adaptation,* New York, 1974, Basic Books.

Morley WE et al: Crisis: paradigms of intervention, *J Psychiatr Nurs* 5:537–538, 1967.

Phifer JF: Psychological distress and somatic symptoms after natural disaster: differential vulnerability among older adults, *Psychology and Aging* 5(3):412–420, 1990.

Rappoport R: Normal crises, family structure, and mental health, *Fam Process* 2:68, 1963.

CHAPTER 22

Interactive Therapies and Methods of Implementation

Mary Magenheimer Webster

Attending Paying attention to what a client is saying.

Boundary The definition and separation of the self from others through the clarification of limits and extent of responsibilities and duties of one's self in relationship to others.

Countertransference Feelings the nurse has toward the client as a natural part of the therapeutic relationship.

Identified client In family therapy the member of the family (or group) whose behavior is seen as causing the problem for the family (or group).

Norms The standards of behavior, attitudes, and, at times, perceptions that a group has for its members; norms represent the shared expectations of appropriateness in behavior.

Roles The socially expected behavior patterns usually determined by an individual's status in a particular group. Peplau (1952) identified four roles for the psychiatric nurse: (1) resource person, (2) counselor, (3) surrogate, and (4) technical expert.

Safety The sense of security developed within the therapeutic relationship when the responsibilities and expectations of each party are clearly defined. Safety develops from knowing the boundaries of a relationship and acting within them.

Themes The recurring patterns of interactions the client experiences in relationships with self and/or others.

Therapeutic milieu An environment designed to promote emotional health that is based on the assumption that clients are active participants in their own lives and therefore need to be involved in the management of their behavior and environment.

Therapeutic relationship A personal relationship that is established to help one of the participants deal more effectively and maturely with some difficulty in life. It is a goal-directed, client-centered, and objective relationship.

Transference Feelings the client has toward the therapist and the helping relationship, which truly belong to significant people in the client's life and are transferred to the therapeutic relationship.

Trust The reliance on the truthfulness or accuracy of the therapeutic relationship developed through a congruency between the therapist's words and actions.

- Compare the concepts of boundary, safety, and trust development as they relate to individual, milieu, family, and group therapy.

- Discuss the processes that support the various phases of therapy.

- Identify personal characteristics and attitudes that affect one's ability to function as a psychiatric nurse.

- Describe the appropriate tasks for individual, milieu, family, and group therapy and discuss ways in which the nurse promotes these tasks.

I nteractive therapy implies one's therapeutic interaction with an individual, a family, or a group. This is not a new concept for nurses. Much of nursing's work involves interacting with the client to provide healing measures. The nurse changes a dressing on one client to assist wound healing or provides antibiotics to help another client to fight an infection. The nurse also manages the many types of equipment required for the client's treatments. All this can be viewed as one individual providing treatment (or therapy) for another. This work, however, entails the nurse doing something very visible for the client. Nurses use their hands and actively do something that the client can see. Much of the nurse's speech is used for teaching, assessing the client's status, or exchanging pleasantries.

In contrast, much of the work of psychiatric nursing is initially "invisible." Beginning students often complain that there is "nothing to do" in a psychiatric setting, since hands-on treatments are few. Some individuals become confused about and even frustrated with their roles as psychiatric nurses, or with the delivery of psychiatric nursing care.

The beauty, as well as the challenge, of psychiatric nursing is that the nurse's very self is used as the therapeutic agent. The nurse's words and interactions are designed to assist the client to heal psychically and emotionally. Just as it took time and experience to learn to change dressings, give medications, and manage equipment, so too it takes time to use oneself and one's words as healers.

The reader should not assume that the nurse involved in interactive therapy needs to be a psychotherapist. A psychotherapist is generally an advanced clinical practitioner with specialized credentials in the area of psychotherapy. Nurses can be therapeutic interactively without being licensed psychotherapists.

It is essential to examine assumptions regarding the nurse-client relationship in psychiatric nursing. This chapter discusses the role of the nurse with clients in a therapeutic psychiatric environment.

THE THERAPEUTIC RELATIONSHIP

The goal of nursing has always been to promote health. Mental health is defined as the "forward movement of personality and other ongoing human processes in the direction of creative, constructive, productive, personal, and community living" (Peplau, 1952, p. 12). The psychiatric nurse needs to recognize that every interaction has the potential to promote the health of the client. Indeed, psychiatric nurses have an obligation to use their skills within a therapeutic relationship to promote and maintain health.

Social versus Therapeutic Relationships

The therapeutic relationship is unique in the world of human interactions. It stands apart from other types of relationships in its focus, purpose, and enactment. Beginning practitioners frequently act in ways that are associated more with a social relationship than with a therapeutic one. A social relationship is with friends and acquaintances, and it exists for the mutual satisfaction of those involved. Its duration, focus, and intensity vary according to the participant's wishes; it is a subjective relationship.

In contrast to the social relationship, the **therapeutic relationship** exists to help one of the participants, the client, deal more effectively and maturely with some difficulty. It is viewed as a personal relationship where "two people come to know each other well enough to face the problem at hand in a cooperative way" (Peplau, 1952, p. 9). The nursing functions in a therapeutic relationship are (1) to assist the client in identifying emotionally felt difficulties, and (2) to apply knowledge of the principles of human relations to the problems or issues that arise at all levels of experiences (Peplau, 1952). This requires nurses to understand themselves and their behavior well enough to be objective and capable of focusing on their clients' needs; this is discussed further in the section on self-development.

Roles in the Therapeutic Relationship

Roles are the socially expected behavior patterns determined by an individual's position or status in a particular group or relationship. The psychiatric nurse enacts several educational and therapeutic roles during various phases of the therapeutic relationship. Peplau (1952) has identified four roles: (1) *resource person,* who gives specific information to clients, thus allowing them to understand situations or procedures; (2) *counselor,* who listens to the client's experience and assists in clarifying feelings associated with it; (3) *surrogate,* whom the client casts into roles of past relationships (parent, sibling, spouse, teacher), perhaps needing clarification of feelings; and (4) *technical expert,* who can navigate the complexities of the health care system.

Aspects of the Therapeutic Relationship

The therapeutic relationship is goal-directed, client-centered, objective (Fortinash and Holoday-Worret, 1995), and involves transference and countertransference.

Goal direction in a relationship implies a purpose for the relationship's existence. The overall goal of any therapeutic relationship is to assist the client to move toward health by becoming more self-responsible (Kennedy, 1977). Each individual is unique, however, and specific goals need to be defined for each person. Most people desire the relief of uncomfortable symptoms (i.e., anxiety, depression, suicidal thoughts, outbursts of anger, feelings of unworthiness). The therapeutic relationship is initiated to help the individual deal with offending symptoms in a way that is more conducive to health. It is a highly focused relationship, with both participants agreeing to direct their energies toward achieving the identified goal. This also implies that the relationship has limits: it exists to meet certain defined goals, not to meet all the client's needs. This concept of boundaries will be discussed in a later section of this chapter.

Client-centered implies that the relationship is focused on the client; it is the client's goals, reactions, coping strategies, and growth that are at the center of the relationship. The therapeutic relationship requires that nurses turn their attention to another for a while and suspend their preoccupations with events in their own lives, in order to experience a client's sense of being (Kennedy, 1977). This does not mean that the nurse's reactions and sense of self are not important; it means they are not the focus of the relationship. The nurse's sense of self and reactions to the client are crucial to the work of a psychiatric nurse. By paying attention to one's own reactions and being able to sort them out, the nurse will gain knowledge of the client's interpersonal dynamics. This is some of the most difficult work in psychiatric nursing: to recognize one's own reactions and to use this information in a way that will assist the client to grow toward emotional health.

Objectivity is required on the part of the nurse. Objectivity implies an analytical approach to the subjective experience. In other words, it requires nurses to be aware of their feelings and reactions to being with clients rather than to just responding to clients on a personal level. For instance, perhaps a client is acting in a way that makes the nurse increasingly angry. It would not benefit anyone if the nurse were to snap back at the client in anger, because this may simply mirror similar experiences the client has had with many others in the past; it will not bring the client any closer to the goal of more healthful interactions. Instead, nurses should deal with their own reactions in a way that allows them to be of use therapeutically.

Transference refers to the feelings the client has toward the nurse and the helping relationship. These feelings truly belong to the significant people in the client's life prior to the therapeutic relationship with the nurse, and are transferred and played out again in the therapeutic relationship. Consequently, nurses must avoid responding as if clients' feelings are directed at them personally; such feelings are evoked by what the nurse represents to the clients. This is the surrogate role Peplau refers to. For instance, clients who behave in ways that made the nurse angry in the previous example may be responding to their nurses as if they were overintrusive parent figures. Perhaps the only way that the client could attain any separateness was to push the nurse away with anger, a pattern the client still continues. Thus, nurses who behave as if the feelings were actually directed toward them would personalize the situation and miss an opportunity to be therapeutic. By responding more objectively, nurses could help clients to begin to recognize a pattern. Instead of responding in anger, nurses could make open-ended comments, opening the door for clients to explore their feelings. By being objective, the nurse allows the client to take a step beyond the act itself, and begin to talk objectively about it rather than merely respond in the same way again and again.

Countertransference is defined as the feelings the nurse has toward the client. These feelings may be positive or negative and are a natural part of a therapeutic relationship. Problems arise only when the feeling is discounted because it upsets, surprises, or embarrasses the nurse in some way. Nurses need to recognize, identify, and accept these feelings; otherwise they will influence the nurses responses to clients, whether or not this is apparent (Kennedy, 1977). For example, nurses who are attracted to, or feel contempt for, their clients may be horrified about having these feelings, knowing as they do that the relationship is a professional one. Nurses may respond by keeping their distance from clients and treating them superficially to distance themselves from their feelings. Thus, no work is accomplished in the therapeutic relationship because it is dominated by the nurse's personal concerns.

Personal Qualities of Effective Helpers

There is growing recognition that the personal qualities of effective helpers are as significant in their promotion of growth in others as the methods they use (Brammer, 1993). Effective helpers express a positive view of peo-ple's ability to solve their own problems and manage their own lives. In addition, they tend to view people as dependable, friendly, and worthy. Effective helpers tend to identify with people rather than things, demonstrate a capacity to cope, and are willing to reveal their thoughts rather than conceal them (Brammer, 1993). Helpers care for themselves and others. A helper must balance a sense of strength and maturity with the humility and vulnerability that come from experiencing life's problems. It is this vulnerability that assists in the building of trust (Brammer, 1993).

PREPARATION FOR INTERACTIVE THERAPY
Self-Awareness

It is clear from the preceding discussion that the psychiatric nurse needs a strong sense of self or at least the willingness to develop one. The term *sense of self* refers to self-awareness or self-knowledge. This is necessary because nurses must be able to separate their own subjective beliefs from the facts. Self-awareness implies a recognition of one's thinking, values, conflicts, interaction styles and attitudes, and an awareness of how these can influence interactions with clients. The nurse need not be perfect—obviously such a goal cannot be achieved even over a lifetime. It is necessary, still, that the nurse have a commitment and an openness to self-exploration.

There are many ways for the nurse to do this work. Many schools of therapy require therapists to undergo ongoing personal therapy. Not only does this assist developing therapists with resolving issues/conflicts in their own lives but also makes them sensitive to what their clients are experiencing. Other avenues for self-exploration are support groups, value clarification work, role-playing, and individual supervision. The staff at one state hospital participated in a simulation game in which they shared the common experience of temporarily being inpatients, as a way to influence their attitudes toward those with mental illness (Cosgray et al, 1990). After the simulation experience, postgame discussion reflected recurring feeling among the staff of powerlessness/helplessness and anger/hostility. The staff "reached consensus about the need to treat patients with respect and dignity" (Cosgray et al, 1990).

Self-reflection is an appropriate first step. Nurses can assess their values, attitudes, and orientation by asking themselves some general questions. Again, the point of this is not to conform to any preconceived notion of a therapist. This self-assessment will simply increase the nurses' self-awareness of so that they will best be able to use that awareness therapeutically and not minimize their own work.

Areas for Self-Assessment
NEED TO BE LIKED

It is important to assess the need to be liked. The need to be accepted and valued can be so strong that it can paralyze the nurse in interactions. For example, the nurse is at risk for becoming hurt or angry if the client acts in an angry or hostile manner. Or, the nurse may hesitate to comment, for fear that the client would be offended in some way and consequently think less of the nurse. With time and experience the nurse learns that the key to an effective approach is simply to be comfortable with the other person. This arises out of a sincere effort to attend to the client's words and listen carefully to that experience. In fact, rapport will develop best when nurses focus on their clients so much that they forget their own need to be liked (Kennedy, 1977).

BEING JUDGMENTAL

Another area to evaluate is being judgmental. Judgments are the quick stereotyping of people so as to fit them into categories to ease one's own interactive experience. Forming judgments is also a survival skill that allows us to decide issues of emotional safety quickly. Often these judgments are based on a few life experiences and tend to be generalized in others. Thus someone who reminds the client in some way of a favorite aunt would tend to be judged favorably even before the client gets to know the person as an individual. Culture also influences the ways in which people are viewed. The portrayals of individuals or groups in the media, for instance, affect one's judgment of them. The end result of this is stereotyping, as a result of which individuals lose a personal identity and are clumped into a collective group. Such judgments have no place in a therapeutic relationship that focuses on the individual. Judgments produce labels that only serve to distance people. Although it is unrealistic to expect anyone to rid themselves of their judgments completely, psychiatric nurses should at least be aware of their judgments and how they affect relationships. Nurses must be able to suspend judgments of clients so that they can focus on their clients' individuality and experiences, and remain open to learning (Kennedy, 1977). As Peplau (1952, p. 31) has written, "Nursing symbolizes the acceptance of people as they are and assistance in times of stress."

RESPONSIBILITY

Another critical area is the assumption of responsibility. It is necessary for psychiatric nurses to clarify their own understanding of who is responsible for what in the therapeutic relationship. There are areas of nursing where the outcomes depend solely on nursing performance (e.g., the absence of sepsis around a surgical wound, the administration of medication, or the proper rate of fluid replacement via an intravenous infusion). All these administrations involve the nurse *doing* something for the client. As noted before, many beginners in psychiatric nursing feel the need to *do* something visible. Consequently, they tend to ask too many questions rather than listen to clients, and to give advice rather than assist clients with their own problem solving. Closely related to this need to do something is the issue of patience. Many nurses want or expect to see rapid results and tend

to become impatient with the time it takes for psychiatric work to progress. Again, when impatience is a problem, the nurse may take over by becoming overly bossy or judgmental, both of which are nontherapeutic and potentially destructive.

Thus, it is important that psychiatric nurses be clear about their responsibility to their clients. It is not up to the nurse to define the area, direction, or time frame of growth for the client but rather to further the client's own work along those lines and to support the client in the work of therapy. "Real support arises from entering into the experience of other persons, being able to stand there with them as they explore themselves, and not in backing away when the experience threatens to become hard on us" (Kennedy, 1977).

POTENTIAL FOR HUMAN GROWTH

This also requires the psychiatric nurse to have some confidence in the client's ability to grow, learn, and make changes. Nurses need to assess their own assumptions about the potential for human growth. Nurses can assess these symptoms by evaluating their own personal needs for sympathy and protection (Fortinash and Holoday-Worret, 1995). If nurses believe that they need to be protected from life experiences, they may assume that they do not have the capabilities to deal with life and that it is not possible to develop them. Hence, the need for protection exists. Nurses who feel this way about themselves may tend to generalize this life stance to their clients. They may tend to protect their clients from the challenges of psychological growth, rather than assist them in moving through the challenges to achieve growth.

These areas of self-assessment are not meant to be a complete list. Psychiatric nurses will find themselves examining their values and attitudes anew with each client. They will examine their assumptions about dependence, responsibility, competence, and intimacy (or closeness), to name a few. Self-examination (autodiagnosis) is an ongoing process because each phase of life and each situation is unique.

Concerns Experienced by the Nurse

It has been noted that student nurses generally have three concerns: self-consciousness about enacting the role, fears and fantasies about what constitutes professional behavior, and uncertainty about how to proceed technically with clients (Denton, 1987). Student psychiatric nurses generally demonstrate these anxieties by worrying about their choice of words. They often fear saying "the wrong thing" that may damage the client permanently. They may become awkward about using words, and fret over finding the right word or correct way to speak. This hyper–self-awareness is probably a result of the process of beginning to learn to use the self in a therapeutic manner. As such, this self-consciousness is part of the normal learning process. This attention to words also extends to the nurse's perception of the client. Students tend to focus solely on the content (or words). By focusing on words only, student nurses can miss the richness of the nonverbal information presented by the client, and may neglect to follow up on a tone of voice or special look on the client's face.

Psychiatric nursing is not only about words. It is about therapeutic relationships and focusing on another individual. When nurses are aware of the work occurring at each phase of the relationship, they can consciously use a variety of skills to promote the desired change in the client. When the focus is on the work, words can be used more fluidly as a tool. This does not diminish the use of language as an important tool. More experienced practitioners will use sentence structure and word choice as a way of analyzing the client's thought processes.

An important aspect in the development of trust and safety is the nurse's manner or behavior. Nurses must outwardly model or demonstrate their attention to the client. This counseling skill is called **attending** and includes all the ways in which therapists demonstrate to

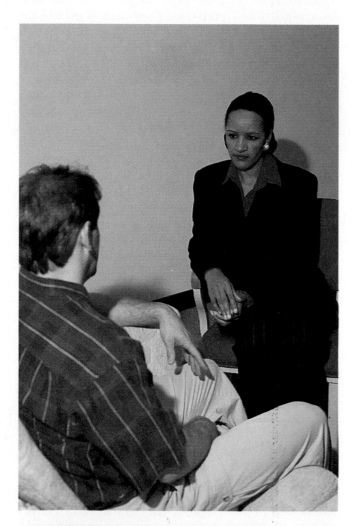

Figure 22-1 This therapist's nonverbal behaviors—relaxed posture, slight forward lean, and good eye contact—indicate openness, acceptance, and interest in the client.

(Copyright 1995, © Cathy Lander-Goldberg, Lander Photographics.)

clients that they are heard; clients are thus encouraged to express feelings and experiences.

The nurse shows this attention nonverbally and verbally. *Nonverbal behaviors* include a relaxed posture indicating openness and acceptance, and with a slight forward lean demonstrating interest (Fig. 22-1). The nurse maintains good eye contact, "seeing" the client. It is important not to simply stare or glare at the client since this is an aggressive behavior, but rather to meet the client's eyes in a relaxed, comfortable manner, occasionally looking away. *Verbal behaviors* associated with attending demonstrate careful listening and include open-ended questions, paraphrasing, reflection of feelings, summarization, and allowing clients to set their own pace (see Chapter 5).

Perhaps the easiest way for nurses to demonstrate attending skills toward clients while earning their trust is for them to enact the qualities of genuineness, respect, and empathy. *Genuineness* has been defined as verbal and behavioral congruence and authenticity. *Respect* is defined as unconditional positive regard and is noted to be conveyed through consistency and active listening. *Empathy* implies seeing the situation from the client's point of view, yet remaining objective. The empathic nurse can intervene to assist clients in their understanding of a situation, and suggest appropriate avenues for change (Fortinash and Holoday-Worret, 1995).

DEVELOPMENT OF A THERAPEUTIC RELATIONSHIP

Establishing a therapeutic relationship is not magic; it requires hard work and the skillful application of knowledge. Beginners in interactive therapy are often so concerned with the content of the session that they overlook the basic concepts at work in every therapeutic relationship. These concepts are boundary development and maintenance, safety development, and trust development. The concepts apply to the individual therapeutic relationship as well as the family and group processes although they are expressed in different ways. These three concepts are tightly interwoven, each affecting the other.

Boundary

The term **boundary** refers to the definition of an entity. The boundaries of a country define its shape, size, and location in relationship to other countries. Each country negotiates for itself in various kinds of social interactions. Boundaries serve to separate and define entities at the point where the entity interacts with others.

In psychological terms, boundaries refer to the definition and separation of the self from others. They serve to define the responsibilities and duties of one's self in relationship to others. This is an extremely important concept in working with psychiatric clients whose sense of self is often unclear in some way. Very often psychiatric clients do not have a sense of what constitutes their own responsibility and will ask nurses to do things that are not the nurse's responsibility. Consequently, nurses must have a clear sense of self and of their role to prevent collusion with the client in this way. For example, consider the following: a nurse and client have been engaged in an interaction trying to identify the source of the client's agitation. They finally arrive at a point where the client identifies feeling angry with someone else about an earlier incident. In order to resolve this, the client suggests that the nurse discuss the incident with the other person so the person becomes aware of the effect of his or her action. A nurse complying with this request would be in the middle of a confusing situation, that of conveying another person's emotional reaction. If, however, nurses in such a situation are aware of their role of furthering the client's sense of self (and its attendant responsibilities), they decline to shuttle information and instead assist the client in finding a way to accomplish this task.

Boundaries refer to acting in ways that are appropriate to role and self. Consequently, it is essential for nurses to have a clear sense of what constitutes their responsibilities and what the client's responsibilities are. Maintaining safe boundaries does not necessarily mean therapeutic touch cannot be used as a way to communicate caring (Gagne, 1994). Touching a client in a therapeutic manner, such as gently placing a hand on a client's forearm, when trust has been established can enhance a therapeutic relationship. The nurse will decide when therapeutic touch is appropriate for each individual client.

Safety

Safety is the sense of security within the therapeutic relationship. A clear sense of boundaries is essential to developing a sense of safety in the therapeutic relationship. Safety comes from knowing what the expectations are and what one's responsibilities are in meeting those expectations. In other words, safety develops from knowing what the boundaries of the relationship are and acting within them. By defining the structure of the therapeutic relationship, clients are safe to experiment within these boundaries while knowing that there are definable limits. All individuals need to feel safe when experimenting with new ways of being; this is especially true of psychiatric caregivers and their clients.

This is similar to a student preparing for an examination. Knowing that the examination is limited to Chapter 20, for example, leaves the student free to explore and concentrate on Chapter 20 without fear that issues from other chapters will be included. Similarly, if the client knows the relationship will be limited to client growth and the furthering of self-understanding, the client is free to focus on that work without being distracted by other concerns (e.g., sexuality, popularity, or competition).

Consequently, part of the nurse's role in a therapeutic relationship is to enhance safety, by acting consistently within the defined boundaries. It is confusing and dangerous for the clients if a nurse should introduce social elements into a therapeutic relationship in an attempt to be "friendly." Nurses should act within the boundaries of their role by assisting the client to focus on the assigned task and explore new options for growth, healing, and understanding.

Trust

As the nurse exercises the concepts of boundary and safety, trust develops within the nurse-client relationship. **Trust** is the reliance on the truthfulness or accuracy of the relationship. Trust develops when there is a congruence between words and actions. If nurses consistently do what they say they will, the client is free to work on the given task in ever-expanding ways. For many clients the relationship with the caregivers may be the most trusting one in their lives. As nurses continue to model their responsibilities in maintaining a trusting relationship, clients can begin to trust themselves and their reactions more. Trust is essential to the development of a sense of self.

A note of caution is necessary: acting in a trustworthy manner does not imply that conflicts will not occur. Trust does not imply agreement, only consistency. If the client makes an inappropriate demand, the nurse is not expected to meet it to maintain trust. (In fact, trust could be damaged when a nurse meets a demand that is inappropriate for the relationship.) Trust does not develop from doing everything the client asks; trust develops from doing what one said one would do.

These three concepts of boundary development and maintenance, safety development, and trust development are the foundations of every therapeutic relationship. The nurse constantly works to develop these in each relationship; it is "invisible work." Within the net of these three concepts, the nurse works with the client in a goal-directed, objective, and client-centered way, using a variety of skills such as listening and feedback.

PHASES OF THE THERAPEUTIC RELATIONSHIP
Orientation Phase

The orientation phase is the first phase of the therapeutic relationship. It occurs when clients enter the system and are full of the tension and anxiety associated with their own needs, in addition to those generated by exposure to a new and uncertain situation. Successful orientation is essential in assisting the client to combine these experiences (rather than to split them away in some manner—repression or dissociation) so as to be able to participate fully in the therapeutic relationship (Peplau, 1952). Orientation serves to define and clarify the relationship: the formulation of the client's issue or conflict, the purpose or goal of the work, and the relationship between the client and the nurse. The major "invisible work" of the orientation phase is boundary formation. The nurse works to assist clients to clarify their impression of the problem, thus defining the scope or boundary of the work. In addition, the nurse assists the client to function within the relationship, to have questions answered, needs expressed, and sincerity developed (Peplau, 1952), thus defining the scope or boundaries of the relationship itself.

Boundary development is done in specific ways. Nurses initially approach clients as strangers (Peplau, 1952) and must work to define themselves as allies and helpers. In introducing themselves to clients, nurses must state their purposes clearly. It is important that when speaking with new clients (strangers), nurses say whatever is appropriate for clients to hear, without using slang terms or incomplete remarks (Peplau, 1952). For example, if meeting a depressed client on an inpatient unit, the nurse could say: "Hello, I'm Mary Webster. I'm your nurse. I'll be working with you while you're here, to help you get used to the hospital and to look at the areas in your life that are troubling you." This introduction serves to identify the relationship as therapeutic and defines the nurse's role as a helping professional. Student psychiatric nurses are frequently vague in their introductions to the client (Sayre, 1978). They may say, "I'd like to help you," or "You're interesting to me." Vague introductions do not work because they do not address the formation of the boundary. The purpose of the introduction is to begin to define the scope of the work and of the relationship.

The next step of the introduction builds on this boundary definition by defining when the work can be done. This may be as formal as a contract for a scheduled outpatient appointment or as simple as an agreement. The nurse on an inpatient unit could say, "Normally, I'll be able to meet with you individually for 20 minutes a day after lunch. Since we're just getting started, I'd like to spend more time with you now to get acquainted. Would that be all right with you?" This serves to further define the time boundaries. Now the nurse has defined the purpose of the relationship (i.e., orientation to the hospital and work on the troubling issues) and the time frame (i.e., "now" and "20 minutes a day"). The specifics will vary with different clients and in different settings; the words will vary with the nurse's personality. These variances are to be expected and encouraged. For instance, when first meeting a frightened, psychotic client, it is important to speak simply and briefly. The nurse could say, "My name is Mary. I'm your nurse. I will be here today to help keep you safe." This also defines the nurse's role and time frame. However it is done or said, each introduction must frame the boundaries for the nurse's role, the scope of the work, and the time frame for doing the work.

WORK OF THE ORIENTATION PHASE

The work of the orientation phase is to help the client become a full participant in the therapeutic process by developing safety and trust. It has been noted that trust and security (or safety) are the first level of any interpersonal experience (Fortinash and Holoday-Worret, 1995). To do this the nurse must follow through on the agreements made in the introduction. As noted earlier, safety comes from knowing and meeting one's responsibilities, and trust develops from congruency between words and actions. Simply put, nurses must meet their own defined responsibilities to clients in a congruent manner and work so as to encourage clients to do the same. As Peplau has noted, "A relationship that is useful to the client is one in which what is expected of him is made clear and adhered to consistently, . . . one in which he is treated with understanding and respect as a person" (Peplau, 1952).

This is done in specific ways. The nurse needs to be dependable by being punctual and by being willing to discuss aspects of the contract (i.e., length of meetings, location, confidentiality of information, roles of nurse and client, and other specifics) (Fortinash and Holoday-Worret, 1995). The nurse's remarks initially need to be simple and clear to orient the client to the situation.

In addition, the nurse models focusing on clients and their concerns to assist them to formulate goals. This is done by helping the client define the issue* and then *listening very carefully.* Nurses should listen to what clients say about their own lives (the content) and observe how clients present this information (the process). Questions should be asked to further both the nurse's and the client's understanding of the client's experience. For example, a client may be describing the death of a parent and the subsequent breakup of the family (this is the content, i.e., *what* is said). Yet the client may relate all this information in a matter-of-fact way (this is the process, *how* it is said). The nurse's response should be one that will broaden the client's knowledge of the experience. For example, the nurse could comment, "Please tell me more about what this was like for you." Or the nurse may simply reflect back an important key statement†. Rather than interpreting, nurses should encourage clients to recognize their own feelings (Peplau, 1952). Both these responses serve to focus client's and expand their experiences. Questions are focused on clients' experiences and open-ended to allow clients to expand and clarify their thoughts.

RESPONSES IN ORIENTATION

Very often psychiatric clients have not been able to "tell their story." Families may develop their own lore around issues, and the "family myth" is difficult to challenge.

---

*(or the reason for the hospitalization, or the source of the client's unhappiness, or what would make a difference, etc. Again, it is not a matter of specific words so much as the direction of the nurse's focus on the client.)

†A key statement is one that is continually brought up by the client in conversation; or one that the client stresses or emphasizes; or words that are *not said* or deliberately omitted even though the topic is a known problem or conflict, given the client's history.

Friends may tire of the story or respond in a socially appropriate way. As a result, clients have no one to tell their story to and thus the story gets "stopped" at a certain point and is never allowed to reach a conclusion. Consequently, many of the emotions are also "blocked" and never worked through to resolution. The nurse's work in orientation is to help the client continue the story.

Although some clients are open to continuing their story, others do not welcome this opportunity or even know how to use it. There is a great deal of anxiety whenever one ventures beyond the known social conventions. When the client begins to challenge "the family myth" or the socially acceptable ways of dealing with aspects of the story, anxiety may be manifested in several ways. The client may test the nurse in some way, such as being late for meetings, ending them early, or questioning their usefulness. The client may focus on the nurse personally by questioning the nurse's competence, showing sexual interest, or attempting to shock the nurse through profanity, confrontation, or sharing bizarre experiences or behavior (Fortinash and Holoday-Worret, 1995).

The nurse needs to observe this behavior sensitively and objectively as both data about the client's interactive style and as a level of the client's anxiety. The nurse responds in role by focusing the client on the therapeutic work. For instance, to a client who demonstrates withdrawal, unusual behavior, or silence after being asked a question, the nurse could say, "That seems to be a difficult question for you right now. We don't have to talk about it now if you'd rather not." Or, to a client who continually focuses on the nurse rather than focusing on self, the nurse could say, "It seems difficult for you to talk about yourself." In both cases the nurse acknowledges the client's situation and refocuses on the therapeutic relationship.

ASSESSMENT

In addition to establishing the relationship, the orientation phase provides the nurse the opportunity to assess the client.

Themes.   The psychiatric nurse listens for themes that run throughout the client's stories. **Themes** are recurring patterns of interactions that the client experiences. Examples of themes are: every close relationship ending in anger; clients doubting their abilities at every turn; clients blaming others for life situations and taking no responsibility themselves; clients portraying themselves as victims. Themes are the underlying dynamics of many encounters. It is important to discern these patterns, and it takes time to do so. The patterns become more evident as the work progresses; the client may or may not be aware of them.

Themes are often linked to the client's problem areas. Clients are usually aware of their problem areas and can assist in identifying them. Generally clients can give the nurse some idea of what would make the situation

"right" for them (i.e., their thoughts about what is unhealthy for them and what would "fix" it). For instance, the agitated borderline client may say, "I just want everything to be all right." The housewife in crisis may say, "I just can't do it all any more." The psychotic client may speak of voices, tormenting him from which he wishes relief; the suicidal client may just want to die. Only catatonic clients will be unable to verbalize any goal at all; other clients will give some clue to their understanding of their situation. The function of psychiatric nursing is to accept this understanding and work in ways that will safely create opportunities for the client to learn healthy ways of assessing and achieving appropriate parts of the goal. Together the client and the nurse can prioritize the problem areas on which to work.

Observations.   The human mind can process language much faster than the human mouth can speak it. As a result, the brain is not fully occupied when simply listening to another. Psychiatric nurses can enhance their effectiveness by using this "extra brain power" to make observations about clients and the relationship between them. The nurse could make note of the client's affect and demeanor, noticing whether either changes when certain topics are discussed and in what way. The nurse also listens for what is *not* said: the major players in the client's life who are not part of the story; the absence of feelings, reactions, or thoughts. The nurse notes the manner of the client's relationship toward seeing it as a prototype for other relationships. Finally, nurses need to listen and identify their own feelings evoked in the relationship with the client. These feelings provide valuable information about the client's interactive style. The nurse must assess the client's mood, cognitive functioning, and potential for suicide or homicide.

Strengths.   One of the most important aspects of the orientation period is to assess the strengths and positive aspects of the client's personality. These healthy parts of the individual can be used to heal the more problematic areas. If the work of psychiatric nursing is to move the client toward health, then it is wise to know "the allies." Much of the work of psychiatric nursing is to expand and enlarge the healthy aspects of a person's personality while minimizing the dysfunctional aspects.

There is a story of the work of the great hypnotherapist, Milton Ericson, which emphasizes this point. Ericson was working at a V.A. hospital for clients with chronic mental illness. One of the clients was convinced he was Jesus and had for years acted as such. Ericson approached the client and said, "I hear you've had some experience as a carpenter." When the client acknowledged this was so, Ericson asked for some assistance with a minor woodworking project. The client agreed to assist. Over time, Ericson increased the complexity, functionality, and time frame of the woodworking projects, thus expanding the boundaries of the functional aspect of the personality. The client became less delusional and more reality-oriented as time passed. Ericson found the functional part in all the client's dysfunctional behavior and worked to expand it.

It is a skill to assist clients to use their own strengths in ways that benefit them. Together, the psychiatric nurse and the client identify these strengths. It is helpful for clients to view themselves as more than the sum of their problems. Such an expanded self-view may be the first step toward altering clients' self-perception and increasing their objectivity; it will assist them as they begin to engage in problem solving.

Nursing Care Plan. Once the assessment is completed, the nurse identifies the client's problems, nursing diagnoses, and outcome criteria; formulates the nursing care plan; implements the plan with nursing interventions; and evaluates the efficacy of the care plan, modifying it as needed (Fortinash and Holoday-Worret, 1995).

In summary, the work of the orientation phase is to (1) define the boundaries of the therapeutic relationship (i.e., identification of the work to be completed, and the relationship between client and nurse and the time frame; in effect, the "contract" between the nurse and the client); (2) begin the development of safety and trust by acting congruently within the defined boundaries; (3) complete the nursing assessment of the client; and (4) formulate the nursing care plan.

Working Phase

There is no clear ending to the orientation phase or beginning to the next phase, known as the *working phase.* The phases of the relationship overlap. As the working phase begins, the boundaries of the relationship have been established and the client acts within these boundaries. Safety and trust have also developed to the point that the client is willing to risk further exploration of issues. The nurse and the client have come to know each other well enough to be able to cooperate in dealing with a problem.

There are two parts to the working phase:

- Understanding the problem
- Assisting clients to translate this understanding to actions that work to their benefit

UNDERSTANDING THE PROBLEM

Part of understanding the problem is nurses working to facilitate both their understanding of their clients' position as well as the client's own understanding. Sometimes this is called *problem-formulating.* To do this, nurses ask open-ended questions designed to promote clients' recognition and integration of their own experiences, and perhaps gain a new perspective on them. In this part of the work the nurse functions very much in the counselor roles as described by Peplau. Counseling acknowledges that self-renewal, repair, and awareness come from within the individual. The function of the nurse counselor is to assist the individual's self-directed learning in ways that promote health and integration of experience (Peplau, 1952).

Necessary skills for this phase of work are careful listening and open-ended, nonjudgmental responses. The nursing response to a client's statement must not obstruct the possibility of identifying feelings or thoughts that assist clients in learning about themselves (Peplau, 1952). For example, consider the homemaker in crisis mentioned earlier. She had stated, "I just can't do it all anymore." The nurse's goal is to further the client's understanding of her own situation. Evaluate the following conversations to see which statement accomplishes this task.

CONVERSATION #1

Client: "It's overwhelming. I can't do it all anymore."

Nurse: "We all have bad days."

Client: "I've had a string of them."

Nurse: "Then they must be almost over. Hang in there."

Client: "Thanks. I will."

CONVERSATION #2

Client: "It's overwhelming. I can't do it anymore."

Nurse: "I'm not sure I understand. What's it?"

Client: "My life."

Nurse: "Your whole life is overwhelming?"

Client: "No, well, yes. There's so much to be done."

Nurse: "You have a lot to do?"

Client: "I'll say. I take care of the kids and the house and my husband is never around to help out."

Nurse: "You're taking care of the kids and the house without much help?"

Client: "Much help? NO help! He's never there for me, always out doing something while I'm stuck at home with his kids from his first marriage."

Nurse: "What's that like for you?"

Client: "It makes me mad! I'm not his slave."

Nurse: "So, you're angry about this?"

Client: "Sometimes; sometimes I think it's more than I deserve. My first marriage was pretty bad."

Nurse: "It sounds like you have more than one feeling about this."

In the first example, the nurse closed any chance for exploration by injecting her own viewpoint as a reassurance. The client could justifiably assume herself to be a self-pitying whiner. Most likely the client will keep further "failings" from this nurse. In the second example, however, the nurse was simply open to exploring the client's reality with her. Her questions provided focus for this work of exploring but did not limit the client's responses, thereby allowing the client to begin to gain perspective on her situation.

To further demonstrate nursing responses that promote the client's understanding of the situation, consider the following example of the suicidal client.

Client: "I just want to die."

Nurse: "You're thinking about death very seriously."

Client: "Yes. It would take care of everything."

Nurse: "You're seeing death as a solution."

Client: "Yes."

Nurse: "I'm not sure I understand. Tell me more."

Client: "About what?"

Nurse: "About death as a solution."

Client: "Well, the insurance money would pay off my debts and my wife would have money to live on."

Nurse: "You're thinking it would be a financial benefit to your wife."

Client: "Yes. She'd probably be happier, too . . . without me. I'm not worth much these days."

Nurse: "You think your wife would be happier if you were to die."

Client: "Yes . . . well, not right away, of course. She'd be sad . . . but she'd get over it . . . find somebody worthy of her."

Nurse: "It sounds as if you think highly of her."

Client: "Oh, yes! I don't know why she puts up with me, though. I've been terrible to be around."

Nurse: "You sound puzzled that she could love you even during this difficult time."

In this case, the nurse did not argue against the client's solution of suicide but explored the dynamics behind it. The questions/statements also help to introduce different perspectives to the client (the fact that he is worthy of love even during his depression and the possibility that the depression is time-limited).

Further exploration with both these clients would serve to clarify the patterns of thinking and acting that contribute to their dysphoria. This is crucial information. It is the meaning of the behavior, mood, or thoughts perceived by the client that offers the nurse clues to determine which needs must be met (Peplau, 1952). The nurse obtains this information as purely as possible without contaminating it. To do this, the nurse acts as a neutral sounding board so that clients can voice their views in a relationship that is safely defined and nonjudgmental (Peplau, 1952).

SAFETY DEVELOPMENT

It is during the working phase of the relationship that the concepts of safety and boundaries become important again. As noted earlier, safety comes in knowing what the expectations are in a given situation, as well as one's responsibilities in meeting those expectations. Clients sense

in some way that they are expected to tell their story; this may cause them a good deal of anxiety. The nurse assists the client by setting the pace to prevent the client from becoming overwhelmed (Peplau, 1952). By evaluating the client's anxiety level, the nurse ensures that the client does not become overly anxious in the process but instead moves at a pace with which the client feels safe.

Another part of understanding the problem involves the client and nurse determining what sorts of things trigger the maladaptive response. The nurse can help clients determine whether their reactions are a global response to any stressor or whether certain situations set them off or make them worse. This is important to know because it helps the nurse to assist the client in developing effective responses. In order to learn to deal in effective and healthy ways, the client needs to be aware of those situations that produce unhealthy responses. For example, suicidal clients noted earlier may experience what Beck calls *overgeneralization* (see Chapter 5) and tend to generalize their worthlessness to all situations. A homemaker may find that she manages the normal routine without undue distress but becomes overwhelmed when "extra" tasks are added (i.e., the car breaks down, a child gets sick, an organization requests volunteer time, etc.).

Both these situations could require different strategies. The nurse could select to do cognitive work with the client with depression, and stress reduction and assertiveness work with the homemaker.

The nurse's teaching must be appropriate to each client's plan of care; this teaching can be by both instruction and experience. For instance, the nurse must educate the clients about their diagnosis or the effects of any medications they may be receiving. This is done by evaluating clients' current levels of knowledge and then using their experience with their symptoms or medications to expand their levels of understanding. In other instances the nurse may have to teach the client new skills, such as the relaxation response, stress reduction techniques, assertiveness training, and cognitive work.

TRANSLATING UNDERSTANDING INTO ACTION

The second part of the working phase is to assist clients to translate their expanded understanding of the situation into behavioral changes or actions that promote health. There are many ways to do this, depending on the client's situation and the nurse's theoretical perspective. One aspect common to all client situations is that the behavioral changes are practiced in the "here and now." The client actually attempts behavioral change in the clinical situation with nursing support. For example, perhaps the suicidal man has learned that his days are much worse when he does not get out of bed in the morning. Together with the nurse he has identified a behavioral pattern in which he stays in bed isolated from his wife, reflects on his worthlessness, and becomes more despondent as the day goes on. This pattern has been repeated on the unit. The client and the nurse have decided to evaluate whether a change in this pattern would effect a change in his self-perception; they decide to test this by having the client get out of bed promptly in the morning and interact with at least one person at breakfast. (This would be consistent with a cognitive therapy approach.)

The homemaker has discovered an inability to say "no" to requests or to ask for any assistance at all. On the unit she is very helpful to other clients, caring for them and deferring her own needs. After learning some assertiveness skills, she and the nurse devise a plan in which she has to say "no" to three requests made of her and to ask for help once. In both cases the nurse continues to help the client to clarify feelings associated with the task and integrate the experience into their lives.

Working in the "here and now" is always possible. Beginners will often focus on the situation outside of the therapy as if it is a separate entity. If nurses focus on the problem situation as one occurring outside the client they serve to assist clients in dissociating it from their experiences (Peplau, 1952). However, the nurse's function is to assist clients to see that the locus of control is within themselves and that they have or can learn the skills to deal with that and other situations. Clients must experience this to learn it.

ROLES

Much of this learning is done within the client's relationship with the nurse, and it requires a sensitivity to the different roles that clients assign nurses. As noted earlier, clients will often respond to nurses *as if* they were someone else from a previous relationship. This unconscious pattern occurs when the client's situation reactivates feelings that were generated in a prior relationship (Peplau, 1952). The ill and needy client may respond to a female nurse *as if* she were a mother; the borderline client may view the nurse as a tyrant when she defines rules and limits; the client with low self-esteem may respond to the nurse as an authority figure, and so on. In addition, the client will anticipate the nurse's behavior to correspond to that of the earlier role model. The nurses' functions are to assist clients to recognize the likenesses and differences between the nurse and the earlier role model and to assist clients to get to know the nurse as a person just by being natural (Peplau, 1952).

In a way, the client is stereotyping the nurse into a predetermined manner of being. This is most likely to be a pattern the client repeats in many instances. By doing so, clients limit their own actions and reactions to those in the original experiences. This repetitive pattern of interacting is limited and can serve to reinforce maladaptive behavior. As nurses gradually reveal their own individuality they demonstrate the variety of human responses to their clients who are then free to explore their own various responses.

For example, imagine the homemaker in a creative group at which she accidentally spills the paint. She seems horrified by this and begins to clean it up frantically. The nurse approaches her.

Client:	"I'm so sorry! I'm so sorry! I can't believe how clumsy I've been! I can't do anything right."
Nurse:	(Recognizing that the client seems to want the nurse to participate in this "critical parent" stance): "Are you expecting me to criticize you?"
Client:	"Well, you should. I've made a mess of things. Don't you see what I've done?"
Nurse:	"What I see is that you had an accident and you're cleaning it up. That looks like being responsible to me. Can I help you at all?"
Client:	"No, it's almost done. The spill wasn't that big."
Nurse:	"I appreciate your taking care of it."

By being natural and sharing her viewpoint, the nurse provided the client with an important learning experience. The nurse did not respond in the anticipated critical way, but instead offered her own point of view.

From the nurse's viewpoint the client was acting responsibly. The client may have never considered this since her self-perceptions were locked in a self-critical mode, a pattern she enacted in the here-and-now in the presence of the nurse. The nurse used the opportunity to reject the critical role the client attempted to assign her and to acknowledge the client's strength.

The psychiatric nurse recognizes that *every* interaction provides an opportunity to be therapeutic.

TRUST DEVELOPMENT

In the preceding scenario, the nurse promoted trust between herself and the client by congruent words and actions. As noted earlier in this chapter, trust develops when there is congruence between words and actions. The nurse had agreed to work with the client's concerns. By being aware of the roles the client cast upon her, yet refusing to interact as her mother, sister, teacher, or wife, but only as herself, the nurse fulfills her part of therapeutic relationship by focusing on the client's issue of assuming criticism.

As clients learn to trust the nurse's genuineness and experience the nurse's acceptance, they begin to trust their own genuineness. This is one of the remarkable healing features of an effective therapeutic relationship: as clients experience trust and safety in the relationship, they begin to incorporate these elements into their sense of self. Eventually the client will develop an understanding of the situation, its causes, some skills for dealing with it, and some self-confidence to enact those skills. It is then time to terminate the therapeutic relationship.

Termination Phase

Terminating relationships is not generally done effectively in many Western cultures. There is a tendency to ignore, belittle, or hasten terminations in relationships, whether superficial or intimate. Termination is often a difficult phase in therapy as well. Because it represents an "ending" and is consciously or unconsciously associated with death, termination brings out many fears and anxieties in people. Termination forces one to come to terms with the limits of the relationship and therefore acknowledges the limits of life itself. In a more concrete sense, termination is the real loss of the nurse for the client. The relationship ends and the client must face life without the external support of the nurse. But life is nothing if not full of contrasts. At the same time that endings are being acknowledged, so are accomplishments, growth, and individuality. It is as if the ending of a relationship emphasizes the very being of the individuals who created the relationship. The work of the psychiatric nurse during the termination phase is to assist clients to acknowledge both these realities and to integrate them into their personalities. The *therapeutic work* is the acknowledgment of the formal closure of the boundaries of the relationship, and the transfer of safety and trust to the client.

PRIOR TO TERMINATION

As noted earlier, termination work begins during the introductory phase. The nurse defines the time frame for the therapeutic relationship to exist. The inpatient nurse may state: "*While you are in the hospital,* we will be working together." The outpatient nurse may say: "During the 6 weeks of this program . . ." The nurse defines the time frame of the work during the initial meetings and thus begins to prepare the client for the eventual end of the relationship. In addition, the work of the relationship has been clearly defined during the introductory period, and specific goals have been identified. Thus, the relationship has been defined by time limits and desired outcomes.

The nurse must also continue to acknowledge the end of the relationship during the working phase. Comments like, "While we're still working together . . ." or "During the time we have remaining . . ." reinforce the given time boundary and assist the client to get used to the idea of termination.

It is also effective to acknowledge the client's growth or accomplishments toward goal achievement or attainment as they occur during the working phase. By noting movement toward goal achievement, the nurse marks the client's progress and reinforces the concept that the relationship exists to accomplish certain things. Such comments also promote the combining of trust and safety in clients by allowing them to see that they can begin to trust themselves to be effective in certain areas of their lives, and consequently feel safer.

As clients begin to do more for themselves, the nurse can transition to the termination phase by spacing contacts incrementally further apart to allow clients more time to "stand on their own" according to their ability to do so. This gives clients the opportunity to support themselves gradually, and the nurse acknowledges this.

During the transition to the termination phase (and during termination itself), new or intense topics should not be introduced. This is a time of solidifying gains and acknowledging the work accomplished. If other issues exist, they may be acknowledged as areas for future work. It is unfair to the client to raise issues that cannot be resolved within the time that remains.

RESPONSES IN TERMINATION

As the reality of termination dawns, the clients may respond in a variety of ways depending on their personality and coping skills. Some may deny the occurrence or imminence of separation. Clients involved in denial will try to make plans to visit the nurse after discharge or will ask about making arrangements to "drop by" the hospital some time. It is as if by guaranteeing future contact, they can deny the impact of the current separation. Other clients will minimize the importance of the relationship and may make comments comparing the nurse to other supportive people in their lives, as if discounting the work done and the importance of the nurse to the accomplishment of that work. Another common reaction is anger. The client may express anger at the nurse, the institution, or other clients, in an attempt to cover the pain of separation. The client may experience the termination as a rejection, which may activate old feelings of inferiority or negative self-concept. Some clients may attempt to avoid the whole situation through premature discharge or noninvolvement in groups. Others may regress as if to demonstrate their continuing need for the nurse, stemming from their perceived inability to deal with life on their own. A few clients may actually attempt suicide in order to keep the nurse involved. Finally, some clients will accept the termination and demonstrate some perspective on their various reactions (Fortinash and Holoday-Worret, 1995). Careful review of these various reactions will remind the reader of the stages of grief (denial, anger, bargaining, and acceptance; see Chapter 27). This is not surprising when termination is viewed as a loss.

NURSE'S ROLE IN TERMINATION

As noted earlier, the American culture does not deal with endings well. Consequently, few clients have a frame of reference for handling this crucial aspect of life. The nurse has the unique opportunity to assist the client in a successful separation and ending, allowing the client to transfer this knowledge to the next situation. To do this the psychiatric nurse must model effective parting for the client. The first step is for the nurse to clearly understand the goal of termination, which is to dissolve the therapeutic relationship while assuring the client of an improved ability to function independently (Fortinash and Holoday-Worret, 1995).

The second step is for the nurse to have a clear understanding of the dynamics of loss (see Chapter 27) and how these concepts affect the client and the nurse. For instance, it is important that the nurse not respond to the client's anger or regression in a personal manner but instead continue to work to help clarify the client's feelings and reactions.

Preparing to terminate the therapeutic relationship takes time. A general rule is that one-third of the entire length of the therapeutic relationship should be spent on termination issues. Although this may not always be possible, given the current system of health care, it does emphasize the importance of this aspect of care.

As noted earlier, termination is addressed initially and throughout the relationship. Termination begins formally when the client has accomplished the appropriately defined goals and has improved to a higher level of self-sufficiency. The nurse then begins the process of parting with the client, and of modeling successful endings.

To do this the nurse acknowledges the upcoming ending of the relationship and engages the client in open discussions of his or her feelings in this regard. The nurse continues to be accepting and nonjudgmental even if the client verbalizes hostility, apathy, or sadness. By accepting the client's response, the nurse acknowledges that there are myriad human reactions to loss and implies the normalcy of the client's response. This then allows clients to accept and experience their own reactions (instead of defending them) and to view them as part of the whole process.

The nurse helps the client acknowledge the gains made during the course of their work together. It is often useful to review the course of the hospitalization/relationship, acknowledging the client's distress at the beginning, the significant learning that has taken place, and the demonstrated changes in behavior. Although most of this is done by the client, nurses also share their perceptions of the work. This sharing is incredibly powerful, and nurses need to express themselves positively to continue to promote health. The nurse's emphasis is on summarizing the important learning and the aspects of the client's growth. The nurse also shares what she has learned while working with the client. Again, this must be stated positively. Clients are often surprised that nurses "learn" something from being with them, since their focus is rightfully on themselves.

When nurses share with the client how they benefited and learned from the relationship, they reinforce the client's effectiveness and self-worth. (After all, the client must have done *something* if the nurse benefited from the relationship.) The nurse also models the positive influence people can have on each other.

A realistic and natural part of any discussion of termination is the disappointment about what was not achieved. This will be a major part of the work for some, whereas for others it will be a mere footnote. In either case, the topic of things not achieved should not be avoided. Such a discussion provides the opportunity to help the client gain a perspective on the nature of human growth—mainly, that growth continues throughout life. Frequently, the clients and nurses who are most disappointed at termination are those who set goals that are unrealistic or inappropriate to the time frame. Examples are clients who expect to be functioning optimally in all areas of their lives at the time of discharge and nurses who wish to have all their clients become self-actualized during the course of therapy. An important part of termi-

nating is to acknowledge what has not been accomplished and to make tentative plans on ways to accomplish these goals outside the relationship.

Nurses, like clients, need to express their own mixed-feelings about the separation. For example, "I also feel sad that this relationship is ending, and I am happy about the work we've accomplished," is a statement that helps clients normalize any reactions they may experience.

Even with the best preparation, most clients are anxious at the time of discharge or termination of therapy due to fears about their own ability to cope on their own. A list of available community resources will be helpful to the client in the transition to the community. It is important that clients know "the door has not been closed" and that help is available whenever needed.

THERAPEUTIC MILIEU

The therapeutic milieu is the environment designed to promote health. Since its earliest days nursing has recognized the importance of the environment or milieu to healing. Indeed, Florence Nightingale defined her work as organizing the environment to allow the body to heal. The same principle holds true in psychiatric nursing.

The psychiatric unit is a social system in its own right with clients at various points of length of stay, each with their own agenda, interacting and meeting unique personal and social needs. As such, the milieu can be seen both as a large work group with the definitive task of healing, and a community with all the tasks of communal living. The psychiatric nurse is a constant in this system, interacting with clients and staff in a variety of ways. These interactions are very significant and greatly assist in creating the atmosphere or culture of each particular psychiatric unit.

Historical Development

Maxwell Jones developed the concept of the therapeutic community in the 1950s. His goal was to design an entire culture that would promote healthy personalities (Jones, 1953). Jones's goal for patients was one of improved behavior, and he was one of the first to act on the knowledge that the hospital environment affects the symptoms, behaviors, and progress of clients.

Since the 1950s this work has been expanded and revised, although the language has changed from *therapeutic community* to the French term *therapeutic milieu,* meaning environment or setting. Thus, a **therapeutic milieu,** much like a *therapeutic relationship,* is an environment designed to promote health. It is also an environment designed to provide corrective or healing experiences that enhance the client's coping abilities. A milieu can be hierarchical or democratic, open to problem solving or rigid in its application of rules. The environment can foster individual responsibility or behavioral control. It is one of the challenges of psychiatric work to use this environment in a conscious manner to promote the healthy functioning of individuals and the group as a whole. The nurse, who is involved in most of the activities on the unit, is key to effective milieu development.

Principles of Milieu Therapy

In order to be effective, the nurse must understand the underlying assumptions of milieu therapy and promote its principles. The basic underlying assumption of milieu therapy is that *clients are active, not passive, participants in their lives.* This implies that clients "own" their behavior and environment and consequently need to be involved in the management of both. In the milieu, human beings are seen as independent. Distortions, conflicts, and inappropriate behaviors are dealt with in the here-and-now and in the context of their impact on others. Peers are assumed to be necessary for the learning that comes from various interactions, as well as the potential healing effect of peer pressure. The principles of milieu therapy are the following:

- to promote a fundamental respect for individuals (both clients and staff)

- to use the opportunities for communication between client and staff for maximum therapeutic benefit

- to encourage clients to act at a level equal to their ability and to enhance their self-esteem

- to promote socialization

- to provide opportunities for client to be part of unit management (Herz, 1969; Jones, 1953).

The nurse's function is to act in ways that consistently promote these goals.

Boundary, Safety, and Trust Development in a Milieu

The concepts of boundary, safety, and trust are of assistance in formulating this task just as in formulating the

therapeutic relationship discussed earlier. At this level, however, they are expanded to meet the needs of a kind of community, which is the psychiatric unit.

BOUNDARY

As mentioned earlier, boundaries serve to define functions and consequently imply responsibility. The psychiatric nurse must clarify boundaries for clients. It is not easy for anyone to walk into a new culture (such as a psychiatric unit) and make sense of it. It is considerably more difficult if that person is experiencing the cognitive or emotional stress of a psychiatric disorder. By defining functions and tasks of the various groups and activities offered on the unit, the nurse promotes the opportunity for each group or activity to be used efficiently. Appropriate task completion is essential for health.

For example, most units have some type of meeting for staff and client that is designed to orient clients to the staff, activities of the day, and any issues of communal living. This is frequently called the *community* or *contact meeting,* and provides an excellent opportunity for boundary definition because one of its purposes is the orientation of clients. This roughly correlates to the orientation phase in the development of a therapeutic relationship. Introductions and explanation of purpose and role are needed, only now these introductions address the relationship of the client to the unit and staff, rather than the individual therapist.

All too often, the community meeting is reduced to superficial introductions of the members (clients and staff), and a cursory schedule of activities. A rich opportunity to help clients structure their time and focus their work is wasted.

Consider the effects of these two examples of community meetings. In this first example, the nurse leader does little to define the structure, or purpose, of the work.

EXAMPLE 1 (NONTHERAPEUTIC)

Comments

Leader defines function of the meeting as introductory	**Leader:**	"OK. This is community meeting and we usually introduce ourselves. I'm Casey, the nurse. I'll be passing out meds today."
Clients follow defined function of introductions	**Client:**	"I'm Sue."
	Client:	"Carl."
	Client:	"Mike."
	Client:	"Peggy."
	Client:	"Lynn."
	Client:	"Carol."
	Staff:	"I'm Judy. I'm the O.T. I'll see most of you at my group."
Leader offers minimal assistance in organizing	**Leader:**	"OK. The schedule of groups is posted on the board. Who are the contacts?"
Leader does not define function of contacts	**Judy:**	"I'll be working with Carl, Peggy, and Lynn today."
	Leader:	"And I'll work with the rest."

Leader uses "stuff," a vague term that does not focus group to work	**Leader:**	"Any questions about unit stuff?"
	Lynn:	"I still don't have hot water in my room."
Leader does not allow for group problem solving	**Leader:**	"I know. Engineering's working on it. Anything else?" —PAUSE— "OK? Meeting adjourned."

On the surface, boundaries were addressed in a cursory way. The nurse defined one of her functions (med giving) and informed the clients that groups would be formed. Clients picked up on this role-modeling and responded with cursory information of their own. It is difficult to see how they could understand unit organiza-

tion to function effectively within it. A rich opportunity was missed.

Now, consider the difference in tone and expectations when boundaries and tasks are more clearly defined as in the following example:

EXAMPLE 2 (THERAPEUTIC)

Leader defines purpose of meeting	**Leader:**	"Good morning. It's Tuesday, June 14, and this is our community meeting. This is the meeting where we get ourselves organized for the day and take care of any business that comes up just from so many people living together."
Leader provides structure for task	**Leader:**	"Let's do first things first and introduce ourselves and what we do here."
Leader defines tasks and explains how clients can use her in this role	**Leader:**	"I'm Casey and I'm one of the nurses. I'll be passing out the medications today, so if any of you have questions about your medications, please see me. I'll also be leading the Process Group and I'll tell you more about that later."
Leader provides structure	**Leader:**	(To each client) "Would you please introduce yourself to everybody and say something about yourself?"
	Client:	"Well, I think everybody knows me. I'm Sue. I've been here since Friday. I'll probably go home Wednesday or Thursday."
	Client:	"I'm Carol. I don't know if I'll ever go home."
	Client:	"I'm Mike. I'm Carl's roommate and he snores! So loud!"
Leader focuses on task	**Leader:**	"Please say something about yourself."
	Client:	"I'm tired. I'm not sleeping well."
	Leader:	"Thanks."
	Client:	"I'm Peggy. I just came in yesterday and I've met a few of you. This is a real nice place."
	Client:	"I'm Lynn. I've got nothing to say."
	Client:	"I'm Carol. Uh—I don't like to talk in front of people."
Leader models acceptance	**Leader:**	"I appreciate your effort."
	Staff:	"I'm Judy. I'm the occupational therapist. I'll be leading the 9 A.M. and 2 P.M. groups today in the activity room. I also want to meet with you, Peggy, to get to know you and make some plans with you about how you can best use occupational therapy. Could you meet with me after the meeting to set up a time?"
	Peggy:	"Sure."
	Leader:	"Thanks for your introductions."
Leader defines role and how to use contact person to promote task accomplishment	**Leader:**	"Each one of the staff acts as a contact person for each of you. A contact is the person who is working with you for the day. You can talk to your contact about anything that concerns you. I'll be the contact person for Sue, Mike, and Carol. Judy will be the contact person for Carl, Mary, and Lynn. Any questions so far?"
Leader promotes self-responsibility by telling clients how to meet their own needs	**Leader:**	"Let me introduce today's schedule to you. It's posted on the bulletin board if you forget the times. We mostly want to tell you about the activities."

	Judy:	"From 9 A.M. to 10 A.M. is roles group. This group helps you look at the different parts you play in your various relationships. It's a good place to look for patterns that reoccur in your life. I will be the leader."
Leader defines purpose	**Leader:**	"You have free time until 10:30 A.M. From 10:30 A.M. to 11:30 A.M. is process group. This is the group I'll be leading. This is the group where we pay attention to how we communicate with each other. It's a good place to look at any problems you may be having communicating with other people. Lunch is at 11:45 A.M., and at 1 P.M. you have a choice of taking a walk (if you have privilege to do so) or playing a game like Bingo here on the unit. From 2 P.M. to 3 P.M. is the activity group that Judy leads. This is where you can make something. It's a good opportunity to look at how you approach doing a task. At 3:30 P.M. we go home and the evening staff will meet with you to go over the evening schedule and staffing. Any questions?"
Client uses information and responds to cooperative style modeled by leaders	**Carl:**	"Do we have to play Bingo? I hate that game."
	Leader:	"No, that was just what came to mind. Actually, as a group you can choose any game you'd like at that time."
Leader supports client initiative, clarifies the situation, and models acceptance of question asking	**Leader:**	"Thanks for asking. It helps us to make ourselves clear and share understanding of what happens here on the unit."
Leader reiterates ways to be self-responsible	**Leader:**	"Any other questions about the schedule?" —PAUSE— "It's a lot to remember. If any questions come up during the day, check the schedule on the bulletin board or see your contact person."
Leader continues providing structure	**Leader:**	"I think we can move to the last piece of business for this meeting and that's to deal with any issues that come up whenever so many people live together. Anything you want to bring up?"
Leader promotes interaction	**Lynn:**	"I still don't have any hot water."
	Leader:	"I heard about that from night staff again. It's been a while, hasn't it?"
Leader clarifies information	**Lynn:**	"Three days and nothing is happening."
	Leader:	"Well, actually something is happening. Engineering found that the valve is broken and they're waiting for a replacement."
Group follows up on problem solving (probably based on leader's earlier modeled acceptance and encouragement to be self-responsible)	**Lynn:**	(Sarcastically) "Great! They're waiting and I don't have any hot water."
	Sue:	"No hot water at all?"
	Lynn:	"Well, my shower works but I don't have any hot water in my sink to wash up. I don't want to take a whole shower just to wash my face."
	Mike:	"Why don't you just wet your washcloth in the shower?"
	Lynn:	"That's what I've been doing, but I get soaked and my clothes get soaked."
	Sue:	"Well, I don't mind if you want to use my sink for washing up, as long as you ask first."
Clients have clarified their action appropriate to their role	**Lynn:**	"Really? Thanks. I'll do that."
Leader clarifies her action appropriate to her role as staff member	**Leader:**	"That worked out . . . I'll see what engineering can do today, Lynn."
	Lynn:	"Thanks."
	Leader:	"Any other issues?"
	Mike:	"The radio is broken."
	Carl:	"No, it's not broken, just out of batteries."
Leader shares information not available to clients and offers solution	**Leader:**	"We keep batteries at the desk. Mike, would you bring the radio to the desk after this meeting and we'll see what new batteries can do."
	Mike:	"Sure."
Leader acknowledges contribution	**Leader:**	"Thanks. What else?"

	Peggy:	"I just don't know what to do about my son. He never listens to me anymore. He used to be such a good kid and now I just worry all the time."
Leader acknowledges issue and ways to work on it while keeping group focused to accomplish task of this meeting	**Leader:**	"Peggy, this sounds very important to you and something I know you'll want to work on while you're here. Process group or role or even a talk with your contact would be good places to talk about that; that's their purpose. In this meeting we try to handle the nuts and bolts of living on this unit."
	Peggy:	"I'm sorry."
Supportive and accepting approach	**Leader:**	"It's OK. It takes a bit of time to learn how to use this place and what all the meetings are for. It sounds like you have a good idea of some of the issues you want to work on."
	Peggy:	"Oh, yes!"
Leader continues to focus client on task of meeting to promote goal accomplishment	**Leader:**	"That's how it starts. Any questions about living here?"
	Peggy:	"You mentioned that you would be passing medications? I know I'm on some. Where do I go?"
Leader models self-acceptance of faults	**Leader:**	"Thank you. That's an important point and I forgot to mention it."
Leader provides further clarification on unit structure	**Leader:**	"Medications are passed at the medication cart at 9 A.M., right after this meeting, and again at 1 P.M. The evening shift will pass them out at 5 P.M. and 9 P.M. Not everyone gets medications at all these times. If you'd like I can meet with you after this meeting to see when you get your medicine."
	Peggy:	"Thanks. I'd like to do that. There's so much."
Supportive comment from peer	**Sue:**	"Don't worry. You'll get used to it."
	Peggy:	Smiles at Sue.
	Leader:	"Anything else?"
	Mike:	"I don't know if I should bring this up."
Leader continues to focus on task appropriateness	**Leader:**	"Does it have to do with the business of living together?"
	Mike:	"Yes."
	Leader:	"Then this is the place."
	Mike:	"OK then—well, I like Carl, don't get me wrong, but I can't sleep with his snoring and I don't think that's healthy for me."
	Carl:	"I do snore. I've heard that all my life."
Leader makes supportive and educational comment	**Leader:**	"Sleep is important to being able to function. Any solutions?"
	Mike:	"Well, I'd like a new room."
	Leader:	"That would be a great solution, but we don't have another room, and with our current mix of males and females we can't do any swaps."
	Lynn:	"Well, it's not fair! He should be able to sleep, for God's sake. This is a hospital."
Leader models reality orientation and acceptance of limits	**Leader:**	"I couldn't agree with you more. But a hospital has its limits, too. Apparently right now there is limited bed space. So we have to figure out a solution with what we've got."
	Lynn:	"Isn't this ridiculous! What can we do? Sleep in shifts?"
Leader keeps group focused on task of problem solving and does not allow group to degenerate into gripe session	**Leader:**	"There's one idea on the table. Any others?"
	Peggy:	"Maybe he could get a bed on another unit?"
	Mike:	"Well, I actually have an idea that might work."
	Leader:	"What is it?"
	Mike:	"Well, I was wondering if I could sleep in the quiet room, as long as it wasn't in use."

	Leader:	"What do you all think?"
	Group:	Murmurs assent.
Leader supports client initiative and provides link to other shifts as appropriate for staff member role	**Leader:**	"That's a very workable solution, Mike. I'll tell the evening and night staff and you can start tonight."
Leader promotes functional communication by assisting in message completion	**Mike:**	"Thanks!" (To Carl): "No hard feelings?" (No response.)
	Leader:	"Any hard feelings, Carl? Mike wants to know."
	Carl:	"No hard feelings. Like I say, this is an old problem."
	Leader:	"OK, anything else?" —PAUSE— "It seems like we've taken care of a lot of business. Thanks for your contributions here. If there are no objections, this meeting is adjourned."

What a different meeting and tone! The first meeting had a rather superficial feeling, whereas this one actually facilitated movement toward the stated goals of introductions, orientation, and organization. In addition, the psychiatric nurse has had the opportunity to assess the general tone of the milieu—for example, Peggy seemed somewhat bewildered and Lynn appeared angry. This information will be extremely useful to the rest of the staff as they interact with the clients throughout the course of the day. In effect, the clearly defined boundaries greatly assist the nurse in becoming oriented to the tone of the unit and the status of the clients. This information will help the nurse to organize the day while considering the clients' needs.

Boundaries continue to be addressed throughout the day: groups are introduced, duties of staff and patients are defined, and responsibility for various actions is acknowledged. Just as boundaries provide structure for individual work by defining the work, its limits, and time frame, so do boundaries in the milieu.

SAFETY

Safety and trust are developed in a similar manner as well. As noted earlier, safety is developed by knowing what one's responsibilities are in a given situation, and trust develops through actions that are consistent with an individual's or group's stated intent. It is important that these issues be addressed in terms of the milieu. To feel safe, clients need to know what is expected of them in their role as clients. Do they make their own beds or not? Are they called to group or expected to arrive at the stated location on time? Do they go to a certain spot to get meds or are meds delivered? How do they contact a staff member if they want to talk?

The psychiatric staff may not inform clients of their responsibilities, thinking that these expectations are obvious. By addressing these issues in a timely manner, however, The staff is able to ensure that safety is promoted and work may proceed more quickly.

Development of safety is addressed consistently throughout a client's stay through this clarification of ex-

pectations and responsibilities. This clarification of responsibilities is often necessary as it relates to other clients. Often, psychiatric clients will attempt to "help" other clients in certain ways. One client may "help" another by doing a task for him; another may "help" by stating the other's case in a difficult interpersonal interaction. Such "help" is usually "unhelpful" because it violates the boundaries of each individual's responsibilities (completing a task, speaking for one's self). Safety is promoted by clarifying what each member's tasks are and are not and assisting all clients to meet their appropriate responsibilities.

As an example of this, consider the following scenario that occurs on the same day as the community meeting just outlined.

Peggy:	(to nurse) "I need to find a blanket."
Nurse:	"We keep them on the line cart."
Peggy:	"Along with the pillowcases and sheets?"
Nurse:	"Yes. It sounds like you're making a bed. I thought you had already done that."
Peggy:	"Oh, I have done mine. I just wanted to help Mike out and make up the quiet room for him."
Nurse:	"How did you decide to do that?"
Peggy:	"Oh, it's just my way. I'm always doing things like that for people."
Nurse:	"How does that work for you?"
Peggy:	"Pretty well; people always ask me for help, so I know I'm needed."
Nurse:	"So, you're always needed."
Peggy:	"Yes, and always tired."
Nurse:	"It gets tiring doing things for other people."
Peggy:	"Yeah, I don't know any other way, though."
Nurse:	"So, you're doing the same thing here that you do outside?"
Peggy:	"Yes."

Nurse: "I wonder what would happen if you just took care of yourself and your needs here, and let others do the same for themselves. Do you think Mike can make his own bed?"

Peggy: "He's grown, I don't see why not."

Nurse: "Do you think you can let him make his own bed and do his own work?"

Peggy: "I suppose I could, but it would be so different."

Nurse: "It is a different way for you, to let each person do his own work. Are you willing to try it?"

Peggy: "OK."

Nurse: "Let me know later on what it's been like for you."

In this scenario, the nurse was able to turn a casual question into a therapeutic conversation, using this interaction to reinforce the boundaries of personal responsibility (each does own task), focus Peggy on her work (exploring self-defeating patterns), and promote safety by clarifying the expectations of each person's work. The nurse functioned within the role of a nurse in the milieu by: (1) performing within the role to use communication for therapeutic benefit, (2) assisting the client to function within the limits of self-responsibility, (3) promoting the appropriate self-functioning of each client, and (4) demonstrating respect for both the client and the process.

TRUST

Trust in a milieu is nurtured in a similar manner: the promotion of consistency between words and actions. Again, the nurse acts in a consistent manner to achieve defined purposes. For instance, nurses who say that they are medication nurses work to achieve the stated objectives: they pass the medications on schedule and are available to answer questions about the medications. Nurses who say they will orient a new client to the unit follow up by actually doing so.

More subtle, however, is the accomplishment of the overall goal of promoting a functional milieu that fosters self-responsibility, growth, and clear communication patterns. Nurses are involved in creating this type of milieu each time they interact with clients and staff. In the preceding conversation between Peggy and the nurse, the nurse used a client's casual question to more clearly define areas of responsibility for both Peggy (the client) and her peers. Psychiatric nurses must be aware of the various goals of the therapeutic milieu and their own role in facilitating trust; they must then work in a consistent manner to promote trust as a major goal of milieu work.

Working effectively in a milieu is some of the most challenging work for the psychiatric nurse. Each nursing interaction affects the milieu in some way. The challenge, then, is to make every interaction a therapeutic one. This is accomplished by acting in a manner that promotes the achievement of identified therapeutic goals within the milieu.

GROUP THERAPY

Humans spend much of their time in some form of group interaction. We are raised in family groups, participate in work groups at all ages, and socialize in formal or informal group settings. Much of our "humanness" is defined in our interactions with others. Before looking specifically at the use of groups as a form of therapy, it would be helpful to examine some universal characteristics of all groups.

The Group as a Microcosm

Groups offer individuals the opportunity to interact with other individuals in a meaningful way. Groups provide the opportunity for self-definition through human interaction and task accomplishment. All groups have a task or purpose; family groups are for mutual nurturance and support (especially in caring for offspring); work groups are designed to accomplish or produce certain defined tasks; social groups of various types exist to foster interactions. Each group functions as a microcosm, or miniature universe, reflecting its own specific group culture and set of values. People interact within this microcosm to meet their own needs.

Roles

In order for the group to do its work, specific duties need to be accomplished. These duties are formulated into roles. Individuals enact roles based on their own personal dynamics and group needs. Roles are described as either *ascribed* or *achieved*. Ascribed roles are based on certain intrinsic characteristics which are beyond a person's control, such as age or sex; *achieved* roles are based on a person's achievements through interests, education, and talents (Sampson and Marthas, 1990). Examples of achieved roles are teacher, nurse, musician, and athlete. Achieved roles are played out in relation to other roles; thus, in order to fulfill the role, a parent needs a child, a teacher needs a student, a nurse needs a client, and so on.

Roles exist in all groups and are related to the group's main issues of (1) accomplishing its defined task and (2) maintaining member relations (Sampson and Marthas, 1990). Special roles develop in the group to deal with these issues. A *task specialist* is someone within a group who works toward accomplishing the group's defined task. A *social specialist* is someone who maintains relative harmony in member relationships throughout the group process (Sampson and Marthas, 1990). Members enact these roles and others based on personal preference and group need. Roles that serve the individual's

---

Box 22-1   Individual Functions within a Group

Roles Involving Task Functions

Initiator: proposes new ideas, directions, tasks, methods.

Elaborator: expands on existing suggestions, develops the group's plans further.

Evaluator: critically evaluates ideas, proposals, and plans, examining the practicality of proposals and the effectiveness of procedures.

Coordinator: helps to pull together ideas and themes, to clarify suggestions that have been made, and to help various subgroups work more effectively together toward their common goals.

Roles Involving Group Maintenance Functions

Encourager: offers praise to and agrees with other members; communicates acceptance of others and their ideas and an openness to differences within the group.

Harmonizer: mediates conflicts and disagreements that crop up, trying to relieve or reduce tension within the group.

Compromiser: seeks a position between contending sides; seeks a compromise that all parties can accept.

Roles Involving Primarily Personal, Individualistic Functions

Aggressor: acts negatively, with hostility toward other members; criticizes others' contributions; attacks the group and its members.

Recognition-seeker: calls attention to own activities; boasts; redirects things toward self.

Help-seeker or confessor: uses the group as a vehicle either to gain sympathy or to achieve personal insight and self-satisfaction without consideration for others or the group as a whole.

Dominator: asserts authority and seeks to manipulate others so as to be in control of everything that happens.

---

personal needs rather than the group's are referred to as *individual functions;* Box 22-1 summarizes these roles.

Norms

Norms are the group's standards of behavior, attitudes, and perceptions of their members. They represent the shared expectations of appropriateness in behavior (Sampson and Marthas, 1990). Norms serve certain purposes for groups. One major function of norms is to allow a group to act in a fairly coordinated manner to accomplish its goals and tasks. In this way norms fulfill a *task function.* Norms also fulfill a maintenance function by regulating maintenance issues around attendance, conflict resolution, and personal relations. Finally, norms serve a *social reality function.* Much of what we "know" to be true has been socially determined. Overall, group norms provide a framework for the interpretation of data (Sampson and Marthas, 1990).

Norms vary in content, extent, and explicitness. Norm *content* refers to the extent to which the norm covers aspects of the member's life. For instance, it is the norm among some Roman Catholics not to eat meat on Friday; it is the norm for some Buddhists to never eat meat (the latter is a more extensive norm).

Explicitness refers to how obvious or clear the norms are. *Overt* norms are the usually stated expectations for behavior known to all members, such as groups always beginning and ending at a specific time (Northouse and Northouse, 1992). *Covert* norms are often practiced but not defined; they are a shared understanding about appropriate behavior rather than being verbally acknowledged, such as members sitting in the same place at every group session (Northouse and Northouse, 1992). Frequently a new member will conform with the explicit (overt) norms of a group quickly, but take more time to discover and understand implicit (covert) norms (Sampson and Marthas, 1990).

Norms can be *enabling* (assist the group in accomplishing its work) or *restrictive* (hinder movement toward goal accomplishment).

Universal Tasks

Finally, all groups must deal with the issues of group life: forming, working, and ending. Often this work is unknown to the group, but work in human relations theory implies that it is always being addressed. During the forming phase, group members deal with issues of joining a group. They wrestle with questions of how to join a group and issues of pairing with other group members. Acceptance/rejection by group members, issues of sexual attractions, and position within the group are also addressed at some level. During the group's working phase, task accomplishment is emphasized. The group deals with issues of leadership, completion, competence, and trust. At the final or termination stage, the group deals with issues that apply to endings, such as death, loss of the group, grief, separation, loneliness, and limitations.

These issues underlie all group processes and are always being addressed by the group, even if only at an unconscious level.

Types of Groups

Groups in the health care setting vary according to whether they are *content oriented* or *process oriented*. Content refers to the discussion of goals and tasks. Process refers to the discussion of interpersonal relations. Although all groups contain both elements, they vary with the degree of emphasis given (Northouse and Northouse, 1992).

Task groups focus on content issues: defining the tasks and what work is needed to accomplish them. It is rare, however, to find a group that is totally task oriented. There is generally some processing going on among members. Examples of task groups are committees formed to develop clinical or critical pathways or to monitor quality improvement.

Process groups focus on relations among members and their communication styles or patterns. Therapy groups designed to discuss client issues on an inpatient psychiatric unit fall into this category.

Finally, there are the *mid-range* groups that combine both functions of task and process. Many support groups with the emphasis on education and adjustment fall into this category (Fig. 22-2).

Aspects of Group Therapy

Groups, like milieus, function as social communities, and individuals tend to function in groups as they do in other parts of their lives. Likewise, individuals' behavior in group therapy will imitate their behavior in other group settings. A key assumption of group therapy is that psychopathology has its source in disordered relationships (Yalom, 1974). The goal of the therapy group is to help individuals develop more functional and satisfying relationships. Because the individual dysfunction is demon-

strated in the group, the task of the group is to assist members to understand their patterns of interacting within the group so as to be able to generalize to the larger arena of life outside the group. To do this, members must: (1) get information on how they present themselves to others, (2) assess whether their fixed patterns are realistic to continue in the current situation, (3) discover previously unknown parts of themselves (strengths, skills, abilities, desires), (4) gradually try new behaviors within the safety of the group, and (5) accept ultimate responsibility for the way they live (Yalom, 1974).

COHESIVENESS

In order to accomplish these goals, group members need to work together. The degree to which this occurs is called *cohesion:* the sense of "we-ness" that a group experiences which acts as a bond between group members. Cohesion has been associated with positive group outcomes: increased interactions; norm conformity and goal-directed behaviors; and member satisfaction (Northouse and Northouse, 1992). Factors that influence group cohesiveness are summarized in Table 22-1.

THERAPEUTIC FACTORS

Researchers have attempted to define the factors of a group process that have a positive effect on its members. In order to be effective as a group leader, the nurse must have an appreciation of these therapeutic factors of group therapy to be able to promote them. Yalom identifies 11 curative factors, which are listed in Box 22-2.

Inpatient Groups

In order to effectively lead an inpatient group, the psychiatric nurse must be aware of the various factors influencing the group so as to develop a style that is respon-

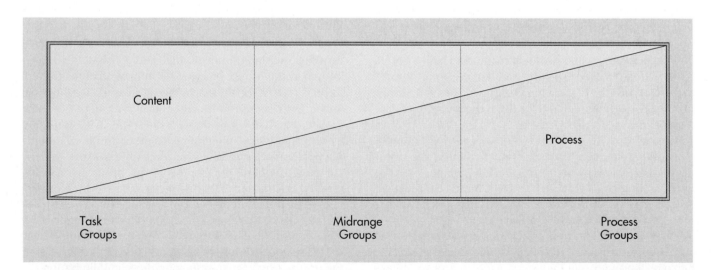

Figure 22-2 The emphasis on content and process in different types of groups. Psychiatric nurses are most involved with the process groups therapy.

(Adapted from Loomis M: *Group process for nurses,* St. Louis, 1979, Mosby.)

TABLE 22-1	Factors that influence group cohesiveness
Group goals	Clear goals, based on similar member values and interests, motivate members to seek or maintain group membership.
Similarity among members	Members are frequently attracted to other members who share similar values and beliefs. There are some instances, however, in which people are attracted to those who are dissimilar in values and attitudes.
Type of interdependence among members	Groups that function in a cooperative versus competitive manner tend to have higher cohesion among members.
Leader behavior	For the most part, democratic styles of leadership are associated with higher group cohesiveness than are other styles of leadership (e.g., autocratic).
Communication structures	Decentralized communication structures, characterized by increased member interaction, are associated with higher morale and increased satisfaction among members.
Group activities	Members who are asked to perform group activities they believe are beyond their capabilities will feel less attraction toward the group, whereas members who believe group activities are within their capabilities will feel more attracted toward the group.
Group atmosphere	Members are frequently attracted to groups that help them feel valued and accepted.
Group size	Group size should match the number of members needed to complete the task. Larger groups, in which the group size interferes with group goals, can decrease cohesiveness.

From Cartwright D: *The nature of group cohesiveness*. In Cartwright D, Zander A, editors: *Group dynamics: research and theory*, ed 3, New York, 1968, Harper & Row.

sive to the unpredictable conditions of inpatient group therapy.

The turnover of clients in today's psychiatric hospitals is rapid. This means it is probable that group membership will not be constant from one meeting to the next. It is likely that one or more members will be new to the group, while others will be ready to leave. Thus, some members may be in totally different phases of the group process (e.g., orientation, working, termination). This has critical implications for how group routines and dynamics are played out and carried over from one group to the next. Rapid turnover may compromise group cohesion. This greatly affects safety development within the group. Because it is rare for all group members to share a single specific diagnosis, the variety of disorders also affects group safety and cohesiveness. Generally, all the clients on a unit will attend all the groups. Therefore, different levels of functioning and presentation will be represented, which may be frightening to some group members and may affect cohesion and safety development.

The clients are inpatients and, by definition, fragile. They are often frightened, confused, and disorganized. Again, the creation of safety and structure becomes important. Many clients are unmotivated. They attend group sessions because they "have to" by unit rules, but it would not be their choice. The nurse leader must find ways to make the group relevant for them and their needs. There is often too little time to prepare the clients for the group experience. Staff may frequently be too busy to effectively orient the clients to the group. This implies that all too often the orientation must happen within the group.

Another issue affecting inpatient group therapy is varying leadership. Not only does the membership vary, so does the leadership based on staff scheduling. This affects the continuity of routine as well as safety development.

Another consideration related to staffing is that the clients see the group leader in a variety of roles throughout the day. The nurse may be their contact person, their medication nurse, and part of the treatment team, in addition to leading the group. It would be easy for clients to confuse these various roles. Consequently, leaders have the responsibility to clarify their roles and functions in the group.

Finally, there is little time for the more subtle aspects of psychiatric treatment. Clients are generally preoccupied with seeking relief from their despair and are not interested in subtle nuances. This implies the work must be direct, effective, and limited in scope to accomplish goals. In summary, the membership of an inpatient group requires leadership that provides orientation and continuity of group norms, defines the structure and limits of the group, promotes safety development, clarifies the relevant group task, and assists the group's accomplishment of that task.

The careful leader will recognize the need for boundary definition, safety, and trust development as just noted. These concepts must be expanded to create a therapeutic relationship at the group level. Instead of applying these concepts to individuals, the nurse leader must now apply them so they are useful to the unique requirements of group functioning. This is accomplished in some specific ways, as are summarized in the Table 22-2 on page 524.

TABLE 22-2   Summary of inpatient group considerations

Considerations of inpatient group work	Clients' requirements	Nurses Technique Functions of Nurse	Nurse's Stlye to Promote function	Promote function
High severity of distress in group members caused by • personal distress • secondary anxiety of hospitalization • rapid turnover • little preparation • many roles of therapist	Defined structure to work within	Lessen the ambiguity of therapy situation through clarification of details:	Provide boundaries: Room Time frame Orientation • expectations for behavior (therapist's and client's) • sequence of group • norm clarification	Firm, explicit, and active Explain actions Model contradictory feelings and solicit feedback
Brief duration of therapy Provide opportunity to explore (not necessarily resolve) questions of interpersonal relation-	Goals that can be achieved: • how am I seen by others? • how does my behavior Finding a safe arena to try new behaviors	Enhance client strengths by: • discouraging self- • acknowledging contributions	Support client by: • modeling feedback • providing positive interpretation • showing relevance of interactions to life outside hospital	Model respect as shown by: • being supportive, constructive, and accepting feedback • using data as learning opportunity • acknowledging client's contributions during summary statement
Group exists as part of a larger whole: • client is member of unit milieu • group session is only one of many groups	Facilitating client-to-client relations	Problem identification	Promote direct communication • client to client • abstract to specific Questions support furthering of relationships • what aspect of behavior gets in way of ideal relationship?	Modeling of openness, selective self-disclosure, risk-taking
	Avoiding and managing stress	Conflict management	Immediate intervention Promoting resolution, objectivity, and learning	

Box 22-2 Yalom's Curative Factors of Group

1. *Instill Hope:* Group members are at various points of the health continuum. Those who are not coping well can gain hope from those who have benefited from the group experience.

2. *Universality:* Members come to learn they are not unique or alone in their discomfort. They learn that others have reactions and thoughts similar to their own.

3. *Imparting Information:* Both formal and informal learning occur in groups. Some groups such as AA and medication-education or symptom recognition groups are designed specifically to impart information. Through groups designed to assist with interpersonal dynamics, members learn about the effects of their interactions on group dynamics.

4. *Altruism:* By and large, members of groups give credit to the other group members for their support and insight. Members view their improvement as related to the work done by all group members. By learning they can be useful, members experience an improved sense of self-value.

5. *Corrective Recapitulation of the Family Group:* As noted earlier, people act as they were taught to act in their families. As is often the case with psychiatric clients, these patterns are dysfunctional and the client continues to repeat these dysfunctional patterns in all interactions. Group therapy provides the opportunity for these patterns to be identified, evaluated, and changed.

6. *Development of Social Techniques:* By interacting with others, members can improve their social skills. Members will often give each other feedback on their reactions to each other's interpersonal style. This enriches member recognition of the various effects of their style on others and gives them opportunities to choose and practice styles that are more in keeping with their goals.

7. *Imitative Behavior:* Very often group members are "caught" or trapped in ways of interacting because they cannot conceive of another way. In a group situation members are able to see how others interact and can choose to model their behavior on those of other group members or the therapist. By looking at options, group members get the help they need to dissolve their rigid behavioral styles and become more flexible in their interactions.

8. *Catharsis:* Catharsis is the release of intense emotions. Psychiatric clients are often hesitant to express these emotions for fear that they will be too overwhelming for anyone to handle and that the consequence of expressing them would be grievous. In group therapy, members learn how to express these emotions and experience the immediate relief catharsis can bring. In addition, members learn that they and the group have survived the expression of emotions without calamity.

9. *Existential Factors:* All human beings must deal with one basic issue of existence: that we are ultimately alone despite the presence of others. Psychiatric clients (and others) may tend to be unrealistic in their expectations of human relationships, thinking that with the perfect mate, friend, or family all feelings of "aloneness" would vanish. In group therapy, members learn that feelings of loneliness can be decreased by human companionship, but not completely eliminated. By not reaching for what is unattainable, members may be able to enjoy what is attainable.

10. *Cohesiveness:* This is one of the most powerful benefits of an effective group. Many members experience extreme isolation from others in their daily lives and consequently experience a feeling of disconnectedness from others. By being part of a group that is achieving its stated goals, members experience a sense of "belonging," a feeling of being part of a "whole" that is greater than each individual self.

11. *Interpersonal Learning:* In groups designed to examine interpersonal relationships, the members learn to identify, clarify, and modify maladaptive behaviors.

From Yalom ID: *The theory and practice of group psychotherapy*, New York, 1974, Basic Books.

Group Boundaries

Boundaries refer to the definition of structure surrounding task, group norms, roles, and time. In working with groups, boundaries between people also must be defined clearly. Not only must members' responsibilities to self and others be clarified, but their obligation to task accomplishment must also be defined. In other words, guidance ought to be given to help group members understand how to work together to accomplish a specific task.

In expanding the concept of boundary to group work, location must be added. Previously the concept of spatial boundaries was identified as the inpatient unit. In group work, an area must be defined as the specific location for the group to do its work. As Yalom (1974) notes, an externally imposed structure is the first step to the internal structure needed by the frightened, confused, and disorganized inpatient. Therefore, the group leader needs to provide clear spatial boundaries for the group. The ideal space is a comfortable room with a door that can be closed when the group begins and opened when the group session ends. This provides not only for privacy of the group but also for a visual reminder of structure. Everyone in the group should be able to see each other (a further expansion of the therapeutic relationship); chairs should be arranged in a circle. This structure will serve to promote the task of interaction in the group. If the clients cannot see each other, they will tend to speak only to the nurse (Yalom, 1974). The space should be the same consistent from group to group. Group size is also a consideration. The ideal number for an inpatient process group is 6 to 10 clients (Yalom, 1974). This number allows for enough interactional material for processing, yet is small enough for all members to interact.

Linked to the concept of spatial boundary is that of temporal or time boundary. The group needs a definite time to begin as well as to end work. The best way for this to occur is for the leader to model promptness. The leader should be in the room ready to begin work at the appointed time. It is also the leader's responsibility to ensure that the group meet its tasks within the appointed time frame, and ends on time. The leader must recognize that the effective life span of the group is one group meeting long. Because of the rapidly changing membership it is unlikely that the same group members will ever meet twice, therefore the leader must provide a beginning, middle, and ending structure to every group.

Perhaps the greatest opportunity for the leader to define group structure and boundaries is in the introductory comments to the group. As in developing a therapeutic relationship with an individual, the introduction serves to clarify:

- the role of the nurse
- the role of the client
- the tasks of the group
- the ways to accomplish these tasks
- the time frame for accomplishing these tasks

An example of such an introduction follows (adapted from Yalom, 1974).

Orientation to names Defining spatial and time boundaries Defining a leadership function	"Hello, I'm Mary Webster and this is the daily therapy group. We meet in this room every day for 1 hour, from 10 AM to 11 AM. I'll keep track of the time and make sure we end on time.
Task definition Limits of work defined	"The purpose of this group is to help members understand their problems better and to learn more about the way they communicate with others. I know there are many different reasons why people come into the hospital, and you may not want to talk about some of these reasons in a group.
Restating task	"But one thing almost everybody here has in common is some unhappiness in their relationships with people who are important to them. What groups do better than any other form of therapy is help people understand more about their relationships with others.
Tasks definition (and method to accomplish)	"One of the ways we'll work on this task is to look at relationships that may go on between people in this room. We're not very different inside the hospital than we are outside of it, so the better we can understand relationships that happen here, the better we'll understand the important relationships outside the hospital.
Information boundary addressed Confidentiality issue to promote safety	"You'll be learning a lot about yourself and other people while you're in the group. It's very natural to want to share what you learn with your family and friends, but confidentiality is of utmost importance. We ask you to pass on the valuable information but to keep the names of the people or other identifying information confidential. This information is only for group members and staff.
Consistent explicit sequence (provides for method to accomplish task)	"As I mentioned before, the group lasts 1 hour. We start by going around the group and asking each member to say something about the kinds of problems they're having in their lives, that they'd like to work on in group. Then we'll talk about as many of those as possible. We save the last 10 minutes or so, to check in on everybody again, about how they feel and what kind of work they saw happening, and to finish up any leftover business."

This type of structured and consistent introduction serves many purposes:

- Provides an orientation to new members as to the purpose and sequence of the group, thus relieving some anxiety.
- Facilitates the transfer of norms from one meeting to the next even in the absence of returning members.

- Defines the work of the group (i.e., relating to others) in relevant terms.
- Sets limits (i.e., not every problem is appropriate for group discussion).
- Defines the role of the nurse implicitly, as the one with the sense of group tasks and appropriateness, and explicitly, as timekeeper and organizer.

The introduction alone, however, will not meet all the boundary issues. The group leader must actively continue to work to shore up the boundaries and structures of the group, throughout the meeting, by using an active, focused style of leadership that promotes task accomplishment. Yalom (1974) suggests that clients are reassured by a leader who is firm, explicit, decisive, and also shares the reasons for her actions.

Thus, the leader of an inpatient group will actively identify group themes, focus discussion on learning from relationships within the group, share her ambivalence and thinking about difficult decisions she makes within the group, and maintain a consistent order to the group. Her choice of actions, directions, and words are consistent with the goal of furthering learning about relationships.

SAFETY AND TRUST

Safety has been defined in terms of knowing what is expected of one's self in a given situation. As has been mentioned earlier, in group situations this concept must be expanded to knowing what is expected in relationship to others. In this example, it is expected that group members explore their relationships with each other to understand their outside relationships better. Recognizing that psychiatric clients may have tumultuous relationships with others, the group leader strives to maintain a safe and supportive environment in which to do the work. In group work, as in other forms of the therapeutic relationship, safety is developed when the nurse demonstrates a personal acceptance or valuing of each member, treats each member with respect, and empathizes with each one's situation as much as possible within the boundary context. The nurse works to reinforce the client's strengths, and encourages higher-level behavior (Yalom, 1974). The nurse models these safety-promoting behaviors by acknowledging each client's contributions openly to the group and by taking each client seriously. These tasks are often accomplished by providing a framework for the group to understand the client's behavior, discouraging self-defeating behavior before anger builds in the group, and acknowledging at some point each client's contribution to the group. The nurse must actively intervene if a client is being verbally attacked by another, and use the opportunity to promote reflection on relationships, appropriate to the group's goal. The leader consistently works to help the members meet their responsibilities to each other in a safe and nonthreatening manner.

FAMILY THERAPY
Definition

Family therapy is a unique form of group therapy in that it deals with the most intimate of all groups, the family. Families are given the tasks of raising children within the expectations of the culture and of providing support and nurturance for its members. A well-functioning family is reflected in a collaborative power structure, an acceptance of the individuality of its members, mutual affection, and an ability to adapt to social change. Generally, families present for therapy when they are experiencing some difficulty in accomplishing these tasks. These difficulties frequently arise at times of transition for the family: births, deaths, marriage, changes in finances, illness, divorce, and the major growth transitions from childhood to adulthood.

The identified difficulty is generally expressed by one member of the family experiencing symptoms. Most often, a child develops certain symptoms such as school failures, drug abuse, acting-out behavior, withdrawn or passive behavior, or sexual promiscuity. This behavior is usually of great concern to the parents, who initiate therapy. At times, however, the parents may be coerced into treatment by the various social systems with which the child interacts such as schools, judicial organizations, and social welfare agencies. Often, these bodies will define the behavior as a problem and recommend therapy, even against parental wishes. Thus, not everyone comes to family therapy willingly.

The child's behavior is usually seen as the child's problem by the parents who assume that the family will become functional again once the child's problem is "fixed." Thus, the child is seen as the **identified client,** that is, the one whose behavior is causing the problem. Occasionally, an adult is the identified client. For example, the problem may be seen as the mother's drinking or the father's absenteeism, and the family belief is that once this behavior (or person) is "fixed," the family will be fine.

Theoretical Perspective

Family therapists view the behavior of the identified client as merely relaying a message about the overall functioning of the family in general. Instead of seeing the "identified client" as the cause of the family's distress, the family therapist sees that person more as the "symptom carrier" for the family. The process of family therapy is geared toward the family as a whole rather than toward any individual member.

Family therapy is based on systems theory. A family is seen as a system that will strive to maintain homeostasis or balance. Consequently, even if the identified client's behavior were to change, systems theory predicts that another symptom would develop in another member in an attempt to maintain the previous balance of a dysfunctional system. A dysfunctional system cannot tolerate health in one member; the entire system must be made functional in order to restore health.

Goals

The goal of family therapy is to relieve the family's pain and to promote functional nurturing of its members.

Satir (1972) has identified four areas that cause a family to be troubled. These areas are the following:

- self-worth or the feelings and ideas one has about one-self

- communication styles in the family, which can be indirect, vague, and dishonest

- the rules the family uses to define behavior as well as the way the rules are negotiated

- the links to society (the way the family relates to institutions outside the family)

The goals of family therapy, therefore, are the following:

- to foster higher self-worth in family members

- to promote communication that is direct, clear, specific, and honest

- to create rules that are flexible, humane, and responsive to varying needs

- to link with society in a way that is open and hopeful (Satir, 1972)

Settings

Family therapy can be conducted in a variety of settings. It most often occurs in a nurse's office in a structured, formal outpatient setting. Families can be seen in the hospital as well, when the "identified client" is admitted. It is difficult to complete the work of family therapy on an inpatient basis, however, and arrangements must be made for follow-up family therapy after discharge.

One of the most valuable settings from the nurse's point of view is the home. The home provides the nurse with much information about the family's unique interactive style. For example, the use of space, the objects valued, and the interaction within the home (as opposed to the office) may reveal a great deal about the family dynamics. A family can be seen as a single unit or groups of families can be seen together, which is called *multiple family therapy,* in which four or five families meet weekly with a nurse to discuss common issues. This form of therapy works well with families dealing with isolation and lack of familial or community support. Several couples can also be seen at a time in couples therapy to work on ways to strengthen the marital relationship.

Basic Concepts of Family Therapy

As noted earlier, the family is a special kind of group. It has defined tasks, roles for its members, norms, and communication patterns. As with other groups, difficulties arise when any one of these aspects is jeopardized in some way. Nurses working as family therapists assess several areas of family functioning.

ROLE CONFUSION

According to the traditional concept of family roles, the parents form the primal unit. They are the authority figures in the family making rules for behavior and decisions for family survival. The parents are seen as a unit. Children are seen as dependents and are given less authority in decision making. As the children grow in age, judgment, and decision-making ability, they are granted more independence and participation in the decision-making process. At times, family members may not be able to fulfill their roles properly, and dysfunctional patterns occur. Examples of role confusion follow:

- A parent dies and the oldest same-sex child takes over the role functions of the deceased parent.

- A child becomes ill, and, in an attempt to support the child, the family revolves around the desires of the ill child—in effect making the child the central authority figure.

- A couple is unhappy with their relationship, and each forms a strong alliance with one of the children, thus negating the spousal unit as the primary unit of the family.

Nurses working with a family evaluate how the family enacts their various roles, and the effects this enactment has on the members.

TASK CONFUSION

The family's tasks are to raise children and provide support and nurturance for its members. This is not always easy to accomplish. As noted earlier, families experience stress at times of transition because of a family's uncertainty about how to perform its tasks during transition points. Examples of this are the following:

- The birth of a new child: the family struggles to adjust to meeting the needs of the baby while continuing to meet the needs of other family members.

- The transition of a child to a teenager: the family must allow increasing separation and individuation and support the growing person in his new tasks.

- The geographic move of a family: the family task is to link to the resources of the community, but the family finds it difficult to locate these resources in a new community.

The nurse will assess the family's ability to meet its tasks and identify areas of difficulty.

COMMUNICATION

Communication, both verbal and nonverbal, is the way family members develop trust and love and nurture one another. In order to do this, both verbal and nonverbal messages must match (see Chapter 7). Family members develop unique ways of communicating with each other as a way of establishing family norms, accomplishing tasks, and enforcing roles. These patterns generally become firmly established, and grown children often continue to use patterns learned in their family of origin.

Nurses examine the communication patterns of the family in several ways. A basic question to answer is: "Who has the right to say what to whom and in what situation?" This question addresses the issues of authority, family position, and content (i.e., what is talked about and what is not). For instance, can the child question a rule laid out by the parent? Can the husband and wife voice their differing opinions? Can they do so in front of the children? Is there a "family secret" that no one discusses?

Nurses also analyze the family's "double messages" or messages that conflict on the verbal and nonverbal levels. The nurse may ask: Does the family express one value verbally, but act in ways that discourage the purported value? For example, does the family say that it wants to hear what a member has to say, but then go on to interrupt, become angry, or pay no attention when that member is speaking? Do the parents say they are open to negotiating family rules but then discount every option suggested? The nurse thus seeks to discern patterns in communication that make it difficult for the family to accomplish its tasks.

Therapeutic Process

Although the family is usually seen in therapy as a unit, occasionally the nurse may wish to work with one member on a particular issue, or perhaps meet with the couple to strengthen their bond. This is consistent with the systems theory viewpoint that a change in one part of the system will precipitate other changes. The overall goal, however, is to decrease the family's pain and increase its abilities to perform its tasks. Because communication is the link between all family members and the family's ability to perform its tasks, attention is always paid to the communication pattern of the family with the goal of changing the family system of interaction (Yalom, 1974).

In general, the process begins when the family makes contact with the nurse. It is important to note which family member makes the actual contact, since this may be the most motivated member. The family usually presents in disarray, its members frequently demoralized, frustrated, and angry. They have tried every solution they can think of but continue to have problems, so they must seek assistance either by their own choice or as prompted by the school or the judicial systems.

Initial meetings are often chaotic as the family demonstrates their way of "being" to the nurse. They frequently demonstrate their mixed messages and confusion; feelings of helplessness and loss of control are common.

The nurse seeks to focus the family's disorganized energy and information toward manageable tasks. Goals for therapy are set by family members. The nurse listens to all the family members as well as watching their interactions in order to determine the structure and dynamics of the family situation. Nurses consider the family's presenting problems when making assessments to help the family clarify issues. Problems related to roles, tasks, and norms are discussed, with the nurse providing a perspective that the family may lack. Frequently the nurse will educate the family on functional communication patterns. The nurse will assist the family with communication within the session and may assign "homework" for them to further their practice. Patterns of communication are identified and evaluated as to their usefulness.

The family is frequently encouraged to make changes in its routine. For example, if a family is always together, they may be encouraged to interact with the community more. Such an expansion of their social network would serve to decrease their overdependence on each other and provide other outlets for their individuation. On the other hand, if a family is rarely together its members may be encouraged to spend an evening together for the sake of learning how to support each other and to communicate needed information.

As in other therapeutic relationships, the nurse must be seen as caring and responsive to the needs of the client. In this case the client is a family, and consequently the nurse must be careful to be responsive to each family member and not fall into an alliance or conspiracy with one member over another.

Summary of Key Concepts

1. The nurse in the therapeutic relationship acts as a resource person, counselor, surrogate, and technical expert for the client.

2. To be an effective counselor, a nurse must continually assess personal values and attitudes.

3. The basic concepts a nurse must develop in each therapeutic relationship are boundary development and maintenance, safety development, and trust development.

4. The orientation phase of the relationship serves to define the client's issue or conflict, the goal of the work, and the relationship between the client and the nurse.

5. In the working phase, the nurse demonstrates understanding of the client's problem and assists in finding beneficial coping actions.

6. The termination phase involves helping the client to acknowledge gains already made and progress yet to be made.

7. The basic purpose of milieu therapy is to make clients active, not passive, participants in their lives.

8. Group therapy allows clients to define themselves through human interaction and task accomplishment.

9. Family therapy promotes the health and functionality of the whole family system.

REFERENCES

Brammer LM: *The helping relationship: process and skills,* Boston, 1993, Allyn & Bacon.

Cartwright D, Zander A, editors: *Group dynamics: research and theory,* ed 3, New York, 1968, Harper & Row.

Cosgray E et al: A day in the life of an inpatient: an experiential game to promote empathy for individuals in a psychiatric hospital, *Arch Psychiatr Nurs* 6:6, 1990.

Denton PL: *Psychiatric occupations therapy: a workbook of practical skills,* New York, 1987, Little, Brown.

Fortinash KM, Holoday-Worret PA: *Psychiatric nursing care plans,* ed 2, St Louis, 1995, Mosby.

Herz MI: The therapeutic milieu: a necessity, *Intl J Psychiatr* 7:209, 1969.

Jones M: *The therapeutic community,* New York, 1953, Basic Books.

Kennedy E: *On becoming a counselor,* New York, 1977, Seabury Press.

Northouse P, Northouse L: *Health communication: strategies for health professionals,* Norwalk, Conn., 1992, Appleton & Lange.

Peplau HE: *Interpersonal relations in nursing,* New York, 1952, GP Putnam's Sons.

Sampson E, Marthas M: *Group process for the health professions,* New York, 1990, Delmar Publishers, Inc.

Satir V: *Peoplemaking,* Palo Alto, Calif. 1972, Science & Behavior Books, Inc.

Sayre J: Common errors in communication made by students in psychiatric nursing, *Perspect Psychiatr Care* 5:175–183, 1978.

Yalom ID: *The theory and practice of group psychotherapy,* New York, 1974, Basic Books.

CHAPTER 23

Psychopharmacology and Other Biologic Therapies

Jay Sherr

Adverse drug reaction An unintended effect of a medication resulting in severe unwanted symptoms or consequences.

Agranulocytosis A drop in the production of leukocytes, specifically the neutrophil cell line, leaving the body defenseless against bacterial infection.

Akathisia Literally, not sitting. A syndrome caused by dopamine-blocking drugs characterized by both motor restlessness and a subjective feeling of inner restlessness.

Antagonist A chemical that results in inhibition of activity of the target receptor.

Anticholinergic delirium Toxic effects of anticholinergic drugs characterized by confusion, perceptive disturbances, sleep disturbance, increased or decreased psychomotor activity, and change in level of consciousness. Also called atropine psychosis, this syndrome may present as a psychotic state.

Extrapyramidal symptoms (EPS) The collective term used to describe the motor side effect of dopamine-blocking medications. EPS includes acute dystonia, akathisia, parkinsonism, and tardive dyskinesia.

Metabolite The result of biotransformation of a drug.

Neuroleptic Literally, to clasp the neuron, the term used to describe what are now called the typical antipsychotic medications.

Neuroleptic malignant syndrome (NMS) A rare but potentially lethal toxic reaction to dopamine-blocking drugs that presents with a constellation of symptoms, including fever, autonomic instability, increased muscular rigidity, and altered mental status.

Psychotropic Literally, mind nutrition, the term used to describe drugs that affect the central nervous system.

Serum level monitoring The process of obtaining blood samples to determine drug concentration.

Side effect An undesired nontherapeutic and often predictable consequence of medication. Frequently diminishes with time. Contrast with *adverse drug reaction*.

Sustained release Medications designed to provide slow controlled dissolution that allows longer dosing intervals.

Tardive dyskinesia (TD) A syndrome of abnormal involuntary movements occurring after months or years of treatment with drugs that block dopamine type 2 receptors. Often described as oral, buccal, lingual masticatory movements, they can occur throughout the body.

- Describe and discuss the pharmacologic issues related to antipsychotic medication therapy.
- Describe and discuss the pharmacologic issues related to antidepressant medication therapy.
- Describe and discuss the pharmacologic issues related to mood stabilization therapy.
- Describe and discuss the pharmacologic issues related to anxiolytic and hypnotic medication therapy.
- Describe and discuss pharmacologic issues related to stimulant medication therapy.
- Explain nonpharmacologic modalities related to the treatment of individuals with mood disorders.
- Explain the nursing issues related to psychopharmacology and nonpharmacologic treatment modalities.

Although humanity has suffered from major mental illnesses throughout history, it is remarkable that truly effective treatments have only been available since the middle of the twentieth century. The impact of effective pharmacologic treatment has been striking. Prior to the advent of chlorpromazine and thioridazine in the 1950s, the permanent inpatient population in mental institutions in the United States was approximately 500,000. These individuals had thought disorders so severe that they could not reside outside of a structured institutional setting. With the advent of pharmacologic interventions, the number of hospitalized clients was dramatically reduced to about 200,000 within 10 years. This decrease demonstrated the effectiveness of antipsychotic medications. Sadly, it also demonstrated that efficacy varied greatly from client to client. Millions continued to suffer from mental disorders that included psychotic symptoms, mood, anxiety, and other related disorders.

PSYCHOPHARMACOLOGY
Mode and Mechanism

Even when most effective, medications for major mental disorders primarily treat symptoms, but have little or no effect on the underlying pathophysiology. All drugs have both a *mode* and *mechanism of action*. The mode of action describes what the drug does to the body, while the mechanism of action is defined specifically by how the drug works to affect symptoms, cure disease, or cause **side effects,** the undesired, nontherapeutic, and often predictable consequences of medication that frequently diminish with time. Often, much is understood about the mode of action for psychoactive drugs, but the mechanism of action is frequently unclear. For example, it is known that lithium affects noradrenergic, serotonergic, and dopaminergic neuronal systems, but this knowledge does not specifically define how lithium helps control manic behavior.

Mode and mechanism of actions on multiple systems contribute to a wide variety of side effects that can be substantial and, in some cases, life-threatening. The ideal drug would be specific and curative, convenient and economical, and have minimal side effects. Since the ideal drug does not yet exist, the process of pharmacologic treatment is always one of compromise. A goal of psychopharmacologic treatment is to provide maximum efficacy (efficiency) and minimum toxicity in a form the client is willing and able to take and can afford.

Psychotropic Pharmacotherapy Assessment

The safe and effective use of psychotropic pharmacotherapy (use of drugs that affect the central nervous system) depends on an accurate assessment of the client's condition. In addition to taking into account both psychiatric and somatic diagnoses, a continually updated problem assessment prior to administering medication includes answering these questions:

- What is the etiology of current symptoms?

- How severe is the problem?

- Why now?

Etiology is important because identification of the origins of a problem can lead to focused treatment of potentially correctable causes. For example, electrolyte imbalances or hyperthyroidism may underlie psychotic behavior. Also, understanding symptom severity guides one to decisions regarding rapidity of treatment. For example, nurses may need to decide the route of administration based on how imminent of a risk a client's current behavior presents.

A client's symptoms must always be assessed in the context of "why now?" For example, a client who has been treated for several days with an antipsychotic medication may develop increasing psychomotor agitation. The physician needs to assess if this is due to worsening psychosis, perhaps implying additional medication, or if the client is developing akathisia. Optimal use of medications carefully considers not only the diagnosis, presenting signs and symptoms, and the specific drug used but also the context of administration.

When assessing clients prior to or during pharmacotherapy, it is necessary to incorporate information from both drug-related and client-related variables before initiating interventions. Common drug- and client-related variables are described in Box 23-1. Drug-related variables include pharmacologic characteristics of available dosage forms. Client-related variables include those factors about the individual that may facilitate, hinder, or interact with medication therapy. Correlation of drug- and client-related variables promotes optimization of therapy for an individual client. The success of psychopharmacological therapy depends on 1) the optimal integration of the anticipated medication effects with the client's personal, physical, and psychosocial dimensions, and 2) the nurse's assessment of the client's response to psychopharmacologic therapy and the communication of this data to the prescriber. **Psychotropic** literally means "mind nutrition." It is used to describes drugs that affect the central nervous system.

Box 23-1   Variables Affecting Drug Therapy

Drug-related variables

- Mode/mechanism of action

- Available dosage forms—oral (solid, liquid, sublingual), parenteral

- Bioavailability of various formulations

- Onset, peak, and duration of action

- Serum half-life

- Method of elimination from the body (hepatic or renal)

- Side effects/toxicities (both predictable and idiosyncratic)

- Cost (drug price, administration, and monitoring costs)

Client-related variables

- Diagnosis

- Other disease states (cardiovascular, liver, renal disease)

- Age

- Weight

- Anticholinergic susceptibility

- History of side effects

- Previous response

- Family history of response

- Willingness to comply/insight into illness

- Financial and/or health insurance

- Support systems

TYPICAL ANTIPSYCHOTICS

Major advances in science are often perceived as the result of coincidence or chance. What really occurs is that an individual with a prepared mind and a willingness for hard work observes something new and unusual. Rather than discarding what does not quite fit the norm, the well-trained observer wonders about the nature of such phenomena and investigates further. Chlorpromazine was discovered in this manner, when Henri Laborit, a French neurosurgeon, was searching for medications to decrease anxiety in preoperative clients. He noted that chlorpromazine caused a "beatific quietude" and recommended it to his psychiatric colleagues for use with agitated clients. In 1951 Delay and Deniker began to use chlorpromazine and observed that their psychiatric clients became more manageable (Deniker, 1990). They also quickly noted side effects that reminded them of Parkinson's disease, a motor disorder known to affect motor neurons. Thus, they coined the term **neuroleptic,** from the Greek, meaning "to clasp the neuron." In 1954 chlorpromazine (Thorazine®) became the first effective antipsychotic available in the United States. Current antipsychotic medications available in the United States are listed in Table 23-1.

Antipsychotics can be divided into two basic types: typical and atypical. Since the introduction of chlorpromazine, no antipsychotic was demonstrated to be more effective than any other until the introduction of clozapine (Clozaril®) in 1989. Until then it was the side effect profile that distinguished differences among what are now called typical or classical antipsychotics, e.g., Haldol. Atypical antipsychotics, e.g., clozapine (Clozaril®) and risperidone (Risperdal®), are characterized by an improved response of negative symptoms and a reduced propensity to cause extrapyramidal side effects.

TABLE 23-1   Antipsychotic medications

Generic name	Trade name	Potency*	Usual dose (mg/day)	Comments
PHENOTHIAZINES				
Aliphatics				
Chlorpromazine	Thorazine®	100	60–2000	IM is painful
Piperazines				
Fluphenazine	Prolixin®	2	2–40	available as immediate release injectable and as 25mg/mL decanoate
Perphenazine	Trilafon®	10	8–64	
Prochlorperazine	Compazine®	15	15–150	
Trifluoperazine	Stelazine®	5	2–80	
Piperidines				
Mesoridazine	Serentil®	50	50–500	
Thioridazine	Mellaril®	100	50–800	no injectable form
Thioxanthenes				
Chlorprothixene	Taractan®	100	100–1600	
Thiothixene	Navane®	4	5–60	
Butyrophenone				
Haloperidol	Haldol®	2	1–100	available as immediate release injectable and as 50mg/mL and 100mg/mL decanoate
Dibenzoxapine				
Clozapine	Clozaril®	50	50–900	tablets only
Loxapine	Loxitane®	10	20–250	
Dihydroindolone				
Molindone	Moban®	10	15–225	no injectable form
Benzisoxazole				
Risperidone	Risperdal®	2	4–16	tablets only

All are available as tablet or capsule, liquid, and parenteral except as noted.

*Expressed as chlorpromazine equivalents.

Indications

Antipsychotics (neuroleptics or major tranquilizers) are effective in treating the symptoms of psychosis. Clients with schizophrenia, schizophreniform disorder, schizoaffective disorder, and delusional disorder may benefit from antipsychotic medications. Exacerbations of psychosis and hospitalizations may be prevented with continued medication use. Psychosis from secondary causes, such as electrolyte or hormonal imbalances, drug abuse, brain tumors, mania, or depression with psychotic features, may also benefit from short-term antipsychotic treatment while the underlying disorder is being treated.

The symptoms of psychosis are varied but have been organized into two main groups: positive and negative. Positive symptoms are associated with increased mental and physical activity. Negative symptoms are related to decreased mental and physical activity. See Chapter 13 for more information about the symptoms of psychosis.

Goals of Therapy

Antipsychotic medications are used to decrease psychotic signs and symptoms, including hallucinations, delusions, and feelings of paranoia. In assessing clients, symptoms at baseline and throughout treatment, it is important to document specific behaviors that demonstrate psychotic symptoms.

The overall goal in treatment of a psychotic client is to return control to the individual. Since these are powerful drugs, it is important to remain sensitive to the potential for their use in controlling the client. Over-medication places control of the individual in the hands of the clinician. Thus, the goal of returning control to the individual is achieved through monitoring specific psychotic symptoms and improvement in the client's ability to provide self-care.

Mode of Action

All known antipsychotics are dopamine receptor blockers. The drug occupies the dopamine receptor on the post-synaptic neuron, and blocks endogenous dopamine from having its effect. Classical antipsychotic potency has been related to its D_2 receptor affinity (Baldessarini, 1990). D_2 receptors are confined primarily to four major

areas of the brain: the mesolimbic and cortical pathways, the nigrostriatal tracts, and the tuberoinfundibular tracts. The nigrostriated pathway begins in the substantia nigra and ascends to the caudate nucleus and the putamen in the extrapyramidal system. The tuberoinfundibular tracts originate in the arcurate nucleus and terminate on the median eminance. This is the site where dopamine blockade can cause increased prolactin release, resulting in gynecomastia (enlarged breasts in men) and galactorrhea (leakage from nipples). The mesolimbic pathway projects from the mesencephalon to the anterior limbic brain and is believed to play a major role in positive psychotic signs and symptoms. Dopamine receptor blockade in the limbic brain, which may contain excess dopamine during psychosis, would relieve positive symptoms. A reduced level of dopamine in mesocortical pathways is thought to contribute to negative signs and symptoms of schizophrenic disorders. Blockade of dopamine receptors in the cortex would then potentially make negative symptoms worse (Davis et al, 1991).

D_2 receptor blockade is also responsible for many of the side effects of antipsychotics. Blockade in the nigrostriatal tracts causes neuroleptic-induced pseudo-parkinsonism, (bradykinesia, stiffness, and tremor) and dystonic reactions (muscle spasms in the tongue, jaw, eyes, and neck). Akathisia and tardive dyskinesia appear to be related to D_2 receptor blockade. These phenomena, collectively known as extrapyramidal symptoms (EPS), are discussed in detail below. The tuberoinfundibular pathway mediates hypothalamic control of endocrine function. Dopamine blockade in this area causes increases in prolactin resulting in gynecomastia and galactorrhea (breast development and milk expression, respectively).

Atypical antipsychotics also block dopamine receptors. However, the specific reasons for the improved efficacy against negative symptoms and reduced EPS are as yet unclear.

Antipsychotic drugs vary greatly in their affinity for other receptors, resulting in additional side effects secondary to receptor blockade. Histamine (H_1) blockade causes sedation, cholinergic blockade causes anticholinergic side effects, and alpha (α) blockade causes hypotension and reflex tachycardia. Side effects caused by receptor blockade and the antipsychotic medications are listed in Table 23-2.

TABLE 23-2   Side Effects associated with receptor blockade

Dopamine$_2$	Histamine$_1$	Cholinergic	Alpha$_1$	Serotonin$_2$
EPS	Sedation	Dry mouth	Orthostatic hypotension	Weight gain
Prolactin	Weight gain	Blurred vision	Reflex tachycardia	GI upset
		Sinus tachycardia		Sexual dysfunction
		Constipation		
		Impaired memory/cognition		

Thus, it is important to understand the receptor-specific characteristics of the different medications, because these characteristics can help predict both the efficacy and side effects likely to be observed.

Clinical Use and Efficacy

Although important and effective medications, antipsychotics are also the most toxic drugs used in psychiatry. The lowest possible effective dose should be used for the shortest amount of time.

Target symptom response varies with time. Positive symptoms are the most responsive. Symptoms such as combativeness, hostility, psychomotor agitation, and irritability are often relieved within hours. Affective symptoms, anxiety, tension, depression, inappropriate affect, reduced attention span, and social withdrawal may take 2–4 weeks to respond. Cognitive and perceptive symptoms such as hallucinations, delusions, and thought broadcasting may take 2–8 weeks to respond. The most negative symptoms—poor social skills, unrealistic planning, poor judgment and insight—respond slowest and least. Many clients have fixed hallucinations and delusions that respond minimally to medications. Given the varied time course of different symptoms, it should be kept in mind that increases in medication dose will not hasten the relief of slow-responding symptoms.

Antipsychotic therapy may be started using divided doses, three or four times a day. This is a useful approach in determining a client's ability to tolerate a medication and to minimize the initial impact of side effects. Once an effective total daily dose has been established and the client has had time to develop tolerance to side effects, the medication is often reduced to once or twice a day. Reduced frequency of administration increases the likelihood of compliance with the regimen.

In general, antipsychotics are well-absorbed from the GI tract. They are extensively metabolized in the liver. Half-life varies highly between individuals but is usually between 20–40 hours in adults with steady state being reached in 4–7 days. **Serum level monitoring,** obtaining blood samples to determine drug concentration, is not routinely useful. Serum level monitoring may be revealing in specific situations, including lack of response to normal doses after 6 weeks, severe or unusual adverse reactions, clients on multiple medications, the physically ill, and as a check for compliance.

Medication Forms
LIQUID

Most antipsychotic medications are available in liquid form. One of the most troubling symptoms of psychotic disorders is lack of insight. A client who believes that he or she is not sick will have little motivation to take medication and may be resistive to drug treatment. Such clients may "cheek" tablets or capsules in efforts to avoid medication. Liquid concentrates may be given at the initiation of therapy to help assure compliance.

INJECTABLE

Immediate-release injectable forms of antipsychotic medications are available for psychiatric emergencies. Single IM injections can often be rapidly effective for clients who present an imminent danger to self or others but refuse oral (PO) medication. Rarely, repeated injection every hour until the client is calm, a technique called rapid tranquilization, is used. This technique is associated with increased risk of acute dystonic reactions and neuroleptic malignant syndrome (NMS) (a potentially lethal toxic reaction to dopamine-blocking drugs) and therefore must be used judiciously. The simultaneous use of a benzodiazepine may help clients regain control more quickly. Haloperidol and lorazepam (Ativan®), in combination, have been used for this purpose (Battaglia et al, 1992).

In the United States, two antipsychotics are available as long-acting injections. Haloperidol decanoate (Haldol Decanoate 50® and Haldol Decanoate 100®) and fluphenazine decanoate (Prolixin Decanoate®) are commonly given as monthly or biweekly injections, respectively. By linking the active drug molecule to a decanoate chain and dissolving it in sesame oil, a slow release of medication is achieved when given as deep IM. The half-lives of haloperidol decanoate and fluphenazine decanoate are approximately 21 days and 14 days, respectively. These sustained-release drugs may increase overall compliance and are useful in clients who are reluctant to take medications every day (Glazer and Kane, 1992).

An important consideration in the use of the decanoate injections is monitoring these medications in an outpatient setting. Conversions from oral to injectable doses are always approximations, since the exact degree of bioavailability varies substantially between clients. The long half-life of these drugs results in steady state serum levels not being obtained until 2–3 months after injections are initiated. Thus, loss of efficacy or increases in side effects can develop over time as serum levels fall or rise toward steady state. Clients need to be educated about this and encouraged to report any problems to their physicians. Clients also need to be examined for local irritation and sterile abscess at the injection sites which can result from repeated injections.

Toxicity of Typical Antipsychotics

The side effect profile differentiates typical antipsychotic drugs. The low-potency drugs are more likely to cause sedation and hypotension, while the high-potency drugs tend to cause more extrapyramidal symptoms (EPS). These drugs vary greatly in the amount of anticholinergic side effects they cause. The severity of these effects—dry mouth, blurred vision, tachycardia, urinary retention, constipation, and disorientation/delirium—vary greatly between individuals. Note that the drugs more likely to cause EPS have less anticholinergic side effects; those drugs with the most anticholinergic effects have relatively less EPS. EPS is often treated with adjunctive anti-

TABLE 23-3 Adjunctive medications used to treat extrapyramidal symptoms

Generic name	Trade name	Equivalent dose (mg)	Dose range (mg)	Dosage forms (all available as tablets unless noted)
ANTICHOLINERGIC				
Benztropine	Cogentin®	1	1–8	injectable
Trihexyphenidyl	Artane®	2	2–15	capsule-extended release, elixir
ANTIHISTAMINE				
Diphenhydramine	Benadryl®	50	50–400	capsules, liquid, injectable
DOPAMINE AGONIST				
Amantadine	Symmetrel®	N/A	100–400	capsule and liquid only

cholinergic drugs. Therefore, it is likely that the relatively reduced EPS caused by the low-potency drugs is due to the anticholinergic profile of the low-potency drugs.

Extrapyramidal Side Effects

The dopamine blockade of antipsychotics can cause a variety of movement-related side effects collectively known as **extrapyramidal symptoms (EPS).** These side effects are troublesome to clients and are a major cause of noncompliance. EPS presents as acute dystonia, neuroleptic-induced pseudo-parkinsonism, akathisia, and tardive dyskinesia. The unifying factor in the presentation of these side effects is disruption of normal motor activity.

ACUTE DYSTONIA

Acute dystonia is muscular spasm that may occur in up to 10% of clients. Taking the client by surprise, this painful and often frightening reaction may affect different muscle groups. Symptoms may present as blepharospasm (eye closing), torticollis (neck muscle contraction pulling the head to the side), oculogyric crisis (severe upward deviation of the eyeballs), and/or opisthotonos (severe dorsal arching of the neck and back). Severe presentations involving the tongue and/or laryngospasm can result in dysphagia (difficult swallowing) and jeopardize the airway.

Fortunately, anticholinergic drugs are rapidly effective. Mild presentations may be treated with oral anticholinergic drugs. Severe, painful presentations will benefit from the rapid onset of IM treatment. Benztropine (Cogentin®) 2mg IM and diphenhydramine (Benadryl®) 50mg IM are commonly used and may be repeated in 30 minutes, if the symptoms have not resolved.

NEUROLEPTIC-INDUCED PSEUDO-PARKINSONISM

Dopamine and acetylcholine exist in balance in the brain. Dopamine blockade in nigrostriatal pathways results in relative cholinergic predominance that produces clinical symptoms. Neuroleptic induced pseudo-parkinsonism presents with tremors, bradykinesia/ akinesia (slowness, absence of movement), cogwheel rigidity (slow, regular muscular jerks), postural instability, hunched posturing, shuffling gait, loss of associated movements, masked facies (loss of mobility in the facial muscles), hypersalivation, and drooling. Pseudo-parkinsonism affects as much as 15% of clients. Symptoms generally start 5–30 days after initiation of therapy.

Anticholinergic drugs or dopamine agonists are usual treatments for pseudo-parkinsonism. Some of the same medications used to treat idiopathic parkinson's disease (degradation of dopamine neurons in the substantia nigra) are useful for relieving symptoms of neuroleptic-induced parkinsonism. Table 23-3 lists drugs ordinarily used as adjunctive treatments to counteract extrapyramidal symptoms. Anticholinergic medications are generally used initially, unless contraindicated. Acute closure (sometimes called narrow angle) glaucoma is an absolute contraindication.

Relative contraindications include dehydration, cardiac arrhythmias, and benign prostatic hypertrophy (BPH). Signs and symptoms of dehydration may be exacerbated by anticholinergic medications. Anticholinergics frequently increase the pulse rate. Clients with existing cardiac arrhythmias may be at increased risk as heart rate increases. Clients with existing BPH may have increased difficulty initiating urine flow when treated with anticholinergics. Older clients and clients on additional medications with anticholinergic effects must be monitored with particular diligence. Excess anticholinergic medication can result in urinary retention requiring catheterization; paralytic ileus; and memory problems with confusion, disorientation, and delirium (that can resemble psychosis). The latter, sometimes called **anticholinergic delirium,** may present with a full spectrum of anticholinergic effects, including blurred vision, mydriasis, tachycardia, tachypnea, diminished bowel sounds, and mental status impairment. This syndrome remits with anticholinergic medication discontinuation but can be treated with a cholinergic agonist. When anticholinergics are contraindicated or not tolerated, dopamine agonists can be helpful. Amantadine (Symmetryl®) is frequently used. Amantadine facilitates the release of dopamine and thus aids in the restoration of dopamine/ acetylcholine balance. The risk in using dopamine agonists is that excess can worsen psychosis. This is seldom seen when amantadine doses are 200mg/day or less. Amantadine is eliminated by the kidneys; therefore, clients with renal dysfunction are at increased risk of accumulating amantadine and worsening their psychosis.

Clients should be counseled that in most cases anticholinergic side effects, whether from primary medications (e.g., high-dose, low-potency antipsychotics) or adjunctive medications (e.g., benztropine-Cogentin,® trihexyphenadyl-Artane®), will diminish over several weeks. This gradual reduction of effect is called tolerance. Most clients develop substantial tolerance to the parkinsonian side effects of antipsychotic medications within three months. Thus, trial reductions of adjunctive medications will simplify medication regimens, reduce the potential for drug interactions, and improve compliance.

AKATHISIA

Akathisia literally means "not sitting" and presents with subjective and objective components. The objective symptoms of akathisia, namely motor restlessness, pacing, rocking, and foot tapping, are common. Most clients with akathisia complain of inner restlessness described as tension, irritability, and the inability to sit still or lie down. However, clients with akathisia may not have or cannot verbalize these feelings of inner disquiet. Although some clinicians believe that virtually all clients receiving typical antipsychotics experience some form of akathisia, it clearly occurs in approximately 25% of those treated.

Differentiating between akathisia and the psychomotor agitation/ irritability of worsening psychosis can be difficult. This differentiation is important because akathisia responds best to dose reduction. Misinterpretation of akathisia as psychomotor agitation or anxiety (secondary to psychosis) could result in increasing the dose of antipsychotic. This would result in worsening the akathisia. Conversely, worsening psychosis interpreted as akathisia could result in the inappropriate reduction of needed antipsychotic medication, resulting in continued or worsened symptoms, prolonged hospital stays, increased risks to clients and staff, and needless adjunctive medications. The nurse must assess the client thoroughly and report observations to the prescriber.

Akathisia may respond to a reduction of the antipsychotic medication. When this is not clinically practical— for instance, when most psychotic symptoms are responding well—anticholinergics and beta-blockers are the most common adjunctive treatments (Adler et al, 1993; Dumon et al, 1992). Anticholinergic treatment is often disappointing. Benztropine (Cogentin®) may be beneficial at relatively high doses of up to 6 mg daily, but many clients cannot tolerate the high dose. Beta-blockers may be the most effective adjunctive treatment; up to

160 mg daily of propranolol (Inderal®) or 80 mg daily of nadolol (Corgard®) have been found useful.

TARDIVE DYSKINESIA (TD)

Tardive dyskinesia (TD) literally means late-occurring, abnormal movements. Although classically described as oral, buccal, lingual, masticatory movements (tongue thrusting and writhing, lip pursing and smacking, facial grimaces and chewing movements), these choreoathetoid (rapid, jerky, and slow-writhing) movements may first occur anywhere in the body. Arm, finger, leg, feet, and truncal movements are often noted. Less commonly, involvement of muscles in the swallowing reflex or the diaphragm can lead to choking or respiratory compromise. The client is frequently unaware of the potentially irreversible movements.

The movements wax and wane over time. Thus, family members and providers who spend a lot of time with clients are frequently the first to report abnormal movements. Although these abnormal involuntary movements are generally not seen before at least six months of antipsychotic treatment, they may be seen substantially earlier or after years of treatment. The overall incidence of TD appears to be approximately 4% per year while taking antipsychotics.

Clients on a stable antipsychotic regimen who develop abnormal involuntary movements and then have their antipsychotic discontinued have about a 50% probability of having permanent abnormal movements. Clients who must remain on drugs are even more likely to have permanent abnormal movements.

Prevention of TD is important because there are no truly effective treatments for TD. Formal monitoring procedures should be performed at least every six months while on antipsychotics.

The pathophysiology of TD is only partially understood and involves complex interactions of multiple neurotransmitter systems. When these antipsychotic drugs block dopamine receptors, over time, the neurons manufacture more dopamine receptors, a process called upregulation or super-sensitivity. If the drug is suddenly removed, increased numbers of dopamine receptors are exposed to endogenous dopamine, resulting in increased abnormal movements. Dose reduction can cause a temporary increase in severity of movements that gradually subside as neurons readjust to the absence of dopamine-blocking drugs.

Withdrawal dyskinesia presents as TD-like movements that occur with antipsychotic dose reduction. Typically these movements fully resolve in two weeks to two months. Withdrawal dyskinesia is most common and most severe in children. Conversely, increasing the dose of antipsychotic, and covering more dopamine receptors, will usually cause a reduction in abnormal involuntary movements. This strategy furthers the toxic process that originally brought about the movements and will eventually result in a return of the movements. Thus, increasing the dose merely "masks" TD and is not an acceptable treatment. Benzodiazepines may be a useful treatment in TD, but response is usually temporary, lasting only several months. Some clients with severe TD have been treated with clozapine (Clozaril®) with benefit (Tamminga et al, 1994a).

NEUROLEPTIC MALIGNANT SYNDROME (NMS)

Kinross-Wright first described the syndrome in 1958, and Delay and Deniker named it **neuroleptic malignant syndrome (NMS)** in 1968. Researchers have suggested that cases of NMS were for years underreported or misdiagnosed (Caroff et al, 1991; Gurrera et al, 1992). The reported incidence of NMS is approximately 0.5%–1.4% of the population who receive antipsychotic medications (Pope et al, 1986). NMS is a potentially fatal idiosyncratic reaction to antipsychotics and is characterized by muscular rigidity, hyperthermia, altered consciousness, and autonomic dysfunction. Laboratory findings can include leucocytosis (15,000–30,000 cells/mm^3), elevated creatine phosphokinase (may be > 3000 IU/mL), and myoglobinuria. NMS may occur any time during treatment but is more frequent shortly after initiation of antipsychotics or dose increases. There are other factors that may predispose development of NMS. Rapid administration of a high-potency antipsychotic (rapid tranquilization) and an increased number of intramuscular injections increase the risk of NMS.

The underlying pathophysiology associated with NMS remains unclear. There exists a relationship to the blockage or depletion of dopamine in the basal ganglia (which also causes extrapyramidal symptoms). This blockade is also associated with the generation of heat through muscle contraction and through effects in the hypothalamus, which controls central thermoregulation (heat dissipation).

NMS may develop within hours after taking antipsychotic medications or after years of exposure. It may present as mild and self-limiting or fulminate progressively over 48–72 hours. Early recognition and treatment may minimize potentially fatal complications that include myocardial infarct, hepatic failure, disseminated intravascular coagulation (DIC), and pulmonary edema. Rapid destruction of muscle tissues (rhabdomyolysis) releases large amounts of myoglobin that can be seen in the urine as myoglobinuria. In extreme cases, myoglobin can saturate the serum, which results in crystallization in the kidney and causes renal failure or permanent renal impairment.

The first and most important step in the treatment of NMS is discontinuation of the antipsychotic. Hydration and cooling are also of paramount importance. A muscle relaxant given IV has been used to reduce the sustained muscle rigidity and thereby reduce fever and the results of muscle tissue breakdown. The dopaminergic drugs e.g., bromocriptine (Parlodel®), amantadine (Symmetryl®), and anticholinergics have also been used.

Clients who require continued antipsychotic treatment are usually changed to an antipsychotic with a different chemical structure using low starting doses and slow titration (incremental adjustment of dose to allow for tolerance to side effects). Whenever possible, reinitiation is delayed until two weeks after symptoms have subsided. The resolution of NMS is related to clearing the antipsychotic from the body. Therefore, the long half-life depot antipsychotics (haloperidol decanoate, fluphenazine decanoate) are avoided in clients with a history of NMS.

Other Side Effects

Antipsychotic medications are associated with a wide variety of additional side effects. Some of these effects are an extension of the known pharmacology of the agents, while other effects are idiosyncratic and unpredictable. Dopamine blockade can lead to gynecomastia and galactorrhea. Small breast pads may be useful for those suffering from galactorrhea. Amenorrhea occasionally occurs in women soon after antipsychotics are first started. Most commonly, one or two cycles are missed before normal cycles resume. Weight gain from unclear mechanisms is common, although molindone (Moban®) may be associated with weight loss. Incontinence is more common in older clients. Impaired temperature regulation can put clients at risk for hypothermia in winter and hyperthermia in the summer. Seizures caused by these agents in clients without any seizure history are well documented. Clients with a seizure history or current seizure disorder must be monitored closely when started on these drugs. All of these agents can reduce the seizure threshold, but this is more common with the low-potency agents (e.g., chlorpromazine-Thorazine® and thioridazine-Mellaril®).

The low-potency agents are more commonly associated with a variety of problems. Electrocardiographic changes (conduction delays) are more common with thioridazine and chlorpromazine. Sudden death via unknown mechanisms, while extremely rare, is more common with low-potency agents. Rare cholestatic jaundice presenting two to four weeks after beginning therapy is more commonly associated with a phenothiazine. Photosensitivity, dramatically increased predisposition to sunburn, may last a month after drugs are stopped. Liberal use of hats and sunscreens are advised before sun exposure. High doses of thioridazine can lead to pigmentary retinopathy and permanent blindness. Sexual dysfunction is vastly underreported but likely affects approximately 25% of treated clients. Up to one-third of males on thioridazine may experience retrograde ejaculation. Complaints of impaired erection are also common. Both men and women may complain of inhibition of orgasm. When side effect problems persist, dose reduction, switching to another drug, and adding an adjunctive agent need to be considered in context. The severity of the problem, the current benefit the client is receiving, other drugs the client is taking, and any other psychiatric and somatic conditions affecting the client must all be evaluated to determine the best intervention.

ATYPICAL ANTIPSYCHOTICS

Psychopharmacologic agents that avoid the major problems associated with typical antipsychotics have long been sought. The term *atypical antipsychotic* has been applied to drugs that have an improved negative symptom response and minimal EPS. A number of such agents are in development, but clozapine (Clozaril®) and risperidone (Risperdal®) are the only atypical agents currently marketed.

Clozapine

The arrival of clozapine created a great deal of excitement in the psychiatric community. It is the first antipsychotic to demonstrate a significantly greater improvement of negative symptoms compared to typical antipsychotics. Clozapine brought substantial improvement in symptoms and quality of life to many individuals who failed to adequately respond to typical antipsychotics. Numerous side effects, including potentially fatal agranulocytosis and extremely high cost, tempered the enthusiasm of many. Regardless, clozapine is the first major advance in the pharmacotherapy for major psychosis in almost 40 years.

INDICATION

Clozapine is indicated for use in treatment of refractory schizophrenia. Clozapine is the only drug that has demonstrated an improved response in treatment refractory clients (Hagger et al, 1993; Kane et al, 1988; Meltzer et al, 1993). Treatment refractory is defined as a failure to respond to two antipsychotics of different chemical classes given at doses of 800 chlorpromazine equivalents a day for at least six weeks. Clozapine has restricted indication because of the risk of agranulocytosis. Although not FDA indicated, clozapine is sometimes useful in schizoaffective disorder (McElroy et al, 1991), bipolar disorder, and severe tardive dyskinesia (Tamminga, 1994a) when standard treatments have failed.

MODE OF ACTION

The pharmacologic reasons for clozapine's unique effects are unclear. Clozapine, like typical antipsychotics, blocks dopamine receptors. Clozapine also has considerable serotonin ($5HT_2$) blockade. Still, the specific reasons for the unique clinical response to clozapine remain elusive. Current investigations are centering on the ratio of serotonin to dopamine blockade as well (Lichter, 1993; Pickar et al, 1992). Clozapine has less penetration into the striatum where EPS is caused as compared to the typical antipsychotics. Thus, there is minimal EPS. Blockade of other receptors, including histamine, alpha, and cholinergic receptors, causes substantial side effects.

CLINICAL USE AND EFFICACY

The recommended starting dose of clozapine is 12.5 mg. This dose reduces the risk of orthostatic hypotension and syncopal episodes, an unusual first-dose effect. This effect may be more common in clients who have had benzodiazepines in the previous seven days. Gradual titration is necessary because of hypotension, tachycardia, and sedation, which generally diminish over several weeks. Most clients respond in the 300 mg–600 mg/day range, usually given as bid or hs. Evaluation of response to clozapine may take 12–24 weeks. Due to the risk of agranulocytosis, clients must have blood drawn for white blood cells (WBC) every week. Clients may only receive a seven-day supply of medication at a time and must have an adequate WBC ($> 3,000$ cells/mm^3) prior to receiving the next seven-day supply. Typically, responding clients gradually demonstrate improvements in socialization and thought organization. Although positive symptom response may be diminished with clozapine use, it is the improved response in negative symptoms and improvement in disorganization that most distinguish clozapine. In robust responders, the psychological effects of recovering from chronic schizophrenia can be dramatic, and many of these clients can demonstrate continuous improvement. However, clients who gain insight into their illness and develop organization in their thoughts may be rapidly confronted with the seriousness of their previous mental state and an awareness of the consequences of their illness. Such clients may suffer serious depression and dysphoria.

SIDE EFFECTS

Agranulocytosis.   Life-threatening **agranulocytosis** develops in approximately 1% of clozapine-treated clients. The greatest risk period is the first six months of treatment (Alvir, 1994), and risk peaks at approximately three months. But cases have also occurred after two years of treatment. Recovery is usually complete if the drug is stopped before clinical symptoms of infection appear. Weekly monitoring of WBC is required as long as treatment continues.

Agranulocytosis is not dose related. Reductions in WBC serious enough to endanger clients require discontinuation of the drug. WBCs should include a white cell differential each week for at least the first 18 weeks to six months of treatment. The differential will determine the percentage of different types of leucocytes in the blood. Clients with WBCs below 2000 cells/mm^3 less than 1000 must discontinue clozapine immediately, and these clients can *never* receive clozapine again. Clients with WBCs between 2000 and 3500 should be monitored closely. Often, additional WBCs are drawn during the week if clients have intermediate values or have had a sudden decrease from their normal values.

Seizures. Seizures are a dose-related side effect and the main reason clozapine's maximum daily dose is 900 mg. Overall seizure incidence is approximately 3%. These generalized seizures may respond to dose reduction. The antiseizure medication valproate, most commonly administered as Depakote®, may be added if needed. Carbamazepine (Tegretol®), also an antiseizure medication, is avoided because of its propensity to reduce white blood cell counts. Myoclonic jerking may precede seizures and may indicate the need to hold or reduce the total daily dose.

Miscellaneous. Other common side effects caused by clozapine include sedation, tachycardia, hypotension, GI upset, benign hyperthermia, anticholinergic effects, and sialorrhea (hypersalivation). Although most side effects diminish substantially with time, fatigue and sedation can be quite persistent. Fatigue can be overwhelming during the titration phase for some clients. Tachycardia with increases of 25 beats/min or greater may also persist and is sometimes treated with beta blockers. Some clients may complain of a vague burning in the stomach, which is relieved by food, and resultant weight gain can be significant. During the first three weeks of therapy, some clients develop a mild fever for a few days. This benign hyperthermia remits on its own and has no clinical consequence. Acetaminophen can be used to provide comfort.

Clozapine has moderate anticholinergic effects, but, paradoxically, there is approximately a 30% incidence of sialorrhea (hypersalivation). When sialorrhea is persistent and problematic, dose reduction or the addition of anticholinergics may help. Anticholinergics should be added with caution because of the risk of anticholinergic delirium, particularly in the elderly and individuals with a bowel impaction.

Clozapine is a drug with great potential benefits and risks. Rapid changes in clozapine dose can be serious. Sudden discontinuation of clozapine can result in serious rebound psychosis and anticholinergic rebound (e.g., nausea, vomiting, diarrhea). Noncompliance for more than a few days and abrupt reinstitution of the previous dosage (commonly 300 mg/day–600 mg/day) could result in syncopal episodes, orthostatic hypotension, or seizures. Thus, while clozapine is indicated for treatment refractory clients, an individual's ability to comply is important. This overall response results not only in medication compliance but also in clients remaining in treatment. It is important to note that slow, gradual improvement, particularly in negative symptoms, occurs over at least several months. Clients may continue to improve throughout the first year.

The difference between the atypical antipsychotic clozapine and the typical antipsychotic haloperidol can be dramatically demonstrated using Positron Emission Tomography (PET) scan techniques as illustrated in Figure 23-1.

Risperidone

Risperidone (Risperdal®) is a landmark drug in psychiatry. It was the first marketed drug designed specifically with the structure of CNS receptors in mind. One portion of the molecule was designed to block the dopamine receptor, and another portion was designed to block serotonin receptors. This elegant work is the result of a gradually developing understanding of the very nature of the brain and of schizophrenia.

INDICATION

Risperidone, like the typical antipsychotics, is indicated in the treatment of major psychotic disorders. Unlike clozapine, risperidone has not yet been demonstrated to have an improved response rate in the treatment refractory client population.

MODE OF ACTION

Risperidone blocks both serotonin and dopamine receptors. It is speculated that the improved negative symptom response and lack of EPS at lower doses are due to this combination of receptor blockade. Risperidone also has mild alpha blockade and histamine blockade, resulting in some risk of orthostatic hypotension and sedation, respectively (Borison et al, 1992). It does not significantly block cholinergic receptors.

CLINICAL USE AND EFFICACY

Like other antipsychotics, risperidone is well absorbed and may be taken with or without food. The starting dose in adults is 1 mg bid. Unless limited by side effects, the dose may be increased by 1 mg bid each day to an initial daily dose of 4 mg–6 mg/day. In geriatric clients, whose metabolism is slower than younger adults, dosing should be halved, starting at 0.5 mg bid and titrating to 1.5 mg bid. The optimal dose of risperidone for most clients will be 4 mg/day–8 mg/day. Increasing doses of risperidone result in increased EPS and a potential loss of the improved negative symptom response. It seems that as doses of risperidone are increased beyond 8 mg/day, it appears more like a typical antipsychotic. The time course of response may be slightly quicker than with typical neuroleptics, but this has not been clearly demonstrated at this time.

Risperidone may be of particular benefit in clients who have responded poorly to typical antipsychotics and in those who have suffered from unacceptable EPS.

SIDE EFFECTS

EPS is a dose-related side effect of risperidone. Side effects noted include insomnia, agitation, headache, anxiety, rhinitis, somnolence, tachycardia, and weight gain.

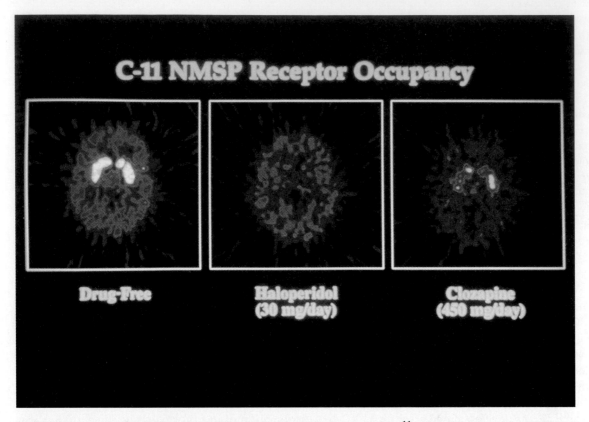

Figure 23-1 A transaxial PET scan image at the level of the basal ganglia. C^{11} N-methylspiperone (NMSP) is a radioactive tag that binds, and thus highlights, dopamine type-2 (D_2) receptors. The three panels are from the same 36-year-old man with schizophrenia. In the first panel, he is drug-free, and the D_2 rich basal ganglia is highlighted by the NMSP. Note the absence of NMSP in the next panel, six weeks later on haloperidol 30 mg/day with 85% of his basal ganglia D_2 receptors occupied with haloperidol. Finally, on clozapine 450 mg/day, only 37% of the D_2 receptors are occupied by drug. While his psychosis was responsive to both medications, motor side effects were considerable on haloperidol and absent on clozapine.

(From Tamminga CA et al, Maryland Psychiatric Research Center, University of Maryland, Baltimore, Md.)

The risk of orthostatic hypotension is minimized by starting doses not greater than 1 mg BID. Some cardiac conduction delay (widening QT intervals) has been noted but is unlikely to be problematic unless there is an existing arrhythmia. Like typical antipsychotics, it causes hyperprolactinemia, increased serum prolactin in the blood that can result in increased breast development and milk expression. The potential for risperidone to cause tardive dyskinesia is unknown. Therefore, clients should be monitored for tardive dyskinesia, as with typical antipsychotics.

CONCLUSION

Since the 1950s when the first truly effective medications for the treatment of major psychotic disorders became available, antipsychotic drugs have remained a double-edged sword. The great benefits have been counterbalanced by serious toxicities such as neuroleptic malignant syndrome and tardive dyskinesia. Also, a significant portion of the schizophrenic population has remained refractory to treatment. Atypical antipsychotic medications in development herald a new era in treatment, with im-

proved efficacy and reduced or absent extrapyramidal side effects. However, as tardive dyskinesia and NMS were not predicted when chlorpromazine and thioridazine were introduced, these new medications may contain unanticipated side effects and adverse reactions. The astute physician may observe a new level of efficacy but must remain alert for unanticipated toxicities.

ANTIDEPRESSANTS

The first modern antidepressant medication, marketed in 1958, was imipramine. This tricyclic compound is a modification of the structure of the antipsychotic chlorpromazine. The reason imipramine and similar drugs are called *tricyclics* can be readily seen by the three-ring chemical structure of the compounds (see Figure 23-2). Dr. Roland Kuhn, a Swiss psychiatrist, originally administered imipramine to clients with schizophrenia and found no clinical efficacy. Astute observation and the persistence of Dr. Kuhn, who proceeded to study imipramine in clients with depression, quickly lead to proving imipramine's efficacy in the treatment of depression.

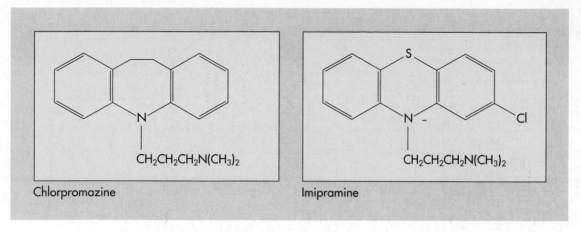

Figure 23-2 Chlorpromazine and imipramine are referred to as tricyclics because of their three-ring chemical structure.

This success served as the catalyst for the search for additional antidepressant medications exhibiting improved efficacy and reduced side effects. At the same time, advances in the understanding of the role of serotonin in depression pointed toward a new class of antidepressants, the selective serotonin reuptake inhibitors (SSRIs).

Indications

As their name implies, antidepressants are indicated in the treatment of major depressive disorders. However, research has indicated the use of antidepressants in a wide variety of disorders, such as enuresis, eating disorders, and anxiety disorders.

Mode of Action

The biogenic amine hypothesis of depression proposes that depression is caused by a reduced quantity or function of the catecholamine neurotransmitters norepinephrine and/or serotonin.

Antidepressant drugs affect the fate of the neurotransmitters norepinephrine (NE) and/or serotonin (SR). Presynaptic neurons synthesize NE and SR, which are incorporated into vesicles. Action potentials cause the vesicles to release their contents into the synapse. Normally, once released from the vesicles, the neurotransmitter crosses the synapse to impact receptors on the post-synaptic neuron. Most of the released neurotransmitter is taken back up into the pre-synaptic neuron in an effort to conserve this valuable resource. There, it re-enters the synthesis process and is incorporated into vesicles for future use. The cyclic antidepressants partially block the re-uptake of NE and SR. Initially, this re-uptake blockade results in increased amounts of neurotransmitter in the synapse. The increased amount of neurotransmitter in the synapse is associated with a reduction in the number of receptors on the post-synaptic membrane. This change

in receptor density, called down regulation, can take several weeks to occur and is temporally associated with antidepressant response (Figure 23-3). In clients who have failed to respond to an antidepressant more specific for one neurotransmitter, it is rational to switch to a drug more specific for the other neurotransmitter.

The pathophysiology of depression remains elusive. It is unlikely that a single theory will explain the etiology of depression. The efficacy of medications and the ability to measure interneuronal effects give important clues toward understanding the causes of depression. It is likely that there are multiple causes of depression. A single, underlying process has not been identified, and the cause of depression remains unclear.

CYCLIC ANTIDEPRESSANTS
Clinical Use and Efficacy

Approximately 70% of clients with major depression will respond to antidepressant therapy (Andrews, 1994). One individual may respond better to one drug rather than another. Likelihood of response is not predictable based on the presenting symptoms of depression. Thus, initial selection of an antidepressant is based on the client's history and how the anticipated side effects of the drug interact with the client's specific physical and psychiatric status. See Box 23-1 for common client-related variables.

Antidepressant drugs are well absorbed, and there is extensive first-pass metabolism. Initial doses and dosage ranges are listed in Table 23-4. Cyclic antidepressant dosing begins with low doses to allow the client time to tolerate the side effects. The most common reason for failure to respond to cyclic antidepressant treatment is inadequate dose or duration of therapy. This can result from a prescriber's reluctance to prescribe enough, in an effort to avoid serious toxicity, or from client noncompliance secondary to side effects. Serum levels may be most useful when monitoring imipramine (Tofranil®), desipramine

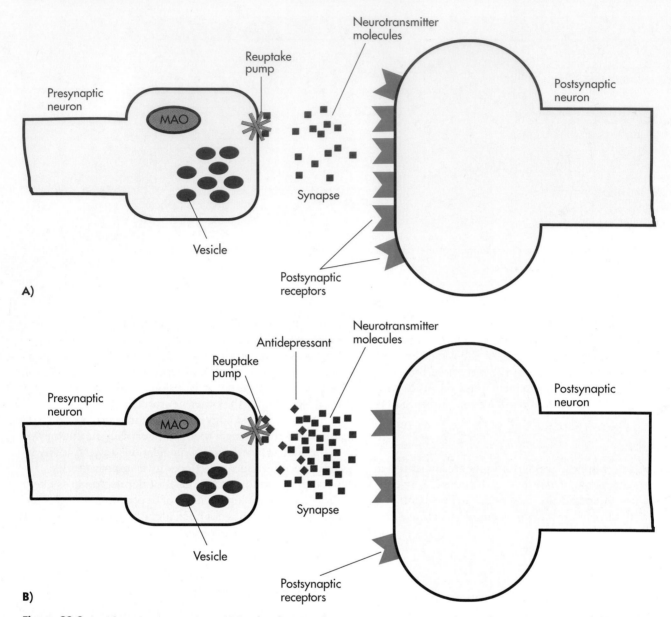

Figure 23-3 Antidepressant response. A) In the depressed state, sparse amounts of neurotransmitter are available in the synapse of a depressed person. B) With treatment, the reuptake of neurotransmitter is blocked by the antidepressant drug (in red). The result is increased amounts of neurotransmitter in the synapse, and, finally, after several weeks, the postsynaptic receptors have decreased (i.e., down regulated), which is associated with resolving depression. For the sake of clarity, this drawing omits numerous receptors and postsynaptic intracellular mechanisms that may ultimately prove important components of the pathophysiologic substrate of depression and antidepressant response.

(Norpramin®), and nortriptyline (Pamelor®). Target symptom response in depression is gradual, usually occurring over several weeks. The time course of response to antidepressant therapy is summarized in Box 23-2.

Clients should be advised early of potential side effects and that therapeutic response will take some time (Pollack, 1987). Clients and families often become impatient when suffering from the side effects of medication while the original symptoms remain. Compliance is often facilitated when there is a discussion with clients and families about expectations regarding medications. There are times

when the depression has resolved, and the side effects remain. It is therefore important to communicate that compliance with medication after the depression has cleared is vital. Letting clients know that side effects will diminish with time or that there are management alternatives also helps ensure compliance for the total duration of therapy.

When clients have been on therapeutic doses for three or four weeks and are not demonstrating clinical improvement, changing medications may be indicated. Adjunctive medications in partial and nonresponding clients are sometimes useful.

TABLE 23-4   Antidepressant dosing

Generic (trade name)	Starting dose (mg/d)	Maintenance dose (mg/d)
CYCLIC ANTIDEPRESSANTS		
Tricyclics		
amitriptyline (Elavil®, Endep®)	25–50	100–300
desipramine (Norpramin®)	25–50	100–300
imipramine (Tofranil®)	25–50	100–300
nortriptyline (Aventyl®)	25–50	100–300
protriptyline (Vivactil®)	10	15–60
doxepin (Sinequan®)	25–50	100–300
trimipramine (Surmontil®)	25–50	100–300
maprotiline (Ludiomil®)	50	100–225
clomipramine (Anafranil®)	25	100–250
tricyclic dibenzoxazepine		
amoxapine (Ascendin®)	50	100–400
triazolopyridine		
trazodone (Desyrel®)	50	150–500
nefazodone (Serzone®)	200	300–600
MONOAMINE OXIDASE INHIBITOR		
phenelzine (Nardil®)	15	15–90
isocaroxzid (Marplan®)	10–30	10–50
tranylcypromine (Parnate®)	10	10–40
SEROTONIN SPECIFIC		
fluvoxamine (Luvox®)	50	100–300
fluoxetine (Prozac®)	5–20	20–80
paroxetine (Paxil®)	10–20	20–50
sertraline (Zoloft®)	50–100	50–200
INDOLAMINE		
bupropion (Wellbutrin®)	200	300–450

Use about 1/2 the dose for the elderly.

Box 23-2   Time Course of Response to Antidepressants

Symptom Remission

First week

- decreased anxiety
- improved sleep
- patient often unaware of these changes

One to three weeks

- increased activity, sex drive, self-care
- improved concentration, memory
- psychomotor retardation resolves

Two to four weeks

- relief of depressed mood
- less hopelessness
- suicidal ideation subsides

"First break" (meaning the first episode of major depression) treatment should continue for 6–12 months. Many clinicians are treating recurrence of major depression for at least five years, and lifelong treatment may be indicated for some clients (APA, 1993). Decisions regarding duration of treatment need to consider the severity of the depression and the history and risk of suicidal gestures. Major depression with psychotic features is often treated by adding an antipsychotic. As the depression resolves, the psychotic symptoms will also clear and the antipsychotic can be discontinued.

Side Effects

These drugs are routinely associated with increased sedation and anticholinergic effects. These effects are directly related to the degree of histamine and cholinergic receptor blockade of each drug. The secondary amine drugs, nortriptyline, protriptyline, and desipramine, are less sedating and less anticholinergic than the tertiary amines amitriptyline, imipramine, trimipramine, and doxepin. Clients often complain about these side effects, and they are a significant cause of noncompliance. These sedating and drying effects, so-called "nuisance" side effects, generally diminish with time. Over time, cyclic antidepressants are associated with substantial weight gain.

A wide variety of side effects may be caused by CNS receptor activity, allergy, or from unclear mechanisms. Whenever possible, the best way to treat problematic side effects is to remove the offending agent. Of course, this is not always possible. Allergies excluded, most side effects will substantially diminish with time. When they do not diminish, a variety of interventions can be offered to help clients who are demonstrating adequate efficacy and are continuing to suffer from bothersome side effects. Interventions for helping clients with both initial and persistent side effects are listed in Table 23-5. Do not underestimate the significance of "minor" side effects. Constipation, particularly in the elderly, can lead to paralytic ileus, bowel obstruction, and the need for hospitalization. Noncompliance due to "minor" side effects can lead to relapse and increased suicide risk.

One of the most serious side effects of antidepressants is directly related to its efficacy. During the gradual response of depressive symptoms, clients may demonstrate increased energy and physical activity while suicidal ideation remains. It is in this intermediate stage of response, often the second week of therapy, that clients may be at the highest risk to act on self-destructive thoughts. Careful monitoring is essential as clients begin to emerge from depression (APA, 1993).

Tricyclic antidepressants are associated with significant cardiac toxicity. All tricyclics cause a dose-related widening of EKG intervals. It is unfortunate that medications effective in the treatment of depression can also be fatal in overdose.

While helping clients rise from depression, antidepressants can sometimes elevate mood beyond the desired effect. In clients with bipolar disorder, it is not uncommon for antidepressants to "push" clients into mania. A first episode of mania sometimes occurs during antidepressant therapy (Pickar et al, 1984).

Monoamine Oxidase Inhibitors (MAOIs)

Iproniazid, an antitubercular drug in the 1950s, was a monoamine oxidase inhibitor (MAOI). Some patients receiving iproniazid were noted to become euphoric. This observation ultimately lead to the use of MAOIs as antidepressant agents. The use of MAOIs has been limited as a result of the side affects and dietary modifications. Thus, investigation for antidepressant agents continued.

MODE OF ACTION

The neurotransmitters norepinephrine, serotonin, and dopamine are chemically described as monoamines. In the CNS, these molecules are synthesized inside the presynaptic neuron. Maintenance of cellular homeostasis requires a mechanism to degrade monoamines. Monoamine oxidase (MAO) is an enzyme found in the mitochondria of cells that participates in the normal process of degradation of these amines. MAOIs are drugs that inhibit this enzyme. This inhibition initially results in increased availability of these neurotransmitters. As with other antidepressants, these initial neurotransmitter increases result in post-synaptic receptor down regulation that is temporally related to antidepressant response.

CLINICAL USE AND EFFICACY

MAOIs are indicated in the treatment of atypical depression, major depression without melancholia, or depressives disorders resistant to tricyclic antidepressants. Atypical depression is characterized by hypersomnia, hyperphagia, anxiety, and the absence of vegetative symptoms. In addition, MAOIs have been used with variable success in the treatment of other disorders such as certain anxiety disorders, eating disorders, and some pain syndromes (for example, migraines).

The MAOIs are rapidly absorbed, liver metabolized, and have average half-lives of approximately 24 hours. A majority of individuals metabolize MAOIs relatively slowly. This metabolic difference among individuals results in wide variation with respect to required doses for efficacy and sensitivity to side effects at a given dose (Johnstone, 1973). There is no clinically available test for this metabolic rate. Thus, many clinicians begin MAOI therapy with a 10 mg or 15 mg test dose and monitor vital signs and complaints of side effects closely before beginning titration.

Contraindications to the use of MAOIs include cerebrovascular defects, major cardiovascular disease, and pheochromocytoma (tumor of the adrenal medulla). The elderly do not tolerate MAOIs well, and use is uncommon in individuals over age 65. MAOIs have been known to worsen symptoms of Parkinson's disease, induce manic states in bipolar clients, and exacerbate psychotic symptoms in schizophrenics. Diabetics may require adjustment of their hypoglycemic medication. MAOIs are contraindicated in pregnancy.

The use of MAOIs requires additional considerations. As with cyclic antidepressants, initial dosing must be titrated to give clients time to tolerate side effects. Table 23-4 lists initial and maintenance dosing ranges. Clients on MAOIs must comply with a tyramine-restricted diet and must studiously avoid stimulant medications to avoid the risk of a potentially fatal hypertensive crisis. Thus, the client's ability to comply with dietary and medication restrictions is an important consideration prior to initiating therapy. Response to therapy may take 3–6 weeks. Except in emergencies, discontinuations should be tapered.

SIDE EFFECTS

Orthostatic hypotension is a common initial and sometimes persistent side effect of MAOIs. Dangling feet on rising, changing positions slowly, support stockings, and

TABLE 23-5   Side effects of antidepressants with nursing interventions

Side effect	Nursing interventions
ANTICHOLINERGIC EFFECTS	
Dry mouth	Offer sugarless gum and candy, artificial saliva. For persistent problems treat with pilocarpine 1% rinse and spit (4 drops of 4% pilocarpine and 12 drops water) or bethanecol (Duvoid®, Urecholine®) 5 mg sublingual or 10–30 mg qd-bid.
Blurred vision: disturbance of presbyopia (near vision), far vision usually preserved	Ask if vision prescription current; try pilocarpine 1% eye drops, or bethanecol 10–30mg tid.
Urinary retention	When not caused by benign prostatic hypertrophy (BPH), may be treated with bethanecol 10–30 mg tid.
Constipation	Prevention: encourage fluids (medication givers may offer), fruits and vegetables, mild physical exercise (walks). Bulk-forming laxatives (e.g., Metamucil® 1–2 tablespoons-ful qam, or docusate 100 mg qd-bid). Avoid stimulant laxatives when possible; if needed, limit duration to avoid laxative dependence. Or bethanecol 10–30 mg qd-bid.
Anticholinergic delirium (also known as atropine psychosis)	Monitor for agitation restlessness, psychotic signs and symptoms, myoclonic jerking. May occur with or without peripheral anticholinergic signs. Hold anticholinergic drugs. Physostigmine 5 mg IV can rapidly reverse but requires life-support backup and cardiac monitoring.
ALPHA BLOCKADE	
Orthostatic hypotension	Consider other contributing factors such as low-salt diets, restricted fluid intake, dehydration. Antihypertensive medications may exacerbate. Advise client to change positions slowly, dangle feet one minute in sitting position when rising from prone, sit immediately when lightheaded. Offer support hose, exercise to strengthen calf muscles to improve venous return.
SEXUAL DYSFUNCTION	Obtain a clear history that the complaint does not predate the depression or medication use.
Decreased libido	Neostigmine 7.5–15 mg 30 minutes prior to anticipated intercourse.
Impaired erection	Often an anticholinergic problem, change to less anticholinergic drug or try bethanecol.
Priapism	Rare disorder associated with trazodone. Prolonged painful nonsexual erection. Medical urgency treated with epinephrine injections to the corpus cavernosa. May require surgical intervention leading to permanent impotence.
Impaired ejaculation	May require switching drug. Try Neostigmine 7.5–15 mg 30 minutes prior to antici-pated intercourse.
Inhibition of orgasm	Less serotonergic drug. Try cyproheptadine 4mg qd. Note that cyproheptadine, a serotonin antagonist, has caused loss of antidepressant efficacy in some clients.
HEMATOLOGIC	
Agranulocytosis	Exceedingly rare allergic reaction usually occurring in the first three months of treat-ment. Monitor for fever, sore throat, mucosal ulceration, weakness. Discontinue drug, change to a different chemical class.
Petechia, ecchymosis, easy bruising, bleeding	Associated with SSRIs affect on platelet. May occur with normal or decreased platelet counts. Discontinue drug. Monitor CBC, dizziness, lightheadedness.
OTHER	
Weight gain	Associated with cyclic antidepressants and MAOIs. Recommend diet and exercise. Diuretics (e.g., hydrochlorothiazide for edema).
Weight loss	Associated with SSRI; rarely clinically significant.
Tremor	Advise caffeine may exacerbate. Determine degree of interference with daily activities. Propranolol 10–20 mg tid-qid may be useful.
Antidepressant withdrawal	Anticholinergic rebound can result in GI upset, cramps, diarrhea. Educate client on potential withdrawal symptoms. When discontinuing, taper slower over several weeks. SSRI withdrawal symptoms include nausea, lightheadedness, dizziness, faint-ness, fatigue, parasthesias, flu-like syndrome. Taper slowly.

Andrews JM, Nemerov CB: Contemporary management of depression. *Am J Medicine* 97(6A):24S–32S, 1994 and adapted from Pollack MH, Rosen-baum JF: Management of antidepressant-induced side effects: a practical guide for the clinician. *J Clin Psychiatry* 48(1):3–8, 1987.

increased fluid and salt intake can be effective treatments. A caffeinated drink in the morning may be useful as long as vital signs are monitored initially. Edema, sexual dysfunction, and weight gain are also common and can lead to drug discontinuation. Complaints of insomnia occur with all MAOIs. Moving the last dose of the day to an earlier time may be helpful. Complaints of confusion or feeling drunk may indicate an excessive dosage. Although these drugs do not have direct effects on cholinergic receptors, anticholinergic-type side effects (e.g., dry mouth, urinary hesitancy, constipation) are seen. Parasthesias (numbness, prickling, tingling feelings) may be caused by MAOI-induced pyridoxine (vitamin B_6) deficiency and is treated with oral pyridoxine (Goodhart et al, 1991).

Avoiding certain foods is essential when clients are taking MAOIs. Dietary tyramine is a precursor in the synthesis of norepinephrine. In the presence of an MAOI, foods high in tyramine (an amino acid by-product formed by the bacterial breakdown of tyrosine in fermented foods) can lead to a sharp increase in available norepinephrine and potentially fatal hypertensive crisis. Box 23-3 lists some foods that may interact with MAOIs. Tyramine is not the only factor in food that can interact with MAOIs. For instance, fava beans contain dopamine, which can affect blood pressure in the presence of MAOIs. Previously, dietary restrictions for MAOIs were extensive and made compliance unlikely. Estimates of compliance with an MAOI diet have been as low as 40%. Yet, for several reasons, there are not an overwhelming number of MAOI hypertensive reactions. Foods, different brands of prepared foods, and a client's susceptibility to this interaction all vary widely. For instance, while a cup of coffee may elevate blood pressure and cause headaches in some clients, others on MAOIs benefit from a cup of coffee as an adjunct to treat hypotension on awakening. Thus, client education should consist of simple, clear, written and verbal instructions to absolutely avoid certain foods. Warnings of other foods that may cause problems in some clients or when taken in large quantity should be reviewed. Dietary restrictions should be maintained for two weeks after MAOIs are discontinued. All clients need to know the warning signs of hypertensive crisis, which include headache, stiff neck, sweating, nausea, and vomiting. Clients with such symptoms should seek medical attention immediately.

Many drugs can also interact with MAOIs and can lead to a hypertensive crisis or dangerous hypotension. These drugs are listed in Box 23-4. Many over-the-counter medications may be dangerous when taken with MAOIs, including diet pills, nasal decongestants, asthma medications (including inhalers), and cough suppressants (dextromethorphan). Literally hundreds of over-the-counter and prescription combination products under many different brand names contain sympathomimetics that are unsafe to use with MAOIs. Therefore, every client on an MAOI must be educated to consult a physician, dentist, nurse, or pharmacist prior to taking any additional medication. Although hypertensive events are generally more dangerous and more common, the response to a sympathomimetic medication or dietary indiscretion can be hypotension rather than hypertension. Whether a hypo- or hypertensive reaction ensues is a function of the overall adrenergic tone of the client and is not predictable.

Treatment for hypertensive crisis may be started with nifedipine (Procardia®, Adalat®) 10 mg. Absorption from oral administration is extremely rapid, and reductions of blood pressure may be seen in a matter of minutes. Vital signs should be monitored every 10–15 minutes until stable. Other therapies that have been used include the alpha-adrenergic blocker.

Clients who fail to respond to a non-MAOI antidepressant should usually wait at least two weeks before starting on an MAOI. An important exception to this is fluoxetine (Prozac®). Due to the long half-life of fluoxetine and

---

Box 23-3 Dietary Restrictions for Clients on MAOIs

Prohibited

- aged cheeses
- ripe avocados
- ripe figs
- anchovies
- bean curd/fermented beans
- broad beans (fava/Italian)
- yeast extracts and yeast derived vitamin supplements
- liver
- delicatessen meats (especially sausage)
- pickled herring
- meat extracts (Marmite, Borvil)
- fermented foods
- chianti and sherry

Allowed with Moderation

- beer and ale (*tyramine content varies with brand and can be especially high in imported beers and some nonalcoholic beers*)
- white wine/distilled spirits
- cottage cheese, cream cheese
- coffee (< 2 cups day)
- chocolate
- soy sauce (tyramine content varies with brand)
- yogurt and sour cream
- spinach, raisins, tomatoes, eggplant, plums

Box 23-4   Drugs to Avoid When Taking MAOIs

Antiasthmatics
    theophylline and inhalers containing epinephrine or Beta-agonists, e.g., albuterol (Proventil®, Ventolin®)

Antihypertensives
    methyldopa (Aldomet®), guanethidine (Ismelin®), reserpine

Anesthetics with epinephrine

Allergy, Hayfever, Cough and Cold Products, Decongestants, Diet Pills
    (Many combination over-the-counter products. Look for inclusion of phenylpropanolamine, ephedrine, phenylephrine, dextromethorphan.)

Buspirone (Buspar®)
Meperidine (Demerol®)
Serotonin Selective Reuptake Inhibitors
    fluoxetine (Prozac®), sertraline (Zoloft®), paroxetine (Paxil®), fluvoxamine (Luvox®), nefazodone (Serzone®)

Yohimbine (Yocon®)

Understanding and Applying
RESEARCH

Delgado PL et al: Serotonin function and the mechanism of antidepressant action, *Arch Gen Psychiatry* 47:411–418, 1990.

The role of serotonin in depression was demonstrated by an important study by Delgado et al. They examined a group of 21 hospitalized clients with depression medicated with a variety of antidepressants and whose depression had remitted. These clients were placed on tyrosine-free diets. Tyrosine, an essential amino acid, is required in the diet. In the brain, the synthesis of 5-HT is limited by the availability of tyrosine. When deprived of all tyrosine for 24 hours, two-thirds (14/21) of the clients in the study rapidly became depressed. Some became suicidal. Depression quickly remitted when tyrosine was restored to the diet. This is the first study to demonstrate that for some depressed clients, a functional serotonin system is required for antidepressant efficacy.

It is not yet possible to predict which depressed clients are more likely to respond to an SSRI versus a more adrenergic cyclic antidepressant. However, studies such as this, which are beginning to elucidate more precisely how the depressed brain responds to medication, are bringing us closer to understanding the underlying etiology of depression and more effective means to treat it.

---

its active metabolite norfluoxetine (approximately 7–10 days), clients discontinuing fluoxetine should wait at least 5 weeks before starting an MAOI.

Serotonin Selective Reuptake Inhibitors (SSRIs)

There has been an explosion of research and interest in the role of serotonin in depression in recent years, such as the study in Understanding and Applying Research above. Important findings include:

- In some depressed clients, reduced serotonin and its major metabolite 5-hydroxy indole acetic acid (5-HIAA) are found in the cerebral spinal fluid.

- Reduced serotonin has been noted in the brains of depressed suicides.

- Blood platelet serotonin receptors are altered in some clients with depression.

- All known SSRIs are clinically effective antidepressants (Risch and Nemeroff, 1992).

MODE OF ACTION

As their name implies, SSRIs act primarily to block the reuptake of serotonin. These drugs, listed in Table 23-4, have minimal direct effects on other receptors, including cholinergic, adrenergic, and histamine systems (Cole, 1992; Dechant, 1991; De Wilde et al, 1993; Wilde et al, 1993).

CLINICAL USE AND EFFICACY

Serotonin specific (selective) reuptake inhibitors now comprise more than half of all antidepressant use. The huge success of the SSRI antidepressants, starting with the release of fluoxetine in 1988, is due to several factors. The side effect profile is relatively mild compared to other antidepressants (Richelson, 1991). There is minimal cardiac toxicity, eliminating the need for ECGs. Serum levels are not clinically useful to determine dose or monitor for toxicity. Dose titration is minimal, and in the treatment of major depression the starting dose is also the maintenance dose for the majority of clients. Finally, all SSRIs currently on the market are comparatively safe in overdose. When taken as a single agent, SSRI overdoses are serious and can cause seizures, but complete recovery is common.

SSRIs are absorbed from the GI tract relatively slowly, and peak serum concentrations are obtained in 4–10 hours. All marketed SSRIs have serum half-lives averaging 15–24 hours, except fluoxetine (Prozac®). Fluoxetine's half-life in adults averages 2–3 days and its active metabolite norfluoxetine has a half-life of 7–10 days. This means that frequent dosage adjustments of fluoxetine are not generally warranted. Elimination can be substantially longer in older clients and those with hepatic disease where norfluoxetine half-lives of 14–21 days are well documented. Also, it is not possible to abruptly discontinue fluoxetine. This has important implications for drug interactions. A minimum five-week wash-out before MAOI use is required. Clients switched to a cyclic antidepressant must be started on low doses and titrated slowly, because remaining fluoxetine can inhibit metabolism of the cyclic antidepressant and yield toxic serum levels (Vaughn, 1988).

SIDE EFFECTS

Common initial side effects of SSRIs include nausea, drowsiness, dizziness, headache, sweating, anxiety, insomnia, anorexia, and nervousness. These are generally milder and more tolerable to the client than the sedation and anticholinergic effects of cyclic antidepressants. Often these are substantially more tolerable within a few weeks. Although all SSRIs share these side effects, the susceptibility of an individual to a particular agent varies. Paroxetine (Paxil®) may be slightly anticholinergic and more sedating than other SSRIs (Tulloch and Johnson, 1992). These medications, particularly fluoxetine, have been associated with insomnia. This also diminishes significantly with time but can be persistent in some clients. Dose reduction should be considered before adding an adjunctive agent for sleep. Trazodone (Desyrel®) 50 mg is sometimes used.

Fluoxetine may cause more agitation and anxiety, but this may be a dosing issue, since the commonly used 20 mg starting dose is too much for many clients. Sometimes SSRIs, and most commonly fluoxetine, can cause substantial anxiety and restlessness that appears to be a form of akathisia. These symptoms warrant close scrutiny because akathisia is associated with increased aggression and suicide. All SSRIs have been linked to occasional EPS.

A great deal of publicity has surrounded fluoxetine (Prozac®) and the risk of increased suicidal ideation when taking fluoxetine. This reaction was first described in a case report of six clients during fluoxetine's premarketing studies (Teicher, 1990). Paradoxical increased suicidal ideation has been reported for virtually all antidepressants (Damluji and Ferguson, 1988; Fava and Rosenbaum, 1991). Unfortunately, popular media sensationalism has blown this risk way out of proportion. This jaded perception continues to persist in the minds of many individuals despite considerable scientific evidence to the contrary. Prozac® has become a cultural icon, and stories of benefits and risks have reached mythic proportions. Clients should be allowed to express feelings about this medication regimen. Noncompliance can result from unaddressed concerns.

An often overlooked side effect of SSRIs is sexual dysfunction. As many as 20%–40% of clients may suffer from loss of libido, erectile dysfunction, ejaculatory dysfunction, or anorgasmia. Clients are often reluctant to discuss these issues. Therefore, sensitive inquiry can reveal side effects that could lead to noncompliance and a relapse of depression. Side effects and considerations to treat antidepressant sexual dysfunction are found in Table 23-5.

Other Agents

In recent years, antidepressant medications with a variety of chemical structures and varied modes of action have appeared on the market. These agents are not easily characterized into groups and thus are discussed individually below.

Clomipramine (Anafranil®) was the first drug indicated for the treatment of obsessive-compulsive disorder (OCD) in the United States. Clomipramine has been used in Europe to treat depression for more than a decade. It is structurally a tricyclic and shares the anticholinergic, sedative profile of these agents. The most serotonergic of the cyclic agents, clomipramine can cause GI upset, sweating, insomnia, and nervousness typical of these agents. It must be titrated to effective doses like the tricyclics. The starting dose is 25 mg/day, and the maximum daily dose is 250 mg. This drug does have an increased risk of causing seizures by lowering the seizure threshold. Fluoxetine (Prozac®) and fluvoxamine (Luvox®) are also FDA-indicated drugs for the treatment of OCD (Pigot et al, 1990; Wilde et al, 1993). However, the use of fluvoxamine in depression is still under investigation.

Bupropion (Wellbutrin®) has a somewhat different mechanism of action in that it blocks the reuptake of dopamine while having only minimal reuptake effects on norepinephrine (Ferris, 1993). Yet, bupropion has demonstrated efficacy against depression. It has a mild side-effect profile, causing less sedation, anticholinergic, and cardiac conduction side effects than TCAs. The most common side effects are agitation and insomnia. The starting dose is no greater than 75 mg tid. Bupropion can cause dose-related seizures. Therefore, it must never be dosed greater than 150 mg at one time; when the maximum dose is required, the recommended regimen is 150 mg tid. Depressed individuals with a history of bipolar disorder taking bupropion need to be assessed for symptoms of mania.

Venlafaxine (Effexor®) is the first of a new class of antidepressants that significantly block the reuptake of both serotonin and norepinephrine (Montgomery, 1993). Venlafaxine has mild dopamine reuptake blockade effects. It is rapidly absorbed and has a short half-life of approximately five hours. Its active metabolite has a half-life of 11 hours. Because of the short half-life, venlafaxine is dosed two or three times a day, starting at 75 mg, either 37.5 mg bid or 25 mg tid. Preliminary data suggest that outpatient clients have responded to doses between 75–225 mg/day while hospitalized; presumably more severely depressed clients may require the maximum dose of 375 mg/day.

Venlafaxine has side effects similar to SSRIs and may have mild anticholinergic-like effects. Nervousness and anxiety sometimes seen at lower doses may resolve at higher doses. Hypertension, increased diastolic blood pressure to greater than 90 mm/Hg and greater than 10 mm/Hg over baseline, is a dose-related side effect and an indication to reduce the dose or discontinue the medication.

Conclusion

Depression is a common and potentially deadly illness. Pharmacotherapy for depression, while effective, has many liabilities. Tricyclics are deadly in overdose. MAOIs require dietary discipline and particular vigilance for drug interactions. SSRIs cause sexual side effects many clients may be reluctant to discuss and that may lead to noncompliance. Nurses should know efficacy and toxicity of these agents. Moreover, teaching clients what to expect is a crucial component in helping to maintain safety, compliance, and optimal therapeutic response.

LITHIUM

Lithium is the simplest possible drug, a single ion. This single ion has had purported medical uses for more than 100 years. In the late nineteenth century, lithium was used as a treatment for gout, seizures, and as a sedative. Around this time, Trousseau in France and Carl and Fritz Lange in Denmark reported efficacy of lithium in mania and depression, respectively. In the early 1900s, fashionable spas touted lithium waters as healing and rejuvenating. Actually, these "lithia" waters contained only rare traces of lithium with inconceivable medical benefit. Unfortunately, in the United States in 1949 lithium was given to some cardiac clients as a salt substitute. The subsequent toxicity resulted in some deaths and cast a pall on the use of lithium. Interestingly, that same year in Australia, John Cade, in noting that guinea pigs given lithium became sluggish, wondered if lithium would help his agitated and manic clients. His astute observation resulted in the rediscovery of Trousseau's observation, that lithium had a specific effect in his manic clients.

Indications

Since Cade first used lithium in the treatment of bipolar disorder in 1949, it has remained one of the most effective psychotropic medications . Approximately 70–80% of clients with bipolar disorder respond to lithium in the treatment of both acute manic episodes and maintenance treatment (Baastrup et al, 1970; Prien, 1992). Lithium is also commonly used in the treatment of schizoaffective disorder and as an adjunct to antidepressant therapy in depression. It has also been used in treating impulse control disorders, self-injurious behaviors in conduct disorder, pervasive developmental disorder, and mental retardation.

Mode of Action

Lithium affects the neurotransmitters of multiple systems, including dopamine, norepinephrine, serotonin, acetylcholine, and GABA. These effects are modest; none of them has been directly linked to lithium's efficacy in bipolar disorder. Promising research suggests that lithium may work inside the neuron by interfering with guanine nucleotide (G-protein) binding (Manji et al, 1995). G-proteins may be thought of as signal transducers or chemical messengers inside the cell. The effects of many endogenous substances and drugs that impact receptors are subsequently manifest through the intracellular actions of G-proteins. Thus, the effects of neurotransmitters may be altered by lithium's effects on this signal transduction system. Future research in clarifying lithium's effects on G-proteins holds great promise in leading to a better understanding of the pathophysiological nature of bipolar disorder.

Clinical Use and Efficacy

Lithium's most important clinical feature is its narrow therapeutic index. Because serious toxic effects can occur with small increases in lithium plasma concentrations, conscientious monitoring is required. Lithium is rapidly absorbed from the gastrointestinal tract and is widely distributed throughout the body. Lithium is not metabolized and is excreted primarily by the kidney. Its clearance is directly proportional to the glomerular filtration rate. The average half-life is 24 hours in adults and 36 hours in geriatric clients. Due to the potential for toxicity, rigorous baseline laboratory monitoring is common. Conventional prelithium baseline monitoring is shown in Box 23-5. Baseline values are vital in the assessment of both acute and chronic lithium toxicity.

Starting doses for clients with normal renal function are generally 900–1200 mg/d in divided doses. Available lithium products are shown in Table 23-6. Sustained release lithium may be useful in clients who persistently

---

Box 23-5   Lithium Baseline Monitoring

- Vital signs
- Weight
- BUN/creatinine
- Electrolytes
- Thyroid function tests
- CBC with differential
- Urinalysis
- Electrocardiogram*
- Pregnancy test

*For those older than age 40 or with a history of cardiovascular disease suffer GI upset. The slow absorption of sustained-release lithium preparation results in 12-hour post-dose serum lithium levels that are approximately 30% higher than those obtained with immediate-release products. Subsequent dose adjustments are based on lithium plasma concentrations. Clients with normal renal function will reach steady state in 4–5 days, which is when first serum levels should be obtained. It is common to obtain levels earlier in clients with impaired renal function or in those prone to lithium toxicity. Routinely monitored serum lithium levels should be obtained 12 hours after the previous dose.

TABLE 23-6 Lithium products

Generic	Trade name
CAPSULES	
150 mg lithium carbonate	
300 mg lithium carbonate	Eskalith®, Lithonate®
600 mg lithium carbonate	
TABLETS (SCORED)	
300 mg lithium carbonate	Eskalith®, Lithane®
EXTENDED RELEASE TABLETS	
300 mg lithium carbonate	Lithobid®
450 mg lithium carbonate	Eskalith CR®
SYRUP	
lithium citrate syrup	Cibalith-S® Syrup
8 mEq per 5 mL*	

*300 mg of lithium carbonate = 8.12 mEq of lithium

The therapeutic range for lithium is customarily defined as 0.5–1.2 mEq/L measured 12 hours after the last dose. Acute mania may require plasma levels as high as 1.2–1.5 mEq/L. Maintenance treatment serum levels are lower. Recent studies suggest that relapse and hospitalization are reduced by plasma levels of 0.8–1.0 mEq/L in adults (Gelenberg et al, 1989). Geriatric clients may respond well to lower levels (0.4–0.6 mEq/L). Older clients are generally more sensitive to the neurotoxic effects of higher doses.

During maintenance, lithium is usually dosed two or three times a day. It has been suggested that once-a-day dosing at bedtime can reduce side effects, such as polyuria. Once-a-day-at-bedtime dosing is practical when the total daily dose is 1500 mg/day or less. Larger single doses often result in significant GI upset.

In the treatment of mania, initial response to lithium may take a week or longer. Therefore, concomitant antipsychotic therapy is often added temporarily to assist with the acute treatment of psychotic arousal symptoms (e.g., agitation, irritability, insomnia). Manic symptoms such as euphoria, grandiosity, pressured speech, flight of ideas, and hypersexuality may take somewhat longer to respond. Lithium alone may be effective to treat depression in individuals who are, in reality, bipolar but have not had their first manic episode. Low-dose lithium therapy (e.g., 300 mg bid) can be effective in treating major depression as an augmenting agent to antidepressant therapy.

Side Effects

Continuous monitoring for signs and symptoms of toxicity is a requirement for the safe use of lithium. Lithium side effects can be divided into those occurring early in

Box 23-6 Lithium Serum Levels and Side Effects

Transient effects and mild toxicity
- fine tremor
- GI upset
- mild polyuria, polydipsia
- muscle weakness, lethargy

Persistent effects
- fine tremor
- mild polyuria, polydipsia
- increased white blood count
- nontoxic goiter, hypothyroidism
- exacerbation of psoriasis
- acne
- alopecia
- weight gain

Effective acute treatment and prophylaxis—0.5–1.2 mEq/L

Moderate toxicity—lithium level > 1.5 mEq/L
- coarsening of tremor
- reappearance of GI symptoms
- confusion
- sedation, lethargy

As levels increase
- ataxia
- dysarthria
- mental status deterioration

Severe toxicity—lithium level > 2.5 mEq/L
- seizures
- coma
- death
- cardiovascular collapse

therapy and those that tend to persist. Box 23-6 delineates these side effects. Most early onset symptoms resolve or diminish considerably but persist to a lesser extent in many clients.

A variety of problems caused by lithium may yield to simple interventions. Lithium-induced hypothyroidism is treatable with thyroid supplementation and is reversible if lithium is discontinued. Weight gain with lithium may be greater than 10 Kg but will respond to diet adjustments. Mild leucocytosis is benign and does not require treatment. Acne may be treated with benzoyl peroxide or erythromycin topical solutions. Exacerbation of psoriasis can be serious and may require discontinuation of lithium treatment.

Lithium's effects on cardiac function are generally mild and of little consequence. Lithium may substitute for potassium in ion channels in the heart. EKG changes resemble those seen in hypokalemia, but usually these are benign. Despite this, idiosyncratic cardiotoxicity is rarely observed, and the astute clinician must remain alert. Baseline and yearly ECGs are advisable in clients over age 40 or those with cardiac disease. Lithium can cause sinus node depression and should be avoided in clients with sick sinus syndrome.

Lithium is generally avoided in pregnancy, especially in the first trimester, due to a possible low incidence association with Ebstein's anomaly, a cardiac malformation (Jacobson, 1992; Schou, 1973). Often, low doses of a high-potency antipsychotic agent is substituted if drug treatment is required during pregnancy. When the behavioral toxicity and/or physical health risks of being manic while pregnant clearly outweigh the risks of lithium use, extra monitoring must be performed due to changes in renal function during pregnancy. Lithium should be discontinued several days prior to delivery. Nursing mothers should not use lithium.

The polyuria caused by lithium is a mild nephrogenic diabetes insipidus. When persistent and problematic, this polyuria can be treated with amiloride 5–10 mg/day, a potassium-sparing diuretic. Contrary to popular belief, even with long-term treatment, lithium is rarely toxic to the kidney unless plasma levels rise (Schou et al, 1988). Permanent damage to nephrons and subsequent loss of renal function can occur with substantially elevated lithium levels.

Many side effects of lithium toxicity are dose-related (see Box 23-6). If a client on stable lithium therapy experiences a return of some of his or her original transient side effects, this may be an indication of impending lithium toxicity. Gastrointestinal complaints and coarsening of the fine lithium tremor should result in examining plasma lithium levels. If these dose-related warning signs were reliable, there would be little need to monitor serum levels. Unfortunately, sometimes seizures or cardiovascular collapse are the first signs of lithium toxicity. For this reason, particular attention should be paid to factors that expose clients to the risk of lithium toxicity.

Because lithium is excreted primarily by the kidney, factors that affect sodium and water metabolism are intimately linked to lithium elimination. Stable diets, whether high or low in sodium, are not problematic. It is the change in dietary salt intake that will affect lithium levels. Addition of salt to the diet will result in lower lithium levels and possible loss of efficacy. Less salt in the diet or conditions that cause sodium loss, such as fever or dehydration, will increase lithium levels. For example, clients leaving the hospital and returning to a substantially different diet at home may be at increased risk for lithium toxicity.

As lithium levels rise, CNS toxicity becomes more pronounced. Clients who become ataxic, dysarthric, or have any change in mental status should be evaluated immediately for lithium toxicity.

Conclusion

For more than 40 years, lithium has been the most effective psychopharmacologic agent in the treatment of bipolar disorder. Although extensively studied, the exact mechanism of action remains a mystery. Because of a narrow therapeutic range and side effects, the search for alternative treatments continues. Currently, two anticonvulsant agents, valproate and carbamazepine, have been used as alternatives to lithium. This is addressed in detail below. Today, lithium remains the drug of choice in the treatment of bipolar disorder.

ANXIOLYTICS AND HYPNOTICS

The sensation of extreme anxiety triggers the "fight or flight reaction." This reaction elicits a series of observable physical changes or responses. The client's emotionally charged response may include dramatic physical symptoms, such as chest pain or pressure with radiation to the shoulder and arm, rapid heartbeat or palpitations, and shortness of breath. This syndrome is not a new malady of the twentieth century, and documented reports of it are found from the Civil War in the 1860s.

Today, symptoms such as these often motivate people to seek medical treatment. Once underlying somatic medical causes are ruled out, a variety of treatment alternatives is available. Commonly, comprehensive treatment involves a combination of psychotherapy and adjunctive pharmacotherapy.

Sleep is commonly reported to be disrupted in anxiety. In the treatment of anxiety disorders, the appropriate initiation and maintenance of sleep are intrinsically related to the use of a variety of compounds with sedative properties. Whether the medication is being used as an anxiolytic (anti-anxiety) or a hypnotic, the effect of sedative agents on sleep requires consideration.

Barbiturates
INDICATIONS

Historically, barbiturates were the primary agents used to treat anxiety and insomnia. Their use in anxiety predates the advent of benzodiazepines. However, almost all barbiturate use has been replaced by benzodiazepines, which are safer and more effective anxiolytics and hypnotics.

Barbiturates have several disadvantages. First, they are not good anxiolytics and provide mostly sedation. As hypnotics, tolerance develops rapidly in many clients. Thus, therapeutic and toxic doses converge with continued use. In acute overdose, barbiturates can be fatal when taken as a single agent. Death occurs secondary to respiratory depression, which is exceedingly rare for benzodiazepines.

All barbiturates have the potential to be habit-forming. Barbiturates induce hepatic enzymes and can thus result in increased metabolism, decreased serum levels, and reduced efficacy of other hepatically cleared drugs, including cyclic antidepressants, anticonvulsants, anticoagulants, and some cardiac medications. Barbiturates can also interfere with oral contraceptives, and alternative methods of birth control should be used if barbiturates are added to the regimen.

MECHANISM OF ACTION

The mechanism of action of barbiturates is unknown. Researchers have found that the mesencephalic reticular activating system is remarkably sensitive to barbiturates. It is likely that barbiturates diminish neuronal responsiveness. Unlike benzodiazepines, as doses increase, barbiturates reduce the respiratory drive and mechanisms responsible for the rhythmic character of respiration. Barbiturates are differentiated primarily by their pharmacokinetic half-lives. Amobarbital has the shortest-acting half-life, and phenobarbital has the longest. Half-lives and usual dosages are listed in Table 23-7.

Despite their liabilities, barbiturates still retain some legitimate uses. Barbiturates may be used as hypnotics in clients who have failed benzodiazepine therapy. Phenobarbital is still used occasionally in the treatment of seizure disorders. IV amobarbital is used in the narcoanalysis, a technique of medication-induced mental relaxation/hypnosis, that may help properly prepared clients address suppressed memories and emotions.

Benzodiazepines
INDICATIONS

Benzodiazepines are one of the most widely used classes of medications in all of medicine and have a variety of indications. In general medicine, they are used for preoperative relief of anxiety and for sedation, light anesthesia, and to induce anterograde amnesia (an inability to remember events that occurred after ingesting the medication) for perioperative events (King, 1992). They are used in higher doses as skeletal muscle relaxants. Diazepam (Valium®) is used intravenously to treat status epilepticus, and oral clonazepam (Klonopin®) is indicated for the treatment of Lennox-Gastaut seizures. Ben-

zodiazepines are frequently used as hypnotics to treat insomnia and in the management of anxiety disorders.

Although indicated as hypnotic and antianxiety agents, benzodiazepines are commonly used in a broad array of settings. There is limited evidence that benzodiazepines may be useful in the treatment of some clients with mood disorders. Clonazepam (Klonopin®) has been used with some success in the treatment of bipolar disorder and as an adjunct to lithium in partially responsive clients (Sachs, 1990). Akathisia may be treated with benzodiazepines. Chlordiazepoxide (Librium®) has long been used to treat the acute signs and symptoms of alcohol withdrawal. Catatonic clients are sometimes aroused by benzodiazepines. Finally, lorazepam (Ativan®), along with antipsychotics, has become a standard in the treatment of psychotic agitation in emergency situations.

MECHANISM OF ACTION

Gamma aminobutyric acid (GABA) is the primary inhibitory neurotransmitter in the brain. Receptors, dubbed benzodiazepine receptors, serve as chloride ion gates. GABA interacts with these chloride ion channels to allow chloride ion into neurons, thus hyperpolarizing the neuron and reducing the firing rate. In the presence of a benzodiazepine, the activity of GABA is enhanced, resulting in further opening of the chloride ion channel and a further inhibition of neuronal activity.

GOALS OF THERAPY

In the treatment of anxiety, medications are best viewed as an adjunct to therapy. During drug treatment, clients may find relief from their symptoms which allows them to benefit from a variety of psychotherapies. Some clients may require maintenance treatment with antianxiety agents. Target symptoms of anxiety and panic should be clearly identified.

The goal of therapy in the treatment of sleep disorders is the (re)establishment of normal sleep patterns. Again, short-term intervention is the standard of care.

CLINICAL USE AND EFFICACY

The benzodiazepines are the drugs of choice for the treatment of anxiety and sleep disturbances. All benzodiazepines have anxiolytic effects. A particular benzodiazepine may be sedative at low doses, provide improved relief from anxiety at higher doses, and be a hypnotic at even higher doses. The available benzodiazepines are listed in Table 23-7. This table points out the speed of oral absorption, the elimination half-lives, active metabolites, and relative potency of the agents.

The main difference between benzodiazepines is in their pharmacokinetic profiles and potency. Thus, the rational use of benzodiazepines is derived from applying effects of their pharmacokinetic differences to the clinical setting. When used for the treatment of acute anxiety or agitation, rapid oral absorption is desirable; whereas, in the chronic treatment of an anxiety disorder, rapid oral

TABLE 23-7 Hypnotic and anxiolytic agents

Generic name	Trade name	Approved indication	Approx. benzodiazepine equivalency (mg)	Active metabolite	Usual dosage range (mg/d)	Half-life hours
BARBITURATES						
amobarbital	Amytal®	hypnotic	na	—	100–200	8–42
butabarbital	Butisol®	hypnotic	na	—	50–100	34–42
pentobarbital	Nembutal®	hypnotic	na	—	100–200	15–48
phenobarbital	Luminal®	hypnotic	na	—	100–200	80–120
secobarbital	Seconal®	hypnotic	na	—	100–300	15–40
BENZODIAZEPINES						
alprazolam	Xanax®	A, AD, P	0.5	no	0.75–4 ANX. 4–10 PANIC	12–15
clonazepam	Klonopin®	LGS	2.5	no	1–6*	20–50
clorazepate	Tranxene®	A	7.5	yes	7.5–90	20–80
chlordiazepoxide	Librium®	A, AW, PS	10	yes	25–200	5–30
diazepam	Valium®	A, PS, SE	5	yes	2–40	20–80
estazolam	Prosom®	hypnotic	2	no	1–2	10–15
flurazepam	Dalmane®	hypnotic	15	yes	15–30	8–40
halazepam	Paxipam®	A	20	yes	20–160	10–20
lorazepam	Lorazepam®	A, PS	1	no	0.5–10	10–20
oxazepam	Serax®	A, AD, AW	15	no	30–120	5–20
prazepam	Centrax®	A	10	yes	20–60	20–80
quazepam	Doral®	hypnotic	2	yes	30–50	30–50
temazepam	Restoril®	hypnotic	15	no	15–30	10–20
triazolam	Halcion®	hypnotic	0.25	no	0.125–0.25	1.5–5
NONBARBITURATE, NONBENZODIAZEPINE						
chloral hydrate	Noctec®	hypnotic	na		500–2000	8–11
ethchlorvynol	Placydyl®	hypnotic	na		500–1000	18–20
diphenhydramine	Benadryl®	hypnotic	na		25–100	3–9
doxylamine	Unisom®	hypnotic	na		25–100	8–12
zolpidem	Ambien®	hypnotic	na		5–10	1.5–4
buspirone	Buspar®	A	na		10–60	2–4

*dosed up to 20 mg/day for seizure

A = anxiety, AD = anxiety associated with depression, AW = alcohol withdrawal LGS= Lennox-Gastaut syndrome (seizures) P = panic disorders, PS = psychotic disorders, SE = status epilepticus.

absorption is less important. Parenteral and concentrate forms of some benzodiazepines are sensitive to light and temperature, and significant degradation may occur if left at room temperature for more than a few hours. For example, liquid lorazepam should be refrigerated until immediately prior to use to prevent degradation.

There is an additional absorption issue important with benzodiazepines. Once in the bloodstream, the drug must be absorbed into the brain. The two benzodiazepines absorbed the fastest from the blood are diazepam (Valium®) and alprazolam (Xanax®). This rapid penetration into the brain is the likely reason for the "buzz" effect commonly reported for these two drugs. People who do not abuse drugs often find this "buzz" unpleasant and may report feeling spacey, out of it, or disconnected.

Benzodiazepine should be started at low doses and gradually increased as needed to achieve clinical response. There is a rapid onset of clinical efficacy once an appropriate dose is achieved. In anxiety disorders, some reduction of anxiety may be apparent almost immediately. The antianxiety effect, with initial dosing, may not last as long as the serum half-life would suggest. This is probably due to the drug redistributing out of the brain. With continued dosing, steady-state brain levels and sustained efficacy are achieved. For the treatment of anxiety, benzodiazepines are usually dosed at bedtime or BID. Only occasionally is TID dosing required.

Ideally, hypnotics should be rapidly absorbed and thus have a short onset of action and a short elimination half-life so that next-day carry-over effects such as sedation and impaired cognition would be minimized. Realistically, individuals may experience sedation "hangover effect" the next day.

As with antianxiety treatment, hypnotic pharmacotherapy should be for as short a time as possible. Medication should be an adjunct to help clients (re)establish a regular sleep pattern. Along with improved sleep, hygiene techniques taught to the client, benzodiazepines should be used for 7–10 days and discontinued. Clients who require longer pharmacotherapy are at greater risk to develop rebound insomnia and anxiety on drug discontinuation.

SIDE EFFECTS

Unwanted sedation is the most common side effect of benzodiazepines and affects at least 10% of clients. Sedation may diminish with time or a decrease in dose. Clients should always be counseled not to drive or use dangerous machinery when initiating these drugs. This is important even in clients taking hypnotic medications at bedtime only. Next-day, or carry-over, sedation can affect driving as well as result in cognitive dysfunction that can affect work or school performance. Dizziness and ataxia occur less frequently and are more common in the elderly and physically debilitated. A paradoxical excitability, hyperarousal, or increase in aggression may be seen.

However, these side effects are rare and may be more common in children and in the elderly with organic brain disease. Clients with chronic obstructive pulmonary disease or sleep apnea may develop clinically significant respiratory impairment.

Benzodiazepines may be teratogenic and should not be used during pregnancy. If used during the third trimester and immediately prior to delivery, newborns may develop withdrawal reactions. Benzodiazepines are secreted in breast milk in sufficient concentrations to cause symptoms such as dyspnea, bradycardia, and drowsiness in nursing infants.

When used for more than brief periods, the accumulation of active metabolites can be clinically significant. During this time clients may gradually develop increasing sedation, decreased cognitive functioning, and even ataxia. This is especially true in the elderly population and clients with hepatic dysfunction. Even for drugs without active metabolites, clients on these potent drugs should be monitored closely for ataxia and risk for falls.

Abuse and Withdrawal of Benzodiazepines and Barbiturates

Prior to any use of either benzodiazepines or barbiturates, the clinician must consider their abuse potential. Use of these agents in clients with a history of substance abuse, particularly in the outpatient setting, must be carefully considered. Barbiturate intoxication presents with confusion, drowsiness, irritability, hyporeflexia, ataxia, and nystagmus. More serious overdoses can result in coma. Intoxication with benzodiazepines does not generally present with nystagmus (Roy-Byrne and Hommer, 1988). Barbiturate overdose can easily result in death from respiratory depression and is especially dangerous in the presence of alcohol and/or other CNS depressant drugs. Benzodiazepines as single-agent overdoses are not usually life-threatening. However, a possible benzodiazepine overdose must always be taken seriously because it is often unclear in the clinical situation if other medications are present. As with barbiturates, benzodiazepine overdose is potentially fatal when combined with alcohol or other CNS-depressant agents.

Physical withdrawal symptoms can occur anytime these drugs are taken continuously for more than two weeks and occur in almost half of clients who have taken these drugs for more than four weeks. Accordingly, drug discontinuation should be gradual. The most severe withdrawal symptoms are experienced by clients who have been taking high doses for long periods of time and suddenly stop taking the drug. Long half-life drugs tend to have milder withdrawal phenomena, while short half-life drugs are associated with more severe withdrawal. Barbiturate withdrawal symptoms occur more often and are generally more severe than with benzodiazepines. Withdrawal presents as a hyper-arousal state, including anxiety, irritability, insomnia, fatigue, muscle aches, tremors, sweating, and difficulty in concentrating. These signs and symptoms closely resemble the original sleep or anxiety complaints. The nurse communicates the client's response to the detoxification protocol with the treatment team.

Nonbenzodiazepines

The first nonbenzodiazepine anxiolytic is buspirone (Buspar®). Buspirone is indicated for the treatment of anxiety disorders—specifically, generalized anxiety disorder. It is notable for its mild side-effect profile. Common side effects include dizziness, headache, drowsiness, and lightheadedness. The CNS sedation and cognitive impairment occur much less frequently than with other anxiolytics. Clients whose anxiety responds to buspirone may report that they do not feel like they are taking a drug. That is, they now feel normal, their symptoms are relieved, and they are without side effects. It is important to note that the antianxiety effects of buspirone begin to occur gradually over the first two weeks of therapy and full efficacy may not be apparent for 3–6 weeks. For this reason, some individuals can become impatient waiting for the drug to work, particularly if they are under a great deal of stress. Further, many clients have previously been treated with a benzodiazepine whose antianxiety effects begin almost immediately. Thus, clients who hold the same expectations for buspirone may require education about the gradual onset of efficacy to remain motivated and compliant with treatment.

Buspirone's mechanism of action is unknown. It is a partial agonist at the serotonin receptor (Eison et al, 1986). This means that it stimulates the receptor but not as much as serotonin. Overstimulation of serotonin receptors has been hypothesized to cause anxiety. Thus, buspirone's partial agonist activity may restore more "normal" serotonergic tone in anxiety disorders. At high doses, buspirone can block the dopamine receptor. It is unknown at this time if prolonged use at high doses may result in the development of abnormal involuntary movements.

Safer and commonly used hypnotics for the treatment of short-term insomnia include chloral hydrate (Noctec®) and the antihistamines diphenhydramine (Benadryl®), doxylamine (Unisom®, Nitetime Sleep-Aid®, and Sleep 2-Nite®).

The first of a new class of hypnotics is zolpidem (Ambien®). Zolpidem is indicated for the short-term treatment of insomnia and is a schedule IV controlled substance.

Zolpidem's mechanism of action is different from that of benzodiazepines. The GABA chloride ion channel has several different binding sites. While zolpidem interacts with the benzodiazepine receptor, this selectivity for only part of the benzodiazepine receptor results in quite a different effect profile. Zolpidem, unlike benzodiazepines, does not have anticonvulsant or myorelaxant

effects (Sanger, 1987). Sleep studies have revealed that zolpidem does not suppress REM sleep. Further, abrupt discontinuation in clients taking zolpidem for up to 30 days has resulted in little rebound insomnia (Lader, 1992; Scharf et al, 1991).

The most common side effects are drowsiness and dizziness. At doses greater than 10 mg (the maximum recommended dose), the incidence of nausea and dizziness increases dramatically (Merlotti et al, 1989). This suggests that although zolpidem is potentially habit-forming, it will not be popular with substance abusers.

Conclusion

Hypnotics and anxiolytics, while effective agents, can produce their own set of clinical problems. First, the appropriate duration of therapy is often unclear. Also, even gradual discontinuation can result in a recurrence of the original signs and symptoms. Lastly, an addictive potential must often be considered.

ANTICONVULSANTS IN PSYCHIATRY

The use of terminology to group medications by the description of a drug's initial indication, while useful, can at times be misleading. Such drugs may have vastly different chemical structures, pharmacokinetics, modes of action, side effects, and, in the case of anticonvulsants, a variety of uses as well. Two anticonvulsants originally used in the control of seizure disorders, carbamazepine (Tegretol®) and valproate (Depakene® and Depakote®), are being used with increasing frequency in the treatment of psychiatric disorders.

Indications

Carbamazepine has long been used in the treatment of simple partial, complex partial, and tonic-clonic seizures, while valproate has been indicated for only the latter and in absence of seizures. Recently, valproate received FDA approval for the initial control of acute mania (Bowden et al, 1994). All other uses of these agents for psychiatric indications are based on the scientific literature and medical standards of care. Bipolar disorder is the best studied indication. While lithium currently remains the drug of choice, both valproate and carbamazepine have been used effectively. The broad scope of research into potential uses for these agents in psychiatry is summarized in Table 23-8. Studies have examined these two drugs in various mood and anxiety disorders. Carbamazepine does not appear to have a role in panic disorder, while valproate has had little effect on unipolar depression.

Mode of Action

The mode of action of these agents on psychiatric neurobiology is uncertain at this time, although several issues are clear. The effects of these agents in psychiatric

TABLE 23-8 Anticonvulsants in psychiatry

Potential use	Carbamazepine	Valproate
Bipolar disorder	XX	XX
Unipolar depression	X	—
Aggression/dyscontrol syndromes	XX	X
Panic disorder	—	X
PTSD	X	X
substance withdrawal	XX	X

XX = documented efficacy for some clients; X = some potential usefulness but more study is needed — = usefulness not demonstrated.

disorders appear to be separate from their antiseizure mechanisms. Valproate and carbamazepine work via different mechanisms. For example, valproate has mild effects on CNS GABA receptors, while carbamazepine does not. It appears likely that these drugs have substantial effects on the inner chemistry of neurons via pathways known as second messenger systems (Post et al, 1992). Second messenger refers to a broad variety of intracellular chemical reactions that influence both the metabolism and action potential transmission of neurons. Stimulation or inhibition of receptors on the cell membrane is one way of affecting second messengers systems. Some drugs (e.g., carbamazepine, valproate, and lithium) appear to affect second messenger systems directly. The study of these systems in health and disease and the effects of drugs on these systems are leading toward greater understanding of the pathophysiology of psychiatric disease.

Goals of Therapy

The goals of therapy for mood and anxiety disorders have been described previously. However, the role of anticonvulsants in the pharmacotherapy of chronic aggression has not been addressed. Anticonvulsants were first used to treat aggression after the relationship between seizure disorders and aggression was noticed (Monroe, 1970). One important step in titrating the medication is to objectively note the type of aggression (e.g., verbal and/or physical, against self, inanimate objects, or others) and the frequency of the occurrences over time both before and after medication changes.

Clinical Use and Efficacy

It is a mistake to think of both of these agents as similar in efficacy because they are both anticonvulsants. Bipolar clients who have failed to respond to lithium and sub-

sequent treatment with one of these anticonvulsants may eventually respond to the other anticonvulsant. Usually, these drugs are titrated gradually to allow for tolerance to side effects. Baseline monitoring after a medical history and physical examination includes electrolytes, liver function tests, complete blood counts, EKG, and pregnancy testing. Valproate is teratogenic and is associated with neural tube defects—most commonly spina bifida—and should be avoided in pregnancy.

VALPROATE

Valproate is available in several dosage forms as different salts of valproate. Valproate is the common compound that is measured in the plasma. Depakene® is the trade name for both an immediate-release tablet and a liquid concentrate. Depakote® is an enteric-coated capsule with a slower release. Depakote® sprinkles are capsules that contain coated particles that can be taken intact or pulled apart and sprinkled on food. The half-life averages 6–16 hours. Serum levels should be monitored and dosing adjusted accordingly. There may be a response threshold because response to valproate is rarely seen with serum levels less than 50 mcg/mL (McElroy et al, 1992). Efficacy is generally found with levels of 50–120 mcg/mL, although levels up to 150 mcg/mL may be useful in the treatment of acute mania. An exception to the initial titration of these agents is the use of a so-called loading regimen of valproate in the treatment of acute mania. Given as Depakote® 500 mg TID, acutely manic clients can frequently tolerate this aggressive dosing without the GI upset and sedation often seen. With this regimen some acutely manic clients may respond within three days, more than twice as fast as with standard lithium therapy (Keck et al, 1993).

CARBAMAZEPINE

Carbamazepine has a unique pharmacokinetic profile. Initially it has a half-life of approximately 36 hours. However, carbamazepine induces its own metabolism. That is, in the presence of the drug, the liver gradually manufactures more of the enzymes that metabolize carbamazepine, which results in faster metabolism. After 4–6 weeks, the approximate half-life is 24 hours. For this reason, clients on carbamazepine are not at steady state for at least one month after a dosage change. When used to treat the signs and symptoms of substance withdrawal, dosing is low (200 mg–400 mg/day) and the duration of therapy is brief. For other indications the starting dose is usually 200 mg twice a day and may be taken with meals to reduce GI upset. The average dose is titrated to about 1000 mg/day in divided doses, but dosage requirements vary widely and should be guided by serum levels. Efficacy for psychiatric indications is associated with serum levels of 7–12 mcg/mL, although some clients become overly sedated or ataxic at serum levels greater than 7 mcg/mL.

Side Effects

VALPROATE

Gastrointestinal complaints, nausea and vomiting, anorexia, dyspepsia, and diarrhea are the most common side effects of valproate. GI complaints usually occur early and usually subside with continued treatment. Persistent complaints can be treated with dose reduction, a switch to sprinkles, or H_2 blockers (e.g., ranitidine [Zantac®]). Initial somnolence is common. Minor liver enzyme elevations (less than three times normal) may occur. Regardless, in the presence of substantial therapeutic benefits, valproate is usually continued in the face of minor liver enzyme elevations (McElroy et al, 1992). Tremor is common. If tremor persists and is a problem, propranolol (Inderal®) has been used effectively. Weight gain with and without increased appetite may occur. Hair loss, usually transient, affects approximately 10% of clients. More serious but less common side effects include thrombocytopenia, coagulopathies, pancreatitis, edema, and hepatic failure. Hepatic failure is a greater risk in children under the age of 10 and in clients on other anticonvulsant drugs. Liver enzymes should be monitored closely.

CARBAMAZEPINE

During the initiation of carbamazepine therapy, clients may complain of sedation, lethargy, GI upset, and blurred vision. These side effects tend to diminish with time and are the primary reason for dose titration. Mild fluid retention and edema may occur. Liver enzyme elevations similar to those with valproate occur, and periodic liver enzyme monitoring is the standard of care for both drugs.

Carbamazepine causes a predictable suppression of the white blood cell count (WBC). In most cases this reduction is benign and will stabilize at 10%–15% below baseline levels. Thus, the WBC is monitored at baseline and periodically after treatment is initiated. Agranulocytosis, a life-threatening absence of white blood cells, is associated with carbamazepine but is extremely rare and should not be confused with the mild neutropenia. Similarly, a mild reduction in platelets (thrombocytopenia) is usually not clinically significant.

Ataxia is a sign of carbamazepine toxicity usually associated with increased serum levels. Nurses should consider holding the dose of carbamazepine in a client with ataxia. Urticaria, pruritic, and erythematous rashes occur occasionally. These rashes may be mild and self-limiting but must be evaluated closely and monitored continuously.

Conclusion

Although the use of anticonvulsants in psychiatry is rapidly increasing, with the exception of valproate in the treatment of acute mania, unequivocal evidence of efficacy is not always available. Side effects and toxicity can be substantial. Thus, clear expectations of response and well-defined target symptoms must be specified before pharmacotherapy is begun.

STIMULANTS

Indications

The use of stimulants in psychiatry has a checkered history. Before the advent of antidepressant medications, stimulants were used to treat depression. In the 1950s these drugs were widely prescribed to reduce appetite in the treatment of obesity. Failure to achieve lasting weight loss and the high abuse liability of these drugs have substantially curtailed this practice. Today, stimulants are used in psychiatry primarily to treat attention-deficit hyperactivity disorder (ADHD). Drugs used to treat ADHD include methylphenidate (Ritalin®), dextroamphetamine (Dexadrine®), and pemoline (Cylert®). Methylphenidate and dextroamphetamine are schedule II drugs, and pemoline is a schedule IV drug. Stimulants are also used in the treatment of narcolepsy and less commonly in withdrawn and apathetic states in the elderly.

Mode of Action

Stimulants are used in the treatment of ADHD. The exact pathophysiology of ADHD is not known, but it clearly involves both dopamine and norepinephrine. All of the stimulants block the reuptake of dopamine and norepinephrine. Dextroamphetamine also blocks serotonin reuptake and blocks the enzyme monoamine oxidase. In higher doses, dextroamphetamine also facilitates release of dopamine and norepinephrine. Methylphenidate affects dopamine and norepinephrine reuptake more and affects release less than dextroamphetamine. Pemoline's reuptake effect appears to be greater for dopamine than for norepinephrine. The ascending reticular activating system is particularly affected by the psychostimulants.

Goals of Therapy

Clients with ADHD suffer from increased motor activity, impulsiveness, and inattention. The goal of pharmacotherapeutic treatment is to decrease motor activity and impulsivity. However, optimal treatment integrates medication use and behavioral interventions.

Clinical Use and Efficacy

While both methylphenidate and dextroamphetamine are effective in the treatment of ADHD, methylphenidate is used more often. Many clinicians suggest that optimal therapy should involve sequential trials of both methylphenidate and dextroamphetamine to determine which offers better effect in a particular individual (Calis et al,

TABLE 23-9 Stimulants				
Drug name	Dosage forms	Starting dose mg/day	Average (maximum) daily dose	Half-life (hours)
Dextroamphetamine (Dexadrine®)	5, 10 mg tablets 5 mg/5 mL elixir 5, 10, 15 mg sustained-release tablets	2.5–10	10–20	8–12
Methylphenidate (Ritalin®)	5, 10, 20 mg tablets 20 mg sustained-release tablets	5–10	20–30	1–2
Pemoline (Cylert®)	18.75, 37.5, 75 mg tablets 37.5 mg chewable tablets	18.75–37.5	56.25–75	9–14

1990). Both drugs are rapidly absorbed, and some therapeutic efficacy may be initially noted almost immediately. Full effects are often seen in two or three days. Dosage forms, half-lives, and starting and maintenance doses are listed in Table 23-9. The short half-lives of methylphenidate and dextroamphetamine can result in a return of symptoms in the afternoon or evenings. Thus, dosing is often with breakfast, again at midday, and in the afternoon when symptoms begin to break through. Dosing later in the day may increase the potential for insomnia. Pemoline's longer half-life allows for once-a-day dosing.

Side Effects

These three medications cause many similar side effects. GI upset, nausea, cramps, and anorexia are common. Initial GI symptoms often diminish with time. Lack of appetite for several hours after dosing may persist. Weight loss and growth suppression have been reported for all three stimulants. Dosing strategies that include drug holidays (e.g., school days only or periods off medication in the summer) allow for a correction of the growth suppression and result in children remaining within normal physical growth and development guidelines. All of these medications are occasionally associated with headache, dizziness, nervousness, irritability, and, rarely, emotional lability and psychosis. When these side effects are persistent, dose reduction or changing medication is a useful tactic.

Emergence of tics may be observed. Tics may diminish with dose reduction. However, these medications are often initiated in children during ages when the tic disorder Tourette's syndrome may first emerge. Whether tics are a part of Tourette's syndrome or not, their presence may make it difficult to use stimulants at any dose, and alternative ADHD treatments (e.g., antidepressants) may need to be tried.

There are differences in side effects between methylphenidate, dextroamphetamine, and pemoline. Both of the former can cause palpitations, tachycardia, and increases in blood pressure, although these are seldom clinically significant. Nonetheless, these medications are sympathomimetics, and cardiac status, particularly hypertension and tachyarrhythmias, should be monitored at baseline and with dose titration. Pemoline has been occasionally associated with liver toxicity, usually during the first three months of therapy (Pratt and Dubois, 1990). Thus, baseline and periodic monitoring of liver function tests are warranted.

Conclusion

There is a great deal of public misunderstanding about the use of stimulant medication. An urban myth, that stimulants cause brain damage, is unsubstantiated but persists in some areas. Families must be provided with accurate information about anticipated efficacy and side effects. Optimal therapy involves the client, family, teachers, and clinicians working together.

OTHER BIOLOGIC THERAPIES

Electroconvulsive Therapy (ECT)

HISTORICAL PERSPECTIVE

Electroconvulsive therapy (ECT) was first used as a treatment modality in 1934 to "cure" psychotic disorders by inducing convulsions. Throughout the years, ECT has been a topic of much controversy, some of which can be linked to the criticism of consumer groups. As a result of this criticism, ECT fell into disfavor and was rarely used. Used appropriately, ECT can be an effective therapy for many clients who have not responded to other treatment modalities.

ECT is not a new innovation. Paracelsus, a sixteenth-century Swiss physician, gave camphor to induce convulsions as a method of treating lunacy. This intervention also was used by von Auenbrugger in 1764. However, Auenbrugger's treatment was to ameliorate symptoms of mania. The "modern era" of convulsive therapy dates back to von Meduna's original work with a client who had been in a catatonic stupor for four years. In 1934,

Meduna administered the injection of camphor oil to a client with schizophrenia, which resulted in a remarkable recovery after a series of treatments. Inspired by that success, Meduna administered the convulsive treatment to an additional 26 clients of which 13 demonstrated considerable improvement.

Reports of the success of the new therapy spread and served as an impetus to explore additional methods to induce convulsions. This investigation lead to the examination of electrical stimulus as a seizure-induction agent. By 1938 Cerletti and Bini achieved worldwide notoriety after administering 11 separate transcerebral treatments to a client with schizophrenia who demonstrated a full recovery from his illness (Abrams, 1988). It is unlikely that this client would be diagnosed with schizophrenia by today's standards, but the relative safety and potential efficacy of the procedure opened an entirely new treatment technique in psychiatry.

Even though modern ECT bears little resemblance to early ECT, there remains a stigma attached to its use. Confusion regarding the current practice of ECT is due to the lack of accurate information. Media versions of ECT portray barbaric methods of psychiatric treatment regimens.

Nurses play an integral role in the use of ECT by providing accurate education to client and family to ameliorate fear and prevent distortions regarding the use of ECT. Nurses must fully understand the indications, contraindications, procedures, and side effects of ECT to educate, monitor, and support the client recommended for ECT and his or her family.

MODERN ECT

ECT is a safe and effective treatment for major depression. The most appropriate candidates are clients experiencing a major mood disorder. Melancholic, delusional, and psychotic depression tend to respond well to ECT. Other indications for ECT include previous positive results from ECT, clients who cannot tolerate side effects of antidepressants, acute suicidal ruminations and behavior, and clients in danger of fluid and electrolyte imbalances secondary to inability to eat or drink due to severe depression. ECT has also been used in the treatment of mania, severe catatonia, and schizophrenia unresponsive to antipsychotic medications. ECT is also considered in the first trimester of pregnancy when pharmacotherapy is contraindicated.

Absolute contraindications include clients with space-occupying lesions with increased intracranial pressure. Risk factors to be considered are clients with recent myocardial infarction, aneurysms, acute respiratory infection, cardiac arrhythmias, organic syndromes, thrombophlebitis, and narrow-angle glaucoma. ECT is not indicated for clients with a diagnosis of drug dependence, personality disorder, reactive depression, and paranoid schizophrenia.

Prior to and after the procedure, the client and family require education. Informed consent, which nurses frequently witness, can only be obtained after the client is thoroughly educated. Consent is given prior to treatment and authorizes the physician to perform it. The consent discusses the purpose of the treatment, the proposed number of treatments, and risk factors associated with ECT. Preliminary baseline tests (CBC, SMA, urinalysis, EKG, and physical exam) are obtained.

Today, the client may receive ECT on either an inpatient or outpatient basis. A typical ECT procedure is as follows. Clients scheduled for the procedure are fasted overnight (NPO) and are routinely prepared for an operative procedure (i.e., clients are asked to empty bladder and remove jewelry, dental work, and nail polish). Approximately 30 minutes prior to the procedure, the client receives an IM atropine injection, typically 0.5 mg. This will reduce secretions and protect against vagal bradycardia, which can occur after application of the stimulus. In the ECT suite, blood pressure, cardiac, and EEG monitors are placed to assess vital functions. Wherever ECT is given, emergency equipment, including oxygen, suction, and cardiac arrest cart must also be available. Staff attendance includes at minimum a psychiatrist, anesthetist, and nurse. A short-acting anesthetic and a muscle relaxant are given IV. Muscle paralysis prevents increased movement to decrease the risk of fracture or injury. A mouthguard and 100% oxygen is administered. Once anesthesia and paralysis are obtained, the ECT electrodes are placed. For bilateral ECT, electrodes are placed on the anterior portion of the client's temples; in unilateral ECT, the electrode is placed on the anterior portion of the client's nondominant temple (i.e., right handed-right temple). Once the electrodes are placed, a brief electrical stimulus (usually less than two seconds' total duration) is applied. The body does not move, and the seizure is confirmed by EEG monitoring. The client wakes in a few minutes, and oxygen is discontinued. The client is monitored closely for any respiratory distress and excess secretions that may need to be suctioned. The client remains in a recovery room, usually 1–3 hours, until vital signs are stable and the client is alert, oriented, and able to walk without assistance. The client may now eat and resume normal activity. Some clients may feel sleepy and return to bed.

Side effects most associated with ECT are headache and memory loss. Clients who experience headache may be given mild analgesia and instructed to rest. Memory impairment tends to be more pronounced with bilateral treatment. It can be quite severe during the course of treatment but generally improves significantly after completion of a series of treatments. The nurse will reorient clients and offer support and reassurance to those who are distraught regarding the memory loss. It is important to remember, especially with clients suffering memory loss, that client teaching will require repetition throughout the course of treatment. Nurses will allow clients to ventilate fears while offering support and education to assist in decreasing anxiety expressed in relation to ECT.

Seasonal Affective Disorder and Phototherapy

Alterations in mood have been related to seasonal changes in some individuals. Research indicates that attacks of mania are more frequent in the summer (Rosenthal et al, 1983). Conversely, statistics indicate that the incidence of depression is more common in late fall. In 1981 Aschoff made an environmental observation noting that, in the least industrialized countries, seasonal variation in mood disorders was greater than in industrialized nations (Aschoff, 1981). He hypothesized that factors such as artificial light, central heating, and adherence to a work day based on clock hours opposed to available natural light may reduce risk for affective episodes. Seasonal variation was increased in temperate climates and not in the north, as one might expect. Environmentally, this pattern correlated with clear sunshine and not with length of day, thus implicating brightness and duration of light in affecting mood.

Seasonal changes in time and duration of daylight trigger many changes seen in the behavior of various organisms. Artificial light has been used in industry to bring plants into bloom out of season, to increase productivity in egg-laying chickens, and to breed animals out of season. Bright, full-spectrum light may improve the productivity and irritability of shift workers whose work schedules force a discordance between "normal" sleep patterns and natural sunlight. Thus, multiple observations suggest that phototherapy is potential treatment for seasonal affective disorder (SAD) (Lewy et al, 1986; Rosenthal et al, 1985; Terman et al, 1986).

Researchers have investigated seasonal depression. The depression usually begins in November and is characterized by hypersomnia, anergia, carbohydrate craving resulting in weight gain, decreased libido, social withdrawal, and suicidal thoughts. This depression lifts in March and may be followed by hypomania in spring (Kukopulos and Reginaldi, 1973).

Investigators of SAD have noted some biological markers may be more common in clients with this disorder. Altered sleep architecture has been observed on sleep EEGs (Rosenthal et al, 1983). Prolactin and melatonin, two hormones that have seasonal rhythms, are often abnormally high in clients with SAD.

Clinical trials have yielded several generalizations regarding the effectiveness of phototherapy. Often up to 80% of clients have been rated as much improved with phototherapy (Lewy et al, 1986; Rosenthal et al, 1985). The light used must be several times brighter than that which is usually encountered during indoor activities. Typically, clients are exposed to eight four-foot fluorescent bulbs at a distance of three feet. Light administration in the middle of the day is as effective as early morning or late at night. Effective treatment regimens require at least two hours of light exposure; greater effectiveness may be seen with four hours of exposure. The therapeutic effect appears to be mediated by the quantity of light that strikes the eyes and not the skin.

Response to phototherapy can be quite rapid. Some clients report improvement with 1–2 treatments, and maximum benefit may be seen in 4–7 days. Conversely, relapse with the withdrawal of light is reported to be just as rapid.

The mechanism of action of phototherapy, like the mechanism underlying SAD, is not clearly understood. Investigations into these issues, as well as practical devices and procedures to provide light therapy to clients, are active areas of investigation.

Summary of Key Concepts

1. Both typical and atypical antipsychotics block dopamine receptors, but atypical antipsychotics have an improved efficacy against negative symptoms. Despite the high toxicity of antipsychotics, for many clients their benefits outweigh their risks.

2. Symptom response to antipsychotics varies. The order of response time from quickest to slowest follows: positive symptoms, affective symptoms, cognitive and perceptive symptoms, and negative symptoms.

3. Neuroleptic malignant syndrome (NMS) is a potentially fatal reaction to typical antipsychotics and must be recognized early to minimize fatal complications. However, NMS is often misdiagnosed as heat stroke, pneumonia, or lethal catatonia.

4. Seventy percent of clients with major depression will respond to antidepressants. The 30% failure rate is generally due to inadequate dose or duration of therapy.

5. Although antidepressants may cause increased energy and physical activity, suicidal ideations continue. Clients are at the highest risk to act on harmful impulses during the second week of therapy.

6. Pharmacotherapy for depression has many liabilities. Thus, knowledge of toxicity and efficacy is essential to achieve optimal therapeutic response.

7. Because response to lithium may take a week or longer, concomitant antipsychotic therapy is often used to decrease acute psychotic symptoms.

8. Anxiolytics and hypnotics such as benzodiazepines are an adjunct to therapy. Short-term (7–10 day) intervention is the standard treatment.

9. Withdrawal symptoms from barbiturates closely resemble the original sleep or anxiety complaints.

10. Although barbiturates and benzodiazepines are commonly used, they have a highly addictive potential that must be considered.

11. Use of anticonvulsants should occur only with clear response expectations and well-defined target symptoms.

12. ECT, despite common consumer beliefs, is a safe and effective treatment for major depression.

13. Phototherapy has been found to be effective for clients with seasonal affective disorder (SAD).

REFERENCES

Abrams R: *Electroconvulsive therapy,* New York, 1988, Oxford University Press.

Adler LA et al: A controlled comparison of the effects of propranolol, benztropine and placebo on akathisia: an interim analysis, *Psychopharmacol Bull* 29(2):283–286, 1993.

Alvir JM, Lieberman JA: A reevaluation of the clinical characteristics of clozapine-induced agranulocytosis in light of the United States experience, *J Clin Psychopharm* 14(2):87–88, 1994.

American Psychiatric Association: Practice guidelines for major depressive disorder in adults, *Am J Psychiatry* 150 Supplement: 1–26, 1993.

Andrews JM, Nemeroff CB: Contemporary management of depression, *Am J Medicine* 97(6A):24S–32S, 1994.

Aschoff J: Annual rhythms in man. In *Handbook of behavioral neurobiology,* New York, 1981, Plenum Press.

Baastrup PC et al: Prophylactic lithium: double-blind discontinuation in manic-depressive and recurrent depressive disorders, *Lancet* 2:326–330, 1970.

Baldessarini RJ: Drugs and the treatment of psychiatric disorders. In Gilman AG et al, editors: *Goodman and Gilman's the pharmacologic basis of therapeutics,* ed 8, New York, 1990, Pergamon.

Battaglia J et al: Rapid tranquilization of agitated psychotic patients in the emergency room. Presented at *New Clinical Drug Evaluation Unit,* Boca Raton, Fla., May 1992.

Borison RL et al: Risperidone: clinical safety and efficacy in schizophrenia, *Psychopharmocol Bull* 28(2):213–218, 1992.

Bowden C et al: Efficacy of divalproex vs lithium and placebo in the treatment of mania, *JAMA* 271:918–924, 1994.

Calis KA et al: Attention-deficit hyperactivity disorder, *Clin Pharmacy* 9:632–642, 1990.

Caroff SN et al: Neuroleptic malignant syndrome: diagnostic issues, *Psychiatric Ann* 21(2):130–147, 1991.

Cole J: New directions in antidepressant therapy: a review of sertraline, a unique serotonin reuptake inhibitor, *J Clin Psychiatry* 53(9):335–340, 1992.

Damluji NF, Ferguson JM: Paradoxical worsening of depressive symptomatology caused by antidepressants, *J Clin Psychopharm* 8(5):347–349, 1988.

Davis KL et al: Dopamine in schizophrenia: a review and reconceptualization, *Am J Psychiatry* 148:1474–1786, 1991.

Dechant KL, Clissold SP: Paroxetine—a review of its pharmacodynamic and pharmacokinetic properties and therapeutic potential in depressive illness, *Drugs* 41(2):225–253, 1991.

Delgado PL et al: Serotonin function and the mechanism of antidepressant action, *Arch Gen Psychiatry* 47:411–418, 1990.

Deniker P: The neuroleptics: an historical survey, *Acta Psychiatr Scand* 82 (Suppl. 358):83–87, 1990.

De Wilde J et al: A double-blind, comparative, multi-center study comparing paroxetine with fluoxetine in depressed patients, *Acta Psychiatr Scand* 87:141–145, 1993.

Dumon JP et al: Randomized, double-blind, crossover, placebo-controlled comparison of propranolol and betaxolol in the treatment of neuroleptic-induced akathisia, *Am J Psychiatry* 149:647–650, 1992.

Eison AS et al: Review of its pharmacology and current perspectives on its mechanism of action, *Am J Med* 80(Supp 3B):1–9, 1986.

Fava M, Rosenbaum JF: Suicidality and fluoxetine: is there a relationship, *J Clin Psych* 52:108–111, 1991.

Ferris RM, Cooper BR: Mechanism of antidepressant activity of bupropion, *J Clin Psychiatry* Monograph 11(1):2–14, 1993.

Gelenberg AJ et al: Comparison of standard and low serum levels of lithium for maintenance treatment of bipolar disorder, *NEJM* 321(22):1489–1493, 1989.

Glazer WM, Kane JM: Depot neuroleptic therapy: an underutilized treatment option, *J Clin Psychiatry* 53:426–433, 1992.

Goodhart RS et al: Phenelzine-associated peripheral neuropathy, clinical and electrophysiologic findings, *Aust N Z J Med* 21:339–340, 1991.

Gurrera RJ et al: A comparison of diagnostic criteria for neuroleptic malignant syndrome, *J Clin Psychiatry* 53:56–62, 1992.

Hagger C et al: Improvement in cognitive functions and psychiatric symptoms in treatment-refractory schizophrenic patients receiving clozapine, *Biol Psychiatry* 34:702–712, 1993.

Jacobson SJ et al: Prospective multi-center study of pregnancy outcome after lithium exposure during the first trimester, *Lancet* 339:530–533, 1992.

Johnstone EC, Marsh W: The relationship between response to phenelzine and acetylation status in depressed patients, *Proc R Soc Lond* (Bio)66:947–949, 1973.

Kane J et al: Clozapine for the treatment schizophrenic, *Arch Gen Psychiatry* 45:789–796, 1988.

Kane JM, Marder SR: Psychopharmacologic treatment of schizophrenia, *Special Report: Schizophrenia* 113–128, 1993.

Keck PE et al: Valproate oral loading in the treatment of acute mania, *J Clin Psychiatry* 54:305–308, 1993.

King DJ: Benzodiazepines, amnesia and sedation: theoretical and clinical issues and controversies, *Human Pharmacol* 7:75–87, 1992.

Kukopulos A, Reginaldi D: Does lithium prevent depression by suppressing manias? *Int J Pharmacopsychiatry* 8:152–158, 1973.

Lader M: Rebound insomnia and newer hypnotics, *Psychopharmacology* 108(3): 649–658, 1992.

Lewy AJ et al: Treatment of winter depression with light. In Shagass C et al, editors: *Biological psychiatry,* vol 6, New York, 1986, Elsevier.

Lichter JB et al: A hypervariable segment in the human dopamine receptor D_4 (DRD4) gene, *Human Molecular Genetics* 2(6): 767–773, 1993.

Manji HK et al: Signal transduction pathways, molecular targets for lithium's actions, *Arch Gen Psychiatry* 52:531–543, 1995.

McElroy SL et al: Clozapine in the treatment of psychotic mood disorders, schizoaffective disorder and schizophrenia, *J Clin Psychiatry* 51:411–414, 1991.

McElroy SL et al: Valproate in the treatment of bipolar disorder: literature review and clinical guidelines, *J Clin Psychiatry* 12: 42S–52S, 1992.

Meltzer HY et al: Cost effectiveness of clozapine in neuroleptic-resistant patients, *Am J Psychiatry* 150:1630–1638, 1993.

Merlotti L et al: The dose effects of zolpidem on the sleep of healthy normals, *J Clin Psychiatry* 9(1): 9–14, 1989.

Monroe RR: *Episodic behavioral disorders,* Cambridge, Mass., 1970, Harvard University Press.

Montgomery S: Venlafaxine: A new dimension in antidepressant pharmacotherapy, *J Clin Psychiatry* 54:3:119–126, 1993.

Pickar D et al: Clinical and biologic response to clozapine in patients with schizophrenia, crossover comparison with fluphenazine, *Arch Gen Psychiatry* 49:345–353, 1992.

Pickar D et al: Mania and hypomania during antidepressant pharmacotherapy: clinical and research implications. In Post RM, Ballenger JC, editors: *Neurobiology of mood disorders,* Baltimore, 1984, Williams and Wilkins.

Pigot TA et al: Controlled comparison of clomipramine and fluoxetine in the treatment of obsessive-compulsive disorder, *Arch Gen Psychiatry* 47(10):926–932, 1990.

Pollack MH, Rosenbaum JF: Management of antidepressant-induced side effects: a practical guide for the clinician, *J Clin Psychiatry* 48(1):3–8, 1987.

Pope H et al: Frequency and presentation of neuroleptic malignant syndrome in a large psychiatric hospital, *Am J Psychiatry* 143(10):1227–1233, 1986.

Post RM et al: Mechanism of action of anticonvulsants in affective disorders: comparisons with lithium, *J Clinical Psychopharmacol* 12:23S–35S, 1992.

Pratt DS, Dubois RS: Hepatotoxicity due to pemoline: a report of two cases, *J Pediatr Gastroenterol Nutr* 10:239–241, 1990.

Prien RF: Maintenance therapy. In Paykel E, editor: *Handbook of affective disorders,* London, 1992, Churchill Livingston.

Quitkin FM et al: Response to phenelzine and imipramine in placebo non-responders with atypical depression, *Arch Gen Psychiatry* 48:319–323, 1991.

Richelson R: Side effects of old and new generation antidepressants: a pharmacologic framework, *J Clin Psychiatry* Monograph 9(1):13–19, 1991.

Risch SC, Nemeroff CB: Neurochemical alterations of serotonergic neuronal systems in depression, *J Clin Psychiatry* 53(10, Suppl): 3–7, 1992.

Rosenthal NE et al: Antidepressant effects of light in seasonal affective disorder, *Am J Psychiatry* 142:163–170, 1985.

Rosenthal NE et al: Seasonal variation in affective disorders. In Wehr TA, Goodwin FK, editors: *Biological rhythms and psychiatry,* Pacific Grove, Calif., 1983, Boxwood Press.

Roy-Byrne PP, Hommer D: Benzodiazepine withdrawal: overview and implications for the treatment of anxiety, *Am J Med* 84(6):1041–1052, 1988.

Sachs GS: Use of clonazepam for bipolar affective disorder, *J Clin Psychiatry* 51(5, Suppl):31–34, 1990.

Sanger DJ et al: The behavioral profile of zolpidem, a novel hypnotic drug of imidazopyridins structure. *Physiology and Behav* 4:(2)39–1987.

Scharf MB et al: Dose response effects of zolpidem in normal geriatric subjects, *J Clin Psychiatry* 52:77–83, 1991.

Schou M: Effects of long-term lithium treatment on kidney function: an overview, *J Psychiatr Res* 22:287–296, 1988.

Schou M et al: Lithium and pregnancy, I: report from the register of lithium babies, *British Med J* 2:135–136, 1973.

Tamminga CA et al: Clozapine in tardive dyskinesia: observations from human and animal model studies. *J Clin Psychiatry* 55(9, Suppl B):102–106, 1994a.

Teicher MH et al: Emergence of intense suicidal preoccupation during fluoxetine treatment, *Am J Psychiatry* 247(2):207–210, 1990.

Terman M et al: Bright light treatment of seasonal affective disorder, *New Research Abstracts,* 139th Annual Meeting of the American Psychiatric Association, 1986.

Thomas H et al: Droperidol versus haloperidol for chemical restraint of agitated and combative patients. *Ann Emerg Med* 21(4):407–413, 1992.

Tulloch IF, Johnson AM: The pharmacologic profile of paroxetine, a new selective serotonin reuptake inhibitor, *J Clin Psychiatry* 53(Suppl 2):7–12, 1992.

Vaughn DA: Interaction of fluoxetine and tricyclic antidepressants, *Am J Psychiatry* 145:1478, 1988.

Wilde MI et al: Fluvoxamine: an updated review of its pharmacology and therapeutic use in depressive illness, *Drugs* 46(5):895–924, 1993.

Wysowski DK, Barash D: Adverse behavioral reactions attributed to triazolam in the food and drug administration's spontaneous reporting system, *Arch Intern Med* 151:2003–2008, 1991.

CHAPTER 24

Adjunct Therapies

Theresa Williams

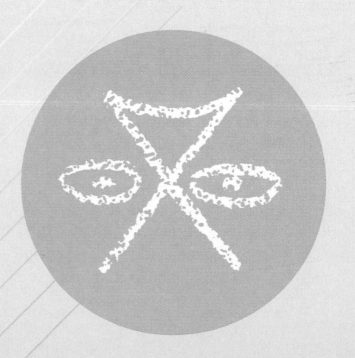

Adjunct therapy Action-oriented process with the primary intention of fostering adaption and productivity in order to minimize pathology and promote the maintenance of health.

Art medium Material or technical means of artistic expression.

Art therapy The use of artistic activities, such as painting and clay modeling, in psychotherapy and rehabilitation.

Closure Also called sharing; the last stage in a psychodrama or movement/dance therapy experience in which the experience is processed (verbally and nonverbally), and insight and a sense of completion are promoted.

Double The individual in psychodrama who operates as the "inner voice" of the protagonist to express repressed thoughts, feelings, and conflicts.

Enactment The action portion in psychodrama in which a scene or sequence of scenes is portrayed.

Mirroring A technique in psychodrama and movement/dance therapy in which one individual imitates the behavior patterns of another to show the person how other people perceive and react to him or her.

Movement Kinesthetic behavior in which individuals communicate by the use of body motions rather than formal language.

Movement/dance therapy The use of movement to promote increased awareness of the body and changes in feeling states, cognition, and behavior.

Music The science or art of assembling or performing intelligible combinations of tones in an organized, structured form.

Music therapy The use of the music to provide a variety of listening and participatory experiences adapted to the needs of the individual clients, such as an opportunity for nonverbal communication, shared experience, emotional expression, relaxation, and nonthreatening enjoyment.

Occupation The goal-directed use of time, energy, interest, and attention to foster adaption and productivity, to minimize pathology, and to promote the maintenance of health.

Occupational therapy The application of goal-directed, purposeful activity in the assessment and treatment of individuals with psychological, physical, or developmental disabilities.

Protagonist The individual in psychodrama who presents and acts out his or her emotional problems and interpersonal relationships.

Psychodrama A form of psychotherapy in which an individual reenacts life situations in order to examine subjective experiences, promote insight, and alter specific behavior patterns.

Recreation To create again by some form of play, amusement, or relaxation.

Recreational therapy The use of recreational activities as an integral part of the rehabilitation or therapeutic process. The purpose is to increase enjoyment of life, stimulate activity and self-expression, enhance socialization, and counterbalance self-concern.

Theme development The part of movement/dance therapy in which a specific issue or feeling is actively being explored.

Warm-up A stage of psychodrama and movement/dance therapy that focuses on introducing group members, increasing the comfort level, and determining the theme or issue to be addressed.

- Distinguish between occupational, recreational, art, music, psychodrama, and movement/dance therapies.

- Describe common settings where adjunct therapies are found and give examples of therapeutic activities for each modality.

- Identify the goals and objectives of adjunct therapies when used for specific DSM-IV diagnoses.

- Compare and contrast adjunct therapies with traditional verbal therapies.

- Describe effective nursing roles for each of the adjunct therapies.

Adjunct therapies, also known as expressive, experiential, or activity therapies, include occupational therapy, recreational therapy, art therapy, music therapy, movement/dance therapy, and psychodrama. The techniques involved in these modalities become therapeutic when the primary intention is to increase the client's awareness of feelings, behavior, perceptions, cognitions, and sensations. The "action" in these therapies can be physical and/or imagined. Although nurses will not lead the adjunct therapy exercise, they are valuable assets to the therapist. Nurses work closely with these various therapies. Thus, it is important to have an understanding of them.

HISTORICAL PERSPECTIVES

Adjunct therapies date back to early Greek, Roman, and Egyptian times when, as early as 2000 BC, exercise and the arts were found to be healing, especially for melancholia that we know today as depression. However, it was not until the increased moral treatment of people with mental illness in the eighteenth and nineteenth centuries that these activities became widely recognized and used in therapeutic settings. In the present, although adjunct therapies at times are discounted as diversionary "extras," they are generally recognized as therapies in their own right. They parallel verbal therapies and act as "catalytic agents giving impetus to the development of relationships and intrapsychic experiences used by the therapist and client to illuminate or alter pathology" (American Occupational Therapy Association, 1972).

Adjunct therapists provide services to children, adolescents, adults, and elderly of all functional levels and diagnostic categories. They can be found in a broad range of therapeutic settings, including general psychiatric hospitals, nursing homes, psychosocial and physical rehabilitation centers, homeless shelters, clinics, public and private schools, group homes, correctional centers, home health agencies, community mental health centers, day care centers, and private practices.

In many situations, the use of adjunct therapies becomes advantageous over verbal therapies because they are not limited by the constraints of linear verbal communication such as the reporting of past occurrences or projected future events, censorship of thoughts and fantasies, or use of the many defense mechanisms. Instead, these therapeutic modalities allow the client to be expressive on multiple levels at once, including the physical, the emotional, and the symbolic levels. They also allow the client to demonstrate conflicts, strengths, and limitations, both developmental and psychological, and to resolve the conflicts and developmental issues in the present with the support of the therapist. Additionally, the creative process is recognized as curative because it involves that part of oneself that problem-solves, experiences hope, and connects with the internal and external world. These expressive experiences also allow the client to be viewed as a whole person, rather than being identified by pathology and subsequent depersonalization.

Special considerations must be made by a nurse before deciding to participate in or to direct experiential work. Most of the methods described in this chapter require that the primary facilitator receive some degree of formal training and supervised experience. Adjunct therapists generally specialize in one specific field, namely occupational, recreational, art, music, dance, or psychodrama therapy, and have received formal training within a supervised internship that often leads to a master's degree. They are also usually registered or certified by a national association representing their area of expertise.

The Role of Nursing in Adjunct Therapy

In deciding to use these methods, nurses must assess whether they have sufficient skills or the interest or ability to obtain the skills necessary to facilitate the use of the particular modality. Nurses may vary in their degree of comfort with specific techniques (for example, being physically active or directive with a client). Even if one is uncomfortable with directing or participating, it is still beneficial for the nurse to become familiar with the specific therapies in order to recommend them to the primary physician and to support the contributions of all treatment team members. When there is a comfort level but not enough expertise to direct a particular adjunct

therapy experience, the nurse's participation can still be extremely valuable, adding an additional trained observer to the group, as well as decreasing many clients' inhibitions by participating with enthusiasm and interest. Most therapists expect to be approached by the nurses prior to the session to inquire about the treatment goal, the theme of the specific activity, and how the nurse can best participate in the process.

As the reader becomes familiar with each modality and its objectives, it will become obvious that there is an overlapping of treatment goals. A team approach using as many combined therapies as possible has proven to be the most effective and efficient approach for many of the acute diagnoses. This variety allows the client to explore the same problem or symptom from many different perspectives and increases opportunities for the client to use a therapeutic strategy that is comfortable, familiar, and safe to resolve conflicts and experience successes.

OCCUPATIONAL THERAPY

Occupational therapy (OT) was developed in the twentieth century by Adolf Meyer, a neuropathologist, who realized the importance of viewing the individual holistically and creating balance in productivity, self-care, and leisure. Despite this awareness, the use of occupational therapy services was limited primarily to the physically disabled throughout World wars I and II. It was not until the 1950s that intrapsychic issues were incorporated into occupational therapy services when it was recognized that radical treatment alone was not sufficient for an illness that also impaired social skills. At that time, the emphasis was placed on the integration of the client into social settings and the appreciation for activities as therapy. Presently, occupational therapy focuses on the assessment of task performance, cognitive functioning, and psychosocial development. Treatment is directed toward recognizing strengths, minimizing weaknesses, and adapting to change.

The American Occupational Therapy Association defines occupational therapy as "the application of goal-directed, purposeful activity in the assessment and treatment of individuals with psychological, physical, or developmental disabilities" (American Occupational Therapy Association, 1972). The word **occupation** means "the goal-directed use of time, energy, interest, and attention, to foster adaptation and productivity; to minimize pathology; and to promote the maintenance of health" (Kaplan and Sadock, 1995).

Like nurses, occupational therapists treat physical dysfunction as well as psychosocial impairment. Generally, the assessment and treatment services of occupational therapy in mental health include the following:

1. **Task-oriented treatment using creative modalities such as crafts.**
   Observing and directing a client's approach to a project provide occupational therapists with data about

levels of concentration, impulsivity, frustration tolerance, and problem solving that can be used to assess skill or provide the client feedback about progress.

2. **Living skills involving self-care and maintenance.**

   Clients with psychiatric diagnoses may not tend to personal hygiene when decompensating. Occupational therapists, along with nurses, provide the time, supplies, and encouragement to teach or reestablish good habits of personal grooming and general health.

3. **Independent living skills through psychoeducational groups.**

   Using didactic material, discussion, or creative media, clients learn to recognize past behaviors as maladaptive and begin to develop more effective skills in areas of communication, stress management, and adjustment to change.

4. **Sensorimotor skills, including neuromuscular, sensory-integrative activities, and therapeutic exercise.**

   Movement groups improve functional performance, increase relaxation, and are often designed to include a memory or other cognitive component.

5. **Discharge planning and community re-entry.**

   May include integration through community outings, information about resources, or outpatient treatment in a partial hospitalization program.

6. **Prevocational assessment.**

   When and if appropriate, may involve conducting a client interview, interest inventory, and the supervision of work-related tasks.

Clinical Example: Occupational Therapy

A 35-year-old divorced, unemployed female is hospitalized for depression on a psychiatric unit. Her hospitalization was prompted by an overdose of prescription medication. She has two adolescent children. She held jobs for a short time in food service but has not worked for 10 years. She overdosed on prescription medication because her negative thoughts led to self-destructive behavior. She has a DSM-IV, Axis I diagnosis of schizoaffective disorder, depressive type.

ASSESSMENT

1. Impaired social-interpersonal skills.

2. Low self-concept and self-confidence.

3. Low cognitive functions, i.e., poor concentration, limited problem-solving abilities, and limited frustration tolerance.

4. Low adaptive capacities, i.e., difficulty completing tasks of daily living and tasks necessary for effective parenting or return to work.

5. Poor sensorimotor/psychomotor functioning.

OCCUPATIONAL THERAPIST'S TASKS AND OBJECTIVES, AND THE NURSE'S ROLE

- Separate self-care and maintenance tasks into small, manageable steps specific to hygiene, dress, makeup, and laundry.
  Nurse's Role: Collaborative effort with occupational therapist, including brief daily contact with the client to provide encouragement and reinforce feedback regarding these tasks.

- Provide task-oriented craft group to address concentration, planning, and sequencing of tasks, self-confidence, and problem-solving skills. Additionally, to allow for reality testing and increase tolerance for socialization.
  Nurse's Role: Provide encouragement, support, and role modeling.

- Provide educational groups to help the client recognize and use more effective coping techniques.
  Nurse's Role: Provide similar teaching on an individual basis, and support changes in behavior.

- As acute symptoms decrease, meet with the client to assess and assist in setting goals for current occupational role. Suggest possible avenues including a parenting class and a gradual return to work process.
  Nurse's Role: Encourage discussion with the client regarding occupational roles and choices and discharge planning. Assist in reality testing.

RECREATIONAL THERAPY

As far back as 2000 B.C., Egyptians used games, songs, and dances as therapy, specifically noting their benefits with melancholia (depression). At the turn of the century, Florence Nightingale introduced recreational services to hospitalized soldiers. She came to appreciate the significant therapeutic value of such services as she observed that clients involved in the care and feeding of pets experienced increased feelings of self-worth and self-esteem. During World War I, the American Red Cross used recreation services in hospital settings. In the 1920s and 1930s, recreation programs began appearing in state mental hospitals and schools for individuals with mental retardation. It wasn't until World War II, however, that recreation services began to be recognized as legitimate, curative therapy that could be used to meet specific medical goals and objectives.

During that time, mental health professionals began to realize the disadvantages and limitations of the sterile hospital environment. Psychiatric hospitals were known to limit their services to physical exams, balanced meals, pharmacology, and a "safe place to rest." Not only did this stress-free environment prevent an accurate observation of the client's coping skills and adaptive skills but it also promoted the depersonalization of the client. "The hospitalized client tended almost inescapably to be depersonalized—to be regarded as an instance of pathology rather than an afflicted and suffering being with all of the sensitivities, needs, hopes and discouragements" (Haun, 1965).

Recreation can be thought of as creating again, or refreshing oneself, by some form of play, amusement, or relaxation. Play can also be a powerful tool for venting aggression, and games provide a repetitive motor discharge that serves as an effective device for achieving motor mastery in children and recalling this success as adults. Within the regressive elements of play, there are also limits and structures set by the rules of the game.

Recreational therapy (RT) is generally practiced by trained professionals and incorporates the active process of demonstrating and applying observable skills within the curative elements of play. The four primary goals of recreational therapy are:

1. Provide clients with structured, "normal" activities of daily living.

2. Assist clients in developing leisure skills and interests suitable to their lifestyles.

3. Augment verbal psychotherapy and other adjunct therapies.

4. Assist clients in bridging the gap between the hospital and the community.

The recreational therapist selects an activity based on the treatment goals, taking into account the client's functional abilities, physical requirements, degree of coordination, tolerance for social involvement and interaction, and the level of difficulty of the activity. Some of the activities that might be prescribed are arts and crafts, audiovisual activities, dances, hobbies and special interest programs, musical activities, nature and outing activities, cooking sessions, special events, sports, and games (see Figure 24-1).

Clinical Example: Recreational Therapy

Presented to the recreational therapist is a mixed adult population in an inpatient psychiatric setting with a variety of DSM-IV, Axis I diagnoses including: major depressive disorder, severe without psychotic features, schizophrenia, chronic undifferentiated type, and bipolar disorder, most recent episode, mixed.

ASSESSMENT

1. Difficulty expressing emotions in a safe and socially acceptable way.

2. Ineffective social-interpersonal skills.

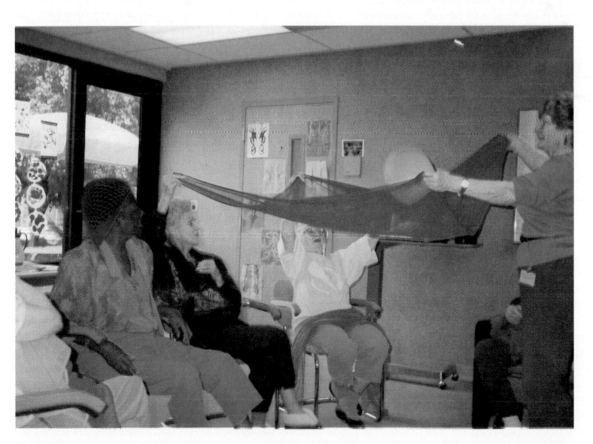

Figure 24-1 Balloon toss. Several clients and a therapist are holding a scarf as a vehicle to toss a balloon. This activity has several purposes: it provides an opportunity for cooperative effort to keep the balloon afloat, it stimulates the senses with colors, and it provides physical exercise.

(Courtesy Charter Behavioral Health Center, San Diego, Calif.).

3. A tendency toward isolation.

4. Low self-concept and lack of self-confidence.

5. Difficulty acting independently, including accepting responsibility and problem solving.

RECREATIONAL THERAPIST'S ACTIVITY AND OBJECTIVES, AND THE NURSE'S ROLE

• Plan a unit dance with the highest-functioning clients and assign specific preparation tasks to foster independence, responsibility, and problem-solving skills. These tasks include decorating the craft room, preparing snacks, selecting music, and designing a flyer to announce the dance to the staff and other clients on the unit.

  Nurse's Role: Demonstrate enthusiasm, encouragement, and support and assist clients with problem-solving these tasks through role modeling.

• Provide a safe, "normal" environment for clients, to decrease isolation and increase the opportunity to practice appropriate social skills.

  Nurse's Role: Engage the clients in a discussion regarding the upcoming dance, thus promoting anticipation and modeling social interaction.

• Encourage participation in dancing styles that clients are familiar with or can easily learn, to increase self-confidence and social contact, and provide an outlet for emotions through movement, spontaneity, and play.

  Nurse's Role: Encourage clients to participate in the dancing; involve the more timid clients by dancing with them; engage lower-functioning clients who are on the periphery by sitting with them and conversing whenever possible.

• Provide the clients with a safe, enjoyable activity that will promote fun and mental health.

  Nurse's Role: Role-model healthy enjoyment in response to recreation.

ART THERAPY

Throughout history, art has been an important means of expression. In prehistoric times, symbols and images were the primary forms of communication. In 2500 B.C., the Greeks used stone carvings to represent their gods. The early Christian church used paintings and sculpture to educate and stimulate intense emotion in people who were predominantly illiterate.

It was not until 1922, however, that art was additionally appreciated for representing inner psychologic processes when Hans Prinzhorn put together a collection of artwork from asylum clients in Europe. Art was also recognized as a bridge between the client's inside and outside world when Sigmund Freud described the unconscious and its expression in imagery, especially in dreams. Freud often provided his clients with paints to re-create their dreams because they had difficulty de-

scribing dream images in words alone. As Freud wrote, "Part of the difficulty of giving an account of dreams, is due to our having to translate these images into words. 'I could draw it,' a dreamer often says to us 'but I don't know how to say it.'" (Freud, 1963). Carl Jung (1964) took the symbolism in artwork a step farther when he realized that art gave form to the conscious and the unconscious. Jung observed that many symbols crossed over cultures and generations, which suggested that a "universal unconscious" was being communicated in art.

Art therapy was formalized in the United States as a therapy in its own right in the 1940s. Margaret Naumburg and Edith Kramer were two leaders of this movement. The American Art Therapy Association was organized in 1965.

Naumburg, influenced by Sigmund Freud, viewed art therapy from a psychoanalytic perspective. She recognized the art experience as a release of unconscious material and encouraged her clients to engage in free associations about their artwork (Naumburg, 1966). Edith Kramer, on the other hand, concentrated on the creative process itself as curative. She believed that art paralleled life, and in art, life could be "practiced," "changed," and "repeated," without negative consequences.

Elinor Ulman expanded the scope of art therapy for psychotic clients by increasing directiveness and focusing more on building defenses against unconscious material. Ulman saw art therapy as ". . . a way to bring order out of chaos-chaotic feelings and impulses within, the bewildering mass of impressions from without. It is a means to discover both the self and the world, and to establish a relation between the two" (Ulman and Dachinger, 1975).

Art therapy is defined by the American Art Therapy Association (1965) as follows:

Art therapy includes a range of endeavors facilitated by a therapist trained in visual arts and behavioral science: one is the use of art as a non-verbal means of communication and expression using various art media that, in conjunction with the individual's verbal associations and explorations, enable diagnostic assessment and planned therapeutic interventions related to understanding and working through emotional problems and conflicts; and involvement in the artistic process itself is therapeutic through the age-old power of the arts to alleviate distress, problem-solve, reduce physical or psychological impairment, reconcile conflict and promote positive development in the individual.

Art therapy can be viewed from many of the same schools of thought as verbal therapies. The most common theories applied are psychoanalytic, gestalt, developmental, and behavioral. Despite the range of theories, it is generally agreed by art therapists that art allows for diverse elements of experience to be communicated simultaneously in a single expressive way.

The **art medium,** or art materials generally used, require little or no technical knowledge, and artistic training is not necessary. In fact, as developmental theorists have observed, healthy people physically and intellectually progress naturally through stages of artistic development up to the age of 12, without any artistic training or talent. For example, children between the ages of 0 and 1 scribble, and children between the ages of 9 and 12 deal in "schemas," or repeated symbols. Viktor Lowenfield (1970) observed and documented these stages, adding further insight and validity to the interpretation of art. In fact, the level at which a client draws can be extremely valuable information in determining his or her intellectual capacity as well as the age of emotional or cognitive injury. For example, a verbally articulate and high-functioning adult may appear comfortable working with the art materials until a theme about relationships is introduced, at which time the art style regresses to age 5. This would suggest issues regarding relationships that began at the age of 5.

It is critical that the client's diagnosis and level of functioning be taken into consideration when selecting the art materials to be used because some medium, such as finger paints and clay, promote regression, while pencils and marking pens promote defenses against regression. In other words, a client with obsessive-compulsive disorder might be encouraged to progress from pencils to paints and to a larger piece of paper, while a client with schizophrenia would be given more structured materials such as colored pencils, marking pens, and a defined space within which to draw.

The primary goals of the art therapist are to:

- Provide a safe environment free of judgment and censorship for the expression of feelings, cognitions, and unconscious material.
- Select a medium that will promote the therapeutic balance between regression and the use of healthy defenses.
- Encourage clients to verbally share their artwork with the therapist, individually, or with a group, to increase insight and promote a connection with others.
- Provide a creative experience as an outlet for emotions, cognitions, and perceptions.
- Expose clients to art materials in order for them to benefit from the curative qualities of color and design.

Clinical Example: Art Therapy

A group of ten adolescent boys and girls, ages 14–17, being treated in an adolescent residential treatment facility, present with a range of DSM-IV, Axis I diagnoses that include major depressive disorder, moderate, and conduct disorders.

ASSESSMENT

1. Difficulty expressing thoughts and emotions in a safe and productive way.
2. Impaired social-interpersonal skills.

3. Low self-esteem.
4. Difficulty with issues of separation, individuation, and identity.
5. Poor problem-solving skills.
6. Low impulse-control and low frustration level.
7. Limited insight and awareness of problems.

ART THERAPY ACTIVITY SESSION AND OBJECTIVES, AND THE NURSE'S ROLE

- Materials provided are liquid paint tempura, pastels, self-hardening clay, watercolors, colored marking pens, pencils, erasers, and white drawing paper of varying sizes. The variety of materials for this group allows for a wide range of expression and an opportunity for the therapist to observe the level of defenses used.
  Nurse's Role: Assist art therapist in putting out the materials and observe the clients as they interact with the materials. Which materials do they select? Are they using these materials appropriately?

- The art therapist may provide a theme for the clients to draw. For example, the therapist may say, "Draw a picture of yourself in a box and show how you would get out of the box. The box can be any size or shape and made out of any material you choose. You can get out of the box any way you choose." This theme addresses problem-solving skills, both in dealing with the blank piece of paper and with the theme of getting out of the box. Also, working individually with the art promotes individuation and, as with all art production, a healthy outlet for expression of thoughts and feelings.
  Nurse's Role: The nurse may participate in the art production, providing his or her own drawing. This can be beneficial in reducing the level of anxiety within the group, as well as serving as another means for the nurse to connect with the clients.

- The group is told at the outset that anything they put down on paper is acceptable. For example, at the beginning of each session, the therapist may state, "There is no right or wrong, good or bad, or censorship here." This establishes a safe, judgment-free environment that allows for increased self-expression. This unconditional acceptance also enhances self-esteem by providing a successful experience.
  Nurse's Role: Support the nonjudgmental environment by not commenting on the artistic value of the art productions or influencing their content by suggesting additions or deletions. Rather, the nurse's most important contribution is to treat all art productions with merit and value, even a blank piece of paper presented as a finished product.

- Clients are encouraged to verbally share their finished products with the group. The art therapists leads a discussion exploring the metaphor of the box as a problem and the act of getting out of the box as representation of how the clients solve their problems. This promotes further awareness and appreciation of the content of the artwork.

Nurse's Role: Participate in discussion by sharing any honest observations or feelings elicited by each client's artwork, without judgment, and valuing all expression (for example, "When I look at your picture I see . . ." or ". . . I feel . . ."; "I wonder if . . .").

- Following the art therapy session, the art therapist will assess the artwork for additional information regarding intellectual capacity, level of depression, elements of suicidal ideation, impulse control, and defenses used.

  Nurse's Role: Share *any* observations with the art therapist.

MUSIC THERAPY

Music can be found in every culture throughout history. Although originally used in rituals and ceremonies for religious and curative purposes, music has come to be recognized as both a science and an art. In our contemporary society, music is used to achieve ambiance in the home, in restaurants, in places of business, and in shopping malls. It creates mood in movies. It is an entertainment medium in its own right. And it is an accompaniment for dance. Since the eighteenth century, music has been documented as effecting healing, and it was used during both World Wars I and II as therapy with wounded soldiers.

Music is defined as "the science or art of assembling or performing intelligible combinations of tones in organized structured form, with infinitive varieties of expression possible, depending on the relation of its several component factors of rhythm, melody, volume and tonal quality" (Gaston, 1957).

Music becomes **music therapy** when it is used to bring about a specific change in the person who listens to it or performs it. "The responses will be neurophysiological, endocrinological, psychological, and sociological. . . We react through our own interpretations, integrated through our own experiences, augmented by our own emotional feedback system, which makes it even more forceful and meaningful" (Gaston, 1957).

Music therapy allows for an immediate experience within a defined structure, promoting both self-organization and social connection. The music medium is selected based on the client's age, the level of cognitive functioning, and the client's ego strength. The therapeutic process may incorporate recorded music, song writing, movement and music, or the use of instruments that allow the client to create music easily, with little or no formal training. For music to be universally accepted by a diverse group of people, it must contain neutral sounds instead of recognizable tunes embraced only by a specific age group. Technically, the musical qualities should be characterized by a slow tempo; a slow irregular, and unpredictable rhythm; and a certain homoge-

nous monotony throughout (Goddaer and Abraham, 1994).

Clinical Example: Music Therapy

Six adult clients attending a day treatment program are admitted to the program with DSM-IV, Axis I diagnosis of major depression.

ASSESSMENT

1. Difficulty expressing feelings verbally.
2. Poor interpersonal skills.
3. Low self-esteem.
4. Tendency to isolate and avoid conflict.
5. Low attention span and difficulty with concentration.
6. Difficulty taking responsibility for own actions and feelings.

MUSIC THERAPY ACTIVITY AND OBJECTIVES, AND THE NURSE'S ROLE

- Direct each member of the group to select a song that describes how he or she feels, and another song that describes how he or she would like to feel. This allows each person to individually explore his or her own feelings in a nonverbal, nonthreatening way.

  Nurse's Role: Participation in the activity to decrease group anxiety and model healthy behavior.

- Play each member's song for the group and encourage discussion, to provide further awareness and identification of feelings, catharsis of feelings, increased spontaneous verbalization, decreased isolation, and increased attention span.

  Nurse's Role: Provide nonjudgmental validation of feelings and modeling of interpersonal social skills.

MOVEMENT/DANCE THERAPY

Dance has been used throughout history for celebration, worship, mourning, and healing. Movement/dance therapy is often described as the oldest of the expressive therapies, with many of its concepts taken from the Classical Greeks, and the religious and healing application of dance from the Orient.

In the early twentieth century, Isadora Duncan developed a framework by which modern dance and movement/dance therapy are defined. Duncan's basic concept was that "physical movement is the natural, biological reaction of man to inner emotion or 'the soul' . . . " (Rosen, 1974). Movement/dance therapy was formally described in the United States by in 1942 Marion Chase. Chase recognized **movement** as a direct expression of the self through the body, promoting increased awareness of the body and changes in feeling states, cognitions, and behavior. She also noted that this increased awareness of the body in space allowed distorted body image perceptions to be confronted and corrected.

Movement/dance therapy is defined as "a therapeutic modality in which . . . individuals are encouraged to express emotion, work off tensions, develop an improved body image, and achieve greater body awareness and social interaction through rhythmic exercises and responses to music" (Goldenson, 1984) (see Fig. 24-2).

The movement/dance therapist initially observes the client's movements as they reflect psychologic difficulties. The therapist then presents themes to alter the movements, thereby affecting the emotions and cognition. The flow of the session is established as the movement therapist facilitates the client's spontaneous movements and connects them to the movements of others with such methods as **mirroring** the action, extending it, changing it, or moving in opposition to it. This linking of material is based on the movement therapist's assessment of the process as it unfolds. There are three parts of this process:

1. The **warm-up** heightens the client's awareness of his or her physical and emotional state and increases comfort with movement. The warm-up focuses on introducing group members, increasing the comfort level, and determining the theme or issues to be addressed.

2. The **theme-development stage** explores specific issues or feelings.

3. In **closure,** the experience is processed verbally and nonverbally to promote insight and a sense of completion.

As Marian Chase recognized, "Those who have been helped are the ones who know what happened" (Charklin, 1975).

Clinical Example: Movement/Dance Therapy

Six female clients in a partial hospitalization eating disorders program, with DSM-IV, Axis I diagnoses of anorexia nervosa or bulimia nervosa, were prescribed a weekly movement therapy group.

ASSESSMENT

1. Low self-esteem.

2. Distorted body image.

3. Experience of detachment from the body.

4. Inability to identify and express feelings and cognitions in a healthy manner.

5. Poor interpersonal and social skills.

6. Difficulty with spontaneity.

7. Self-deprecating thoughts and low tolerance for error.

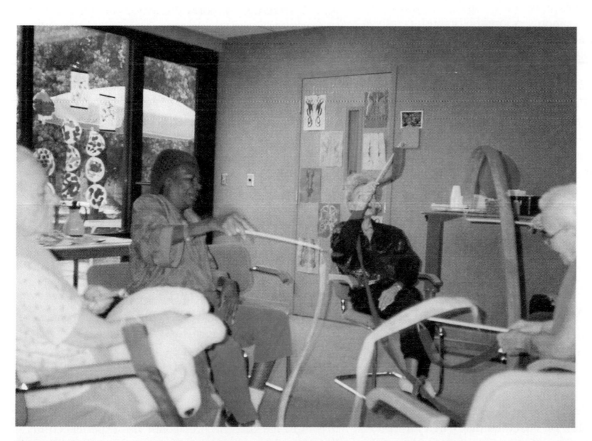

Figure 24-2 Wands with colorful material attached to the end are used to provide exercise, stimulate the imagination, and provide sensory stimulation through the vivid colors.

(Courtesy Charter Behavioral Health Center, San Diego, Calif.)

8. Poor definition and implementation of physical, sexual, and internal boundaries.

MOVEMENT THERAPY ACTIVITY AND OBJECTIVES, AND THE NURSE'S ROLE

- A *warm-up* exercise is presented with relaxation techniques that include lying on mats and using diaphragmatic breathing to relax. The clients are encouraged to note any specific tension in their bodies and to observe any emotions. This experience decreases anxiety and promotes body awareness and attention to feelings.
  Nurse's Role: Participate actively in the relaxation exercise to decrease the client's resistance and anxiety.

- The clients are presented with a theme regarding boundaries and are instructed to select one partner to explore the issues of defining and defending boundaries. A towel is given to one member in each pair and told that the towel "belongs" to her alone. The partner is instructed to attempt to take the towel away and claim it as hers. This experience allows the emotional and kinesthetic (movement) experiences of defending that which belongs exclusively to the individual, whether the towel represents physical, sexual, or internal boundaries. Self-esteem is also increased as the client is presented the opportunity to successfully "take a stand" in his or her own defense. Also, it allows for an increased awarenes of the body and its strength, and promotes spontaneity and creative problem solving.
  Nurse's Role: Observe and encourage those individuals who display passivity, ambivalence, or difficulty maintaining boundaries. Note the various attempts, effective or ineffective, by the clients to defend their boundaries. Be prepared to participate if modeling or an additional partner is needed.

- The theme is followed by closure in the form of an open discussion in which each client is encouraged to talk about the experience and problem-solve alternative ways to deal with the situation.
  Nurse's Role: Share observations honestly, draw the quiet or withdrawn client into the discussion whenever possible, and acknowledge when a client has taken a risk and validate his or her efforts.

PSYCHODRAMA

Psychodrama was developed in the early 1900s by Jacob L. Moreno, a Romanian psychiatrist, and grew out of the principle that play is therapeutic. In 1934 he founded the Psychodrama Institute in Beacon, New York. Moreno viewed people as "natural role players" and believed that health was promoted from the spontaneous expression of many diverse roles. He observed that when this spontaneity is curtailed, the self cannot emerge, and growth and change are not permitted to take place.

Psychodrama is a form of therapy that " . . . uses a wide range of action methods to examine one's subjective experience and to promote constructive change through the development of new perceptions, behaviors and connections with others" (Hornyak and Baker, 1989).

Psychodrama uses dramatic techniques to "act out" the emotional problem. The drama includes six operational aspects, which are listed in Box 24-1.

Clients may use this modality to reenact past situations, address present dilemmas, or explore future expectations and fantasies. Addressing these problems in the "here and now" allows for increased awareness of the problems and an opportunity to actively work them through. The primary goal of psychodrama is to provide an experience that allows behavior to become "visible and measurable, then reintegrate the behavior" into the client's unconscious (Landy, 1986). Further, Moreno focused on developing spontaneity, increasing a repetoire for responding to new situations and resolving repressed emotions from the past.

There are three parts of a psychodrama:

1. In the **warm-up,** the group is prepared by introducing the members to each other, and the protagonist and situation are chosen.

2. In the **enactment,** or action portion, one scene or a sequence of scenes is portrayed.

3. The **sharing** promotes discussion among the group members about the enactment, as well as the individual experiences and reactions to the process (Fleshman and Fryrear, 1981).

Psychodrama is a powerful form of therapy. Therefore, the techniques need to be applied carefully with

---

Box 24-1   Elements of a Psychodrama

1. The **protagonist,** usually the client—the individual who presents and acts out his or her emotional problems and interpersonal relationships.

2. The **auxillary ego,** or **alter ego,** chosen by the protagonist from the group to portray significant others in the life of the client.

3. The **director** or **psychodramatist.**

4. **Doubles,** who operate as the "inner voices" of the protagonist to express repressed thoughts, feelings, and conflicts.

5. The **group,** which provides observation and support and benefits from its own catharsis and identification.

6. The **space,** which can symbolize any environment or time that the protagonist has experienced or imagined.

specific attention given to the level of functioning and ego strengths of the clients in the group. For example, fantasy and emotionally charged expression can be used for high-functioning, nonpsychotic groups, while reality-based role-play is best used when working with clients with schizophrenia or even clients with borderline personality disorder.

Clinical Example: Psychodrama

Eight men and women, ranging from ages 24–40, are participating in an outpatient group for unresolved grief. All the group members have lost a significant family member. A 32-year-old woman is identified during the warm-up as the protagonist. She is a single woman who has struggled with major depression, single episode, and bulimia nervosa since the untimely death of her mother to cancer when the client was 18 years old. The woman describes her grief and her regret that she arrived too late to the hospital to say good-bye to her mother before she died.

ASSESSMENT

Unresolved grief resulting in the following:

1. Denial
2. Guilt
3. Repressed anger
4. Depression
5. Isolation and withdrawal
6. Difficulty with interpersonal relationships

PSYCHODRAMA ACTIVITY AND OBJECTIVES, AND THE NURSE'S ROLE

- During the warm-up, the protagonist is encouraged to choose someone to act as her auxiliary ego (her mother) and other group members to act as doubles ("inner voices") to help her verbalize her repressed thoughts, feelings, and conflicts. A hospital stage is set, and the other group members position themselves where they can observe unintrusively. The client describes how her mother would have been expected to respond (for example, nurturing, withdrawn, hostile, responsive, etc.). As the protagonist talks about her loss and sets the scene for the enactment, she is addressing denial and increasing contact with others.
  Nurse's Role: Assist director in determining who the protagonist will be by observing who speaks first in the group or appears most tense or anxious, and invite him or her into the preliminary warm-up discussion.

- The enactment allows the protagonist to have the dialogue with her mother that she was unable to have before her mother died. The client is encouraged to tell her mother anything she wishes, especially those things that have felt unfinished. This is an opportunity

for guilt and anger to be resolved and the grieving process to finally be initiated.
Nurse's Role: It is possible that the nurse will be asked to participate in the enactment, either as the auxiliary ego or as a double. It is important that participation is honest and sensitive to the grieving process.

- The closure involves discussion with the protagonist, auxiliary ego, doubles, and group members regarding feelings and thoughts resulting from the enactment. Feedback and observations are also made at this time. This is an opportunity for the therapist to assess the degree of movement in initiating the grieving process for the protagonist, as well as for other group members. The therapist also uses this time to help the group move out of the intense feeling state, and reinstate a healthy distance from the experience.
  Nurse's Role: Observe if the clients appear anxious or withdrawn, or markedly upset, and encourage them to process their reactions within the group. "Normalize" their reactions whenever possible by relating them to the stages of grief, using reflective and empathic listening skills.

Summary of Key Concepts

1. Adjunct therapies, also known as expressive, experimental, or activity therapies, include occupational, recreational, art, music, movement/dance, and psychodrama.

2. The primary intention of adjunct therapies is to increase the client's awareness of feelings, behavior, perceptions, cognitions, and sensations.

3. Adjunct therapies are used in a variety of therapeutic settings.

4. It is important for the nurse to become familiar with specific adjunct therapies in order to recommend one to the primary physician and to support all members of the treatment team.

5. Occupational therapy focuses on assessment of task performance, cognitive functioning, psychosocial development, recognizing strengths and improving weaknesses, and adapting to change.

6. The nurse's role in occupational therapy includes daily contact with clients to provide encouragement, support, role modeling, assisted teaching, and to encourage discussion and reality testing in self-care and maintenance tasks.

7. Recreational therapy incorporates the active process of demonstrating and applying observable skills within the curative elements of play to assist clients in developing leisure skills and interests suitable to their lifestyles.

8. The nurse's role in recreational therapy is to demonstrate enthusiasm, encouragement, and health enjoyment, as well as assisting the client through role

modeling and interaction for recreational tasks that foster independence, responsibility, and problem-solving skills.

9. Art therapy, the use of art as a nonverbal means of communication by an individual, can increase understanding in working through emotional problems and conflicts.

10. The nurse's role in art therapy can be to put out materials and observe clients use those materials, as well as to participate in the clients' projects and provide support and discussion by sharing honest observations and not commenting on artistic values or influencing the content through suggestion.

11. Music therapy is used to bring about specific change in the client and allows for an experience within a defined structure, thus promoting self-organization, social connection, and expression.

12. The nurse's role in music therapy may be to participate in the activity, to decrease anxiety, to model healthy behavior, and to provide nonjudgmental validation of feelings.

13. Movement/dance therapy encourages individual expression of emotion to work off tensions, develop improved body image, and achieve body awareness and social interaction through rhythmic exercises and responses to music.

14. The nurse's role in movement/dance therapy may be to participate in the activity, observe and encourage all clients with honest observations, and to promote discussion when possible.

15. Psychodrama uses spontaneous expression and dramatic techniques to act out emotional problems to promote health through the development of new perceptions, behaviors, and connections with others.

16. The nurse's role in psychodrama may be to assist, participate in, and encourage participation of clients and to listen and relate their reaction.

REFERENCES

American Art Therapy Association. Baltimore, 1965.

American Occupational Therapy Association: Occupational therapy: its definition and function, *Amer J Occupational Therapy* 26:204, 1972.

Charklin H: *Marion Chase, her papers,* Columbia, Md., 1975, American Dance Therapy Association.

Fleshman B, Fryrear JL: *The arts in therapy,* Chicago, 1981, Nelson-Hall.

Freud S: "Dreams," *New introductory lectures on psychoanalysis,* vol XV, London, 1963, The Hogarth Press.

Gaston E: Factors contributing to responses in music. In *Book of proceedings,* Kansas City, Kansas, 1957, National Association for Music Therapy.

Gaston E: *Music in therapy,* New York, 1968, Macmillan.

Goddaer J, Abraham IL: Effects of relaxing music on agitation during meals among nursing home residents with severe cognitive impairment, *Arch Psychiatric Nur* 8(3): 150–158, June 1994.

Goldenson RM, editor: *Longman dictionary of psychology and psychiatry,* New York, 1984, Longman.

Haun P: *Recreation: a medical viewpoint,* New York, 1965, Teachers College.

Hornyak LM, Baker EK: *Experiential therapies for eating disorders,* New York, 1989, Guilford Press.

Jung CG: *Man and his symbols,* New York, 1964, Doubleday.

Kaplan HI, Sadock BJ: *Comprehensive textbook of psychiatry,* ed 6, Baltimore, 1995, Williams and Wilkins.

Landy RJ: *Drama therapy: concepts and practices,* Springfield, Ill., 1986, Charles C. Thomas.

Lowenfield V, Brittain WC: *Creative and mental growth,* ed 5, New York, 1970, Macmillan.

Naumburg M: *Dynamically oriented art therapy: its principles and practice,* New York, 1966, Grune & Stratton.

Rosen E: *Dance in psychotherapy,* New York, 1974, A Dance Horizons Republication.

Ulman E, Dachinger P, editors: *Art therapy in theory and practice,* New York, 1975, Schocken Books.

Nursing Implications for Contemporary Issues

Wawa Aba
ASHANTI, WEST AFRICA

The seeds of the owawa tree that are represented by this symbol are extremely hard. The symbol infers that hardiness and a sense of purpose can assist individuals to overcome difficult events, situations, and circumstances. The chapters in Part Six discuss significant contemporary issues that can have psychiatric implications.

CHAPTER 25

Survivors of Violence

Joan Urbancic

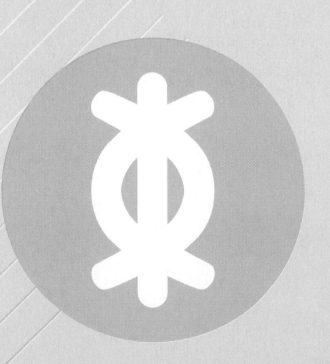

Battered wife Women who are abused physically or mentally by their male intimates or those with whom they have been intimate.

Childhood incest Any type of exploitative sexual experience between relatives or surrogate relatives before the victim reaches the age of 18.

Child neglect Harm or threatened harm to a child's health or welfare by a parent, legal guardian, or any other person responsible for the child's health or welfare through either failure to provide adequate food, clothing, shelter, or medical care; or by placing the child's health or welfare at unreasonable risk.

Child physical abuse Inflicted injury to a child that can range from minor bruises and lacerations to severe neurological trauma and death. Psychological abuse is also included.

Child psychologic abuse Rejection, degradation/devaluation, terrorization, isolation, corruption, exploitation, denying essential stimulation to a child, or unreliable and inconsistent parenting.

Elder abuse Includes psychological or emotional neglect, psychological or emotional abuse, violation of personal rights, financial abuse, physical neglect, or direct physical abuse to persons over 65 years of age.

Machismo Compulsive masculinity characterized by a male's excessive need to control and dominate his wife at all costs.

Social learning theory Bandura's theory that aggression is not instinctual, but a learned behavior.

Transgenerational violence When violence within the family is an accepted everyday occurrence, a natural, normal component of family living.

- Analyze various theories of family violence for application to nursing practice.
- Discuss conditions that discourage a battered woman from leaving her violent situation.
- Discuss the role of "control" in the etiology of domestic violence.
- Compare the child physical offender with the child sexual offender.
- Describe the common characteristics of victims of family violence.
- Apply the nursing process in the care of victims of family violence.
- Construct examples of how women who are raped are revictimized by society.

Violence in the United States has become a major concern of contemporary American society. According to the Federal Bureau of Investigation (1985), the United States has the highest murder rate among advanced capitalist countries (7.9 per 100,000). One million American residents die each year as a result of intentional homicide or suicide. The primary cause of death for both black and white male teenagers in the United States is gunshot wounds; suicide is the third leading cause of death among children and adolescents. France's death rate from trauma is 66% of the U.S. rate, whereas that of the Netherlands is 39% of the U.S. rate.

The perpetrator of interpersonal violence is often believed by the public to be a drug-addicted male or someone who has gone berserk. Most often the public believes the potential attacker is a stranger to the victim. In reality, interpersonal violence is usually committed by someone the victim knows well—a close friend or family member. The belief that people are safe in their own homes and that family violence is rare is a myth that is difficult to dispel. A women is much more likely to be beaten, raped, and/or murdered by a partner or ex-partner than a stranger. In a significant study, Straus and Gelles (1986) reported that one out of eight intact couples had an incident in which the husband was physically aggressive toward his wife in the last year. One-third of these aggressive

579

acts were severely abusive and included such behaviors as punching, kicking, choking, beating, or using a knife or gun.

Reports of child abuse and neglect by parents or other caretakers exceed two million a year (American Humane Society, 1988). Children are much more likely to be sexually abused by a family member than by someone unknown to them. The same holds true for elder abuse. Each year one million elderly are typically abused by their own children or spouses (Straus and Gelles, 1986). Thus family members are at much greater risk of being abused by another family member than they are by a stranger. Family violence is multicausal and highly complex. Usually it is insidious in onset and occurs together with a variety of interrelated factors. Despite the many contributing factors, it is the sociocultural attitudes toward women, children, and the elderly and the value placed on violence to solve problems that underlie and support family violence.

Straus et al, (1980) have noted that a marriage license is really a hitting license. The U.S. Commission on the Causes and Prevention of Violence (Stark and McElroy, 1970) found that one in four men and one in six women believed that hitting between married couples was valid at times. The respondents in this same study also believed that children need "strong" discipline. Thus, there is strong societal support for violence in the family.

Because of beliefs about the privacy and sanctity of the family, interfamilial violence generally remains hidden; nurses, doctors, and other health care professionals maintain the dark secret of family violence by their conspiracy of silence. This is true despite the heavy media attention given to family violence in recent years.

The most dramatic examples of failure by health care professionals to address family violence are reflected in studies that have examined battered women's experiences when seeking health care services. In general, these studies (Drake, 1982; Goldberg and Tomlanovich, 1985; Kurz, 1987; Warshaw, 1989) have reported a lack of assessment, intervention, and responsiveness by doctors and nurses in the treatment of battered women. In a qualitative study, Kurz documented the subtle blaming and rejection of battered women by nurses and other personnel in emergency room settings.

Recently the Joint Commission on Accreditation of Healthcare Organizations (JCAHO) has mandated policies and procedures for the assessment, treatment, and referral of victims of violence. Following the JCAHO mandate, in 1992 the American Medical Association took steps to recognize and intervene in domestic violence by developing guidelines for practice.

Thus, awareness is developing that the growing problem of family violence must be addressed on multiple levels. Because nurses interact with families and individuals in a wide variety of settings, they have frequent opportunities to identify and intervene therapeutically with victims of family violence. One wonders why nurses have often failed to be therapeutic with victims of family violence in the past. Some explanations state that lack of knowledge, stereotypes, prejudices, and poor role models are factors. King and Ryan (1989) found that 18% of nurses in their study reported being victims of physical and emotional abuse, and another 28% reported abuse among family members. Nurses are certainly not exempt from violence in their own lives; to confront violence in the lives of others may be too painful a reminder of what has occurred in the histories of many nurses. Thus, it may be less painful to deny the existence of family violence than to confront it.

This chapter will discuss the various types of family violence: wife battering, child physical and sexual abuse, and elder abuse. Although it is recognized that domestic violence may at times be mutual, the woman is typically the victim. Most important, repeated studies have indicated that women usually do not initiate the violence and when they are violent toward their partners, it is usually in self-defense. Because of their lack of power and authority in the family, women are much more vulnerable to battering and abuse. Dobash and Dobash (1979) claim that the type of violent abuse that is repetitive, extending and escalating over time with minimal or no motivation and characterized by forced control, is limited to the male abuse of females.

DEFINITIONS OF VIOLENCE AND ABUSE

A major problem in the field of family violence has been the difficulty in developing useful and clear definitions of violence and abuse. Some researchers have defined violence on the basis of physical injury only; others insist that mental injury must also be included in the definition. Severe psychological abuse can often occur without visible physical symptoms; therefore, it is critical to use a broad, holistic approach in the assessment of family violence.

Still others argue for a definition that would consider the intent of the abuser. Gelles and Cornell (1990) point out that if a father shoots a gun at his child but misses, his behavior would not quality as violent by many definitions. Thus, these researchers maintain that harmful acts, whether they result in physical injury, should be included in the definition of violence and abuse.

There is sharp disagreement on whether spanking constitutes violent and abusive behavior. Many parents use spanking at least occasionally. Gelles and Cornell (1990) have suggested making a distinction between "so-called normal" acts of force such as spanking versus harmful acts of violence. However, the question continues to be: What is harmful? Such determinations may be significantly different from one cultural group to another.

THEORIES OF FAMILY VIOLENCE

The following discussion focuses on a number of models that attempt to explain family violence (Box 25-1). Although some models have better explanations than others, no single model is able to fully explain family violence. Various statistics on family violence are listed in Box 25-2.

The Psychiatric/Mental Illness Model

This model focuses on the individual characteristics of the abuser or victim to explain the phenomenon at hand. Thus, the person who severely injures an innocent child is said to be psychotic or mentally disturbed. It is interesting to note that when the victim is a battered woman, she (rather than the abuser) is the focus of attention and is judged to be mentally defective (masochistic) for remaining with the abuser. Only recently has the spotlight turned to examining the characteristics of the abuser instead of placing blame on the victim. Some psychiatrists continue to maintain that battered women are masochistic and choose to remain in an abusive relationship in order to satisfy their unconscious need for punishment. Thus, within the psychiatric model—defects in the individual (abuser or victim), such as mental illness, alcohol, drugs, and personality disorders—are seen as being the causative factors in family violence. Interventions would focus on changing the personality characteristics of the person, and factors outside the individual would not be a focus within this model. The psychiatric model is very popular and commonly used because it is comforting for society to believe that it is the "abnormal or deranged" person who abuses others or chooses to remain in an abusive relationship. Because most people do not consider themselves mentally ill, they do not question their potential for abuse or examine their behavior if they are abusive.

In reality, only a small percentage of abusers have been found to possess characteristics that indicate some type of psychopathology. Gelles and Cornell (1990) reported that there is no consistent evidence for a psychopathological profile for abusive parents. Batterers and their victims were not found to be significantly different from the rest of the population in terms of mental illness (Campbell and Humphreys, 1993). No evidence has been found to support the theory that women remain in abusive relationships because they are masochistic.

Social Learning Theory

Social learning theory is based on aggression research by the psychologist Albert Bandura (1973). This model combines components of behavioral and sociological theories. In Bandura's model, aggression is not viewed as instinctual but rather as learned behavior. Although Bandura does recognize neurophysiologic structures that produce aggressive behavior, he maintains that these biologic mechanisms are dependent on appropriate stimulation in order to be activated, and even when these mechanisms are activated, aggressive behavior remains under cognitive control.

Bandura's research demonstrates that children learn how to behave by observing the role models in their own families. Values, attitudes, and behaviors are shaped and developed by significant others in a child's life. Thus, the manner in which parents cope with stress, anger, and frustration becomes a powerful lesson for the impressionable and innocent child.

Because family role models are usually the ones that a child has most exposure to, the child assumes that the family behavior is normal and acceptable even though it may be highly violent and abusive. Physical discipline by parents gives the message to the child that punishment is necessary to enforce rules and gain compliance. In this sense, the use of violence or physical force is reinforcing because of the power obtained from its use. Besides role modeling in the family, children learn aggressive behavior through direct experience, practice, and observation of other mediums of violence.

Box 25-1   Etiologic Theories Related to Family Violence

Psychiatric/mental illness model

Social learning theory

- Aggression as a learned behavior—not instinctual
- Family role modeling
- Desensitization to violence through repeated exposure via the media

Sociological theory

- Unemployment
- Poverty
- Crime
- Teenage pregnancy
- Isolation

Anthropological theories

- Sexual inequalities
- Social organization
- Cultural patterning

Feminist theories

- Explanatory utility of constructs of gender and power
- Analysis of the family as a historically situated institution
- Importance of understanding and validating women's experiences
- Employing scholarship for women

Box 25-2 Epidemiology for Family Violence

Battered women

- 1.8 million wives in the United States are abused every year by their husbands

- Between 25% and 50% of all women are abused by their intimate partners at least once

- 20%–25% of women who seek treatment in emergency rooms are there because of battering injuries

- 2%–8% of these women identified abuse as the cause of their injuries

- 7%–17% of pregnant women experience physical abuse by their partners

Child physical abuse

- Physical abuse of children has increased 58% from 1980 to 1986

- 2 million children are seriously abused each year by their parents and caretakers

- Of these, 1,000 die from results of these injuries

- 25% of the 2 million abused children are physically abused, 20% are sexually abused, 55% are neglected

- 25% of the 2 million abused children are under age 5, 60% are between ages 5 and 14

- Children under age 3 are at a greater risk for fatal abuse than older children

- Abused and neglected children are at a greater risk for later delinquency, adult criminality, and violent crimes than nonabused or nonneglected children

Sexually abused children

- 50% of psychiatric clients have histories of physical and sexual abuse

- The average age at which child incest begins is age 6, with an average duration of 7 years

Rape

- Only one in 10% to 20% of rapes are reported to the police

- Over 90% of rape victims are women

- 20% of college women are raped at some time during their college careers

- The most common age group for rape victims is 16–25 years

- In 84% of rape cases, the victim is acquainted with the offender

- Only 5% of rapists were psychotic when they raped

- In 90% of rape cases, victims and perpetrators are of the same race

- 51% of males in a study reported that they would rape if they were certain they would not be punished

---

Support for social learning theory is seen in repeated generational patterns of family violence. Although exposure to family violence does not guarantee that the pattern of violence will be repeated in subsequent generations, it does increase the child's risk of using violent behavior in adulthood.

Much has been written about the influence of television, films, music, and other media to promote violence. Campbell and Humphreys (1993) described multiple studies supporting the contention that violence in the media (1) encourages aggressive behavior through modeling, (2) unsuppresses aggressive acting-out behaviors by repeated exposure, and (3) desensitizes people to violence around them. The desensitization to violence results in people becoming apathetic or unimpressed with the impact of violence on others. These research studies also suggested that repeated exposure to media violence increases feelings of insecurity, distrust, and suspiciousness. Bandura (1973) and other researchers who replicated his studies acknowledge that the vast majority of people do not act out the violence that they observe in the media. However, for the majority of heavy viewers of television violence, the world becomes a dangerous, unsafe place. Believing that the world is unsafe may predis-

pose people to misinterpret social cues and respond as though they are under attack even when they are not.

Sociological Theory

Sociological models recognize the influence of neurophysiological and psychological factors, but their focus is on the environmental and socioeconomic forces that underlie violence. Like social learning theorists, sociologists reject the notion that aggression is instinctual. According to these theories, conditions such as unemployment, crime, poverty, isolation, teenage pregnancy, and stress are the major concern in addressing violence in families. Many sociologists view violence in families as gender neutral, believing that both sexes play a role in the problem. Feminists criticized this stance because it minimizes the impact of male domination and power as a cause.

A wide variety of sociological theories abounds. Nye (1979) has noted that family violence is more common in (1) societies that lack legal or normative structural sanctions against the violence, (2) families that do not have extended family members available or nearby for formal and informal support, and (3) single-parent rather than in two-parent homes. Gelles and Cornell (1990) maintain

that violence occurs in families because it "can" occur. The challenge is to provide social controls by increasing the consequences of violence (imprisonment, fines, loss of status in the community, loss of family) and decreasing the rewards (power and control over family members).

Anthropological Theories

Cultural attitudes and definitions of abuse and violence can vary significantly from one society to another. Some societies may view particular behaviors by its members as violent; other societies may not. This lack of agreement on the perception of violence and abuse makes it difficult to establish a universal definition of family violence that will be culturally acceptable by various societies. Despite this lack of consensus on definitions, it is recognized that a number of nonviolent societies exist (Campbell, 1985; Eisler, 1988). Anthropological theories explain family violence in terms of various cultural influences such as sexual inequality, social organization, and cultural patterning. According to Campbell and Humphreys (1993), nonviolent societies tend to be more egalitarian (consisting of human equality) than hierarchical (consisting of social and political classes) in sex roles and ethnic group arrangements. Males and females cooperate more and have greater interdependence in their work roles, which extend to child care.

Feminist Theories

Multiple studies exist to demonstrate that batterers are characterized by an excessive need to control and dominate their wives at all costs. Campbell and Fishwick (1993) use the concept of **machismo,** or compulsive masculinity to explain wife abuse and violence against women. Although machismo is not the direct cause of family violence and wife abuse, it is helpful in understanding some of the complex factors that contribute to violence. According to these two researchers, violence is a central component of male social standing in Western culture. Male heroes are "Rambo" and "James Bond" types who are able to achieve success, admiration, and acceptance through machismo. Their relationships with women are characterized by disdain, control, dominance, and the treatment of women as commodities and sexual objects. Typically the male with high machismo believes it is his right and responsibility to control and beat his wife and children because they are his property to do with as he pleases. Campbell and Fishwick (1993) define machismo as "male attitudes and behavior arising from and supported by the patriarchal social structure that express sexism and male ownership of women, glorify violence, emphasize virility, and despise gentleness and the expression of any emotions except anger and rape" (p. 85).

Attitudes of machismo are linked with traditional patriarchal values that have a long and enduring history in the United States and have been the underlying basis for violence against women (Campbell and Fishwick, 1993). Barbee (1992) has described how men use culture, custom, and tradition as excuses for the continuation of violence against women. In particular, she described the combined impact of racism, sexism, and patriarchy on the African-American woman. The patriarchal cultural argument seems to be that if wife beating has been the tradition in a particular cultural group, then the male is not responsible because he is merely carrying on that tradition.

Although there are multiple feminist perspectives on family violence and wife abuse in particular, there are also basic areas of agreement. Bograd (1988) states that feminists are interested in asking the questions, "Why do men beat their female partners, and what purpose does this behavior satisfy for society at a given time?" Feminists are interested in men as a group rather than in examining the characteristics of specific males. Feminists also strongly believe that wife abuse must not be subsumed under such terms as *family violence* or *spouse abuse* because such language obscures the reality that, in the great majority of domestic violence cases, it is the woman who is battered. With generic terms the issues of power and control are not given the focus they must have in order for the dynamics of woman battering to be understood (Bograd, 1988).

THE BATTERED WOMAN

Battering is the most common cause of injury to women in the United States. Studies have reported that between 25% and 50% of all women are abused by their intimate partners at least once (Tilden and Shepherd, 1987). Although some women escape from their abusive partners, many remain in violent relationships in which the violence gradually escalates in frequency and severity.

Sampselle (1992) cautions nurses to be aware that one out of every ten women in any health care setting is a victim of abuse by her intimate mate. In emergency rooms the incidence is even higher. Of women who seek treatment in emergency rooms, 20%–25% are there because of battering injuries. Studies that have examined these emergency room records retrospectively reveal that only 2%–8% of women were identified as abused on their medical records (Campbell and Fishwick, 1993).

Among pregnant women, 7%–17% experience physical abuse by their partners. Effects of physical abuse on the pregnant woman are direct or indirect. Direct effects include low birth weight, preterm labor, preterm infants, and infant injury and death. Bohn and Parker (1993) report that indirect effects of physical abuse have a more profound effect on women's health than direct effects. Indirect effects include chronic pain, depression, high anxiety, use of drugs and alcohol, or suicide attempts by the women to escape their violent situations.

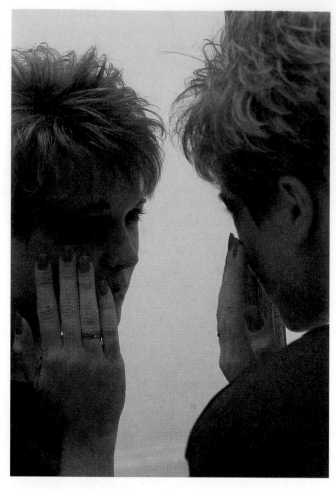

Figure 25-1 Physical abuse is the most common cause of injury to women in the United States. Battering occurs in all ethnic, religious, and socioeconomic groups. Although the batterer is unprovoked, the woman is made to feel it is her fault.

(Copyright © Cathy Lander-Goldberg, Lander Photographics.)

A number of studies have been done on battered women and their experiences with the health care system (Brendtro and Bowker, 1989; Drake, 1982; Goldberg and Tomlanovich, 1985; Kurz, 1987; Stark et al, 1979). These studies have documented: (1) the failure of doctors and nurses to make direct inquiries about how the women received their injuries even when women wanted to provide this information, (2) subtle blaming and negative labeling of the women, and (3) unnecessary or inappropriate medication such as tranquilizers. In an extensive survey of battered women who had sought support from various health care and helping professionals, Brendtro and Bowker reported in 1989 that "battered wives find health care services to be less effective than any other formal source of help, including the clergy, lawyers, police, district attorneys, social service and counseling agencies, women's groups and battered women's shelters" (p. 170).

Definition of the Battered Wife

The term **battered wife** is used in this chapter to mean women who are battered by their male intimates or those with whom they have been intimate. This includes ongoing and past relationships. Indeed, women are in greatest danger when they attempt to leave the controlling mate. Although it is recognized that violence exists between gay couples, this discussion focuses on the most common type of domestic violence, that of male abuser and female victim.

Abuse of the battered woman is not limited to physical abuse. For example, one survivor lived under the constant threat of a loaded gun pressed to her temple by her abuser but never received a bruise on her body. Such psychological abuse is devastating. Other battered women report that over time the physical abuse actually ends, but profound psychological abuse continues. This happens because the threat of violence so terrorizes the woman that the threat alone becomes the controlling force. For this reason, advocates for battered women define domestic violence as physical, psychological, and sexual abuse primarily directed at women by men for the purpose of maintaining power and control over the woman (Box 25-3).

Battered women represent all ethnic, religious, and socioeconomic groups. However, women from middle and upper socioeconomic groups can more easily hide their abuse. Material resources allow middle-class and upper-class women to be seen by a private physician who is more likely to keep their secret and frequently ask no questions. Other resources that may be available are members of the extended family who may agree to provide temporary shelter, summer homes to which the woman may retreat, and the financial support needed for the woman to leave the battering spouse and go to a hotel for a few days. The extended family of women with-

---

Box 25-3   Controlling Behaviors of the Abuser

1. Economic abuse—strict control of money (even when she earns it), food, clothing, transportation, and other resources

2. Sexual abuse—includes marital rape and forcing her to participate in sex against her will

3. Threats and intimidation including threats of taking the children from her or hurting them or other family members

4. Threatening to injure or kill family pets

5. Isolating her from any support system including her family, friends, and health care professionals

6. Constantly demeaning and insulting her

7. Intentionally breaking objects to terrorize her

out financial resources is often itself financially overburdened and thus unable to help. Such women do not possess the finances that would allow them to stay in a hotel for a few days. Consequently, most of the women seen in shelters for battered women are those without other options.

The Batterer

Too often the batterer is portrayed as a male who has temporarily lost control, usually under provocation. This loss of control is frequently blamed on alcohol or drugs. However, batterers abuse their partners while drunk or sober, and typically use drunkenness as an excuse. In reality, the object of the abuse is control. Despite numerous studies on the characteristics of the batterer, no evidence exists to support the belief that the typical batterer is an alcoholic or is mentally ill. Usually they are described by fellow workers as average, normal males, and they give no hint of the abusive behavior they mete out in the privacy of their own homes. Few batterers have criminal records or have physical altercations with others outside their homes. Indeed, such physical abuse against a stranger would result in arrest and incarceration. But the privacy of the homes has protected the batterer and continues to do so as society turns a blind eye. Batterers have learned that there are few if any consequences to their abusive behaviors. Indeed, the privacy and secrecy in which abuse toward women occurs is one of the main reasons why abuse continues.

THE NURSING PROCESS

■ ASSESSMENT

Assessment of the battered woman must begin with the nurse's critical examination of his or her own beliefs and biases about battered women. For example, a nurse who feels that the woman has brought the problem on herself for not leaving the abusive relationship will communicate this attitude, consciously or unconsciously, to the battered woman. Thus, nurses who act out of their own attitudes may result in the revictimization of battered women.

Because holistic assessments are the foundation of the nursing process, culture is an important consideration in that assessment and the subsequent treatment plan. Culture often defines how the battered woman will interpret and respond to the violence that has been committed against her. Understanding the battered woman's culture is also critical for developing a treatment plan for her.

Culture is also an important determinant of whether the battered woman seeks assistance from community resources such as the police and shelters. Women from some ethnic groups are very isolated and unaware of community resources for abuse or are suspicious of caregivers outside their own cultural group, fearing ostracization by their cultural group if they reach out to the broader community. Most battered women's shelters are making a concerted effort to reach out to women of all colors and ethnic groups. When caring for a client from a minority culture, it is the nurse's responsibility to learn about the client's culture in order to provide culturally sensitive care. Questions about the woman's culture are appropriate but must be presented in a sensitive, respectful manner so that the woman understands the nurse's concern in learning more about the woman's values and customs in order to provide effective, holistic nursing care.

An understanding of culture is equally important when working with the male batterer. Before treatment strategies can be planned for the abuser, his cultural attitudes and beliefs must be acknowledged and respected. However, no cultural beliefs and traditions can be accepted or tolerated at the expense of another person's health and well-being. Barbee (1992) suggests that the defense of abusive behaviors as being culture bound serves to maintain the status quo of patriarchy.

Because physical abuse of women by their partners is not uncommon, it is critical to ask about physical, sexual, and emotional abuse in the histories of all women. Battering during pregnancy (Bohn and Parker, 1993) is one of the major causes of complications during pregnancy, and nurses should assess for it. Even elderly widows may have serious unresolved issues relating to abusive relationships with their deceased husbands. Many battered women will report a myriad of physical problems without disclosing the source of violence. Because they have been programmed to believe that they somehow provoked the violence, battered women feel guilty and ashamed. Nevertheless, if asked directly and under appropriate conditions, most women will disclose the nature of their injuries. These conditions include being respectful and sensitive to the woman's disclosures and informing her that she is not at fault and that no human being has the right to abuse another. In addition, the nurse must provide a safe environment that is conducive

Nursing Care in the Community

Survivors of Violence

Survivors of trauma may be of any age, gender, or nationality. They share a bond in that their ability to enjoy fully functional lives has been altered by a disruptive event, be it molestation as a child, rape as an adult, or armed conflict in war. The event may involve family members or strangers, be life-threatening or totally demeaning, and the responses of family, friends, or society may be problematic.

The nurse in the community setting, who works with such a disparate group of clients, must be extremely flexible and accepting. As in other emotional disturbances, the presence of a strong supportive network is critical. Debriefing a traumatic incident requires a team effort in which the nurse may play a role as the individual counselor hearing every detail, or as the group facilitator helping the victims begin to repattern their lives and social interactions. The relationship will be on a longer-term basis than a crisis intervention in the controlled hospital environment.

Getting to the truth of such a situation is often difficult, as there may be a molester, rapist, or batterer involved who may still be threatening the survivor and even anyone who helps him or her. Nurses may feel angry at or fearful of the perpetrator and must carefully monitor their own reactions to the situation in order to establish trust and keep communication lines open. Other professions, including child protective services or the police, may be-

come involved, and communication channels must be clear and overt. There is no margin of error when dealing with such a potentially volatile situation as a parent molesting a child or a husband battering his wife.

Survivors of combat are often diagnosed with post-traumatic stress disorder. These persons have often led lives estranged from mainstream society and complicated by drug/alcohol abuse. They often respond with anger to any type of help offered and require prolonged, specialized counseling before they are willing to participate in group therapy. The community nurse may encounter these persons in homeless shelters or living on the street. The nurse must be able to tolerate frequent rebuffs before any sort of therapeutic relationship can be established. Patience and an appropriate sense of humor in a tense situation may often be the keys to interaction.

The nurse in the community may encounter victims with a strong sense of entitlement, who will emphasize their victimization to get special treatment. These individuals will quickly exhaust even the most patient mental health professional. Often such clients must be offered what is available and be told that no more will be forthcoming, despite their distress or anger. These situations often require a concerted effort from other disciplines, so that one person does not have to bear the brunt of the client's irritation.

---

to disclosure. The first step is to separate the woman from her abuser. On many occasions it will be obvious that the woman's partner is determined not to be separated from her. Nevertheless, separation must occur even if it means calling security personnel for assistance.

In the assessment and history-taking, it is recommended that the nurse begin with the least personal questions and gradually move to more personal ones. Questions should be simple and direct. The Nursing Research Consortium on Violence and Abuse has developed a simple four-item questionnaire that was adapted by Campbell and Humphreys (1993) for general history-taking format (Box 25-4).

When women do come forward with current physical trauma, a delay in seeking treatment and/or an illogical explanation for the injury are cues that may indicate abuse. Abused women often seek treatment for indirect effects of their violent relationships. Their complaints may reflect the stress of these violent relationships and/or residual pain from past injuries. Past health history may indicate frequent accidents and other traumatic injuries such as lacerations, bruises, and fractures. Spontaneous abortions, attempts at suicide, and substance abuse may also be reported.

Other potential indicators of wife abuse may be identified in the family history. Potential indicators that relate to the woman's partner include: very strict disciplinarian who believes in physical punishment, abuses children, abuses alcohol and drugs, is extremely possessive and

---

Box 25-4　General Case History Questions for the Abused

1. Have you ever been emotionally or physically abused by your partner or someone important to you?

2. Within the last year, have you been hit, slapped, kicked, or otherwise physically hurt by someone? If yes, by whom and how many times?

3. Within the last year, has anyone forced you to have sex? If yes, who, and how many times?

4. Are you afraid of your partner or anyone else listed above?

(From Nursing Research Consortium on Violence and Abuse, 1993)

CLINICAL ALERT !

Women who seek treatment for indirect effects of their violent relationships often have vague complaints and appear depressed, anxious, and chronically fatigued. They often wear clothing that conceals bruises or other injuries.

CLINICAL ALERT !

Nurses should consider abuse as the cause of injury when women complain of sleep and appetite disturbances; elimination problems; chronic head, back, and pelvic pain; anxiety symptoms such as heart palpitations, dizziness, and dyspnea; and have a history of taking tranquilizers as pain medication.

Box 25-5   Physical Indicators of Possible Wife/Partner Abuse

General appearance

Anxious and frightened, depressed and passive, ashamed and embarrassed, poor eye contact, looks to partner for answers, partner does all the talking, partner exhibits smothering and extremely possessive behavior, and weight problems

Skin

Contusions, bruises, abrasions, and minor lacerations; scars; burns, particularly on breasts, arms, abdomen, chest, neck, face, and genitals

Musculoskeletal

Fractures and sprains (skull, facial bones, and extremities); dislocated shoulder; and evidence of old fractures

Genital/Rectal

Evidence of vaginal/anal rape such as bruising, edema, and bleeding; also evidence of direct kicks or punches

Abdominal

Internal bleeding or other injuries; chronic pelvic pain

Neurological

Post-traumatic stress disorder, hyperactive reflexes, chronic headaches and backaches, paresthesias from old injuries

---

jealous, has history of violence in his family of origin, is unemployed, and seeks to isolate family members. Box 25-5 presents the most important physical examination indicators of wife abuse.

When the battered woman discloses being abused or when the abuse is medically established, the crime must be reported to the proper authorities. The nurse or some other advocate needs to remain with the woman when she is interrogated by police.

When taking information from the woman, the nurse must accurately document whatever statements the woman makes. Open-ended questions that reflect what the woman is disclosing should be used whenever possible so that she feels in charge of the interview. Documented information must include the name of the abuser and when and how the abuse occurred. When possible, the nurse should record the exact words of the woman, because such documentation is very powerful legally. The nurse must also ask if the abuser hits the children. Protective services must be notified if the children have been abused.

A complete physical examination must be performed on any woman who is suspected of being battered. This includes a neurological examination and x-rays, if necessary, to determine the existence of previous injuries. A detailed description of the woman's injuries must be documented in the narrative, and a body chart diagram should be used to indicate the location and type of injury. The woman must be asked if she was forced into sexual acts against her will and examined for anal and vaginal tears. If there is a possibility of marital rape, the rape protocol should be followed and the evidence collection kit used. Assess the woman for sexually transmitted diseases. In addition, all laboratory and x-ray results need to be documented. According to the American Medical Association Guidelines on treatment of domestic violence (Flitcraft, 1992), at least two photographs of each trauma area should be taken, although a signed informed consent must first be given by the woman. One set of photographs will be placed in the woman's record with identifying data—date, woman's name, hospital number, and name of photographer—listed on the back. Because of the possibility of future legal proceedings, the nurse should request a safe address to which the second set of photographs can be mailed.

It is crucial to reassure the woman that all documentation is confidential and that her husband is not permitted access to it without her permission. Retaliation by the batterer is always a major concern for the abused woman. The woman also needs to understand that she has the right to access her records and that they will be valuable to her in child custody cases or if she chooses to file charges against the abuser.

Campbell and Fishwick (1993) caution against the use of such terms as *abuse* and *battering* because many

Nursing Assessment Questions

Battered Women

1. We often see women who have been hurt by their partners. Is your partner responsible for your injuries?
2. Has your partner ever hurt you in the past?
3. Have you noticed any pattern to the violence, such as an increase in frequency and severity?
4. Does he threaten to use or has he ever used a weapon to hurt you?

abused women do not have this image of themselves. Direct questions such as "Did someone hit you?" are more helpful. It is also important to understand that the woman may love her partner and desperately want to believe him when he promises it will never happen again.

It is imperative to assess the woman's potential danger in cases of domestic violence. Thus, information about the pattern of abuse and whether it has increased in severity and frequency is vital. Other critical signs that indicate increased risk are whether the abuser has a weapon, has been violent outside the house, is a substance abuser, has been stalking the woman, and has threatened suicide/homicide. At times, the woman herself may be contemplating suicide. It is well documented that the battered woman is at greatest risk of harm when she tries to leave her abuser; therefore, the woman must become aware of this risk and the nurse must assist her to develop a safety plan. Such a plan typically involves providing the woman with phone numbers of nearby shelters, crisis lines, and community resources. The woman should also be referred to the local crime victims' compensation board.

■ ■ ■ NURSING DIAGNOSES

The nursing diagnoses identified below are a sample of those that are relevant to the case study on Nina. They are based on information identified in the case study. However, all nursing diagnoses are formulated from information obtained during the assessment phase of the nursing process. The accuracy of the diagnoses depends on a careful, in-depth assessment. Based on the information provided, can you identify additional nursing diagnoses?

Nursing Diagnoses

Pain related to injuries sustained by battering as evidenced by difficulty breathing deeply and sleeping (multiple fractures)

CASE STUDY

Nina was brought to the emergency room by her husband to whom she has been married for 10 years. Her husband was very attentive to her, spoke reassuringly, and appeared very concerned about Nina's condition. According to her husband, a day ago Nina slipped as she was getting out of the bathtub. When she slipped she bumped her head on the faucet and then fell on her arm. As her husband spoke, Nina sat quietly with her head down. She cradled her right arm and appeared to be in severe pain. Her right eye was red and swollen shut and she seemed to have some difficulty breathing. Despite protests from her husband, the nurse interviewed Nina separately in a private consultation room. Although the nurse inquired directly whether Nina's husband had beaten her, Nina denied the abuse. A complete physical and neurological examination was performed by the physician and a series of x-rays taken. When Nina returned from x-ray she was told that she had fractures of the wrist, facial bones, and several ribs. In addition, Nina was informed that the x-rays indicated multiple old healed fractures of the ribs and pelvic girdle. The nurse spent time explaining to Nina how unlikely it was for her injuries to have resulted from a fall in the bathtub. The nurse also reassured Nina that nothing she could have done would deserve such abuse. Nina finally acknowledged that her husband had abused her but insisted she had no intentions of leaving him because he was a good husband. She further stated that the only time her husband was abusive was when she failed to fulfill her domestic responsibilities, thereby provoking him into losing his temper and beating her. Nina has no children or family nearby except for a younger sister who is currently overwhelmed with her own family problems. Nina is psychologically and economically dependent on her husband and without any other means of financial or psychological support.

Critical Thinking and Assessment

1. What is the first priority for the nurse who suspects abuse when assessing a woman?
2. How should the nurse respond to the shame, guilt, and self-blame of the battered woman?
3. What should a nurse do if she feels herself becoming angry and rejecting with a battered woman who is in denial about being battered?
4. If you suspected that your neighbor were in an abusive situation, what signs would you look for in their relationship?

Risk for further violence; risk factors: present and past abuse by husband

Anxiety and fear related to threat of further battering in the future

Ineffective family coping related to abuse by husband and denial by wife

No diagnosis in DSM-IV is currently appropriate for the battered woman. Some researchers and clinicians maintain that post-traumatic stress disorder is an appropriate diagnosis for many battered women who are repeatedly and severely abused (Ammerman and Hersen, 1992). The battered woman syndrome is a description of what happens over time to the battered woman. This syndrome, as described by Walker (1989), has been allowed in courtrooms in all states as a defense in cases in which battered women have murdered their abusers.

■ ■ ■ OUTCOME IDENTIFICATION

The following outcome criteria are derived from the nursing diagnoses identified in the case study on Nina. These outcomes are the expected behaviors that Nina will demonstrate as a result of implementation of the care plan and nursing interventions. Stabilizing Nina's physical condition and securing her safety are the immediate short-term goals. Nina will also require long-term goals and nursing interventions to assist her in making enduring changes in her life-threatening situation.

Outcome Identification for Battered Women

Client will:

1. Report a decrease in pain as a result of injuries sustained by her abuse.

2. Demonstrate no difficulty breathing and feel more relaxed.

3. Demonstrate less fear and anxiety by being able to realistically discuss her abuse and explore possible options for resolving it with the nurse.

4. Verbalize an awareness of her increasingly dangerous situation because the abuse has occurred in the past and continues to increase in intensity over time.

5. Discuss with the nurse the implications of her remaining in the present abusive situation, her spouse, and other family members, and explore alternative means of family coping.

6. Demonstrate an awareness of this need for safety by taking steps to protect herself in the future.

7. Explore the possibility of pursuing litigation against her husband and requesting a restraining order if her husband is not jailed.

8. Devise plans to secure her safety in case of future threats of abuse.

9. Take advantage of community resources that increase her self-esteem and independence and become involved with an outreach group for battered women.

■ ■ ■ ■ PLANNING

The plan of care for any victim of violence focuses on addressing critical physical problems, securing the immediate safety of the victim, examining the implications of the abuse on the woman and other family members, and discussing future plans for safety. In the case of a battered woman such as Nina who acknowledges the abuse only when confronted by the nurse, it is critical to explore all possible options because she may need to use them in the future. All goals are developed through the collaboration of nurse and client with the full realization that any effort to impose one's own beliefs on the battered woman is doomed to fail. Instead, the battered woman needs assistance to believe that she is capable of making appropriate decisions for herself—even if it means that she decides to return to her abuser. It is only through empowerment, not threats and intimidation, that the woman is most likely to develop the strength to make growth-producing decisions independently.

■ ■ ■ ■ ■ IMPLEMENTATION

Once the battered woman's physical condition has been stabilized, it is critical to assess her future safety and explore her fears, anxieties, and concerns. Despite an obvious need to leave the battering situation, the woman may strongly believe that she has no other option except to return. If the woman chooses to return to the batterer, it is important to respect this decision. Making a decision to leave the batterer is usually a gradual process. However, it is critical that the woman realize that she has options. The nurse may serve as the key factor in a beginning awareness that other options do exist.

Today all states have laws that provide some level of protection for victims of domestic violence, and there is a definite trend across the country to pass further legislation to ensure this protection. However, in reality there is a large gap between the actual laws and their implementation by the police and criminal justice system. In some localities police are mandated to arrest the abuser if there is probable evidence of violence. In many states the police must provide the battered woman with information on local shelters, domestic violence crisis lines, and her legal rights. However, the police may not always respond appropriately, so it is important that the nurse inform the battered woman of her legal rights.

Nursing Interventions

Primary prevention for wife abuse begins with identifying families at risk and changing societal views toward wife abuse. Nurses must become more knowledgeable about factors such as poverty, drugs, and unemployment, which increase the risk of domestic violence, and work with other members of the community to establish public policy and programs to address these issues.

Secondary prevention of wife battering involves early case finding and decisive intervention. Specific nursing interventions will be determined by the stage that the battered woman is in, since a woman in denial about the abuse will require a different strategy than one who is determined not to return to the relationship. In relationships where the abuse is just beginning and is mild, it may be possible to work with the couple when both partners choose to do so. In these cases, the male generally accepts all responsibility for the abuse, and the counseling focuses on preventing any further abuse.

Tertiary prevention is required when the woman has been repeatedly abused (as was Nina). In such cases, the focus is on assisting the abused woman to overcome the physical and psychologic effects of the abuse and prevent future abuse. Because the abuser frequently threatens and harasses the woman when she attempts to leave, it may be very difficult for her to follow through. Fre-

quently these women will seek assistance from local shelters where they receive safety and counseling. Nurses are often in the position to provide support and counseling to battered women in shelters. The nursing interventions identified in the table below relate to the case study describing Nina, who requires tertiary prevention measures in an emergency department setting.

■ ■ ■ ■ ■ ■ EVALUATION

Evaluation is a critical component of the nursing process. It is especially important to evaluate the battered woman, because inadequate or inappropriate nursing interventions may result in more serious abuse or even death. Nurses who work in settings where battered women seek treatment must be knowledgeable about responses of women to battering in order to evaluate nursing interventions. Once a complete nursing care plan is developed, the evaluation will be based on achievement of the outcome criteria.

Nursing interventions for battered women

Nursing interventions	Rationales
Report abuse to police.	Provide for safety.
Provide medications to relieve pain and anxiety.	Relieve her pain and reduce anxiety.
Discuss validity of her anxiety.	
Encourage Nina to discuss events leading to past and present abuse.	Reduce her guilt and shame.
Point out the increasingly violent nature of her marital relationship and concern for her safety.	
Insist that no person has the right to abuse another.	
Explore effectiveness of current coping skills and suggest additional skills.	Increase her independence and effective coping skills.
Focus on strengths, endurance, and abilities.	Increase her self-esteem.
Discuss destructive societal expectations of women.	
Discuss frequency of wife abuse among women like her.	
Explore family and/or friends as support possibilities.	Increase her awareness of potential support.
Discuss potential for using community resources, e.g., shelters and/or hotlines and police.	
Describe current laws on domestic violence.	Increase her awareness of abuse implications.
Explore implications of pressing charges against husband.	
Explore meaning of potential relationship loss.	
Explore various options for the future.	Identify long-term goals.
Provide fact sheet on domestic violence.	
Provide referrals.	
Develop a safety plan with critical papers, money, clothing, and other essentials to be set aside for emergency exits.	
Offer to be available for further questions.	(Provide continuity of care)

CHILD PHYSICAL ABUSE

In 1988 the National Center on Child Abuse and Neglect reported that physical abuse of children has increased by 58% from 1980 to 1986. Recently it was reported that *each year* approximately two million children in the United States are seriously abused by their parents and caregivers, and at least 1,000 deaths result from these injuries (American Humane Society, 1988). Of the two million abused children, 25% are physically abused, 20% sexually abused, and 55% are neglected. A quarter of abused children are under 5 years old, and about 60% are between 5 and 14 years old (see Box 25-2 for other statistics). Besides physical violence and neglect, many children suffer severe psychological consequences from exposure to violence among family members. This issue is only beginning to gain attention from nurse researchers and social scientists.

In the 1940s, the identification of abused children was dramatically facilitated by the introduction of x-ray technology. At this time some physicians began to notice patterns of healed fractures in small children. However, it was not until 1962 when the classic article, "The Battered Child Syndrome" (Kempe et al) was published that child abuse was thrust into the public consciousness. Soon afterward, four groups developed model legislation for child abuse: the U.S. Children's Bureau, the Children's Division of the American Humane Association, the American Medical Association, and the Council of State Governments. In 1974 the U.S. government established the National Center on Child Abuse and Neglect. By that time mandatory reporting requirements for child abuse and neglect were instituted by all 50 states.

Humphreys and Ramsey (1993) reported that most child physical abuse is classified as moderate in severity and includes physical injuries such as bruises and depression and emotional distress, which is not severe enough to warrant medical attention. Therefore, most children who are physically abused do not come to the attention of emergency room doctors and nurses; instead, they must be identified at clinics, schools, and through the efforts of community health nurses.

Social science research indicates that the majority of parents have used physical punishment to discipline their children. Gelles and Cornell (1990) claim that spanking is the most common form of family violence in the United States. Parents tend to discipline their children the way they were disciplined in youth. It is difficult to change repeated generational patterns of family discipline even though social science research has found no potential benefit from physical punishment as discipline and much to condemn it. Herman (1992) described the child who is chronically abused as one who learns to adapt to the unpredictability of the abuse by developing a seething state of frozen watchfulness and a core belief of innate badness since they believe that they are to blame for the abuse. Many times the abused child attempts to compensate for these feelings of badness by striving to be the perfect child.

Definitions of Child Abuse and Neglect

Definitions of child abuse and neglect vary from state to state and among clinicians and researchers. The American Medical Association (Berkowitz et al, 1992) defined **child physical abuse** as "inflicted injury to a child that can range from minor bruises and lacerations to severe neurologic trauma and death". In many states, child abuse is defined as actual or threatened physical violence.

Definitions of neglect are also problematic because people may define "adequate" in a variety of ways. Ammerman and Hersen (1992) have reflected on the difficulties of defining child abuse and state that "arriving at a universally accepted operational definition of maltreatment has proven to a dilemma that is virtually insurmountable". This is primarily because the definitions have such wide application that many parents and institutions would be viewed as abusive in the United States. Nevertheless, it is clear that nurses and other health care professionals must conduct holistic assessments and search for psychologic as well as physical trauma, because even abuse that leaves no physical scars can disrupt normal growth and development of children in profound ways.

Inherent in all physical abuse is a psychologic component. Briere (1992) described eight parent/caretaker behaviors that comprise his definition of **child psychological abuse:** rejecting, degrading/devaluing, terrorizing, isolating, corrupting, exploiting, denying essential stimulation or availability, and unreliable and inconsistent parenting. Since psychological abuse impacts later psychosocial functioning, it is imperative to recognize its potential for long-lasting trauma and develop interventions to address it.

Theoretical Frameworks of Child Abuse and Neglect

There is no single theory that explains the cause of child abuse. It is generally recognized that many complex interacting factors place children at risk for abuse. Box 25-6 summarizes the various theories of child abuse and neglect.

The Abused Child

Younger children, especially those under age 3, are at a greater risk for fatal abuse than older children. Younger children are more fragile than older ones, which accounts for their increased risk of fatality caused by abuse. Earlier studies reported that premature, handicapped, and developmentally disabled children were also at

Box 25-6   Etiologic Theories Related to Child Abuse

Biological theory

- Parents who were abused as children are at risk for abusing their own children

Social learning theories

- Family teaching and accepting violent behavior
- Glorifying violence in the media
- Accepting violence in families, schools, churches

Environmental theories

- Socioeconomic class
- Unemployment
- Stressful life events

higher risk; however, recent studies have not found this association (Gelles and Cornell, 1990).

Data from a national study by the National Center for Child Abuse and Neglect (1988) indicated that child abuse actually increases as a child gets older and plateaus by age 14. However, although this study found no gender differences for neglect, the incidence of abuse differed significantly in males and females; females were more likely to experience physical, emotional, and sexual abuse than males.

In a discussion of the long-term consequences of childhood abuse, Gelles and Cornell (1990) reported that abused and neglected children are at greater risk for later delinquency, adult criminality, and violent crimes than matched controls. Abused and neglected children also have more intellectual deficits, learning disabilities, drug and alcohol abuse, and psychiatric problems.

The Child Physical Abuser

Research on the characteristics of child physical abusers have described them as immature, lacking self-esteem, having unrealistic expectations of children, poor impulse control, and minimal or no external support systems. Males and females are equally likely to be abusers. However, in fatal child abuse cases the mother's boyfriend is most commonly identified, followed by the natural mother and the natural father (Humphreys and Ramsey, 1993).

When analyzing the equal likelihood of males and females being child abusers, the fact that the mother is frequently the only adult in the household needs to be considered. Even in two-parent homes, the mother usually spends more time with the children than the father. When the data are adjusted for the situations in which no male caregiver is present, mothers account for only one-third of the abuse (Humphreys and Ramsey, 1993).

The Nurse's Attitude in Child Abuse

Nurses working in settings in which they may encounter abusive families must take time to assess their own attitudes and feelings before interacting with such families. Humphreys and Ramsey (1993) described three typical reactions by the nurse: (1) horror that parents could abuse their children, (2) denial of the abuse, and (3) fantasies of saving or rescuing the child. None of these responses is helpful to the child, family, or nurse because each interferes with meeting the therapeutic needs of the child and the family and prevents the nurse from providing effective nursing care.

Nurses must accept that most families, given the necessary conditions, have the potential for abusing and neglecting their children. This assumption will promote effectiveness on the primary prevention level because it will enable the nurse to be alert to the possibility of abuse and neglect.

THE NURSING PROCESS ■ ■ ■ ■ ■ ■ ■ ■ ■ ■ ■ ■ ■ ■ ■

■ ASSESSMENT

The following discussion focuses on the nurse's responsibilities in making a holistic assessment of the abused child. The areas of assessment will cover physical and emotional abuse and neglect of the child. Assessment of the sexually abused child will be covered in the next section of this chapter.

History

It is the nurse's responsibility to identify abuse and neglect and intervene in a nonjudgmental and nonthreatening manner. An open, honest attitude with parents is much more likely to gain cooperation and trust than a hostile, blaming one. Direct honest questions are necessary.

CLINICAL ALERT   **!**

All states require nurses or other health care professionals to report any suspicions of child abuse to protective services. Failure to do so may constitute a misdemeanor.

Humphreys and Ramsey (1993) pointed out that it is not the nurse's role to judge whether a crime has been committed or to punish or discipline abusive parents. It is the nurse's role to report the case if there is a suspicion of abuse and assist parents to learn new skills so that they are able to provide a healthy, safe, and nurturing environment for their children.

The nurse needs to be aware of group process principles and avoid an environment that projects a superior/inferior relationship with the parents during history-taking. The usual history-taking format is used, after a brief introduction to the parents on the purpose of the interview and its format. Typically the history format will first focus on parental concerns, general family history, and finally the present concern. This progression moves from least to most threatening and offers the nurse the opportunity to establish rapport with the parents before requesting information about the most sensitive issue, the possibility of abuse.

When taking the history, the nurse needs to be alert to discrepancies between parental history of the child injuries and physical findings. An example of a discrepancy could be the parents' claim that they have no knowledge of how a child broke his femur. Fractures of the femur are not typical accidental injuries, and, without some history of significant trauma such as a car accident, child abuse should be suspected. Other clues include parental delay in seeking treatment for the child's injuries, failure to use hospitals closer to home, the child's history of multiple past injuries, reluctance by parents to give a history, or discrepancies between the histories given by both parents. To identify inconsistencies, each parent should be interviewed separately. Whenever possible, children should also be interviewed separately from parents, although even then they will often deny abuse in an effort to protect their parents out of loyalty or fear of retaliation.

It is extremely helpful to observe the parent-child relationship while taking the history. The history-taking also allows the nurse to model appropriate child-rearing skills and allows the parents to express their fears, concerns, and problems.

All physical findings should be documented on the child diagram in the history form, and direct quotations of the parents should be included whenever possible (Box 25-7). Today photographs are being used more extensively, although they are not a substitute for a detailed

Nursing Assessment Questions

Parents Who Are Suspected of Child Abuse

1. Is there anything in particular you would like to share about your child or your family as we begin this history?
2. Does your child have any particular health or behavior problems?
3. Have any of your other children ever had similar injuries?
4. How did your child receive these injuries?

---

history and physical exam. State laws vary on authorization for taking photographs without parental consent; therefore, nurses who work in settings that provide care for children should be familiar with state laws in this regard.

■ ■ NURSING DIAGNOSES

The nursing diagnoses below refer to the case study about Marilee on page 595. They must include the parents because the identified client is an infant who is totally dependent on her parents for care and nurturance. Therefore, the following diagnoses relate to both parents and child. Multiple nursing diagnoses may be identified; the ones listed below are a partial sample. Nursing diagnoses are formulated from information obtained during the assessment phase of the nursing process. The accuracy of diagnoses depends on a careful, in-depth assessment.

Family-Related Diagnosis

Altered Parenting, Related To: inexperience with caregiving, unrealistic expectations, marginal family adaptation, social isolation, lack of resources, and poverty.

Child-Related Diagnosis

Sensory/Perceptual Alterations, Related to cerebral trauma effects (subdural hemorrhage)

Fear, Related to responses of physical and emotional abuse

Anxiety, Related to responses of physical and emotional abuse

■ ■ ■ OUTCOME IDENTIFICATION

Outcome criteria for Marilee are derived from the diagnoses that were formulated for her and her parents. These outcomes are the expected behaviors that Marilee

---

Box 25-7   Child Abuse and Neglect—Possible/Actual Physical Indicators

General appearance

- Excessive fearfulness and watchfulness
- Disheveled and malnourished
- Failure to thrive

Multiple injuries

- Suspicious if no history of significant trauma

Skin

- Unexplained bruises, welts, and scratches in various stages of healing (different colors)
- Regular patterns of bruises and welts such as bite marks or marks from electrical cords
- Untreated infected wounds
- Lacerations from rope burns especially on neck, wrists, ankles, and torso
- Bruises on buttocks, genitalia, thighs, side of face, trunk, and upper arms are suspicious

Burns

- Cigarette burns (small round) (infected insect bites resemble cigarette burns)
- Immersion burns (even boundaries that are glove-like, sock-like, or symmetrical; accidental burns are asymmetrical with splash marks)
- Patterned burn marks (e.g., from an iron or grill)

Fractures

- Fractures in infants younger than age 1 are suspicious
- Fractures of femur, humerus, posterior ribs, skull, and long bones and any uncommon fractures are suspicious

Head injuries

- Leading cause of death among abused children; skull fractures and subdural hematomas are suspicious
- Shaken Baby Syndrome may result in brain hemorrhages or contusions without external signs of injury
- Alopecia caused by hair pulling

Abdominal injuries

- Ruptured liver or spleen
- Ruptured blood vessels
- Kidney, bladder, or pancreatic injuries
- Injuries to jejunum or duodenum

Injuries to eyes, ears, nose, and mouth

- Includes a wide variety of injuries including missing teeth, bruising, perforation of tympanic membrane, epistaxis and nose fractures, retinal hemorrhage or detachment corneal abrasions, and periorbital hematomas

Other types of abuse/neglect

- Munchausen's syndrome by proxy
- Deprivational syndromes

---

and her parents will demonstrate as a result of the implementation of the care plan and the nursing interventions.

For Marilee, the first priority is the short-term nursing goal of stabilizing her critical physical condition, the subdural hemorrhage, which resulted when she was vigorously shaken by her father. This outcome will be demonstrated by Marilee's renewed ability to respond to stimuli—that is, Marilee will be able to respond to sounds, sights, touch, motion, and smell at the same developmental level she had before she was injured. She will recognize her parents, be able to ambulate, and tolerate a light diet.

The nursing diagnoses of fear and anxiety related to Marilee's abuse will involve long-term nursing goals of helping her to reestablish trust in her father.

Outcome Identification for an Abused Child

Client will:

1. Demonstrate this trust by being receptive to her father and not exhibiting any fear of him. This outcome will depend on her father's outcome.

Outcome Identification for an Abusing Parent

Client will:

1. Learn positive parenting skills and use them consistently with his daughter.

2. Attend parenting classes to improve his knowledge and understanding of normal child growth and development.

3. Cooperate with protective services, which will be investigating him for the alleged abuse.

■ ■ ■ ■ PLANNING

In all cases of child abuse, the primary concern is the health and safety of the child. Because Marilee is experiencing a medical crisis, the first priority is to stabilize her physical condition. Then steps must be taken to secure her short- and long-term safety and to support the family in meeting these goals. Because the child's future health and safety depends on her family, the nurse must establish a trusting relationship with the family and collaborate on developing mutually acceptable goals. These

CASE STUDY

Eighteen-month-old Marilee was brought into Southside Hospital emergency room by her parents, Betty and Jim Brown. Although the Browns live on the north side of town, they chose to bring their daughter to the Southside Hospital. Marilee was unconscious when she arrived at 7 AM. The physical exam revealed no external signs of trauma on the body except for bruises on the child's upper arms that resembled grip marks. The Browns reported that Marilee was put to bed the night before in the usual manner, but that they were unable to rouse her this morning. The Browns were unaware of any trauma or significant event that could account for their daughter's unconscious state. Both parents were teenagers and clearly agitated about their infant daughter's condition. Mr. Brown refused to have his wife interviewed separately from him. During the interview and history-taking, Betty sat across the room crying softly while Jim answered the nurse's questions. The young people stated that they were estranged from their own parents and rarely saw them. Mr. Brown is currently unemployed.

Critical Thinking and Assessment

1. What is the first priority for the nurse and health care team in this scenario?

2. Why would this young couple be at high risk for child abuse?

3. How would you build trust with this young couple?

4. If you suspect child abuse, how would you protect the future safety of this child?

5. Why is an understanding of child developmental stages a critical component of effective parenting?

goals may be difficult to achieve in child abuse cases, because many parents firmly believe that "sparing the rod spoils the child." However, children are sometimes punished because parents are ignorant of normal child development and interpret the child's inability to meet parental demands as obstinacy or disobedience. Classes in basic child growth and development are a critical component in addressing the needs of families who abuse or neglect their children. Child discipline and anger control classes also are important in preventing future child abuse.

■ ■ ■ ■ ■ IMPLEMENTATION

All too frequently in cases of child abuse, the child's physical trauma will be treated but the underlying problem of the abuse will not be addressed. Hospitals and agencies that provide primary care are currently mandated by the Joint Commission of Accreditation of Health Organizations to identify clients who are victims of abuse and to provide treatment and referrals for them and their families. This mandate usually requires a concerted and collaborative effort by the health care team. The nurse is usually in an optimal position to coordinate this effort. In particular, the nurse needs to (1) secure the physical and psychological safety and health of the child, (2) assist the parents to understand the consequences of their abusive behavior, and (3) develop strategies with the parents to prevent any recurrence of abuse.

When nurses plan interventions for abusive families, they must go beyond the focused family and think in terms of primary prevention for all families, that is, from families that appear normal through high-risk families. Potential settings for educating and identifying parents are hospital obstetric and pediatric units, emergency departments, substance abuse programs, health clinics, schools, churches, and the community at large. Because of their access to families in their own homes, community health nurses are in an excellent position to assess, teach, and model parenting skills and to intervene on the primary prevention level before child maltreatment occurs. Specific nursing interventions will be dependent on the setting in which the nurse and family interact.

Nursing Interventions

Primary prevention is focused on identifying families at risk and implementing interventions directed at preventing any onset of abuse. For Marilee, the nursing interventions will occur on the secondary prevention level because abuse has already occurred—the present focus is on addressing the current crisis and preventing future occurrences of abuse. Tertiary prevention for child abuse is directed at rehabilitating the abused child who has suffered irreversible damage. The goal is to maximize the future potential of the child within the constraints of the existing damage. In tertiary prevention the child is removed from the home because the child's safety cannot be secured there. The nursing interventions listed in the table on page 596 focus on secondary prevention for Marilee, an 18-month-old infant with a subdural hemorrhage caused by shaken baby syndrome. The nursing setting is the hospital emergency department.

■ ■ ■ ■ ■ ■ EVALUATION

Because the nursing care of this family will proceed after hospital discharge, the nursing evaluation will continue throughout the nursing involvement with the family. Evaluation will focus on the family achievement of identified goals. A final evaluation will be conducted when the public health nurse determines that the family has achieved its goals and is at minimal risk for child abuse.

Nursing Interventions for the physically abused child

Nursing interventions (secondary prevention)	Rationales
Develop trusting relationship with parents.	Provide environment for parents that facilitates their sharing sequence of events leading to abuse.
Be direct and open, but supportive.	
Obtain a holistic history, including stresses and problems the family is experiencing.	
Explore how events that led to abuse might be altered in the future.	Problem-solve and educate on how to avoid similar scenarios in the future.
Explore alternative strategies for child care problems.	
Discuss basic child growth and development.	
Provide parents with basic materials on child growth and development.	
Have parents apply child development principles.	
Discuss need for parenting classes.	
Discuss strategies for anger control.	
Discuss reporting laws on child abuse.	Gain parental agreement to cooperate with protective services.
Explain child welfare function of protective services.	
Take steps to inform protective services.	
Observe parent-child interactions unobtrusively.	Role-model providing care and support for child.
Involve parents in child care during hospitalization when appropriate.	
Discuss physical impact of abuse with parents.	Have parents verbalize their understanding of abusive behavior on child.
Discuss short- and long-term psychologic effects of child abuse.	
Provide referral to postdischarge public health child nursing.	Support parents in the prevention of future abuse.
Public health nurse will coordinate services and monitor parental progress.	
Public health nurse will role-model and assist parents to apply principles learned in parenting classes in their own lives.	Involve parents in child care classes.
Public health nurse will reinforce positive parenting skills.	
Have father discuss how he will maintain anger skills.	Demonstrate anger control skills.
Teach mother to intervene if father exhibits negative parenting.	
Assist parents to develop social support systems.	Prevent isolation of problem and expand support system.
Explore community resources with family.	

INTRAFAMILIAL SEXUAL ABUSE OF CHILDREN (INCEST)

The most commonly cited study of the incidence of childhood sexual abuse is derived from Diane Russell's work (1986) with a random sample of 953 women. Russell found that approximately one-third of her sample had been sexually abused as children; 16% of this sample had been incestually abused by a relative before the age of 18. Wyatt's 1985 study corroborated Russell's results with female subjects. Other studies have reported that 15%–20% of male children have been sexually abused (Briere, 1992; Jacobson and Herald, 1990).

Throughout the following discussion on childhood sexual abuse, the pronoun "she" will be used in reference to the child victim although it is recognized that male children are also victims of sexual abuse (as cited above). Also, the term *sexual abuse* will be used inter-changeably with *incest* since most childhood sexual abuse is perpetrated by someone the child knows and trusts (Courtois, 1988). Therefore, many researchers argue that most childhood sexual abuse is incestual.

Multiple studies have indicated that approximately 50% of psychiatric clients have histories of physical and sexual abuse. Although many studies indicate that childhood sexual abuse is a core issue in mental health disorders, the effects of sexual abuse are frequently compounded by concurrent severe physical and emotional abuse.

Many experts insist that sexual abuse is the worst kind of child abuse because it is hidden and therefore more difficult to detect and address. The vast majority of children who have been sexually abused will demonstrate no physical evidence of having been abused—their trauma is primarily psychological. Conversely, physical abuse of children is much easier to identify because it is more visible and easier to document.

Definition of Intrafamilial Sexual Abuse

The definition of **childhood incest** used here is any type of exploitative sexual experience between relatives or surrogate relatives before the victim reaches 18 years of age (Urbancic, 1993). Exploitative actions involve behaviors that the perpetrator uses to achieve sexual gratification with the child. This includes disrobing, nudity, masturbation, voyeurism, fondling, digital or object penetration, and oral, anal, or vaginal penetration.

In the typical incestual relationship the abuse begins very gradually with gentle fondling and gradually escalates over time, often progressing to vaginal or oral penetration. Initially some children may derive pleasure and gratification from the attention and the sexual activity and may actually seek the abuser out. It must be remembered that children are capable of experiencing sexual pleasure when stimulated sexually. Many times children feel very special to be the object of such focused attention, particularly if their emotional needs have not been met by others and the sexual activity provides them with feelings of pleasure, love, and attention. However, despite the enjoyable aspects of the abuse, the child usually feels confused and shamed and may find that the pleasurable memories of the abuse become the basis for serious guilt and shame in adulthood. Such feelings can be difficult to overcome because the adult survivor believes that he or she gave consent and does not view the activity as abusive. Thus, it cannot be overemphasized that the adult is always the responsible person—regardless of how the child responds. It is the adult's task to nurture, set boundaries, and teach age-appropriate behaviors rather than exploit children for his own sexual gratification.

Historical and Theoretical Perspectives on Incest

Since the late 1970s and early 1980s, research on childhood sexual abuse has increased; currently there is an explosion of research on the topic. Many researchers have attempted to explain the basis of the traumatic effects of childhood sexual abuse. Most have incorporated the diagnosis of post-traumatic stress disorder or various aspects of psychological trauma into their conceptual model. Some researchers have used a cognitive model and maintained that if the traumatic events are not processed and neutralized, they cannot be stored in distant memory. Instead, these traumatic memories remain in active memory, and the person has to make a constant effort to defend against them through a variety of cognitive defense mechanisms. Burgess et al (1987) termed this effort to defend oneself from traumatic memories *trauma encapsulation.*

Carmen and Rieker (1989) and Briere (1992) propose models similar to the Burgess model that explain the traumatic effects as efforts by a defenseless child to cope in the best way possible. The cognitive defense mechanisms include denial, repression, disassociation, splitting, and compartmentalization. There is no doubt that these defenses are helpful and adaptive in coping with the trauma of the abuse during childhood; however, the same defenses become entrenched in adulthood and are counterproductive, often becoming the basis for mental health problems.

Characteristics of the Incestual Family

Research on intrafamilial sexual abuse indicates that these families are highly dysfunctional, although overtly they may appear quite normal. Studies have not found a correlation with incest and such characteristics as socioeconomic status, culture, race, and ethnicity; rather, incest seems to cross all boundaries.

Within incestual families, multiple forms of abuse are likely to be present, including physical and other forms of psychological/emotional abuse. Most incestual families are described as enmeshed or endogenous, which means that they are relatively isolated from those outside the family and tend to focus most of their energies on relationships within the family. Boundaries are poorly defined and are characterized by excessive dependency on each other for physical, social, and psychological needs. Role reversals often occur with the abused child assuming a caretaker role for the parents and other family members. However, it must be emphasized that no single pattern can accurately describe the complexity of the incestual family.

OFFENDERS

Characteristics of offenders are primarily based on research of those cases examined within the criminal justice system and usually were more serious abuse cases. Most cases of sexual abuse are never reported, so these criminal cases are not widely representative. Most research has also focused on father (or stepfather) and daughter abuse because the dyad of adult-male and female-child is by far the most typical kind of childhood sexual abuse pattern. Finkelhor and Browne (1986) reported that 95% of female child abuse and 85% of male child abuse is perpetrated by males. Therefore, for the sake of simplicity, the female child and adult male will be most commonly referred to in this discussion of childhood sexual abuse.

The most common description of the abuser is that of the socially immature introverted male who has difficulty relating to adults and is more comfortable with children. Justice and Justice (1979) claim that the majority of abusers fall within this category. Such an abuser is referred to as a *symbiotic offender.*

The abuser may be married, have children, and even appear outwardly normal in adjustment; however, it is likely that he has difficulty establishing relationships outside the family and is extremely dependent on his family to fulfill his psychologic needs. He strongly believes that it is his right to have his needs met by family members. Justice and Justice (1979) claim that the symbiotic abuser may be introverted, tyrannical, and/or alcoholic.

Great concern has been expressed in recent years because the age of offenders has continued to drop. More juveniles are being identified as offenders, and they demonstrate more violent behavior than the typical adult offender. In addition, more of these juvenile offenders are prepubescent and include female offenders (whose numbers are growing).

In general, there is no universal description by which the child sexual offender can be recognized. Usually the offender is someone the child knows and trusts, rather than a stranger. They are not mentally ill, but many have a history of being sexually abused as children.

Characteristics of the Nonoffending Parent

When the abuser is the father, the mother has typically been blamed for failing to satisfy her husband's psychologic and sexual needs; of being rejecting and dominating; and of expecting her daughter to assume the lover role with the father and be caretaker to both parents. The literature has also blamed the mother for being absent when the incest occurred, even if she was working to support the family. In addition, when the child discloses the abuse to the mother, it has been claimed that the mother commonly denies that the abuse occurred or blames the child for initiating or encouraging it.

Although these have been common themes in literature, little or no research exists to support these contentions. In fact, recent research suggests that the majority of nonoffending mothers believe their children and take steps to protect them by notifying protective services (Conte and Berliner, 1988; Mannarino and Cohen, 1986). In a 1993 study by Deblinger et al, mothers of children who were sexually abused by partners were more likely to be battered by the abusive partners than were mothers of children abused by other relatives or nonrelatives. These researchers thus suggest that it is more appropriate to view these battered mothers as secondary victims of abuse rather than as colluders and deniers. In addition, it was found that the vast majority of mothers believed their children's reports of abuse.

In the author's clinical practice (Urbancic, 1993), many nonoffending mothers are initially shocked and ambivalent about their children's disclosure of sexual abuse. It is especially devastating to the woman if she loves and trusts her partner, since she must now cope with her partner's betrayal in addition to her child's violation and traumatization. It is much simpler and less painful to believe that the abuse did not occur. Never-

theless, many mothers who are initially in shock experience a process involving a crisis of disbelief and/or ambivalence, followed by gradual acceptance and eventual dedication to healing their children's trauma as well as their own. It is probably most accurate to recognize that a variety of scenarios exist in relation to the nonoffending mother; it is inappropriate to try to categorize the complexity of the nonoffending mother according to any particular pattern or description.

Sexually Abused Children

Most of the research on child victims of sexual abuse has been directed toward female children; much less is known about the male child victim. Typically the incest victim is the oldest daughter in the family, and often when she is able to extricate herself from this role, the next daughter replaces her. Some research indicates that the average age at which the incestual relationship begins is 8 or 9 years. However, in Urbancic's study (1993) the average age of the child when the incest began was 6 years, with an average duration of 7 years. Often, the secret is never revealed, but at other times the child may tell a close friend or trusted relative. The child may disclose the incest during a family argument in which her acting-out behavior is being criticized by her parents. Although acting-out behavior by the child is common, there is no unique pattern of behavior that indicates the presence of abuse; indeed, sometimes the victim is a model child in every way.

Effects of Sexual Abuse on Children

Briere (1992) and Herman (1992) have emphasized that frequently physical, psychologic, and sexual abuse are combined, and the resulting combined effects are extremely traumatic. However, Briere and Herman emphasize that even when the effects of other abuse are considered and analyzed in research studies, sexual abuse effects are still significant and usually a key issue. This is a crucial point, because some writers have discounted the trauma of childhood sexual abuse insisting that the chaotic family, not the sexual abuse, is the core problem. Nevertheless, it is important to use a holistic view in the assessment and treatment of abused clients and address whatever abuse issues are salient to the client.

Recently an extensive review of the literature was reported by Kendall-Tackett et al, (1993). After reviewing 45 studies, these researchers concluded that no single core of symptoms exists as a common denominator among those who had been sexually abused as children. Instead, a multitude of symptoms have been identified. Symptomatology seems to be dependent on a complex blend of factors: developmental age of the child when the abuse occurs, maternal support, individual coping skills, positive influences that could neutralize the abuse, severity of abuse, duration, frequency, relationship of the abuser, and degree of force.

The literature review by Kendall-Tackett et al (1993) indicates that childhood sexual abuse has serious repercussions that are reflected in a wide variety of symptoms and pathological behaviors. The most common symptoms are sexual acting-out behaviors and post-traumatic stress disorder. Other commonly experienced symptoms and behaviors in the abused children include anxiety, fear, depression, somatic complaints, aggressive antisocial behavior, withdrawn behavior, school learning problems, and hyperactivity. Sexual acting-out behaviors are evidenced by a preoccupation with sexual play with dolls and other children, inserting objects into anal and vaginal openings, compulsive masturbation, sexual knowledge beyond age appropriateness, and promiscuity. Since many of the symptoms are developmentally specific, the researchers caution about generalizing all symptoms across all age groups.

Long-Term Effects of Childhood Sexual Abuse: Adult Survivors

Just as there is no specific profile for the sexually abused child, neither is there one for the adult survivor. In the recent past, most survivors of childhood sexual abuse reported being treated by multiple therapists before finding one who effectively identified and facilitated the survivor's recovery process (Urbancic, 1993). With the explosion of clinical literature, training workshops, and research, it is hoped that this scenario is rapidly changing. A growing awareness that people can heal from childhood sexual abuse is reflected in the use of the term *survivor* rather than *victim* by professionals and those who have been abused. A survivor is viewed as a person who has discarded the helpless victim mentality in favor of an attitude of empowerment in which she acts on the belief that she is capable of overcoming and recovering from the trauma.

Clinicians and researchers have categorized the long-term effects of childhood sexual abuse in a variety of ways. Jehu (1992) has identified the most common psychosocial problems of survivors who seek treatment as post-traumatic stress reactions, self-damaging behavior, mood disturbances, interpersonal problems, and sexual difficulties, including rape, prostitution, compulsive sexuality, and confusion about sexual orientation.

For many survivors of childhood sexual abuse, post-traumatic stress disorder (PTSD) is a reality characterized by a reexperiencing of the trauma via flashbacks and recurrent dreams. Other symptoms of PTSD include numbing or constricted affect, memory problems, difficulty concentrating, irrational guilt and shame, constant vigilance, sleep problems, and anxiety attacks. The traumatic memories can be experienced through the senses of smell, touch, taste, sight, or sound. Thus, the survivor may experience an overwhelming sense of terror when some cue in the environment triggers such a sensory memory. A common example is that of the survivor who is exposed to someone who resembles her abuser and so experiences an overwhelming sense of fear, panic, and dread. Because she is unaware of the connection between her powerful reaction and this person being a trigger to her abusive childhood experience, she is unable to give a logical explanation for her reaction and may fear that she is "going crazy."

On many occasions survivors will report recurring physical symptoms for which no organic cause can be found. Recently clinicians, researchers, and survivors have begun to relate many of these symptoms to specifics of the abuse. These symptoms are referred to as *body memories*. Approximately 35% of Urbancic's 1993 sample of adult survivors reported symptoms that could be categorized as body memories. Women who reported being forced into oral sex tended to report such symptoms as absent gag reflex, teeth clenching, difficulty swallowing, and severe biting of the inside of the mouth. Women who were penetrated vaginally or rectally often report pelvic or rectal pain or severe pain on intercourse. Other body memories were represented by symptoms such as heavy pressure on the chest and difficulty breathing (abuser lying on top of child) and periodic numbness of the hand (hand that masturbated abuser).

In the same study, most survivors reported having difficulty trusting others, feeling isolated, different, depressed, vulnerable, and helpless. Most also complained of feeling deep shame, guilt, and very low self-esteem. About 20% of the women reported dissociative and depersonalization experiences, panic attacks, and agoraphobia. Thus, a wide variety of symptoms are reported by adult survivors of childhood sexual abuse, leaving no doubt that there can be and often are serious repercussions from such experiences.

■ ASSESSMENT

As with the assessment of other victims of violence, nurses should begin by assessing their own assumptions, beliefs, and attitudes about childhood sexual abuse. Nurses who believe that the child is responsible in any way for the sexual abuse will find it difficult to be supportive toward the child. The nurse needs to be comfortable when speaking with the child about the abuse so that an attitude of discomfort is not conveyed. Children are very adept at picking up nonverbal cues, and the nurse's discomfort may be interpreted by the child as a sign that she should not talk about the abuse or that she is disbelieved.

As with all nursing assessments, a holistic approach is essential. Because the trauma of childhood sexual abuse is highly complex and dependent on multiple interacting factors, it is important to gain as much information as possible without subjecting the child to unnecessary and repetitive probing and questioning. Most often the nurse will encounter the sexually abused child in an emergency department or outpatient clinic to which the mother or other caretaker brings the child to determine whether sexual abuse has occurred. Whenever a suspicion of childhood abuse occurs, a complete physical examination must be done.

The primary focus is to establish a trusting relationship so that the child is as comfortable as possible in relating relevant events and cooperating with the physical examination. It is important to assess the relationship between the caretaker and the child to determine if the child is more comfortable with or without that person present. In most cases younger children will not want to be separated from this caregiver; older children, however, may be too inhibited to speak openly in front of the caregiver for a variety of reasons, such as fear of being blamed by family members, being disbelieved, or being perceived as instrumental in the family breakup. Sometimes children may retract their disclosure in an effort to protect their abuser, with whom they may have a love/hate relationship. Finally, the developmental age of the child is an important factor in the ability to successfully provide data about the abuse; the younger the child, the less ability the child has to describe events and understand the interviewer's questions.

The majority of children who have been sexually abused will not display any physical signs of abuse because the most common type of abusive activity is fondling, which seldom has any physical manifestations. The occurrence of oral copulation or mock intercourse is also difficult to physically document unless the child is examined within a short time after the activity. Giardino et al (1992) reported that even serious physical injuries from sexual abuse can heal without any significant residual signs. Evidence such as enlargement of the hymenal orifice alone is not conclusive for proving sexual abuse. Thus, it is very difficult to demonstrate physical signs of sexual abuse.

In addition to the lack of physical evidence, the sexually abused child may display no signs of emotional trauma and may deny, retract, and be inconsistent in her description of the abuse. Caretakers often interpret this behavior to mean the abuse did not occur and that the child is lying. The significance of absent physical or emotional signs must be clearly explained to the child's caretakers.

Conversely, multiple emotional/psychologic indicators may be present, but because many of these signs can also reflect other problems their presence alone is not conclusive that sexual abuse has occurred. The diagnosis of sexual abuse is difficult and challenging because there is no single profile or set of symptoms that guarantee its presence. Many of the following signs and symptoms must be viewed as potential indicators of sexual abuse only, whereas others are highly probable indicators. Detailed psychosocial protocols and guidelines for health care professionals who interview and evaluate children for sexual abuse have been developed by the American Professional Society on Abused Children (APSAC Task Force, 1990). Guidelines for evaluation of physical signs of sexual abuse have been published by Giardino et al (1992). The indicators in Box 25-8 are derived from these two sets of guidelines and this author's experience.

As noted earlier, there is no single profile or set of signs and symptoms that indicates the presence of sexual abuse, and in some cases there is an absence of obvious indicators. However, when caretakers look back at the child's behavior after the disclosure of the abuse, they are often able to identify signs and symptoms that seemed to have no significance at the time.

Clearly, the meaning of any child's acting-out behavior needs to be explored. Such behavior in abused children usually reflects the anger, confusion, and sense of betrayal that the child is experiencing and unable to discuss. Although many abused children are able to act out their feelings through rebellious and delinquent behavior, others withdraw, blame themselves, become guilt-ridden, and continuously try to be a "better" or "good" child. Such children may function at a high level in school and even be praised for what appears to be mature behavior because they often take on adult caretaker roles at home. Finally, some children with abusive histories do not exhibit signs of trauma during childhood but rather manifest them later in life; others seem to escape trauma from abuse throughout their lives. As previously discussed, the presence of sexual abuse trauma depends on a wide variety of complex factors; in particular, the degree to which the child receives validation, protection, and support after disclosure is crucial to the resolution of trauma.

Box 25-8 Possible/Probable Physical, Behavioral, and Psychosocial Indicators of Childhood Sexual Abuse

General appearance

- Varies from normal to anxious, fearful, and depressed

Probable physical exam indicators

- Bruises, lacerations, or bite marks on breasts, neck, buttocks, extremities, and oropharynx
- Presence of sexually transmitted disease including HIV
- Presence of adult pubic hair and semen
- Edema, abrasions, petechiae and erythema of genital area
- Lacerations to vagina or anus
- Alterations and/or enlargement of hymenal orifice
- Dysuria due to periurethral trauma
- Rectal fissures, chafing and erythema, bruising, lacerations, and perianal scarring
- Semen in the oropharynx and/or nasopharynx
- Scar tissue of labia minora, hymenal membrane, and anus

High-risk family history indicators

- Substance abuse in caretakers
- History of abuse in parents
- Domestic violence

- Inadequate impulse control/mental illness in caretakers
- Alleged offender with sexual dysfunction and/or poor coping, poor social skills
- Socially isolated family
- Sexual abuse of sibling

Behavioral indicators

- Disclosure and spontaneous discussion of the abuse
- Preoccupation with drawing genitals or anxious avoidance of anything to do with genitals/sex
- Inappropriate sexual play behavior with dolls or other children, compulsive masturbation, inserting objects into vagina and/or anus, sexualized kissing, fondling genitals of others, and imitating intercourse
- Dissociation
- Avoidance of particular people, school/learning problems

Possible psychosocial indicators

- Increased anxiety, fears, depression, poor self-esteem
- Multiple somatic complaints
- Signs of post-traumatic stress disorder
- Antisocial behavior, promiscuity, substance abuse
- Running away, self-destructive behavior

The assessment of child sexual abuse should include a physical examination, interviews with the child and family members, outside information from sources such as teachers and baby-sitters, and possible psychological tests if needed. Psychological testing of the child can be helpful in assessing general functioning, memory, and developmental level.

Many researchers and clinicians are working on protocols for interviewing sexually abused children of different developmental ages. Some have developed protocols to use with dolls, puppets, drawings, and other play therapy methods to facilitate disclosure in the child.

In general, the interview with the child should take place in an environment in which the child can feel safe and comfortable. As with all sensitive topics, the questions evolve from the least sensitive and positive topics to the most sensitive and direct ones. Initial questions are meant to gain the child's trust and to assist the child to relax and be spontaneous. The developmental age of the child is a critical factor in the type and level of questioning used; therefore, all techniques must be modified according to the child's needs. Small children may have

difficulty with nondirect, open-ended questions. Interviewers must be extremely cautious *not* to use leading questions such as "Daddy likes to tickle your bottom, doesn't he?"

The nurse's role is to provide comfort and safety for the child. Thus, the immediate physical and psychologic needs of the child must be determined and addressed. Once these needs have been addressed, it is always important for nurses and other health care professionals to determine whether the child will be safe if returned to the home. Some sexual abuse may constitute an emergency situation because of severe physical trauma to the child. In such a case the physical condition must be stabilized as soon as possible, while remembering that the child will be in great pain and very frightened. Most often the abuse will involve fondling rather than physical injury.

Eventually, the child must be asked directly about the existence of sexual abuse. In a nonemergency situation the following sample questions could be used with a small child whose father, stepfather, or other male caretaker is suspected of the abuse.

Nursing Assessment Questions

Sexually Abused Children

1. Who do you like to play with best of all?

2. What kind of fun things do you and (name) do together?

3. What kinds of games do you and (name) play when Mom isn't around?

4. Are there any games that you and (name) play that you don't like?

CASE STUDY

Suzy, a 5-year-old female, was brought to the emergency room by her mother and stepfather, Mr. and Mrs. Jones, because she was bleeding from the vagina. Mrs. Jones reported that she was bathing Suzy in the tub when the phone rang. She then left Suzy for a few minutes to answer the phone. Mr. Jones claims that he went in to check on Suzy when he heard her crying and found her standing in the tub crying and bleeding from the vagina. Mr. and Mrs. Jones maintained that when Suzy tried to get out of the tub, she slipped and injured herself on the tub faucet. No one else was in the home at the time of the accident. Suzy was obviously distressed and unable to give a history. She clung to her mother and would not allow anyone, including the father, to touch her. On physical examination Suzy was found to have lacerations of the hymenal membrane and vaginal wall, trauma to surrounding perineal area, and old scarring.

Critical Thinking and Assessment

1. What are the possible mechanisms for the injury that Suzy received?

2. How would you best prepare Suzy for her physical examination?

3. What kind of questions and comments would be appropriate for and helpful to Suzy at this time?

4. How can the nurse structure the environment so that Suzy will feel safer?

■ ■ NURSING DIAGNOSES

The following nursing diagnoses are based on data identified in the case study on Suzy. Nursing diagnoses are formulated from the information obtained during the assessment phase of the nursing process. The accuracy of diagnosis depends on a careful, in-depth assessment.

Pain related to trauma and injuries sustained from sexual abuse

Anxiety and fear related to threat of further abuse

Risk for violence: risk factors—sexual abuse by father (increased chances of recurrence and possible prior incidents of sexual abuse with daughter)

Ineffective family coping related to sexual abuse behaviors by father, and mother's possible denial as noted by inability to protect her daughter

■ ■ ■ OUTCOME IDENTIFICATION

Outcome criteria for Suzy are derived from the identified nursing diagnoses. These outcomes are the expected behaviors that Suzy and her mother will demonstrate as a result of the implementation of the plan of care and the nursing interventions.

For Suzy, the first priority is addressing the physical trauma of the sexual abuse, which is the hymenal and vaginal laceration and localized trauma to the perineal area. Presence of scar tissue indicates prior abuse. Depending on the extent of damage and bleeding, Suzy may require surgical repair of her injuries. Therefore, based on her plan of care, the first nursing goal will be focused on stabilizing Suzy's physical condition. The second priority regarding nursing goals is to ensure that the abuse will not recur and that the child will be protected in the future.

Outcome Identification for Child Sexual Abuse

Child will:

1. Report a decrease in pain and anxiety.

2. Verbalize an awareness that she will be protected in the future and that no one will be allowed to injure her again.

3. Discuss her present perceptions, distortions, and fears with the nurse.

Child and parent will:

1. Follow through on referral sources for herself and her family. Because Suzy's abuse was ongoing and severe, she will require an individual therapist.

2. Participate in individual or group therapy. Many organizations exist that conduct groups for survivors, nonoffending parents, offenders, and siblings of families with sexual abuse. All family members need to be assessed for the level of their therapy needs.

3. Mother will attend parenting classes because she will require assistance in learning how to nurture, support, and protect her daughter in the future.

No specific diagnosis exists in the DSM-IV manual for childhood sexual abuse. Many adult survivors have been identified as experiencing post-traumatic stress disorder, but symptoms for both children and adult survivors of abuse vary greatly, and no single profile has been identified that would clearly describe sexual abuse survivors.

■ ■ ■ ■ PLANNING

The plan of care for the abused child begins with stabilizing the child's physical needs, securing the child's safety, and addressing the child's psychologic needs. Because the child depends on the parents for the continuation of these goals outside the hospital, the family system must also be assessed. In the case study on Suzy, the father is the suspected abuser; therefore, it must be clearly established that the alleged abuser will not have access to his daughter, and that the mother is capable of nurturing and protecting her child in the future. A police and protective service report must be completed by the attending staff.

■ ■ ■ ■ IMPLEMENTATION

Nurses need to be educated about the signs and symptoms of childhood sexual abuse so that they are able to recognize and take swift action in all potential cases. Since the child's safety is critical, nurses should be knowledgeable about the laws in their state and the policies and procedures of their institution for caring for all survivors of abuse, especially children, who are the most vulnerable. In severe cases such as Suzy's, the father will be removed from the home. The nurse is often the coordinator who ensures that protective services and law enforcement agencies are notified and that treatment referrals are made and followed through on. Usually treatment is ordered by the court after investigations by protective services and the criminal justice system are conducted.

Types of long-term treatment will depend on the child's developmental level and the mother's potential for supporting and protecting the child in the future. Play therapy is often used with a younger child who may have difficulty verbalizing feelings about the abuse. Group therapy with other young children is also very useful because common fears and misperceptions can be addressed. As the child is able to repeatedly address these fears and misperceptions, they will gradually be resolved. Group therapy with children is also a powerful modality for teaching them self-assertive behavior and how to protect themselves in the future.

■ ■ ■ ■ ■ ■ EVALUATION

Ongoing evaluation of the client and family outcomes reveals the efficiency of the nursing interventions and is critical toward ensuring that the child is protected and supported while recovering from the trauma of the abuse. In addition, an ongoing evaluation of the caregiver is needed to determine if this person is following through with the plan of care and to address any problems that may arise. A reliable evaluation of the mother's motivation and ability to support and protect her child requires both short- and long-term assessment. Sometimes the mother may become involved with another partner who is at high risk for child abuse. Thus, the mother must be able to confront her own behavior and the decisions she makes in regard to the safety of her children.

Nursing interventions for the sexually abused child

Nursing interventions	Rationales
Call police and protective services.	Provide for safety needs.
Provide medication prn; reassure child that she is safe and that no one will hurt her again.	Relieve Suzy's pain and anxiety.
Encourage her to talk about fears and concerns.	Allow expression of feelings.
Reassure her that she is not to blame and that her father did a bad thing to hurt her.	Reduce guilt.
Verify that appropriate agencies have been notified and will follow through.	Coordinate contact of appropriate agencies.
Document mother's responses in terms of supporting child and being committed to protecting child in the future.	Assess and strengthen mother's coping abilities.
Provide support and educate about potential resources (e.g., treatment centers, role of social services and criminal justice system).	
Educate mother about the signs and symptoms of abuse that Suzy may exhibit and how to support her.	
Assess the mother for her ability to cope with possible feelings of grief and betrayal.	

ELDER ABUSE

Elder abuse is the last area of family violence to break through public awareness. Because it is the most recent family violence phenomenon to gain public attention, it is also the least researched. In the past 10 years a growing body of knowledge has developed on the issue of elder abuse and that dispelled some of the earlier beliefs about this type of family violence. The first medical publication about elder abuse appeared in the *British Medical Journal* in 1975. In this article Burston described the phenomenon of "granny battering." The emerging belief was that elder abuse was the result of stressed caregivers who occasionally became overwhelmed and beat their unruly parents. Victim blaming was implicit in this explanation. Just as the abused child and battered woman are blamed for provoking or somehow initiating the abuse, so too the elderly "asked for it."

Because of demographic changes in the United States, an increasing number of elderly people live much longer and account for a greater proportion of the population. This large block of elderly citizens has caused a heightened public interest in the concerns of the aged. Elderly citizens have also become more active politically with organizations such as the American Association for Retire Persons (AARP) and the Grey Panthers. However, because so many elderly are isolated and dependent on the people who abuse them, it has been difficult to accurately describe and explain the parameters of this hidden problem.

Even when abuse is clearly documented, the elderly frequently refuse to acknowledge it. As with other victims of abuse, the elderly feel too ashamed and guilty to disclose the abuse and frequently believe that somehow they provoked or deserved it. Because their abusers are frequently family members the elderly may hesitate to report abusive incidents for fear of possible institutionalization or loss of their cherished homes. Furthermore, as with the battered woman and the abused child, the elderly person may have strong feelings of affection and loyalty to his or her abuser. Gelles and Cornell (1990) claim that only one in four cases of elder abuse is reported by the victims themselves.

Definition of Elder Abuse

Six major categories of elder abuse are commonly identified (Sengstock and Barrett, 1993). These are:

1. Psychologic or emotional neglect
2. Psychologic or emotional abuse
3. Violation of personal rights
4. Financial abuse
5. Physical neglect
6. Direct physical abuse

Psychologic neglect involves ignoring or consistently failing to address the concerns of the elderly person. Psychologic abuse includes isolating the elderly person, threatening their safety in some way, inducing fear, and being verbally assaultive. Elderly persons' rights are violated when they are forced to act against their will. An example of such a violation would be forcing elders to move into nursing homes against their will. Financial abuse is characterized by theft or misuse of the elder's money, property, or other possessions. Physical neglect involves the failure to provide the basic necessities of daily living for the elderly person. Sengstock and Barrett (1993) claim that the major difference between direct abuse and neglect is that, in neglect, there is no intent to injure. Finally, direct physical abuse is described as deliberate actions to injure the aged person. These may include such actions as beatings, punches, sexual assaults, and threats with an actual weapon.

The Abused Elder

The elderly abused person has been defined as over age 65. There are no other specific characteristics because the elderly abused person can be male or female, healthy or unhealthy, and competent or incompetent. In terms of severity, abuse of wives by elderly husbands was found to be more severe than that inflicted by wives on husbands.

The Abuser

The earlier image of elder abuse was that of a white elderly female being abused by her middle-aged, overwhelmed caregiver daughter. However, recent research indicates that the person most likely to abuse the elderly is someone who lives with them—a son, daughter, or spouse. This contention is supported by the research of Pillemer and Finkelhor (1988) who found that spouses were the most frequent abusers and that elderly people who lived alone were abused only 25% as often as those who lived with others. Although the abuse typically occurs in the person's home, it is not uncommon for relatives to visit and abuse their elderly relatives in nursing homes. As with other types of abuse, the typical pattern in elder abuse is one of gradually increasing violence and frequency.

In child-to-parent abuse, sons and daughters are equally likely to abuse the elderly. Sons are more likely to inflict physical abuse, whereas psychologic abuse or neglect is more commonly committed by daughters.

Theories of Elder Abuse

Although there are many theories that seek to explain elder abuse, no single theory is completely adequate (Box 25-9). Sengstock and Barrett (1993) identified three main foci for theories on elder abuse: abuser characteristics, situational stress, and family relationships. Pillemer (1986) identified five risk factors for elder abuse, which can be articulated within the theoretical foci of Sengstock and Barrett. These factors are (1) psychopathology of the abuser, (2) external stress, (3) dependency, (4) social isolation, and (5) transgenerational violence.

Elder abuse is frequently compared to child abuse because in both cases neglect is such a common issue. However, with elder abuse, the elder continues to have the rights of an adult unless declared incompetent by a judge. Therefore, decisions cannot legally be forced on the elder as they can on a child. Elders have the right to choose to remain in a particular environment even when it is obvious that they are being abused or neglected.

Box 25-9 Etiologic Factors Related to Elder Abuse

Biologic factors

- Psychopathology of the abuser

Social learning factors

- Dependency (financial and relational)
- Social isolation
- Transgenerational violence

Environmental factors

- External stress

THE NURSING PROCESS ■ ■ ■ ■ ■ ■ ■ ■ ■ ■ ■ ■ ■ ■ ■ ■

■ ASSESSMENT

As with other types of family abuse, it is critical to interview the elder apart from the caregiver. In the hospital it is quite easy to simply assert that hospital policy mandates clients be seen alone. If the nurse is conducting the interview at home, it may be much more difficult to gain access to the elder; nurses may even jeopardize their own safety by insisting on privacy. In these cases suspected abusers need to be assessed for their potential to harm nonfamily members. This assessment needs to determine whether the abuser is a substance abuser or has a history of mental illness and/or violence, since these factors may further compromise the nurse's safety. Sometimes another person in the family who is trusted may provide an opportunity to visit the elder while also providing security for the nurse. Visiting with another nurse is always an option, but at no time should nurses intentionally place themselves in dangerous home-visit situations.

It is not uncommon for both abuser and abused to maintain secrecy about the abuse. As with other types of family violence, abusers frequently threaten their victims with harm if they disclose the reality of their lives. However, even without threats of retaliation, a great deal of time often lapses before the abused elderly are comfortable disclosing their mistreatment. Their reluctance is usually due to shame, self-blame, or fear of abandonment, institutionalization, and serious consequences for the abuser. Sengstock and Barrett (1993) stated that

some elderly victims are unable to report their abuse because it is too devastating to accept the reality of being abused by a loved one.

Box 25-10 identifies physical indicators of actual or potential elder abuse. Many of these symptoms are present with normal aging. Therefore, as with other types of family violence, the nurse must do a comprehensive assessment and consider the physical symptoms within the broader context of the person's life history.

In addition to the above signs and symptoms, the elderly may experience abuse by being overmedicated,

---

Nursing Assessment Questions

Abused Elderly Persons

1. Are you happy living with your ———?
2. Tell me about your financial assets and how they are managed?
3. Who do you turn to when you are feeling down?
4. How are family disagreements handled in your household?
5. Has anyone ever hurt you or touched you when you didn't want to be touched?

Box 25-10   Physical Indicators of Actual or Potential Elder Abuse/Neglect

General appearance

- Anxious, fearful, and passive
- Poor eye contact
- Looks to caregiver for answers
- Poor hygiene and inappropriate dress
- Underweight or malnourished
- Physically handicapped
- No glasses, false teeth, or hearing aid despite need

Skin

- Contusions, abrasions, burns, and scars in various stages of healing
- Decubitus ulcers, urine burns
- Rope marks

Abdominal/rectal

- Distended
- Internal bleeding
- Fecal impactions

Musculoskeletal fractures

- Evidence of old healed fractures
- Current fractures and sprains
- Limited range of motion
- Contractures

Genital/urinary

- Vaginal lacerations, bruises, and infections
- Urinary tract infections

Neurologic

- Slurred speech
- Confusion

CASE STUDY

Eighty-year-old Marjorie Jones was brought, anxiously holding her chest and gasping for breath, to the emergency room by her daughter and son-in-law. Marjorie is currently on medication for congestive heart failure. She is underweight, dehydrated, without dentures, and has poor hygiene. When asked about her missing dentures, she reported that they were lost for quite a few months and no one was able to find them. After receiving medical treatment to stabilize her heart condition, Marjorie began to feel better and was able to give a brief history to the nurse in the privacy of her hospital room.

Marjorie appeared depressed, withdrawn, and had difficulty making eye contact. She reported that because of her inability to maintain her own apartment any longer, she had moved in with her daughter and son-in-law 18 months ago. Until that time Marjorie had a full life with her widowed friends and social activities. She had had a part-time housekeeper since her husband died 5 years ago and was able to maintain her independence quite well until she developed congestive heart failure.

Marjorie reported that life is quite different for her now that she is no longer independent. She stated that she is having a difficult time adjusting to being "so dependent and misses her friends." She denies ever being hurt by anyone. Gradually through gentle questioning, Marjorie admits having difficulty living with her daughter and son-in-law because of their alcohol abuse. While neither has harmed her physically, they have discouraged Marjorie's friends from visiting her and have continually demanded exorbitant room and board payments. Recently, she has begun to notice that some of her jewelry is beginning to disappear. Marjorie is left alone for long periods, sometimes for an entire weekend, which is frightening to her because she is physically unable to provide for her own needs and has no access to the telephone. In addition, she periodically becomes dyspneic and experiences chest pressure.

Critical Thinking and Assessment

1. What is the first priority for the nurse in the care of an elderly person who may be a victim of abuse, neglect, or exploitation?
2. What is the best way to assist an elderly client like Marjorie to disclose feelings, concerns, and fears?
3. What type of mistreatment has Marjorie been experiencing from her daughter and son-in-law?
4. What characteristics require assessment of Marjorie's daughter and son-in-law?

socially isolated, and threatened with physical punishment if their behavior is not deemed appropriate.

Besides possible physical signs and symptoms of elder abuse and neglect, it is also necessary to assess the elder for signs of exploitation and/or abandonment. Signs of exploitation include complaints by the elder or evidence of misuse of their money, loss of control over their finances, material goods taken without consent or approval, and unmet financial needs that are inconsistent with their actual financial status. Signs of abandonment include reports by the elder or evidence of being left alone and helpless for extended periods of time without adequate assistance.

▪ ▪ NURSING DIAGNOSIS

The following nursing diagnoses are based on the assessment data gathered by the nurse who interviewed and examined Marjorie. These diagnoses represent a few of the possibilities that might be relevant for similar cases. Nursing diagnoses are formulated from the information obtained during the assessment phase of the nursing process. The accuracy of diagnoses depends on a careful, in-depth assessment.

Decreased cardiac output and activity intolerance related to change in health status (congestive heart failure)

Moderate to severe anxiety related to change in health status and role functioning

Ineffective family coping related to alcohol abuse by caregivers and caregiver role strain

Personal identity disturbances related to changes in health status and role functioning

No diagnosis in the DSM-IV is currently appropriate for the abused elderly person.

▪ ▪ ▪ OUTCOME IDENTIFICATION

Outcome criteria for this section are based on the nursing diagnoses derived from the case study on Marjorie, as described earlier. These outcomes are the expected behaviors that someone like Marjorie would demonstrate or achieve as a result of the implementation of the plan of care and the nursing interventions. Because Marjorie came to the emergency room for severe cardiac distress, the first nursing priority is stabilizing her congestive heart failure so that she can regain normal cardiac output as evidenced by normal vital signs, freedom from chest pain and dyspnea, and decreased anxiety and fear. The remainder of Marjorie's nursing diagnoses relate to her psychosocial needs, including her depression. Because of her change in health status and her dependency on exploitative and neglectful caregivers, Marjorie is feeling helpless, frightened, and depressed.

Outcome Identification for Elder Abuse

Client will:

1. Explore options that may exist in relation to her home situation. Because Marjorie is an adult, she cannot be forced to leave her children's home or press charges against them. If there are mandatory reporting laws in Marjorie's state, her children's abusive behavior will have to be reported.

2. Verbalize feelings about her change in health care status, her dependency on her children, the treatment she has received from them, and available options for dealing with these concerns.

▪ ▪ ▪ ▪ PLANNING

As with other victims of family violence, securing safety is a major aspect in the plan of care for the abused elderly. In the case of Marjorie, stabilizing her congestive heart failure had to be achieved before her abusive home situation could be assessed and a plan of care for this aspect of her life established. Because most states have mandatory elder abuse reporting laws, it is critical that nurses and other health care professionals remain open to the possibility of elder abuse whenever there are potential indicators for it. As noted earlier, the elderly person will often deny the existence of the abuse; therefore, it is necessary to establish a trusting relationship with elderly clients to facilitate disclosure. Sengstock and Barrett (1993) suggest that the establishment of trust is the most critical component in planning the care of the abused client. In particular, they warn about being critical of the abuser because the elderly are most likely to strongly defend their loved ones, despite the abuse they have experienced. Since nurses have time constraints in such settings as emergency rooms and clinics, it can be difficult to establish the trust necessary to facilitate disclosure by the abused elderly client. Nevertheless, often it will be the nurse who is in the best position to assess and identify the abused client. Thus, the plan of care should include taking time to communicate concern, compassion, and a desire to explore options and resources that can determine whether clients disclose critical information or continue to suffer in silence.

▪ ▪ ▪ ▪ IMPLEMENTATION

As in other cases of family violence, the nurse will often be called on to function as the coordinator of care. In Marjorie's case, the nurse may need to work closely with the social worker to develop and implement the plan of care. Since the nurse has frequent opportunities to discuss Marjorie's problems with her, she will be a key person in assisting Marjorie to identify her feelings, recognize her strengths, realistically assess the situation, and explore all possible options before making decisions. Thus, the nurse is in a position to address the total biopsychosocial, spiritual, and cultural needs of the client.

Nursing Interventions

As previously mentioned, nursing interventions will be focused on meeting the biopsychosocial, spiritual, and cultural needs of the client. Thus, the nurse can assist Marjorie to accept the limitations of her congestive heart failure while encouraging her to optimize her self-care

---

Nursing interventions for the abused elderly

Nursing interventions	Rationales
Monitor response to decreased cardiac output. Monitor response to medications. Provide reassurance and support. Educate about medications and limitations.	Support return of normal cardiac output.
Monitor for increased depression and suicide potential. Explore with the client the reasons for feelings of helplessness and grief. Discuss capabilities and strengths. Explore options relating to increased control. Explore ways to increase self-care.	Reduce sense of helplessness and grief; increase feelings of control.
Explore feelings related to family abuse.	Increase awareness of feelings related to abuse by family.
Explore options for remaining with family versus alternate living arrangements. Coordinate referrals. Show respect for client's decisions.	Increase awareness of options relating to living arrangements.
Evaluate motivation for seeking and using assistance. Evaluate coping skills. Evaluate substance abuse. Evaluate willingness to acknowledge and work on family problems.	Evaluate family for motivation and ability to provide care in the future.

---

abilities. At the same time, it is very important to help Marjorie learn about the community resources available to her in terms of maximizing her mental and physical health. Marjorie will require assistance dealing with the guilt and shame she feels about being a burden to her daughter and son-in-law and the abuse they mete out. A plan must be made with the family if Marjorie insists on remaining with them. This plan must clearly explain the family's obligations, Marjorie's rights, and the consequences of future abusive or neglectful behavior. As Marjorie's care requirements increase, the potential for greater abuse increases proportionately. Thus, ongoing monitoring and evaluation are necessary, and these tasks are becoming more important for nurses as they provide ever-increasing amounts of care for elderly clients in their homes.

The home health care nurse must be prepared to provide counseling, referrals, support, and education to elderly citizens and their families. Sometimes the caregiver may be in desperate need of stress management techniques, general information on the aging process, basic nursing care principles, and community agencies that provide assistance to the elderly. Providing such support may dramatically ease the burden of caring for the elderly relative and prevent the occurrence of abuse and neglect.

■ ■ ■ ■ ■ ■ EVALUATION

Evaluating the effectiveness of the outcomes and nursing care plan for the elder who has been abused is important because the abuse may continue and even escalate if the elderly person chooses to return to the abusive environment. In a situation like Marjorie's, the potential for escalating abuse is significant because she will probably require increasing assistance from dysfunctional caregivers who are at high risk for continuing the abuse owing to their substance abuse. However, nurses are frequently not in a position to follow up on clients once they leave the hospital.

Sengstock and Barrett (1993) claim that certain clues can be helpful in determining whether the nursing interventions will be successful. These include the willingness of the elderly person to acknowledge the abuse, the willingness of the elder and the abusive family members to accept outside interventions, and/or removal of the elder from the abusive environment. Although many resources for the elderly exist in most communities, the family cannot be assisted if they deny the existence of the abuse. Like the battered wife, an elderly person may experience multiple occasions of abuse before gradually making the decision to leave the abusive environment.

RAPE

In recent years, much energy and attention has been devoted to the public discussion of rape. Two recent rape cases involving high-profile males were especially prominent in the media (Mike Tyson and William Kennedy Smith). Recently Congress held hearings on sexual assault in the U.S. Navy Tailhook event and on sexual assault incidents in the Air Force. As a result of the growing public concern about female sexual assault and feminists' demands for action to prevent this violence, many states have passed laws to protect rape victims and to prosecute rapists more aggressively.

The National Institutes of Mental Health has also responded to the call for action by increasing funding for rape research. In addition, stronger federal policies for prosecuting perpetrators of sexual harassment and assault have forced corporations and universities to develop policies and procedures for addressing sexual harassment and sexual assault.

Despite these positive steps in recent years to support victims, prosecute offenders, and prevent sexual assault, victim blaming persists. Instead of placing blame on the rapist where it belongs, victims are blamed and revictimized in myriad ways. The following scenarios are common examples of victim blaming and revictimization.

- If a woman cannot provide evidence of resisting a rapist, she is often accused of consenting to the sexual activity.
- If she was drinking, she is often viewed as causing her own rape.
- If she dressed "sensually" or was out late at night, she was "looking for it."
- If she acted friendly to him, she "led him on or seduced him."
- If he spent money on her, she "owed" it to him.

No one has the right to verbally or physically force another into sexual activity against his or her will. If a person says "no," that means "no," even if he or she said "yes" first, then changed his or her mind later.

Definition of Rape

The traditional legal definition of rape is forced penile-vaginal penetration against the will of the woman. In the last few years this traditional definition has been expanded by most states and the federal government to include cunnilingus, fellatio, anal intercourse, or any intrusion of any part of a person's body (Koss, 1993). Nonconsent involves physical force, the threat of physical force, or the inability of the victim to consent for reasons such as age, developmental disability, or intoxication.

Estimating the prevalence of rape is difficult because most rapes are not reported, and research studies that attempt to report accurate figures are based on a variety of definitions, screening questions, and samples that are not always representative of the population. Koss (1993) emphasized that failure to report rape is a much greater problem than false reports of rape. False reports of rape are projected at 2%, the same rate as for other crimes. Conversely, only one in 10%–20% of rapes is reported to police (Botash et al, 1994).

Prevalence studies on completed rape generally range from 20%–25% (Koss, 1993; Russell, 1984; Wyatt, 1985). Koss reported that women who are incarcerated and those with a history of psychiatric inpatient treatment have a much higher prevalence of reported rape. It is also recognized that males have a much lower rape prevalence than females. In a national crime survey conducted by Jamieson and Flanagan (1989), over 90% of rape victims were women. Koss concludes that the United States have a major rape problem.

Twenty percent of college women are raped at some time during their college careers. This is consistent with the statistic that the most common age group for rape victims is women ages 16 to 25. In 84% of rape cases the victim is acquainted with the offender. Thus, rape by a stranger is the exception rather than the rule (Warshaw, 1988).

Rather than in dark alleys, rapes most commonly occur on dates or at parties and other social functions. Although society may believe that rapists are "sick or psychopathic," research has failed to find support for such general personality patterns. Abel et al (1980) found that only 5% of rapists were psychotic when they committed rape. Indeed, a growing body of research indicates that many males are sexually aggressive and force their partners into sex. A common male attitude is that women exist to satisfy males, and therefore consent is unnecessary. Scully and Marolla (1993) discussed several decades of research on male sexual aggression and concluded that such behavior is viewed as "normal." By not addressing the sexually aggressive behavior of many males and maintaining the myth that all rapists are psychotic, society avoids its responsibility to examine most rapes within the context of learned and socially sanctioned male behavior.

Characteristics of a Rapist

A common myth about rapists is that most are black. Botash et al (1994) reported that most perpetrators and victims are white; in 90% of cases, victims and perpetrators are of the same race.

Although research has focused on individual characteristics of rapists rather than group behavior, in recent years more attention has been focused on fraternities on college campuses as a rape-prone social context. Martin and Hummer (1993) in their study on fraternities and rape on campus concluded that fraternities provide a physical and sociocultural context that encourages the sexual coercion of women. These researchers acknowledge that not all fraternity men are rapists; nevertheless, they insist that because of the type of man recruited, the social expectations of these organizations, and the lack of university or community supervision, the occurrence of rape is a probability in fraternities. Martin and Hummer dismiss the notion of peer pressure as an excuse and suggest "that fraternities create a sociocultural context in which the use of coercion in sexual relations with women is normative and in which the mechanisms to keep this pattern of behavior in check are minimal at best and absent at worse". They also report that fraternity men acknowledge using alcohol as a weapon to gain sexual mastery over reluctant women and that the prim and proper sorority girl is particularly prized as a sexual trophy. In another study by Malamuth et al (1980), 51% of male respondents reported that they would rape if they could be certain of not being punished.

Effects of Rape on the Victim

Many rape victims experience devastating effects from their rape. In the past, rape was frequently viewed as unwanted sex with few if any negative consequences. Today society is much more aware of the serious short- and long-term effects of rape.

In a literature review of the psychological consequences of rape, Resick (1993) reported that 1 month after the rape, a majority of women continued to experience significant fear, depression, sexual dysfunction, and social adjustment problems. After 2 or 3 months, the symptoms of most women began to improve. However, 1 year after the rape, many victims continued to experience these symptoms when compared to a control group of women who had not been raped. About one-third of the women continued to experience distress 3 to 6 years after the rape. Resick reported that the symptoms in this latter group of the women became chronic and generally involved post-traumatic stress disorder, depression, anxiety, sexual dysfunctions, and social adjustment problems. In addition, rape victims reported feeling more anger, hostility, and confusion than nonvictims and were more likely to use alcohol and drugs.

Not all women experience long-term serious effects from being raped. Many factors can account for these differences among rape victims, but much more research is needed before the interrelationships among these factors can be understood (Resick, 1993). Currently, research evidence is unclear as to whether demographic factors such as age, socioeconomic status, and race have a significant effect on rape trauma. However, prior psychological functioning and life stressors have been reported to be important in the development of long-term effects from rape. Women with mental health problems, revictimization, and multiple-incident revictimization seem to have more difficulty overcoming long-term effects of rape. Resick reported that preassault, assault, and postassault factors may all influence the psychological functioning of the rape victim.

Thus, although victim responses are varied, rape is a traumatic experience and its victims require immediate attention and support from health care professionals. Evidence of the rape must be gathered and documented, laboratory tests for pregnancy and sexually transmitted diseases performed, and the victim referred to an experienced counselor or rape crisis center.

As with victims of family violence, nurses are often in a position to assist victims of rape. It is encumbent on the professional nurse to accept responsibility for becoming knowledgeable and skillful in assisting rape victims. This assistance may take a variety of forms including identification, support for disclosure, as well as therapeutic interventions to facilitate recovery of this often-neglected population.

Summary of Key Concepts

1. Violence and abusive behavior is a major public health concern.

2. Because they assume many roles in a variety of settings, nurses are in a prime position to advocate and intervene for victims of violence.

3. Interpersonal violence is more likely to be done by someone the victim knows.

4. Battering is the most common cause of injury to women in the United States.

5. Domestic violence is generally defined as physical, psychologic, and sexual abuse primarily directed at women by men for the purpose of maintaining control and power.

6. Emotional and psychologic abuse can be just as devastating as direct physical abuse.

7. Most child physical and sexual abuse is perpetrated by an adult known to the child.

8. Actions that ensure protection and safety for the victim are the most important nursing interventions in abuse situations.

9. Elder abuse is becoming a greater public concern as the number of elderly persons in the population is growing.

REFERENCES

Abel G, et al: Aggressive behavior and sex. *Psychiatr Clin North Am* 3: 133–141, 1980.

American Humane Society: *Highlights of official child neglect and abuse reporting—1986,* Denver, Colo., 1988, American Humane Association.

Ammerman RT, Hersen M: *Assessment of family violence: a clinical and legal sourcebook,* New York, 1992, Wiley & Sons.

APSAC Task Force: *Guidelines for psychosocial evaluation of suspected sexual abuse in young children,* 1990.

Bandura A: *Aggression: a social learning analysis,* Englewood Cliffs, N.J., 1973, Prentice Hall.

Barbee EL: *Ethnicity and woman abuse in the United States.* In Sampselle C, editor: *Violence against women,* New York, 1992, Hemisphere.

Berkowitz CD, et al: American Medical Association diagnostic and treatment guidelines on child physical abuse and neglect. *Arch Fam Med,* 1:187–197, 1992.

Bohn D, Parker B: *Domestic violence and pregnancy.* In Campbell J, Humphreys J, editors: *Nursing care of survivors of family violence,* St. Louis, 1993, Mosby.

Botash AS, et al: Acute care for sexual assault victims, *Patient Care* 28:112–137, 1994.

Bremner RH, editor: *Children and youth in America: a documentary history,* vols 1–2, Cambridge, Mass., 1970, 1971, Harvard University Press.

Brendtro M, Bowker LH: Battered women: how can nurses help? *Issues in Mental Health Nursing* 10:169–180, 1989.

Briere J: *Child abuse trauma,* Newbury Park, Calif., 1992, Sage.

Bullock L, McFarlane J: The birth weight/battering connection, *Am J Nurs* 89(9): 1153–1155, 1989.

Burgess A, et al: Child molestation: assessing impact in multiple victims (part 1), *Arch Psychiatr Nurs* 1:33–39, 1987.

Campbell JC: The battering of wives: a cross-cultural perspective, *Victimology* 10:174–185, 1985.

Campbell JC, Fishwick N: Abuse of female partners. In Campbell JC, Humphreys J, editors: *Nursing care of survivors of family violence,* St. Louis, 1993, Mosby.

Campbell JC, Humphreys J: *Nursing care of survivors of family violence,* St. Louis, 1993, Mosby.

Carmen E, Rieker PP: A psychosocial model of the victim-to-patient process, *Psychiatr Clin North Am* 12:431–443, 1989.

Conte J, Berliner: The impact of sexual abuse of children: empirical findings. In Walker LE, editor: *Handbook on sexual abuse of children,* New York, 1988, Springer.

Courtois C: *Healing the incest wound,* New York, 1988, Norton.

Deblinger E, et al: Psychosocial characteristics and correlates of symptom distress in nonoffending mothers of sexually abused children, *J Interpers Viol* 8:155–167, 1993.

Dobash RE, Dobash RP: *Violence against wives,* New York, 1979, The Free Press.

Drake VK: Battered women: a health care problem in disguise, *Image* 14:40–47, 1982.

Eisler R: *The chalice and the blade: our history, our future,* San Francisco, 1988, Harper & Row.

Federal Bureau of Investigation: *Crime in the United States,* Washington, D.C., Government Printing Office, 1985.

Finkelhor D, Brown A: The traumatic impact of sexual abuse: a conceptualization, *American Jour of Orthopsych* 55, 530–541, 1986.

Flitcraft AH: American Medical Association diagnostic and treatment guidelines on domestic violence. *Arch Fam Med* 1:39–47, 1992.

Gardner R: *The parental alienation syndrome and the differentiation between fabricated and genuine child sex abuse,* Cresskill, N.J., 1987, Creative Therapeutics.

Giordino A, et al: *A practical guide to the evaluation of sexual abuse in the prepubertal child,* Newbury Park, Calif, 1992, Sage.

Goldberg WG, Tomlanovich MC: Domestic violence victims in the emergency department, *JAMA* 251:3259–3264, 1985.

Henderson J: *Incest.* In Freedman AM, Kaplan HI, Sadock BS, editors: *Comprehensive textbook of psychiatry,* Baltimore, 1975, Williams & Wilkins.

Herman J: *Trauma and recovery,* New York, 1992, Basic Books.

Humphreys J, Ramsey AM: *Child abuse.* In Campbell J, Humphreys J, editors: *Nursing care of survivors of family violence,* St. Louis, 1993, Mosby.

Jacobson A, Herald C: The relevance of childhood sexual abuse to adult psychiatric inpatient care. *Hosp Commun Psychiatr* 41:154–158, 1990.

Jamieson KM, Flanagan TJ: *Sourcebook of criminal justice statistics-1988 (NCJ-100899),* Washington D.C., 1989, US Department of Justice, Bureau of Justice Statistics.

Jehu D: Adult survivors of sexual abuse. In Ammerman R, Hersen M, editors: *The assessment of family violence,* New York, 1992, Wiley.

Justice B, Justice R: *The broken taboo: sex in the family,* New York, 1979, Human Sciences Press.

Kempe CH, et al: The battered child syndrome, *JAMA,* 181:17–24, 1962.

King MC, Ryan J: Abused women: dispelling myths and encouraging intervention. *Nurse Practitioner,* 14:47-58, 1989.

Koop CE, Lundberg GD: Violence in America: a public health emergency, *JAMA* 267: 3075–3076, 1992.

Koss MP: Detecting the scope of rape, *J Interpers Viol* 8:198–222, 1993.

Kurz D: Emergency department repsonses to battered women: resistance to medicalization, *Soc Probl* 34:501–513, 1987.

Malamuth N, et al: Testing hypotheses regarding rape: exposure to sexual violence, sex difference, and the 'normality' of rapists, *J Res Pers* 14:121–137, 1980.

Mannarino AP, Cohen JA: A clinical-demographic study of sexually abused children, *Child Abuse Neglect* 10:17–23, 1986.

Martin PY, Hummer RA: *Fraternities and rape on campus.* In Bart PB, Moran EG, editors: *Violence against women,* Newbury Park, Calif., 1993, Sage.

National Center on Child Abuse and Neglect: *Study of national incidence and prevalence of child abuse and neglect: 1988.* (Contract No. 105-85-1702). Washington, D.C., 1988, U.S. Department of Health and Human Services.

Nye R: *Choice, exchange, and the family.* In Burr WR et al, editors: *Contemporary theories about the family,* New York, 1979, The Free Press.

Pillemer KA: Risk factors in elder abuse: results from a case-control study, in Pillemer KA and Wolff, editors, *Elder Abuse: Conflict in the family,* Dover, 1986, Auburn House.

Resick P: The psychological impact of rape, *J Interpers Viol* 8:223–255, 1993.

Russell, D: *Sexual exploitation,* Beverly Hills, Calif., 1984, Sage.

Russell D: *The secret trauma,* New York, 1986, Basic Books.

Sampselle CM: *Violence against women,* New York, 1992, Hemisphere.

Scully D, Marolla J: Riding the bull at Gilley's: convicted rapists describe the rewards of rape. In Bart PB, Moran EG, editors: *Violence against women: the bloody footprints,* Newbury Park, Calif, 1993, Sage.

Sengstock MC, Barrett AA: Abuse and neglect of the elderly in family settings. In Campbell JC. Humphreys J, editors: *Nursing Care of Survivors of Family violence,* St. Louis, 1993, Mosby.

Stark E, et al: Medicine and patriarchal violence: the social construction of a private event, *Intl J Health Serv* 9:461–493, 1979.

Stark R, McElroy J: Middle-class violence, *Psychology Today* 4:52–65, 1970.

Straus MA, Gelles RJ: Societal change and change in family violence from 1975 to 1985 as revealed by two national surveys, *J Marr Fam* 48:465–479, 1986.

Straus MA, et al: *Behind closed doors: violence in the American family,* Garden City, N.Y., 1980, Anchor.

Tilden VP, Shepherd P: Battered women: the shadow side of families, *Hol Nurs Pract* 1(2):25–32, 1987.

United States Department of Health and Human Services, Public Health Service: *Healthy People 2000: national health promotion and disease prevention objectives,* DHSS Publication No. (PHS) 91-50212. Washington, D.C., 1990, U.S. Government Printing Office.

Urbancic J: *Intrafamilial sexual abuse.* In Campbell J, Humphries J, editors: *Nursing care of survivors of family violence,* St. Louis, 1993, Mosby-Year Book.

Urbancic J: The relationship between empowerment support, mental health self-care, well-being, and incest trauma resolution in adult female survivors, Doctoral dissertation, Wayne State University, *Diss Abstr Intl* 54: 1896B, 1992.

Walker LE: Psychology and violence against women, *Am Psychol* 44(4):695–702, 1989.

Warshaw C: Limitations of the medical model in the care of battered women, *Gender Sociol* 3:506–517, 1989.

Warshaw R : *I never called it rape,* San Francisco, 1988, Harper & Row.

Weinberg SK: *Incest behavior,* New York, 1955, Citadel.

Wyatt GE: The sexual abuse of Afro-American and White-American women in childhood, *Child Abuse Neglect* 9:507–519, 1985.

CHAPTER 26

Suicide

Mary Ann Barbee
Pamela Bricker

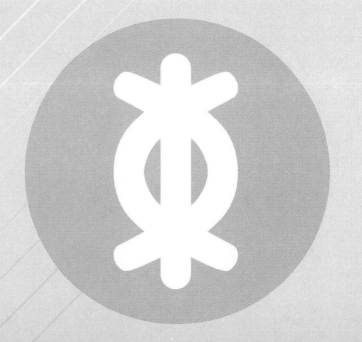

Cognitive rigidity   The inability to adequately identify problems and corresponding solutions.

Comorbidity   The co-occurrence of two or more disorders in the same individual at the same time.

Conscious suicidal intention   A state of awareness characterized by a desire to bring about one's own death.

Imminence   The likelihood that an event will occur within a specific time period.

Lethality   The potential for causing death related to the level of danger associated with the suicidal plan, along a continuum from low to high probability (for example, aspirin overdose versus a gunshot wound to the head).

Parasuicidal behavior   Suicidal gestures and attempts that are unsuccessful and of low lethality (for example, superficial cutting of the wrists).

Perturbation   A determination of an individual's level of distress, developed by Shneidman and rated on a scale of 1–9. Refers to how upset, disturbed, perturbed the individual is.

Suicide   The act of taking one's own life.

Suicide ideators   Those persons who experience suicidal thinking on a consistent basis.

Suicidology   The scientific and humane study of human self-destruction.

Unconscious suicidal intention   A state outside of awareness during which persons engage in risk-taking behaviors that have a high likelihood of causing their deaths.

- Discuss the scope of suicide by age, gender, ethnicity, socioeconomic status, and familial factors.

- Compare and contrast biological, psychological, and sociological theories regarding the etiology of suicide.

- Distinguish between suicidal ideation, gesture, threat, attempt, and successful suicide.

- Discuss key elements in the assessment of suicide risk.

- Apply the nursing process for suicidal clients and their families.

- Construct a nursing care plan for a client admitted to the psychiatric care unit with depression and suicidality.

S uicide, the act of taking one's own life, is a major public health and mental health problem in the United States. It is among the leading causes of death for youth between ages 15 and 24. The suicide rate for the elderly population is growing faster than for any age group.

Suicidal thoughts, threats, and attempts often precede clients' search for mental health treatment in a variety of settings. Imminent risk for suicide is one of the leading criteria for medical care of clients admitted to psychiatric hospitals. Health professionals in all disciplines increasingly are called on to assist with assessing suicidal risk and ensuring that clients receive prompt intervention to provide physical and psychologic safety. Nurses are positioned strategically to contribute to these efforts by the nature of the broad scope of their practice in multiple health care settings.

HISTORICAL AND THEORETICAL PERSPECTIVES

World history includes many references to suicide as a religious, psychologic, or social phenomenon. Suicide was considered both a spiritual offense and a legal offense against the king in Europe dating back to 673 A.D. Those who committ suicide were not allowed a Christian burial, and all of their possessions were forfeited to the king unless it was determined that a suicide was a result of madness or physical illness (Celo-Cruz, 1992). Shakespeare wrote of suicide in *Romeo and Juliet* and *Macbeth.* Suicides increased following the Wall Street crash in 1929 and during the Great Depression as people took their own lives rather than face financial ruin and humiliation. Japan's kamikaze pilots of World War II elevated suicide to a high cultural level as they sacrificed their lives for their country and their religious principles.

Throughout history, suicide has served as a solution to the disappointments and obstacles that people have faced. It was not until the late 1800s that pioneers such as Durkheim, a sociologist, and Freud began to study the phenomenon from theoretical viewpoints.

Sociological Theory

Durkheim, in his classic work of 1897, classified the social and cultural aspects of suicide into four subtypes: anomic, egoistic, altruistic, and fatalistic. He defined *anomic suicides* as acts of self-destruction by individuals who have become estranged from important relationships in their groups, especially as related to their standards of living (for example, the suicides after the 1929 crash of the stock market). *Egoistic suicides* were characterized as those deaths of individuals who are influenced by a group to turn against their own conscience (for example, the devout Catholic adolescent who commits suicide after undergoing an abortion forbidden by her religion). Durkheim described *altruistic suicides* as those self-inflicted deaths based on obedience to a group's goals that override the person's own best interests (for example, the kamikaze pilot incidents). Finally, he defined *fatalistic suicides* as a deaths resulting from excessive regulation (for example, the suicides of felons who hang themselves in prison to escape oppression) (Durkheim, 1951).

Psychoanalytic Theory

Freud viewed suicide from a psychoanalytic viewpoint. At the 1910 psychoanalytic meeting on suicide in Vienna, he and Stekel described self-destruction as hostility directed inward toward the internalized love object (Freud, 1920; Stekel, 1967). These early formulations ignored other critical feeling states, such as shame, hopelessness, helplessness, worthlessness, and fear. Later, Freud incorporated many accompanying psychologic and sociological clinical features, such as guilt into his views about suicide (Litman, 1967). Freud identified three features he believed made each individual somewhat vulnerable to suicide:

1. The death instinct.

2. The splitting of the ego when the individual is unable to assume mastery over his or her instincts and has to conform to others' wishes or die.

3. The influence of group institutions such as family and society, which require compliance from each member of the group through guilt (Litman, 1967).

Psychoanalytic theorists who followed Freud have added their own perspectives to the notion of suicide (Weiss, 1966). Menninger described several sources of suicidal impulses: the wish to kill, the wish to be killed, and the wish to die. Jung postulated that the suicidal person held an unconscious wish for spiritual rebirth after feeling that life had lost its meaning. Adler identified the importance of inferiority, narcissism, and low self-esteem in suicidal acts. Horney believed suicide was a solution for one who experienced extreme alienation of self as a result of great disparity between the idealized self and the perceived psychosocial self (Weiss, 1966).

Interpersonal Theory

Sullivan broadened the theoretical knowledge base of suicide by emphasizing the importance of interpersonal relationship factors. He observed that persons can never be isolated from the interactions of significant people in their lives (Sullivan, 1931). Therefore, Sullivan believed, the suicidal act should be understood within the context of the perceptions of the suicidal person by his or her significant others. He viewed suicide as evidence of failure to resolve interpersonal conflicts (Sullivan, 1956).

These classical sociological, psychodynamic, and interpersonal theories formed the foundation for the major contemporary etiologies that followed in the 1960s.

ETIOLOGY

The contemporary, scientific, and humane study of suicide, called **suicidology,** began in the early 1960s when several important events occurred (Shneidman, 1969):

1. There was an increase in the number of suicide prevention centers from 3 in 1958 to more than 100 in 1968.

2. The Center for Studies of Suicide Prevention was established at the National Institute of Mental Health in 1966.

3. The American Association of Suicidology was founded in 1967.

4. *The Bulletin of Suicidology,* the first professional journal devoted to the study of self-destruction phenomenabegan, publication in 1967.

5. The 1910 Viennese psychoanalytic meetings on suicide were reconvened at the first annual conference of the American Association of Suicidology in Chicago in 1968. Shneidman and his colleagues led the proceedings in the discussion of innovations in the prevention of suicide.

Biologic

The structure and chemistry of the brain have been studied most thoroughly in relation to affective or mood disorders (for further information see Chapter 12). Neurotransmitters, or certain chemicals in the brain that regulate mood, have been identified, e.g., *serotonin, dopamine, norepinephrine,* and *gamma amino butric acid.* Recently, research with adults suggests that irregularities in the serotonin system are found in suicidal patients. In a 1994 study by Nielson and colleagues, the major metabolite of serotonin, 5-hydroxyindoleacetic acid (5-HIAA), which is found in cerebrospinal fluid, was studied in conjunction with the genotype, tryptophan hydroxylase (TPH). This was the first report "to implicate a specific gene in the predisposition to a behavior (suicidality) in impulsive, alcoholic violent offenders postulated to be regulated by serotonin (Nielson et al, 1994). (See Understanding and Applying Research below.)

Currently there are no medications that specifically affect suicidal behavior. However, medications that regulate serotonin levels are effective in the treatment of mood disorders that often accompany suicidal ideation.

Understanding and Applying
RESEARCH

Nielsen D et al.: Suicidality and 5-hydroxyindoleacetic acid, concentration associated with tryptophan hydroxylase polymorphism, *Arch GEn Psychiatry* 51:34–38, 1994.

Family and twin studies have suggested a genetic component to certain antisocial and suicidal behaviors. This study found that the genotype tryptophan hydroxylase (THP) was a factor influencing the neurotransmitter serotonin and its principal metabolite 5-hydroxyindoleacetic acid (5-HIAA), found in the cerebrospinal fluid, and suicide attempts.

The THP genotype was found in 56 impulsive and 14 nonimpulsive Finnish alcoholic violent offenders and in 20 healthy volunteers with no mental disorders. All subjects were evaluated for documented histories of severe suicide attempts. THP analysis and 5-HIAA concentration levels in the cerebrospinal fluid were obtained by investigators unaware of the subjects. A significant association of the THP genotype with violent offenders who had histories of severe suicide attempts was found. If replicated, the findings of this study could lead to an improved ability to identify individuals at risk for suicide and to suggest pharmocologic or genetic interventions. This information could assist nurses in improving their assessment of clients for suicidal risk and in determining the most appropriate interventions.

Another psychologic factor is the neurobiologic correlation of depression and suicide. Suicide is most often correlated to depression, and as depression resolves suicide risk diminishes. According to Cummings (1993), the dimensions of depression can be correlated with alterations in specific areas of the brain.

- *Mood:* sadness and dysphoria are associated with limbic lesions that can be moderated with dopamine.

- *Affect:* separate motor systems of the limbic and brain stem regions of the brain influence control of the face and facial expressions, and the muscular responses associated with emotional affect, for example, crying.

- *Motivation:* changes in the pleasure response, which is moderated by dopamine and dopamine antagonists, are correlated to motivational levels.

- *Cognitive content:* frontal lobe dysfunction is thought to be related to feelings of hopelessness and worthlessness, both of which are precursors to suicidal thoughts.

The explosion of knowledge in psychobiology requires that nurses integrate the psychophysiologic aspects of illness with the behavioral sciences in their own nursing practice. Trygstad (1994), in a descriptive study of the perceived psychobiological learning needs of psychiatric nurses, identified five areas of focus. They are listed in Box 26-1.

Future research in psychobiology as it relates to suicidal behavior may begin to overshadow the contributions of the more traditional fields of psychology and sociology.

Psychologic

Intrapsychic and interpersonal theories continue to dominate the psychologic view of suicidal behavior. Contemporary etiologies include

- self-directed aggression or self-destruction as an act of murder directed at the love object toward whom the person feels ambivalent, leading to states of isolation and loneliness;
- death as an atonement for wrongdoings;
- death as a way to recapture the lost love object;
- suicidal death as a secondary result of the major depressive processes.

Most psychodynamic theorists following Freud theorized that depression followed the loss of a significant love object and led to feelings of helplessness, hopelessness, guilt, and diminished self-esteem. Suicide can serve as a way to end those painful feeling states (Toolan, 1974). This model emphasized the functioning of the psyche and the reporting of subjective experiences. Case studies of individuals and a small series of similar cases were examined to identify the mental mechanisms that led to suicide attempts or completions (Andreasen, 1984).

Cognitive theory adds to the understanding of suicidal episodes by emphasizing the role of particular thought patterns: negativism, self-worthlessness, and a bleak view of the future. **Cognitive rigidity,** the inability to identify problems and solutions, has been hypothesized as a factor in suicide when accompanied by stress (Rudd et al, 1994).

Shneidman (1985) developed the term **perturbation,** defined as a determination of an individual's level of distress and rated on a scale of 1–9. Perturbation refers to how upset, disturbed, or perturbed the individual is. Shneidman, building on his 35 years of work as a suicidologist, lectured about the common psychologic features of suicide (1985). He defined suicide as a "response to an inner decision that the pain is unendurable, intolerable, and unacceptable. It is an unwillingness to endure that pain rather than the pain itself." He outlined the 10 psychologic commonalities of suicide from his studies. They are listed in Box 26-2.

Additionally, the development of behavioral approaches based on learning theory contributed to the understanding and treatment of mental health problems. Interventions for suicidal ideation based on learning theory are directed toward decreasing unpleasant events and increasing pleasant events. Tension-reducing relaxation techniques, stress management skills, and rehearsal of problem-solving techniques are valuable adjuncts to reducing depression and suicidal behavior (Lewinsohn and Mischel, 1980).

Sociological

Contemporary sociologists have reinforced Durkheim's earlier work on suicide. Contemporary social scientists have supported the idea that alienation from social groups after disruption of family, community, or social re-

---

Box 26-2   Psychologic Commonalities of Suicide

1. The common *purpose* of suicide is to solve a problem. The health care professional must assist the suicidal person to identify the life problem that needs to be solved or changed.
2. The common *goal* of suicide is the cessation of consciousness, i.e., death.
3. The common *stimulus* of suicide is intolerable psychological pain, along with the decision not to experience that pain.
4. The common *stressor* in suicide is frustrated psychological needs, such as achievement, affiliation, aggression, autonomy, dominance, harm avoidance, shame avoidance, nurturance, order, or play.
5. The common *emotions* of suicide are helplessness and hopelessness.
6. The common *cognitive state* is ambivalence.
7. The common *perceptual state* is constriction with pain, frustration of needs, and helplessness.
8. The common *action* of suicide is aggression or exiting the scene.
9. The common *interpersonal act* is the communication of intention.
10. The common *consistency* in suicide is lifelong patterns of failure, stress, duress, and threats to self-esteem.

---

lationships leads some individuals to attempt or commit suicide (Maris, 1985; Richman, 1986).

Sociologists Hoyer and Lund found empirical support for Durkheim's notion that marriage and parenthood lead to a lower suicide mortality rate for women in a prospective study of almost 100,000 women from 1970–1975 in Norway (1993).

Thus, the findings of sociological studies provide added dimensions to the biologic and psychologic explanations of suicidal behavior. A more holistic approach is to consider a biopsychosocial model that integrates all these schools of thought in explaining such complex human concepts as suicide (Box 26-3).

EPIDEMIOLOGY

Prevalence

Suicide and suicidal behavior are found among persons of all ages (including young children), among both sexes, and among all ethnic groups and socioeconomic levels. Wilson reported that suicide accounts for nearly 1% of all

Box 26-3   Etiologic Factors Related to Suicide

Biologic

- The neurotransmitters—principally serotonin, dopamine, norepinephrine, and GABA—have been linked through extensive research to emotional responses.

- Serotonin plays a major role in regulating mood and impacts the occurrence of depression and suicidality.

- Genetic influences are being found; a specific gene has been implicated in the predisposition to suicide.

- Others have found that dimensions of depression, such as mood, affect, motivation, and cognitive content, are correlated to alterations in specific brain structure.

Psychologic

- self-directed aggression
- unresolved interpersonal conflicts
- negativistic thinking patterns
- a reduction in positive reinforcement

Sociological

- isolation and alienation from social groups
- biopsychosocial influences

deaths in the world. The Hungarians and Finns have suicide rates 2–3 times those of the United States and most of Europe. Interestingly, that figure holds true even when persons of those nationalities emigrate to other countries, suggesting some biologic influence (Wilson, 1994). Currently in the United States, there are slightly more than 30,000 suicides annually, or 1 suicide every 17 minutes, with 12 of every 100,000 Americans killing themselves. Suicide is the eighth leading cause of death in the United States (AAS, 1993).

AGE

The two most vulnerable age groups for suicide are the elderly and youth, ages 15–24 years.

Elderly. Rates of suicide are highest among the older population, 65 years and above. Elder adults have suicide rates 50% higher than the nation as a whole. In 1987, older white males had a suicide rate of 46 deaths per 100,000 population. The prevalence rate for older Caucasian males is substantially higher than for African-American males, Caucasian females, and African-American females. (U.S. Senate Committee on Aging, Federal Council on Aging, and U.S. Department of Health and Human Services, 1991). Figure 26-1 shows that white males 85 years and older are most at risk, with a suicide rate of 72 deaths per 100,000.

Shneidman suggests that the high suicide rates among the elderly represent the failure to adapt to significant losses, the inability to endure emotional pain, and pessimistic attitudes toward the aging process related to loneliness, illness, rejection by family and society, sud-

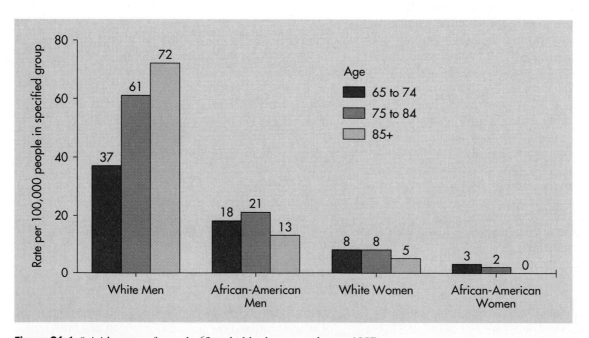

Figure 26-1 Suicide rates of people 65 and older by age and race, 1987.

(From National Center for Health Statistics. *Health, United States, 1989,* DHHS Pub. No. (PHS)90-1232, Washington, D.C. 1990, Department of Health and Human Services.)

den termination of meaningful work, disruption of long-standing relationships, and feelings of emptiness. As the population ages and seniors become the dominant subgroup, suicide may increasingly become a major public health problem (Shneidman, 1985).

Youth. Young people ages 15–24 have a suicide rate approximately 200% higher than in the 1950s. The rates have stabilized since the 1970s. However, suicide now ranks as the third leading cause of death for youth, behind accidents and homicides (AAS, 1993). Currently the rate is about 6000 suicides a year with 400,000 teenagers attempting suicide a year. As many as 11% of all high school students have made at least one suicide attempt.

While there are few studies related to suicide rates for children under the age of 15, some statistical and anecdotal studies have chronicled successful suicide attempts in this age group. Children as young as two and one-half years have attempted suicide. In 1985 there were 278 suicide deaths of children 5–14 years of age in the U.S. (Valente, 1989).

GENDER AND ETHNICITY

National suicide rates tend to obscure the importance of gender and ethnicity in defining the scope of suicidal behavior. Caucasian suicide rates are approximately twice those of non-Caucasian rates as a whole. While the high suicide rates of older Caucasian males have been highlighted, it is important to note that suicide rates for African-American men have tripled during the past 25 years among the 85+ age group. This increased rate of suicide among the oldest African-American men rivals the increased rate among young men ages 15–24 for both races (Monk, 1987).

After older white males, African-American young adult males have the next highest rate of suicide. Males commit suicide at rates three to four times those of females. While Figure 26-1 indicates that Caucasian and African-American women have comparatively low completed suicide rates, females have the highest rate of suicide attempts (Valente, 1989). Females have been found generally to make three to four times as many attempts, and the female Hispanic suicide attempt rate is higher than that of any other ethnic minority group in the United States (Heacock, 1990).

African-Americans and Hispanics rank below the midrange when compared to the suicide rates of other reporting nations of the world. In the United States, Hispanic and Asian rates of suicide are similar to those of Caucasians. However, there are very few publications detailing the incidence of suicide among Hispanic youth. One article points out that the Hispanic population is not homogeneous and what may be characteristic of one subgroup may not be of another. For example, rates vary among Puerto Ricans, Dominicans, Cubans, and Mexican-Americans (Smith et al, 1985). Zayas, in an early study, noted that several cultural factors have bearing on suicide attempts among Hispanic adolescent females: socioeconomic disadvantages, traditional gender roles, socialization, acculturation, cultural identity, and intergenerational conflict (Zayas, 1978).

Another infrequently studied ethnic group is Native Americans. This oversight is particularly alarming in that Native Americans are often noted to be the ethnic group with the highest suicide rates in the United States, according to the American Association of Suicidology. As with Hispanics, there are great tribal group differences, and Shore demonstrated that suicide rates for certain tribes varied from higher to lower than that of the general population (Shore, 1975). May and Dizmang stressed that suicide in Native Americans was largely a problem within the male adolescent subgroup (May and Dizmang, 1974). Epidemiological research focusing on Native American suicide factors warrants a higher profile.

SOCIOECONOMIC STATUS

Suicide crosses all socioeconomic levels. In fact, studies show that poverty and unemployment contribute to high suicide rates and, conversely, that a high gross national product per capita and a high quality of life with associated stresses also contribute to suicidal behavior. Yang et al studied the sociological and economic theories of suicide and found that high unemployment rates positively related to suicide rates. They argued that people's expectations of decreased future income because of unemployment led to an increased probability of suicide (Yang et al, 1992). Marshall found a correlation between increased suicide rates and decreased income status among older Social Security recipients (Marshall, 1978).

Zayas noted that socioeconomic disadvantages such as poverty, substandard housing, unemployment, crime, victimization, poor health care, and poor education contributed to the high rate of suicidal behavior among Hispanics (Zayas, 1978). By contrast, Lester demonstrated that nations with a higher quality of life and income also had higher suicide rates but for different reasons. A high quality of life leaves fewer external events on which to blame one's misfortune and failures, and thus inner-directed aggression may occur (Lester, 1984). Yang and colleagues postulated that economic prosperity produces a social environment that is conducive to suicidal behavior: urbanization, often a by-product of prosperity, leads to a decline in social cohesion or an increase in social isolation, and a quickened pace of life increases stress for individuals (Yang et al, 1992). Thus, both economic well-being and poverty can create circumstances leading to the choice of suicide as a solution to stressful events.

FAMILIAL INFLUENCES

Suicidal behavior is frequently a symptom of prolonged and progressive family disruption and dysfunction. Additionally, significant changes in the family such as divorce; death of a spouse, parent, or child; and social isolation contribute to high suicide rates (Blazer, 1989).

The family is most influential in the lives of children and adolescents and contributes to the incidence of suicidal behavior in those age groups. A suicidal adolescent may feel estranged from family members and may experience rejection and a loss of love. Actual physical or psychologic loss, as in death, separation, or emotional distancing from the family, is thought to be one of the most significant factors in the high incidence of adolescent suicides (Husain, 1990).

There is a familial predisposition to suicide in that many suicidal adolescents often have histories of suicidal behavior among their immediate and extended families. Those adolescents who completed suicide more often lost their mothers by suicide prior to their own deaths than did those who attempted suicide. Tishler and colleagues suggest that suicidal behavior among many family members serves as a means of communication or as a language that is understood when other forms of communication fail. Suicidal behavior becomes a learned familial adaptation to problems and stressors (Tishler et al, 1981).

Familial cultural values also are strong factors in suicidal behavior. For example, in Hispanic families, family honor and family centeredness and cohesiveness are variables that buffer against suicidal behavior or contribute to it. Hispanic youth may experience conflict between traditional Hispanic values and the values of the dominant culture. Intergenerational tension, language barriers, and role conflicts may contribute to mental health problems. Those adolescents who can relate positively to the main culture and still have positive relationships with their family members who have more traditional values are often sheltered from such problems.

Co-occurrence with Related Health Issues

Suicidal behavior is strongly associated with the occurrence of psychiatric disorders and other health-related problems. Psychiatric illness, alcohol and other drug use and abuse, and medical illnesses are important adjuncts to suicidal events.

PSYCHIATRIC DISORDERS

The presence of a diagnosable mental illness increases the risk for suicide, regardless of age. Miles (1977) reviewed more than 100 longitudinal studies of psychiatric clients and concluded that nearly all suicides committed in the United States were committed by persons with a mental disorder. Others concur that the comorbidity of mood disorder and substance abuse with suicide is very high. Most investigators report that suicide risk secondary to a mental disorder is higher in men than in women (Monk, 1987).

Depression. The single best predictor of suicidal thinking is the presence of a mood disorder. Research indicates that 30%–70% of all completed suicides were related to depression. Other studies indicate that 10%–15% of completed suicides were committed by persons specifically diagnosed with major depressive disorder. Depression is a major factor for persons *attempting* suicide as well (Arato et al, 1988).

Schizophrenia.   Another diagnostic category linked with suicide is schizophrenia. Suicide is the leading cause of premature death in that population, with an estimated 10% incidence of suicide in the first 10 years of the illness and a 15% lifetime incidence (Nyman and Jonsson, 1986). One study reported that clients with schizophrenia expressed high levels of subjective stress and feelings of hopelessness, loneliness, and dissatisfaction with social relationships (Cohen et al, 1990). Since schizophrenia most often has its onset in late adolescence or early young adulthood, the high-risk period for suicide is in the 20–30 year age group. This population must be carefully evaluated and reevaluated for suicide risk, particularly during the first 10 years of the illness.

Panic disorder.   There is controversy among views of a co-occurrence factor with panic disorder and suicide attempts. Some studies indicate there is a high comorbidity of suicidal behavior with panic disorder, major depression, and substance abuse (Lepine et al, 1993). Others report that panic disorder is an independent risk factor for suicide or suicidal behavior (Weissman et al, 1989). Others assert there is evidence to support panic disorder as a risk factor for suicide and suicide attempts (Sakinofsky et al, 1991) and in conjunction with phobias and obsessive-compulsive disorders. (See the Clinical Alert box below.)

Some researchers have concluded that clients with panic disorder have an increased risk for suicide attempts comparable to clients with major depression and are at greater risk than persons without a psychiatric disorder (Johnson et al, 1990).

ALCOHOL AND OTHER DRUGS

Of special clinical relevance is the high incidence of concurrence of the use of alcohol and other drugs with suicidal behavior. In a clinical review of eight clients who

> ## CLINICAL ALERT   !
>
> Conflicting findings among researchers may lead nurses and other clinicians to overlook the possible lethality of clients with panic disorder, obsessive-compulsive disorder, and phobias. A careful suicide assessment is required to ensure that this possibility is considered.

committed suicide less than 60 days after discharge from one of two psychiatric hospitals from 1988 to 1993, all had been drinking or using other drugs at the time of the completed suicides (Barbee, 1993).

One study of 93 outpatient clients who completed suicide found that the majority of them were young, male, had a history of drug and alcohol abuse, and had a primary diagnosis of depression. Of the outpatient clients who completed suicide, 62% used drugs compared to 18% of all outpatient clients (Earle et al, 1994). In another study of 44 youths who completed suicide, 25% had used alcohol weekly, 11% used marijuana weekly, 14% used marijuana daily (Litman and Farberow, 1986). Drugs contribute to poor, impulsive decisions that can lead to high-risk, self-injurious behaviors. A high percentage of alcohol- and drug-related automobile accidents among teens may be suicide attempts (Barbee, 1993).

Research related to the role that alcohol and drugs play in suicidal behavior is somewhat conflicting. Mellick, et al, (1992) conducted a study focusing on completed suicides of 84 elderly white males in Iowa. The men were found not to have been addicted to drugs and did not have a strong reliance on drugs. These findings contradict the 1976 study by Miller that Mellick and colleagues were replicating. In contrast, Miller's original findings indicated a statistically significant difference between completed suicides and controls in that the former group was addicted to or had a strong reliance on drugs (Miller, 1979). Conflicting results from these studies may result from the the under-reporting and under-diagnosing of alcohol and drug problems among the depressed elderly.

MEDICAL ILLNESSES

Physical health problems have been identified as a component of the profile for persons at risk for suicidal behaviors because of their co-occurrence with depression. The Medical Outcomes Study, one of the first major national studies to link medical illnesses and depression (Wells et al, 1989), found that the physical and social dysfunctions associated with depression are greater than with most chronic medical conditions. Depression is thought to cause as much physical and social impairment as that of chronic heart disease. Depressed persons perceived their current health as poor and experienced greater body pain. In comparison with chronic illness, the physical functions of depressed clients were found to be worse than those of clients with hypertension, diabetes, arthritis, and gastrointestinal and back problems. When depression and a medical condition such as advanced coronary artery disease coexisted, the client was noted to suffer nearly twice the loss of social functions than when either condition existed alone. Suicide risk also was noted to increase in such coexisting conditions (Gonzales et al, 1985).

A complicating factor is that these clients often seek medical care for their health problems, and the coexistence of a depressive disorder is overlooked or missed. A study of 93 completed outpatient suicides found that physical health problems were reported for more than half the clients who committed suicide. The mean age of the sample was 42 years. The most common problem identified was obesity (14%), followed by heart disease and hypertension (10%), diabetes (8%), asthma (8%), loss of hearing or sight (8%), severe acne or abscess (6%), arthritis (5%), ulcer or stomach problems (4%), epilepsy (4%), and HIV seropositivity (3%) (Earle et al, 1994). (See Box 26-4).

Physical health problems often enhance the emotional pain experienced by suicidal persons and may contribute to the decisions to end their lives. Nurses play a critical role in assessing clients for depression and suicidal risk when they present in medical-surgical health care settings. Alerting the health care team to these findings may help to avert suicide attempts and deaths.

Erroneous Beliefs about Suicide

Despite the numerous studies done on suicide, the massive efforts to educate people about suicide risk and the efforts of mental health advocacy groups to break the stigmatized silence about suicidal behavior, erroneous beliefs and myths still exist. It is important to highlight several long-standing erroneous beliefs that can contribute to errors in judgment when assessing for suicidal intent. These beliefs are summarized in Table 26-1.

CLINICAL DESCRIPTION

The assessment of suicide risk is an important skill for the professional nurse practicing in all clinical settings. Merely voicing a concern about a client's possible suicidality to other members of the health care team is no longer an adequate or safe response. The nurse needs to use interviewing skills to talk directly with the client and family about suicide during the initial nursing assessment and at points of reassessment in the treatment process. Being alert to past medical history and psychiatric history of suicidal behavior gives the nurse clues in identifying areas for further inquiry.

This section highlights the background information needed to complement the assessment phase of the nursing process. Definitions of the five levels of suicidal behavior are given in Box 26-5 and risk factors are discussed.

Often the five levels of suicidal thought or action are described collectively as "suicidal behaviors," yet it is very important to be specific in naming the types of thoughts and/or actions in the nursing assessment with clear descriptions or examples so that others may judge the level of intent themselves.

Box 26-4 Epidemiology of Suicide

Age, gender, and ethnicity

- Of the 30,000 completed suicides in the United States annually, the majority are white males of all ages.

- The two subgroups most at risk are youth ages 15–24 years, with African-American males 19–24 years increasing at the fastest rate, and Caucasian elderly males over age 65, with the 85+ group increasing at the fastest rate.

- Native American adolescent males and Hispanic females are high-risk groups among ethnic minority populations.

- Females in general attempt more suicides than males.

Socioeconomic and familial factors

- Suicide crosses all socioeconomic levels.

- Affluent, educated, overachievers are as vulnerable to suicide as people at the poverty level who are unemployed, undereducated, living in substandard housing, and often the victims of crime.

- Prolonged family disruption and familial predisposition to depression and suicide biologically, or as a learned behavior from other family members, contribute to the incidence rates.

- Family turmoil, disturbed parent-child relationships, physical and sexual abuse by family members, and hostile and rejecting parental attitudes have been found to promote suicidal behavior.

Co-occurrence with related health issues

- Suicidal behavior is strongly associated with psychiatric disorders.

- Mood disorders, substance abuse, schizophrenia, and panic disorders have a co-occurrence with high-risk suicidal behavior.

- Depression remains as the single best predictor of suicide risk in all ages.

- Suicide is the leading cause of death during the first 10 years of the course of schizophrenic illness.

- The research is mixed on the correlation of suicide with panic disorders, but it is thought by most to be associated with suicide risk, especially when panic disorder co-occurs with OCD or phobias.

- Independent of another specific psychiatric diagnosis, alcohol use and abuse are highly correlated with most suicidal acts, especially among youth. It is underdiagnosed and underreported among the elderly.

- Similarly, chronic physical illness contributes to suicidal behavior. Physical health problems, such as heart disease, hypertension, obesity, and diabetes were found in more than half the outpatient clients who committed suicide in several studies. The elderly are particularly prone.

CLINICAL ALERT !

A sudden change in affect for the better or a dramatic lifting of depression may be an indication that the person may have resolved ambivalence about living or dying and has made the decision to commit suicide. Increased energy and the ability to concentrate and plan facilitate the suicidal actions. Be alert.

CLINICAL ALERT !

Adolescents who completed suicides experienced the loss of their mothers by suicide prior to their own deaths more often than those who attempted suicide. A careful family history and a record of previous attempts are critical to the thoroughness of the nursing assessment and the determination of suicide risk.

Of special note is that young children and older adults are less likely to have an explicit plan, thus making the assessment of risk more difficult.

Risk Factors for Suicide

Nurses should use a knowledge of risk factors to assist in assessing intent and lethality. Risk factors based in part on key points from the epidemiologic findings discussed earlier in the chapter are presented in Box 26-6.

Lethality Assessment Factors

In addition to the suicide risk factors the assessment of **lethality,** the potential for causing death related to the level of danger associated with the suicide plan, must be considered. **Imminence** (the likelihood that an event will occur within a specific time period), intent, and the method chosen and its accessibility are often the three determinants that indicate the level of lethality and the extent of interventions required for safety.

IMMINENCE VERSUS NONIMMINENCE

The determination of imminence is critical. If persons are imminently in danger of killing themselves, rapid action must be taken. Determination of imminence, however, is subjective and at best is a clinical judgment based

TABLE 26-1   Erroneous beliefs and facts about suicide

Erroneous belief	Fact
1. People who talk about suicide won't commit suicide.	1. Most people communicate directly about their suicidal intent verbally, in writing, through artwork, and behaviorally through previous suicide attempts. These are all high risk indicators of suicidal intent. Manipulation is not usually a factor. Treat all messages of intent seriously.
2. People who are serious about committing suicide don't give clues.	2. Most suicidal people give warnings of their intent by giving away possessions, wrapping up business affairs, isolating from friends, demonstrating increased incidence of accidents, being preoccupied about death in writing, music, and art, and making self-deprecating comments related to worthlessness and hopelessness.
3. Young children don't commit suicide.	3. There were 278 suicide deaths of children between the ages of 5 and 14 in 1985 in the United States. Consider all threats from young children seriously. Remember, suicidal behavior is the leading precipitating event for the psychiatric hospitalization of young children.
4. An improved mood means the suicide crisis is over.	4. Persons who completed suicide often showed improved mood and energy prior to their deaths. It is thought that the improved mood and energy level mean the person's ambivalence has ended and he or she has made the decision to commit suicide.
5. Only people with the diagnosis of depression kill themselves.	5. While depression is the single best indicator of suicidal risk, some people who commit suicide are not diagnosed as depressed. At risk are those with schizophrenia, substance-related disorders, panic disorder, post-traumatic stress disorder, obsessive-compulsive disorder, and the manic phase of bipolar disease. Some people don't exhibit a specific mental disorder at all; for example, an elderly male who commits suicide after learning he has terminal cancer. Clients with the above diagnoses may experience depressed feelings, however.

Box 26-5   Five Levels of Suicidal Thought

The following terms are used often in clinical settings to describe the five levels of suicidal thought or action.

1. **Suicidal ideation.** Direct or indirect thoughts or fantasies of suicide or self-injurious acts expressed verbally or through writing or artwork without definite intent or action expressed. May be veiled or expressed symbolically.

2. **Suicide threats.** Direct verbal or written expressions of intent to commit suicide but without action.

3. **Suicide gestures.** Self-directed actions that result in no injury or minor injury by persons who neither intended to end their lives nor expected to die as a result, but were done in such a way that others would interpret the act as suicidal in purpose, for example: minor scratches on the wrist with a plastic knife.

4. **Suicide attempts.** Serious self-directed actions that may result in minor or major injury by persons who intend to end their lives or cause serious harm to themselves. Gestures and attempts that are unsuccessful and of low lethality are often called **para-suicidal** behavior.

5. **Completed or successful suicides.** Deaths of persons who ended their lives by their own means with conscious intent to die. However, it is important to note that some suicides may occur based on *unconscious* intent to die, for example, engaging in high-risk activities.

---

on the professional's experience, knowledge base, and intuition. The specifics of the suicide plan often offer clues as to when the individual will be ready to act.

Some mental health professionals arbitrarily define imminence as the likelihood that the person will engage in suicidal behavior within the next 24 hours. A specific plan, access to lethal measures, behaviors that signal a decision to die, and admission of wanting to die suggest imminent risk for the client. Those who refuse treatment and are at high risk can be placed on an involuntary hold-and-treat status by a qualified person, usually for 72 hours, depending on specific state statutes, judged to be imminently dangerous to themselves. This allows clinicians to hospitalize these individuals for an evaluation of

---

Box 26-6 Risk Factors for Suicide

1. **Age.** Persons most at risk for suicide are youth ages 15–24 and older adults ages 65 and over, with those 85 years and over the most vulnerable.

2. **Sex.** Men by far have a greater incidence of completed suicides. Women have a higher rate of suicide attempts and gestures.

3. **Race/ethnicity.** Suicide rates for Caucasians are twice those of non-Caucasians. However, rates for African-American men over age 85 are increasing faster than any other group. Second most at risk are young African-American and Native American males.

4. **Physical and emotional symptoms.** High-risk indicators are serious depression, significant changes in weight, serious sleep disturbances, extreme fatigue and loss of energy, self-deprecation, anger, feelings of hopelessness, and preoccupation with themes of death and dying. Remember that serious depression is often the precursor to suicidal behavior.

5. **Suicide plan.** The presence and the nature of the suicide plan is one of the most critical factors in assigning suicide risk. A plan clearly signals forethought and intent and often helps determine the level of lethality. Plans that are more precise, detailed, and explicit about the method to be used in the suicide act indicate high risk. If the method described is highly lethal (for example, a gunshot to the head versus an overdose of pills) and if the method is readily available, the risk is elevated even more. Add alcohol and other drugs, poor impulse control, and limited time for rescue attempts, and the risk reaches a critical level. Plans often include instructions regarding the distribution of possessions and may mention the intent to join a deceased loved one in afterlife, especially if the loved one had committed suicide.

6. **History of previous attempts.** The majority of persons who complete suicides have made previous suicide attempts.

7. **Social supports and resources.** The availability of a support system for a suicidal person often determines the outcome of an emotional crisis. This "life line" of caring, support, confrontation, and limit-setting, as appropriate from family, friends, and community resources, assists suicidal persons in choosing other alternatives in solving their problems. Real or perceived lack of support systems or failure to use the support system that is available increase the risk for suicide significantly.

8. **Recent losses.** One of the major emotional determinants of suicidal behavior is real or perceived losses, separations, or abandonments. Unresolved grief reactions can lead to depression and suicidal behavior.

9. **Medical problems.** Persons who suffer painful, debilitating, acute or chronic conditions, or terminal illness are of special concern for suicide risk.

10. **Alcohol and other drugs.** These substances are often lethal companions to suicidal acts. Drugs may lower inhibition, heighten depression, and quicken impulsivity. It is generally thought that at least 50% of adolescents were legally drunk at the time of their deaths by suicide, and an even higher percentage had a history of recent alcohol or other drug abuse.

11. **Cognition and problem-solving ability.** The inability to identify problems and corresponding solutions adequately greatly contributes to the choice of suicide as a solution to problems.

---

risk and to determine appropriate treatment recommendations. These clients' rights are protected in order to prevent exploitation and punishment. Those judged not to be imminently in danger of hurting or killing themselves may choose less restrictive treatment options such as partial hospitalization programs or outpatient programs. Any suicidal thoughts or behaviors, whether ideation, threat, gesture, or attempt, indicate an emergency situation and require prompt assessment (Bongar, 1991). Suicide risk and imminence usually decrease after support systems are established for those at risk and the cry for help has been answered.

IDEATION VERSUS INTENT

Ideation, or thinking about suicide without clear intent, places a person at lower risk than a person who intends or proposes to die through a suicidal act. There are two categories of intention, conscious and unconscious.

Conscious suicidal intention is usually characterized by various aspects of awareness:

- awareness of the outcomes or anticipated results of the suicidal behavior

- awareness of other's responses to suicidal threats or attempts

- awareness of the lethality index of the chosen method

- awareness of rescue possibilities, i.e., part of the plan includes various avenues of rescue or the plan is designed so that rescue is difficult or remote; the latter is a more lethal attribute than the former (Farberow, 1980)

Unconscious suicidal intention is often more difficult to assess because it requires a higher level of skill and knowledge of psychodynamic theory. Often, there is a cluster of symptoms characteristic of the dynamics of self-destruction: depression, anxiety, guilt, hostility, and dependency, along with fantasies symbolic of death, hurting others, killing self, failure, and hopelessness. The motivation to hurt or kill oneself is outside of awareness yet is often expressed by extreme risk-taking behaviors. For example, some platform parachutists who jump from low heights off stationary objects such as buildings, towers, or cliffs may have unconscious wishes to hurt themselves or end their lives under the guise of an "extreme sport." Others may seek dangerous occupations such as skyscraper workers, bridge builders, and high-wire artists without nets as metaphors for suicidal wishes. Some persons may place themselves in dangerous, vulnerable situations that result in their deaths at the hands of others, for example, victim-precipitated homicides. Some psychiatric clients unconsciously manipulate others through suicidal threats or attempts and unconsciously arrange to be found or rescued. Unfortunately, the rescue plans may fail, resulting in completed suicides.

Fawcett wrote about the importance of the communication of intent among suicidal persons. He found that 50%–70% of higher-risk persons who completed suicides communicated their intent in advance, often only to their significant other. The group that was at moderate risk of suicide communicated by threatening suicide to family members or health care providers (Fawcett et al, (1969).

Nurses should carefully observe and listen for direct and indirect communication regarding clients' suicidal intent. Listen not only for the words, but for the underlying themes that the words refer to or symbolize. Suicidal intent accompanied by suicidal imminence represents a high level of lethality.

CHOSEN METHOD AND ACCESSIBILITY

The third determinant of lethality is perhaps the most critical. The method and its availability determine the outcome of the suicidal behavior. One is more likely to seriously injure or kill oneself if there is an easily accessible means or method.

Persons who complete suicides tend to engage in only one high-lethality act through violent methods: using firearms (the most prevalent high-lethality method used in the United States), piercing of vital organs, hanging, jumping from high places, and carbon monoxide poisoning. Men who complete suicides are more likely to select more violent means and use guns or knives or hang themselves; women are more likely to jump from high places or overdose. Nonfatal attempters tend to engage in multiple, low-lethality acts and use self-poisoning by pill ingestion (the most common method for suicide attempts), followed by wrist cutting. These methods allow time for rescue because of the slowness of their physiologic actions. Most who attempt will use the same method for repeated suicide attempts.

Boyd and Moscicki noted that accessibility to dangerous weapons raises the suicidal risk. They observed that the use of firearms increased in proportion to the increase in youth suicide rates. The most rapid increase in firearm suicides has been in the 15–24 age range (Boyd and Moscicki, (1986).

Suicidal clients in psychiatric hospitals or on psychiatric units in general hospitals are high suicidal risks. Hospitals report a wide range of 20–90 completed suicides per 100,000 client years. The most vulnerable periods for attempts are within the first 24 hours after admission and as discharge approaches. Close observation is required as clients move from one suicide precaution level to another. Remember that a sudden brightening of affect or lifting of depression may signal that the client has resolved his or her ambivalence about living or dying, has made the decision to commit suicide, and is awaiting the opportunity. Some clients have attempted or completed suicide while they were not on suicide precautions at all. Observation of all clients at least every 30 minutes, whether or not they are suicidal, is vital in detecting early clues to self-destructive behavior.

Hanging is the most prevalent suicide method used in hospital settings and is a lethal one. Sharp objects are usually not available to clients, as part of the safety program of the unit. However, sheets, towels, belts, cords, plastic garbage bags, shoe strings, and articles of clothing have been used to create nooses. Other clients may "cheek" their psychotropic medications and use them later in overdose attempts. Some chronically suicidal clients who sneak sharp objects into the hospital are prone to cutting attempts, usually of the wrists or antecubital areas of the arms. Clients diagnosed with borderline personality disorders or dissociative disorders are prone to these attempts. Searching the client on admission and when returning from off-ground passes are important safety interventions to detect contraband such as razors, knives, pieces of glass, and aluminum cans.

It is not possible to prevent all suicides, even in the most secure facilities such as psychiatric hospitals and jails, but close observation and continued reassessment of suicidal risk minimize the chances of completed sui-

CLINICAL ALERT !

Asking suicidal clients and their family members about their access to dangerous weapons must be a part of the nursing assessment. Many will verify that there are guns and other dangerous weapons in the home that are easily accessible. If the clients are experienced in firearms use—for example, policemen, military personnel, or hunters—the risk for suicide rises sharply. Provisions must be made at the end of the assessment to secure the weapons and have family and friends remove them from the home or from automobiles and trucks. Usually, a physician's order is required before dangerous weapons are returned to the at-risk client.

cides. Mental health professionals have an obligation to protect clients from harming themselves.

PROGNOSIS

Suicidal behavior is a treatable mental health problem. The prognosis for many suicidal clients is related to the severity of their accompanying mental illness. Since most suicidal behavior is correlated closely with major depressive disorders, effective treatment of depression results in a rapid reduction in suicidal risk. The majority of clients with depression who are treated with antidepressant medications demonstrate increased improvement or complete remission of their depressive symptoms, according to the Clinical Practice Guidelines (U.S. Department of Health and Human Services, 1993). Clients with schizophrenia and panic disorder who maintain therapeutic blood levels of the prescribed psychotropic medications also have a favorable response and a positive outcome related to reduction in suicide risk.

DISCHARGE CRITERIA

Discharge criteria are necessary guides for both client and nursing staff and lead toward a completion of treatment goals. The admission assessment establishes the groundwork for discharge criteria. Without an accurate, thorough, and knowledgeable assessment and appropriate treatment plan, effective interventions and timely discharge activities can be delayed. Discharge criteria help to establish time frames in which goals are achieved, designate areas of responsibility and accountability by way of documentation, and meet specific institutional, professional, certifying, legal, or funding requirements.

Discharge criteria for the suicidal client must include:

- indications that the client is no longer imminently suicidal
- determination that the client's living environment is safe for his or her return
- a consistent, available support system for the client to access if feeling self-destructive

THE NURSING PROCESS ■ ■ ■ ■ ■ ■ ■ ■ ■ ■ ■ ■ ■ ■ ■ ■

■ ASSESSMENT

The nursing assessment is a critical step toward ensuring the client's safety. Accurate assessment, continuing throughout the course of hospitalization, helps the nurse provide appropriate intervention and discharge planning. Determining an individual's risk for self-harm requires a thorough evaluation of factors that contribute to suicidality, e.g., a mental status examination and an evaluation of the client's support resources.

The initial assessment helps determine the presence of specific risk factors. Noting the presence of symptoms does not necessarily mean that a client is suicidal. However, recognizing a cluster of certain symptoms within a given time frame is necessary to accurately assess suicidal intent. (See Nursing Care in the Community on page 627.)

When assessing client's potential for suicide, the nurse will observe for the following:

1. *The observable behavior of the client*
   A calm client may be highly suicidal, while an agitated client may not be dangerous. While appearances can be deceiving, increased perturbation, Shneidman (1985), often signals an imminent suicide attempt and is characterized by impulsivity, restlessness, excessive motor agitation, and a brightening of affect. With

some clients, however, withdrawal, apathy, irritability, and immobility may intensify with suicidality.

Suicides do occur in hospitals. It is important that nurses consistently monitor a suicidal client's behavior, affect, and interactions with others. Lethality levels can increase during hospitalization, particularly as depression lifts and discharge becomes imminent.

2. *The history from the client*
   Careful scrutiny will sometimes reveal precipitating events that contribute to current self-destructive thoughts. It is important to determine why the client is feeling suicidal at this time. In gathering the client's history, the nurse may identify self-defeating coping patterns and past experiences that have negatively affected the client's self-esteem. Making note of significant anniversary dates may help to predict a future suicide attempt.

3. *Information from friends or relatives*
   Useful information regarding the client's history can be obtained from friends or relatives. Often, it is helpful to interview the client and family together and separately, in case the friend or relative is hesitant to speak openly in front of the client. The nurse should assess how family members and friends feel about the client's suicidal behavior. Family members who are an-

Nursing Care in the Community

Suicide

There are a few guidelines that everyone working in mental health learns. Every individual who admits to depression is immediately overtly assessed for suicidality and the ability to make a no-harm contract with his or her mental health professional. Evaluation is based on the lethality of the plan and the availability of the means to carry it out. This is standard procedure. The community mental health nurse has a distinct advantage in the process, being able to offer access to the mental health system, and often having personal knowledge of the client's family and lifestyle. The nurse's availability on an extended basis may help to establish credibility with clients, so that agreements are based on relationship and trust.

It is important to consider the individual in the context of daily life, which is also an advantage of being in the community. The elderly individual who lives alone may be at high risk for suicidal acts, as are young persons newly diagnosed with a major psychiatric illness. Assessment can be made, not only on the basis of the client's demographics, but also from interviews with the persons in the client's support system. Notations that should be included in an evaluation are appearance of the vegetative signs of depression, as well as religious orientation, personal habits, and medication compliance. The capability of the client, especially the ability to organize, is important. Those who seem to be improving are often at increased risk, as they are better able to plan a more lethal attempt. Other elements that must be considered as risk factors are the disinhibiting effect of some medications and the mind-altering influence of substance abuse.

Assessment of suicidality remains a baffling issue in the community, because many clients want the security of the hospital psychiatric unit and have found that expressing suicidal intent will get them through the doors. They have become experts at using the system to get what they feel they need without making an effort to change themselves. The mental health nurse must recognize ongoing abuse of the system.

On the other hand, preserving life is a central duty of the community mental health nurse. No matter how often the client has used suicidality as a ploy to enter the hospital, each situation must be individually evaluated and all options must be explored. The nurse's most significant role is as an advocate for the client. Sometimes the human contact and focused attention, along with a personalized no-harm contract, will make a difference in the client's feeling of despair, isolation, and subsequent suicidal behavior. At times a partial hospitalization or day treatment program will give enough individual support. However, occasionally, nothing short of hospitalization will be effective in persuading the client that suicide is not the solution to problems.

gry, disgusted, or frustrated with the self-destructive client may actually provoke the client to complete a plan of suicide.

4. *Past history of suicidal gestures or attempts*
   The suicide attempt is often used as a way of coping with painful feelings. People who have used this coping style in the past are at greater risk for using it again.

5. *The mental status exam*
   Disturbance in concentration, orientation, and memory suggest possible organic brain syndrome, which may reduce the client's impulse control and increase the potential for self-harm. Disturbance in thought processing, evidenced in command hallucinations, places the client at greater risk to act destructively.

6. *The physical examination*
   A physical examination should always be conducted when there are obvious signs and symptoms of substance abuse (for example, impaired attention, irritability, euphoria, slurred speech, unsteady gait, flushed face, psychomotor agitation, needle tracks), previous suicide attempts (for example, scars on wrists), or debilitating medical conditions.

7. *The nurse's intuition*
   The nurse's own feelings of uneasiness, anxiety, or unexplained sadness may be the only clues that a seemingly calm client is barely able to refrain from acting on suicidal impulses. Although these feelings may be described as intuition, research suggests that "intuitive feelings" tend to be based on previous experiences in similar client-care situations (Aguilera, 1994). Nevertheless, if the nurse does not "feel right" about a client, this important source of information should not be ignored.

Nurses can use the assessment tool in Figure 26-2 to determine risk for suicide.

Regarding the case study about John on page 627, the nurse knew the first task of assessment was to make psychological contact with the client. She planned to listen to how John viewed his situation and then communicate her understanding of his thoughts and feelings. The nurse realized that it was important to establish rapport and trust with John. She believed that the client-centered approach, developed by Rogers would facilitate open communication and, in turn, assist her in more accurately assessing a suicide risk (Rogers, 1961).

NURSING SUICIDE RISK SCREENING SCALE

Name _____   Age _____   Sex _____   Date _____

Evaluator _____   Screening Score _____

Lethality Level	Low 1	2	Moderate 3	4	High 5	Score
AGE	0–4	5–14	15–25	25–49	50+	
SEX		Male	Male	Female/Male	Male	
RACE		Hispanic, Asian African-American Women	African-American	Urban African-American, Caucasian	Native American, Caucasian over 65	
EMOTIONAL SIGNS AND SYMPTOMS	Stress-related, transient emotional problems		Presence of psychiatric illness physical, emotional exhaustion	Symptoms of major depression, panic attacks, schizophrenia	apathy, despondency, hopelessness, preoccupation with death	
SUICIDE PLAN	Ideation without plan	Ideation vague plan, no means to carry out, rescue plan	Plan, previous low-level attempt, rescue plan	Explicit plan, previous high-level attempt, less immediacy	Lethal plan, means, intent to die, previous high-level attempt, no rescue plan	
SOCIAL SUPPORT, RESOURCES	Friends, family	Friends, family	Family, history of suicide in nuclear or extended family	Withdrawal from family or friends	Isolated, lives alone	
RECENT LOSS OR CHANGES		Success, promotion, increased obligations	Health, job problems, loss of self-esteem	Divorce, separation	Death of loved one, anniversary date of significant loss	
MEDICAL PROBLEMS				Debilitating illness	Terminal illness	
ALCOHOL, OTHER DRUGS				Prescription medication availability	Alcohol or other drug use/abuse	
COGNITION, PROBLEM SOLVING ABILITY		Ineffective coping skills	Problem solving impaired	Cognitive rigidity	Limited divergent thinking, hopelessness	
METHOD		Limited knowledge or access to pills or wrist-cutting	Availability of lethal prescriptions	Guns, knives, jumps, hangings, CO poisoning	Weapons in home, knowledge of use	

SCORING

High Risk Level	-	25–40
Moderate Risk Level	-	15–24
Low Risk Level	-	0–14

Total Score _____

Figure 26-2 Nursing suicide risk screening scale.

(Developed and copyright © by Bricker P and Barbee M)

CASE STUDY

John, age 24, had been hospitalized at age 18 after overdosing on tricyclic antidepressants. At the time, John's suicide attempt seemed linked to the end of a two-year relationship with his girlfriend. Since the initial episode of major depression, John successfully graduated from college and, following the sudden death of his father, returned home to live with his mother. Soon, however, he began to feel frustrated and inadequate when unable to find employment commensurate with his educational background and intellectual capabilities. John was forced to accept a part-time position that paid minimum wage and lacked benefits. When his steady girlfriend suddenly relocated to another state, he felt rejected and abandoned.

John's mother, who noticed he had become more withdrawn, was concerned that John might be self-destructive. After finding a loaded pistol lying on a table alongside John's bed, John's mother phoned the local mental health crisis intervention program to discuss her concerns about her son's behavior. While talking with the intake nurse, she added that John had recently instructed her to donate his body organs to medical science if "anything should happen" to him.

The nurse requested that John come to the center for an immediate assessment to determine his risk for suicide.

Critical Thinking and Assessment

1. What information did the nurse gather during the phone conversation with John's mother that alerted her to his need for an immediate suicide assessment? Why is this information pertinent to suicide ideation?

2. What other factors will the nurse consider when assessing John's risk for suicide during the face-to-face evaluation?

3. Identify one factor noted in the assessment that may help reduce John's risk for self-harm.

The nurse used empathic listening techniques by listening for both facts and feelings (i.e., what happened and how the client felt about it). The nurse demonstrated caring and interest by using reflective statements so that John knew the nurse had heard what he had been saying.

When feelings were obviously present but not yet expressed, the nurse would gently comment, "I sense how upset you are by the way you are speaking. It seems like you are also angry and frustrated about what has happened."

Psychologic contact is not always made solely through verbal communication. Sometimes, nonverbal, physical contact is quite effective. A gentle touch on the forearm,

or placing an arm around a shoulder, can have an important calming effect and signify human concern as well.

The nurse demonstrated concern for John by offering him a tissue when his eyes filled with tears. The nurse not only recognized and acknowledged his feelings but also responded in a calm, controlled manner, resisting the tendency to become anxious, angry, or depressed because of the intensity of the client's feelings.

During the assessment of John, the nurse included the Questions in the Nursing Assessment box below.

Nursing Assessment Questions

Suicide

1. What does the client understand about why his mother suggested he come to the center for a mental health assessment?
   (To determine if the client will validate his mother's concerns or deny that a problem exists.)

2. What was John's intention in having a loaded gun lying next to his bed? Did he intend to kill himself or someone else?
   (Asking directly about a client's intentions can decrease anxiety and feelings of humiliation and shame.)

3. Has John taken antidepressants or mood-stabilizing medications in the past? currently?
   (Have medications used in the past been effective at improving John's mood and lowering his lethality level? Does he have access to other lethal means of suicide?)

4. When was the last time John used alcohol or other drugs? When was he last intoxicated?
   (Clients who use alcohol and other drugs are in higher risk to complete a suicide attempt. Increased impulsivity, disorientation, and confusion that often accompany drug and alcohol use place people at higher risk for suicide.)

5. With whom does John share his feelings?
   (To determine if John has a trusted and reliable support system. If so, the lethality level could be lower.)

6. What were the circumstances surrounding his father's death? Is there a history of depression or suicide on either side of John's family?
   (To determine the nature of John's father's death, family history of depression, or family style of coping, all of which increase the risk of suicide.)

7. The nurse asked John's mother: How do you feel about John's thoughts of suicide?
   (To determine if John's mother is a support resource for him.)

Following a suicide attempt, an individual may continue to be at high risk for attempting suicide again. When clients are admitted to hospitals following a suicide attempt, ongoing assessments are necessary to determine whether the person continues to be at high risk.

■ ■ NURSING DIAGNOSIS

Suicidal clients are frequently admitted to psychiatric units, emergency rooms, and intensive care units of general medical hospitals. Suicide attempts can occur prior to or during hospitalization. Hangings, medication overdoses, and jumps from high places are frequent methods of suicide in hospitals. An accurate nursing diagnosis, based on a thorough, ongoing assessment, is necessary when identifying and prioritizing the client's needs for nursing interventions.

A complete nursing diagnosis is individualized and related to the client's behaviors and nursing needs. Validation of the nursing diagnosis with the client is required. However, the client may deny suicidal intent or the need for extra precautions. In the case of the diagnosis of *risk for violence: self-directed,* caution is recommended in determining the level of risk. It is best to err on the side of caution than to allow serious injury or death to occur.

NANDA Diagnoses Related to Suicide

Primary diagnosis:

> Risk for violence: self-directed

Secondary diagnoses may include:

> Ineffective individual coping
> Hopelessness
> Powerlessness
> Chronic low self-esteem
> Altered thought processes
> Social isolation
> Defensive coping

Collaborative Diagnoses

Clients with chronic mental illness are at higher risk for suicide. Several medical diagnoses include a group of symptoms that relate to the nursing diagnosis, *risk for violence: self-directed.*

Major depression and bipolar disorder are affective disorders that may include the symptoms of suicidal ideation, plans, gestures, and recurring suicide attempts.

Schizophrenia, with associated psychotic features such as delusions and command hallucinations, can also manifest in life-threatening behaviors. Hostile voices may direct the client to kill himself or herself.

Mental disorders due to a medical condition (such as substance abuse) may involve increased suicide risk if the client is repeating negative or self-defeating patterns. The client may be subject to an increased potential for

---

COLLABORATIVE DIAGNOSES

DSM-IV Diagnoses*	NANDA Diagnoses**
Major depression, single episode	Risk for violence, self-directed
Major depression, recurrent	Ineffective individual coping
Major depression, with psychotic features	Hopelessness
	Powerlessness
Bipolar disorder	Impaired social interactions
	Chronic low self-esteem
	Altered thought processes
Schizophrenia	Altered thought processes
	Social isolation
	Defensive coping
Mental disorders due to a medical condition	Altered thought processes
	Impaired social interactions
	Self-care deficit

*Reprinted with permission from *Diagnostic and statistical manual of mental disorders,* ed 4, Washington, D.C., 1994, American Psychiatric Association.

**Reprinted with permission from *NANDA nursing diagnoses: definitions and classifications, 1995–1996,* Philadelphia, 1994, North American Nursing Diagnosis Association.

---

self-directed violence when attempting to deal with stress by using alcohol or other drugs, demonstrating impulsive behavior, or having limited adaptive responses, mood swings, or confusion.

Indirect, self-destructive behaviors, sometimes identified as passive forms of suicide, are exhibited in the medical diagnoses of anorexia nervosa, bulimia nervosa, and noncompliance with medical treatment.

■ ■ ■ OUTCOME IDENTIFICATION

Outcomes are derived from the nursing diagnosis and are defined as anticipated, expected client behaviors or responses that are achieved as a result of nursing interventions. Outcomes must be stated in clear behavioral or measurable terms.

Outcome Identification for Suicide

The client will:

1. Remain safe and free from self-harm.

2. Verbalize an absence of suicidal ideation/plan/intent.

3. Verbalize a desire to live and list several reasons for wanting to live.

4. Agree to maintain a signed "no self-harm contract" with the nursing staff, attending psychiatrist, or individual therapist for a specified length of time. Agree

to inform staff immediately if suicidal feelings/thoughts recur.

5. Display brightened affect with broad range of expression and spontaneity and cheerful content of speech that reflects a hopeful, optimistic attitude.

6. Initiate social interactions with peers and staff (individually and in groups).

7. Use effective coping methods to counteract feelings of hopelessness.

8. Express a sense of self-worth.

9. Meet own needs through clear, direct methods of communication.

10. Verbalize more realistic role expectations and goals for meeting them.

11. Demonstrate absence of psychotic thinking (e.g., delusions, command hallucinations directing self-harm).

12. Make plans for the future that include follow-up psychotherapy and prescribed medication compliance.

■ ■ ■ ■   PLANNING

The nurse's awareness of a client's risk for suicide and the recurrent nature of suicide attempts warrant a plan of care aimed at saving lives and restoring biopsychosocial stability. The plan of care for the suicidal client emphasizes a reduction in the risk of self-destructive behaviors by monitoring client behaviors and providing a safe environment, promoting the client's feelings of self-worth and hope, improving coping skills, limiting social isolation, and building self-esteem.

NURSING CARE PLAN ■ ■ ■ ■ ■ ■ ■ ■ ■ ■ ■ ■ ■ ■

Tiffany, a 15-year-old, was admitted to the adolescent psychiatric unit of a local community hospital after her nurse therapist assessed that she was imminently suicidal. Over the past year, Tiffany had become preoccupied with wanting to die. She reported she had overdosed on analgesics and antibiotics three times in the past six months, but never told anyone and did not seek medical attention. She reported that she made her first suicide attempt when she was 10 by self-inflicting lacerations to her wrists with a razor blade. Within the past year, she cut her wrists five or six times. Tiffany complained that she felt helpless to change her relationship with her mother with whom she felt alienated and misunderstood. She reported poor school performance, increased irritability, morbid thoughts, decreased appetite, periods of insomnia, low self-esteem, and a history of sexual abuse by a babysitter's boyfriend when she was eight.

During her weekly therapy session, Tiffany announced to her therapist: "I am no longer willing to honor our contract not to harm myself. Nothing is changing at home. My mother hates me and doesn't want me in her life. My stepdad is the only person mom really cares about outside of herself. I hate how I look, and I hate how I am. I saved most of the pain pills my doctor gave me when I injured my leg." Laughing, she added, "I think there's enough to really put me out of my pain this time."

When questioned further, Tiffany admitted she was planning to kill herself. She indicated that she didn't know exactly when she would attempt to do so but promised, "I am not going to wait much longer."

To provide for her immediate safety, the nurse therapist ordered Tiffany's admission to the hospital.

DSM-IV Diagnoses

AXIS I	Major depression; recurrent adjustment disorder
AXIS II	Developmental reading disorder; Borderline personality traits
AXIS III	Fractured left tibia; healing
AXIS IV	Severe: two overdoses, self-inflicted wrist lacerations, persistent morbid thinking, severe depression, dysfunctional family relationships
AXIS V	GAF = 10-current GAF = 35-past year

Nursing Diagnosis: Risk for violence: self-directed. Risk factors: dysfunctional family relationships, ineffective coping style, low self-esteem, effects of sexual abuse, verbalized intent to die, history of several previous suicide attempts, lethal suicide plan, severely depressed mood.

Client Outcomes	*Nursing Interventions*	*Evaluation*
• Tiffany will verbalize an absence of suicidal ideation, intent, plan.	• Check client and room for potentially dangerous items and observe for any secretive behavior. *Protecting the client from self-destructive behavior promotes safety and gives message of caring and concern.*	• On the third day of hospitalization, Tiffany told her primary nurse that she wants to live. She reported that suicidal ideation had ceased by the fifth day of hospitalization.

NURSING CARE PLAN

Client Outcomes	Nursing Interventions	Evaluation
• Tiffany will express a desire to live and will list several reasons for wanting to live.	• Support Tiffany in developing a hopeful attitude. Reinforce her efforts at positive self-evaluation, self-control and goal-setting to *promote self-esteem and provide hope for change.*	• The client is looking forward to summer vacation. She has accepted a job as a veterinarian's assistant. She now identifies her appearance and intelligence as positive attributes.
• Tiffany will make plans for the future that include identification of a viable support system and a daily plan for structured activities with friends and family, routine exercise, weekly therapy sessions, and medication compliance.	• Encourage Tiffany to list people she will contact for support and help her develop a daily plan of structured activities that include a health care regimen. *Additional support and success-oriented activities will increase client's sense of self-worth, decrease feelings of alienation, and lessen suicide risk.*	• Tiffany developed a weekly plan of activities which includes a health care regimen and a part-time job. She listed her mother, stepfather, and two friends as people she will talk with.

Nursing Diagnosis: Ineffective individual coping, related to negative thinking patterns, self-defeating behaviors, disturbance in self-concept, multiple stressors, and ineffective support system, as evidenced by self-destructive behaviors, lack of assertive communication, impaired judgment and insight, misdirected anger, and social isolation.

Client Outcomes	Nursing Interventions	Evaluation
• Tiffany will demonstrate improved coping skills by: • discussing feelings and needs assertively. • taking responsibility for feelings and not blaming others. • making a written list of healthy coping skills to use in times of increased stress. • keeping a daily journal of thoughts and feelings related to her relationships. • engaging in efforts to socialize with peers and reestablish communication with family.	• Teach cognitive and behavioral techniques to assist Tiffany in limiting negative thought patterns and self-defeating behaviors and using more realistic self-evaluations. Encourage attendance at all psychoeducation groups. Review journal daily. Point out any self-defeating thoughts. Role-model assertive communication. *Therapeutic modalities can help client to identify and replace self-defeating thoughts and behaviors with an improved, healthy coping style.*	• Tiffany directly confronted her feelings with others in group, individual, and family therapy. • Tiffany labeled and challenged her "thinking errors" in journal work, owned responsibility for her feelings/actions, and progressively stopped accusing or blaming others.

NURSING CARE PLAN

Nursing Diagnosis: Ineffective family coping, related to highly conflicted family relationships, enmeshed relationship with mother, hostile relationship with stepfather, ineffective communication and parenting skills, as evidenced by distancing behaviors toward client, inability to set consistent limits, and inappropriate parent-child boundaries.

Client Family Outcomes	*Nursing Interventions*	*Evaluation*
• Family will attend all scheduled family therapies and parents' support group where they will discuss their feelings of fear, guilt, and frustration related to Tiffany's suicide attempts.	• Encourage parents to actively participate in Tiffany's treatment. Routinely update parents on any changes in Tiffany's behaviors. Encourage Tiffany and parents to directly confront their feelings. Role-model effective listening skills and assertive communication. *Demonstrating involvement in Tiffany's treatment will convey a message of caring and concern and parents' willingness to make needed changes.*	• Parents attended all family groups. Mother planned one afternoon each week for special time with Tiffany. Parents openly discussed feelings with the client and each other. They asked for referral to a parenting skills workshop.
• Parents will demonstrate willingness to listen to daughter's concerns and self-doubts. Parents will praise Tiffany when she engages in healthy coping behaviors.	• Apprise parents of any changes in Tiffany's behavior. Provide support and reassurance when Tiffany's mood and/or behavior fluctuate. Discuss warning signs of impending decompensation such as increased irritability, isolation, failure to maintain medication regime, and depressed mood. Inform parents of risk factors following hospitalization, for example, significant losses or disappointments that forewarn decompensation. Reinforce attempts at improved communication and parenting skills. *Maintaining supportive communication with families enhances client's support resources, decreases family members' anxiety, and promotes healthy coping.*	• Parents reassured Tiffany when she voiced self-doubts. Parents requested involvement in parents' aftercare group following Tiffany's discharge.

■ ■ ■ ■ ■ IMPLEMENTATION

Primary nursing responsibilities involve the prevention of suicide. The nurse must recognize and effectively intervene in the potentially lethal behaviors of clients at risk. This process involves a continuing assessment of lethality factors to determine the client's risk level, while working with the client to restore hope, connect with support resources, and develop positive alternatives to assist in improved coping.

Nursing Interventions

The following interventions must be consistently implemented with all hospitalized suicidal clients.

1. *To provide safety and prevent violence*

   a. All unit precautions for preventing suicide should be strictly enforced. This includes vigilantly maintaining a safe environment by:

   - routinely counting silverware and all other sharp objects before and after the clients' use.

   - having awareness of the clients' whereabouts at all times.

   - providing one-to-one supervision for the client as warranted, based on assessment of current lethality level.

   - planning so that the unit is always covered by experienced staff, especially at staff meal times, breaks, vacations, change of shift, or unit staff meetings (times during which most suicides occur in hospitals).

   - providing a roommate for the suicidal client.

   - requesting that visitors clear all gifts with staff.

   - searching the suicidal client for drugs, sharp objects, cords, and other potential weapons following the client's return from pass.

   - thoroughly assessing the client prior to any passes to determine current risk level.

   - encouraging the client to sign a "no suicide" contract for a specified length of time, which is reviewed during hospitalization and prior to discharge, and renegotiated prior to its expiration to indicate to the client the nurse's caring, concern, and consistent follow-through.

b. Being mindful that most suicides occur within 90 days post-hospitalization, the nurse must reinforce with families, guardians, social services, or legal authorities the necessity of removing any possible weapons (for example, guns, or drugs) in the person's home environment to a safe location prior to the client's return home.

c. Because working with suicidal clients is emotionally draining and anxiety-producing, the nurse must help create a supportive environment for self and other staff which includes daily supervision and informal discussions regarding feelings about suicide, death, hostility, anger, depression, and other painful feelings. Developing an ongoing relationship with a suicidal client is an intense experience in which the client and nurse each examine their feelings about the meaning of life and death. It is an opportunity for the nurse to share a commitment to life, hope, and caring for another person. Receiving support and supervision will enable the nurse to develop this kind of intense, caring relationship so that both the nurse and the client will experience less anxiety and have increased energy to work toward hope and health.

2. *To assist in development of improved coping skills*
Nurses use specific techniques which include nonjudgmental, empathic listening, encouragement, tolerance of expression of painful effect, a flexible response to the client's needs, and consistent limit-setting.

The nurse encourages the client to focus on strengths rather than weaknesses so the client becomes aware of positive qualities and capabilities that have helped with coping in the past. Nurses provide learning opportunities for improved coping by introducing the client to therapeutic modalities that assist in more positive thinking. By replacing or substituting irrational, self-deprecating thoughts, beliefs, and images, the client becomes more capable of viewing life realistically and rationally.

Nurses help reduce the overwhelming effects of problems by helping clients prioritize their concerns. This is done by breaking them down into more manageable parts. The nurse can assist in this process by:

- encouraging the client to list problems from most to least urgent.
- supporting the client in finding immediate solutions for the most pressing problems.
- postponing finding solutions to those problems that do not require immediate remedy.
- encouraging the client to delegate problem solving to others when appropriate.

- helping the client to acknowledge problems that are beyond control.
- identifying, defining, and promoting healthy adaptive behaviors with clients.
- encouraging continuance of healthy behaviors when improved coping strategies are demonstrated (positive reinforcement).
- encouraging the client to discuss the feelings generated by ineffectively coping (for example, frustration, anger, inadequacy).
- affirming the client's rational decisions which have been based on accurate judgment.
- reinforcing the client's attempts to make independent decisions.
- acknowledging the client's demonstrated willingness to implement improved coping behaviors such as assertive communication.
- responding to delusional statements by stating the reality of the situation without arguing with the client's reality.

3. *To enhance family and social support systems*

- Enlist the family as allies in the client's treatment. Family attendance at psychoeducation groups and family therapy are crucial components in helping the client to work through and understand complex and toxic family structures, systems, and dynamics that may contribute to the client's suicidal feelings.
- Determine the degree of available family support which contributes to overall risk management. Inform family members about critical signs which the client may exhibit as depression lifts and discharge occurs. Encourage the removal of any lethal weapons from the client's home environment.
- Provide understanding and encouragement when family members express feelings (for example, frustration, helplessness, or guilt) and intense affect.
- Contact social services to assist with any needed vocational and financial support.
- Refer the client to aftercare groups, support groups, and 12-step groups, as warranted.

Additional Treatment Modalities

Depending on the client's diagnosis, pharmacologic intervention is often a primary consideration in the treatment of the suicidal client. Antidepressants, anxiolytics, and antipsychotic medications are frequently used, depending on the client's need, history, and previous response to medication intervention.

Psychotherapeutic interventions may vary and can include insight-oriented techniques, cognitive reframing, and brief, solution-focused crisis interventions.

Electroconvulsive therapy (ECT) may be used with adults whose response patterns reflect a lack of positive response to medication (i.e., "intractible" or "refractory" depression). These adults concurrently present with longstanding histories of severe depression while expressing imminent intent to die. ECT is discussed in detail in Chapter 23.

■ ■ ■ ▪ ▫ ■ **EVALUATION**

An evaluation of the client's response to the plan of care is crucial in working with the suicidal client. An ongoing, all-encompassing process and evaluation considers the accuracy of the nursing diagnosis, the appropriateness of the intervention based on the client's response, and the timeliness with which the intervention occurred. Evaluation helps the nurse target areas of outcome that are critical to the client's continued survival. A client's lack of positive response to nursing interventions may indicate a need to alter the interventions, implement other treatment modalities, or reexamine target dates for completion of outcomes.

Deliberate, conscientious evaluation of a suicidal client's response to nursing interventions that are directed toward promoting safety and biopsychosocial stabilization help ensure the client's continued safety and readiness for discharge.

Summary of Key Concepts

1. Suicide is a major public health and mental health problem in the United States.

2. Durkheim classified four subtypes of suicide relating to social and cultural aspects: anomic, egoistic, altruistic, and fatalistic.

3. Etiologies of suicide include biologic, which deals with chemical imbalances; psychologic, which dominates the understanding of suicide and defines the dynamics of intrapsychic, interpersonal, cognitive and behavioral approaches in explaining suicidal behavior; and **sociological,** relating to influences of social groups that contribute to suicide.

4. Around the world, suicide accounts for nearly 1% of all deaths. The United States reports 30,000 suicides annually.

5. The most vulnerable groups for suicide are the elderly and youth ages 15 to 24. Caucasians and men are more likely at risk for suicide. Suicide crosses all socioeconomic levels.

6. Suicidal behavior is strongly associated with the occurrence of psychiatric disorders and other health-related problems such as depression, schizophrenia, panic disorders, substance abuse, and medical illnesses.

7. Imminence, intent, and method chosen and its accessibility are the three determinants that indicate the level of lethality and the levels of interventions necessary for safety.

8. Suicidal behavior is treatable.

9. Discharge criteria for the suicidal client must include indications that the client is no longer imminently suicidal, that the client's environment is safe to return to, and that a support system is in place for that client to access.

10. The plan of care emphasizes a reduction in the risk of self-destructive behaviors by monitoring the client's behaviors and providing a safe environment, promoting feelings of self-worth and hope, improving coping skills, limiting social isolation, and building self-esteem.

REFERENCES

Aguilera D: Suicide—Theoretical Concepts. In *Crisis intervention—theory and methodology,* ed 7, St. Louis, 1994, Mosby.

Andreasen N: *The broken brain,* New York, 1984, Harper and Row.

Arato M et al: Retrospective psychiatric assessment of 200 suicides, *Acta Psychiatr Scand* 77:454–456, 1988.

Barbee M: Professionally speaking: what are the warning signs for suicidal adolescents? *J Psychosoc Nurs Ment Health Serv* 31:37–41, 1993.

Blazer D: *Suicide risk factors in the elderly: an epidemiological study,* a paper presented at the conference on Suicide Risk in the Elderly, Boston, 1989, Boston Society for Gerontologic Psychiatry.

Bongar B: *The suicidal patient, clinical and legal standards of care,* Washington,

D.C., 1991, American Psychological Association.

Boyd J, Moscicki E: Firearms and youth suicide, *Am J Public Health* 76:1240–1242, 1986.

Celo-Cruz M: Aid-in-dying: should we decriminalize physician-assisted suicide and physician-committed euthanasia? *Am J Law Med* 4:369–394, 1992.

Cohen L et al: Suicide and schizophrenia: data from a prospective community treatment study, *Am J Psychiatry* 147:602–607, 1990.

Cummings J: The neuroanatomy of depression, *J Clin Psychiatry* 54:14–20, 1993.

Depression in primary care: detection, diagnosis, and treatment, a quick reference guide for clinicians based on Clinical Practice Guidelines, U.S. Dept. of Health and Human Services, vols 1,2. In *Psychosoc Nurs Ment Health Serv* 31:19–28, 1993.

Durkheim E: *Suicide,* 1951, *Glencol The Free Press* (originally published as *Le Suicide* in 1897).

Earle K et al: Characteristics of outpatient suicides, *Hosp Community Psychiatry* 45: 123–126, 1994.

Facts about suicide in the USA, Denver, 1993, American Association of Suicidology.

Farberow N, editor: *The many faces of suicide: indirect self-destructive behavior,* New York, 1980, McGraw-Hill.

Fawcett J et al: Suicide: clues from interpersonal communication, *Arch Gen Psychiatry* 21:129–137, 1969.

Fortinash K, Holoday-Worret P: *Psychiatric nursing care plans,* ed 2, St. Louis, 1995, Mosby.

Freud S: Mourning and melancholia, *Collected papers,* London, 1920, Hogarth Press (originally published in Germany in 1917).

Gonzales L et al: Longitudinal follow-up of unipolar depressives: an investigation of predictors of relapse, *J Consult Clin Psychol* 53:461–469, 1985.

Heacock D: Suicidal behavior in Black and Hispanic youth, *Psychiatric Annals* 20:134–142, 1990.

Hoyer G, Lund E: Suicide among women related to number of children in marriage, *Arch Gen Psychiatry* 50(2):134–137, 1993.

Husain S: Current perspectives on the role of psychosocial factors in adolescent suicide, *Psychiatric Annals* 20:122–127, 1990.

Johnson J: Panic disorder, comorbidity, and suicide attempts, *Arch Gen Psychiatry* 47:805–808, 1990.

Lepine J et al: Suicide attempts in patients with panic disorder, *Arch Gen Psychiatry* 50:144–149, 1993.

Lester D: The association between quality of life and suicide and homicide rates, *J Soc Psychol* 124:247–248, 1984.

Lewinsohn P, Mischel W: Social competence and depression: the role of illusory self-perceptions, *J Abnorm Psychol* 89:203–212, 1980.

Litman R: Sigmund Freud on suicide, *Bull Suicidology* 11–23, July 1967.

Litman R, Farberow N: *Youth suicide in California,* 1986, California Department of Mental Health CMV 85-2482. Sacramento

Maris R: The adolescent suicide problem, *Suicide Life Threat Behav* 15:91–109, 1985.

Marshall J: Changes in aged white male suicide: 1948–1972, *J Gerontology* 33:763–768, 1978.

May P, Dizmang L: Suicide and the American Indian, *Psychiatric Ann* 4(9):22–28, 1974.

Mellick E et al: Suicide among elderly white men: development of a profile, *J Psychosoc Nurs Ment Health Serv* 30:29–34, 1992.

Miles C: Conditions predisposing to suicide: a review, *J Nerv Ment Dis* 164:231–246, 1977.

Miller M: *Suicide after sixty: the final alternative,* New York, 1979, Springer Publishing.

Monk M: Epidemiology of suicide, *Epidemiology Rev* 9:51–69, 1987.

Monk M, Warshaur E: Completed and attempted suicide in three ethnic groups, *Amer J Epidemiology* 100:333–345, 1974.

Nielsen D et al: Suicidality and 5-hydroxyindoleacetic acid concentration associated with tryptophanhydroxylase polymorphism, *Arch Gen Psychiatry* 51:34–38, 1994.

Nyman A, Jonsson H: Patterns of self-destructive behavior in schizophrenia, *Acta Psychiatr Scand* 73:252–262, 1986.

Richman J: *Family therapy for suicidal people,* New York, 1986, Springer Publishing.

Rogers C, editor: *On becoming a person,* Boston, 1961, Houghton Mifflin.

Rudd D et al: Problem-solving appraisal in suicide ideators and attempters, *Amer J Orthopsychiatry* 64(1):136–149, 1994.

Sakinofsky I et al: Problem resolution and repetition of parasuicide: a prospective study, *Br J Psychiatry* 156:395–399, 1991.

Shneidman E: Fifty-eight years. In Shneidman E, editor: *On the nature of suicide,* San Francisco, 1969, Jossey-Bass.

Shneidman E: *Definition of suicide,* New York, 1985, John Wiley and Sons.

Shore J: American Indian suicide—fact and fantasy, *Psychiatry* 38:86–91, 1975.

Smith J et al: Comparison of suicide among Anglos and Hispanics in five Southwestern states, *Suicide Life Threat Behav* 15:14–16, 1985.

Stekel W: Suicide and will. In Freidman P, editor: *On suicide,* New York, 1967, International Universities Press.

Sullivan H: Socio-psychiatric research: its implications for the schizophrenia problem and mental hygiene, *Am J Psychiatry* 10:977–991, 1931.

Sullivan H: The manic-depressive psychosis. In Perry H et al, editors: *Clinical studies in psychiatry,* New York, 1956, W.W. Norton and Company.

Tishler C et al: Adolescent suicide attempts: some significant factors, *Suicide Life Threat Behav* 11:86–92, 1981.

Toolan J: Depression and suicide. In Caplan G, editor: *Child and adolescent psychiatry, sociocultural and community psychiatry,* New York, 1974, Basic Books.

Trygstad L: The need to know: biological learning needs identified by practicing psychiatric nurses, *J Psychosoc Nurs Ment Health Serv* 32(2): 13–18, 1994.

U.S. Senate Special Committee on Aging, the Federal Council on Aging, and the U.S. Department of Health and Human Services: *Aging America—trends and projections,* Washington D.C., 1991.

Valente S: Adolescent suicide: assessment and intervention, *J Child and Adolescent Psychiatric Nursing* 2(1):34–39, 1989.

Weiss J: The suicidal patient. In Arieti S, editor: *American Handbook of Psychiatry,* New York, 1966, Basic Books.

Weissman M et al: Suicidal ideation and suicide attempts in panic disorder and attacks, *N Engl J Med* 321:1209–1214, 1989.

Wells K et al: The functioning and well-being of depressed patients, *JAMA* 262: 914–919, 1989.

Wilson D: *The New York Times,* April 9, 1994.

Wright J, Beck A: Cognitive therapy of depression: theory and practice, *Hosp Community Psychiatry* 34:1119–1124, 1983.

Yang B et al: Sociological and economic theories of suicide: a comparison of the USA and Taiwan, *Social Science Medicine* 34:333–334, 1992.

Zayas L: Towards an understanding of suicide risks in young Hispanic females, *J Adolescent Research* 2:1–11, 1978.

CHAPTER 27

Grief and Loss

Charles Kemp
Gay Mallon-Frank

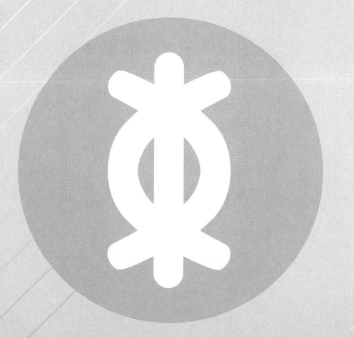

Acute grief The initial response to loss. While diminishing over time, acute grief may last for as long as several years, depending primarily on the meaning of the lost person/object for the survivor.

Anticipatory grief Grief experienced before death or loss occurs, for example, when a loved one has a terminal illness; also called premourning.

Bereavement The state of grieving.

Chronic sorrow Grief in response to an ongoing loss such as chronic illness in a loved one.

Dysfunctional grief Grief that is expressed to a significantly greater or lesser intensity over a significantly longer or shorter time than is culturally expected. It may manifest itself in serious physical and/or emotional disabilities.

Grief The dynamic natural psychologic and physiologic responses to loss. Grief affects physical, cognitive, behavioral, emotional, social, and spiritual aspects of the individual.

Grief work The intense psychologic effort to fully express the feelings associated with grief, understand the relationship with the deceased, and, paradoxically, carry on with essential activities of daily living.

Mourning Feeling or expressing grief or sorrow.

Postvention Grief therapy after the death occurs but before pathology develops.

Social support The presence of other individuals who are able to give understanding, encouragement, and assistance in life, especially during difficult times.

- Discuss four major categories for symptoms of grief.

- Describe three components of the normal grief process.

- Distinguish between symptoms and behaviors of grief and depression.

- Analyze the risk for pathologic grief reactions in selected high-risk clients.

- Discuss the major goals for intervention in acute grief.

- Evaluate the "points of intervention" with respect to intervention efficacy.

GRIEF

Grief is the painful psychologic and physiologic responses to loss. While most commonly associated with the death of a loved one, grief occurs when there is any significant loss, including loss of self-esteem, dignity, or sense of worth. Grief descends on the client newly admitted to a psychiatric hospital, the client who undergoes mutilating surgery, the parents of an infant with birth defects, the child who changes schools, the victim of violence, the nurse who works with victims of violence, the betrayed lover, the person who loses a job or retires. Grief comes to everyone. Most nurses are in daily contact with grief—other people's and their own.

Grief is not an illness that needs to be fixed. It is a normal reaction to loss, and it must be experienced (rather than suppressed) so that healing can occur.

Symptoms of Grief

Grief is most often defined or discussed in terms of symptoms (Cowles and Rodgers, 1991). Few descriptions of the symptoms of grief capture the power or intensity of those symptoms. Sad and lonely feelings after a loved one dies are natural. However, the intensity of the sadness and loneliness is a surprise to many. Lindemann's classic study of grief identified many of the symptoms of grief, including physical distress, preoccupation with the image of the deceased, guilt, hostile reactions, and disruptions in patterns of conduct (Lindemann, 1944). These and other psychologic manifestations can be summarized as follows.

PHYSICAL SYMPTOMS

Physical manifestations of grief include weakness, anorexia, feelings of choking, shortness of breath, tightness in the chest, dry mouth, and gastrointestinal disturbances (Burnell and Burnell, 1989). Fatigue, exhaustion, and insomnia are common. Bereaved persons frequently seek medical assistance for vague symptoms, such as chest discomfort or GI problems, many of which seem to have no physiologic basis. Additionally, while grief is seldom a direct cause of illness or death, there is a clear link between grief and increased vulnerability to physical and mental illness, especially heart disease and depression (Parkes, 1987).

COGNITIVE SYMPTOMS

Cognitive manifestations center on preoccupation with the image and thoughts of the deceased. Some find the involuntary nature and intensity of the preoccupation surprising and distressing. It is not uncommon for the preoccupation to take the form of conversations with the deceased. Especially in the elderly, these conversations may continue for the rest of the survivor's life. Over time, preoccupation usually diminishes, although links with the deceased may be maintained for many years. These links may be in the form of remembrances, such as treasured things, or renegotiated relationships with the deceased. Formerly thought by some to be a symptom that needed resolution, the drive to maintain links between the living and the dead is increasingly recognized as normative behavior (Silverman and Worden, 1992). Indeed, in some cultures, for example, the Chinese and Vietnamese cultures, the failure to maintain formal links is thought to be pathological.

Another common symptom is difficulty concentrating, such as complete lapses of focus or even orientation to time and place. Seeking and longing for the lost person or object are universally experienced. Some grieving people experience hallucinations that are most often described as momentary glimpses of the person who died, or brief auditory messages (two or three words) perceived to be spoken by the deceased. In most cases, hallucinations diminish within a month or two after the loss and thus may be considered as part of the normal grieving process. If hallucinations persist, increase in number or intensity, or become derogatory or threatening (such as beckoning the survivor to join the deceased), they are considered to be negative hallucinations. In such cases, therapeutic interventions, including hospitalization and/or antipsychotic medications, may be indicated.

BEHAVIORAL AND RELATING SYMPTOMS

Behavioral and relating manifestations include disruptions in patterns of conduct, ranging from an inability to perform even basic activities of daily living, to dragging through daily activities, to a restless, disorganized behavior that includes "searching" for that which is lost (Carter, 1989; Lindemann, 1944). The survivor can no longer function well. The old life and patterns lose meaning and satisfaction without the lost object/person, and there does not seem to be a new life or patterns to which the bereaved individual can turn. This loss of relating and meaning is a major etiology of despair or hopelessness.

AFFECTIVE SYMPTOMS

Affective manifestations of grief are often overwhelming, with sadness, guilt, and anger among the most common. Sadness, loneliness, and hopelessness tend to predominate and may (along with other symptoms) meet the criteria for diagnosis of a mood disorder, e.g., major depression or dysthymic disorder. The most common differences between symptoms of **bereavement** (the state of grieving) and major depression or dysthymic disorder are that psychomotor retardation, morbid guilt, and suicidal ideation are less common in bereavement and that affective disorders are of longer duration than bereavement (Nuss and Zubenko, 1992). However, dysfunctional or unresolved grief may result in major depression.

Guilt is a pervasive theme in grief, even in children as young as age 2 (Gibbons, 1992). Many survivors search for their failures or omissions in the relationship. When they find significant mistakes, they magnify whatever small transgressions might exist (Lindemann, 1944). Guilt may be especially troublesome for those whose relationship with the deceased was ambivalent and characterized by unresolved or unexpressed feelings (Burnell and Burnell, 1989). "Survivor guilt" is common among people who go through an intense experience such as war and survive, while others do not. A similar guilt is experienced when survivors feel that they should have died instead of the loved one.

Grief accompanied by sustained loss of self-esteem and ambivalence about living is an indication that suicide risk is increased and help is needed. Anger is common and may be directed outward to the person who died, family members, health care staff, God, or turned inward to self. Anger is generally a response to the anxiety derived from the powerlessness and vulnerability resulting from death of a loved one and other losses. Many survivors think it is wrong to direct anger toward a deceased loved one, and thus turn the anger inward. Anger turned inward may also reflect a survivor's inability to release the lost object or person. To those who have spent a lifetime suppressing anger, these overwhelming and "wrong" or ego-dystonic feelings are distressing and make some people feel they are "going crazy." Some need permission to express anger. If the death itself is not enough to engender anger, tending to such business surrounding the death as funeral preparations may result in anger. Death, usually the greatest and most painful loss in life, is seen by some morticians, lawyers, and others only as a point of vulnerability through which survivors can be exploited for profit. The impulse to use drugs, including prescription drugs and alcohol, may occur. Or if the survivor already uses, the use may increase. Bereaved persons with a history of any sort of drug misuse or mental illness are at risk for recurrence or exacerbation of these problems.

Stages and Process of Grief
STAGES OF GRIEF

Grief is often described in terms of stages. Although there exists variation among the different conceptions, many stage-oriented theories can be summarized as having three basic stages: avoidance, confrontation, and reestablishment. Avoidance includes both the initial denial and also subsequent brief periods of time when the survivor "forgets" then "remembers," with shock and pain, the losses and grief. Confrontation is an often lengthy period of active mourning and includes the previously discussed most acute physical, cognitive, behavioral and relating, and affective manifestations of grief. Reestablishment occurs, not as a distinct stage, but as the gradual decrease of symptoms and adjustment to life without the person or object lost. Stages tend to be neater in theory than they are in reality, and thus may mislead some individuals into thinking that grief is a matter of progressing in an orderly manner through stages and then being finished with grief.

PROCESS OF GRIEF

Characteristics. Rather than considering well-defined stages, it is more helpful to think of grief in terms of a process of common and dynamic responses. Thus, a person might initially respond to the death of a loved one with shock and disbelief, then protest and despair; go through a period of emotionless cognitive activity (planning the funeral, etc.); then experience yearning, despair, and disorganization (sobbing, confusion, wandering); and gradually begin the long, painful, and varied process of rebuilding a life without the person who died. An essential feature of this process is its dynamic, changing nature (Cowles and Rodgers, 1991). Periods of apparently normal functioning, for example, may be interspersed with

---

Box 27-1   Summary of Theories of Grief

Lindemann

Grief is manifested by predictable psychologic and somatic symptomatology. Acute **mourning** (feeling or expressing grief or sorrow) is characterized by somatic distress, preoccupation with the deceased person's image, guilt, hostile reactions, and loss of patterns of conduct. Dysfunctional or "morbid" grief reactions are defined as distortions of some aspect of "normal grief." The duration of grief and the development of dysfunctional grief largely depend on the success with which the mourner works through the grief.

Kubler-Ross

Elisabeth Kubler-Ross's stages of dying (denial, anger, bargaining, depression, and acceptance) are often applied to grief. The initial response to loss may include denial, anger, and bargaining. Denial is characterized by refusal to accept the loss. Anger may initially be directed at health care staff and, later in the process, at the person who died. Bargaining and denial are often mixed in a futile attempt to "reverse reality." Depression tends to be the lengthiest phase and, in dysfunctional grief, may become chronic and meet DSM-IV criteria for major depression. Acceptance of the loss is a gradual process that includes aspects of previous stages. As the grief work progresses, acceptance increases.

Bowlby

Grief and loss are characterized first by numbness in which the loss is recognized, but not necessarily felt as real. Numbness is followed by yearning and searching, in which the loss is still not fully realized. In the third phase,

disorganization and despair, the loss is real, and intense emotional pain and cognitive disorganization occur. Reorganization is the final phase and is characterized by a gradual adjustment to life without the deceased.

Engel

The initial response to loss is shock and disbelief. Awareness of the loss and the meaning of the loss develop during the first year of mourning. Eventually, the relationship is resolved and put into perspective.

Shneidman

Conceptualizing less structure or stages than other theorists in regard to grief, Shneidman views the expression of grief as dependent primarily on an individual's personality or style of living. An individual who goes through life feeling depressed and guilty is likely to grieve similarly. One who avoids emotional investments with others will also tend to try to avoid grief.

Theory synthesis

Grief tends to occur in several phases. The initial response to loss may be shock, numbness, denial, or other attempts to defend against the reality and pain of loss. This initial phase is followed by painful psychologic and physical disequilibrium which, in the case of dysfunctional grief, may last indefinitely. The third phase of resolution or recovery is a gradual process in which "the good days begin to outnumber the bad." Ultimately, while not forgotten, the relationship with the deceased is resolved and put into perspective.

periods of psychologic distress or symptoms (almost indistinguishable from those of major depression). Countless people say, "It seems like I'm doing fine, and then for no reason at all, I start crying" (as if some practical reason were needed in order to justify crying!).

The grief process might include all the above responses or only two or three of them. There might not be a "stage of avoidance," or a period of organized cognitive activity, or little resolution, reorganization, or adjustment to the environment in the absence of the deceased. Moreover, when death is expected, the grief process begins before the person dies. Grief before death occurs is called **anticipatory grief** (Rando, 1988) and is discussed below. Box 27-1 summarizes the major theories of grief.

Grief work. Stages and process are associated with another common characteristic of grief, which is **grief work.** Named first by Lindemann (1944), grief work is the means by which people move through the stages or process of grief. Grief work is both a struggle to avoid despair and a willingness to confront the reality of despair. Thus, within the grief process, the bereaved person must continue to some extent to move forward with the business of life (for example, paying the bills, making decisions) and at the same time being able to express the deep, painful emotions of grieving (Figure 27-1).

Complicating factors. Grief work is complicated by several factors. First, it is extremely painful. Many people are surprised at the intensity and depth of the pain experienced in grieving. There is often a conscious or unconscious attempt to avoid the distress, perhaps by doing such things as throwing themselves back into a busy schedule or taking a long vacation. Second, the work is inherently contradictory. The pain demands expression, but there is often the fear that if the pain is expressed, control over feelings will be lost ("I know that if I start crying, I will never stop"). Third, both emotion-based coping, such as expressing deep, powerful feelings, and problem-solving coping, such as developing strategies for going on with life, are needed to most successfully complete the work (Gass and Chang, 1989). Finally, in most of the Western world, cultural values exist that support avoiding the expression of grief. For example, self-control is highly valued, especially by men (Lindemann, 1944). There is a tendency to try to "rush through" grief and get back to work or get on with one's life. Rituals that helped in individual and community expression of grief are now often brief "celebrations" of the deceased's life or other upbeat and usually brief events. Thus, the expression of grief is limited to what is "appropriate" in public and then what occurs when the bereaved individual is alone with the pain.

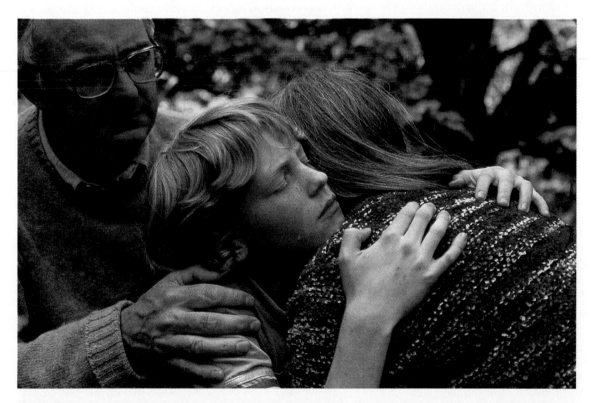

Figure 27-1 Throughout the grief process, it is normal for a bereaved person to express deep, painful emotions.
(Copyright © The Image Bank, Photographer: Mieke Maas.)

Types of Grief

Types of grief include anticipatory grief, acute grief, dysfunctional grief, and chronic sorrow. There is some disagreement about definitions, especially in terms of the time required for resolution of a particular form of grief.

ANTICIPATORY GRIEF

Anticipatory grief, or premourning, is defined as grief associated with anticipation of a predicted death or loss (Shneidman, 1980). Anticipatory grief is generally viewed as an adaptive process that can help resolve relationships and prepare survivors to some extent for the loss. Ideally, the realization that loss is approaching provides those involved an opportunity to work on interpersonal and spiritual reconciliation and to provide support for one another (Rando, 1988). In some circumstances, anticipatory grief provides family and practitioners a preview of the grief to come. Current needs or needs likely to occur after the loss may be identified (McFarland and Gerety, 1993). At other times, however, anticipatory grief is associated with a high incidence of depression (Levy, 1991). Lengthy illness (more than six months), highly ambivalent relationships, premature detachment, and guilt over giving up hope may all lead to later difficulties when anticipatory grief exists (Levy, 1991; Rando, 1988).

ACUTE GRIEF

Acute grief, usually referred to simply as grief, is the prototypical painful experience after a loss. Its symptoms and process are described earlier in the chapter. There is agreement that acute grief is time-limited. However, an issue that has never been satisfactorily resolved is the question of how long acute (or normal) grief lasts (Cowles and Rodgers, 1991). An early theory is that acute grief lasts approximately one year (Shneidman, 1980). More recently, grief is estimated to last for one to two years for spouses and two to five years for parents (Burnell and Burnell, 1989). In some traditional cultures (for example, East Indian) and among some individuals in certain religions (for example, Judaism and Hinduism) grief may be ongoing and not limited by time (Goodman et al 1991).

Many factors other than culture and religion influence the length and intensity of grief, such as the nature of the relationship, manner of death, survivor involvement in care, length of illness, and the presence or absence of hope. Acute grief does not have a clear ending. Gradually the sadness lessens, the pain diminishes, and eventually the mourner moves forward with her or his life (Schiff, 1977).

Within the process of healing and moving on, there are times of acute exacerbation when some situation or event brings back the pain and the mourner again feels overwhelmed with grief. Holidays, birthdays, and other significant milestones are obvious events with the poten-

tial to rekindle the grief. Other precipitants are less obvious, and thus the mourner is unable to prepare for them. For example, a song, an image, or a smell may occur in an unguarded moment, and the sadness returns as powerfully as it was in the initial stages of grief. These moments of exacerbation also decrease over time.

DYSFUNCTIONAL GRIEF

Dysfunctional grief has been described in multiple ways. Lindemann (1944) and a host of contemporary writers and researchers (e.g., Bowlby, 1980; Cowles and Rodgers, 1991; Parkes, 1987) emphasize normative and dysfunctional aspects of grief. In other words, up to some point, grief is "normal"; beyond that point, grief is variously termed "dysfunctional" (McFarland and Gerety, 1993), "pathological" (Burnell and Burnell, 1989), or "complicated" (Wolfelt, 1991). All sources refer to essentially the same phenomenon when describing dysfunctional grief: grief that lasts longer and is characterized by greater disability or other dysfunctional patterns than usual as defined by cultural values. Types of dysfunctional grief (Wolfelt, 1991) include:

- **Absent** or **inhibited grief:** characterized by no expression of grief following significant loss. Suppressed or repressed grief may manifest as chronic physical illness such as ulcerative colitis or rheumatoid arthritis or psychological disability such as major depression.

- **Distorted grief:** characterized by distortion, usually exaggeration, of one or more components of grief, especially guilt and/or anger. Distorted grief may result in significant psychosocial disability such as major depression or legal difficulties following angry or violent outbursts.

- **Converted grief:** similar in nature to a conversion disorder in which preoccupation with the deceased may be exaggerated to the extent that the survivor exhibits symptoms or characteristics of the deceased (Lindemann, 1944).

- **Chronic grief:** unending grief, the symptoms of which may intensify over time. Chronic grief occurs in response to a loss (for example, a death), while chronic sorrow occurs in response to an ongoing loss, (for example, the sorrow of parents with a child with mental retardation).

Dysfunctional grief is often associated with unresolved issues in the relationship with the person who died, coupled with the pain of the loss. Dysfunctional grief is also associated with circumstances that inhibit the expression of grief. Persons who do not deal with their own grief or pain but constantly help others to do so are at risk. This is a familiar situation for nurses and others in "helping professions" (Adams et al, 1992). Other reasons for dysfunctional grief are lack of social support; the "deritualization" of Western culture (for example, mourning periods of one to two days); uncertain loss as in the case of prisoners of war; traumatic loss such as by murder; multiple losses or compound grief (for example, most of a family killed at one time or within a brief period of time); loss that is seldom discussed (for example, rape); undervalued loss such as that felt by some who have an abortion, miscarriage, or other losses that may not be recognized by others as a significant loss; and by the accumulated effects of current grief on past unresolved grief.

CHRONIC SORROW

Only recently described in the literature, **chronic sorrow** is a form of grief that may include characteristics of

---

CLINICAL ALERT !

Persons with the greatest potential for dysfunctional grief have the following characteristics:

- premorbid psychiatric history
- social isolation
- relationship with the deceased characterized by unresolved conflict, ambivalence, e.g., "love-hate"
- relationship with the deceased characterized by enmeshment and a high level introjection, hence difficulty "letting go"
- suppression of grief

---

other forms of grief but differs in several key aspects. First, chronic sorrow is a response to ongoing loss such as chronic illness. Second, persons experiencing chronic sorrow seldom experience disability such as major depression, but typically function at a higher level in activities of daily living than those experiencing other forms of grief (Burke et al, 1992). Persons at risk for chronic sorrow include parents with children who have mental retardation, schizophrenia, or other chronic illness; spouses of persons with long-term chronic illnesses such as multiple sclerosis, alcoholism, or Alzheimer's disease; and persons with disorders similar to the above. It is still undocumented as to what effects on the grief process result when the etiology of chronic sorrow is removed, for example, when the disabled person dies.

Grief and depression are often compared with each other. Astute readers may also notice that grief, especially dysfunctional grief, shares characteristics with post-traumatic stress disorder, particularly in that both invariably involve loss (Table 27-1).

BEREAVEMENT CARE ACROSS THE LIFE SPAN
Prevention
PREVENTION PRIOR TO LOSS

Grief is a universal experience that may come with or without warning and occurs many times and with varying intensity throughout life. The major psychosocial determinants of pathology in grief are a psychiatric history prior to the loss and inadequate **social support** (Nuss and Zubenko, 1992). Other factors that significantly influence grief are multiple losses and lengthy ter-

---

TABLE 27-1   Comparison of grief, depression, and post-traumatic stress disorder (PTSD)

Grief	Depression	PTSD
Process related to loss.	Relatively static or cyclic affective disorder not necessarily related to loss.	Relatively static anxiety disorder related to trauma. Precipitating event is outside the range of usual human experience.
Symptoms usually appear shortly after the loss.	May or may not be associated with an identified loss.	Symptoms often appear years after the trauma.
Depressive symptoms include dysphoric mood of sadness, hopelessness, and despair; anger is common, as are periods of agitation.	Depressive symptoms are similar to but more intense than grief, except that anger is seldom expressed and psychomotor retardation, morbid guilt, and suicidal ideation are more common.	Depressive symptoms are common. Other symptoms include persistent reexperiencing of the trauma (versus preoccupation with image of the deceased, as in grief). Increased arousal is common.
Physical symptoms cover a wide spectrum. Physical sequelae may include heart disease and other chronic illnesses.	Physical symptoms are primarily neurovegetative.	Sleep disturbances may resemble those of grief or depression; hypervigilance is common.
Spiritual beliefs may provide meaning or context.	Spiritual beliefs seldom provide context or meaning	Seldom any relation to spiritual beliefs.

minal illness. It follows, then, that grief is best addressed by the primary promotion of mental health. It is reasonable to believe that children who are wanted and born into supportive and healthy families are less likely to experience dysfunctional grief. At this time, family programs to prevent dysfunctional grief are unlikely to be funded. However, preventive mental programs for families are likely to promote a healthier grief experience among members.

PREVENTION WHEN LOSS IS EXPECTED

A second point at which health promotion or disability prevention should be considered in relation to grief work is in the case of terminal illness or other anticipated loss. Interventions in these situations include assisting individuals and families in working toward personal, interpersonal, and spiritual reconciliation; and not necessarily anticipatory grief. Even in the best of relationships, there are often unresolved issues or areas in which growth is

possible. Whether or not interpersonal issues are addressed, promoting health in this stage of life includes promoting participation of the client and family in care. Clearly, effective participation in care has a positive effect on the grief process after death (although long-term effects are not known for caregivers in Alzheimer's disease, schizophrenia, and other similar chronic illnesses). A variety of means exist for intervention at this point, including individual informal or formal counseling in acute care settings, family support groups, hospice care, and support from religious institutions. Nurses and other health care professionals should address the health needs of family members as well as those of clients. (See Understanding and Applying Research below.)

PREVENTION AFTER THE LOSS

The third intervention point is after the loss occurs. This is known as **postvention** (Shneidman, 1973), often simply called grief therapy. Intervention at this point may be preventive, directed toward addressing existing problems that are interpersonal in nature or related to normative or dysfunctional grief.

Preventive grief therapy is offered as a matter of course to survivors in several circumstances. Hospice programs, for example, typically offer bereavement calls or visits at specified intervals to survivors. Many hospice programs also periodically hold picnics or other activities for bereaved adults or children. Many churches and synagogues hold grief workshops for members and others in the community. These are generally weekend or time-limited groups similar to self-help groups such as I Can Cope.

PROBLEM-ORIENTED GRIEF THERAPY

Problem-oriented grief therapy or postvention is offered when a problem, not necessarily dysfunctional grief, exists or is anticipated (Shneidman, 1980). As in many of life's unavoidable processes, the difficult and painful transitions in normative grief usually respond to understanding and support. Effective grief therapy focuses on emotional responses to the loss and problem solving related to moving forward in life (Gass and Chang, 1989). Emotional issues center around the telling and retelling of the details of the story (the death and surrounding issues) and the history of the relationship, with emphasis on the experience and expression of the feelings, particularly sadness, anger, guilt, or other troubling feelings. In earlier phases of the process, the bereaved person may only recall the positive qualities of the deceased. As the mourner progresses through the grief work, both positive and negative qualities of the deceased and the relationship emerge. Problem-focused strategies address questions of developing support, relationships, and other issues inherent in "the new life" or life after a loved one dies.

Understanding and Applying
RESEARCH

Ferrell JA, Boyle JS: Bereavement experiences: caring for a partner with AIDS, *J Comm Health Nurs* 9(3):127–135.

This study describes the bereavement experiences of gay men who cared for a partner with AIDS. Researchers used a field research design with face-to-face interviews of survivors who were selected on the basis of insight and verbal communication skills. Interviews were tape-recorded and analyzed using *Ethnograph*, a qualitative software program. Two "major conceptual categories" were identified: 1) strategies used to care for partners during the illness (i.e., "themes" such as being committed to care, taking care of self, and dealing with the health care system); and 2) the survivors' bereavement experiences (i.e., themes such as seeking support from others and accepting the loss). Bereavement began with the diagnosis of the partner's HIV infection, was characterized by seeking support of others, and finally, focused on accepting the loss after death. Successful caregiving was linked to decreased risk of complicated bereavement. While limited by a small single-gender sample of subjects (five men), the study identifies an ideal in responding to diagnosis, care, and grief for a partner with AIDS. The study should be replicated with larger and more varied populations. This study indicates that nurses need to counsel the significant others of clients with AIDS about caregiving to reduce complications of bereavement.

In response to frequent overuse of medications to mask grief, some practitioners discourage the use of anxiolytic or antidepressant medications for bereaved persons. However, even in cases of "normal" grief, mourners may require short-term use of these drugs at certain stages of the grief process.

Reassurance is an essential component in grief therapy. The absence of cultural norms for expressing or otherwise dealing with grief results in some people feeling as if their grief is the beginning of "madness." Even though some will not initially believe it, they need to hear from the nurse that their experience is grief and not mental illness.

Interventions in Dysfunctional Grief

In dysfunctional grief, there is often either unresolved grief from the past and/or a preexisting psychologic condition that must be addressed as part of the grief therapy. Thus, therapy includes the issues noted above as well as other interpersonal issues. Often, a central issue in dysfunctional grief is the promotion of the client's ability to express the pain of the grief rather than only the anger or guilt. It is common for bereaved persons to have ill-defined fantasies of catastrophe if their pain is expressed: "If I ever start crying, I will never stop." Clients with dysfunctional grief are at increased risk for suicide or, to a lesser extent, for hurting others. They may also experience physical and mental disorders, as previously discussed.

The client's primary physician, nurse, or other source of primary health care should be involved or at least kept aware of treatment for several specific reasons. First, it is common for such clients to frequently seek medical care, often for vague or difficult-to-evaluate complaints that are actually somatic expressions of grief. Awareness of dysfunctional grief and ongoing therapy may help health care providers avoid unnecessary tests and treatment. Second, there is significant risk of suicide in dysfunctional grief, and an informed health care provider can be alert to suicidal hints, gestures, and attempts to obtain lethal amounts of medications. All health professionals involved in the care of a person with dysfunctional grief should be alert to the possibility of the client seeking help from multiple sources and the potential for lethal medication admixture.

SPIRITUALITY AND GRIEF

All basic spiritual needs or issues may be threatened by the grief experience: meaning, hope, relatedness, forgiveness, and transcendence may fall away and leave the mourner in a spiritual vacuum. The nature of God and previously held beliefs, including any easy answers to life's problems (for example, that faith protects one from pain) are called into question and may not support the reality of the current feelings. Grief may then be experienced as a test of faith, and the awareness or acknowledgment of anger may be interpreted as a personal spiritual failure. While dreams and visions are seen as significant spiritual events in some cultures, they may be discounted as either immaterial or pathologic in the context of Western cultures. There may be reluctance by the grieving individual to discuss these experiences and feelings with family, friends, or clergy. As mourners struggle to find a context for the doubt and confusion that may accompany these experiences, it is important for the nurse to listen with openness to determine how these experiences confirm or challenge the mourner's spiritual and religious beliefs. Some individuals are confirmed in their traditional beliefs; others see the dissolution of their faith; and some find or rediscover a deeper faith.

■ ASSESSMENT

Nursing assessment of a bereaved person is based on knowledge of normal and pathologic aspects of the grief process, influences on the grief process, and the person's resources. Assessment encompasses the following: 1) the grief experience of the mourner; 2) factors that inhibit or promote working through the grief process, including cultural and religious norms; and 3) the mourner's ability to mobilize cognitive, behavioral, and emotional coping strategies and supports. The client's current level of functioning should be assessed, with the understanding that up to a point, impaired functioning is to be expected.

■ ■ NURSING DIAGNOSIS

Nursing diagnosis of grief or problems occurring in grief may be complicated by the more common approach of identifying problems of a physical or psychologic nature and seeking to alleviate the discomfort. The grief process by itself includes discomfort, and attempts to avoid or eliminate the discomfort, no matter how well intentioned, impede the grieving process. Thus, an insightful diagnosis may focus more on the expression of normal feelings (e.g., anger, guilt, sadness) than on what the feelings are. Nursing diagnoses are formulated from the information obtained during the assessment phase of the nursing process. The accuracy of diagnoses depends on a careful, in-depth assessment.

NANDA Diagnoses for Acute Grief

Personal identity disturbance
Situational low self-esteem
Impaired social interaction
Dysfunctional grief
Risk for violence: self-directed
Grieving, dysfunctional: unexpressed
Caregiver role strain

■ ■ ■ OUTCOME IDENTIFICATION

Outcome criteria focus on enhancement of emotional coping skills or methods, i.e., greater expression of feelings of grief; and cognitive and behavioral coping abilities, i.e., strategies to develop more functional patterns of living that are appropriate to changed life circumstances.

Outcome Identification for Grief

Client will:

1. Verbalize absence of suicidal ideations.

2. Express any guilty and/or angry feelings related to the death and grief versus suppression of grief.

CLINICAL SYMPTOMS

Bereavement Disturbances

Physical

In acute grief, physical disturbances include weakness, anorexia, shortness of breath, tightness of the chest, dry mouth, and gastrointestinal disturbances such as constipation or diarrhea, abdominal pain, gas, nausea, and vomiting. Cardiovascular and gastrointestinal problems predominate in chronic grief.

Thinking

These disturbances are often focused on preoccupation with images and thoughts of the deceased. This preoccupation may be so pervasive that the bereaved person is unable to carry on with some activities of daily living. The inability to control the thoughts is distressing to many mourners. In acute grief, these obsessive thoughts are normal; they are simply part of the process. Preoccupation with the deceased that results in significant disruption of daily activities such as one's work, is widely considered pathologic after about one year past the date of death when the deceased was an adult, and two or more years past the date of death when the deceased was a child.

Behavioral and Relating

These disturbances may result from the depressive aspects of grief. People who are bereaved may describe themselves as "stopped," and thus unable to participate in relationships. There is tendency in survivors to ruminate about the death and the relationship with the deceased. In at least the earlier phases of the process, talk of the deceased tends to focus only on her or his "good" qualities and ignore the multifaceted nature of the individual. Many people who are bereaved cry with little apparent provocation, which often results in discomfort for the mourner and others. In chronic grief, the talk of the death and the relationship tends to be repetitive rather than progressive and insightful.

Feeling

These disturbances are primarily those of sadness or depression, anger, and guilt. Cultural norms against "carrying on" inhibit expression of these feelings. People who are bereaved soon learn that "nobody wants to hear your sad story." Sadness, and even feelings of depression, are not considered pathologic unless they persist a year or two past the death, or include suicidal ideation.

Nursing Assessment Questions

Persons Experiencing Grief

1. Describe how it has been for you since your husband died.
   (To determine the risk of pathologic grief and the need for grief therapy.)

2. How have you reacted to other major losses in your life?
   (To establish client's previous coping patterns in response to loss.)

3. Who do you depend on when you are having a hard time as you are now? How do you feel when you ask for help?
   (To identify support system and determine ability to express feelings.)

4. What medications are you currently taking?
   (To determine if client is taking any medications to ease the pain of grief.)

5. How often do you have alcoholic drinks or take other drugs? Has this increased since your loss? How much are you currently taking, and how does it make you feel?
   (To determine usual intake of substances versus use during grief, and how this affects the grief process.)

Do not ask, "How are you doing?" Cultural norms are to respond to such questions with "pretty good," or "okay," or "fine," which are essentially meaningless.

CASE STUDY

Mrs. Jones is 70 years old and lives alone in the apartment she shared with her husband for the past 17 years. Her husband died last month after a two-year struggle with prostate cancer. Since her husband's death, Mrs. Jones has felt sad and depressed. She wants to spend time with others but says, "They are happy and I'm sad, and it's no good for anyone." For the past week, except for "forcing" herself to take her daily walk around the block, Mrs. Jones has spent most of her time alone in her apartment. She has a poor appetite, difficulty sleeping, and feels guilty about "all the things I could have done to help my husband." Most of the other residents in the complex are similar in age to Mrs. Jones, and she is very close to several of them. Mrs. Jones's only son lives in another state and has offered to let her move into a bedroom in his home.

Critical Thinking and Assessment

1. What type of grief is Mrs. Jones experiencing?

2. Identify three of Mrs. Jones's important needs.

3. What personal resources are likely to be most helpful to Mrs. Jones at the present time?

---

3. Express both positive and negative feelings about the deceased versus idealizing the qualities of the deceased.

4. Explore the relationship with the deceased in a multifaceted way that includes both positive and negative aspects.

5. Formulate and implement reasonable plans for adapting life and identified role to present circumstances.

6. Participate in at least one social or community activity each week.

■ ■ ■ ■ **PLANNING**

The plan of care for a person with acute grief consists primarily of 1) supporting mobilization of the person's personal and community resources, 2) providing normative data about the grief process, and 3) supporting the person in her or his grief work. Each of these is discussed below.

Assistance may be needed in mobilizing resources (e.g., family, friends, and spiritual supports) because in-

dividuals often are reluctant to ask for help, and resources often do not know how to provide help. In addition, some of the symptoms of grief (fatigue, sadness, anger, etc.) promote isolation rather than relating. Frequently, if either the bereaved person or her or his support systems can initiate contact, the other will respond appropriately. Too often, however, the mourner and resources exist in isolation, each wishing they knew how to make contact.

Normative data on grief, i.e., explanation of physical, emotional, social, and spiritual difficulties inherent in the grief process, can be provided to both the bereaved and her or his support systems. In a culture that is lacking in ritual and tradition in many ways, grief may sometimes seem mysterious and/or pathologic even by those one might expect to be helpful (for example, clergy). The nurse teaches survivors and others (such as family members) what they might experience in the grief process. Bereavement (survivor) groups are an excellent forum for such teaching.

Supporting the mourner in her or his grief work includes facilitating the mourner's ability to tell how the deceased died and related events, exploring positive and negative aspects of the relationship with the deceased, exploring the deceased's positive and negative aspects, and determining cognitive and behavioral coping strate-

COLLABORATIVE DIAGNOSES

DSM-IV Diagnoses*	NANDA Diagnoses**
Dysthymic Disorder	Situational low self-esteem
Major Depressive	Sleep pattern disturbance
Disorder	Altered thought process
Adjustment Disorder	Fatigue
	Hopelessness
	Powerlessness
	Anticipatory grieving
	Dysfunctional grieving
	Altered role performance
	Personal identity disturbance
	Social isolation
	Impaired social interaction
	Altered family processes
	Risk for violence, self-directed
	Risk for violence, directed at others
	Altered sexuality patterns
	Ineffective individual coping
	Ineffective denial
	Impaired adjustment
	Post-trauma response
	Ineffective family coping
	Spiritual distress

*From American Psychiatric Association: *Diagnostic and statistical manual of mental disorders,* ed 4, Washington, D.C., 1994, American Psychiatric Association.

**From North American Nursing Diagnosis Association: *NANDA nursing diagnoses: definitions and classifications, 1992–1993,* Philadelphia, 1992, North American Nursing Diagnosis Association.

Nursing Care in the Community

Grief and Loss

The grieving process ideally includes community supports. The community mental health nurse can ensure that such supports are in place for a client, as well as personally provide comfort. The nurse in the community must determine the extent of emotional expression the client desires. Sometimes the client may only need companionship. Expressing emotional empathy with the client is not unprofessional.

The nurse should encourage the client to express emotions and memories rather than prescribe medications during initial grief reactions. Since individuals vary in their ability to tolerate emotions, the nurse must be sensitive to the client and the support network to gauge the extent of intervention the client is able tolerate. The client's cultural rituals regarding grief should be respected and encouraged. Spiritual counselors, such as priests or rabbis, can offer a ritualized pattern for the expression and resolution of grief.

Since the grieving process takes varying amounts of time, preset standards and reliance on the concept of well-delineated, consecutive grief stages will have to be adapted to each client. Some clients may have difficulty focusing on their grief, so the process will take longer. A client can appear to have returned to a normal state, while still feeling numb and anguished inside. The nurse must acknowledge the length of the grieving process and educate the family and community in respecting the amount of time necessary for a client's recovery.

---

gies. Assisting with mobilizing resources and providing normative data are also part of support.

The plan of care for a person with dysfunctional grieving focuses on the specific pathology of the client. Normal aspects of grief are also addressed.

Plans can also be directed toward the community. In community-focused planning, the nurse helps churches, synagogues, community centers, hospitals, and other organizations develop self-help groups for bereaved persons. Nurses also serve as facilitators for such groups.

■ ■ ■ ■ ■ IMPLEMENTATION

The first priority in planning care for a person with dysfunctional grief is to reduce the risk for violence toward self or others. The client's physical health may also be a major concern. The plan will include efforts to work toward resolving the grief through emotional, cognitive, and behavioral means. Chemical dependency presents a major barrier to the individual's goal attainment and must

be addressed. Dependence on anxiolytic medications is common. In many cases, such as the one presented in the Nursing Care Plan opposite, the approach can be growth-oriented rather than directed only to treatment of symptoms.

Bereavement care should ideally take place in the community before the client deteriorates to the extent that hospitalization is required.

Nursing Interventions

1. Assess any intent to harm self or others *to ensure safety and prevent violence.*

2. Promote a therapeutic alliance with the client *to encourage healthy expression of grief.*

3. Follow through on all obligations and care with consistency *to promote an orderly predictable environment for the client who is experiencing the chaos of grief.*

NURSING CARE PLAN ■ ■ ■ ■ ■ ■ ■   ■ ■ ■ ■ ■ ■

Mr. Smith and his wife had been married for 41 years when she died 18 months ago from bacterial endocarditis. Since his wife's death, Mr. Smith has become increasingly seclusive. He expresses extreme anger toward the physicians and nurses involved in his wife's care. He keeps his home exactly as it was when Mrs. Smith was alive. He has not disposed of any of her belongings and has renewed subscriptions to magazines that only she read. Both Mr. and Mrs. Smith drank heavily but denied alcoholism. They had no children, and their relationship was characterized by frequent verbal and occasional physical abuse. Mr. Smith continues to drink daily. He complains of heart problems and is angry with his physician who insists that Mr. Smith has only mild hypertension that should respond to dietary changes. Mr. Smith has begun keeping his curtains drawn and denies the need for interpersonal relationships.

DSM-IV Diagnoses

Axis I	Major Depression; Alcohol Abuse
Axis II	None known
Axis III	Hypertension
Axis IV	Severity: 6–extreme (death of spouse): Alcoholism
Axis V	GAF Current: 45 (after death of spouse) Past year: 40

Nursing Diagnosis: Dysfunctional grieving, chronic distorted, related to inability to appropriately express the full spectrum of feelings associated with his wife's death, as evidenced by reclusiveness, anger, and alcohol use.

Client Outcomes	Nursing Interventions	Evaluation
• Mr. Smith will engage in a therapeutic alliance with the nurse.	• Visit Mr. Smith's home at a regular time on the same day once each week for 30 minutes. *Constancy and dependability are essential in developing productive relationships.*	• Mr. Smith agreed to visits.
• Mr. Smith will cease intake of alcohol at least four hours before and during visits with nurse.	• Develop a contract with Mr. Smith in which he agrees to sobriety during visits. *Sobriety is essential to therapeutic relationships and personal growth.*	• Mr. Smith maintained sobriety during visits. • Mr. Smith entered and continued a 12-step or other program intended to promote sobriety.
• Mr. Smith will express angry, sad, and other feelings concerning his wife's death.	• Gradually present Mr. Smith with aspects of his grief experience that will help him uncover his sadness and ambivalence. *Feelings of sadness and ambivalence are threatening to Mr. Smith and should not be introduced too rapidly.* • Recognize the legitimacy of Mr. Smith's anger. Demonstrate acceptance and understanding of the ambivalence and other feelings such as sadness and confusion. *Anger is the means by which Mr. Smith may be expressing other feelings not yet in his awareness. Facilitating other feelings helps to better manage anger and promote resolution of grief.*	• Mr. Smith expressed sadness, confusion, ambivalence, and other feelings in addition to anger. • Mr. Smith accepted the validity of anger and feelings other than anger that may have been hidden behind the expression of anger and rage.
• Mr. Smith will discuss his hopes (fulfilled and unfulfilled) and his disappointments about his relationship with his wife.	• Assist Mr. Smith in reviewing his relationship with his wife and the hopes each one held, including those that were fulfilled and those that led to disappointments. *Although Mr. Smith's problems are attributed to his wife's death, they are also, to a great extent, attributable to his relationship with his wife and his difficulty coping with the loss of his wife.*	• Mr. Smith discussed his relationship with his wife in realistic terms (neither idealized nor all negative) and expressed both positive and negative feelings about their relationship.
• Mr. Smith will grieve in a functional manner for his wife, their relationship, and for himself.	• Facilitate Mr. Smith's linking together all his feelings and responses related to the relationship with his wife, to his life, and to his current dysfunctional behavior. *This is the full expression of grief.*	• Mr. Smith fully expressed his grief.

NURSING CARE PLAN ■ ■ ■ ■ ■ ■ ■ ■   ■ ■ ■ ■ ■ ■ ■

Nursing Diagnosis: Social isolation, related to seclusive behavior patterns secondary to unresolved grief, as evidenced by refusal to engage in interpersonal relationships.

Client Outcomes	Nursing Interventions	Evaluation
• Mr. Smith will agree to regular visits in his home with the nurse.	• Adhere to 30-minute time limit for visits; be prompt according to schedule. *Structure in care increases order, understanding, and predictability. It will also help Mr. Smith to develop cognitive coping strategies, such as making realistic plans for the future.*	• Mr. Smith tolerated visits and eventually remarked that he looked forward to them.
• Mr. Smith will participate in one social activity weekly. (Alcohol should not be served or available).	• Give Mr. Smith choices of time-limited social activities that are likely to be enjoyable and convenient for him. *Activities that are enjoyable and sociable are more likely to be repeated; too many choices are likely to be overwhelming; time limits will reduce anxiety.*	• Mr. Smith followed through by attending activities and expressed a favorable response.
• Mr. Smith will participate in the termination phase of the relationship by increasing his social activities and continuing in his recovery from alcoholism.	• Include Mr. Smith in plans for increasing his social activity as the relationship is terminated. Together, the nurse and Mr. Smith should write a schedule for termination that decreases the frequency of visits and ultimately ends the visits. *The therapeutic alliance progresses from collaboration between the nurse and client to the client achieving independence.*	• Mr. Smith participated in planning for termination, initiated additional social activities, and continued in his recovery.

4. Facilitate the expression of feelings related to the loss *to help the client understand and accept his or her grief responses.*

5. Introduce the possibility of other feelings related to the loss, such as anger, frustration, and despair *to help the client acknowledge feelings that may be part of the grief process in order to deal with them.*

6. Help the client understand the relationship between self and the lost object/person *to assist the client in moving beyond grief responses and in recognizing the meaning of the relationship to the lost object/person.*

7. Discuss meanings within the relationship such as hopes fulfilled, disappointments, and strengths and weaknesses *to view the content of the relationship in a holistic and realistic manner.*

8. Assess the client's degree of ambivalence toward the loss. *The client who continually blames self for the loss and cannot resolve guilt is prone to suicide and may require further grief counseling.*

9. Promote interactions with others *to keep the client from spending prolonged periods of time alone, and help the client return to a normal routine.*

10. Ensure that the client does not spend long periods of time alone, even after the initial grief period. *The client needs to be continually observed for signs of despair and hopelessness throughout the grief process because, as the client returns to a higher* *level of energy and activity, he or she may still be prone to suicide and may be more likely to act on suicidal ideations.*

Additional Treatment Modalities

An interdisciplinary approach consisting of nurse, psychiatrist, psychologist, social worker, occupational therapist, and other health care providers is not usually necessary, although community resources including clergy are an important part of care. Because of the frequency and vagueness of physical complaints, the most important discipline other than nursing is the client's general practitioner or other source of primary care.

■ ■ ■ ■ ■ ■ EVALUATION

The nurse evaluates the client's increasing ability to express feelings and to develop effective coping strategies such as increasing social interactions. It is important for the client to express the full spectrum of feelings that are 1) associated with the loss and 2) related to the relationship with the deceased. Expressing feelings only about the loss itself is not sufficient for successful progress in grief work. The nurse should remember that grief is a normal response to loss, and the feelings associated with grief are necessarily painful. The key to successful grief work depends on the individual's understanding of the relationship with the deceased. When that occurs, the client is able to continue the work of investing in new relationships.

CASE STUDY

Mr. and Mrs. Mason have a 26-year-old son, Jim, who has chronic undifferentiated schizophrenia. Jim lives at home most of the year, except when he is admitted to the state hospital two to three times a year. Jim has never worked, has no friends, is withdrawn most of the time, has violent episodes about once a month, and is noncompliant with medications. The Masons have tried different hospitals (they no longer have any insurance coverage for Jim), a variety of antipsychotic medications, different therapists, prayer, and "alternative therapies." Nothing has changed the course of the illness. Mr. Mason works long hours at an auto parts store, and Mrs. Mason stays home with Jim. Mr. and Mrs. Mason began seeing the clinical nurse specialist from the state hospital community outreach program. Their chief complaints as a couple and individually are overwhelming feelings of hopelessness and physical and mental exhaustion. The clinical nurse specialist diagnosed their problem as caregiver role strain, related to chronic sorrow, as evidenced by caregiver withdrawal from community life in order to care for their son with chronic schizophrenia. The nurse implemented a plan of care that includes 1) weekly couples counseling, 2) regular family support group in a community facility, 3) biweekly home visits by an outreach staff member to assist Jim with medication compliance.

Critical Thinking and Evaluation

1. Do you think Jim will experience significant improvement in his disorder? Why or why not?

2. Part of the care is directed to the parents. Why are they also receiving care instead of Jim alone, since he is the one who has mental illness?

3. Discuss potential success in relation to this plan. Are the Masons likely to achieve happiness as a result of receiving care? Why or why not?

4. Discuss each of the following feelings that family members sometimes experience regarding relatives with chronic mental illness: anger, sorrow, love, and despair.

Summary of Key Concepts

1. Grief encompasses all spheres of being. Symptoms of grief include physical, cognitive, behavioral, and affective manifestations.

2. Although grief is commonly presented in stages, it is more efficacious to conceptualize grief in terms of a dynamic process.

3. Grief may be classified as anticipatory, acute, dysfunctional, and chronic sorrow. Types of dysfunctional grief include absent or inhibited, distorted, converted, and chronic.

4. The potential for dysfunctional grief is decreased in situations such as a healthy family life, providing care for the person who is dying, community-oriented bereavement programs, and therapy provided for persons at risk.

5. Therapy for individuals experiencing dysfunctional grief includes facilitating expression of suppressed feelings, mobilizing cognitive and behavioral coping skills, dealing with unresolved aspects of the relationship, and encouraging reentry into socialization.

REFERENCES

Adams JP et al: Accumulated loss phenomenon among hospice caregivers *Am J Hospice and Palliative Care* 8(3):29–37, 1992.

Bowlby J: *Loss: sadness and depression,* vol 3, *Attachment and loss,* New York, 1980, Basic Books.

Burke ML et al: Current knowledge and research on chronic sorrow: a foundation for inquiry, *Death Studies* 16:231–245, 1992.

Burnell GM, Burnell AL: *Clinical management of bereavement: a handbook for healthcare professionals,* New York, 1989, Human Sciences Press.

Carse JB: *Death and existence,* New York, 1980, John Wiley & Sons.

Carter SL: Themes of grief, *Nurs Res* 38(6): 354–358, 1989.

Cowles KV, Rodgers BL: The concept of grief: a foundation for nursing research and practice, *Res in Nurs and Health* 14(2): 119–127, 1991.

Engel G: Grief and grieving, *Am J Nurs* 64:93–98, 1964.

Freud S: Mourning and melancholia. In Strachey J, editor: *The standard edition of the complete psychological works of Sigmund Freud,* vol 14, London, 1917, Hogarth Press.

Gass KA, Chang AS: Appraisals of bereavement, coping, resources, and psychosocial health dysfunction in widows and widowers, *Nurs Res* 38(1):31–36, 1989.

Gibbons MB: A child dies, a child survives: the impact of sibling loss, *J Pediatr Health Care* 6(2):65–72, 1992.

Goodman M et al: Cultural differences among elderly women in coping with the death of an adult child, *J Geront* 46(6):321–329, 1991.

Kubler-Ross E: *On death and dying,* New York, 1969, Macmillan.

Levy LH: Anticipatory grief: its measurement and proposed reconceptualization, *Hosp J* 7(4):1–28, 1991.

Lindemann E: Symptomatology and management of acute grief, *Am J Psychiatry* 101:141–148, 1944.

McFarland GK, Gerety EK: Grieving. In Kim MJ et al, editors: *Pocket guide to nursing diagnoses,* ed 5, St. Louis, 1993, Mosby.

Nuss WS, Zubenko GS: Correlates of persistent depressive symptoms in widows, *Am J Psychiatry* 149(3):346–351, 1992.

Parkes CM: *Bereavement: studies of grief in adult life,* ed 2, Madison, Conn., 1987, International Universities Press.

Rando TA: *Grieving,* Lexington, Mass., 1988, Lexington Books.

Schiff HS: *The bereaved parent,* New York, 1977, Crown Publishers.

Shneidman ES: *Deaths of man,* New York, 1973, Quadrangle/The New York Times Book Company.

Shneidman ES: *Voices of death,* New York, 1980, Harper & Row.

Silverman PR, Worden JW: Children's reactions in the early months after the death of a parent, *Am J Orthopsychiatr* 62(1): 93–104, 1992.

Wolfelt AD: Toward an understanding of complicated grief: a comprehensive overview, *Am J Hosp and Palliative Care* 8(2):28–30, 1991.

CHAPTER 28

Persons with AIDS

Gwen van Servellen

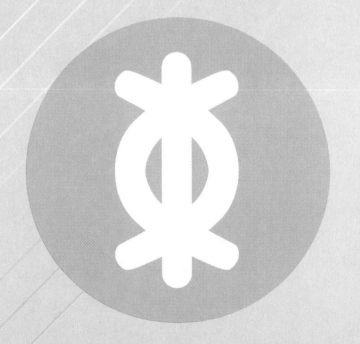

Antiretroviral therapy The use of drugs, such as AZT, ddI, and ddC. These drugs, often administered to clients via drug trials, treat the major opportunistic diseases associated with AIDS. Treatment with antiretroviral therapy can significantly impact the progression of AIDS by preventing opportunistic infections.

AIDS Dementia Complex (ADC) A progressive neurological syndrome caused by a subacute chronic HIV encephalitis. Cognitive impairment indicative of damage to the central nervous system is evidenced in these clients.

CD$_4$ count The CD$_4$ lymphocyte count (T4 cell count) is the most commonly used marker to determine HIV progression. HIV attacks CD$_4$ cells that help fight infections.

Opportunistic diseases Diseases that commonly appear in AIDS clients, especially when their T-cell count drops; they include cytomegalovirus mycobacterium and Kaposi's sarcoma.

- Discuss the threat of HIV disease as a public health problem.

- Examine the risk of psychiatric and psychologic morbidity for those coping with HIV disease.

- Distinguish between adjustment disorders and AXIS I mood disorders in people with HIV disease, using the criteria of severity of symptoms, treatment, and prognosis.

- Examine behavioral characteristics of those persons placing themselves at high risk for the acquisition of HIV.

- Discuss why persons practicing high-risk behaviors may have difficulty changing these behaviors.

- Apply the nursing process for persons with AIDS.

This chapter will identify and discuss the skills and knowledge needed to provide care to clients experiencing the neuropsychiatric and psychosocial aspects of human immunodeficiency virus (HIV) and acquired immunodeficiency syndrome (AIDS). To understand the consequences of HIV disease on the mental and emotional functioning of clients and their families, it is important to first define HIV disease.

HIV disease has been identified by the U.S. Department of Health and Human Services as the foremost public health problem in the nation. AIDS, the advanced stage of illness in HIV disease, is fatal. HIV disease is characterized by a defect in the natural immunity against disease, especially against certain opportunistic infections and AIDS-related cancers, e.g., Kaposi's sarcoma (KS) or non-Hodgkin's lymphoma. While individuals in the symptomatic state are identifiable by a specific set of signs and symptoms, those who are infected but asymptomatic may go undiagnosed for long periods of time. Unfortunately, the infected asymptomatic individuals are capable of transmitting the disease to others, even if they remain asymptomatic for a long time. Due to this fact, HIV disease is unquestionably a serious public health threat.

Both clinical and research evidence indicate that HIV infects the brain and results in central nervous system impairment in some individuals. In addition to the troublesome neuropsychologic and neuropsychiatric consequences of HIV, many more if not all individuals with asymptomatic HIV and AIDS, as well as those who perceive themselves at high risk for infection, and their families and significant others experience a wide range of psychosocial needs. All of them need help in varying degrees in order to cope with psychologic symptoms that are a result of the AIDS epidemic. While this includes care and counsel to those infected, it also includes information and counseling services to those who need to change high-risk behaviors or to regain or maintain low-risk activities. Since sexual transmission and infection through needle exchange in drug abuse are the primary modes of transmission, efforts to change behaviors effectively are exceedingly complex. They involve curbing behaviors that are not easily discussed or readily changed. Since African-Americans and Hispanics are disproportionately represented in the AIDS community, focus on culture-specific needs of these groups related to the prevention and treatment of HIV is needed.

Feelings of anxiety and depression in persons with AIDS (PWAs) are of concern to clinicians caring for individuals with HIV disease for a variety of reasons. First, these conditions are negative-affective states reflective of subjective distress. In turn, this subjective distress can significantly alter clients' quality of life in the short and long term. And these conditions, when present as enduring clinical syndromes, present with behavioral, somatic, and cognitive features (in addition to affective symptoms) that impact clients' health status and ability to follow medical treatment protocol. These include negative affect, irritability, decreased energy and lethargy, altered performance, restlessness and/or interrupted sleep, feelings of helplessness, punitive and self-accusatory evaluations, and persistent fear and worry. These conditions further tax clients' resources and affect their quality of life. Perhaps most serious is the risk of suicide. While suicide in this population is understandable, suicides among AIDS clients are believed preventable risks and should be addressed. Life-threatening illnesses increase the incidence of depression and suicide (see Understanding and Applying Research at right). Although some debate exists regarding exact figures, higher rates of depression and suicide risk appear to be associated with HIV infection (Marzuk et al, 1988). In light of available and appropriate pharmacologic therapy and concomitant counseling and/or social support, relief from depression is possible (Buck and Duffy, 1993; Rabkin et al, 1994).

In HIV as in other life-threatening illness, for example, advanced cancer, somatic symptomatic health status carries both primary and secondary implications for quality of life and functional performance. Symptoms have a di-

Understanding and Applying RESEARCH

Rabkin JG et al: Suicidality in AIDS long-term survivors: what is the evidence? *AIDS Care* 5(4):401–411, 1993.

Fifty-three homosexual men who were enrolled as clients at the Gay Men's Health Crisis Center in New York City and had an AIDS-defining opportunistic infection at least three years prior were surveyed with a 25-page semi-structured interview. A structured clinical interview based on DSM-III-R criteria, as well as the Karnofsky Performance Status rating scale, the Brief Symptom Inventory, Beck Hopelessness scales, Wortman Social Support scale, and Rand Corporation Physical Abilities Battery was also conducted. The purpose of the study was to investigate the prevalence of suicidal ideation and attempts, thoughts about living and dying, and the maintenance of hope in a sample of long-term AIDS survivors.

The results of this study indicate that there are low rates of current syndromal mood disorders (6%) or psychiatric distress. While thoughts about death and wishes to die were reported by a significant portion of the men, they were thought to be context-specific, occurring almost exclusively during serious illness and often accompanied by severe pain or at times of bereavement. Only 2 men out of 53 had made a suicide attempt after being diagnosed with AIDS, and both had a history of prior (pre-AIDS) suicide attempts.

While anger is a prominent affect, hopelessness is not, despite the experience of the protracted biologic and psychologic stress associated with AIDS. Overall, the researchers found a high level of positive psychologic health independent of HIV illness, stage, or degree of illness-induced physical limitations. Nurses can use this information to be more aware of the situations and stages that promote risk of suicide.

rect effect on quality of life but also an indirect effect through the process of secondary appraisal. These symptoms in and of themselves can be perceived as threatening. Likewise, their consequences, e.g., deficits in role performance, functional decline, and altered social activities, are also felt to be as threatening. Adaptation at this stage of HIV disease requires realignment of goal-related activities in order to achieve a positive emotional state. When viewed as outside the individual's control, this decline leads to anxiety. Symptoms can also be perceived as stable (recurrent) and global (affecting many outcomes important to the individual). To the extent that one or more symptoms are perceived as uncontrollable, stable, and global, their presence may produce a depressed mood state which, if intractable and/or continues untreated over time, may develop into clinical depression.

EPIDEMIOLOGY OF HIV/AIDS

The Centers for Disease Control (CDC) composes a quarterly HIV/AIDS Surveillance Report. This report identifies the numbers of full-blown AIDS cases in the U.S. reported to the CDC, but it does not reflect the total number of infected individuals.

As of December 31, 1993, the cumulative number of AIDS cases reported to the CDC was 361,164 (CDC, 1994). Adult and adolescent cases (these groups are combined) totaled 355,935; 311,578 cases occurred in males, and 44,357 occurred in females. During this same period, 5228 cases were reported in children (youth under age 13 at the time of diagnosis). The total number of deaths caused by AIDS was 220,736, which included 217,917 adults and adolescents and 2819 children. Of these cases, the highest number was reported in the Caucasian population (181,157). AIDS was second most prevalent among African-Americans (114,868). The two reported primary means of exposure were men having sex with men (193,152 cases) and injecting drug use (87,259 cases). Among children (under 13 years) the majority were exposed by a mother with or at risk for HIV infection (4637 of the 5228 cases).

The five states leading in number of AIDS cases among residents during this period (through December 31, 1993) were as follows:

- New York: 68,454
- California: 65,753
- Florida: 35,378
- Texas: 24,904
- New Jersey: 20,171

The five leading metropolitan statistical areas reporting the highest number of AIDS cases among residents were:

- New York City: 58,815
- Los Angeles: 22,798
- San Francisco: 18,142
- Miami: 10,919
- Washington, D.C.: 10,168

In conclusion, the data on cumulative AIDS cases reported to the CDC reveal that AIDS occurs in children, adolescents, and adults. Males and females are disproportionately represented, with more cases reported in males. Caucasians and African-Americans have reported the most cases in the U.S. to date. The risk behaviors reported most frequently in cases to date (among adults and adolescents) are IV drug use and men having sex with men.

While these generalizations are valid and informative, they have limitations. They do not reveal the characteristics of those currently infected with HIV disease; they merely reveal cases of full-blown AIDS. Because of this limitation, it is difficult to discern future trends. Prevalency rates, specifically with respect to infection rates, reveal more of the picture. Two groups of particular concern to researchers and clinicians are adolescents and women.

Recent research reveals that women and men differ in mortality and morbidity. More specifically, these differences include the following:

1. Decreased survival among women with AIDS. It is unknown whether differences in survival are a result of later diagnosis, poor access to care, increased susceptibility to HIV immunosuppression, or a combination.

2. There are gender-related differences; one is the incidence and severity of cancer, particularly cervical neoplasia among women. Also, there is some evidence to suggest that women are generally more immunologically reactive than men, and that gender-specific hormones may influence susceptibility and course of symptomatology in these women.

3. The number of psychosocial stressors present in women with AIDS are thought to be greater and could prove to inhibit access to care and overall management of symptomatology. Lower socioeconomic status (a largely unemployed, government-assisted group), preexisting feelings of powerlessness, and child care demands place these women in exceedingly compromising situations. Consideration for the social and psychologic state of these women is paramount in helping them manage their symptomatology and experience relief from emotional distress. The majority of these women are single parents. They have many concerns about the care and welfare of their children within the context of their own illness, particularly when they are the sole provider and caretaker.

The increasing numbers of women with HIV suggest a greater risk for incidences of AIDS-related malignancies. While 40% of all clients with AIDS have one or more malignancies, the incidence of AIDS-related cancers is expected to increase. The result of this trend further complicates the lives of persons with HIV. Cancers resulting from HIV serve as an immediate cause of death, but also as a source of great morbidity (Levine, 1993).

ETIOLOGY OF EMOTIONAL DISTRESS IN HIV DISEASE

In establishing the basis for emotional distress in HIV disease it is important to understand various etiologic departures. Psychoneurologic and psychosocial theories will be discussed as they explain the etiology of emotional distress in HIV disease. If clients exhibit major mental illnesses such as schizophrenia, bipolar disorder, and borderline personality disorder, these conditions will not be addressed. The focus is on mood and cognitive disorders relating to HIV diagnosis. The primary DSM-IV diagnoses for review are adjustment disorders with anxiety, depression, and/or disturbance of conduct.

Neuropsychiatric Factors

Soon after the discovery of AIDS, nurses and physicians were puzzled not only by the frequency of cognitive impairment among hospitalized clients, but also by the severity of the cases.

The profound dementia noted in some AIDS clients seemed disproportionate to the clinical condition, laboratory values, and gross neuropathologic findings present in these clients (Perry and Markowitz, 1986). To confound this discovery even more, the histories of many of these clients revealed that psychologic and cognitive problems predated signs of immune deficiency. It is now known that HIV has a direct effect on the central nervous system and causes a subacute encephalopathy. Cortical atrophy and ventricular dilatation have been shown on CT scan, indicating possible permanent and significant damage to the central nervous system (Perry and Jacobsen, 1986).

With this knowledge of histopathology, accurate diagnosis of cognitive and affective changes in PWAs can be made. Changes in mood could be evidence of exogenous depression or represent signs of AIDS-related dementia. Even with organically based changes, the signs and symptoms can be subtle, and laboratory findings may not immediately point to irregularities. The insidious emotional problems tend to mimic functional disorders. And initially, the neurologic examination, laboratory values, electroencephalogram, cerebrospinal fluid, and computerized axial tomography (CT scan) of the brain, may appear normal. Additionally confusing is that many of these high-risk and sometimes socially impaired individuals have psychosocial stresses that can explain the emotional distress they exhibit. Differential diagnosis is aided by seropositivity, the absence of a premorbid or family history of psychiatric illness, positive signs on neuropsychologic testing, and signs of organicity (e.g., imbalance, tremor, avoidance of complex tasks, and sensitivity to drugs and alcohol). While AIDS dementias vary, they can generally be categorized into two primary types: a dementia chiefly characterized by moderate signs of depression, and a more acute psychotic presentation. The first of these is evidenced in apathy, withdrawal, fatigue, hypersomnia, weight loss, anorexia, psychomotor retardation, and subtle cognitive deficits. The acute psychotic presentation can include delusions, hallucinations, psychomotor agitation, mania with grandiosity, and profound cognitive impairment.

When clients' impairment is determined to be organically based, the influence of psychosocial phenomena may be present, but is not the initial target for intervention. Rather, clients with AIDS-related dementia are treated like clients with other organically based dementias.

In summary, AIDS clearly carries the potential for neuropsychiatric complications and is believed to act directly on the central nervous system. This has been labeled the **AIDS Dementia Complex (ADC),** and includes behavioral symptoms such as organic psychosis, apathy, social withdrawal, dysphoric mood, and regressed behavior. Cognitive changes include forgetfulness, loss of concentration, confusion, slowness of thought, and motor deficits that may include loss of balance, leg weakness, and deterioration of handwriting. It is confounding that many of these clients are also abusing alcohol and/or cocaine and other drugs, and are frequently undergoing severe stress. There are multiple potential reasons for much of this symptomatology. Cocaine psychosis may closely resemble and mask psychosis caused by HIV (Shaffer and Costikyan, 1988).

Psychosocial Factors

With HIV disease there is a spectrum of disorders in which psychosocial, particularly stress-related disorders, are important. Essentially, four categories of individuals may need intervention.

First, there are *those who believe they are at risk for HIV but have not gone for testing.* These individuals are "the worried well," some of whom experience ongoing stress, assuming they are indeed seropositive. They tend to exaggerate their risk, rather than deny it. They may display low self-esteem, anxiety, uncertainty, and at times irrationality. They may appear somewhat histrionic and indecisive. They may offer clues to their concern, indicating a desire for help. Still, their fear of being seropositive may prevent them from taking care of themselves and confronting their irrationally based concerns.

The second category of individuals needing attention are *those who are asymptomatic but are HIV+.* Although one tends to think of HIV as an acute fatal illness, most clients are either asymptomatic or symptomatic, but don't meet the criteria for full-blown AIDS. Even those who have been symptomatic may remain highly functional between symptomatic episodes. After a prolonged incubation period of months or years, most clients will go on to develop AIDS-related symptoms and AIDS. Of primary concern to the individuals is the uncertainty that is with them on a day-to-day basis.

The third category of individuals are *those who are symptomatic but have not yet developed an AIDS-defining condition.* Early in the epidemic, these clients were diagnosed with ARC (AIDS-Related Complex). Symptomatic individuals are not acutely ill but tend to suffer from various AIDS-related conditions, e.g., fatigue, fever, night sweats, and nausea.

In studies of symptomatic versus asymptomatic HIV disease, persons with symptoms were reported to exhibit more distress. It is this group that seems to wait in dread of a drop in their **CD$_4$ count,** or a diagnosable malignancy that would usher in fears of impending demise. The CD$_4$ lymphocyte count (T4 cell count) is the most commonly used marker to determine HIV progression. HIV attacks CD$_4$ cells that help fight infection. The increased dependency in these individuals has been attributed to a "state" phenomenon and not a characterologic condition. Many of these clients exhibiting dependency, helplessness, and anxiety would not display these characteristics if not for their HIV disease.

The final category of individuals suffering directly from HIV disease is *clients with full-blown AIDS.* The clinical course of many AIDS-related conditions may be quite varied. Kaposi's sarcoma, a malignant neoplastic vascular proliferation in immunocompromised AIDS clients, for example, may present as a slowly progressive disease over many years, or a rapidly fulminant progression over weeks to months. It is estimated that in the absence of other conditions, the median survival is approximately 31 months, while the presence of an opportunistic infection, for example, cytomegalovirus (CMV), ushers in a median survival of only 7 months (Levine, 1993). Available data on the client's disease course, immune status (current CD$_4$ count), and general health status can offer a clearer prognosis for clients. The depression these clients experience may not be simply a normal grief response about having a fatal illness. For some individuals, a pathologic process characterized by alienation, irrational guilt, diminished self-esteem, and pronounced suicidal ideation may be present.

The data about suicidal ideation and numbers of suicide attempts in PWAs has been limited. Studies suggest that suicide is a common occurrence in AIDS clients and that suicidal ideation is high (Brown and Rundell 1989; Frierson and Lippmann, 1988; Glass, 1988; Kiezer et al, 1988; Marzuk et al, 1988; Plott et al, 1989). Increasing evidence suggests that declining physical health status may increase suicide risk. With declining physical health status, hopelessness ensues. Hopelessness is seen as an important risk factor for both suicidal ideation and suicide.

CLINICAL DESCRIPTION

The primary DSM-IV diagnostic condition addressed here is adjustment disorder. Adjustment disorders are coded according to the subtype that best characterizes the predominant symptoms. Diagnoses include:

Adjustment Disorder
with depressed mood
with anxiety
with anxiety and depressed mood
with disturbance of conduct
with disturbance of emotions and conduct

unspecified, referring to maladaptive reactions to psychosocial stressors that are not classifiable as one of the specific subtypes listed above

Note that while PWAs may also display other psychiatric disorders (for example, a major depressive episode and/or psychoactive substance abuse), adjustment disorders with anxious and/or depressed mood are more commonly diagnosed in these clients, especially in outpatient clients. This diagnosis pertains to their reaction to having a fatal illness. Other disorders generally refer to conditions that predated **seroconversion.** AIDS clients have reported previous psychiatric histories. The exact rate of previous psychiatric illness and/or substance abuse in HIV-infected individuals is not known, but it is believed to be higher than for some community samples.

Two additional diagnostic categories are important in assessing these clients: bereavement reaction and organic manifestations related to HIV disease. While diagnostic assessments may vary, substance abuse, bereavement reactions, and organicity are frequently seen as comorbid conditions in these clients whose Axis I diagnosis is either major depressive episode or adjustment disorder with mixed emotional features. Specific HIV-related problems observed on psychiatric hospital admissions are anxiety and depression over deteriorating physical health status, social rejection related to HIV seropositive status, increased drug use as a response to HIV seropositivity, shame/guilt concerning stigmatized sexual practices, guilt or fear over having put others at risk (including fear of retribution), and homicidal ideation toward the presumed party who infected the client.

PROGNOSIS

The prognosis for resolution of anxiety and depression in PWAs is not well-documented. Scientists who study the emotional effects of this disease attempt to isolate crisis points where psychosocial stressors or other precipitants can lead to depression, anxiety, and other psychiatric problems.

Since HIV is a chronic stressful life event depicted by a series of physical, functional, and psychosocial losses, anxiety and depression are likely to occur intermittently and relate to the psychologic pain accompanying different phases of the disease process. Some experiences may be severe enough to precipitate a dysphoric mood and/or a crisis (Duffy, 1994). While the concept of "crisis points" seems to be applicable to this population, several important points should be made.

The experience of AIDS as a crisis is highly individualized. Some clients struggle with the disease, and this struggle is evident. Other clients with HIV cope well and even seem to take a new lease on life. Not everyone will experience a confirmed diagnosis of seropositive status as a crisis. Thus, caution should be used in predicting emotional distress, the crisis points that will occur, and any outcomes of the process of adapting to HIV disease.

■ ASSESSMENT

The psychosocial assessment of a PWA with a medical diagnosis of adjustment disorder, anxiety, and/or depression requires a thorough appraisal of primary and secondary nursing diagnoses. In PWAs the emotional and behavioral symptoms that occur develop in response to the stress of having, or being diagnosed with, a general medical condition.

The clinical assessment that enables nurses to derive pertinent nursing diagnoses must be all-inclusive. Identifying data, current symptoms, and history of the present problem (anxiety, depression, and/or conduct) must all be addressed. Specific data about sleep patterns, appetite, and change in weight are important in assessing severity of mood disturbance. Details about previous psychiatric contacts (both outpatient and hospitalizations), including precipitating events, will establish any preexisting psychiatric illnesses that may place the client at risk for future episodes.

Data about the client's family unit and current social network is extremely relevant. A description of the family unit of origin, including the family's history of traumatic events, migration, and cultural factors, will help to sensitize providers to the contextual nature of the PWAs' responses to their illness. This same data about current relationships is also critical because they influence ways in which clients cope with AIDS and the availability of coping resources.

Social history information is of general importance, but there is certain data for PWAs that holds special significance. Current social activities, history of (and current) sexual practices, and history of significant relationships are important. In many cases, PWAs are not only living with the personal threat of HIV, but they are also dealing with the possibility of placing others at risk. A diagnosis of HIV positivity brings with it an array of responsibilities to those these clients have been intimate with. Finally, in assessing emotional distress in PWAs, a thorough mental status exam should be conducted as part of the assessment process, because of the prevalence of neuropsychiatric complications.

A final area of assessment is the client's previous and current suicidal or homicidal tendencies, and tendency for violent behavior. As previously noted, severe medical problems place people at risk for suicide. Anger and rage may be manifested by PWAs through violent behaviors, homicidal threats or gestures directed at those believed to be the source of infection, and occasionally toward society at large. PWAs with disturbances of conduct may violate the rights of others, social norms, or even commit minor infractions of the law.

■ ■ NURSING DIAGNOSIS

Nursing diagnoses are formulated from the data gathered by the nurse during the assessment phase of the nursing process. The accuracy of nursing diagnoses relies on the careful, comprehensive assessment of the client's history, presenting symptoms, behavior, and responses to actual and potential life stressors. The reliability of all informants, whether the sources are clients themselves, their significant others, and/or previous data from charts during this phase, is extremely important. Multiple sources of data can confirm information and ensure appropriate diagnoses.

NANDA Diagnoses for Persons with AIDS

Risk for violence: self-directed or directed at others
Ineffective individual coping
Hopelessness
Powerlessness

CASE ● STUDY

Rocio is a 29-year-old Hispanic woman married to José who is reported to be bisexual and HIV+. In February of this year, Rocio was diagnosed HIV+ with symptomatic HIV disease. She is positive for AIDS-related fatigue, fevers, nausea, diarrhea, dyspnea, and wasting syndrome. A thorough gynecologic examination reveals that Rocio is in the early stages of cervical dysplasia. The nurse practitioner in the women's clinic asked to have her evaluated by the psychiatric team. She is five months pregnant and has three additional children under age five. Rocio and José are illegal aliens who have resided in the United States for one and one-half years. Their primary language is Spanish. When questioned about her pregnancy and her personal health, Rocio sobbed uncontrollably. She explained that she is really worried about her children and what will happen to them. She has not told any friends or family that she is HIV+, because she is ashamed and worried that they would not be kind to her children if they knew her diagnosis.

Critical Thinking and Assessment

1. What are the client's most immediate problems or needs related to her HIV diagnosis?

2. What assessment data reflect the client's sensitivity to her diagnosis?

3. Why might the client be reluctant to seek the social support she needs?

4. What stressors could contribute to the anxiety and depression she is exhibiting?

Self-esteem disturbance
Social isolation
Anxiety
Fear
Noncompliance
Ineffective denial
Defensive coping

■ ■ ■ OUTCOME IDENTIFICATION

Outcome criteria are derived from the nursing diagnoses and are the expected client responses to be achieved.

Outcome Identification for Persons with HIV/AIDS

Client will:

1. Verbalize absence of suicidal ideation and plans.
2. State reduced frequency/intensity of feelings of hopelessness and powerlessness.

COLLABORATIVE DIAGNOSES

DSM-IV Diagnoses*	NANDA Diagnoses**
Adjustment Disorder With Depressed Mood	Risk for violence: self-directed or directed at others
	Ineffective individual coping
	Hopelessness
	Powerlessness
	Self-esteem disturbance
	Social isolation
With Anxiety	Ineffective individual coping
	Anxiety
	Fear
With Mixed Anxiety and Depressed Mood	Ineffective individual coping
With Disturbance of Conduct	Risk for violence: self-directed or directed at others
	Ineffective individual coping
	Noncompliance
	Ineffective denial
	Defensive coping

DSM-IV diagnoses of With Mixed Disturbance of Emotions and Conduct, and Unspecified, are not addressed here, given the overlap with the previous diagnostic subtypes.

*Reprinted with permission from *Diagnostic and statistical manual of mental disorders,* ed 4, Washington, D.C., 1994, American Psychiatric Association.

**Reprinted with permission from *NANDA nursing diagnoses: definitions and classifications, 1995–1996,* Philadelphia, 1994, North American Nursing Diagnosis Association.

---

3. Engage in a therapeutic alliance with staff to evaluate coping options.
4. Initiate social interactions with others with HIV/AIDS (both individually and in groups) to gain information and support about coping effectively with HIV/AIDS.
5. Identify barriers or problems that may precipitate exacerbation of the experience of anxiety and/or depression (for example, perception of inadequate social support or perception of powerlessness over physical symptoms).
6. Verbalize clear, goal-directed, short-term plans that are achievable and problem-solution focused.

■ ■ ■ ■ PLANNING

The nurse's awareness of the complexities of living with HIV disease is extremely critical in deriving an appropriate plan of care for the client and the client's family.

For clients who are diagnosed with adjustment disorders, the nurse considers a plan of action that will promote the following: prevent violence toward self; help clients address concerns in a coherent, goal-directed, problem-solving manner; increase social networking that will provide needed information and comfort; monitor adverse effects of stressors on clients' current level of adaptation; and use staff in an effective therapeutic alliance when social supports diminish or cannot provide the technical expertise the client requires.

■ ■ ■ ■ IMPLEMENTATION

The challenges of working and intervening with PWAs are considerable and multiple. Families and caregivers also are greatly affected and often devastated by both the client's diagnosis and the functional and neuropsychiatric responses to the disease. Therefore, it is important that families and significant others are considered and included in the interventions when appropriate and with the consent of the client.

For example, clients whose significant others are encouraged to engage in problem-solving coping methods (versus emotion-focused coping) may be more helpful to clients who are trying to minimize the emotional burden of their disease. Significant others need to be taught about the disease, its course, and what can be expected at various crisis points. Support groups for caregivers of PWAs are available and appreciated by significant others dealing with issues of bereavement, fear of contagion, and the stress of care-giving. Support networks of a less formal design also exist to provide assistance for PWAs and their loved ones, through newsletters and drop-in centers.

AIDS clients have numerous symptoms; consequently, these clients require multiple interventions addressing various aspects of their spiritual, psychosocial, and physical well-being. The interventions discussed here are largely in the psychosocial domain and they are directed toward altering maladaptive individual coping and treat-

NURSING CARE PLAN

Steve, a 32-year-old Caucasian homosexual male, formerly a travel agent, has been retired for two years due to complications from AIDS. He has a history of depression since his early twenties for which he received outpatient counseling. He sees his physician regularly; currently he has esophageal candidiasis and wasting syndrome. He came to this clinic appointment expressing a great deal of hopelessness about his future. He stated that he didn't want to live anymore and that he was tired of fighting AIDS. When asked if he had a suicide plan, he stated he could make it quick and fatal, e.g., jumping out a window of a 15-story building.

Nursing Diagnosis: Powerlessness, related to responses to course of HIV disease and symptoms, as evidenced by verbalization of suicidal thoughts and plans, inability to forecast a positive future, verbalization of powerlessness as a result of physical decline and decreased functioning.

Client Outcomes	*Nursing Intervention*	*Evaluation*
• Steve will verbalize absence of suicidal ideation and plans.	• Identify with Steve goals and aims relating to his life tasks, despite prognosis. Contract with Steve to avoid acting out with suicidal gestures or attempts *to facilitate the client's adaptive coping responses and decrease feelings of loss of control; to help support Steve's goal.*	• Steve progressively states optimism about achieving goals within his anticipated life span.
• Steve will verbalize increased feelings of personal competence and self-efficacy in relation to managing his symptoms.	• Identify, with Steve, options he has in controlling his emotional and physical distress (e.g., stress management strategies and ways to cope with fatigue and diarrhea) *to counteract feelings of helplessness which, if not abated, result in hopelessness.*	• Steve identifies and begins to implement new strategies for coping with his symptoms. He verbalizes feelings of competence, as identified in main outcome.
• Steve will develop a therapeutic alliance with staff.	• Engage Steve in an active problem-solving approach addressing each stressor and discussing appropriate coping options/strategies *to evaluate Steve's coping options/methods.*	• Steve regards the nurse as a facilitator and supportive resource. Initiates discussion of stressors and options.
• Steve will initiate social interactions with others with HIV to gain information and support.	• Offer referrals to Steve regarding support groups and particularly voluntary home care services to PWAs *to help Steve gain information and support.*	• Steve attends support group of his choice or identifies at least one other person with AIDS that he can talk to on a weekly basis.
• Steve will identify barriers or problems associated with exacerbation of his anxiety/depression.	• Assist Steve to review what precipitating events and/or thoughts increase his anxiety/depression *to avoid such events, when possible, through increased awareness.*	• Steve expressed awareness of recurring stressors that worsen his anxiety and depression.
• Steve will verbalize goal-directed plans that are both achievable and problem-solution focused.	• Assist Steve in formulating goals that are realistic and achievable. These should be directed toward improving quality of life, and reducing stressors in day-to-day living *to decrease frustration and increase success through goal attainment.*	• Steve articulates 2–3 short-term goals he can realistically commit to with respect to his present condition.

ing impaired social interactions. Many nursing interventions for symptoms of HIV disease parallel interventions used with symptoms associated with other illnesses, particularly life-threatening cancers. People with HIV, however, experience other complications, for example, dealing with stigma, estrangement from their family of origin, and inadequate medical intervention. These factors are related to emotional distress and negatively impact treatment. Successful coping with symptoms is a priority in maintaining these clients' quality of life.

The primary category of intervention in the psychosocial domain is facilitating adaptive coping to the multiple stressors the client will confront. Interventions for effective or adaptive coping to offer clients hope, increase self-worth, and reduce anxiety and feelings of powerlessness are the following:

- maintain or improve their quality of life
- control or contain their feelings of fear, anxiety, grief, guilt, depression, and helplessness
- maintain or enhance a sense of self-worth and positive self-esteem
- avert a state of hopelessness and powerlessness
- satisfactorily adapt their relationships as they are confronted with various stages of dependency on others
- maintain physical functioning within capacity

Along these lines nurses can also intervene to help clients cope adaptively to their phase of illness.

In terms of maintaining or improving clients' quality of life, nurses can intervene to alter the physical discomfort and psychosocial isolation clients experience. They can teach clients to handle pain and fatigue caused by their illness and/or treatment. In doing this, they are also helping the client to exert control and minimize feelings of helplessness.

Social support networks are important to the AIDS client. Without them, social isolation and loneliness can occur. Also, disengagement is a normal process in adjusting to physical decline. The nurse needs to help the client preserve those relationships with friends and family who are capable of meeting the client's dependency needs. Loss of role functioning is usually very painful to a client but even more so when supportive relationships do not exist for the client.

Containing feelings of anxiety, helplessness, grief, guilt, depression, and fear is also important to maintaining the client's quality of life. Helping the client become informed about the illness and treatment will lessen the anxiety many clients experience because it relieves stress associated with uncertainty surrounding the disease. However, the nurse needs to consider that some clients are not comforted by instruction they are receiving because they do not understand the information and need further clarification.

Supporting clients when they are confronting the multiple losses concomitant with their disease is helpful in treating clients' feelings of grief and depression. These losses include deterioration of physical abilities and functions; and loss of roles, income, and social relationships. Loss of dignity related to declining health may also occur. The client's distress may be reduced if nurses anticipate losses, prepare clients for coping and supplement clients' resources by providing them with knowledge of financial and medical assistance.

Helping the client maintain or enhance a sense of self-worth and avert a state of powerlessness and hopelessness in the face of this devastating disease requires thoughtful consideration about the ways clients are affected by their disease. Sometimes the nurse will teach the client how to respond to the curiosity of others. Hiding one's illness and minimizing its effects can be adaptive because it helps clients live as normally as possible despite their symptoms and effects of treatment.

Assisting the client in preserving relationships requires both direct and indirect intervention. Nurses can help clients understand reasons for reactions of family and friends. Less directly, they can assist these informal caregivers by teaching them how to respond to the client's illness and treatment. AIDS caregivers usually are concerned about contagion of the disease. Providing factual information to these caregivers may decrease any tendency of these supportive others to withdraw due to fear of getting AIDS themselves. In cases where clients are sexually active with partners, nurses need to monitor, teach, and support them in adhering to safe sexual practices. The role of the nurse in dealing with persons with AIDS in the community is summarized in the Nursing Care in the Community box on page 663.

A final important category of intervention is related to treatment of acute and subacute syndromes associated with cognitive impairment. The AIDS Dementia Complex (ADC) is a syndrome that includes cognitive, motor, and behavioral manifestations. Initial symptoms are usually memory impairment and concentration difficulties. These symptoms can be overlooked and are frequently confused with symptoms associated with depression. However, clients may complain of forgetfulness, "slowed thinking," and difficulty concentrating when engaged in conversations, watching TV programs, or reading. In some cases, poor balance and coordination occur early on. As this syndrome progresses, with no chance of reversal, clients may become dependent on others for completion of activities of daily living. Clients' observation of declining functioning frequently causes emotional distress and social isolation. Early signs of inability to concentrate and lapses in short-term memory are within the client's awareness although they may not always be described by the client.

Many clients and their caregivers fear the development of dementia. They may have observed friends who were exceedingly compromised by ADC in all areas—cognitive, motor, and behavior. Additionally, AIDS dementia is not easily identified, and symptoms can wax and wane. This fact can cause a great deal of uncertainty and anxiety about one's diagnosis and evidence of decline. For this reason, early thorough assessment and teaching the client and caregivers about signs and symptoms are extremely important interventions leading to the client's ability to cope adaptively and avert severe states of helplessness and hopelessness.

Researchers have been hopeful that some of the antiretroviral therapies, e.g., AZT, ddI, and ddC, may help AIDS clients with ADC to regain some of their lost facul-

Nursing Care in the Community

Persons with AIDS

The continued epidemic of AIDS in gay and heterosexual communities presents challenges and opportunities for community mental health nurses. As health care becomes a more integrated managed care system constrained by capitation, the role of community mental health nurses is changing. No longer bound to the traditions of the past, these nurses are becoming an integral part of community-based care for a variety of AIDS clients.

The market trend continues for more home health agencies along with major pharmaceutical companies to provide in-home care to AIDS clients. In-home care services cut down on the high costs associated with hospitalization. In the home, many of these clients receive direct care via home health nurses. Pharmaceutical companies are providing IV therapy such as Total Parental Nutrition (TPN) along with antibiotics, antiemetics, and hydration delivered by a PICC line. Other agencies may provide maintenance functions for clients, such as various AIDS projects, related organizations, and self-help groups.

What is the role of community mental health nurses in a managed care arena? To work successfully with AIDS clients, the nurse must confront the self about personal attitudes, beliefs, and values about AIDS, gay lifestyles, and sexuality. Also, a thorough knowledge of AIDS and its psychosocial issues associated with the initial HIV+ diagnosis, progression to AIDS, its chronicity and sequelae, and eventual death is essential.

Nurses can offer much to clients with AIDS. Counseling, brief supportive therapy, and just being a caring presence make a difference. Anxiety and depression must be anticipated, dealt with, and worked through. Social support, available financial resources, housing needs, and possible job loss are other issues to consider. Perhaps one of the most important aspects will be working with the client's partner, lover, and/or family. Instruction in safe sex is paramount. The potential for suicide should be of concern. The nurse must be prepared to work collaboratively with other health professionals. Teamwork in coordination of services, medication adherence, physician appointments, clinic visits, and referral to other community-based services will enhance the quality of care for AIDS clients who are often invisible in the community.

ties. **Antiretroviral therapy** is the use of certain drugs to treat the major opportunistic diseases associated with AIDS. **Opportunistic diseases** are diseases that commonly appear in AIDS clients, especially when their T-cell count drops. Whether these symptoms are reversible and what level of cognitive improvement can be made are the subjects of ongoing study.

Nurses working with AIDS clients who also have dementia will participate in the neuropsychiatric assessment of their clients by recording problems with memory, attention span, and concentration. They will provide support to the client, family, and friends who are assuming client care. They may refer the client to day care, home care or respite care, depending on the client's functional status and needs. With clients such as these, it is important to help them and their families remember treatment and medication schedules. This may include checklists, bulletin boards, pillbox alarms, and other plans to promote self-care potential and ease the burden of care for significant others.

Additional Treatment Modalities

Nursing interventions contribute significantly to the client's ability to cope effectively with HIV disease. But it is important to keep in mind that other disciplines and therapies play a critical role in the client's disease course. Currently accepted treatments of adjustment problems in PWAs parallel those for other populations with adjustment disorders. However, there are important key differences addressed in this section that include particulars about pharmacologic intervention, the preferred format for individual counseling, psychosocial support networks specific to PWAs and their significant others, and the use of adjunct therapies, for example, occupational and recreational therapies for stress reduction.

Pharmacologic Intervention

Psychotropic medications can be useful in the treatment of clients with HIV. There are no medical reasons to avoid their use. The most commonly used psychotropic medications with HIV clients experiencing moderate to severe distress are antidepressants and anxiolytics.

Antidepressant medication can be prescribed if the client manifests a significant depressed condition. Sometimes an antidepressant is initiated prophylactically when new uncontrollable stressors are anticipated. Anxiolytics are prescribed in daily dosages or PRN to curb the client's anxiety. The choice of antidepressant or anxiolytic and dosage of the medication will often depend on the client's neurovegetative symptoms and underlying physical illness. For example, for an agitated client with gastroenteritis who is also having difficulties with diarrhea due to the disease or complications from treatment, an antidepressant medication with more anticholinergic action may be the best choice. This medication will diminish diarrhea and provide a mild sedation. In addition to the individual's overall health status and specific emotional distress, the age of the client is important. Children and adolescents are generally treated with lower doses of psychotropic medications.

Alternative Therapies

Alternative therapeutic programs for PWAs include many traditional and nontraditional therapies aimed at reducing stress and increasing chances of long-term survival. The stress of HIV disease is chronic and may persist over long periods of time with acute exacerbations. Dependency on psychotropic intervention alone is not the answer. Attention is drawn to recommended alternative actions.

There are well-documented techniques, for example, stress reduction, relaxation, and cognitive restructuring techniques, that are extremely useful to many persons at various stages of HIV disease. These include stress management strategies and progressive relaxation exercises that nurses can teach clients to help them cope more effectively. Manuals and self-help books as well as short workshops are available to teach clients these techniques. Some of these instructional aids are also on videotape.

The individual's desire to control emotional distress through diet and exercise must be recognized. It is therefore important to recommend proper exercise and healthy nutrition as general guidelines for addressing stress-related illnesses, such as depression, cancers, and heart disease.

PWAs must be cautioned that HIV-infected bodies are different from disease-free systems. Weight loss generated by diet changes and exercise is usually more of a problem than a desired goal. Unnecessary calorie depletion and calorie burning should be kept at a minimum. The recommendation for exercise should focus on moderation with the major goal of exercise geared to strength building and resistance training. Adding muscle mass is a

good thing; burning calories is not. Specific recommendations for diet therapy are not well-established. What is known is that there is a relationship between nutritional status and survival. In a study by Guenter et al, the nutritional status of persons with HIV infection who were treated with recent therapies (including antiretroviral agents) predicted their survival, even after adjusting for age and CD_4 counts (Guenter et al., 1993).

■ ■ ■ ■ ■ ■ EVALUATION

If nursing interventions are successful, the client will show significant signs of improvement in coping ability. Nurses are expected to evaluate changes in client mood, behavior, and functional abilities. Clients' understanding of their illness and treatment should also be evident. A large part of the treatment of persons with HIV is individualized teaching to help them regain or maintain a sense of control over their symptoms and disease.

Effective coping should be evidenced in the outcome criteria addressed in the treatment plan. That is, clients should demonstrate an ability to contain uncomfortable feelings of fear, anxiety, guilt, grief, and depression. Because their ability to manage their symptoms should have improved, their sense of self-worth and self-esteem should be enhanced. Relationships with others, especially those in caregiver roles, should have been strengthened by the added instruction and support of the nurse. The client should demonstrate a realistic level of hope despite the downward course of the illness, due to the nurse's efforts to help the client find meaning in life and set small, realistic goals. While clients will not experience a high level of wellness, they should experience a quality to their life based on increased feelings of cognitive, behavioral, and decisional control. Helping clients achieve a sense of control helps the client avert high levels of anxiety and depression, and may also be vital to the ability to sustain physical health.

Summary of Key Concepts

1. HIV disease is considered by the U.S. government to be the foremost public health problem in the country.

2. Persons may be infected with HIV but may be asymptomatic for long periods of time.

3. AIDS is the advanced stages of HIV disease and is fatal.

4. AIDS occurs in all age groups and ethnicities.

5. IV drug use and male homosexual activity are the most frequently reported risk behaviors for AIDS to date.

6. The primary DSM-IV diagnosis for emotional distress associated with HIV and AIDS is adjustment disorder.

7. Nursing assessment and interventions should be done in collaboration with the PWA and significant others.

8. Alternative therapy techniques such as stress reduction, relaxation, and cognitive restructuring have been found to be useful to many clients in various stages of HIV disease.

REFERENCES

Brown G, Rundell J: Suicidal tendencies in women with Human Immunodeficiency Virus infection, *Amer J Psychiatr* 146: 556–557, 1989.

Buck B, Duffy VJ: The use of psychotropic medications in outpatient AIDS care, *AIDS Patient Care* 7(4):203–206, 1993.

Centers for Disease Control: *HIV/AIDS surveillance report/public information data set, data through December 31, 1993,* Atlanta, August 1994, U.S. Dept. of Health and Human Services.

Duffy VJ: Crisis points in HIV disease, *AIDS Patient Care* 8(1):28–32, 1994.

Frierson RL, Lippmann SB: Suicide and AIDS, *Psychosomatics* 29:226–231, 1988.

Gala C et al.: The psychosocial impact of HIV infection in gay men, drug users and heterosexuals, *Br J Psych* 163:651–659, 1993.

Glass RM: AIDS and suicide, *JAMA* 259: 1369–1370, 1988.

Guenter P et al: Relationships among nutritional status, disease progression and survival in HIV infection, *J Acquired Immune Deficiency Syndromes* 6:1130–1138, 1993.

Kieger K et al: AIDS and suicide in California, *JAMA* 266:1881, 1988.

Levine AM: AIDS-related malignancies: the emerging epidemic, *J National Cancer Institute* 85:1382–1397, 1993.

Marzuk PM et al: Increased risk of suicide in persons with AIDS, *JAMA* 259: 1333–1337, 1988.

Pergami A et al: The psychosocial impact of HIV infection in women, *J Psychosomatic Research* 37(7):687–696, 1993.

Perry S, Jacobsen P: Neuropsychiatric manifestations of AIDS-spectrum disorders, *Hosp & Comm Psychiatr* 37:135–142, 1986.

Perry S, Markowitz J: Psychiatric intervention for AIDS-spectrum disorders, *Hosp & Comm Psychiatr* 37:1001–1006, 1986.

Plott RT et al: Suicide of AIDS patients in Texas: a preliminary report, *Texas Medicine* 85:40–43, 1989.

Rabkin JG et al: Effect of imipramine on mood and enumerative measures of immune status in depressed patients with HIV illness, *Amer J Psychiatr* 151(4):516–523, 1994.

Shaffer HJ, Costikyan DS: Cocaine psychosis and AIDS: a contemporary diagnostic dilemma, *J Substance Abuse Treatment* 5:9–12, 1988.

CHAPTER 29

Psychologic Aspects of Physiologic Illness

Ruth N. Grendell

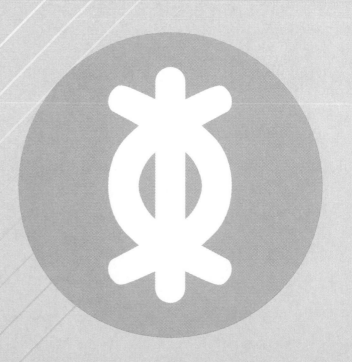

Adaptation A constant, ongoing process occurring along the time continuum that includes the dimensions of health and illness, beginning with birth and ending with death. Adaption involves both cognitive and physiologic neural-chemical-endocrine processes.

Coping What a person does in response to interruptions caused by stress or stressful events.

Hardiness A sense of mastery or self-confidence needed to appropriately appraise and interpret health stressors.

Sick role A set of social expectations that an ill person meets such as 1) being exempt from usual social role responsibilities, 2) not being morally responsible for being ill, 3) being obligated to "want to get well," and 4) being obligated to seek competent help.

Stress 1) A term that refers to both a stimulus and a response. It can denote a nonspecific response of the body to any demand placed on it, whether the causal event is negative (a painful experience) or positive (a happy occasion). 2) A state produced by a change in the environment that is perceived as challenging, threatening, or damaging to the person's dynamic equilibrium. 3) The wear and tear on the body over time. 4) Psychologic stress has been defined as all processes, whether originating in the external environment or within the person, which demand a mental appraisal of the event prior to the involvement or activation of any other system.

- Discuss the influence of mind-body interrelationships on wellness and health promotion.

- Describe the impact of mind-body interrelationships during physiologic illness or disease.

- Identify major physiologic and psychosocial stressors.

- Define the concepts of stress and adaptation.

- Describe the processes involved in mind-body response and adaptation to stress (cognitive appraisal, autonomic nervous system responses, and coping mechanisms).

- Describe the role and influence of social support in the adaptation to stress.

- Design a plan of care that incorporates interventions for psychosocial and physiologic needs for an individual with a health care problem.

For centuries humans have been considered parts of separate systems or units—the body, mind, and spirit. In Western civilizations, ancient healers of the body were "bleeders" or "bile examiners"; the mind was treated by magicians and alchemists; spiritual needs were the province of orthodox religions (Pelletier, 1977). This practice continues up to modern times as physicians treat physical illness, psychiatrists deal with mental disorders, and the clergy attend to spiritual needs. There is still a strong tendency to consider a human as a complex system composed of many interconnecting subsystems. The total person is, then, a sum of the individual parts.

Holistic health care emphasizes health promotion and prevention of illness. This perspective cuts across disciplines, and individuals are viewed as total beings. In addition to physical findings, health care providers are interested in the influence of cultural and genetic factors, past and current experiences, family structure, role functions on the person's perception of health and illness, and use of coping mechanisms. In this perspective, human beings are more than the sum of their parts. Each person is perceived as uniquely separate from another human being.

Individuals are encouraged to take active responsibility for their own health and participate in the recovery process when illnesses do occur. It is imperative that health care providers consider the dynamic interactions between mental and physical processes in maintaining equilibrium and in the disorders that result from imbalances.

HISTORICAL OVERVIEW OF THE MIND-BODY-SPIRIT CONNECTION

The mind-body-spirit connection has been a subject of interest for centuries. How human beings perceive and respond to environmental stimuli was as intriguing to early philosophers as it is to modern-day scientists. Today's interpretation of these connections is founded in both Eastern and Western scientific and philosophical perspectives.

Western Philosophical Perspectives

Before the early Greek philosophers began their quest for truth, the meaning of human existence, and the meaning of wisdom, all physical events were explained by supernatural causes. People believed that the whims of the various gods dictated all things. The sun rose and ran its course each day, seeds sprouted and produced grain, lightning flashed and thunder rolled, disasters occurred, and illness struck and people died—all because the gods willed such things to happen. Even today, some people attribute their health, tragedy, or illness to the hands of fate.

EARLY GREEK PHILOSOPHERS

These beliefs were first challenged by the Greek philosopher Thales who suggested that the cause of events might exist within "nature" or within the situation itself (Christian, 1990). The hypothesis was reinforced by the great fifth-century Greek philosophers Socrates, Plato, and Aristotle. Rather than halt his search for the truth, Socrates declared that "an unexamined life was not worth living." Perhaps human beings *were* more than puppets of the gods!

Aristotle also believed that humans were more than reactors to the environment. Although he used the principles of logic and the "five senses" to gather empirical data about the biologic world, he also used a comprehensive approach to gain new insights about events in nature and human behavior. Later, Hippocrates, known as the father of medicine, treated the body, mind, and spirit.

DARK AGES

Unfortunately, much of the enlightenment achieved through these earlier philosophers was lost during the Dark Ages (A.D. 500–1000) when the religious doctrines of a powerful church prohibited the study of the mind. The mind was then considered to be closely associated with the spirit or soul and thus became the exclusive province of the church. The belief in mind-body dualism maintained popularity as seventeenth- and eighteenth-century scientists continued to view human beings as passive receptors to external environmental events.

MIDDLE AGES

During the Middle Ages, St. Augustine influenced philosophical views by introducing his beliefs that all events were directed by God and that the supreme goal of man was to be in mystical union with God. St. Thomas Aquinas, inspired by the writings of Aristotle, argued that the act of reasoning was needed as well as the act of faith for humans to live in harmony with the Creator. However, religious leaders of the day ruled out reasoning as a criterion for seeking religious truths.

SHIFT IN PHILOSOPHICAL THOUGHT

In the 1600s there was a radical shift away from belief in supernatural causes of events back to natural causes. Reason and logic again gained precedence. René Descartes, a French philosopher and mathematician (1596–1650), considered the body a machine that should be logically studied in the same manner as other machines. His premise was that the mind housed thoughts, consciousness, and soul but had no way to come directly in contact with reality; therefore, the mind was inaccessible to study. In contrast, he stated that behavior was observable and could be interpreted. The separation of mind and body stayed in vogue until Sigmund Freud (1856–1939) reintroduced the connecting tie between them.

BIOMEDICAL MODEL

The foundation for the biomedical model was laid in the nineteenth century when scientists discovered microbes as the origin of many diseases. This cause-effect model separated the person into many systems and subsystems that added up to the sum total; it was conducive to studying and explaining the body functions.

FACTORS CONTRIBUTING TO A CHANGE IN PHILOSOPHY

The biomedical model, however, did not explain function or disease of the mind or interpret the interactions between mind, spirit, and body. Scientists discovered that some people exposed to pathogens did not become ill, and these findings led researchers to challenge the existing theory and to explore other possible influencing causes.

A broader perspective of factors contributing to disease was achieved through epidemiologic studies that portrayed the general events preceding morbidity and mortality of individuals. The strong possibility of a connection between the mind, spirit, and body in health and illness encouraged further investigation. The following discussion of Eastern philosophy and practices provides the background for understanding some of the subsequent changes in Western sciences.

Eastern Philosophical Perspectives

ANCIENT PHILOSOPHIES AND PRACTICES

Contributions from the Eastern philosophies have gained increasing prominence with the merging of world cultures. Western scientists have learned that other societies consider health to be a balance of mind-body interaction and have for centuries practiced healing rituals that treat the whole person. These rituals often include the family and community as part of the healing process.

Buddhism. In Buddhism, founded in India around 500 B.C., the 'self' is an illusion. Human existence is considered to be a continual cycle of life, death, and rebirth, with each life determined by the previous lives. Individuals strive to become detached from material things to rid themselves of pain and suffering and finally reach nirvana, the state of perfect peace.

There are several branches of Buddhism. Perhaps the most influential is Zen Buddhism, which is now practiced primarily in Japan. Followers of Zen believe in attaining spiritual enlightenment through meditation and self-discipline. This mind-body state, termed *satori,* embraces an intense alertness accompanied by a deep sense of inner calmness.

Confucianism and Taoism. The Taoist religion is also currently practiced in many Eastern countries. In contrast to Confucian followers who emphasize social conformity, Taoist followers profess a preference for a simple, spontaneous way of life that is close to nature and incorporates meditation, special diet, and breath control. A Taoist proverb states: "When you have a disease, do not try to cure it. Find your center, and you will be healed" (Moyers, 1993).

Hinduism. Hinduism is a mixture of many religions and philosophies involving deities, reincarnation, and how life should be lived. The law of karma states that every action, no matter how small, exerts an influence on how the soul will be born in the next reincarnation. Hindus believe that this process continues until the person has achieved spiritual perfection, or *nirvana.* (Note the similarity to Buddhist beliefs.) The practice of yoga is probably the best known of the six schools of Hindu philosophy and has been introduced to the Western world as a method of coping with stress. The purpose of yoga is to help bring an integration of body, mind, and spirit.

Blending of Eastern and Western Philosophies

Therapies associated with Eastern philosophies such as meditation, self-hypnosis, biofeedback, acupuncture, and acupressure—all formerly considered unconventional treatments by mainstream Western medicine—have been introduced into current health care plans (see Figure 29-1). Acupressure—pressure applied to specific acupuncture points of the body—is sometimes prescribed to relieve muscle tension and fatigue.

These alternative techniques have been accepted by many in the Western world. They have been used in the pursuit of a healthy lifestyle and as options to the use of drugs or surgery, and/or combined with traditional medicine as aids in coping with stress and illness.

DISCOVERY OF ENDORPHINS

A major breakthrough in understanding the mind-body connection resulted when Pert, a molecular biologist, isolated the opiate drug receptor in the brain in the mid-1980s (Groer, 1991; Moyers, 1993). This led to the discovery of endogeneous morphines (endorphins) and other chemical communicators released by the brain, the immune and endocrine systems, and other parts of the body. It was discovered that molecules released from one part of the body are diffused to the surface of every cell in the body, providing instructions for action. Pert labeled these complex interactions as a "psychosomatic communication network." Scientists now "theorize that these neuropeptides and their receptors are the biochemical correlates of emotions" (Moyers, 1993). Pert believes that the residence of the mind is in the body as well as the brain.

The peptides, endorphin and enkephalin, have been shown to relieve pain by the same mechanism as morphine and other narcotics. The use of placebos, acupuncture, and transcutaneous nerve stimulation are thought to release endorphins and thus aid in pain relief. Mental imagery, music, and humor have been reported to serve as distractions from the person's focus on the pain and stress (Black and Matassurn-Jacobs 1993; Selye, 1976; Smeltzer and Bare, 1992; Pelletier, 1977; and Simonton et al, (1978) have demonstrated the effectiveness of these methods with cancer clients, and others with life-threatening illnesses.

PSYCHONEUROIMMUNOLOGY

Psychoneuroimmunology (formerly termed psychosomatic medicine) is concerned with the impact of emotional and psychologic disturbances on neural and organic function and subsequent ailments such as cardiovascular disease, gastric ulcers, ulcerative colitis, asthma, migraine, dermatologic manifestations, arthritis, and cancer. This branch of medicine is also concerned with the beneficial effects of mind-body connections in promoting wellness and recovery from illness and disease.

Solomon first coined the term *psychoneuroimmunology* (PNI) in 1964. In several studies conducted by Solomon and others, there were indications that immune response to disease was closely associated with emotions and attitudes toward stress (Glaser and Glaser, 1991; Groer, 1991).

Psychoneuroimmunology spans the disciplines of nursing, medicine, sociology, and psychology. The three

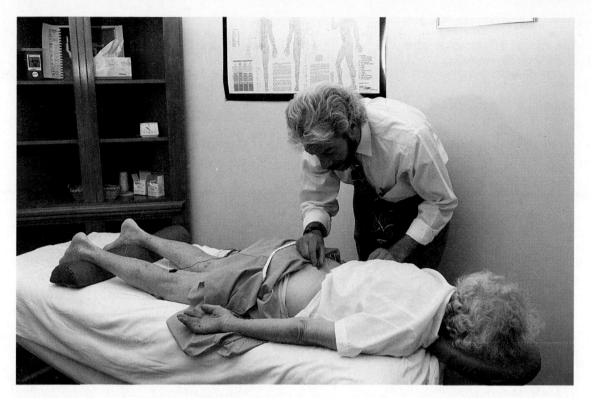

Figure 29-1 Acupuncture is a health practice with a basis in Eastern philosophy that has gained increasing acceptance in traditional health care.

(Copyright © Cathy Lander-Goldberg, Lander Photographics.)

processes of cognitive, neuroendocrine, and antibody formation by cellular and humeral (blood and plasma) immune systems are studied as a total network. Much of the research has been concerned with immunodepression. Mental imagery is believed to aid in the release of chemicals in the brain and alter the immune system. Studies have been done on the beneficial effects of meditation and hypnosis on allergies and viral infections. Additional research is needed in other areas of the wellness-illness states (Groer, 1991). Neuroimmunology is discussed in further depth in Chapter 5.

STRESS AS AN ETIOLOGIC FACTOR IN ILLNESS

A large body of literature exists on the relationship of **stress,** a nonspecific response of the body to any positive or negative demand placed on it, and the potential for illness. However, stress and its sources are often difficult to identify. Several research studies have been conducted across populations on the effects of various life events, for example, bereavement, divorce, clinical depression, chronic stressors, academic stress, and mental and physical illnesses. Studies have also shown that persons do not always adapt positively to disasters such as earthquakes, floods, and war (Glaser and Glaser, 1991). Box 29-1 depicts examples of many stress factors that are linked to physiologic, psychologic, and emotional re-

sponses or behaviors. Box 29-2 describes several indices of stress.

Illness has been labeled as an unexpected stressful event in individuals' lives that can interrupt them from fulfilling their usual tasks or roles. Illness is often perceived to be a major crisis (Benner and Wrubel, 1989).

A number of factors are now being considered as causes of illness and determinants of an individual's response (Kozier et al, 1992). "The intensity of the stress response depends on a combination of 1) intensity of stimulus, 2) duration of stimulus, and 3) perception of control over the stimulus" (Phipps et al, 1995). The perception of control is also influenced by the person's cultural background, values, and beliefs. Other factors that may influence the response are the individual's past experiences with the stressor or similar stressors and the capacity for **coping,** what a person does in response to interruptions caused by stress or stressful events.

Theories on Effects of Stress on Mind and Body Interactions

Several theories have been developed to explain the impact of stress as a *response,* as a *stimulus,* or as a *transaction.* Selye's theory (1976) demonstrates the nonspecific body response to any form of stress; Nuernberger (1981) believes there is a response beyond the arousal of the sympathetic nervous system. Lazarus (1984) states

---

Box 29-1   Sources of Physiologic and Psychosocial Stressors

Physiologic stressors

- Infectious agents (viruses, bacteria, fungi)
- Chemical agents (drugs, alcohol, poison)
- Physical agents (heat/cold, radiation, electric shock, trauma)
- Suppressed immune system
- Genetic disorders
- Illness processes
- Aging processes

Psychosocial stressors

- Daily hassles (common frustrations)
- Life events (birth/death, job change, role change, illness)
- Major disasters (earthquake, flood)
- War (manmade)

Effects and response to the stressor are dependent on the individual's perception of the intensity of the stressor and:

- acute/chronic duration of the stressor
- cumulative effect of simultaneous stressors
- sequence of stressors
- severity of stressors
- individual previous experience with stressors
- amount of social support

Box 29-2   Indices of Stress

- Dryness of throat and mouth
- Pounding of heart
- Insomnia and/or nightmares
- Increased urinary frequency
- Muscle tension and migraine headaches
- Pain in neck or lower back
- Loss of or excessive appetite
- Gastrointestinal signs and symptoms:

    "butterflies" in stomach

    cramping, constipation, or diarrhea

    vomiting

    change in menstrual cycle

    body tics or twitches

    flushing, sweating

    nervous cough

- General irritability, hyperexcitation, depression
- Disturbed behavior
- Feelings of unreality
- Easily fatigued, weakness, dizziness
- "Floating anxiety" without knowing exact cause
- Overpowering urge to cry or run and hide
- Easily startled, tension, heightened alertness
- Inability to concentrate, loss of interest
- Forgetfulness
- Increased smoking
- Increased use of drug and/or alcohol
- Accident-proneness
- Repetitive movements—picking at fingernails
- Impulsive behavior, emotional instability
- Nervous laughter
- Stuttering or other speech difficulties
- Hypermotility: pacing, restlessness

---

that the individual's interpretation of the stress determines the degree and type of response. Figure 29-2 depicts an integration of these three theories.

STRESS AS A RESPONSE (SELYE)

Selye's theory, first generated in 1936 during studies with laboratory animals, identified stress as a nonspecific biologic patterned response to some environmental stressor—regardless of what the stressful stimulus might be. He defined the sequence of body responses to a stressor as the General Adaptation Syndrome (GAS). The three major phases are the *alarm reaction,* the *stage of resistance,* and the *stage of exhaustion.*

The stimulation of the sympathetic nervous system is the primary response during the alarm reaction and is often referred to as the "flight or fight" mechanism. The release of endocrine hormones is closely associated with the stimulation of the sympathetic system. During the stage of resistance, the person continues to use sources of energy to adapt to the stressor. The stage of exhaus-

tion is characterized by total expenditure of energy; the person usually becomes ill and may die without replenishment of resources. The condition may also be reversed by the use of external resources such as medication, nutrition, and psychotherapy.

GENERAL INHIBITION SYNDROME RESPONSE TO STRESS (NUERNBERGER)

Nuernberger proposed an additional theory of adaptation to stress in 1981 labeled as the General Inhibition Syndrome or "possum response." This self-protective mechanism is due to the arousal of the parasympathetic

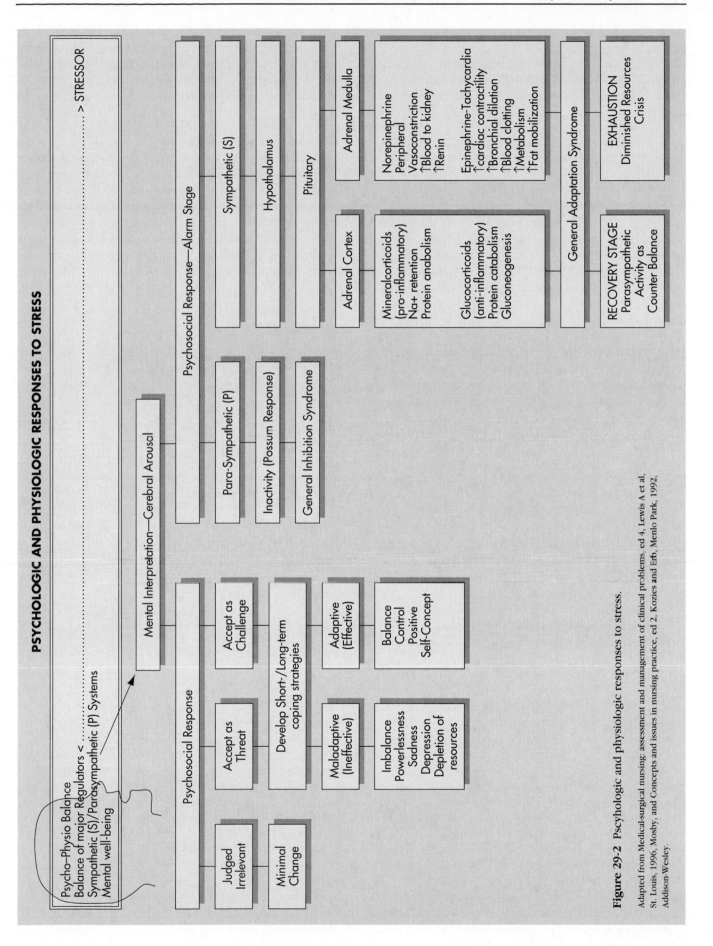

Figure 29-2 Pscychologic and physiologic responses to stress.

Adapted from Medical-surgical nursing: assessment and management of clinical problems, ed 4, Lewis A et al, St. Louis, 1996, Mosby, and Concepts and issues in nursing practice, ed 2, Kozies and Erb, Menlo Park, 1992, Addison-Wesley.

system, the opposing branch to the sympathetic component of the autonomic nervous system. Stress is a reflection of an imbalance between these two systems, and prolonged or intense imbalances can lead to illness. Table 29-1 presents a listing of physiologic illnesses that have been attributed to stress. The imbalance is caused not by the external stressor, but by the individual's perception of threat, pain, or discomfort (Kozier et al, 1992; Smeltzer and Bare, 1992).

STRESS AS A TRANSACTION (LAZARUS)

Transactional theories of stress are based in part on the work of Lazarus, who believed that neither the stimulus nor response theories explained an individual's particular response to stress. The person confronted by a stressor makes a *primary cognitive appraisal* of its intensity. During primary appraisal, stressors can be classified as irrelevant, benign-positive, or stressful. Irrelevant demands often require minimal attention. Benign-positive stressors can be challenges and potential for growth. Stressful demands are perceived as harmful threats or losses. During *secondary cognitive appraisal* of the stressor, the coping methods to use are decided on, whereas reappraisal evaluates whether coping methods have been effective. Stress is viewed as a dynamic state that requires effort in the process of adaptation or coping. **Adaptation** is an ongoing process involving both cognitive and physiologic neural-chemical-endocrine processes.

The individual's sensitivity and vulnerability to the stressor are the determining factors of emotional and behavioral responses. Therefore, what may be an acutely stressful event to one person is not necessarily perceived as stressful by another. Coping mechanisms may also differ and can be effective or ineffective. The stress of daily hassles (minor life events) can be buffered by uplifting daily activities such as reading a good book, prayer and meditation, or spending quality time with friends and family (Carson, 1989; Lazarus and Folkman, 1984; Lewis and Collier, 1996).

Mind-Body Responses to Stress

The mind-body connection is an important factor in the promotion of health and in the recuperative process from an illness. Mental and physical health are closely in-

---

TABLE 29-1   Examples of physiologic and psychologic related effects

Physiologic problem	Related psychologic effects
ACUTE PROBLEM	
Trauma	Anxiety
Surgery (disfigurement or alterations in body processes)	Fear of deformity, mutilation
	Lowered and self-image and self-esteem
Cardiovascular problems	Diminished self-confidence
myocardial infarction	Confusion
hypertension	Shock, unable to make decisions
cerebral vascular accident	Denial
Pain	
Stressful event	
Major disaster (flood, earthquake)	
War	
Life-threatening diagnosis	
CHRONIC PROBLEM	
Progressive effects of acute health problem	Powerlessness (uncertainty of future)
Epilepsy	Depression
Lupus	Suicidal thoughts
Arthritis	Hopelessness
Renal/liver failure	Helplessness
Diabetes mellitus	Chronic fatigue
Post-traumatic stress syndrome	Insomnia
Terminal illness (cancer)	Worry over finances
Aging process/multiple health problems	Decisional conflict
Respiratory-COPD (cystic fibrosis)	
Diminished immune response (AIDS)	

Note: Person may experience one or more psychologic effects with any of the above physiologic problems.

tertwined, as are physical and mental illness. Researchers have discovered several conditioning factors that determine the human response to stress. A person seeking medical help experiences a variety of emotions prior to the actual diagnosis. Often, these individuals will try to hide their emotions, and health care providers must be alert to subtle cues.

Lambert and Lambert (1979, 1985) developed a conceptual framework for studying the impact of physical illness on a person's mental health. The list of constructs includes the impact on a sense of well-being, somatic identity (body image), sexuality, occupational identity, and social roles. The complexity of individuals yields a variety of interpretations of the illness experience. People learn coping mechanisms that aid them in adapting to stress and then apply them to similar situations.

CONCEPT OF HARDINESS

The ability of some people to overcome adversity, to recover from a serious illness against all odds, or to survive severe tragedy has been an area of study for many scientists. The concept of *hardiness* has been introduced as a means for mastering or controlling stressful events (Pollock and Duffy, 1990). **Hardiness** is defined as a sense of mastery or self-confidence needed to appropriately appraise and interpret health stressors. Studies have identified hardiness as a moderating factor on stress and psychologic strain for both men and women in work situations, in survival rates for people with cancer, in lowering blood pressure, and in delaying conversion to AIDS in persons with AIDS-related complex.

Hardiness is not a unitary concept. Some components include commitment to self, an internal sense of control, and perception of stress as a challenge. Persons who exhibit hardiness usually take care of themselves and possess physical and mental health (Kobasa, 1979; Taylor, 1991).

COPING MEASURES FOR STRESS ADAPTATION

Several methods for coping with and reducing stress, some derived from Eastern practices, have been introduced over the years. Exercise and recreation provide a variety of benefits, including increased oxygenation, changes in heart rate, and lowered blood pressure. Additional outcomes may be relaxation, peaceful sleep, distraction from concerns, increased appetite, and a feeling of well-being. Music therapy and humor have also helped to relieve tension and anxiety and reduce aggression. Use of saunas or massage helps individuals to relax and stimulates skin circulation. Pet therapy has been introduced as a means of social interaction to relieve tension and depression. Progressive relaxation, guided imagery, biofeedback, meditation, and yoga are used in states of both health and illness to aid in feelings of calmness and to provide a sense of being in control of life events.

Therapeutic touch (TT) is a term first coined in 1979 by a nurse, Delores Krieger, and is derived from the "laying on of hands" associated with Eastern, European, and religious philosophies. This method is based on a theory that the release of excess energy from the healer helps the ill person in the healing process. Basic concepts of TT are that humans are energy fields constantly influenced by the flow of energy from the environment; illness, disease, or pain disrupts the energy flow patterns. Four steps are used during the therapeutic touch process:

1. The healer "centers" and calms the self through meditation.
2. The healer conducts an assessment for asymmetry of the client's energy flow (heat, cold, pressure, congestion, etc.) by passing hands over the client's body.
3. The healer performs an "unruffling" with a sweeping movement of the hands over the long bones of the body to make the client's energy field more receptive to the transfer of energy from the healer.
4. The healer transfers energy to the client in order to realign the energy field.

Therapeutic touch is a highly complex technique that requires instruction and much practice (Black and Matassarin-Jacobs, 1993; Kozier et al, 1992; Krieger et al, 1979). However, nurses often use the simple act of touch in daily interactions with clients to aid relaxation and to demonstrate interest and caring.

Humor therapy. The renewed interest in implementing nontraditional and holistic methods is often attributed to the contributions of Cousins (1979) through his article titled "Anatomy of an Illness: a Patient's Perspective." The medical community was so impressed with this layman's narrative about his recovery from a debilitating illness (ankylosing spondylitis), using nontraditional methods, that it was accepted for publication in *The New England Journal of Medicine*. Subsequently, the article was expanded into a book.

Cousins attributed his illness to be the result of lowered immunity brought on by extreme stress, and his recovery to the use of humor, vitamin C therapy, the placebo effect of positive thinking, and experiencing love and hope. His own prescription of watching comedy movies produced an anesthetic effect and gave him at least two hours of pain-free sleep. He stated that the chemical changes produced by the brain may be more powerful than any medicine, and he placed great emphasis on the positive influence of having a purpose in life and the will to live—elements of spirituality. Cousins also paid tribute to his physician who permitted him to be an active participant in his care.

Cousins was criticized by some for his report in 1979 on the use of humor as a temporary relief from pain. At that time little was known about the brain's capability of secreting the morphine-like molecules called endorphins and enkephalins (Cousins, 1989). Since that time, humor rooms have been used as a distractive measure in several medical centers across the country (Buxman, 1991; Cousins, 1989). Humor may help the ill person to "reframe" a stressful situation and to examine it from a different, less serious perspective. Rooms have been designed to hold a variety of media such as books, movies, and cartoons to amuse and distract sick children and adults.

Group therapy.   Group therapy began in the 1940s and has experienced several transitions to meet changing clinical needs. In addition to therapy groups for people with acute and chronic psychiatric illnesses, multiple therapy groups have been designed for persons with stress-related conditions such as acute (myocardial infarct) and chronic physical (rheumatoid arthritis) conditions, life-threatening illnesses (cancer), and other health problems. Therapeutic goals of all groups include the development of the participant's positive potential, awareness of own behavior, sensitivity to and acceptance of others, and developing coping skills (Yalom, 1985).

Several studies by Spiegel conducted in 1983–1989 demonstrated the positive relationship of supportive group therapy and self-hypnosis on the recovery and longevity of women with metastatic breast cancer. Women in the treatment group lived twice as long as women who did not participate in the sessions (Glaser and Glaser, 1991; Moyers, 1993). Women in the control group reported that their pain had doubled in intensity, whereas women in the treatment group ranked on a numbered scale an average two-point decrease in pain.

Biofeedback.   Biofeedback is a technique that uses equipment to help people gain voluntary control over striated muscles. It is often combined with controlled breathing techniques and/or meditation. Case histories, primarily for reduction of stress, were first presented in the 1960s (Basmeyrian, 1979). Studies were also conducted in the 1970s regarding the benefits of biofeedback on reduction of hypertension, number of asthmatic attacks, and depression in cancer patients (Pelletier, 1977).

Three basic principles of biofeedback are:

1. Any mental-emotional-body function that can be observed through electrical monitoring and amplification and is perceived through sensory feedback can be controlled by the individual.

2. Every conscious and unconscious change in the mental and/or emotional state influences and is influenced by any change in the physiologic state.

3. A relaxed meditative state enhances voluntary control and increases the individual's awareness of subliminal imagery, sensations, and fantasies (Pelletier, 1977).

A recent nursing research study (Hahn et al, 1993) examined the effects of self-controlled thermal biofeedback combined with progressive muscle relaxation on blood pressure levels of Korean women who had been diagnosed with essential hypertension. (See Understanding and Applying Research below.)

Meditative therapies.   Progressive relaxation techniques were first introduced by Jacobson in 1925–1929 and later modified by Paul. Jacobson's work laid the foundation for biofeedback therapy. The person learns to alternately tense and relax one group of muscles at a time until total physiologic and psychologic relaxation transpires. This technique is frequently combined with mental imagery, biofeedback, and meditation. Mental im-

---

Understanding and Applying
RESEARCH

Hahn Y et al: The effect of thermal biofeedback and progressive muscle relaxation training in reducing blood pressure of patients with essential hypertension, *Image: J Nursing Scholarship,* 25(3):204–207, 1993.

In this study, a combination of thermal biofeedback and progressive muscle relaxation was used. The sample was composed of 19 Korean women ages 30–59 who had been diagnosed with essential hypertension (readings above 140/90 mm Hg), and without complications or on medication therapy. Eleven women in the treatment group received instructions for both biofeedback and muscle relaxation. Eight women in the control group received instructions on muscle relaxation for an eight-week period only.

Systolic and diastolic blood pressures gradually declined over the semiweekly sessions for women in the treatment group. A significant decrease in systolic readings was evident by the second session. There was an average decrease of 20.6 mm Hg for systolic and 14.4 mm Hg for diastolic pressures. However, there was a tendency for increases in both blood pressures for women in the control group.

This study supports previous studies that examined a combination of therapies in the reduction of hypertension. The authors suggested that the results of lowered blood pressure would be effective as long as subjects continued to practice the techniques regularly. The use of these techniques offers nurses an additional therapeutic measure for clients identified with essential hypertension.

agery may consist of visualizing tension as a rope tied in a knot, then relaxed like a limp rubber band as the person tenses and relaxes the muscles (Morris, 1979; Simonton et al, 1978).

Yoga has been practiced since ancient times and consists of meditation, controlled breathing, and an orderly sequence of positions or postures designed to strengthen and stretch the entire body. The branch of yoga involving physical exercises is properly called Hatha yoga. A set of gentle yoga exercises and balanced breathing routines are used in Ayurvedic medicine to simultaneously integrate the whole physiology of mind, body, and breath (Chopra, 1991).

ALTERNATIVE MEDICINE AND THERAPIES

Increased attention given by the general public to alternative medicine and therapies is manifested by the number of articles appearing in popular magazines, journals, and newspapers. Books on these subjects occupy large sections in bookstores. Some of the major alternative methods are chiropractic manipulation, hypnosis, biofeedback, homeopathy, naturopathy, herbal medicines, Chinese methods, and Ayurvedic medicine (see Table 29-2).

Homeopathic medicine. Homeopathic medicine is based on the belief that a drug which will produce certain disease symptoms in a healthy person can provide a cure for a sick person experiencing the same symptoms. Diluted substances are used to elicit a cure; for example, a dilute solution containing poison ivy compound may be prescribed for a skin rash. The medication must be shaken vigorously or "potentized" for the greatest effectiveness as the solution picks up energy from the dissolved substance.

Naturopathy. Naturopathy is a method primarily used by a small group of physicians on the west coast of the United States who use an eclectic selection of alternative therapies—for example, herbs, homeopathy, behavioral modification, and Ayurvedic medicine. A research study conducted in Oregon stated that positive changes in pap smears resulted following these treatment modalities (Abrams, 1994). Naturopathy focuses on self-healing and the integration of psychologic and physiologic based therapies.

Ayurvedic medicine. Ayurvedic (science of life) medicine originated in India and dates back thousands of years. This method may use a combination of the previously described therapies while also employing meditation, massage, herbs, aromatherapy, and biofeedback. The body is viewed as a pharmacy that can make its own natural drugs to heal itself (Carson, 1989). Dr. Deepak Chopra, a principal proponent of Ayurvedic medicine, uses a combination of Eastern and Western medicine to "bring together ancient wisdom and modern science." He states: "The guiding principle of Ayurveda is that the mind exerts the deepest influence on the body, and free-

dom from sickness depends upon contacting our own awareness, bringing it into balance, and then extending that balance to the body." (Chopra, 1991).

Chiropractic. Chiropractic is a method of treating illnesses based on the theory that pressure, strain, or tension on the spinal cord leads to a disturbance in nerve function. X rays are frequently used to determine whether vertebrae are out of alignment. The practitioner uses manipulation to restore proper placement. Chiropractors believe that these methods were known and practiced in ancient times.

Herbal medicine. The use of herbal medicine is an ancient practice worldwide. The rain forests that produce 80%–90% of today's medicines are quickly disappearing, and scientists are conducting an international search for new drugs before these sources are lost. Scientists believe that only 1% of the world's plants have been analyzed, leaving many potential drugs yet to be discovered. In a recent Chinese study, 300 participants with alcoholism experienced an 80% reduction in cravings for alcohol, with no visible side effects, from the administration of a newly discovered extract from a plant called kudzu. One study investigated the effects of the herb on laboratory animals bred to prefer alcohol. A 50% reduction in alcohol consumption was found (Abrams, 1994).

For centuries, the Chinese have diligently studied foods and have placed their highest value on "food herbs." Their formulas are based on the correct ratio or balance of a variety of these healing herbs, which are enhanced by the harvesting and preparation of the herbs at the appropriate time. These mixtures are used as supplements to a well-balanced diet, and are often prescribed in conjunction with daily exercise and positive thinking, in the belief that a balanced body is a result of a balanced life.

INTEGRATION OF NONTRADITIONAL METHODS INTO PLAN OF CARE

Many U.S. physicians describe the alternative therapies as fringe medicine by Western standards. However, some scientists view them as complements to traditional practices and are exploring some of these methods through research to determine what benefits, if any, may be derived from them.

Drug treatments once considered nontraditional folk remedies, for example, digitalis, morphine, and aspirin, are now included in mainstream treatment. Clients should be cautioned regarding overreliance on unproven therapies, which may delay their seeking conventional treatment and make them susceptible to complications such as superimposed infections or advanced disease progression. Clients should also be cautioned about false hope given by nontraditional "healers." The public can be aware of the hazards of any treatment, can ask questions, and can consult with a physician before attempting unproven methods (Abrams, 1994).

TABLE 29-2 Alternative medicine methods

Method	Purpose	Components	Research/Reports
Chiropractic	• Reduce pain caused by disturbance or spine movement or "sublexation" • Peptic ulcer • Menses discomfort	• Manipulation • Exercise • Diet • Acupuncture • Homeopathy	• Decrease in cost for care of back injuries
Acupuncture	• Anesthesia • Chronic pain relief • Substance abuse • Weight reduction	• Fine, hairlike needles inserted under skin at specific points of body	• Decrease in cravings for addictive substances • Pain relief
Acupressure (Shiatsu)	• Chronic pain/illnesses	• Pressure with fingers or small seed on sensitive areas, ears, temples, wrists, etc.	• Assist in treatment of attention deficit disorders in children
Hypnosis/biofeedback	• Chronic pain • Childbirth • Cancer pain • Pre-anesthesia • Depression • Self-regulation of autonomic nervous system	• Imaging/relaxation • Focused concentration • Combination of techniques	• Relief of pain, headache • Diabetes control • Breast cancer survival
Homeopathy	• Alleviate numerous chronic problems that have not responded to traditional treatments	• Minute amount of substances (that are similar to cause of health problem) dissolved in solution	• Anecdotal reports (none validated through research)
Herbal medicine	• Pain reduction • Laxatives • Diuretics • Calming effect • Viral infections • Colon spasms	• Herbal/plant substances (common and rare)	• Alcohol abuse treatment
Naturopathy (West Coast primarily)	• Bolster immune system • Change in lifestyle • Allergies	• Eclectic choice of herbs homeopathy Rx	• Anecdotal reports (none validated through research)
Chinese medicine	• AIDS treatment • Chronic problems • Recovery after traditional interventions	• Herbal treatment • Acupuncture • Acupressure	• Anecdotal reports
Ayurvedic medicine	• Aids own body's healing system • Controls mind/body • Decreases stress response • During chemotherapy for cancer	• Meditation • Massage • Herbs • Aromatherapy • Biofeedback	

PERSONS AT RISK FOR PSYCHOLOGIC-PHYSIOLOGIC INTERACTIVE HEALTH PROBLEMS

Persons with Acute Health Problems

Acute illnesses may suddenly interrupt or curtail a person's activities. There is usually a temporary loss of control over one's life and body. Fear, anxiety, powerlessness, helplessness, hostility, and anger are also common responses to illness. When an illness occurs, the person often asks "Why me?" or "What did I do to deserve this?" Sometimes a person will deny being ill and attempt to continue with his or her usual roles or tasks. This may eventually contribute to complications and result in a prolonged recuperation.

During the recovery stages, the person who experiences lasting effects from an acute problem, for example, a burn or spinal cord injury, must change his or her self-identity and concept of self-worth that has previously been based on physical appearance. Often these people believe that the traumatic experience has made them stronger and better persons. Empathy for others and a renewed religious faith often emerge after the traumatic event and become important facets of life (Lambert and Lambert, 1979).

Persons with Chronic Health Problems

The long-term effects and unpredictability of chronic illness challenge the person's self-esteem, body image, and sexuality; disrupt social relationships; and alter usual role functions within the family, place of employment, and community. A sense of autonomy is frequently lost (Barry, 1989).

Chronic illnesses have been termed as permanent or progressive health problems that require ongoing adaptation on the part of the individuals and their social network. Depression is a common reaction, accompanied by sleep disturbances, lack of appetite, neglect of personal appearance, and fatigue. Chronic conditions affect every aspect of people's lives and require long-term monitoring by health professionals (Lambert and Lambert, 1979; Primomo et al, 1989).

Individuals with chronic illnesses sometimes take on a deviant **sick role.** Instead of wanting to get well, they may use their illness for secondary gains of receiving attention or gaining control over other people and as a means of avoiding responsibilities. These behaviors are frequently the result of anger, fear, or depression (Black and Matassarin-Jacobs, 1993). The "invalid" role can also be the result of self-pity (Lambert and Lambert, 1979). Total rehabilitation from an illness occurs with the return to society and functioning at the individual's greatest potential. To achieve this goal, it is essential to involve family and client in the instructions for recuperation and in the activities that will promote recovery.

Persons with Multiple Health Problems

Multiple health problems are common occurrences as the person's physical and mental systems respond to chronic illness. The person with long-term diabetes mellitus, for example, is at risk of developing complications involving every physiologic system. The person who has a chronic obstructive pulmonary disease frequently has circulatory and cardiovascular problems as well. Complications of COPD lead to respiratory failure, fluid and electrolyte imbalances, depression, and anxiety.

Endocrine imbalances can lead to a variety of disturbances to life-sustaining functions. Individuals with diminished immunity are at risk for a number of complications. Various degrees of psychologic distress accompany all of these conditions (Black and Matassarin-Jacobs, 1993). Any of these physical symptoms may, and fre-

quently do, accompany depression, anxiety, or full psychiatric disorders secondary to the physical disorder.

Elderly Persons

The majority of the aging population in the United States lives independently, and many older citizens are able to enjoy their retirement years. However, the aging process most often brings multiple health problems and threatens independence. Aging produces a gradual decline in multisystem coordination. Changes are cumulative and progressive, and a healthy response to stress is diminished. An elderly person who has adequate cardiac function at rest may be unable to withstand extended exertion, and it may take longer for the heart rate to return to the baseline level; the resistance to an infection may be lowered; the reserve capacity of hormonal and neural regulation can lead to slower reaction time (Phipps et al, 1995).

Mental disorders are a major problem for the aging. Successful psychologic adjustment to aging is dependent on the person's ability to adapt to the multiple stressors, their severity, and change. A positive self-image and finding a purpose or meaning in life are essential components.

Persons Experiencing Pain

There are several definitions of pain. McCaffery and Bebbe (1989) state that "pain is whatever the experiencing person says it is and existing whenever the person says it does." The experience of pain is dependent on many variables such as the person's age, culture, gender, pain tolerance, and the situation itself. Pain is a multidimensional phenomenon involving both physiologic and psychologic components. Physiologic responses to pain include tachycardia, diaphoresis, tachypnea, and fluctuations in blood pressure. Psychologic responses include a pattern of responses to protect oneself from harm. The pain becomes the major focus, and the individual often assumes a protective posture that will guard the painful part. High levels of anxiety are likely to increase the perception of pain, and the person will seek relief by doing such things as pacing back and forth, using restless hand movements, or using drugs and/or alcohol as distractors. Additional psychologic responses are impaired thought processes, changes in sleep patterns, fatigue, tenseness and restlessness, episodes of crying, social withdrawal, and fearfulness of increased intensity or return of pain. Some may fear that the pain is an indication of a progression of the disease (Black and Matassarin-Jacobs, 1993; Doenges and Moorhouse, 1992; Fortinash and Holoday-Worret, 1995).

Persons with Terminal Illness

Spiritual distress is a common response of clients with life-threatening illness as death becomes imminent. Like pain, grief pervades every aspect of the person's existence. Grief is a normal response to loss. Physical alterations in heart rate and blood pressure, as well as changes in mood and affect such as depression, are all manifestations of grief (see Chapter 27). The dying process may extend over several months to a year or more, consisting of many crises and plateaus. Each crisis results in increased anxiety; each plateau invokes a sense of hope.

THE NURSING PROCESS ■ ■ ■ ■ ■ ■ ■ ■ ■ ■ ■ ■ ■ ■

THE NURSING PROCESS IN THE CARE OF INDIVIDUALS WITH PSYCHOLOGIC-PHYSIOLOGIC ILLNESS

The six-step nursing process provides an efficient method for gathering the necessary information, in problem solving, in clinical decision making, and for the delivery of higher-quality, individualized client care. The cyclic nature of the nursing process minimizes errors and omission of important facets of client care through ongoing assessment and evaluation of client responses and reported perceptions, thoughts, and feelings.

The effective use of the nursing process also requires the nurse to have a thorough knowledge of science and theory related to nursing and other disciplines, particularly medicine and psychology (Doenges and Moorhouse, 1992; Lewis and Collier, 1996; Phipps, et al, 1995). The involvement of the client in the nursing process provides a sense of ownership and personal control while enhancing the client's responsibility and commitment to goal achievement.

■ ASSESSMENT

Assessment is one of the most essential components of the nursing process. The nurse uses a variety of resources to collect data about the client's health status. Ideally, the client can provide much of the information. The health history should include questions pertaining to the client's current health problem and its impact on daily activities, social and family support systems, occupation, religion or belief, and ethnic-cultural background. (See Chapter 6)

During the initial interview, the nurse listens to the client's subjective report of symptoms and observes the person's verbal and nonverbal behaviors. When the client cannot provide an accurate report, another resource person can be used (Fortinash and Holoday-Worret, 1995).

The interviewing process continues during the physical assessment performed by the nurse. Often, the nurse is able to clarify previous comments regarding the client's perception of the current health problem. An important feature of the assessment is that it is mutually agreed on by the nurse and the individual client (Fortinash and Holoday-Worret, 1995; Lewis et al, 1996;

Phipps et al, 1995). Information is also obtained from reports of diagnostic tests and procedures, from the client's record, and through consultation with other members of the health care team.

The final phase of assessment is the analysis of data. The information is categorized and organized into a logical format. The nursing diagnoses emerge from this framework and identify the existing needs.

■ ■ NURSING DIAGNOSES

When a conclusion has been made through data analysis, one or more diagnoses are made. The diagnostic statement serves to describe a health problem or need that is responsive to nursing intervention. The statement is phrased to link the problem or need with its etiologic factors. For example, a person may be experiencing moderate to severe anxiety (diagnosis) related to the effects of a myocardial infarct or a possible open heart surgery (source or etiology). Nursing diagnoses can refer to actual or potential health problems and can also be used as etiologies for other nursing diagnoses.

More recently, the concept of wellness and the individual's strengths have been included on the NANDA list of approved diagnoses (NANDA, 1994). The diagnostic statement *family coping-potential for growth* could indicate effective adaptation to change in the family structure due to illness of one member. A statement of specific *health-seeking behaviors* demonstrates an individual's desire to improve the level of wellness.

The diagnostic statement is further validated by coupling the diagnosis with a qualifying factor, for example, anxiety (diagnosis), severe (qualifying factor). Placing the diagnostic statement within the **P**roblem/need, **E**tiology, and **S**igns and symptoms or risk factors (PES) format provides a scientific basis and helps eliminate errors in judgment (Doenges and Moorhouse, 1992).

The client with severe anxiety related to a cardiac condition may be at risk for further alteration in cardiac tissue perfusion, an increase in pain intensity, and impaired gas exchange, which can, in turn, lead to an overwhelming state of anxiety. The client's anxiety may trigger a fear about dying or helplessness and contribute to total unhealthy mind-body responses.

■ ■ ■ OUTCOME IDENTIFICATION

"Outcomes are identified from the diagnoses" (McFarland and McFarlane, 1993). One or more expected client outcomes may be identified for each nursing diagnosis and can be physiologic, psychologic, sociocultural, or spiritual. Expected outcomes should be stated as desirable client health states, specific, and in measurable terms. Outcomes are used to assist in the planning, intervention, and evaluation processes—for example, "The client will be able to express feelings about the effects of the recent myocardial infarction on future lifestyle" and "The client will recognize the relationship between his feelings of anxiety and the occurrence and intensity of pain." Other examples of expected outcomes for the cardiac client would include the increase of the client's knowledge regarding benefits of diet and exercise, and stress reduction techniques.

■ ■ ■ PLANNING

The planning phase includes establishing priority of needs, outcomes derived from the nursing diagnoses, and methods to achieve the stated objectives. The selection of appropriate nursing interventions to achieve the desired physiologic and psychologic outcomes is the next step of the planning phase. Interventions are based on scientific rationale and standards of care and are specific to the identified need.

Discharge planning and future needs are also components of the plan of care. Discharge planning begins when the person enters the health care setting. Continuity of care is essential as the client returns to the home environment. See Nursing Care in the Community on page 000 for specific issues.

■ ■ ■ ■ IMPLEMENTATION

During this phase, the nurse carries out the identified interventions. A carefully constructed plan must also allow for some flexibility. Therefore, the nurse is constantly monitoring the client's total response to the interventions. An analysis of these findings aids in making modifications or revisions to the plan of care.

Time constraints, interruptions, and other factors can limit the effectiveness of the nurse's intervention. Therefore, to assure continuity of care, the implementation phase requires careful and concise documentation and appropriate reporting to other health care team members regarding progress in meeting the desired goals.

■ ■ ■ ■ ■ EVALUATION

This phase determines the appropriateness of the interventions and the client's progress or lack of progress in meeting the expected outcomes. The process requires a continual reassessment. Positive reinforcement and

---

Nursing Care in the Community

Psychologic Aspects of Physiologic Illness

When a person who continues to be somewhat debilitated returns home from the hospital, family dynamics are affected in multiple ways. Even the return of a woman after childbirth may have disruptive effects on a functioning family. The client's perception of his or her level of functioning must be compared with the family's perception of the client's needs. If too great a disparity exists, the client may deplete his or her reserves of strength while trying to live up to expectations. Or the family may try to do too much and undermine the client's sense of autonomy. In either case, the community nurse may act as a facilitator of communication, able to assist each side to have a realistic understanding of the client's medical situation and possibilities. Such an intervention may prevent the further debilitating effects of depression, whether postpartum or due to a weakened condition.

Chronic physiologic illnesses often are not only disabling in themselves but also may inspire such frustration in the client that depression and suicidal behavior often result. This is a disturbing problem for the mental health nurse working in the community. Not only does the client require support and encouragement as a result of physical symptoms, but the nurse must be constantly mindful of the state of the client's mental health. Emotional states are often labile, as physical symptoms vary. The client may present a positive affect to cover unacknowledged depression. Assessment may require probing questions if the client's mood is inconsistent with his or her physical condition. Therapeutic inquiries can often be successfully interjected when offering information about the client's physical condition itself or about medication and potential side effects.

Factors that seem to be important in the client sustaining a relatively positive state of mind are the client's perceived degree of autonomy, his or her successful efforts to reduce stress, and minimal secondary gains from the maintenance of the helpless attitude. The client should always be allowed to do as much as possible for himself or herself with frequent offers of assistance. The client should make decisions as a part of the treatment team and be given as much information as possible about available options. Stress reduction techniques such as imagery or biofeedback should be taught to minimize tension. Physical contact such as hobbies or reading can be explored and encouraged. The nurse should model giving positive attention frequently to encourage interaction and minimize demanding behavior for the routine caregivers.

Box 29-3   Case Study: Woman with Terminal Illness

Anh Huynh, a 68-year-old Chinese/Vietnamese female with metastatic cancer of the cervix, is now in terminal stages after surgery two years ago and radium implant. She was admitted to the hospital for colostomy surgery and pain relief. She has been in the United States approximately 10 years, but does not speak English. Her husband speaks little English; some family members are able to speak, write, and read English. Her religious beliefs are Buddhist, but she has no local affiliation. Her diet consists of typical oriental foods. The figure below depicts several stressors and the phases of the nursing process in outlining the plan of care.

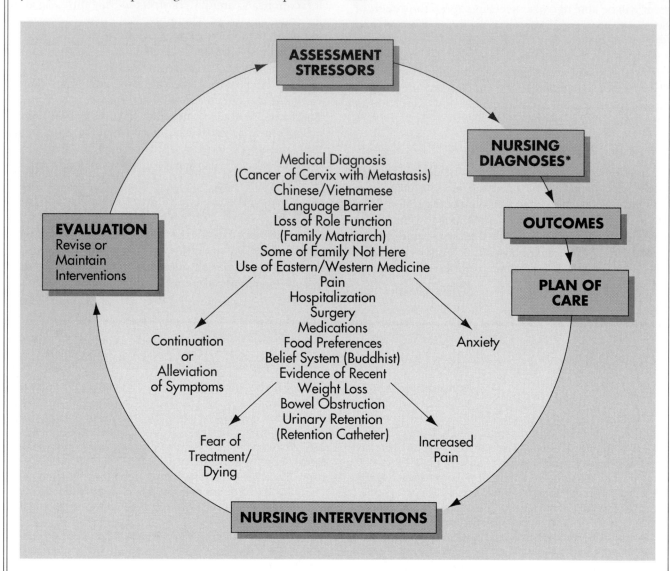

*Nursing Diagnoses include (but not limited to):

- anxiety
- impaired communication
- pain
- knowledge deficit related to diagnosis and treatment
- fear
- powerlessness
- social interaction impaired
- spiritual distress
- body image disturbance
- ineffective individual coping
- altered family processes
- altered nutrition: less than body requirements
- anticipatory grieving
- elimination (urinary and bowel), altered patterns related to metastasis
- risk infection

encouragement are also part of this phase, thus allowing modifications to the original plan if needed.

New problems may arise during the course of rehabilitation. Assessment, new or revised diagnoses, and expected outcomes may be necessary. There may be a need for a referral to physical therapy, the home health nurse, social services, a support group, and so on. Priorities may need to be adjusted to meet the changing needs of care.

Planning for termination of nursing care is started when the desired outcomes have been achieved. Discharge planning for any unmet needs would assure that continued services would be provided. Follow-through measures are taken, and the client and family caregivers are given instructions in methods to enhance the recovery and health status in the future. All members of the health care team, including the client and family, should be informed.

In order to meet this challenge of the evaluation phase, nurses must possess a comprehensive knowledge of the balance and imbalance of human biologic and behavioral responses to stress. In addition, nurses must consider the impact of life events, social and cultural values, and belief systems on the individual in maintaining health and in adaptation to stressful events and illness (McCloskey and Bulechek, 1996; Smith and Selye, 1979).

Summary of Key Concepts

1. For centuries, Western philosophers considered the mind, body, and spirit as separate components or systems. The human being was judged as a sum of the individual parts.

2. Eastern philosophies consider people as one with their environment, not separate from it. Past and present experiences play an important role in human behavior.

3. A blending of Eastern and Western philosophies has brought about a change in health care practices.

4. A strong relationship between stress and illness has been substantiated through theory and research.

5. A person's response to stress is varied and includes an integrated multisystem response of body, mind, and spirit.

Choosing specific nursing interventions for a particular client is part of the clinical decision-making process.

In addressing the psychologic needs of a physiologic illness, nurses must be able to:

- understand the concept of stress
- recognize its manifestations on mind-body interactions
- know which factors alter resistance to stress
- formulate realistic plans to strengthen the positive influencing/coping factors
- implement actions to reduce the individual's stress
- educate the individual about how to control personal stressors, for example, cognitive "reframing" of stressful event, using diversional activities, etc.
- include client in decision making
- provide positive reinforcement for effective coping measures
- recognize own imbalances and incorporate stress reduction measures for self
- promote healthy lifestyle for self

Box 29-3 presents the application of all the steps of the nursing process to a woman with terminal illness.

6. Social support is an essential component in coping with stress and illness, and in facing death.

7. Coping measures can be labeled as effective or ineffective; ineffective coping can result in illness.

8. Certain individuals are at great risk for experiencing psychologic-physiologic health problems. These are related to acute, chronic, or multiple health problems; the elderly, the pain experience, terminal illnesses, and stressful occupations.

9. Current trends in health care demand that nurses and other health care providers be knowledgeable about alternative methods that help clients manage their lives.

REFERENCES

Abrams M: Alternative medicine, *Good Housekeeping* 99–120, February 1994.

American Nurses Association: *Nursing: a social policy statement*, Kansas City, Mo., 1980, American Nurses Association.

Barry P: *Psychosocial nursing assessment and intervention: care of the physically ill person*, Philadelphia, 1989, J.P. Lippincott.

Basmeyrian J, editor: *Biofeedback: principles and practice for clinicians*, Baltimore, 1979, Williams and Wilkins.

Benner P, Wrubel J: *The primacy of caring: stress and coping in health and illness*, Menlo Park, Calif., 1989, Addison-Wesley.

Berne A et al: A nursing model for addressing health needs of homeless families, *Image: J Nursing Scholarship* 22(1):8–12, 1990.

Black J, Matassarin-Jacobs E: *Luckmann and Sorensen's medical-surgical nursing: a psychophysiologic approach*, Philadelphia, 1993, W.B. Saunders.

Burns D: *Feeling good: the new mood therapy*, New York, 1980, William Morrow.

Buxman K: Make room for laughter, *Amer J Nursing* 91(12):46–51, 1991.

Carson V: *Spiritual dimensions of nursing practice*, Philadelphia, 1989, W.B. Saunders.

Chopra D: *Perfect health: the complete mind/body guide*, New York, 1991, Harmony Books.

Christian J: *An introduction to the art of wondering*, New York, 1990, Harcourt Brace.

Clark C: Death beliefs limit life span, *San Diego Union-Tribune* 1, 28, November 4, 1993.

Cousins N: *Anatomy of an illness as perceived by the patient,* New York, 1979, W. W. Norton.

Cousins N: *Head first: the biology of hope,* New York, 1989, E.P. Dutton.

Criddle L: Healing from surgery: a phenomenological study, *Image: J Nursing Scholarship* 25(3):208–213, 1993.

DiVosbugh P: Linking family theory and practice: a family nursing program, *Image: J Nursing Scholarship* 25(3):321–335, 1993.

Doenges M, Moorhouse M: *Application of nursing process and nursing diagnosis,* Philadelphia, 1992, F.A. Davis.

Emery G: *Own your own life,* New York, 1982, The New American Library.

Fawcett C: *Family psychiatric nursing,* St. Louis, 1993, Mosby.

Fortinash K, Holoday-Worret P: *Psychiatric nursing care plans,* ed 2, St. Louis, 1995, Mosby.

Gage M: The patient-driven interdisciplinary care plan, *J Nursing Administration* 24(4):26–35, 1994.

Glaser J, Glaser R: Perspective on psycho-immune response. In Adler R et al, editors: *Psychoneuroimmunology,* San Diego, 1991, Academic Press.

Grendell R: *Relationship of stress and illness for wife caregivers following husbands' cardiac surgery,* 1994.

Groer M: Psychoneuroimmunology, *Amer J Nursing* 91(8):33, 1991.

Hahn Y et al: The effect of thermal biofeedback and progressive muscle relaxation training in reducing blood pressure of patients with essential hypertension, *Image: J Nursing Scholarship* 25(3):204–207, 1993.

Heinrich K, Killeen M: A gentle art of nurturing yourself, *Amer J Nursing* 93(10): 41–44, 1993.

Kobasa A: Stressful life events, personality, and health: an inquiry into hardiness. *Journal of Personality and Social Psychology* 37:1, 1-1-, 1979.

Kozier B et al: *Concepts and issues in nursing practice,* Menlo Park, Calif., 1992, Addison-Wesley.

Krieger D et al: Therapeutic touch: searching for evidence of physiological change, *Amer J Nursing* 79(4):660–665, 1979.

Lambert V, Lambert C: *The impact of physical illness and related mental health concepts,* Englewood Cliffs, N.J., 1979, Prentice-Hall.

Lambert V, Lambert C: *Psychosocial care of physically ill,* ed 2, Englewood Cliffs, N.J., 1985, Prentice-Hall.

Lambert V et al: Social support, hardiness and psychological well-being in women with arthritis, *Image: J Nursing Scholarship* 21(3):128–131, 1989.

Lazarus R, Folkman S: *Stress, appraisal, and coping,* New York, 1984, Springer.

Leidy N: Stress in chronic illness, *Nurs Research* 39(4):230–236, 1990.

Leininger M: *Caring: an essential human need,* Detroit, 1981, Wayne State University Press.

Lewis S et al: *Medical-surgical nursing,* St. Louis, 1996, Mosby.

Lindgren C: The caregiver career, *Image: J Nursing Scholarship* 25(3):214–219, 1993.

McCaffery M, Bebbe A: *Pain: clinical manual for nursing practice,* St. Louis, 1989, Mosby.

McCarthy P: Burnout in psychiatric nursing, *J Advanced Nur* 10:305–310, 1985.

McCloskey J, Bulechek G: *Nursing interventions classification,* ed 2, 1996, St. Louis, Mosby.

McFarland G, McFarlane E: *Nursing diagnosis and intervention,* ed 2, St. Louis, 1993, Mosby.

Mella D: *The legendary and practical use of gems and stones,* 1979, Domel.

Miller J: *Coping with chronic illness: overcoming powerlessness,* Philadelphia, 1983, F.A. Davis.

Morris C: Relaxation therapy in a clinic, *Amer J Nursing* 79(11):128–129, 1979.

Moyers B: *Healing and the mind,* New York, 1993, Doubleday.

Murray R: Home before dark, *Amer J Nursing* 93(11):36–42, 1993.

North American Nursing Diagnosis Association: *Nursing diagnoses: definitions and classification, 1995–1996,* Philadelphia, 1994, North American Nursing Diagnosis Association.

Nuernberger P: *Freedom from stress: a holistic approach,* Honesdale, Penn., 1981, The Himalayan International Institute of Yoga Science and Philosophy.

Pelletier K: *Mind as healer: mind as slayer,* New York, 1977, Dell.

Phipps W et al: *Medical-surgical nursing concepts and clinical practice,* ed 5, St. Louis, 1995, Mosby.

Pollock S, Duffy M: The health-related hardiness scale: development and psychometric analysis, *Nurs Research* 39(4): 218–222, 1990.

Primomo J et al: Social support for women during chronic illness, *J Nurs and Health* 40(13):153–161, 1989.

Rahe et al: A longitudinal study of life changes and illness patterns, *J Psychosomatic Research* 10:355–365, 1967.

Reinhard S: Perspectives on the family's caregiving experience in mental illness, *Image: J Nursing Scholarship* 26(1):70–73, 1994.

Selye H: *Stress in health and disease,* Boston, 1976, Butterworth.

Simonton OC et al: *Getting well again,* Los Angeles, 1978, J.P. Tarcher.

Smeltzer S, Bare B: *Brunner & Suddarth's textbook of medical-surgical nursing,* Philadelphia, 1992, J.B. Lippincott.

Smith MJT, Selye H: Reducing negative effects of stress, *Amer J Nursing* 79(10): 1952–1955, 1979.

Taylor A: *Health Psychology,* New York, 1991, McGraw Hill.

Woods et al: Supporting families during chronic illness, *Image: J Nursing Scholarship* 21(1):46–50, 1989.

Yalom I: *The theory and practice of group psychotherapy,* New York, 1985, Basic Books.

CHAPTER 30

Persons with Chronic Mental Illness

Alwilda Scholler-Jaquish

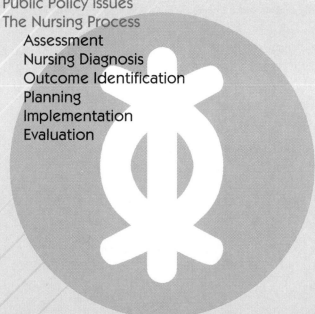

Anhedonia An inability to experience pleasure.

Chronic mental illness A psychiatric disorder that persists over time with remissions and recurrence of severe and disabling symptoms.

Chronically mentally ill Persons who have manifest the symptoms of chronic mental illness.

Chemical restraint The use of psychotropic drugs and sedatives to reduce or eliminate psychiatric symptoms.

Deinstitutionalization The process of returning psychiatric clients to the community, which includes limited admission and commitment policies.

Disaffiliated A person who does not associate with family, friends, or service providers.

Dual diagnosis A term used when the individual has two identified primary psychiatric diagnoses, most commonly used when one diagnosis is drug- or alcohol-related. For example, the person may have both a substance-related disorder and a mood disorder.

Idea of influence A delusional belief that one's thought processes are being influenced by an external source, such as radar, space aliens, or another person.

Institutionalization Placing or confining persons with mental disorders in state-run facilities such as residential treatment programs designed to treat such disorders.

Overselect Behavior commonly noted in children with psychiatric disorders. The child tends to be so specific about the stimuli that he or she selects to respond to, it appears as if there is no response at all.

Parasitic One's total dependence on someone else for one's every need.

Restrictive admission policies A component of the deinstitutionalization process that limits the length of stay until symptoms are under control.

Restrictive commitment policies A component of the deinstitutionalization process that limits commitment to a psychiatric facility for threat to harm self and/or others.

Restrictive environment An environment that restricts the activity of a client to assist the client in regaining control of his or her behavior. The individual may be placed in open-door or closed-door seclusion during periods of extreme agitation, suicidal ideations, or threats of violence to self or others.

Sleep reversal A state in which normal sleeping patterns are reversed; the individual sleeps during the day and is active during the night.

Transinstitutionalization A process in which clients are transferred from one institution to another, such as from a psychiatric hospital to a nursing home.

Underselect The inability of children with psychiatric disorders to select which stimuli is most important; manifested by inappropriate responses to routine events.

- Identify components of deinstitutionalization that have significantly affected people with chronic mental illness.

- Discuss psychologic problems manifested by persons with chronic mental illness and the impact they have on the client and his or her family members.

- Describe several behavioral manifestations of chronic mental illness and how they affect a person's ability to function independently.

- Examine the relationship between poverty, chronic mental illness, and homelessness.

- Distinguish between the behavioral manifestations of people with chronic mental illness in those who have been institutionalized and the young with chronic mental illness who have had few experiences with mental health treatment.

- Apply the nursing process to clients with chronic mental illness.

T he impact of chronic mental illness on the individual, family members, health care providers, and the community is significant. Although any psychiatric diagnosis can result in a disabling condition, most references to **chronic mental illness** (a psychiatric disorder that persists over time with remissions and recurrence of severe and disabling symptoms) address the concerns of the most severely disabled people (Birren et al, 1992; Krauss and Slavinsky, 1982). Persons with chronic mental illness pose some of the most difficult social, medical, and political problems of our time. Each individual with a chronic mental illness will have a different life experience. However, each person lives in a world in which he or she is expected to have relationships with others and provide for shelter and the basic necessities of life. The impact of the degree and frequency of psychiatric symptoms will affect the ability to function effectively in the world in which the person lives. The general public is supportive of the person who recovers from a psychiatric illness and is able to resume normal functions. However, people with chronic mental illness are often shunned by society and isolated from the community (Krauss and Slavinsky, 1982).

Nurses are the health care professionals who have the most frequent and most consistent involvement with the **chronically mentally ill** (persons who manifest the symptoms of chronic mental illness). Few people are so dependent on the compassionate and professional care provided by nurses as persons with chronic mental illness and their families. Nurses help the person with chronic mental illness to develop strategies for coping with emotional and behavioral manifestations of their mental disorder. The individual is supported during times of crisis and encouraged during times of remission. Nurses help family members cope with the challenges of living with a person with the behavioral and emotional manifestations of chronic mental illness.

DEVELOPMENT OF CHRONIC MENTAL ILLNESS

Chronic mental illness is diagnosed when it is believed that the person will have some manifestation of the disease process throughout his or her lifetime. The person with chronic mental illness may experience psychiatric transient and recurrent symptoms. Symptoms of chronic mental illness often are passed off as "odd" behaviors ("That's just her way") without recognition that these behaviors are clues to mental illness. Family members may tolerate a wide range of behaviors without clear understanding that an individual may have a psychiatric illness. Even treatment by mental health professionals in outpatient or inpatient facilities may not clearly identify the chronicity of the person's illness.

Chronic mental illness is often identified in retrospect. By the time symptoms have endured persistently enough for a major mental disorder to be confirmed, the individual may have had several episodes of symptomatic behavior. Looking back at the person's history of behavioral problems and symptoms, a pattern emerges that reveals the chronicity and impact of the mental disorder. Often the episodes were symptoms of a more comprehensive pattern of mental illness (Rawnsley, 1991).

Diagnostic Features

Persons with chronic mental illness have severe and persistent emotional disorders that interfere with their ability to live and function independently. The extent of disability has been defined by the National Plan for the Chronically Mentally Ill (Department of Health and Human Services, 1981). This definition includes disorders that interfere with the individual's ability to perform the activities of daily living, such as personal hygiene and self-care, self-direction, interpersonal relationships, social interactions, learning, recreation, and economic self-sufficiency. The most common chronic mental illness medical diagnoses include schizophrenia, mood disorders, delusional disorders, delirium, dementia, and amnestic and other cognitive disorders, and other psychotic disorders. In children, the most common diagnoses include pervasive developmental disorders, childhood schizophrenia, conduct disorders, and mental retardation (APA, 1994).

Effects of Deinstitutionalization

The Community Mental Health Act of 1965 was passed in response to many societal changes, including the advent of psychotropic drugs and the recognition of the effects of long-term **institutionalization** (placing or confining persons with mental disorders in state-run facilities such as residential treatment programs designed to treat such disorders). A combination of psycho-socio-political changes created the climate for change. From the psychologic perspective, it was clear that long-term institutionalization had negative effects on the client's mental status. New medications allowed for increased control of symptoms and more effective response to psychotherapy.

The federal law included the concept of mental health centers in the local communities. However, little funding was provided, and the number of centers was inadeqate to meet the needs of the numbers of people who were discharged from the mental institutions. Persons with mental illness were sent home to live in the community without appropriate treatment programs, and there were many problems associated with the **deinstitutionalization** process (the process of returning psychiatric clients to the community, which includes limited admission and commitment policies). Families didn't know how to cope, and many of the deinstitutionalized clients wandered away from their homes or residential treatment programs. Residents of local communities did not welcome the development of treatment programs in their neighborhoods for those with chronic mental illness. It has been almost 30 years since deinstitutionalization began, and there is strong evidence that persons with chronic mental illness still receive less care than they need (Aiken et al, 1986).

Young Adults with Chronic Mental Illness

Some of the deinstitutionalization components included restriction of admissions to psychiatric facilities as well as short-term hospital stays (Pepper and Ryglewicz, 1984). These policies have probably contributed to the development of the new phenomenon known as the *young chronically mentally ill*. These adults between ages 18–35 have the most severe, overt pathology. They lack internal controls, rarely take psychotropic medications, and exhibit excessive drug and alcohol abuse (Caton et al, 1989; Fischer and Breakey, 1986; Holcomb and Ahr, 1987).

It has been suggested that substance abuse is a form of self-medication for chronic mental illness. There is an indication that those with mood disorders are more likely to abuse cocaine, those with schizophrenia are more likely to use alcohol for symptom relief, and those with conduct disorders are more likely to abuse heroin and other drugs. Many of those with chronic mental illness are poly-substance abusers (Caton et al, 1989).

PSYCHOLOGIC MANIFESTATIONS OF CHRONIC MENTAL ILLNESS

The person with chronic mental illness will have numerous psychologic manifestations. The specific cognitive or behavioral manifestations may be associated with specific mental disorders as well as the individual's unique life history.

Altered Thought Processes

For the purposes of this chapter, altered thought processes will be considered any disruption in the individual's ability to solve problems and think clearly. Alterations may include hallucinations, delusions, or confusion. The alterations in thought processes may be transient, recurrent, or permanent. The recurrent and transient alterations in thought processes are a major difficulty that persons with chronic mental illness face in establishing independent living arrangements. One example is an **idea of influence,** in which the person believes that his or her thoughts are influenced by an external source.

Persons with chronic mental illness have limited skills in coping with the problems of day-to-day living. They lack skills in communicating their thoughts and emotions to others. Additional stressors can precipitate major disruptions in their ability to cope (Krauss and Slavinsky, 1982).

Chronic Low Self-Esteem

Chronic low self-esteem is a persistent problem for persons with chronic mental illness. Mental illness affects the self-perception and the ability to make sense out of life events. The delusions, hallucinations, and other negative symptoms of mental illness affect their memory, perception, and ability to think clearly. Persons with chronic mental illness are often excluded from social activities because they look and act different from others. They thus see themselves as ineffective and helpless; many are very much aware of their own deviance (Drew, 1991; Gerhart, 1990; Lefley, 1987; Rawnsley, 1991). Persons with chronic mental illness who experience small successes resist making further attempts for fear of failure or expectations that they could do more (Bernheim and Lehman, 1985; Krauss and Slavinsky, 1982).

Loneliness

Whether social isolation is self-imposed or results from avoidance of others, people with chronic mental illness are often lonely people. "Loneliness occurs when the need for intimacy is not met. It renders people emotion-ally paralyzed and helpless" (Copel, 1988). Some elements of loneliness include problems with social relationships, inability to make decisions, and a focus on weakness in self or others. Persons with chronic mental illness are often unable to express their feelings of loneliness and may withdraw further in fear of rejection. They experience a significant amount of distress in attempting to describe their feelings of loneliness. Loneliness is difficult for anyone, yet persons with a chronic mental illness are often unable to make the necessary changes in their lives or behaviors to break out of the experience of loneliness (Copel, 1988).

Hopelessness

People who struggle with major mental illness can experience an overwhelming sense of worthlessness and hopelessness. Worthlessness is an awareness that one's efforts are ineffectual or insignificant. Feelings of worthlessness diminish the person's self-esteem and increase his or her risk of depression.

Hopelessness is a feeling that there are few alternatives or personal choices available to them. The individual is unable to mobilize energy to relieve feelings of futility and despair (Fortinash and Holoday-Worret, 1995).

Depression

Depressive episodes can accompany other mental disorders, making the life of the person with chronic mental illness much more difficult. Depression has been defined as "an emotional state, ranging in severity from mild to severe, characterized by discouragement, sadness, worthlessness, psychomotor retardation or agitation, and varying degrees of inability to care for self" (McFarland et al, 1992).

CLINICAL ALERT !

Secondary depression that can be found following an acute episode of schizophrenia is a significant risk factor for suicide (Drake and Cotton, 1984).

Depression may be related to the individual's awareness that he or she is unable to cope with the world. Persons who develop chronic mental illness as adults and who have experienced relationships and successes in life should be considered at high risk for suicide during depressive episodes. When depression accompanies schizophrenia or Alzheimer's disease, the risk of suicide increases significantly. See Chapter 12 for further discussion.

Suicide

Suicide has been defined as the self-induced annihilation in a person who believes death is the best solution for his or her perceived problem. Suicide attempts in persons with chronic mental illness occur most often in persons with mood disorders or schizophrenia. Although persons with chronic mental illness may express suicidal ideations while in the hospital, they are more likely to commit suicide after they leave the nursing unit (Roy, 1995). However, any person with suicidal ideations or a past history of suicidal gestures should be considered at high risk for a suicide attempt. Chapter 26 discusses this topic in more depth.

CLINICAL ALERT

The return to reality is the stage during which there is frequent loss of hope for ever attaining the kind of life that the client's talents and intelligence entitled him or her to have. For some, this is the period in which successful suicide occurs (Lefley, 1987).

BEHAVIORAL MANIFESTATIONS OF CHRONIC MENTAL ILLNESS

Persons with chronic mental illness often have difficulty in self-care, personal hygiene, independent living, interpersonal relations, and employment. Assaultive behaviors and criminal activity can alienate them from their family and professional mental health services. These behavioral manifestations may be present in young children as well as adults and the elderly. The degree of disability will determine the extent and nature of the individual's behavioral manifestations. Persons with chronic mental illness who are on psychotropic medication in an inpatient setting may not exhibit the extent of disability demonstrated when they leave the hospital and resume living in the community. Persons who are noncompliant with their psychotropic medications may return to problematic behaviors once they return to their previous living situation. It is important to assess the extent and nature of the individual's behavior in the community, as described by the client and his or her family or care-givers.

Activities of Daily Living

Activities of daily living are essential skills needed to live independently. Persons with chronic mental illness often lack basic self-maintenance skills such as personal grooming, table manners, and social interaction skills. Their careless behavior may result from impaired judgment,

CLINICAL ALERT

Careless behaviors in handling cigarettes, sharp instruments, or hot liquids pose safety hazards to persons with chronic mental illness. These behaviors can be attributed to impaired judgment, forgetfulness, neglect of self, or lack of motivation (Bernheim and Lehman, 1985).

forgetfulness, or lack of motivation (Bellack and Mueser, 1986; Bernheim and Lehman, 1985).

The lack of these essential skills interferes with the individual's ability to be accepted in community settings. The inability to function adequately in social settings is a major factor in the poor quality of life that many persons with chronic mental illness experience. Persons with schizophrenia often have poor social skills and are frequently asocial (Bellack and Mueser, 1986).

Independent Living

During the deinstitutionalization process, it was believed that mental deterioration was caused by long-term hospitalization. It was not recognized that many persons with chronic mental illness are not fully capable of living in the community. More important, it was not recognized that such individuals would experience significant exacerbations during the course of their disease process (Belcher, 1991).

Personal survival depends on the person's ability to secure an income, locate a place to live, and maintain interpersonal relationships. Persons who live independently are responsible for obtaining food and clothing, and for maintaining their living space. A large proportion of the people with chronic mental illness are living impoverished existences and rely heavily on others for financial and personal support (Hogstel, 1995; Lurigio and Lewis, 1989).

Employment

Work is a key factor in rehabilitation of persons with chronic mental illness because it provides meaning and organization in their lives. However, many skills are required to obtain a job, such as transportation to the place of employment, completing an application, and negotiating an interview. Persons with chronic mental illness may never have acquired job skills or they may not be able to resume their former occupation. Once they secure a job, many are unable to retain it for a long period of time. The inability to obtain employment is a major difficulty for the psychiatric client and contributes significantly to the person's poor quality of living (see Figure 30-1).

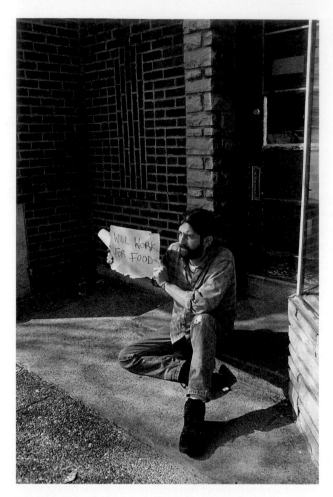

Figure 30-1 Persons with chronic mental illness are often unable to maintain regular employment and must rely on others for support.

(Copyright © Cathy Lander-Goldberg, Lander Photographics.)

Dependent Living with Family

The majority of persons with chronic mental illness live with their families. The person's presence in the home drains financial, emotional, and personal resources. Mental health professionals look to the family as primary support persons for individuals with chronic mental illness. Not all families are healthy enough to cope with the demands of the family member with chronic mental illness. In some cases, the family is dysfunctional and may be unable to provide the necessary supportive roles for the person.

There are persons with chronic mental illness who are married and have had children prior to or during the onset of the severe psychiatric symptoms. A spouse may be repeatedly hospitalized or maintained primarily on an outpatient basis. The unpredictability of mental disorders places an extra burden on the spouse and children. Some persons with mood disorders are able to sustain minimal employment however, they are unable to disguise their pathology from the family members, a dilemma which may be confusing for everyone concerned.

Children of persons with chronic mental illness are often at risk for mental illness themselves. The mental illness of a parent has a significant effect on the child's development. Unstable family life has been correlated with the subsequent development of chronic mental illness in the children. The children may also be at great risk for physical abuse. The home environment and the ability of family members to successfully cope should be evaluated by mental health professionals in any setting (Krauss and Slavinsky, 1982).

The behaviors of persons with chronic mental illness may be passive or hostile. Some individuals are **parasitic** (totally dependent on someone else for their every need), apathetic, and live in self-imposed isolation within the family unit. Others may refuse to take medication and reflect profound hopelessness and despair. Hostile, abusive, and assaultive behaviors may also be directed at family members. **Sleep reversal** (a state in which normal sleeping patterns are reversed and the individual sleeps during the day and is active during the night), running away, poor personal hygiene, and property damage are some of the most frustrating behaviors that disrupt the household (Bernheim and Lehman, 1985; Krauss and Slavinsky, 1982; Lefley, 1987; Steinglass and Horan, 1988).

Sexuality

There are two important dimensions of sexuality in the person with chronic mental illness. First is the normal sexual drive and the inability to discern appropriate sexual responses. Individuals with chronic mental illness may be sexually promiscuous or may be exploited because of their desires for affection and acceptance. Rape is not uncommon in women with chronic mental illness who may be unable to discern inappropriate sexual advances. Pregnancies occur during hospitalization, which result in additional stressors for all concerned. Second, there can be inappropriate sexual acting-out behaviors by persons with chronic mental illness. Individuals may masturbate or expose themselves in ways that are offensive or threatening to others (Bernheim and Lehman, 1985; Issac and Armat, 1990). Efforts to control offensive sexual behavior have included punishment, stigmatization, and chemical castration. The use of Depo-Provera can significantly reduce a male's sex drive and render him medically castrated.

Violent and Criminal Behavior

Persons with chronic mental illness commit a disproportionate number of violent or criminal acts, which reveals lack of judgment and self-control (Isaac and Armat, 1990). Violence by a person with chronic mental illness may pose a danger to family members or care providers. Children may be the targets of verbal and physical aggression. Violent behavior often makes community living difficult if not impossible. There is an even greater risk for violence in persons with a dual diagnosis, for example, when drug and alcohol abuse coexist (Bernheim and Lehman, 1985; Isaac and Armat, 1990; McFarland et al, 1989; Tardiff, 1984).

Many persons with chronic mental illness have had extensive contact with the criminal justice system (McFarland et al, 1989; Tardiff, 1984). People with mental illness commit crimes for a variety of reasons, such as poor impulse control and acting-out behaviors that include disorderly conduct, criminal trespass, disturbing the peace, and trespassing. Other persons with chronic mental illness tend to commit such crimes as shoplifting, petty theft, and prostitution as a means for survival (Lurigio and Lewis, 1989).

There are also those persons with chronic mental illness who commit violent crimes that pose a threat to public safety such as residential burglary, assault, rape, and robbery. Young persons with chronic mental illness who have had little mental health treatment are more likely to be involved in criminal acts of violence.

Many mass murders have been committed by such people who experienced hallucinations or delusions caused by poor impulse control and substance abuse. With the restricted policies for hospitalization, many violent persons are treated for a brief period and then released. Persons with chronic mental illness who commit criminal acts of violence are more likely to be placed in prison than in a psychiatric institution. Even in prison, persons with psychosis are legally allowed to choose whether they will take their medication. The rights of the individual and the goal of freedom of choice collide with the rights of family members to live without the fear of harm to themselves or others (Isaac and Armat, 1990; Lurigio and Lewis, 1989; Tardiff, 1984).

PERSONS WITH CHRONIC MENTAL ILLNESS WHO HAVE SPECIAL PROBLEMS

Within the population of people with chronic mental illness there are subgroups with unique and special problems that affect their ability to respond to psychiatric interventions.

Mentally Retarded Persons with Chronic Mental Illness

Essential features of mental retardation are an IQ below 70 with impairments in adaptive functioning that began before the person was 18 years old (Pipchick, 1994). Be-

havioral patterns include cognitive deficits revealed in concreteness of thinking and neurological dysfunction. Persons with mild to moderate retardation are believed to be more susceptible to mental illness. The conflict between the person's expectations and actual abilities may be a source of lifelong stress. In addition to a variety of personality disorders, the person with mental retardation and mental illness can experience affective as well as psychotic disorders. Depression and psychotic disorders are underreported in the work with people with mental retardation (Szymanski and Crocker, 1989). Treatment for this special population requires an interdisciplinary approach.

Person with Sensory and Communication Impairments

Individuals with sensory deprivations may experience many difficulties communicating with others when they are mentally healthy. The person with chronic mental illness who is sight- or hearing-impaired may be hospitalized much longer and receive less treatment (Dickert, 1991). Cases have been reported where hearing-impaired clients were institutionalized for many years before it became known that the individual's social deficits were not the result of mental illness. Any person with symptoms of chronic mental illness should receive a careful medical evaluation before a final diagnosis is made.

Elderly Persons with Chronic Mental Illness

Elderly persons with chronic mental illness include those who have had mental illness for decades, as well as those whose mental disorder was diagnosed after the individual was over 50 years old. Elderly persons who develop chronic mental illness may have an insidious onset that is not immediately noted by their family members or care providers. Depression is a serious problem in the elderly and requires appropriate intervention to reduce the risk of suicide. Schizophrenia is usually manifested during the early years of a person's life, and there are many people who have grown old with this condition. Nevertheless, schizophrenia may also manifest for the first time after age 45. Family members of elders with chronic mental illness may find themselves becoming a primary caregiver in a most difficult situation (Krach and Yang, 1992; Post, 1995).

Alzheimer's disease and other dementias are the most common causes of mental illness in the elderly. As many as 20% of elderly persons over the age of 80 suffer from some form of dementia. The onset of dementia is insidious and requires careful evaluation and diagnosis. The behavioral changes in the elderly with chronic mental illness are disturbing to spouses and adult children. Family members have concerns about the elder's safety as well as his or her memory loss and disorientation. As the person with senile dementia continues to lose cognitive ability, he or she may strike out in fear at family members who have become strangers. The mental deterioration of the elderly person may precipitate emotional disturbances in the spouse or adult children (Small, 1995).

Substance Abuse

Persons with chronic mental illness who are also dependent on one or more substances are among the most difficult to treat in either psychiatric or substance abuse treatment programs. Persons with a **dual diagnosis** (that is, they have two identified primary psychiatric diagnoses) have a high rate of hospitalization. There are many more persons with mental disorders who also abuse alcohol and drugs than in the general population. The coexistence of drug abuse and mental illness is associated with a more severe course of illness. Substance abuse can distort symptoms as well as diminish impulse control. Persons with a dual diagnosis often have unstable living arrangements and may act out in violent and criminal behavior. They have more difficulty organizing their lives and are prone to homelessness. Persons with chronic mental illness who have a dual diagnosis are more difficult to treat than individuals with one primary psychiatric diagnosis (Caton et al, 1989; Osher and Kofoed, 1989).

CHILDREN AND ADOLESCENTS WITH CHRONIC MENTAL ILLNESS

Chronic mental illness is generally considered a diagnosis that occurs in a person's adult years. However, many chronic mental illnesses have their onset in childhood or adolescence. For the most part, children who develop chronic mental illness at an early age will be severely affected throughout their lives. Many adolescents have manifestations of mental illness that may be recognized retrospectively. Chronic mental illnesses in children and youth have severe, long-lasting, and devastating effects on the children, their families, and society.

Children with Chronic Mental Illness

It is difficult to consider the realities of the children with chronic mental illness. The word *chronic* may refer to the anticipated length of treatment, a diagnostic category, or a set of behavioral patterns (Koret, 1981). Some of the symptoms of children with chronic mental illness include interpersonal problems, inability to learn or achieve at school, and behaviors that differ from the norm or are inconsistent with the child's age. These problems are generally long-standing and severe. It is often difficult to distinguish between behaviors of severely disturbed children and behaviors of those who are hearing-impaired, sight-impaired, or brain damaged (Kauffman, 1981; Koret, 1981; Silver, 1988).

Most children with chronic mental illness have no former level of optimal functioning to which they can return, because the basic components of personality func-

CLINICAL ALERT !

The presence of a child with chronic mental illness provokes affective responses in the parents and family members such as guilt, anger, sadness, frustration, fear and a sense of burden. Parents may become overwhelmed by the needs of the child with chronic mental illness. There is an increased risk of abuse in homes where the family members feel than can no longer cope (Silver, 1988).

tioning have never developed to a level approaching age-appropriate maturity. Unable to develop the prerequisites for growth, children with chronic mental illness tend to have deficits in every area of personality and social functioning (Koret, 1981). Their lives may be filled with frightening thoughts, constant fear of failure, and overwhelming sadness. They may fear their own aggressiveness or that of others. Children with chronic mental illness may frighten other children or even adults, because they may be viewed as real physical threats. These children may be difficult to be around due to their demanding, ungrateful, abusive, aggressive, or morose behaviors (Enzer, 1988).

Psychiatric disorders that occur in childhood include mood disorders, schizophrenia, conduct disorders, and autism (Caton et al, 1989).

The self-concept of children with chronic mental illness is poor as they often view themselves as bad or deficient, and many think of themselves as not entirely human. Their behavioral problems cover a wide range—from almost total withdrawal to acts of aggression toward self or others (Kauffman, 1981).

Adolescents with Chronic Mental Illness

Adolescence is a difficult and tumultuous time for many people. Young people in the midst of life transitions, hormonal changes, and relationship difficulties who also have a psychiatric illness can be challenging to their families and to mental health professionals. Mental illnesses may not be recognized initially as family members attempt to make sense of the young person's behavior. Psychiatric disorders that may appear during adolescence include schizophrenia, mood disorders, bipolar disorder, conduct disorder, and subtance abuse.

HOMELESS PERSONS WITH CHRONIC MENTAL ILLNESS

Many homeless persons with chronic mental illness have been institutionalized. However, an increasing number of the homeless are young people with chronic mental illness with severe psychopathology who also have problems with drugs and alcohol. Social conditions such as poverty and unemployment, combined with persistent mental disorders, often result in homeless persons with chronic mental illness who are unable to maintain stable living arrangements. Homeless persons with chronic mental illness may have a primary diagnosis of substance abuse. A significant number have a dual diagnosis, with one or more additional primary diagnoses (Cohen and Thompson, 1992; Fischer and Breakey, 1986).

Homelessness among people with chronic mental illness has multiple and often unrelated causes such as economic recession, unemployment, cutbacks in federal programs, **restrictive admission policies** (limiting the length of stay for inpatient psychiatric treatment), and a lack of adequate low-cost housing facilities (Baxter and Hopper, 1984; Bean et al, 1987; Belcher, 1991). A disproportionate number of homeless with chronic mental illness are members of racial minorities. The poor minority members with chronic mental illness have only their families or public institutions to provide care. Dependent adults can place such an enormous burden on their families that often the family must ask the person with chronic mental illness to leave. When forced out of their family home, these people often have no place to go except the street (Carter, 1991; Rossi and Wright, 1987).

With the increase in poverty and inadequate housing, the number of homeless women has increased. Homeless women tend to be young mothers with young children (see Figure 30-2), single adults, or older women with overt psychopathology. Even though there has been an increase in homelessness among women, only 15% of all homeless people are female.

It is estimated that 25% of homeless women have a serious mental health problem. One study reported that 41% of the women had a major mental illness such as schizophrenia or mood disorders, and that another 44% percent of the same group demonstrated severe anxiety disorders. Unmarried adult homeless women with chronic mental illness tend to have a history similar to the life experiences of men with chronic mental illness. These women have a high rate of alcoholism or substance abuse coexisting with personality disorders or other mental disorders. They may associate with one or more men for companionship and safety, or they may maintain a solitary existence living in fear of assault and rape. The older homeless women with chronic mental illness are **disaffiliated** (they do not associate with family, friends, or service providers) (Strasser, 1978). These women tend to be the "bag ladies" who carry their personal possessions in plastic bags, shopping bags, or grocery carts (see Figure 30-3). They are more likely to have psychotic disorders that may also be associated with alcoholism.

PROVIDERS OF CARE FOR PERSONS WITH CHRONIC MENTAL ILLNESS

Persons with chronic mental illness may live at home; in a community living arrangement with other persons with mental illness; or in an acute care hospital, psychiatric

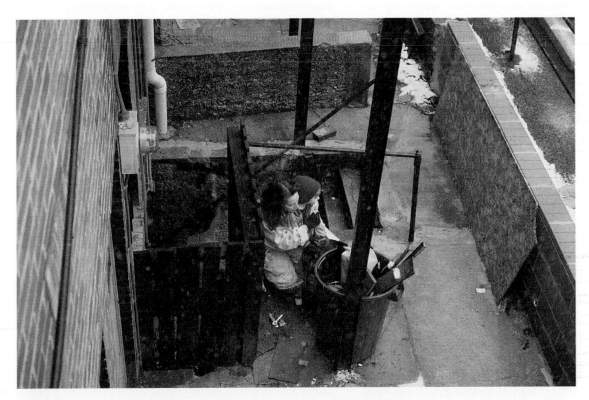

Figure 30-2 Many of the homeless are young mothers with young children.

(Copyright © Cathy Lander-Goldberg, Lander Photographics.)

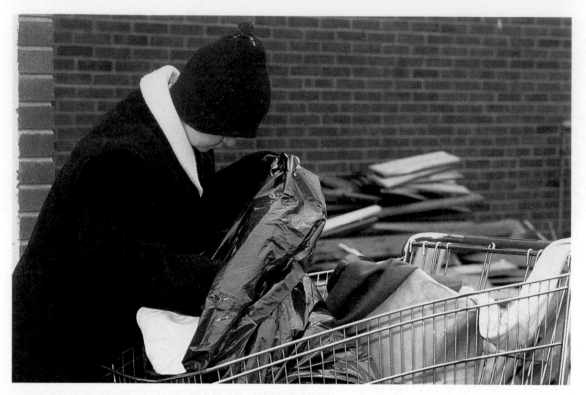

Figure 30-3 Many "bag ladies" suffer from chronic mental illness. They have few or no social supports and carry all their personal belongings with them in bags or carts.

(Copyright © Cathy Lander-Goldberg, Lander Photographics.)

institution, jail, or nursing home. In each case the nature of the care required and the care provided is different. It is important for nurses working with persons with chronic mental illness to be aware of the differences in care available in each of these settings.

Psychiatric Institutions

Despite the impact of deinstitutionalization, state mental hospitals still provide more than 50% of all psychiatric inpatient care. The restrictive policies regarding admission criteria and length of stay result in short-term institutionalization. Short-term care may be stressful and disruptive to clients with schizophrenia who account for the largest number (more than 70%) of hospital admissions in any year. There is a "revolving door" effect with a significant number of clients who are admitted for short-term hospitalization and discharged when symptoms are under control.

General Hospitals

As the state mental hospitals reduced their bed capacity, general hospitals began to increase their number of psychiatric beds (Bellack and Mueser, 1986). Hospital units that had been unlocked began to receive young persons with chronic mental illness as well as acutely ill psychi-

atric clients. Persons with chronic mental illness who were untreated or noncompliant in follow-up care were more likely to be psychotic and violent. They often required **restrictive environments** to protect them from harming themselves or others. A restrictive environment helps a client gain control of his or her behavior. The client may be placed in open-door or closed-door seclusion during periods of extreme agitation, suicidal ideation, or threats of violence to self or others. **Restrictive commitment policies** limit commitment for admission to a psychiatric facility to persons who threaten to harm self or others. These policies have increased the number of persons with severe chronic mental illness who must rely on general community hospitals for care. There are indications that changes in involuntary commitment laws have prevented people with severe mental illness from gaining access to appropriate psychiatric care. General hospital units have become locked wards to house people with chronic mental illness who were a threat to the safety of others (Fischer and Breakey, 1986; Pepper and Ryglewicz, 1984).

Aftercare

Aftercare programs include a variety of community programs and services from partial hospitalization to sheltered living. The kind and type of programs available in a specific community will depend on the size and nature of the community, as well as the community's financial constraints. Outpatient clinics are often associated with acute care hospitals. The size of the outpatient programs and the extent of their services will depend on the availability of reimbursement for services (Surber et al, 1986). Insurance companies may limit the number of days of therapy that they will pay for specific disorders.

A wide variety of community programs have been developed. Some include partial-care services with day care provided in an acute hospital and a return to the individual's place of residence at night. Partial-care programs place their emphasis on improving the capabilities of the persons with chronic mental illness (Marshall and Demmler, 1990). Other living arrangements include lodgings for four or more people. In some situations a manager visits the residence once a day or at other periodic intervals. Some programs provide for a live-in manager who helps the residents resolve interpersonal or household issues.

Homeless Shelters

Other types of community programs that provide services to persons with chronic mental illness include homeless shelters, soup kitchens, and substance abuse treatment programs. These individuals may consistently use the same program or go from place to place. Most service providers for the homeless have restrictions on serving individuals who are actively hallucinating, intoxicated, or displaying threatening acting-out behaviors. Persons who are noncompliant with the provider's rules are often refused admission or forced to leave the facility. Thus, some of the most out-of-touch persons are turned away from the only places that remain available to them. Persons with chronic mental illness who become disaffiliated from family, health care services, and providers for the homeless often suffer the full ravages of untreated mental disorders. Shelters may provide an evening meal, a change of clothes, and a place to take a shower. However, they have no staff or facilities to deal with psychotic or violent homeless people with chronic mental illness.

Foster Care

Foster care can be used as a temporary or permanent way of removing the child, adolescent, or adult with chronic mental illness from an unsafe environment. Children with chronic mental illness may be at risk of abusive behavior from parents or siblings. Adults at risk in their own homes may be removed to foster care to receive appropriate physical care and interpersonal relationships (Green, 1989b).

Nursing Homes

One of the results of deinstitutionalization has been the process of **transinstitutionalization** in which a person is transferred from one institution to another. Nursing homes were never designed to care for the client with chronic mental illness. They do not have psychiatrically trained staff to deal with active psychosis and must rely heavily on **chemical restraint** (the use of psychotropic drugs and sedatives to reduce or eliminate psychiatric symptoms). It is estimated that as many as 750,000 out of 2 million nursing home clients have chronic mental illness (Bellack and Mueser, 1986; Boyd and Luetje, 1992; Mosher-Ashley, 1991). Elderly persons with chronic mental illness who are admitted to or transferred to a nursing home may receive less care than those elders who are alert and aware of their surroundings. The former are at increased risk for behavioral manifestations related to inappropriate types or amounts of medications. Elders with chronic mental illness present the nursing home with the most behavioral problems and require specialized attention from geropsychiatric consultants such as nurses with advanced practice in geropsychiatry. Elders with chronic mental illness are also at risk for physical abuse or neglect from staff in nursing homes where staff members are not prepared or properly supervised.

Prisons and Jails

A large number of persons with mental illness are arrested, which poses serious problems for these individuals as well as for the prison system. Some individuals are arrested for minor offenses and may be held in the local jail. When it is apparent that the offender has chronic mental illness, the person may be referred to a state psychiatric facility for treatment.

Family members may find it necessary to have a relative with chronic mental illness arrested for violent or threatening behavior. In some situations, emergency involuntary admissions require that the violent behavior be witnessed by the persons making the arrest or signing the commitment orders. If that does not happen, the individual may be jailed for his or her mental illness rather than admitted to a psychiatric facility. Many persons with severe mental illness serve long-term prison sentences with a minimal amount of psychiatric treatment.

Family

The majority of people with chronic mental illness live with their families. The family members are key players in providing community mental health services. Family members are elected to assume responsibility for the client with little if any support, few resources, and no appreciation. The behaviors associated with chronic mental illness intrude on the lives of the family members and make extraordinary demands of them. The demands family members experience depend on their physical endurance and emotional health as well as the nature and intensity of their relative's chronic mental illness.

It is important to know that the family structure can provide the greatest support for adults with chronic mental illness. It is, however, a responsible position for the mentally healthy spouse and other family members. The family providers should be referred to self-help groups or for counseling to maintain their emotional stability. The Client and Family Teaching Guidelines below detail information a nurse should provide to the family.

Under any circumstance, it is difficult to live with a family member who has a chronic mental illness, whether he or she is hospitalized, acting out, or in an interval between psychiatric symptoms. Nurses working with persons with chronic mental illness must be aware of the needs and concerns of the family members (Riebschleger, 1991). (See Understanding and Applying Research below right.)

PUBLIC POLICY ISSUES

Nurses have opportunities to make an impact on public policies at the local, state, and national levels. National policies relating to persons with chronic mental illness must address the need for programs that are more flexible, comprehensive, and easier to access. There is a criti-

cal need for coordinated services with consistent financing at the city and state levels. Treatment programs in general, and psychiatric hospitals in particular, must be more creative in their approaches to treating clients with chronic mental illness. Individuals who are clearly unable to care for themselves must not be left to roam the streets without treatment and without access to psychiatric care. Persons who pose a threat to society because of their violent behavior require treatment in appropriate mental health facilities rather than criminal intervention that could worsen their condition.

One of the most acute problems facing persons with chronic mental illness is housing, because they vary in their need for supervised living arrangements. Provisions for housing in a variety of settings could be made available, including adult foster care and residential treatment programs. Adequate low-income housing could be made available for people with chronic mental illness who have low-paying jobs or those who subsist on entitlements alone. The lack of adequate housing is as severe a problem as the unavailability of adequate care (Belcher and DiBlasio, 1990; Lamb and Lamb, 1990).

Client and Family
TEACHING GUIDELINES

Chronic Mental Illness

Caring for a family member with chronic mental illness can be an emotional and physical burden for the caregiver. The nurse needs to educate caregivers not only about how to deal with the problems resulting from the mental illness but also about how to maintain a normal family life in the midst of the illness.

Family members should:

Be able to recognize behaviors and environmental triggers that precede a client's violent episodes.

Develop strategies to protect themselves and others from the client's violent episodes.

Enlist other caregivers to assist in the care of the client so the original caregiver can rest and relax.

Plan specific social activities such as sporting events, trips to the park, or other places of interest. Include the client in these as appropriate, given the client's condition.

Provide concrete directions for the client, using lists and schedules. Provide a consistent time to get up, go to bed, and eat meals. Restrict the client's time in the room alone. Encourage the client to participate in household activities.

Understanding and Applying
RESEARCH

Reinhard SC: Living with mental illness: effects of professional support and personal control on caregiver burden, *Research in Nursing and Health* 17:79–88, 1994.

The purpose of this study was to examine the relationships among professional support, the caregiver's personal sense of control, and his or her sense of burden and well-being. A convenience (random) sample of primary caregivers of persons with chronic mental illness who were enrolled in a community-based rehabilitation program was used for this study. Ninety-four subjects were interviewed using a questionnaire that measured caregiver burden, depression, professional support, and the caregiver's personal sense of control.

The results suggest that most caregivers felt burdened by their responsibilities. There is an indication that caregiver burden is associated with depression. These data lend support to the importance of professional assistance and personal control in explaining differences in family members' burden experiences. The importance of practical advice in helping families manage their situations was consistent with other studies. This advice reduces the sense of burden by enhancing the family's sense of control. Nurses should counsel caregivers to include respite periods in their caregiving role and emphasize the need for support for the caregivers in all their interactions with the family.

Access to care is an increasingly important concern. The individual's ability to access the mental health system may be limited by his or her ability to seek assistance, as well as lack of knowledge. Nurses can play an important role in advocating for increased resources for mental health care. In addition, nurses can educate self-help groups and other community groups about the nature and impact of chronic mental illness. The quality of the available mental health care is also a concern for nurses. Short-term, episodic care is not sufficient to provide adequate care for persons with chronic mental illness. Walk-in mental health clinics could be made available for these clients and their families. The clinics could monitor medication compliance as well as provide individual and/or group psychotherapy. Psychopharmacology alone is not sufficient treatment for persons with chronic mental illness. These individuals must also have access to psychotherapy to assist them with the complexity of their lives and their feelings.

Models for providing mental health services to persons with chronic mental illness vary according to regions of the country and resources available. Lehman (1989) advocates a comprehensive health team approach to address the variety of problems these individuals experience. A treatment team of professionals can provide more and better coordinated services than mental health specialists working independently of one another.

Special programs can be developed for the care and treatment of homeless persons with chronic mental illness. There are strong indications that programs available at locations such as homeless shelters or soup kitchens can be effective means to reach homeless persons with chronic mental illness. Nurse-managed clinics in shelters and soup kitchens allow for easy access to health care professionals (Scholler-Jaquish, 1993). These clinics could serve as a site for the distribution of psychotropic medications to help homeless persons with chronic mental illness increase their compliance with treatment and improve their ability to function in the world.

THE NURSING PROCESS ■ ■ ■ ■ ■ ■ ■ ■ ■ ■ ■ ■ ■ ■ ■ ■ ■

■ ASSESSMENT

When conducting an initial assessment interview with a person with chronic mental illness, it is important to be sensitive to the client's concerns. The establishment of a therapeutic relationship begins with the development of a sense of trust between the nurse and the client. The nurse should explain the nature and purpose of the interview and tell the client where the interview will take place and approximately how long it will last. The nurse must allow for as much privacy as possible. The nurse will use appropriate precautions when interviewing clients with chronic mental illness who have a history of poor impulse control or violent outbursts. Effective assessment will provide the nurse with information about the nature of the client's problems. Clients with chronic

Nursing Assessment Questions

Persons with Chronic Mental Illness

1. When did you first have trouble managing your own life?
   (To determine duration of chronic mental illness disturbances.)

2. What is the place like where you live?
   (To determine the person's current living situation.)

3. Are there times when you hear voices talking to you?
   (To determine the presence of auditory hallucinations.)

4. What are these voices telling you?
   (To determine if the voices are troubling or threatening.)

5. Have there been times when you felt life wasn't worth living?
   (To determine the presence of hopelessness and depression.)

6. Have there been times when you were so excited you could hardly contain yourself?
   (To determine the presence of mania.)

7. Have there been times when you thought about hurting yourself or someone else?
   (To determine patterns of violence to self or others.)

mental illness often have unidentified medical problems or problems that have been neglected as a result of the individual's disordered lifestyle. Thus, it is critical to conduct a thorough assessment of these clients, as each person will present a unique set of nursing problems (Box 30-1).

■ ■ NURSING DIAGNOSES

Nursing diagnosis is a process used to interpret the data collected during assessment phase. Nursing diagnoses are statements that describe an individual's health state or alteration in a person's life processes.

NANDA Diagnosis for Persons with Chronic Mental Illness

Safety and/or health risks

> Risk for violence: self and/or other directed
> Risk for self-mutilation
> Risk for injury
> Self-care deficit: bathing, hygiene, dressing, grooming
> Altered nutrition less than body requirements
> Alterations in health maintenance

Perceptual/cognitive disturbances

> Anxiety
> Fear
> Hopelessness
> Powerlessness
> Chronic low self-esteem
> Sensory/perceptual disturbance (hallucinations)
> Altered thought processes (delusions)
> Impaired problem solving
> Alterations in personal identity
> Fear

Problems in communicating and relating to others

> Impaired verbal communication
> Social isolation
> Impaired social interaction
> Altered growth and development
> Altered sexuality patterns

Disturbances in coping abilities (client and/or family)

> Ineffective individual coping
> Ineffective family coping: disabling or compromised
> Defensive coping
> Ineffective denial

Box 30-1   Assessment of Clients with Chronic Mental Illness

Physiologic Disturbances

Physical integrity

The nurse will examine the client to determine if there is evidence of impaired skin integrity such as abrasions, bruises, lacerations, scars, and needle puncture sites. Abrasions and bruises may indicate that the client with chronic mental illness was subjected to self-inflicted injury or trauma prior to admission. Determine if the injuries are recent or nearly healed and the nature and source of the injuries. When examining abrasions and bruises, it always important to determine if infection or inflammation is present. If there is a history suggestive of trauma or violence, it is important to carefully inspect the client's body surface for additional injuries.

Hormonal/metabolic patterns

Children with chronic mental illness may have inborn errors of metabolism. This information may be obtained through the client's history or from observing the child's physical characteristics. Does the client have a history of diabetes mellitus or kidney disease? Female clients should be assessed for their menstrual patterns. In each of these areas of concern, the nurse will want to know if the client is taking any medications for metabolic or hormonal disturbances.

Circulation

The nurse will assess the client's medical record for indications of neurologic changes and cardiac status.

Nutrition

Assessment of the client's nutritional history and present status is important as many persons with chronic mental illness live a disorganized and confused lifestyle in which their nutritional intake may be significantly altered.

Physical regulation

Assessment of physical regulation will include the client's temperature and the potential for infection. The medication history for persons with chronic mental illness is important. It is necessary to know the nature and type of medications that the client has been prescribed and his or her compliance in taking the medications. Disturbances of the immune system should also be evaluated at this time.

Oxygenation

Assessment of the client's respiratory system will include evidence of dyspnea, cough, or labored breathing. It must be determined if the client smokes, how long he or she has been smoking, and the number of cigarettes smoked each day.

Elimination

It is essential to know if the client has normal elimination habits. The nurse will want to know if the client has difficulties in handling urine or stool, or ritualistic behaviors associated with elimination. The client's urine can also be screened for nonprescription drugs and psychotropic medications.

Box 30-1   Assessment of Clients with Chronic Mental Illness—cont'd

Mobility Disturbances

Activity

The nature and extent of the client's activity provide important information for the nurse. The presence of any physical disability such as paralysis or fractures will affect the development of the nursing care plan. The nurse will want to know if there are gait disturbances, tremors, or ritualistic behavior associated with moving from place to place. The client with chronic mental illness may demonstrate lethargic movements or may be hyperactive and move rapidly from place to place. Lethargy may be related to major depression or catatonic features of schizophrenia. Hyperactivity may be related to agitation associated with anxiety, hallucinations, paranoid delusions, or other mental or neurologic disorders.

Rest

The person with chronic mental illness may have developed sleeping patterns that differ from the norm. They may exhibit sleep reversal, (sleeping during the daytime and being awake during the night). Assess the person's ability to fall asleep and remain asleep. Individuals who have difficulty falling asleep may have symptoms of depression or psychomotor agitation.

Recreation

Individuals with chronic mental illness may have a significant deficit in diversional activities. The person is often so preoccupied with symptoms of his or her mental disorder or the effort to get through each day that he or she leads a dull and uninteresting existence.

Environmental maintenance

The nurse's assessment of the client's ability to manage his or her living arrangement will provide important cues about the plan of care during treatment as well as for discharge planning. If the person lives in a group situation, the nurse will want to know the extent to which he or she participates in maintaining individual and shared living space.

One of the very important components of this section includes assessing the individual's risk factor for injury, violence, and the possession of weapons. Persons with chronic mental illness may be at risk for harming themselves or others. Suicide rates are very high in persons with chronic mental illness, so the nurse will want to assess for suicidal ideations, gestures, or attempts. In assessing suicidal ideations or attempts, the nurse will want to know what method the individual used. Also determine the person's availability of weapons and firearms.

Self-care

The ability of persons with chronic mental illness to perform activities of daily living such as personal hygiene and grooming may be significantly impaired. When these individuals have significant self-care deficits, they may not bathe or clean themselves appropriately.

Communication Disturbances

Verbal communication

In times of illness and stress, bilingual individuals often resort to their native language or may speak in a combined dialect that seems disordered and confused. The presence of speech impairments related to physical defects will provide the nurse with important cues. Verbal symptoms of psychiatric disorders include perseveration, circumstantiality, punning, rhyming, echolalia, mutism, word salad, cryptic language, symbolic references, neologisms, poverty of content, confabulation, and logorrhea.

Nonverbal communication

Nonverbal disturbances include posture, manner of dress, and gestures. Persons with chronic mental illness may crouch on the floor, pace back and forth, or retreat from others. Their ability to make and hold eye contact provides the nurse with important cues. Gestures may include ritualistic movements, striking themselves, or striking out at others. Inappropriate sexual behaviors are also important to note.

Cognitive Disturbances

Orientation

Assessment of the individual's orientation to time, place, and person is essential data for the plan of care. The person with chronic mental illness may be oriented to all three parameters or only one; for example, they may know who they are and where they are, but not the month or year. Mental confusion can be related to the individual's psychiatric disorder, side effects of medications, or physical disorders.

Memory

The nurse will assess the individual's memory to determine if he or she has intact recent and remote memory. The individual's ability to demonstrate abstract or concrete thinking affects his or her ability to understand and communicate effectively.

Perception

The person's understanding of the purpose and nature of treatment should also be assessed. Some persons with chronic mental illness may not be clear about why they have been admitted to an inpatient unit.

Thought processes

The person with chronic mental illness may exhibit one or more thinking disturbances. These may include dereistic and autistic thinking, delusions, thought withdrawal and insertion, thought blocking, thought broadcasting, magical thinking, looseness of association, ideas of reference, flight of ideas, ideas of influence, and tangentiality.

Persons with chronic mental illness may have well-defined delusions such as paranoid delusions in which they believe that a force is attempting to control their mind or

Continued

Box 30-1 Assessment of Clients with Chronic Mental Illness—cont'd

to cause them harm. Obsessional thought patterns may take the form of ritualistic behaviors or may be manifested by an obsessive desire to control or possess another person.

Perceptual Disturbances

Sensory perception

The senses include vision, hearing, taste, touch, and smell. Any of these senses can be impaired by physical and mental disorders. Persons with chronic mental illness may have hallucinations involving one or more senses. The more common hallucinations involve the client's hearing sounds or voices.

Attention

The nurse will assess the client's ability to follow directions as well as verbal and visual cues. Evidence of psychiatric disturbance may include distractibility, hyperalertness, inattention, or selective inattention. The more manic the individual, the more likely he or she will be easily distractible.

Self-concept

The person with chronic mental illness will, almost by definition, have significant disturbances in self-image, self-esteem, and personal identity. Assessment for these disturbances includes statements of negative self-concept and negative self-worth.

Meaningfulness

Persons with chronic mental illness may have difficulty finding meaning in a life that seems purposeless and hopeless. These individuals may express feelings of hopelessness that their life will ever get better. In addition, they may express powerlessness that they are able to effect any change in their life situation. When a person expresses feelings of hopelessness and meaninglessness, it is important to assess for suicidal ideations.

Relating Disturbances

Role

Each person has certain role expectations congruent with societal norms. The assessment of the person's marital status and relationship with parents, siblings, spouse, children, and others provide significant information about the individual's ability to function in society.

Sexual relationships may be difficult for the individual to maintain. There are wide variations in sexual expression among persons with chronic mental illness. Some may exhibit little interest, while others may have difficulty controlling their sexual behavior.

Socialization

Persons with chronic mental illness often have difficulties in maintaining social relationships with others. Their ability to develop a meaningful relationship with people outside their immediate family is often significantly impaired. The age of onset of the mental disorder will affect the individual's ability to socialize with others.

Feeling Disturbances

Comfort

The individual's awareness of pain or discomfort will be affected by his or her physical condition and the presence of any injuries prior to hospitalization. Some individuals with chronic mental illness may not be able to describe their sense of pain or discomfort and must rely on the nurse or others to be aware of changes that could affect their comfort level.

Emotional states

Persons with chronic mental illness may exhibit signs of mood disturbance such as major depression, anxiety, mania, agitation, and fear. The emotional disturbances will be related to the individual's mental disorder(s). Include evidence of the way the individual is coping with emotional disturbance. Anger and aggression may be expressed through sarcasm, fault finding, domineering behavior, and the threat or use of violence.

Problem-Solving Disturbances

Coping

The coping mechanisms of persons with chronic mental illness are often inadequate or inappropriate for the situation. Defense mechanisms that may be exhibited include rationalization, conversion, displacement, regression, introjection, projection, denial, disassociation, symbolization, fantasy, or splitting.

Participation

The individual's ability or willingness to participate in treatment is assessed on admission and on an ongoing basis. Persons with a history of noncompliance may exhibit compliance in a controlled environment. The degree of compliance with the therapeutic regimen can be assessed by nursing observations.

Judgment

Disturbances in judgment are common among persons with chronic mental illness. Impaired thought disorders and disorganized living experiences affect the individual's decision-making ability. These individuals may exhibit indecisiveness or may make poor judgments about themselves and others. The severity of the illness will affect the degree of difficulty the person experiences.

Client and family teaching needs

Knowledge deficit (medication, treatment, symptoms)

Noncompliance (medication, therapy, aftercare)

Altered role performance

■ ■ ■ OUTCOME IDENTIFICATION

Outcome criteria for persons with chronic mental illness include short-term and long-term client behaviors and responses to treatment. Outcomes will be stated in clear, measurable, and behavioral terms, can be identified as expected or anticipated and, whenever possible, will include a time frame in which the client is expected to achieve them. Clients with chronic mental illness vary significantly in the extent and nature of their disorders. The following outcomes are not intended to be all-inclusive for clients with chronic mental illness.

Outcome Identification for Chronic Mental Illness

Client will:

1. Verbalize absence of suicidal ideation or plan.
2. Display consistent, optimistic attitude.
3. List several reasons for wanting to live.
4. Demonstrate self-care appropriate for age.
5. Initiate conversation with staff.
6. Demonstrate effective problem-solving skills.
7. Express sense of self-worth.
8. Demonstrate absence of delusions.
9. Engage positive relationships with significant others or identified support persons.
10. Verbalize feeling in control of self and situations.
11. Make choices regarding management of care.
12. Demonstrate absence of verbal intentions to harm self or others.
13. Demonstrate absence of violent or aggressive behaviors.
14. Communicate with others using appropriate language, tone, and speech pattern.
15. Participate in individual milieu and group activities without disruptions.
16. Demonstrate socially appropriate behavior.
17. Adhere to prescribed facility regimen.
18. Eat adequate amounts of different food groups.
19. Stop talking to self.
20. Seek staff when hallucinations begin.
21. Refrain from harming self or others.
22. Demonstrate reality-based thinking in verbal and nonverbal behavior.
23. Distinguish boundaries between self and others and the environment.
24. Use coping strategies in a functional, adaptive manner.
25. Demonstrate absence of overt confusion.
26. Demonstrate orientation to time, place, and person.

COLLABORATIVE DIAGNOSES

DSM-IV Diagnoses*	NANDA Diagnoses**
Schizophrenia, paranoid type	Sensory/perceptual alterations
Schizophrenia, chronic, undifferentiated type	Self-care deficit Social isolation
Schizophrenia, residual type	Altered thought processes Impaired verbal communication
Schizophrenia, catatonic type	Ineffective individual coping
Mood disorder: Major depression, recurrent	Altered family processes Risk for violence: self-directed
Mood disorder: Bipolar disorder, manic	Impaired social interaction Chronic low self-esteem
Bipolar disorder, depressed	Ineffective individual coping
Bipolar disorder, mixed	Powerlessness
Psychoactive substance abuse disorder (all types)	Hopelessness Self-care deficit Risk for violence: self-directed or directed toward others
Substance dependence Substance abuse	Risk for injury Impaired social interaction Altered thought processes Defensive coping Altered nutrition: less than body requirements Self-care deficits Ineffective denial Ineffective family coping: disabling Risk for injury Risk for violence: self-directed or directed toward others Altered thought processes Impaired social interaction Self-care deficit

*From American Psychiatric Association: *Diagnostic and statistical manual of mental disorders,* ed 4, Washington, D.C., 1994, American Psychiatric Association.

**From North American Nursing Diagnosis Association: *NANDA nursing diagnoses: definitions and classifications 1995–1996,* Philadelphia, 1994, North American Nursing Diagnosis Association.

CASE ⬦ STUDY

Joe was brought to the hospital by a psychiatric nurse who provides consultation to a homeless shelter. The shelter staff asked the nurse to see Joe, who was rocking back and forth on his cot. When the nurse spoke to Joe, he stated his name and date of birth. He said he had been homeless since he was 12 or 13 years of age, adding, "My family thought I was strange, and they sent me away. I found a place to stay in a junkyard. The old man that owned the junkyard let me stay there. He brought me food and let me sleep in a room behind his office. I stayed there until last month when the old man died. I don't have anywhere to go. I can't stand the noise of the radio. The radio plays in my head all of the time. I just wish it would stop."

Critical Thinking and Outcome Identification

1. Identify Joe's most immediate needs.
2. What might the hallucinations be saying to Joe?
3. What nursing diagnoses would be relevant for Joe?
4. What outcome criteria, based on the nursing diagnoses, might be established with Joe?

27. Sit through meals or other activities without agitation or restlessness.
28. Display control of angry, impulsive emotions.

■ ■ ■ ■ PLANNING

The nurse's knowledge and understanding of the complexities of providing care to persons with chronic mental illness are essential in the development of a comprehensive plan of care for the individual client. Each person with chronic mental illness will have his or her own history of mental disorders, previous treatment, coexisting medical illness, and current symptoms. Nursing care will address the acute and long-term needs of the individual and family members when appropriate.

It is important to remember that the individual's altered, disorganized thought process and/or mental deterioration may limit the extent to which he or she participates in the development of a plan of care. Many persons with chronic mental illness have been alienated from their families and live alone or live a homeless existence. For those persons, it may be necessary to include community mental health care providers in the development of the nursing care plan as described in the Nursing Care in the Community box below.

■ ■ ■ ■ ■ IMPLEMENTATION

The plan of care for clients with chronic mental illness will vary depending on the nature of the person's mental disorder, age, and physical health status. While the individual's mental disorder is long-term, the person with

Nursing Care in the Community

Persons with Chronic Mental Illness

The community nurse working with persons with chronic mental illness should encourage an ongoing relationship with the client and support the client's compliance with medication. Clients in the community whose disorders are in remission will have relatively smooth periods of adequate functioning, when it may seem that their disease is well-controlled and that they need only minimal contact with the nurse. During this time their strengths should be assessed and encouraged. However, this period may be deceptive not only for the nurse but also for the client. The client may begin to believe that the need for medication has passed and may discontinue prescriptions without consultation. Unfortunately, when medications are stopped, the person's thought processes often become progressively disorganized. Without a reality check from an aware and supportive person, the client with mental illness may regress to the point of needing involuntary treatment. The nurse in the community must monitor clients effectively, so that acute episodes may be avoided as much as possi-

ble. The nurse must be able to distinguish between chronic low-level functioning and an acute psychotic state. An essential part of the nurse's role is developing a relaxed and trusting relationship with the client and teaching him or her to recognize and report antecedent symptoms, thus facilitating early intervention.

It is important to connect the client to the outside world through meaningful participation in activities such as paid or volunteer work. Many with mental illness live lives of fearful isolation and need encouragement to venture out of their restrictive environments. Clients need to have confidence in long-term, gradually developing relationships, such as with a case manager, who can perhaps draw them into a group of peers for educational purposes. These groups serve multiple functions of social support, corrective feedback, and integration of individuals into the community. The community nurse should focus on supporting the client's efforts within the community, while helping the client to maintain a stable level of functioning.

chronic mental illness will be admitted episodically for treatment of the disease process. General hospitals provide short-term care, while state psychiatric institutions provide longer-term care. Nursing interventions may be applied in either setting. However, achievement of the goals may take much longer for persons with severe mental illness.

Persons with chronic mental illness experience impairment in their physical health, mental status, emotional responses, social status, and spiritual nature. The nurse providing care for the person with chronic mental illness will be challenged to prioritize a plan that addresses the client's most important needs. In addition to the manifestations of the disease process, these individuals need assistance with social interactions, self-esteem, knowledge of the disease process, compliance with the treatment regimen, and discharge planning. Family members or community mental health care providers must be involved in the discharge planning process to maintain a functional status over a period of time.

Nursing Interventions

1. Assess the risk of danger to self and others *to ensure safety and prevent violence.*

2. Encourage the client to alert the staff when self-destructive thoughts occur *to help manage destructive thoughts prior to acting on them.*

3. Orient the client to the milieu and modify the environment *to reduce situations that provoke anxiety.*

4. Provide positive feedback when the client demonstrates self-control *to ensure repetition of functional behaviors.*

5. Seclude the client during periods of high risk for harming self and others *to provide a safe environment.*

6. Educate family members about symptoms of noncompliance with psychotropic medications or exacerbation of the mental disorder *to promote knowledge, which may enhance compliance.*

7. Educate the family in self-protective actions from the client *to ensure family safety.*

8. Provide nonthreatening reality orientation *to decrease the risk of upsetting the client and initiating harmful reactions.*

9. Instruct the client in recognizing harmful or inappropriate behaviors *to increase the client's self-awareness.*

10. Assess for delusions and hallucinations *to determine the level of psychosis.*

11. Interpret the meaning of the hallucination or delusion for the client *to determine the intent.*

12. Instruct the client to alert the staff when hallucinations begin *so the staff can intervene and minimize their impact.*

13. Teach techniques to stop/reduce hallucinations, such as whistling, hand clapping, and loudly telling them to stop *to offer the client strategies to manage hallucinations.*

14. Praise efforts at controlling hallucinations *to reinforce the client's functional behavior.*

15. Work with clients to manage hygiene, grooming, and activities of daily living *to increase self-esteem by improving appearance and giving client the satisfaction of self-help.*

16. Assist in selecting appropriate clothing *to reduce the incidence of ridicule by other clients.*

17. Monitor elimination and bathing patterns and establish a routine *to encourage proper hygiene and prevent injury to bowel and bladder. Clients with psychosis often have trouble attending to activities of daily living.*

18. Set a regular eating schedule *to remind the client when it's time to eat. Clients with psychosis often forget or refuse to eat and could become physically ill.*

19. Supervise food preparation to ensure safety. *Persons with psychosis may be careless in food preparation.*

20. Assist with regulation of sleep/wake patterns *to promote healthy sleep patterns, because clients with chronic mental illness experience irregular sleep/wake patterns.*

    • Provide activities to keep the client awake during the day.

    • Encourage dressing before breakfast and staying awake all day.

    • Promote relaxation at night.

21. Listen actively to the client's verbal and nonverbal communication *to elicit the client's style of communication and to better understand and anticipate the client's needs.*

22. Encourage the client to engage in conversations with others *to promote socialization and decrease isolation.*

23. Teach clients anxiety-reducing techniques when they are experiencing impaired communication *to reduce anxiety when clients are having difficulty expressing themselves.*

24. Praise attempts to speak clearly and effectively *to encourage repetition of the client's clear, expressive behaviors.*

25. Enhance social skills, such as proper communication, eating/table manners, and social activities, *to promote the client's acceptability by others and increase self-esteem.*

26. Act as a role model for effective social interaction *to teach the client effective social skills.*

NURSING CARE PLAN ■ ■ ■ ■ ■ ■ ■ ■   ■ ■ ■ ■ ■ ■ ■

Bill was brought to the emergency room and admitted to the general hospital for psychiatric care. He had been treated in this hospital in the past and also had been committed to the state psychiatric institution three times in the past 10 years.

Bill was the fourth child and appeared to be normal in every respect until he had an onset of psychosis when he was 16 years old. He had lived at home until he was 28 years old and for the past five years had been living periodically in partial-care facilities and supervised residential housing.

When Bill ran out of his antipsychotic medication four weeks ago, he began to be belligerent and threatened another resident, accusing him of stealing his food. When the resident manager tried to intervene, Bill became upset and ran away. His family was unable to locate him until they were notified that Bill was in the emergency room.

Bill had been living on the street and in missions since he ran away. The police had been called to a soup kitchen because Bill was assaultive, noncooperative, and belligerent to the staff and others. Bill fought with the police until they were able to restrain him and take him to the hospital. He had been without antipsychotic drugs for almost one month.

On admission to the unit, Bill was actively hallucinating. His affect was flat, and his movements were slow. When approached by the staff or other clients, Bill ignored them or spoke in a belligerent tone of voice. He has no history of drug or alcohol abuse. He was unkempt, and his clothing was soiled.

DSM-IV Diagnosis

AXIS I   Schizophrenia, Undifferentiated, Chronic with Acute Exacerbation

AXIS II   Deferred

AXIS III Deferred

AXIS IV   Severity of Psychosocial Stressors = 5
          Serious Chronic Illness in Self

AXIS V   GAF past year = 50
          Current = 30

Nursing Diagnosis: Sensory/perceptual alterations, related to change in internal and external stimuli accompanied by impaired ability to respond to stimuli as evidenced by inattention to surroundings, misinterpretation of environment, hallucinations and difficulty maintaining conversations.

Client Outcomes	*Nursing Interventions*	*Evaluation*
• Bill will seek staff when feeling anxious or when hallucinations begin.	• Continuously orient Bill to the nursing unit and to the events and activities that are going on *to present reality*. • Use clear, concrete statements and avoid abstract concepts *to help Bill understand the message*. • Reassure Bill that he is safe and won't be harmed *to begin to trust the environment*.	• Bill sought staff when he was feeling anxious and told them how he was feeling.
• Bill will be able to hold conversations without hallucinating.	• Focus on real events or activities *to reinforce reality and divert Bill's attention from his hallucinations*. • Describe Bill's hallucinatory behavior to him *to facilitate disclosure by reflecting on his behavior*. • Determine stressors that may trigger the hallucinations *to assist Bill to begin to avoid or reduce his hallucinations*.	• Bill held conversations with staff, clients, and family without evidence of hallucinations.
• Bill will refrain from harming himself or others.	• Follow hospital's guidelines for chemical or mechanical restraint or seclusion when Bill is in danger of injuring himself or others *to prevent harm to Bill or others*. • Accept and support Bill's feelings underlying the hallucinations *to convey understanding and reduce anxiety*. • Set limits on Bill's behavior when necessary *to keep the environment safe for all clients*. • Encourage Bill to take medications *to control psychotic symptoms*.	• Bill did not harm himself and was not a threat to others.

NURSING CARE PLAN ■ ■ ■ ■ ■ ■ ■   ■ ■ ■ ■ ■

Client Outcomes	*Nursing Interventions*	*Evaluation*
• Bill will use techniques and activities to manage stress and anxiety.	• Praise Bill's efforts to use techniques to distract from or manage his hallucinations *to promote repetition of positive behavior.* • Provide a consistent, structured milieu *to promote trust, safety, and a sense of well-being.* • Provide group situations in which Bill can learn and practice activities of daily living *to increase feelings of adequacy.*	• Bill demonstrated effective use of techniques to manage his stress and feelings of anxiety prior to discharge.

Nursing Diagnosis: Social isolation, related to negative experiences of aloneness, sensory/perceptual disturbances, as evidenced by running away from the partial-care facility, withdrawal from the environment and others in the environment, noncommunicative, flat affect, and minimal or absent eye contact.

Client Outcomes	*Nursing Interventions*	*Evaluation*
• Bill will say that he is willing to engage in social interaction with others in the environment.	• Engage Bill in meaningful, nonthreatening individual and group interactions every day *to let him know that participation is expected and that he is a worthwhile member of the community.* • Act as a role model for social behaviors in one-to-one and in groups *to help Bill identify appropriate skills.*	• Bill said he was willing to participate in social interactions on the unit.
• Bill will participate in social activities with others on the unit including family, such as meals, games, and crafts.	• Help Bill seek out other clients who have similar interests *to promote more enjoyable socialization.* • Praise Bill for attempts to seek out others with similar interests *to promote continued positive socialization.* • Encourage Bill's family to call him on the telephone and to visit him on the unit. *A strong family network will increase his social contacts and promote self-esteem.*	• Bill participated in social activities on the unit and had social contact with his family.
• Bill will express pleasure derived from social conversations with other clients, staff, and family.	• Provide Bill with graded activities according to his level of tolerance *to gradually expose him to more complex social interactions.* • Provide opportunities for Bill to go on outings *to encourage a variety of more complex social experiences.* • Encourage Bill to engage in social activities that are within his physical capabilities *to provide him with successful social experiences.*	• Bill expressed pleasure in participating in social activities prior to discharge.

NURSING CARE PLAN

Nursing Diagnosis: Impaired verbal communication, related to ineffective use of language in interacting with others, altered thought processes, sensory/perceptual alterations, as evidenced by speaking minimally or not at all for long periods of time.

Client Outcomes	Nursing Interventions	Evaluation
• Bill will communicate his thoughts in a coherent, goal-directed manner.	• Demonstrate a calm, quiet demeanor rather than attempting to force Bill to speak *to demonstrate acceptance of him.* • Actively listen and observe Bill's verbal and nonverbal cues during the communication process *to demonstrate an interest in meeting his needs.* • Anticipate Bill's needs until he is able to communicate effectively *to provide for his safety and comfort.*	• Bill communicated his thoughts and feelings in a goal-directed manner.
• Bill will demonstrate reality-based thought processes in verbal communication.	• Encourage Bill to approach other clients to engage in conversations *to allow him to practice communication skills in a safe setting.* • Assist Bill to listen and engage in actual conversations with staff and other clients in individual and group activities *to encourage him to respond to reality rather than his own autistic thoughts.*	• Bill was able to maintain reality-based verbal communication with staff, peers, and family members prior to discharge.
• Bill will initiate strategies to decrease anxiety and promote meaningful and coherent verbal communication.	• Teach Bill strategies (for example, deep breathing, replacing irrational or negative thoughts with realistic ones, seeking out a supportive person) to use when he initially experiences impaired verbal communication *to decrease anxiety and to promote more functional speech patterns.* • Praise Bill for his attempts to engage in coherent and meaningful conversations with others *to increase self-esteem and promote functional speech patterns.*	• Bill was able to identify and use effective strategies to control his anxiety and to promote effective verbal communication skills prior to discharge.

Nursing Diagnosis: Self-care deficit, related to sensory/perceptual alterations, altered thought processes, as evidenced by withdrawal from reality and impaired ability to perform hygiene tasks, dress, or groom appropriately.

Client Outcomes	Nursing Interventions	Evaluation
• Bill will consistently perform personal hygiene, and groom and dress appropriately.	• Assist Bill with personal hygiene, grooming, dressing, and laundry until he can function independently *to preserve his dignity and self-esteem.* • Establish routines for self-care, adding more complex tasks as Bill's condition improves *to organize his chaotic world and promote success.* • Praise Bill for attempts at self-care and each successfully completed task *to increase feelings of self-worth.*	• Bill performed all self-care activities of hygiene, dressing, and grooming in an appropriate manner prior to discharge.

27. Praise successful social interactions or attempts *to reinforce positive social behavior.*

28. Teach the client and family about the disorder and symptom management *to promote knowledge, which may enhance compliance and reduce guilt.*

29. Arrange private meetings so the family can express special concerns regarding the client *to clarify confusion about the illness and provide opportunities for expression of feelings.*

30. Teach the family to recognize early behavioral signs and symptoms of the client's failure to take medication *to be able to seek early intervention, promote medication compliance, and reduce recidivism.*

Additional Treatment Modalities

Nurses working with persons with chronic mental illness will be involved in collaborative interventions with a variety of mental health specialists. Clients with chronic mental illness require an interdisciplinary approach during hospitalization, for discharge planning, and for follow-up care after discharge.

Psychotropic medications

Psychotropic medications are administered to reduce the client's psychotic behavior and help control anxiety. The most common medications used for clients with chronic mental illness are the antipsychotic drugs.

Medications such as Haloperidol (Haldol) and Loxapine (Loxitane) can be used for both acute episodes of psychosis and long-term management of the client with chronic mental illness. There is a high rate of extrapyramidal reactions with Haldol. Nurses should note any evidence of side effects and report them to the practitioner. Antianxiety and antidepressant drugs are also used for clients with chronic mental illness. See Chapter 23 for further information.

Group, occupational, and other therapies

The client with chronic mental illness will benefit from group therapy in which he or she has an opportunity to enhance communication skills. The group provides an opportunity to interact with others in a safe environment. Nurses and other therapists serve as role models for social interactions.

Occupational therapy can assist the client with chronic mental illness to coordinate movements and express inner feelings through art forms. The client can also learn new dressing, grooming, and homemaking skills. The occupational therapist is an important adjunct to the psychiatric nurse. Recreational therapy and movement or dance therapy can be an important asset in working with the client with chronic mental illness.

■ ■ ■ ■ ■ ■ EVALUATION

The nurse is expected to evaluate changes in client behaviors and responses to treatment and interventions. Outcomes should be stated so that there is a specified time in which the desired behavior will be evaluated. At the time of evaluation, determine if the client has satisfactorily met the desired outcome or made progress toward achieving the outcome. Note the date that the outcome has been achieved and that outcome identification will no longer be active. During evaluation, it may be decided that the original outcome identification is no longer applicable because of changes in the client's condition.

Summary of Key Concepts

1. Chronic mental illness is manifested by acute exacerbations and remissions.

2. Persons with chronic mental illness may have one or more mental disorders.

3. Chronic mental illness affects every aspect of an individual's life.

4. Many chronic mental disorders are first evident during adolescence.

5. Persons with chronic mental illness do not die from their mental disorder and can have the same life span as any other adult.

6. Young adults with chronic mental illness are more likely to live chaotic lifestyles associated with undertreated mental disorders and substance abuse.

7. People with chronic mental illness generally live in impoverished conditions.

8. People with chronic mental illness have normal sexual drives and interests, although they may act them out in inappropriate ways.

9. There is a high rate of suicide among persons with chronic mental illness.

10. Family members of persons with chronic mental illness experience a significant amount of acute and chronic stress.

11. Persons with chronic mental illness can be helped to control hallucinations and delusions.

12. Family members of persons with chronic mental illness can learn how to prevent violence and intervene in sensory/perceptual disturbances.

REFERENCES

Aiken LH et al: (1986). Private foundations in health affairs: a case study of the development of a national initiative for the chronically mentally ill, *Amer Psychologist* 41(11):1290–1295, 1986.

Akiskal HS, Weller EB: Child psychiatry: special areas of interest—mood disorders and suicide in children and adolescents. In Kaplan HI, Sadock BJ, editors: *Comprehensive textbook of psychiatry/V*, vol 2, ed 6, Baltimore, 1995, Williams and Wilkins.

American Psychiatric Association: *Diagnostic and statistical manual of mental disorders*, ed 4, Washington, D.C., 1994, American Psychiatric Association.

Bassuck E, Rosenberg L: Psychosocial characteristics of homeless children and children with homes, *Pediatr* 85(3):257–261, 1990.

Bassuck E, Rubin L: Homeless children: a neglected population, *Amer J Orthopsychiatry* 57(2):279–287, 1987.

Baxter E, Hopper K: Troubled on the streets: the mentally disabled homeless poor. In Talbott JA, editor: *The chronic mental patient: five years later*, Orlando, Fla., 1984, Grune & Stratton.

Bean GJ et al: Mental health and homelessness: issues and findings, *Social Work* 32(5):411–416, 1987.

Belcher JR: Moving into homelessness after psychiatric hospitalization, *J Soc Serv Research* 14(3/4):63–77, 1991.

Belcher JR, DiBlasio FA: *Helping the homeless: where do we go from here?* Lexington, Mass., 1990, Lexington Books.

Bellack AS, Mueser KT: A comprehensive treatment program for schizophrenia and chronic mental illness, *Comm Mental Health J* 22(3):174–189, 1986.

Benda BB: Crime, drug abuse and mental illness: a comparison of homeless men and women, *J Soc Serv Research* 13(30): 39–60, 1990.

Bernheim KF, Lehman AF: *Working with families of the mentally ill,* New York, 1985, W.W. Norton.

Birren JE et al: *Handbook of mental health and aging,* ed 2, San Diego, 1992, Academic Press.

Boyd MA, Luetje V: The individual who is severely and persistently mentally ill: directions for research and practice, *Issues in Mental Health Nurs* 13:207–218, 1992.

Breakey WR et al: Health and mental health problems of homeless men and women in Baltimore, *JAMA* 262(1):1352–1357, 1989.

Brooks GW: Vocational rehabilitation. In Talbott JA, editor: *The chronic mentally ill: treatment, programs, systems,* New York, 1981, Human Sciences Press.

Carter JH: Chronic mental illness and homelessness in black populations: prologue and perspects, *J Nat Med Assoc* 83:313–317, 1991.

Caton CLM et al: Young chronic clients and substance abuse, *Hosp Commun Psychiatry* 40(10):1037–1040, 1989.

Cohen CI, Thompson KS: Homeless mentally ill or mentally ill homeless? *Amer J Psychiatry,* 149(6):816–823, 1992.

Copel LC: Loneliness: a conceptual model, *Psychosoc Nurs* 26(1):14–19, 1988.

Dail PW: The psychosocial context of homeless mothers with young children: program and policy implications, *Child Welfare* 49(4):291–308, 1990.

Dennis DL et al: A decade of research and services for homeless mentally ill persons: where do we stand? *Amer Psychologist* 46(11):1129–1138, 1991.

Dickert J: Examination of bias in mental health evaluation of deaf patients, *Soc Work* 33(3):273–274, 1988.

Drake RE, Cotton PG: Depression, hopelessness and suicide in chronic schizophrenia, *Brit J Psychiatry* 148:554–559, 1984.

Drake RE, Wallach MA: Substance abuse among the chronically mentally ill, *Hosp Comm Psychiatry* 40(10):1041–1046, 1989.

Drew N: Combating the social isolation of chronic mental illness, *J Psychosoc Nurs* 29(6):14–17, 1991.

Enzer NB: The real problem: human pain. In Looney JG, editor: *Chronic mental illness in children and adolescents,* Washington, D.C., 1988, American Psychiatric Press.

Ferguson MA: Psychiatric nursing in a shelter for the homeless, *Amer J Nurs* 89:1060–1062, 1989.

Fischer PJ, Breakey WR: Homelessness and mental health: an overview, *International J Mental Health* 14(4):41, 1986.

Florenzano RU: Chronic mental illness in adolescence: a global overview, *Pediatrician* 18:142–149, 1991.

Forchuck C: Reconceptualizing the environment of the individual with a chronic mental illness, *Issues in Mental Health Nurs* 12:159–170, 1991.

Forte JA: Operating a member-employing therapeutic business as part of an alternative mental health center, *Health and Social Work* 16(3):213–223, 1991.

Fortinash KM, Holoday-Worret PA: *Psychiatric nursing care plans,* ed 2, St. Louis, 1995, Mosby.

Foster GW et al: *Child care work with emotionally disturbed children,* Pittsburgh, 1972, University of Pittsburgh Press.

Gerhart UC: *Caring for the chronic mentally ill,* Itasca, Ill., 1990, F.E. Peacock.

Goodman LA: The prevalence of abuse among homeless and housed poor mothers: a comparison study, *Amer J Orthopsychiatry* 61(4):489–500, 1991.

Green WH: Child psychiatry: special areas of interest—schizophrenia with childhood onset. In Kaplan HI, Sadock BJ, editors: *Comprehensive textbook of psychiatry/V,* vol 2, ed 6, Baltimore, 1995, Williams and Wilkins.

Green WH: Foster care. In Kaplan HI, Sadock BJ, editors: *Comprehensive textbook of psychiatry/V,* vol 2, ed 6, Baltimore, 1995, Williams and Wilkins.

Harris M, Bachrach LL: Perspectives on homeless mentally ill women, *Hosp Comm Psychiatry* 41(23):253–254, 1990.

Hier SJ et al: Social adjustment and symptomatology in two types of homeless adolescents: runaways and throwaways, *Adolescence* 25(100):761–771, 1990.

Hogstel MO: *Geropsychiatric nursing,* ed 2, St. Louis, 1995, Mosby.

Holcomb WR, Ahr PR: Who really treats the severely impaired young adult client? A comparison of treatment settings, *Hosp Comm Psychiatry* 38(6):625–631, 1987.

Isaac RJ, Armat VC: *Madness in the streets,* New York, 1990, The Free Press.

Kauffman JM: *Characteristics of children's behavior disorders,* ed 2, Columbus, Ohio, 1981, Charles E. Merrill.

Koret S: Specialized programs for the chronically mentally ill child. In Talbott JA, editor: *The chronic mentally ill: treatment, programs, systems,* New York, 1981, Human Science Press.

Krach P, Yang J: Functional status of older persons with chronic mental illness living in a home setting, *Arch Psychiatric Nursing* 6(2):90–97, 1992.

Krauss JB, Slavinsky AT: *The chronically ill psychiatric patient and the community,* Boston, 1982, Blackwell Scientific Publications.

Lamb HR, Lamb DM: Factors contributing to homelessness among the chronically and severely mentally ill, *Hosp Comm Psychiatry* 41(3):301–305, 1990.

Lefley JP: Behavioral manifestations of mental illness. In Hatfield AB, Lefley HP, editors: *Families of the mentally ill: coping and adaptation,* New York, 1987, Guilford Press.

Lehman AF: Strategies for improving services for the chronic mentally ill, *Hosp Comm Psychiatry* 40(9):916–920, 1989.

Lurigio AJ, Lewis DA: Worlds that fail: a longitudinal study of urban mental patients, *J Soc Issues* 45(3):79–90, 1989.

Marshall C, Demmler J: Psychosocial rehabilitation as treatment in partial care settings: service delivery for adults with chronic mental illness, *J Rehabilitation:* (2): 27–31, 1990.

Martin J: The trauma of homelessness, *Internat J Mental Health* 20(2):17–27, 1991.

McFarland BH et al: Chronic mental illness and the criminal justice system, *Hosp Comm Psychiatry* 40(7):718–723, 1989.

McFarland GK et al: *Nursing diagnoses and process in psychiatric mental health nursing,* ed 2, Philadelphia, 1992, J.B. Lippincott.

Menninger WW: The chronically mentally ill. In Kaplan HI, Sadock BJ, editors: *Comprehensive textbook of psychiatry/V,* vol 2, ed 5, Baltimore, 1989, Williams and Wilkins.

Morrisey JP, Dennis DL: *NIMH-funded research concerning homeless mentally ill persons: implications for policy and practice,* Albany, 1986, New York State Office of Mental Health.

Mosher-Ashley PM: Attitudes of nursing and rest home administrators toward deinstitutionalized elders with psychiatric disorders, *Comm Mental Health J* 27(4): 241–253, 1991.

Osher FC, Kofoed LL: Treatment of patients with psychiatric and psychoactive substance abuse disorders, *Hosp Comm Psychiatry* 40(10):1025–1030, 1989.

Pepper B: A public policy for the long-term mentally ill: a positive alternative to reinstitutionalization. *Amer J Orthopsychiatry* 57(3):452–457, 1987.

Pepper B, Ryglewicz H: The young chronic patient: a new focus. Talbott J, editor: *The Chronic Mental patient.*

Post F: Geriatric psychiatry: schizophrenia and delusional disorders. In Kaplan HI, Sadock BJ, editors: *Comprehensive textbook of psychiatry,* vol 2, ed 6, Baltimore, 1995, Williams and Wilkins.

Powers JL et al: Maltreatment among runaway and homeless youth, *Child Abuse and Neglect,* 14(1):87–98, 1990.

Price V: Runaways and street youth. In Kneerin J, editor: *Homelessness: critical issues for policy and practice,* Boston, 1987, The Boston Foundation.

Rawnsley MM: Chronic mental illness: the timeless trajectory, *Scholarly Inquiry for Nursing Practice: An International J* 5(3):205–218, 1991.

Riebschleger JL: Families of chronically mentally ill people: siblings speak to social workers, *Health and Soc Work* 16(2):94–103, 1991.

Rossi PH, Wright JD: The determinants of homelessness, *Health Affairs* Spring: 19–31, 1987.

Rotherman-Borus MJ: Serving runaway and homeless youth, *Family and Comm Health* 14(3):23–32,1991.

Roy A: Emergency psychiatry. In Kaplan HI, Sadock BJ, editors: *Comprehensive textbook of psychiatry/V,* vol 2, ed 6, Baltimore, 1995, Williams and Wilkins.

Scholler-Jaquish A: Health care for the homeless: RN to BSN education, *Nurse Educator* 18(5):33–38, 1993.

Silver LB: The scope of the problem in children and adolescents. In Looney JG, editor: *Chronic mental illness in children and adolescents,* Washington, D.C., 1988, American Psychiatric Press.

Small GW: Alzheimer's disease and other dementing disorders. In Kaplan HI, Sadock BJ, editors: *Comprehensive textbook of psychiatry/V,* vol 2, ed 6, Baltimore, 1995, Williams and Wilkins.

Steinglass P, Horan ME: Families and chronic medical illness. In Walsh F, Anderson C, editors: *Chronic disorders and the family,* New York, 1988, Haworth Press.

Strasser JA: Urban transient women. *Amer J Nursing* 78(12):2076–2079, 1978.

Surber RW et al: Effects of fiscal retrenchment on public mental health services for the chronic mentally ill, *Comm Mental Health J* 22(3):215–228, 1986.

Szymanski LS, Crocker AC: Mental retardation. In Kaplan HI, Sadock BJ, editors: *Comprehensive textbook of psychiatry,* vol 2, ed 6, Baltimore, 1995, Williams and Wilkins.

Tardiff K: Research on violence. In Talbott JA, editor: *The chronic mental patient: five years later,* New York, 1984, Grune & Stratton.

U.S. Department of Health and Human Services: *National Plan for the Chronically Mentally Ill,* 1981, Washington, D.C., U.S. Department of Health and Human Services.

Wagner J, Menke E: The depression of homeless children: a focus for nursing intervention. *Issues in Comprehensive Pediatr Nurs* 14(1):17–29, 1991.

CHAPTER 31

Community Mental Health and Home Care

Judith A. Strasser
Maryanne McDonald
Bonnie Neil Spangler

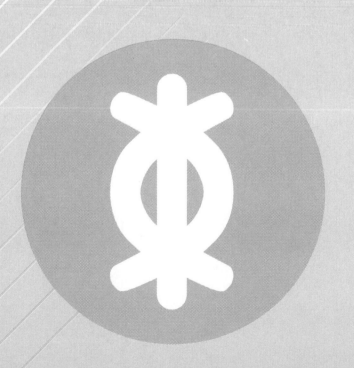

Case finding Methodical and deliberate identification of people of any age who are ill and in need of care or who are at risk for illness and injury.

Collegiality Working within a body of associates or colleagues, e.g., a team of home care providers.

Community-linked health care Care provided by public and/or private partnerships using grant and government funds.

Concentrated care Also called "intensive" care. Home care services delivered during a crisis, usually on a short-term basis, and designed to meet a specific, acute need.

Ethnomethodology The study of people in context or in their own surroundings through inductive, qualitative methods.

Intermediate care Home care services that are short-term and designed to help the client and family achieve a planned, higher level of functioning.

Maintenance care Home care services such as surveillance, client and family education, and emotional support which are provided when the client has reached a stable, higher level of functioning,. Concentrated and intermediate care are performed by skilled providers, and maintenance, by less skilled providers.

Transindividual perspective Looking beyond individuals to the family or community as the unit of care.

- Describe the relationship of the home care delivery system to the larger health care delivery system.

- Discuss the characteristics of home care services.

- Identify the various health care providers who may work in home settings.

- Explain the levels of care available in the home.

- Compare and contrast mental health services in the home and inpatient settings.

- Describe the competencies needed to be a successful clinician in a home care setting.

- Explain the phases of a home care visit.

- Identify cultural aspects to consider during a home visit.

- Analyze the role of case management in mental health home care.

- Discuss home visit safety issues.

- Develop a care plan based on the nursing process for home care settings.

Until the 1960s, most people with mental illness were still seen as a cause for family guilt, shame, and embarrassment, and were consigned to state or private institutions, prisons, or the streets. Some people with severe mental illness were secluded in their homes where they were cared for by family members and attendants for as long as the family could physically, financially, or emotionally deal with the situation.

With the development of antipsychotic medications such as Thorazine and new therapeutic interventions, and with the decreased availability of state institutions more people with mental illness required care in community settings. The community mental health center met some needs of clients with mental illness but did not meet the needs of providers who often worked in isolation from other health centers or hospitals. In many hospitals, care of people with mental illness was not given a high priority, and links with community psychiatric care providers were not always strong. At times this resulted in the alienation of psychiatric clients and their providers from the mainstream of health care delivery.

Today, the emphasis is on community-based or **community-linked health care** (care provided by public and/or private partnerships using grant and government funds), with an attempt to facilitate the maintenance of individuals in the least restrictive and most homelike setting. Such settings include (Figure 31-1):

- the person's own home, living with or supported by family or friends
- a home with a foster family
- a group home
- an adult congregate living facility
- an apartment complex designed for a special population such as the elderly who have mental health problems.

For some individuals, the least restrictive environment may be a nursing home, a correctional facility, or the streets (see Nursing Care in the Community on page 714). All of the preceding living situations can fall under the purview of "home care."

THE MEANING OF HOME

Home symbolizes comfort, security, independence, interdependence, love, nurturing, solace, and the "sweet place" where the heart is. We can feel at home with some people and not with others. Our homes can either

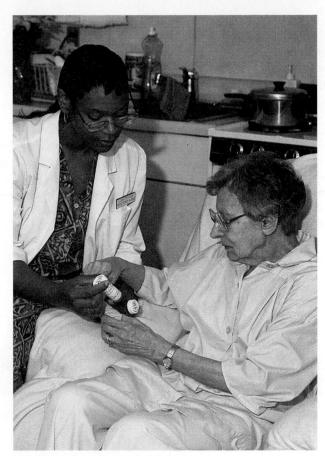

A

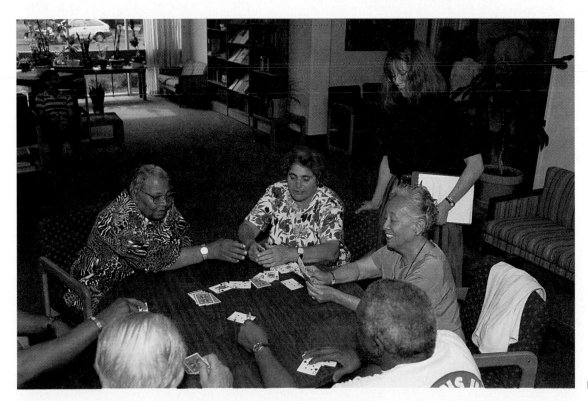

B

Figure 31-1 A, An individual's home, and **B,** a complex for the elderly are two examples of community settings that are within the scope of "home care."

(Copyright © Cathy Lander-Goldberg, Lander Photographics.)

form boundaries for perceived safety from strangers, or they can be wide open to relatives, friends, and neighbors. Bowers' (1992) study of the community psychiatric nurse in the client's home uses an ethnomethodologic approach to examine the home visit. **Ethnomethodology** is an inductive, qualitative method of studying people in context or in their own surroundings. Bowers found that the client-family-nurse interaction is dependent on the home setting. Because the nurse is a visitor in the client's home, the context of care is somewhat like the meeting of friends. The nurse is a visitor or guest, while the client and family or caregiver act as hosts. The home visit is influenced by the family's expectations of usual behavior when a guest visits. This change, from the institutional setting where institutional rules are followed, to the home care setting, requires expanded nursing knowledge and skills. For example, consider the client following a medication regimen. In the hospital,

the nurse administers medications to the client as ordered by the physician. At home, the client is the one who decides whether or not to take the ordered medications and when.

HOME CARE PRACTICE AND THE HEALTH CARE SYSTEM

Home health care practice occurs within the broader context of community health nursing. This has been described by the American Nurses Association (1986) and the World Health Organization (1991). While the community health nurse employs a **transindividual perspective** (looking beyond individuals to the family or community as the unit of care), the home care nurse focuses on the care of an individual in the home setting. Other individuals in the home, and friends or neighbors who are supportive people, are not directly assessed by

---

Nursing Care in the Community

The Correctional Connection

The enigma surrounding the care and control of the criminal, the dangerous, and people with mental illness has historically plagued society. Currently, the emphasis on community-based health care strives to maintain individuals in the least restrictive setting. Unfortunately, due to the persistent and challenging behavior displayed by many offenders with mental disorders, the least restrictive environment may well be a correctional facility or a secure mental health unit.

Nursing practice in this domain reflects the social, political, and economic ideologies of the community at large. Care and treatment of this group are particularly controversial, due to the folklore surrounding the "criminally insane." What constitutes humane care is defined by society and subject to changing convictions regarding offender worthiness. The public is generally not supportive of allotting more than the absolute minimum to the correctional system. Currently a "lock the door and throw away the key" mentality prevails.

The opposing philosophies of custody and caring result in direct implications for the community mental health nurse who chooses to work with an offender population. Nurses constantly "walk the line" between the requirements of security (i.e., protection of society), health care, and client advocacy. Finding the right balance between custody and caring requires ongoing self-evaluation and self-awareness on the part of the nurse.

Therapy issues with this population can be complicated. The orientation phase of the therapeutic relationship is frequently long and tense, and the nurse's sincerity and genuineness are often perceived as qualities to be exploited. Furthermore, clients may view the nursing staff as part of a much hated system and use them as a dumping ground for all their hostilities. Nurses must have a good understanding of the therapeutic nurse-client relationship, with particular attention to therapeutic impasses, transference, and countertransference. Team work is also essential to survival in the correctional milieu. Communication between nurses, other health care professionals, and the correctional personnel is vital to safe and professional practice.

Offenders generally demonstrate poor reasoning abilities and a history of not learning from past mistakes. These attributes, coupled with the stressors associated with mental illness, present the nurse with unique and complex treatment challenges. The nurse's primary focus in working with this group is largely at the tertiary level of prevention. However, nurses are actively involved in a continuum of care that includes both crisis intervention and the rehabilitation of offenders with serious and persistent mental illness. Specialized programming includes suicide prevention, management of self-mutilation, aggressive behavior control, sex offender treatment, and substance abuse management. Through these programs, a crime-free lifestyle is promoted in an effort to prevent the client from reoffending.

Community mental health nurses are also in an excellent position to assume more primary prevention strategies, particularly in relation to interpersonal and domestic violence. Partnerships with a variety of community agencies are necessary to bridge the gap between the judicial system and the mental health care system. These collaborative ventures are not only the answer to primary crime prevention, but also the answer to providing humane quality care to offender clients with mental disorders.

the home care nurse but are viewed as part of the client's support network.

Provider agencies in home care may originate from a hospital, a health maintenance organization (HMO), a health department, or a visiting nurse association (VNA). Spiegel (1987) describes four general agency types: public agencies, combined agencies, nonprofit agencies, and proprietary agencies.

Public agencies are operated by governmental units such as a county or state. Combined agencies are sponsored by multiple groups such as the government and a voluntary agency such as a VNA or voluntary hospital. Nonprofit agencies, which include community hospitals and medical centers, are designed for service; generated income is often designated to help run them. Proprietary agencies are for profit and are privately owned. Public/private partnerships using grant and governmental monies help provide creative, community-based, or community-linked health and welfare projects.

The Home Care System and Services

The home care nurse functions within the scope of preventive treatment and maintenance and generally operates at the third level of prevention, while the community health nurse may function at all three levels during a home visit. The levels of prevention are illustrated in Table 31-1.

Care Providers in the Home Setting

Often, nurses are primary health care providers for the person with mental illness in the home setting. The role of the home health nurse is to help clients regain and maintain optimum mental and physical health to return to their maximum health status. Skills unique to the psychiatric home health nurse include assessment of the clients' mental status and coping skills, establishing therapeutic and trusting relationships, and setting limits and providing structure for clients.

Other professionals may form a part of the health care team, and it is the responsibility of the primary provider to communicate with other members of the care delivery team. Other team members may include the case manager; psychiatrist; clinical psychologist; social worker; medical doctor; clinical pharmacist; psychiatric occupational therapist; community health worker or home visitor; and the physical, respiratory, or occupational therapist.

In addition to the official licensed care providers, family, friends, neighbors, and paid assistants or community workers often assume the role of supportive caregivers to the client and family. These supportive people are also team members, and their roles should be clearly understood by them and by all other team members.

Care providers working in the home often include a master's prepared psychiatric nurse specialist working in the home setting, the home health care nurse, the community health nurse, the practical (vocational) nurse, and/or the nursing assistant. Each of these nursing care providers has different clinical and academic preparation and provides services specific to his or her skills and preparation. The skill required by the coordinator or manager of care is to assure that the right person is in the home setting doing the appropriate activity for the level of skill needed and, collectively, that all providers focus on client problems, needs, goals, and outcomes. Vigilant supervision is necessary to monitor

---

TABLE 31-1   Levels of prevention in the community and type of practitioner

Level of prevention	Practitioner
1. PRIMARY PREVENTION	
• health promotion	Community health nurse
• disease prevention	
• specific protection	
2. SECONDARY PREVENTION	
• case finding	Community health nurse
• early diagnosis and treatment; prevention of complications	Home care nurse
3. TERTIARY PREVENTION	
• care and rehabilitation	Home care nurse

Case finding and referral form an integral part of all professional nursing practice and must be done when the home care nurse becomes aware of a health problem (finds a case) in any household. **Case finding** is the methodical and deliberate identification of people of any age who are ill and in need of care or who are at risk of incurring illness or injury. Referral involves locating and communicating with an appropriate clinical provider concerning the found case. With the found client the nurse may, in some instances, set up the appointment and arrange transportation. Follow-up on the individual's progress with the referral source is a part of the case finding–referral process.

the adequacy of the nursing service and the achievement of outcomes.

Levels of Care at Home

Home care levels have been determined by funding agencies, government agencies, and providers. These levels are based on the type of services (skilled or less skilled) and on the level of client status. Care can be 1) **concentrated** or **intensive,** 2) **intermediate,** or 3) **maintenance,** (when the client is stable and has reached a plateau). Box 31-1 provides a summary of these three levels of care.

NURSE COMPETENCIES AND STANDARDS IN COMMUNITY AND MENTAL HEALTH CARE

The Association of Community Health Nursing Educators (ACHNE), in its 1993 publication titled *Differentiated Practice in Community Health,* identified the skills needed for a nursing care manager in a community setting. The competencies are listed in terms of the three levels of care in community health. The competencies, outlined by the steps of the nursing process, are presented in Box 31-2.

The nurse caring for the psychiatric client at home is responsible for helping the client and family control or manage symptoms and behaviors related to the specified disorders. To do this, the nurse functions both independently and collaboratively. The nurse must be able to assess and monitor mental health status, evaluate the client's response to treatment, collect laboratory specimens and monitor results, instruct the client and family about the illness and coping strategies, and provide supportive psychotherapy. A basic foundation in family and group dynamics as well as in psychiatric disorders is critical for successful home care intervention.

Teaching and communication skills are required in terms of client and family education concerning the specified mental health disorder, coordination of care, and interfamily communication. Interacting with agencies and nonnursing providers to facilitate care is part of the nurse's responsibility.

The nurse in psychiatric home care should have previous inpatient and/or outpatient clinical experience. The nurse must be an independent practitioner with basic medical knowledge and skill. He or she needs a thorough understanding of the health care delivery system and the appropriate care required for each client based on the client's current health status and level of functioning.

THE EFFECTIVE HOME VISIT

The home visit is a therapeutic unit of interaction that involves preplanning, entry, the therapeutic process, exit, evaluation of outcome achievement, a review of process,

---

Box 31-1   Examples of Levels of Home Care

Concentrated or intensive

A client with a long-standing history of depression is newly diagnosed with diabetes and requires insulin twice a day. The home health nurse will visit the client to teach and assess his or her ability to self-administer insulin. Initially, the nurse visits twice a day and gradually decreases visits as the client becomes independent in preparation and administration of insulin.

Intermediate

A client with a long-standing history of schizophrenia has been hospitalized with anemia. The home health nurse will visit two to three times a week, for 8 weeks, to assess physical and mental status, medication regime, nutrition, energy level, and signs and symptoms of bleeding. The nurse will also monitor the client's hemoglobin level. The nurse will discharge the client at the end of 6–8 weeks if the client's mental and physical status has stabilized.

Maintenance

A client with a history of bipolar disorder and COPD for 8 years has received intermediate home health nursing two to three times a week for 8 weeks. During the initial 8 weeks, the nurse assesses physical and mental status, cardiovascular status, activity level, medication regimen, and energy level. By the end of the 8 weeks, the client has reached his or her maximum level of health. However, the nurse is concerned that the client may experience an exacerbation of COPD if home health services are discontinued. The client has been hospitalized six times during the last year. The nurse decides to discontinue intermediate level home care services and initiate maintenance level services. The nurse will visit the client once a week or once every other week for an additional 8 weeks to assess the stability of the client's health. The client will be discharged at the end of 8 weeks if no exacerbation occurs. If the client experiences an exacerbation of illness while receiving maintenance level care, the client will be transferred to the intermediate level of health care.

---

referral, replanning, and closure. Professional nurses have the added task of case finding and referral for other household members and caregivers.

Preplanning

The preplanning phase of a home visit consists of acquiring as much information as possible concerning the client, the client's diagnosis and history, and the clinical plan of care. Planning is conducted before the beginning of the first visit. The client must be prepared for the

Box 31-2   Competencies of the Nursing Care Manager in the Community Setting

Assessment: individuals, families and community groups

1. Perform complex screening procedures and interpret results.

   - mental as well as physical
   - level of stress
   - coping strategies
   - safety

2. Assess health, nursing, and personal care needs of groups of individuals and families.

3. In consultation with the master's prepared community health specialist, conduct community needs assessment through data collection, participation in prioritizing needs, and identifying populations at risk.

Planning: individuals, families, and community groups

1. Participate in planning for community intervention as an interdisciplinary team member.

2. Network with community mental health services and resources.

3. Identify the most appropriate outpatient program for client.

4. Organize nursing activities and delegate less complex level nursing tasks to individuals within their level of competence.

5. In consultation with the community health nurse specialist, develop appropriate health promotion and preventive services at micro and macro levels using data gathered through community assessment.

Implementation: individuals, families, and community groups

1. Assist client access/use community services.

2. Assist client access/use health care services.

3. Establish trusting and/or therapeutic relationship with client and primary caregiver.

4. Establish boundaries of relationship.

5. Set limits.

6. Establish contract with the client regarding the responsibilities of both the client and the nurse.

7. Organize, motivate, and guide other nurses and ancillary personnel in providing health care.

8. Provide direct care and leadership in managing clients with complex or high-risk conditions.

9. Provide case management to a primary case load of clients with complex or high-risk conditions.

10. Deliver health care services to groups, organizations, and communities with a focus on health promotion and prevention.

Evaluation: individuals, families, and community groups

1. Participate in evaluation of outcomes of community-focused care.

2. Monitor the effectiveness of established care plans to individuals, families, and groups, seeking consultation from the master's prepared specialist.

From Association of Community Health Nursing Educators: *Differentiated practice in community health,* Louisville, Ky., 1993, ACHNE.

---

nurse's visit. Usually a phone conversation precedes each visit during which the nurse discusses anticipated plans with the family and sets up a time for the visit. The expected length of the visit is discussed, as well as the nurse/client/family objectives and purpose for the visit. The nurse makes clear his or her expectations for the home visit. For instance, there may be a time set aside for private consultation with the client and a time for family and support persons to be involved.

During the preplanning phase, the nurse needs to recognize that, although the visit is professional, the nurse is still a guest in someone else's home. Moreover, the client being visited may not be the ultimate decision maker when it comes to running the home. The nurse is both a professional and a guest, and the way in which the family and client are approached on the initial visit sets the stage for continued successful visits.

Each home visit is carefully preplanned. This preplanning can be viewed as a mini-plan that contributes to the overall comprehensive plan of care and the long-term client outcomes.

Once the preliminary plan has been developed and the telephone or mail contact has been established, the nurse is ready to conduct a home visit. For the novice home care nurse, it is beneficial to communicate with a more experienced colleague who can function as a mentor, providing supervision and suggestions for improving care. This mentorship is important to the skill development of the psychiatric nurse in a field setting. Since home health practice requires independence, the nurse who is new to this work may find it lonely and lacking a professional support system. If such a support network and/or mentoring system is not in place, it may be up to the nurse to create one.

Entering the Home

The point of entry is the initial point in the therapeutic relationship that sets the tone and starts the nurse and client off on a mutually acceptable course. The nurse's attire is an important preentry consideration. Clothing should be neat and professional, and the nurse should carry some official identification that is readily displayed.

Since the visit is preceded by a phone call, the client may be waiting anxiously for the nurse's arrival. It is a good idea during the first phone contact for the nurse to describe his or her physical appearance and anticipated activities during the visit. Clients may offer to watch for the nurse's arrival. In high-crime areas or during nighttime hours, client and family observance is helpful and illustrates that home care is truly a team effort with clients and families also assuming responsibility.

When entering the home, the nurse must be able to blend the two roles of guest and nurse. For example, most homes have accepted places for family and guests to sit. It may be that guests are offered the most desirable chair, or that some special chair is reserved for a family member of high status or with special needs. The nurse should demonstrate the social skills necessary to ensure a smooth transition for all involved. Once it has been determined where people will sit, a pattern for negotiation is in place. How the client and the identified support persons will participate in the client's treatment and care remains to be decided based on the successful completion of the first steps of the intervention: preplanning and entry.

During the first visit, the nurse attempts to establish a relaxed environment in which to conduct an assessment. The assessment includes a physical assessment, assessment of client and family relationship, and medical and social history. The nurse also discusses the reason for hospitalization and how the client was feeling prior to hospitalization. The nurse explains the services of the agency and the purpose for the nursing visits, and asks the client what he or she expects from the nurse. The length of the visit is determined by the client. If the client shows signs or symptoms of stress or discomfort, the nurse may choose to finish assessment at the next visit. Therefore, it is important to obtain the most important information in the beginning of the visit to establish a plan of care. The nurse reviews the medications with the client to assure that the medications are being taken as ordered.

Functions and Form of the Home Visit

The functions of the nurse making a home visit to a client with a psychiatric diagnosis might include the following:

- provide structure
- establish attainable goals
- monitor medications (the first goal is to take medica-

tions as ordered; if the client is not taking medications, other goals will probably not be realistic)

- monitor client mental status, educating family members and significant others about client status and supportive interventions
- organize complementary interdisciplinary services such as social work or occupational therapy
- help the client and family use health services appropriately
- suggest appropriate client and family referral with team collaboration
- develop and implement the treatment plan with the client and family
- facilitate communication among family members and treatment team members
- communicate visit findings and treatment plan progress to appropriate team members

Within the context of these broad functions, the nurse will determine specific client expected outcomes related to nursing functions and interventions (see Box 31-3).

Documentation of the client plan and progress will accurately reflect the client's condition, the plan of care, and each step in the progress toward the predetermined measurable outcomes. Failure to accurately reflect the client's condition and progress can be detrimental to the

---

Box 31-3   Example of Nursing Interventions for Client Medication Compliance

The nurse reviews the medications with the client. If the client is in a manic phase, he or she may not be able to focus on taking medications several times a day, every day. The nurse will teach the family to administer the medications to the client. If no family members are available, the nurse may pour the medications into a medication box. The medication box is marked Monday through Sunday, and has up to four slots per day. The nurse instructs the client to check the box each day, in the morning, afternoon, and evening, and before going to bed. The nurse checks the medication box during each visit to assess if the client is taking medication as ordered. In cases where the client refuses the medication box, the nurse may assess the client's medications by counting the pills left in the bottles during each visit.

The nurse's goal is to provide as much structure for the client as necessary to reach the goal of taking medications as ordered. The nurse praises the client, even if the client has not taken all of his or her medications consistently. If the client takes 50% of his or her medications, the nurses praises the client and sets the goal for the client to take 75%–100% of medications.

person receiving services, since third-party payment depends on documentation that meets the payer's requirements.

The primary purpose of a home visit generated by client needs will dictate the process of the visit. One skill that must be particularly refined for the home visit is flexibility. Any number of unpredictable occurrences can and do happen. The nurse must be sensitive to changes that occur and be willing and able to modify plans and goals based on observation and insight with regard to the current situation. Skills of observation and insight may be diminished if the nurse experiences anxiety as a result of being unfamiliar with the process of home care. Acquiring good observational skills and insight into the meanings and implications of client and family behavior takes time and adequate guidance.

Previous inpatient experience can provide valuable help to the nurse who is new to home care. A core function of the nurse making a home visit is to create the professional climate for therapeutic interventions to occur. Once the nurse and client are seated in a selected space and at the designated time, a specific interaction occurs. The goal of the interaction is to facilitate an increase in the health of the client. The nurse selects the space and time to use her professional skills to create an opening (the entry), a process (the intervention), and an exit (the closing).

Although the process of the home visit parallels the course of other therapeutic interventions, differences do exist in the area of required social skills: creating a professional space, observation, insight, independent practice, and the professional obligation to refer individuals other than the current client who need health services.

Exiting the Home

Expectations about the length of the home visit should be shared at the beginning of each visit. When the predesignated visiting time is over, it is the nurse's job to make a successful exit. A successful exit implies that work has been accomplished, goals have been achieved, and the client, family, and nurse provider have experienced mutual satisfaction with the process.

A successful exit requires that the client and supporting individuals are left with a clear understanding of the work to be accomplished by the next visit. The visit should conclude on an optimistic note with the client and involved household members looking forward to the next visit and to the specific challenges to be met between visits.

Home visits should end at the designated time, and any manipulative effort by the client or family to extend the visit is addressed the first time it occurs. For example, if the client has been isolative and withdrawn from a spouse, the spouse may welcome the company of a nurse and attempt to bring up new problems during the visit. The nurse must set firm, kind limits and reiterate the designated length of the visit, stating that the new problems will be addressed in subsequent visits.

During the last 5–10 minutes of the visit, the client and support individuals should verbalize the specific goals they will work on in preparation for the next visit. Client and involved family need to describe the strategies they will employ to reach the short-term goal.

Written contracts can also be useful. The nurse states the short-term goal and places it into the long-term plan provided the participants are not already overwhelmed by the short- and long-term challenges. Client and family can better accept the challenges facing them if the nurse helps define positive outcomes as the reward resulting from energy expenditure.

Successfully entering and exiting a home visit is a learned skill that must be adapted to fit each different situation. Just as nurses learn the process of therapeutic intervention, the process of the home visit and the rules of conduct in home settings are learned. Some strategies and skills for preplanning, entry, process, and exit can best be learned in the classroom, and others will be experienced and practiced in the field with professional mentorship.

CULTURAL CONSIDERATIONS DURING THE HOME VISIT

Cultural considerations are taken into account when making a home visit. Culture is learned, shared behavior with expectations about rules of conduct in a given society. When the nurse is working with clients from a culture different from his or her own, it is the nurse's responsibility as a professional to read and learn as much as possible about the beliefs and behaviors of people belonging to the cultural group in question. Talking to professional colleagues who are members of the cultural group in question is also a helpful strategy for learning.

People of every cultural group have expectations about polite and professional behavior, and these expectations vary widely. Since the nurse is a professional guest in the client's home, the nurse will benefit from knowing what the cultural group in question might expect of guests and professionals. Behaviors that the client and family describe as rude or ignorant can be a cause of major communication blocks and may result in a disregard for the nurse's suggestions. This reaction to the nurse can impede the client's progress toward wellness.

Expectations of the "good" guest may include removing one's shoes at the door, partaking of food that is shared with household members, or eating while being observed by one's hosts. Clinical agencies may have rules about accepting food or gifts, and these rules are a part of the culture to which the nurse belongs. The rules must be taken into account, but at times the professional nurse may see fit to discuss the rules with

CASE 📁 STUDY

Mr. Johnson, an 80-year-old man, phoned the home health psychiatric nurse whom he had seen approximately six months prior, requesting additional services. He previously had been seen following an episode of depression complicated with a serious suicide attempt. His current complaint was, "I feel like I'm losing my personality." When further questioned, Mr. Johnson stated he had suicidal thoughts but denied current suicide intent. However, he related that lately he had been feeling despondent and had been withdrawing socially. Mr. Johnson was legally blind secondary to macular degeneration and had limited endurance secondary to chronic obstructive lung disease. He lives alone in a senior high-rise on the eighth floor.

Mr. Johnson's psychiatrist was contacted, and orders were received for an evaluation by a home health psychiatric nurse.

Critical Thinking and Home Health Care

1. On the first home visit, what will the psychiatric nurse need to assess to determine this client's problems/needs?

2. Based on your knowledge of Mr. Johnson's history, what will be most important to assess?

3. What nursing diagnoses might be considered for this client?

4. What data can be used to justify home visits?

5. What information/observations will be used to determine if it is safe for this client to be treated at home?

Box 31-4   Cultural Assessment Categores

Categories to include in a cultural assessment:

• Values
• Beliefs
• Customs
• Social structure factors
• Beliefs and practices about health, health care, and illness
• Customs related to family interactions
• Food ways
• The sick role
• Perceptions about human nature
• Gender
• Time
• Health care systems and communication style and expectations

---

interdisciplinary team members if such rules threaten the success of the therapeutic process. Clients and family members may infer that if the nurse fails to demonstrate even the most basic rules of conduct and politeness, then he or she may not know about the client's health needs. In the area of mental health, if the nurse cannot model what is considered appropriate social behavior, the client and family may not view such a person's advice or suggestions as helpful, in spite of the nurse's professional status.

When working with clients from a different culture, the nurse should conduct a cultural assessment. Tripp-Reimer et al, (1991) present a comparison of cultural assessment guides. Categories for a cultural assessment are presented in Box 31-4.

Once the nurse is familiar with the culture and general expectations of conduct and communication, he or she can adapt when possible. At times, however, familiarity with a culture can be problematic if the nurse general-

izes and/or stereotypes a client who belongs to a specific cultural group. It is important to remember that families or individuals may deviate from their cultural norms. People may belong to more than one cultural group and may exhibit a blended form of cultural belief and conduct. Nurses with an openness and a demonstration of willingness to learn from clients, families, and communities will be the most effective practitioners.

COLLEGIALITY AND COMMUNICATION

Collegiality implies working within a body of associates or colleagues. In home visiting, the colleagues are the team members who work together to provide and monitor client care in the home. They refer the client to other care when a more or less structured part of the health care delivery system is needed. It is important that providers are aware of the identities, roles, and functions of all team members. Home health care often includes the job of coordinating care, an inherent part of the home care nurse's role.

CASE MANAGEMENT

Case management has always been an integral role of the nurse working in the home setting. The case manager assumes a coordinating role and is responsible for overseeing the client's treatment plan. Resources are arranged, and communication channels are kept open. The case manager serves as advocate for the client, monitors payment and available service options, and ensures that the client's care provides the kind of balance between structure and independence that is currently needed and appropriate for the client and family. The nurse case manager should assume a leadership position with regard to long-term planning for people with chronic mental illness. Also, case management should facilitate the best organized use of complementary services, such as occupational therapy or neighborhood visitors.

The goal of case management is to make workable the comprehensive range of home care services so that quality care and supervision are provided in the most appropriate and least structured context.

Case Management and Third-Party Payer Issues

The case manager has the responsibility to assess the client and family's ability to pay for health care services rendered. Many clients are financially compromised, and third-party payers may not pay for all expenses.

In addition to matching payment ability to type of required service, the case manager needs to be aware of specific Medicare regulations. For instance, guidelines for qualified staff state that a psychiatrist must be the primary physician treating the client at home if the client's treatment is based on a psychiatric diagnosis.

There are specific Medicare rules that define homebound status. For example, for the general medical/surgical client, "homebound" may be associated with limited physical mobility. For individuals who have a psychiatric diagnosis, however, symptoms of a mental or emotional disorder will determine homebound status. Homebound status is an important concept to document, since Medicare and other payer regulations prohibit payment for people who are not clearly documented as homebound. Psychiatric diagnoses such as mood and anxiety disorders, schizophrenia and other psychotic disorders, and the dementias, which have resulted in isolation or a functional inability to communicate, greatly contribute to a client's homebound status.

CLIENT COMPLIANCE WITH CARE

Home care nursing provides an opportunity to better understand the client in the context of his or her dwelling. This includes understanding the available supportive people who are important in helping the client more effectively cope with the effects of mental disorders. To successfully manage the symptoms of mental disorders, the client and supportive others need to cooperate as fully as possible with the implementation of the client's plan of care. Compliance implies a yielding concession to the directives being followed. While compliance may be necessary at times, particularly in the area of managing the biologic aspects of mental illness through medication administration, there are other occasions when mutual cooperation is desired. When developing the

long-term treatment plan and desired client outcomes, the client becomes the most active participant. Without the client's involvement, no plan will work. Ultimately, it is the client who must manage his or her own illness. The nurse simply guides, facilitates, and teaches ways to improve care and outcomes.

Client, nurse, and supportive others collectively take responsibility for the care of the client with a defined mental health problem. All participate in the plan of care to achieve known, desired, and anticipated outcomes.

The more that clients and their families understand and participate in the treatment plan and its implementation, the more they will cooperate in the process. The more often cooperation is achieved, the more likely it is that health will be improved.

COMMUNITY VIOLENCE AND HOME VISIT SAFETY

While the fear of community and home violence is real, prevalent media coverage of violent events may promote a level of fear and immobility in individuals that may not be completely justified. Crime and violence, in fact, do occur in homes and neighborhoods and are complicated by use of illegal street drugs; inappropriately prescribed medications; alcohol abuse; and social stressors such as unemployment, work overload, or work deprivation.

Having a working familiarity with neighborhoods in which the nurse works is a valuable asset. Protecting the client, family, and self from injury are primary goals. However, protecting and advocating for safety in the community are also traditional community health nursing interventions.

Keen observation and reporting suspicious behavior in the client's neighborhood to the appropriate authorities may help to protect many people. Suspicious behaviors that may require reporting are listed in Box 31-5.

The suspicious behaviors listed in Box 31-5 do require familiarity with the neighborhood and an alertness to surroundings in order to identify strangers and odd behavior. When reporting suspicious behavior, it is important to provide as clear and detailed a description as possible of the involved person(s): sex, race, age, height, weight, build, hair color and style, eye color, clothing, physical disabilities, or unusual characteristics and speech patterns. A description of vehicles that may be involved should include license plate number; color, make, and year of the car; body style; damage; accessories such as a luggage rack or a special antenna; direction of travel; and number of occupants and their descriptions.

Many clinical agencies have specifically identified safety procedures for home visits that are updated annually as community conditions change. Box 31-6 provides an example of safety procedures from one agency for the home care nurse.

Box 31-5 Suspicious Behaviors to Report During a Neighborhood Home Visit

1. Anyone forcibly entering a car, home, or business.
2. A person running from a home or business.
3. Anyone with a weapon.
4. Someone screaming.
5. A stranger offering children candy or money.
6. An indication that a home or business has been forcibly entered or had its telephone wires cut.
7. A person who is loitering and seems to have no purpose in the neighborhood.
8. A stranger carrying what may be burglary "loot," such as a radio or TV or a full pillowcase or suitcase.
9. Strangers looking into parked cars or into windows of homes, garages, or other buildings.
10. A person who rings the doorbell of a home and then walks around to the rear of the house.
11. Adults loitering around schools, playgrounds, parks, or secluded areas.
12. A stranger entering a neighbor's house when the neighbor is not home.
13. Unusual noise, such as gunfire or breaking glass.
14. Someone selling merchandise at an unusually low price.
15. A car that seems to be cruising an area or driving without lights at night.
16. A car that speeds away from a neighbor's house.
17. Moving, delivery, or maintenance trucks parked at unoccupied homes.
18. A car that has been parked at the same location for several days and is not recognized by people in the neighborhood, particularly if it has out-of-town license plates; or a car that is parked and occupied at an unusual hour.
19. A stranger loading valuable items into a vehicle.

Box 31-6 Safety Procedures for the Home Care Nurse

1. Always submit your visit schedule, update it regularly, and telephone in and out of the office to ensure that the supervisor is aware of your route for the day.
2. Notify the supervisor of any environment in which you feel insecure or threatened so that arrangements can be made for the escort service. All staff members may use the escort service, and its use is strongly recommended during evening and night visits.
3. Be courteous to the residents of the community, but do not engage in solicited conversation that is unnecessary when traveling from your car to the client's residence.
4. Do not enter or remain in homes where alcohol/drug abuse or a threat to the provider's safety is apparent.
5. Telephone clients prior to making home visits to notify them of your anticipated arrival time.
6. Do not carry a pocketbook or any valuable items.
7. Do not wear expensive jewelry or accessories.
8. Keep your car doors locked at all times; never leave valuables or nursing bag visible in your car.
9. If anyone attempts to take your nursing bag or other equipment, do not resist. Leave the area and contact the police and your supervisor immediately.
10. Dress according to the dress code, and you will be identified in the community as a "helper."
11. Beware of suspicious behavior and loitering in certain areas.
12. Do not park your car in an isolated area, i.e., alleys.
13. Leave the home immediately if client/others become argumentative and/or allude to physical or verbal assault/abuse. Telephone your supervisor immediately.
14. Always carry money to make a telephone call, a piece of identification, and your agency identification photograph on your person.
15. Do not accept rides from strangers.
16. Do not enter the home(s) of anyone other than the client's residence.
17. Do not use staircases in high-rise apartment buildings.
18. Never enter a building that is boarded up, appears vacant, or appears structurally unsafe.
19. Do not transport clients, family members, strangers, or client medications in your car.
20. Do not complete your paperwork while sitting in the car.
21. Visit your clients as early as possible during the day before groups of people begin to congregate.
22. Drive to your destination on main streets.
23. Avoid using pay phones.
24. Avoid food "drive-ins" in high crime areas.
25. Avoid bank machines, whether inside or outside the bank or other buildings.
26. Use anticrime devices on your car.
27. Have client or family anticipate your arrival or watch you go to your car.
28. Attend yearly safety seminars.

From Bon Secours Home Health and Hospice: *Safety procedures for the home visit,* Baltimore, 1992, Bon Secours.

RESEARCH IN COMMUNITY MENTAL HEALTH AND HOME CARE NURSING

Participation in research is an integral part of nursing in general and is a critical necessity in home care. Unfortunately, there is currently a clear lack of research about the processes and dynamics of home care. Gubrium and Sankar (1990) were the first researchers to explore the home care experience. They helped to provide some insights into the home as a place of care, patterns of caregiving, and service provision considerations.

Nurses are professionals who monitor and provide care to clients and their families. Moreover, the nurse's role in the client's continuing care gives the nurse a unique opportunity for data collection, evaluation, and reflection concerning the interventions, processes, dynamics, and outcomes of psychiatric care in the home setting. Nursing field notes and impressions could provide a rich and meaningful tool to help health care professionals understand how interventions can be most effective.

NURSING CARE PLAN

A referral was received from Mrs. Lock's psychiatrist requesting a home evaluation by a psychiatric nurse. Mrs. Lock, an 81 year old woman, has a history of hospitalization for major depression, recurrent secondary to seasonal affective disorder. Currently, her husband reports that she is depressed, refuses to eat, and refuses to go to the psychiatrist's office for an evaluation.

Mrs. Lock had assigned her medicare benefits to a managed care HMO to assure payment for services. Authorization to see her had to be obtained from her primary care physician. Approval was received for an evaluation. Then, based on the initial assessment, authorization was received for three additional home visits.

The initial psychiatric nursing assessment of Mrs. Lock revealed the following information. Mrs. Lock demonstrated the following symptoms of major depressive syndrome: 1) pervasive depressed mood accompanied by irritability that had worsened over the previous 4–6 weeks; 2) lack of interest in activities previously found pleasurable; 3) weight loss secondary to poor appetite, sufficient to make all clothing fit loosely; 4) hypersomnia, sleeping 12–14 hours per day; 5) psychomotor retardation with episodes of agitation (she refused to leave her home, spoke little, moved slowly); 6) impaired attention span with poor concentration and inability to problem solve rationally; thought processes were tangential, poorly focused, illogical, and evidenced poor judgment with no insight into her present condition; ability to perform activities of daily living and make routine decisions was severely impaired; 7) frequently expressed a wish to die and feelings that she "can't go on"; however, she denies suicidal thoughts or plans, and there was no history of previous suicide attempt.

Additionally her husband reported that Mrs. Lock had a serious episode of depression every winter for the past 12 years. She had also had a severe post-partum depression following the birth of their daughter when Mrs. Lock was 32 years old. Mrs. Lock's father also had episodes of depression.

Mrs. Lock was generally in good physical health. Current physical complaints included a toothache of several days' duration for which she had refused treatment. She had pain in her left foot secondary to a bone spur. She had a history of leg and ankle edema currently not present. She had a mastectomy two years prior with no apparent complication.

Current medications were Zoloft 100 mg qd, Bumex one qd, K-Dur one qd, and Nolvadex 10 mg bid. Mr. Lock understood the purpose of each medication and was administering each correctly according to prescription. Mrs. Lock showed no side effects.

Mrs. Lock's home met criteria for safe and hygienic conditions. Her caregiver was her husband who was able and willing to care for her but was showing evidence of caregiver stress. It was noted that Mr. Lock had a history of myocardial infarction and that he was concerned and anxious regarding his wife's condition and behavior. His reaction to her behavior and tendency to apologize for her irritability indicated a lack of understanding of disease process and management.

DSM-IV Diagnosis

AXIS I	Major depression, recurrent, severe in conjunction with seasonal affective disorder
AXIS II	None
AXIS III	Edema of ankles and feet, controlled Toothache Bone spur, left foot Status post mastectomy
AXIS IV	Severity of psychosocial stressors: moderate; seasonal change; physical problems
AXIS V	GAF on admission severe-30; GAF within past year-60

NURSING CARE PLAN

Nursing Diagnosis: Knowledge deficit, related to effects of major depression, as evidenced by client/caregiver, failure to report symptoms in timely manner, and failure to institute preventive treatments as previously directed.

Client Outcomes	*Nursing Interventions*	*Evaluation*

• Mr. and Mrs. Lock will demonstrate understanding of the disease process and management of depression by:
  • recognizing signs and symptoms and reporting to physician in timely fashion;
  • complying with recommended treatment, i.e., prescribed medications, exposure to light as scheduled, follow-up visits with physician.
	• Explain basic etiology, course, and treatment for depression in concrete terms. Discuss signs and symptoms of depression and help Mr. and Mrs. Lock identify how symptoms manifest in the client. Stress importance of early recognition of developing symptoms and the importance of timely reporting to physician. *Knowledge of symptoms and behaviors associated with the disorder can lead to early treatment, minimizing of symptoms, and possible prevention.*
	• Identify with the family risk factors that predispose Mrs. Lock to depression: seasonal change, biologic predisposition, and preventive measures, e.g., as hours of sunshine shorten, increase client exposure to direct sun and artificial light. *Knowledge of effective strategies enables family to feel useful.*
	• Reinforce importance of compliance with medication regimen and provide additional instruction regarding action, purpose, and side effects as needed. *Knowledge of medical effects empowers family and increases compliance.*
	• Explain the use of sun-equivalent light in the treatment of seasonal affective disorder. *Increased knowledge improves care and minimizes symptoms.*
	• Establish with Mr. and Mrs. Lock a schedule for daily exposure to direct sunlight and/or artificial sunlight. *Routine and structure ensure compliance.*
		• Mr. Lock became less apologetic regarding his wife's hostile behavior as his understanding of her illness increased. He continued to administer medications as prescribed, and Mrs. Lock took them. With Mr. Lock's prompting, Mrs. Lock complied with a schedule for exposure to direct and artificial light. On the third visit, Mrs. Lock agreed to see her psychiatrist the next week and kept the appointment as scheduled.

Nursing Diagnosis: Risk for self-directed violence. Risk factors: feelings of hopelessness, expressed wish to die, and feeling that she can't go on living.

Client Outcomes	*Nursing Interventions*	*Evaluation*
• Mrs. Lock will not become actively suicidal and will not harm herself.	• Instruct Mr. Lock to assure his wife that he does not want her to die when she expresses a desire to do so. Explain that these verbalizations are a symptom of her depression and will diminish as she gets better *so that Mr. Lock will continue interventions for suicide prevention in the absence of the nurse.* • Instruct Mr. Lock that if Mrs. Lock directly talks about wanting to hurt/kill herself, appears to be making plans to do so, or attempts in any way to harm herself, this should be taken seriously. Mrs. Lock should not be left alone and the psychiatrist should be called immediately *to illustrate the urgency of key statements/behaviors that require immediate interventions.*	• Mrs. Lock did not become actively suicidal during time seen by home health psychiatric nurse.

NURSING CARE PLAN

Nursing Diagnosis: Altered nutrition, less than body requirement secondary to depression, as evidenced by weight loss sufficient to cause clothes to fit loosely.

Client Outcome	Nursing Interventions	Evaluation
• Mrs. Lock will not lose further weight and will regain weight.	• Instruct Mr. and Mrs. Lock • about available nutritional supplements and appropriate use; • how to increase calories without increasing quantity of food; • regarding importance of eating despite lack of appetite; • to purchase scale and to weigh every three days, and report additional loss of greater than two pounds to physician. *Increased knowledge helps the client to maintain adequate nutritional intake.*	• Mrs. Lock's weight stabilized. She had lost 15 pounds over about 7 weeks. She did not lose any more weight.

Nursing Diagnosis: Sleep pattern disturbance related to effects of depression, as evidenced by hypersomnia, sleeping 12–14 hours a day.

Client Outcomes	Nursing Intervention	Evaluation
• Mrs. Lock will gradually return to a normal sleep pattern of 7–9 hours a day.	• With Mr. and Mrs. Lock, establish a sleep schedule that encourages gradually increasing time spent out of bed. *A scheduled routine helps the client balance sleep/wake cycles.* • Establish schedule of simple, routine activities *to structure awake time in order to keep Mrs. Lock alert and occupied.*	• Within 4 weeks, Mrs. Lock's sleep pattern returned to normal.

Nursing Diagnosis: Impaired health maintenance, related to altered thought processes and depressed mood, as evidenced by refusal to visit psychiatrist or dentist or leave her home for an occsional outing.

Client Outcomes	Nursing Intervention	Evaluation
• Mrs. Lock will visit her psychiatrist and dentist, and agree to leave her home for an occasional drive or dinner.	• Instruct Mr. Lock to schedule psychiatrist and dental appointments for Mrs. Lock in a timely manner *to meet her physical needs. Clients with depression often need to rely on others to meet basic health needs.* • Encourage Mr. Lock to take Mrs. Lock for brief rides every day when the weather is nice *to reinforce social and recreational behaviors.*	• Mrs. Lock agreed to go to her scheduled appointments. • On one occasion when they were out for a drive, Mrs. Lock suggested they go for dinner.

NURSING CARE PLAN ■ ■ ■ ■ ■ ■ ■ ■   ■ ■ ■ ■ ■ ■

Nursing Diagnosis: Caregiver role strain, related to wife's severe depression, as evidenced by anxiety expressed regarding wife's condition, irritability toward wife, and apology for wife's behavior.

Client Outcomes	*Nursing Intervention*	*Evaluation*
• Mr. Lock will remain healthy. He will display decreased anxiety and will be able to follow through with home health nurse's instructions.	• Demonstrate positive regard for Mr. Lock by acknowledging his concerns and by reassuring him that his wife's condition will improve *to build trust, offer hope, and reduce anxiety.* • Take Mr. Lock's vital signs and report any abnormal readings to his physician *to demonstrate caring and assess health state.* • Encourage Mr. Lock to spend some quality time by himself and with others. Help to arrange respite caregivers if needed. *Respite is necessary for caregivers to reduce role strain, frustration, and anxiety.*	• Mr. Lock became less anxious as he gained an understanding of his wife's illness. • Mr. Lock gained some comfort by talking to his daughter and close friends and enjoying quality time.

Summary of Key Concepts

1. Mental health services in community and home settings have greatly increased since the 1960s.

2. Community health nurses view the family or community as the unit of care. Home health nurses focus on the care of one individual in the home setting.

3. The home care nurse generally functions at the tertiary level, providing preventive treatment and maintenance care.

4. The phases of a home visit are preplanning, entering the home, nursing care and interventions, and exiting the home.

5. The home care nurse should consider and respect the cultural practices of the client while in the home.

6. The home care nurse should take appropriate safety measures when visiting homes and neighborhoods.

7. The three levels of home care are concentrated, which is provided during an acute crisis; intermediate, which is short-term and helps the client achieve a higher level of functioning; and maintenance, which stabilizes the client at a higher level.

REFERENCES

American Nurses Association: *Statement on essentials of home health care nursing,* Kansas City, Mo., 1986, ANA.

Association of Community Health Nursing Educators: *Research agenda for community health nursing,* Louisville, Ky., 1991, ACHNE.

Association of Community Health Nursing Educators: *Differential practice in community health,* Louisville, Ky., 1993, Association of Community Health Nursing Educators.

Bon Secours Home Health and Hospice: *Safety procedures for the home visit,* Baltimore, 1992, Bon Secours.

Bowers KA: *Case management by nurses.* Washington, D.C., 1992, American Nurses Publishing.

Fortinash K, Holoday-Worret P: *Psychiatric nursing care plans,* ed 2, St. Louis, 1995, Mosby.

Gubrium JF, Aankar A: *The home care experience,* Newbury Park, Calif., 1990, Sage Publications.

Rice R: *Home health nursing practice,* St. Louis, 1992, Mosby.

Spiegel AD: *Home health care,* Owings Mill, Md., 1987, National Health Publishing.

Stulginsky MF: Nurse's home health experience, 1987, *Nursing and Health Care* 14(8):402–407, 1993.

Tripp-Reimer T et al: Cultural assessment content and process. In Spradley B, editor: *Readings in community health nursing,* Philadelphia, 1991, J.B. Lippincott.

World Health Organization: *Primary health care: report of the international conference on primary health care,* Geneva, Switzerland, 1991, WHO.

APPENDIX A

DSM-IV Classification*

NOS = Not Otherwise Specified.

An *x* appearing in a diagnostic code indicates that a specific code number is required.

An ellipsis (. . .) is used in the names of certain disorders to indicate that the name of a specific mental disorder or general medical condition should be inserted when recording the name (e.g., 293.0 Delirium Due to Hypothyroidism).

If criteria are currently met, one of the following severity specifiers may be noted after the diagnosis:
    Mild
    Moderate
    Severe

If criteria are no longer met, one of the following specifiers may be noted:
    In Partial Remission
    In Full Remission
    Prior History

Disorders Usually First Diagnosed in Infancy, Childhood, or Adolescence
MENTAL RETARDATION

Note: These are coded on Axis II.

317	Mild Mental Retardation
318.0	Moderate Mental Retardation
318.1	Severe Mental Retardation
318.2	Profound Mental Retardation
319	Mental Retardation, Severity Unspecified

*Reprinted with permission from the American Psychiatric Association: *Diagnostic and statistical manual of mental disorders,* ed 4, Washington, D.C., 1994, American Psychiatric Association.

LEARNING DISORDERS

315.00	Reading Disorder
315.1	Mathematics Disorder
315.2	Disorder of Written Expression
315.9	Learning Disorder NOS

MOTOR SKILLS DISORDER

315.4	Developmental Coordination Disorder

COMMUNICATION DISORDERS

315.31	Expressive Language Disorder
315.31	Mixed Receptive-Expressive Language Disorder
315.39	Phonological Disorder
307.0	Stuttering
307.9	Communication Disorder NOS

PERVASIVE DEVELOPMENTAL DISORDERS

299.00	Autistic Disorder
299.80	Rett's Disorder
299.10	Childhood Disintegrative Disorder
299.80	Asperger's Disorder
299.80	Pervasive Developmental Disorder NOS

ATTENTION-DEFICIT AND DISRUPTIVE BEHAVIOR DISORDERS

314.xx	Attention-Deficit/Hyperactivity Disorder
.01	Combined Type
.00	Predominantly Inattentive Type
.01	Predominantly Hyperactive-Impulsive Type
314.9	Attention-Deficit/Hyperactivity Disorder NOS

312.8   Conduct Disorder

> *Specify type:* Childhood-Onset
> Type/Adolescent-Onset Type

313.81   Oppositional Defiant Disorder

312.9   Disruptive Behavior Disorder NOS

FEEDING AND EATING DISORDERS OF INFANCY OR EARLY CHILDHOOD

307.52   Pica

307.53   Rumination Disorder

307.59   Feeding Disorder of Infancy or Early
          Childhood

TIC DISORDERS

307.23   Tourette's Disorder

307.22   Chronic Motor or Vocal Tic Disorder

307.21   Transient Tic Disorder

> *Specify if:* Single Episode/Recurrent

307.20   Tic Disorder NOS

ELIMINATION DISORDERS

____.__   Encopresis

787.6   With Constipation and Overflow
          Incontinence

307.7   Without Constipation and Overflow
          Incontinence

307.6   Enuresis (Not Due to a General Medical
          Condition)

> *Specify type:* Nocturnal Only/Diurnal
> Only/Nocturnal and Diurnal

OTHER DISORDERS OF INFANCY, CHILDHOOD, OR ADOLESCENCE

309.21   Separation Anxiety Disorder

> *Specify if:* Early Onset

313.23   Selective Mutism

313.89   Reactive Attachment Disorder of Infancy or
          Early Childhood

> *Specify type:* Inhibited Type/Disinhibited Type

307.3   Stereotypic Movement Disorder

> *Specify if:* With Self-Injurious Behavior

313.9   Disorder of Infancy, Childhood, or
          Adolescence NOS

Delirium, Dementia, and Amnestic and Other Cognitive Disorders

DELIRIUM

293.0   Delirium Due to . . . *[Indicate the General
          Medical Condition]*

____.__   Substance Intoxication Delirium *(refer to
          Substance-Related Disorders for
          substance-specific codes)*

____.__   Substance Withdrawal Delirium *(refer to
          Substance-Related Disorders for
          substance-specific codes)*

____.__   Delirium Due to Multiple Etiologies *(code
          each of the specific etiologies)*

780.09   Delirium NOS

DEMENTIA

290.xx   Dementia of the Alzheimer's Type, With
          Early Onset *(also code 331.0 Alzheimer's
          disease on Axis III)*

.10   Uncomplicated

.11   With Delirium

.12   With Delusions

.13   With Depressed Mood

> *Specify if:* With Behavioral Disturbance

290.xx   Dementia of the Alzheimer's Type, With
          Late Onset *(also code 331.0 Alzheimer's
          disease on Axis III)*

.0   Uncomplicated

.3   With Delirium

.20   With Delusions

.21   With Depressed Mood

> *Specify if:* With Behavioral Disturbance

290.xx   Vascular Dementia

.40   Uncomplicated

.41   With Delirium

.42   With Delusions

.43   With Depressed Mood

> *Specify if:* With Behavioral Disturbance

294.9   Dementia Due to HIV Disease *(also code
          043.1 HIV infection affecting
          central nervous system on Axis III)*

294.1   Dementia Due to Head Trauma *(also code
          854.00 head injury on Axis III)*

294.1   Dementia Due to Parkinson's Disease *(also
          code 332.0 Parkinson's disease on Axis
          III)*

294.1   Dementia Due to Huntington's Disease
          *(also code 333.4 Huntington's disease on
          Axis III)*

290.10   Dementia Due to Pick's Disease *(also code
          331.1 Pick's disease on Axis III)*

290.10   Dementia Due to Creutzfeldt-Jakob Disease
          *(also code 046.1 Creutzfeldt-Jakob disease
          on Axis III)*

294.1 Dementia Due to . . . *[Indicate the General Medical Condition not listed above] (also code the general medical condition on Axis III)*

___._ Substance-Induced Persisting Dementia *(refer to Substance-Related Disorders for substance-specific codes)*

___._ Dementia Due to Multiple Etiologies *(code each of the specific etiologies)*

294.8 Dementia NOS

AMNESTIC DISORDERS

294.0 Amnestic Disorder Due to . . . *[Indicate the General Medical Condition]*

Specify if: Transient/Chronic

___._ Substance-Induced Persisting Amnestic Disorder *(refer to Substance-Related Disorders for substance-specific codes)*

294.8 Amnestic Disorder NOS

OTHER COGNITIVE DISORDERS

294.9 Cognitive Disorder NOS

Mental Disorders Due to a General Medical Condition Not Elsewhere Classified

293.89 Catatonic Disorder Due to . . . *[Indicate the General Medical Condition]*

310.1 Personality Change Due to . . . *[Indicate the General Medical Condition]*

Specify type: Labile Type/Disinhibited Type/ Aggressive Type/Apathetic Type/Paranoid Type/ Other Type/Combined Type/Unspecified Type

293.9 Mental Disorder NOS Due to . . . *[Indicate the General Medical Condition]*

Substance-Related Disorders

[a]*The following specifiers may be applied to Substance Dependence:*

With Physiological Dependence/Without Physiological Dependence

Early Full Remission/Early Partial Remission

Sustained Full Remission/Sustained Partial Remission

On Agonist Therapy/In a Controlled Environment

The following specifiers apply to Substance-Induced Disorders as noted:

[I]With Onset During Intoxication/[W]With Onset During Withdrawal

ALCOHOL-RELATED DISORDERS

Alcohol Use Disorders

303.90 Alcohol Dependence[a]

305.00 Alcohol Abuse

Alcohol-Induced Disorders

303.00 Alcohol Intoxication

291.8 Alcohol Withdrawal

Specify if: With Perceptual Disturbances

291.0 Alcohol Intoxication Delirium

291.0 Alcohol Withdrawal Delirium

291.2 Alcohol-Induced Persisting Dementia

291.1 Alcohol-Induced Persisting Amnestic Disorder

291.x Alcohol-Induced Psychotic Disorder

.5 With Delusions[I,W]

.3 With Hallucinations[I,W]

291.8 Alcohol-Induced Mood Disorder[I,W]

291.8 Alcohol-Induced Anxiety Disorder[I,W]

291.8 Alcohol-Induced Sexual Dysfunction[I]

291.8 Alcohol-Induced Sleep Disorder[I,W]

291.9 Alcohol-Related Disorder NOS

AMPHETAMINE (OR AMPHETAMINE-LIKE)-RELATED DISORDERS

Amphetamine Use Disorders

304.40 Amphetamine Dependence[a]

305.70 Amphetamine Abuse

Amphetamine-Induced Disorders

292.89 Amphetamine Intoxication

Specify if: With Perceptual Disturbances

292.0 Amphetamine Withdrawal

292.81 Amphetamine Intoxication Delirium

292.xx Amphetamine-Induced Psychotic Disorder

.11 With Delusions[I]

.12 With Hallucinations[I]

292.84 Amphetamine-Induced Mood Disorder[I,W]

292.89 Amphetamine-Induced Anxiety Disorder[I]

292.89 Amphetamine-Induced Sexual Dysfunction[I]

292.89 Amphetamine-Induced Sleep Disorder[I,W]

292.9 Amphetamine-Related Disorder NOS

CAFFEINE-RELATED DISORDERS

Caffeine-Induced Disorders

305.90 Caffeine Intoxication

292.89 Caffeine-Induced Anxiety Disorder[I]

292.89   Caffeine-Induced Sleep Disorder[I]

292.9   Caffeine-Related Disorder NOS

CANNABIS-RELATED DISORDERS

Cannabis Use Disorders

304.30   Cannabis Dependence[a]

305.20   Cannabis Abuse

Cannabis-Induced Disorders

292.89   Cannabis Intoxication
          Specify if: With Perceptual Disturbances

292.81   Cannabis Intoxication Delirium

292.xx   Cannabis-Induced Psychotic Disorder

.11   With Delusions[I]

.12   With Hallucinations[I]

292.89   Cannabis-Induced Anxiety Disorder[I]

292.9   Cannabis-Related Disorder NOS

COCAINE-RELATED DISORDERS

Cocaine Use Disorders

304.20   Cocaine Dependence[a]

305.60   Cocaine Abuse

Cocaine-Induced Disorders

292.89   Cocaine Intoxication
          Specify if: With Perceptual Disturbances

292.0   Cocaine Withdrawal

292.81   Cocaine Intoxication Delirium

292.xx   Cocaine-Induced Psychotic Disorder

.11   With Delusions[I]

.12   With Hallucinations[I]

292.84   Cocaine-Induced Mood Disorder[I,W]

292.89   Cocaine-Induced Anxiety Disorder[I,W]

292.89   Cocaine-Induced Sexual Dysfunction[I]

292.89   Cocaine-Induced Sleep Disorder[I,W]

292.9   Cocaine-Related Disorder NOS

HALLUCINOGEN-RELATED DISORDERS

Hallucinogen Use Disorders

304.50   Hallucinogen Dependence[a]

305.30   Hallucinogen Abuse

Hallucinogen-Induced Disorders

292.89   Hallucinogen Intoxication

292.89   Hallucinogen Persisting Perception Disorder (Flashbacks)

292.81   Hallucinogen Intoxication Delirium

292.xx   Hallucinogen-Induced Psychotic Disorder

.11   With Delusions[I]

.12   With Hallucinations[I]

292.84   Hallucinogen-Induced Mood Disorder[I]

292.89   Hallucinogen-Induced Anxiety Disorder[I]

292.9   Hallucinogen-Related Disorder NOS

INHALANT-RELATED DISORDERS

Inhalant Use Disorders

304.60   Inhalant Dependence[a]

305.90   Inhalant Abuse

Inhalant-Induced Disorders

292.89   Inhalant Intoxication

292.81   Inhalant Intoxication Delirium

292.82   Inhalant-Induced Persisting Dementia

292.xx   Inhalant-Induced Psychotic Disorder

.11   With Delusions[I]

.12   With Hallucinations[I]

292.84   Inhalant-Induced Mood Disorder[I]

292.89   Inhalant-Induced Anxiety Disorder[I]

292.9   Inhalant-Related Disorder NOS

NICOTINE-RELATED DISORDERS

Nicotine Use Disorder

305.10   Nicotine Dependence[a]

Nicotine-Induced Disorder

292.0   Nicotine Withdrawal

292.9   Nicotine-Related Disorder NOS

OPIOID-RELATED DISORDERS

Opioid Use Disorders

304.00   Opioid Dependence[a]

305.50   Opioid Abuse

Opioid-Induced Disorders

292.89   Opioid Intoxication
          Specify if: With Perceptual Disturbances

292.0   Opioid Withdrawal

292.81   Opioid Intoxication Delirium

292.xx   Opioid-Induced Psychotic Disorder

.11   With Delusions[I]

.12   With Hallucinations[I]

292.84   Opioid-Induced Mood Disorder[I]

292.89   Opioid-Induced Sexual Dysfunction[I]

292.89   Opioid-Induced Sleep Disorder[I,W]

292.9   Opioid-Related Disorder NOS

PHENCYCLIDINE (OR PHENCYCLIDINE-LIKE)-RELATED DISORDERS

Phencyclidine Use Disorders

304.90   Phencyclidine Dependence[a]

305.90   Phencyclidine Abuse

Phencyclidine-Induced Disorders

292.89   Phencyclidine Intoxication

     Specify if: With Perceptual Disturbances

292.81   Phencyclidine Intoxication Delirium

292.xx   Phencyclidine-Induced Psychotic Disorder

   .11   With Delusions[I]

   .12   With Hallucinations[I]

292.84   Phencyclidine-Induced Mood Disorder[I]

292.89   Phencyclidine-Induced Anxiety Disorder[I]

292.9   Phencyclidine-Related Disorder NOS

SEDATIVE-, HYPNOTIC-, OR ANXIOLYTIC-RELATED DISORDERS

Sedative, Hypnotic, or Anxiolytic Use Disorders

304.10   Sedative, Hypnotic, or Anxiolytic Dependence[a]

305.40   Sedative, Hypnotic, or Anxiolytic Abuse

Sedative-, Hypnotic-, or Anxiolytic-Induced Disorders

292.89   Sedative, Hypnotic, or Anxiolytic Intoxication

292.0   Sedative, Hypnotic, or Anxiolytic Withdrawal

     Specify if: With Perceptual Disturbances

292.81   Sedative, Hypnotic, or Anxiolytic Intoxication Delirium

292.81   Sedative, Hypnotic, or Anxiolytic Withdrawal Delirium

292.82   Sedative-, Hypnotic-, or Anxiolytic-Induced Persisting Dementia

292.83   Sedative-, Hypnotic-, or Anxiolytic-Induced Persisting Amnestic Disorder

292.xx   Sedative-, Hypnotic-, or Anxiolytic-Induced Psychotic Disorder

   .11   With Delusions[I,W]

   .12   With Hallucinations[I,W]

292.84   Sedative-, Hypnotic-, or Anxiolytic-Induced Mood Disorder[I,W]

292.89   Sedative-, Hypnotic-, or Anxiolytic-Induced Anxiety Disorder[W]

292.89   Sedative-, Hypnotic-, or Anxiolytic-Induced Sexual Dysfunction[I]

292.89   Sedative-, Hypnotic-, or Anxiolytic-Induced Sleep Disorder[I,W]

292.9   Sedative-, Hypnotic-, or Anxiolytic-Related Disorder NOS

POLYSUBSTANCE-RELATED DISORDER

304.80   Polysubstance Dependence[a]

OTHER (OR UNKNOWN) SUBSTANCE-RELATED DISORDERS

Other (or Unknown) Substance Use Disorders

304.90   Other (or Unknown) Substance Dependence[a]

305.90   Other (or Unknown) Substance Abuse

OTHER (OR UNKNOWN) SUBSTANCE-INDUCED DISORDERS

292.89   Other (or Unknown) Substance Intoxication

     Specify if: With Perceptual Disturbances

292.0   Other (or Unknown) Substance Withdrawal

     Specify if: With Perceptual Disturbances

292.81   Other (or Unknown) Substance-Induced Delirium

292.82   Other (or Unknown) Substance-Induced Persisting Dementia

292.83   Other (or Unknown) Substance-Induced Persisting Amnestic Disorder

292.xx   Other (or Unknown) Substance-Induced Psychotic Disorder

   .11   With Delusions[I,W]

   .12   With Hallucinations[I,W]

292.84   Other (or Unknown) Substance-Induced Mood Disorder[I,W]

292.89   Other (or Unknown) Substance-Induced Anxiety Disorder[I,W]

292.89   Other (or Unknown) Substance-Induced Sexual Dysfunction[I]

292.89   Other (or Unknown) Substance-Induced Sleep Disorder[I,W]

292.9   Other (or Unknown) Substance-Related Disorder NOS

Schizophrenia and Other Psychotic Disorders

295.xx   Schizophrenia

The following Classification of Longitudinal Course applies to all subtypes of Schizophrenia:

Episodic With Interepisode Residual Symptoms (*specify if:* With Prominent Negative Symptoms)/ Episodic With No Interepisode Residual Symptoms/ Continuous (*specify if:* With Prominent Negative Symptoms)

Single Episode In Partial Remission (*specify if:* With Prominent Negative Symptoms)/Single Episode In Full Remission

Other or Unspecified Pattern

   .30   Paranoid Type

   .10   Disorganized Type

   .20   Catatonic Type

   .90   Undifferentiated Type

   .60   Residual Type

295.40   Schizophreniform Disorder

     Specify if: Without Good Prognostic Features/With Good Prognostic Features

295.70   Schizoaffective Disorder

     Specify type: Bipolar Type/Depressive Type

297.1   Delusional Disorder

     Specify type: Erotomanic Type/Grandiose Type/Jealous Type/Persecutory Type/Somatic Type/Mixed Type/Unspecified Type

298.8   Brief Psychotic Disorder

     Specify if: With Marked Stressor(s)/Without Marked Stressor(s)/With Postpartum Onset

297.3   Shared Psychotic Disorder

293.xx   Psychotic Disorder Due to . . . *[Indicate the General Medical Condition]*

   .81   With Delusions

   .82   With Hallucinations

___._   Substance-Induced Psychotic Disorder *(refer to Substance-Related Disorders for substance-specific codes)*

     Specify if: With Onset During Intoxication/With Onset During Withdrawal

298.9   Psychotic Disorder NOS

Mood Disorders

Code current state of Major Depressive Disorder or Bipolar I Disorder in fifth digit:

1 = Mild

2 = Moderate

3 = Severe Without Psychotic Features

4 = Severe With Psychotic Features

     Specify: Mood-Congruent Psychotic Features/ Mood-Incongruent Psychotic Features

5 = In Partial Remission

6 = In Full Remission

0 = Unspecified

The following specifiers apply (for current or most recent episode) to Mood Disorders as noted:

[a]Severity/Psychotic/Remission Specifiers

[b]Chronic

[c]With Catatonic Features

[d]With Melancholic Features

[e]With Atypical Features

[f]With Postpartum Onset

The following specifiers apply to Mood Disorders as noted:

[g]With or Without Full Interepisode Recovery

[h]With Seasonal Pattern

[i]With Rapid Cycling

DEPRESSIVE DISORDERS

296.xx   Major Depressive Disorder,

   .2x   Single Episode[a,b,c,d,e,f]

   .3x   Recurrent[a,b,c,d,e,f,g,h]

300.4   Dysthymic Disorder

     Specify if: Early Onset/Late Onset

     Specify: With Atypical Features

311   Depressive Disorder NOS

BIPOLAR DISORDERS

296.xx   Bipolar I Disorder,

   .0x   Single Manic Episode[a,c,f]

     Specify if: Mixed

   .40   Most Recent Episode Hypomanic[g,h,i]

   .4x   Most Recent Episode Manic[a,c,f,g,h,i]

   .6x   Most Recent Episode Mixed[a,c,f,g,h,i]

   .5x   Most Recent Episode Depressed[a,b,c,d,e,f,g,h,i]

   .7   Most Recent Episode Unspecified[g,h,i]

296.89   Bipolar II Disorder[a,b,c,d,e,f,g,h,i]

     Specify (current or most recent episode): Hypomanic/Depressed

301.13   Cyclothymic Disorder

296.80   Bipolar Disorder NOS

293.83   Mood Disorder Due to . . . *[Indicate the General Medical Condition]*

     Specify type: With Depressive Features/With Major Depressive-Like Episode/With Manic Features/With Mixed Features

___._   Substance-Induced Mood Disorder *(refer to Substance-Related Disorders for substance-specific codes)*

     Specify type: With Depressive Features/With Manic Features/With Mixed Features

     Specify if: With Onset During Intoxication/With Onset During Withdrawal

296.90   Mood Disorder NOS

Anxiety Disorders

300.01   Panic Disorder Without Agoraphobia

300.21   Panic Disorder With Agoraphobia

300.22   Agoraphobia Without History of Panic Disorder

300.29   Specific Phobia

Specify type: Animal Type/Natural Environment Type/Blood-Injection-Injury Type/Situational Type/Other Type

300.23   Social Phobia

Specify if: Generalized

300.3   Obsessive-Compulsive Disorder

Specify if: With Poor Insight

309.81   Post-traumatic Stress Disorder

Specify if: Acute/Chronic

Specify if: With Delayed Onset

308.3   Acute Stress Disorder

300.02   Generalized Anxiety Disorder

293.89   Anxiety Disorder Due to . . . *[Indicate the General Medical Condition]*

Specify if: With Generalized Anxiety/With Panic Attacks/With Obsessive-Compulsive Symptoms

___.__   Substance-Induced Anxiety Disorder *(refer to Substance-Related Disorders for substance-specific codes)*

Specify if: With Generalized Anxiety/With Panic Attacks/With Obsessive-Compulsive Symptoms/With Phobic Symptoms

Specify if: With Onset During Intoxication/With Onset During Withdrawal

300.00   Anxiety Disorder NOS

Somatoform Disorders

300.81   Somatization Disorder

300.81   Undifferentiated Somatoform Disorder

300.11   Conversion Disorder

Specify type: With Motor Symptom or Deficit/With Sensory Symptom or Deficit/With Seizures or Convulsions/With Mixed Presentation

307.xx   Pain Disorder

.80   Associated with Psychologic Factors

.89   Associated with Both Psychologic Factors and a General Medical Condition

Specify if: Acute/Chronic

300.7   Hypochondriasis

Specify if: With Poor Insight

300.7   Body Dysmorphic Disorder

300.81   Somatoform Disorder NOS

Factitious Disorders

300.xx   Factitious Disorder

.16   With Predominantly Psychologic Signs and Symptoms

.19   With Predominantly Physical Signs and Symptoms

.19   With Combined Psychologic and Physical Signs and Symptoms

300.19   Factitious Disorder NOS

Dissociative Disorders

300.12   Dissociative Amnesia

300.13   Dissociative Fugue

300.14   Dissociative Identity Disorder

300.6   Depersonalization Disorder

300.15   Dissociative Disorder NOS

Sexual and Gender Identity Disorders
SEXUAL DYSFUNCTIONS

The following specifiers apply to all primary Sexual Dysfunctions:

Lifelong Type

Acquired Type

Generalized Type

Situational Type Due to Psychologic Factors

Due to Combined Factors

Sexual Desire Disorders

302.71   Hypoactive Sexual Desire Disorder

302.79   Sexual Aversion Disorder

Sexual Arousal Disorders

302.72   Female Sexual Arousal Disorder

302.72   Male Erectile Disorder

Orgasmic Disorders

302.73   Female Orgasmic Disorder

302.74   Male Orgasmic Disorder

302.75   Premature Ejaculation

Sexual Pain Disorders

302.76   Dyspareunia (Not Due to a General Medical Condition)

306.51   Vaginismus (Not Due to a General Medical Condition)

Sexual Dysfunction Due to a General Medical Condition

625.8   Female Hypoactive Sexual Desire Disorder Due to . . . *[Indicate the General Medical Condition]*

608.89   Male Hypoactive Sexual Desire Disorder Due to . . . *[Indicate the General Medical Condition]*

607.84   Male Erectile Disorder Due to . . . *[Indicate the General Medical Condition]*

625.0   Female Dyspareunia Due to . . . *[Indicate the General Medical Condition]*

608.89   Male Dyspareunia Due to . . . *[Indicate the General Medical Condition]*

625.8   Other Female Sexual Dysfunction Due to . . . *[Indicate the General Medical Condition]*

608.89   Other Male Sexual Dysfunction Due to . . . *[Indicate the General Medical Condition]*

___.__   Substance-Induced Sexual Dysfunction *(refer to Substance-Related Disorders for substance-specific codes)*

Specify if: With Impaired Desire/With Impaired Arousal/With Impaired Orgasm/With Sexual Pain

Specify if: With Onset During Intoxication

302.70   Sexual Dysfunction NOS

PARAPHILIAS

302.4   Exhibitionism

302.81   Fetishism

302.89   Frotteurism

302.2   Pedophilia

Specify if: Sexually Attracted to Males/Sexually Attracted to Females/Sexually Attracted to Both

Specify if: Limited to Incest

Specify type: Exclusive Type/Nonexclusive Type

302.83   Sexual Masochism

302.84   Sexual Sadism

302.3   Transvestic Fetishism

Specify if: With Gender Dysphoria

302.82   Voyeurism

302.9   Paraphilia NOS

GENDER IDENTITY DISORDERS

302.xx   Gender Identity Disorder

.6   in Children

.85   in Adolescents or Adults

Specify if: Sexually Attracted to Males/Sexually Attracted to Females/Sexually Attracted to Both/Sexually Attracted to Neither

302.6   Gender Identity Disorder NOS

302.9   Sexual Disorder NOS

Eating Disorders

307.1   Anorexia Nervosa

Specify type: Restricting Type; Binge-Eating/Purging Type

307.51   Bulimia Nervosa

Specify type: Purging Type/Nonpurging Type

307.50   Eating Disorder NOS

Sleep Disorders

PRIMARY SLEEP DISORDERS

Dyssomnias

307.42   Primary Insomnia

307.44   Primary Hypersomnia

Specify if: Recurrent

347   Narcolepsy

780.59   Breathing-Related Sleep Disorder

307.45   Circadian Rhythm Sleep Disorder

Specify type: Delayed Sleep Phase Type/Jet Lag Type/Shift Work Type/Unspecified Type

307.47   Dyssomnia NOS

Parasomnias

307.47   Nightmare Disorder

307.46   Sleep Terror Disorder

307.46   Sleepwalking Disorder

307.47   Parasomnia NOS

SLEEP DISORDERS RELATED TO ANOTHER MENTAL DISORDER

307.42   Insomnia Related to . . . *[Indicate the Axis I or Axis II Disorder]*

307.44   Hypersomnia Related to . . . *[Indicate the Axis I or Axis II Disorder]*

OTHER SLEEP DISORDERS

780.xx   Sleep Disorder Due to . . . *[Indicate the General Medical Condition]*

.52   Insomnia Type

.54   Hypersomnia Type

.59   Parasomnia Type

.59   Mixed Type

_____.__ Substance-Induced Sleep Disorder *(refer to Substance-Related Disorders for substance-specific codes)*

Specify type: Insomnia Type/Hypersomnia Type/Parasomnia Type/Mixed Type

Specify if: With Onset During Intoxication/With Onset During Withdrawal

Impulse-Control Disorders Not Elsewhere Classified

312.34   Intermittent Explosive Disorder
312.32   Kleptomania
312.33   Pyromania
312.31   Pathological Gambling
312.39   Trichotillomania
312.30   Impulse-Control Disorder NOS

Adjustment Disorders

309.xx   Adjustment Disorder
.0   With Depressed Mood
.24   With Anxiety
.28   With Mixed Anxiety and Depressed Mood
.3   With Disturbance of Conduct
.4   With Mixed Disturbance of Emotions and Conduct
.9   Unspecified

Specify if: Acute/Chronic

Personality Disorders

Note: These are coded on Axis II.

301.0   Paranoid Personality Disorder
301.20   Schizoid Personality Disorder
301.22   Schizotypal Personality Disorder
301.7   Antisocial Personality Disorder
301.83   Borderline Personality Disorder
301.50   Histrionic Personality Disorder
301.81   Narcissistic Personality Disorder
301.82   Avoidant Personality Disorder
301.6   Dependent Personality Disorder
301.4   Obsessive-Compulsive Personality Disorder
301.9   Personality Disorder NOS

Other Conditions That May Be a Focus of Clinical Attention

PSYCHOLOGICAL FACTORS AFFECTING MEDICAL CONDITION

316   . . . *[Specified Psychologic Factor]* Affecting . . . *[Indicate the General Medical Condition]*

Choose name based on nature of factors:

Mental Disorder Affecting Medical Condition

Psychologic Symptoms Affecting Medical Condition

Personality Traits or Coping Style Affecting Medical Condition

Maladaptive Health Behaviors Affecting Medical Condition

Stress-Related Physiologic Response Affecting Medical Condition

Other or Unspecified Psychologic Factors Affecting Medical Condition

MEDICATION-INDUCED MOVEMENT DISORDERS

332.1   Neuroleptic-Induced Parkinsonism
333.92   Neuroleptic Malignant Syndrome
333.7   Neuroleptic-Induced Acute Dystonia
333.99   Neuroleptic-Induced Acute Akathisia
333.82   Neuroleptic-Induced Tardive Dyskinesia
333.1   Medication-Induced Postural Tremor
333.90   Medication-Induced Movement Disorder NOS

OTHER MEDICATION-INDUCED DISORDER

995.2   Adverse Effects of Medication NOS

RELATIONAL PROBLEMS

V61.9   Relational Problem Related to a Mental Disorder or General Medical Condition
V61.20   Parent-Child Relational Problem
V61.1   Partner Relational Problem
V61.8   Sibling Relational Problem
V62.81   Relational Problem NOS

PROBLEMS RELATED TO ABUSE OR NEGLECT

V61.21   Physical Abuse of Child *(code 995.5 if focus of attention is on victim)*
V61.21   Sexual Abuse of Child *(code 995.5 if focus of attention is on victim)*
V61.21   Neglect of Child *(code 995.5 if focus of attention is on victim)*

V61.1   Physical Abuse of Adult *(code 995.81 if focus of attention is on victim)*

V61.1   Sexual Abuse of Adult *(code 995.81 if focus of attention is on victim)*

ADDITIONAL CONDITIONS THAT MAY BE A FOCUS OF CLINICAL ATTENTION

V15.81   Noncompliance With Treatment

V65.2   Malingering

V71.01   Adult Antisocial Behavior

V71.02   Child or Adolescent Antisocial Behavior

V62.89   Borderline Intellectual Functioning
Note: This is coded on Axis II.

780.9   Age-Related Cognitive Decline

V62.82   Bereavement

V62.3   Academic Problem

V62.2   Occupational Problem

313.82   Identity Problem

V62.89   Religious or Spiritual Problem

V62.4   Acculturation Problem

V62.89   Phase of Life Problem

Additional Codes

300.9   Unspecified Mental Disorder (nonpsychotic)

V71.09   No Diagnosis or Condition on Axis I

799.9   Diagnosis or Condition Deferred on Axis I

V71.09   No Diagnosis on Axis II

799.9   Diagnosis Deferred on Axis II

Multiaxial System

Axis I   Clinical Disorders
         Other Conditions That May Be a Focus of Clinical Attention

Axis II   Personality Disorders
          Mental Retardation

Axis III   General Medical Conditions

Axis IV   Psychosocial and Environmental Problems

Axis V   Global Assessment of Functioning

APPENDIX B

American Nurses Association Standards of Psychiatric-Mental Health Clinical Nursing Practice*

STANDARDS OF CARE

STANDARD I. ASSESSMENT

The psychiatric-mental health nurse collects client health data.

STANDARD II. DIAGNOSIS

The psychiatric-mental health nurse analyzes the assessment data in determining diagnoses.

STANDARD III. OUTCOME IDENTIFICATION

The psychiatric-mental health nurse identifies expected outcomes individualized to the client.

STANDARD IV. PLANNING

The psychiatric-mental health nurse develops a plan of care that prescribes interventions to attain expected outcomes.

*Reprinted with permission from *A statement on psychiatric-mental health clinical nursing practice and standards of psychiatric-mental health clinical nursing practice,* Washington, D.C., 1994, American Nurses Association.

STANDARD V. IMPLEMENTATION

The psychiatric-mental health nurse implements the interventions identified in the plan of care.

STANDARD Va. COUNSELING

The psychiatric-mental health nurse uses counseling interventions to assist clients in improving or regaining their previous coping abilities, fostering mental health, and preventing mental illness and disability.

STANDARD Vb. MILIEU THERAPY

The psychiatric-mental health nurse provides, structures, and maintains a therapeutic environment in collaboration with the client and other health care providers.

STANDARD Vc. SELF-CARE ACTIVITIES

The psychiatric-mental health nurse structures interventions around the client's activities of daily living to foster self-care and mental and physical well-being.

STANDARD Vd. PSYCHOBIOLOGICAL INTERVENTIONS

The psychiatric-mental health nurse uses knowledge of psychobiological interventions and applies clinical skills to restore the client's health and prevent further disability.

STANDARD Ve. HEALTH TEACHING

The psychiatric-mental health nurse, through health teaching, assists clients in achieving satisfying, productive, and healthy patterns of living.

STANDARD Vf. CASE MANAGEMENT

The psychiatric-mental health nurse provides case management to coordinate comprehensive health services and ensure continuity of care.

STANDARD Vg. HEALTH PROMOTION AND HEALTH MAINTENANCE

The psychiatric-mental health nurse employs strategies and interventions to promote and maintain mental health and prevent mental illness.

Advanced Practice Interventions Vh–Vj

The following interventions (Vh–Vj) may be performed only by the certified specialist in psychiatric-mental health nursing.

STANDARD Vh. PSYCHOTHERAPY

The certified specialist in psychiatric-mental health nursing uses individual, group, and family psychotherapy, child psychotherapy, and other therapeutic treatments to assist clients in fostering mental health, preventing mental illness and disability, and improving or regaining previous health status and functional abilities.

STANDARD Vi. PRESCRIPTION OF PHARMACOLOGIC AGENTS

The certified specialist uses prescription of pharmacologic agents in accordance with the state nursing practice act to treat symptoms of psychiatric illness and improve functional health status.

STANDARD Vj. CONSULTATION

The certified specialist provides consultation to health care providers and others to influence the plans of care for clients, and to enhance the abilities of others to provide psychiatric and mental health care and effect change in systems.

STANDARD VI. EVALUATION

The psychiatric-mental health nurse evaluates the client's progress in attaining expected outcomes.

STANDARDS OF PROFESSIONAL PERFORMANCE

STANDARD I. QUALITY OF CARE

The psychiatric-mental health nurse systematically evaluates the quality of care and effectiveness of psychiatric-mental health nursing practice.

STANDARD II. PERFORMANCE APPRAISAL

The psychiatric-mental health nurse evaluates own psychiatric-mental health nursing practice in relation to professional practice standards and relevant statutes and regulations.

STANDARD III. EDUCATION

The psychiatric-mental health nurse acquires and maintains current knowledge in nursing practice.

STANDARD IV. COLLEGIALITY

The psychiatric-mental health nurse contributes to the professional development of peers, colleagues, and others.

STANDARD V. ETHICS

The psychiatric-mental health nurse's decisions and actions on behalf of clients are determined in an ethical manner.

STANDARD VI. COLLABORATION

The psychiatric-mental health nurse collaborates with the client, significant others, and health care providers in providing care.

STANDARD VII. RESEARCH

The psychiatric-mental health nurse contributes to nursing and mental health through the use of research.

STANDARD VIII. RESOURCE UTILIZATION

The psychiatric-mental health nurse considers factors related to safety, effectiveness, and cost in planning and delivering client care.

APPENDIX C

Mental Health Organizations

CHAPTER 3   LEGAL-ETHICAL ISSUES

Bazelon Center for Mental Health Law
1101 15th Street NW, Suite 1212
Washington, DC 20005-5002

National Association for Protection and Advocacy Systems
900 2nd Street NE, Suite 211
Washington, DC 20002

CHAPTER 8   CHILDREN AND ADOLESCENTS

American Academy of Child and Adolescent Psychiatry
3615 Wisconsin Avenue NW
Washington, DC 20016

Child Welfare League of America
440 First Street NW, Suite 310
Washington, DC 20001

National Association of Psychiatric Treatment Centers for Children
2920 Brandywine Street NW
Washington, DC 20008

National Organization of State Associations for Children
2219 California Street NW
Washington, DC 20008

Youth Suicide National Center
445 Virginia Avenue
San Mateo, CA 94402
(415) 342-5755

Youth Suicide Prevention
65 Essex Road
Chestnut Hill, MA 02167
(617) 738-0700

CHAPTER 10   THE ELDERLY

American Association of Homes for the Aging
Suite 500, 901 East Street NW
Washington, DC 20004-2037
(202) 783-2242

American Association of Retired Persons
601 East Street NW
Washington, DC 20049
(202) 434-AARP

Foundation for Hospice and Homecare
519 C Street NE
Washington, DC 20002-5809
(202) 547-6586

International Federation on Aging
1909 K Street
Washington, DC 20049
(202) 662-4987

International Senior Citizens Association
1102 South Crenshaw Boulevard
Los Angeles, CA 90019
(213) 857-6434

National Council on the Aging
409 Third Street SW, Suite 200
Washington, DC 20024
(202) 479-1200

CHAPTER 11   ANXIETY AND RELATED DISORDERS

Anxiety Disorders Association of America
600 Executive Boulevard
Rockville, MD 20852
(301) 231-9350

CHAPTER 12   MOOD DISORDERS: DEPRESSION AND MANIA

Depression and Related Affective Disorders Association
Johns Hopkins Hospital Meyer 3-181
600 North Wolfe Street
Baltimore, MD 21205
(410) 955-4647

Depressives Anonymous: Recovery from Depression
329 East 62nd Street
New York, NY 10021
(212) 689-2600

Manic Depressive Association
53 West Jackson Boulevard, Suite 618
Chicago, IL 60654

National Depressive and Manic Depressive Association
730 North Franklin, Suite 501
Chicago, IL 60610
(312) 642-0049

National Foundation for Depressive Illness
P.O. Box 2257
New York, NY 10116

CHAPTER 13   THE SCHIZOPHRENIAS
American Schizophrenia Association
900 North Federal Highway, Suite 330
Boca Raton, FL 33432
(407) 393-6167

Schizophrenics Anonymous
1209 California Road
Eastchester, NY 10709
(914) 337-2252

CHAPTER 14   PERSONALITY DISORDERS
Neurotics Anonymous International Liaison
11140 Bainbridge Drive
Little Rock, AR 72212
(501) 221-2809

Obsessive-Compulsives Anonymous
P.O. Box 215
New Hyde Park, NY 11040
(516) 741-4901

CHAPTER 15   SUBSTANCE-RELATED DISORDERS
Adult Children of Alcoholics, Interim World Service Organization
P.O. Box 3216, 2522 W. Sepulveda Boulevard
Torrance, CA 90505
(213) 534-1815

Al-Anon/Alateen Family Groups Headquarters
P.O. Box 862, Midtown Station
New York, NY 10018

Alcoholics Anonymous (AA)
General Services Office
P.O. Box 450, Grand Central Station
New York, NY 10164

American Council for Drug Education
204 Monroe Street
Rockville, MD 20850
(301) 294-0600

Black Children of Alcoholic and Drug Addicted Persons
c/o National Black Alcoholism Council
417 Dearborn Street
Chicago, IL 60605
(312) 663-5780

Children Are People Too
493 Selby Avenue
St. Paul, MN 55102
(612) 227-4031

Children of Alcoholics
23425 N.W. Highway
Southfield, MI 48075
(313) 353-3567

Children of Alcoholics Foundation, Inc.
200 Park Avenue, 31st Floor
New York, NY 10166
(212) 351-2680

Cocaine Anonymous
3740 Overland Avenue, Suite G
Culver City, CA 90034
(213) 559-5833

Hazelden Foundation
Box 11
Center City, MN 50012
(800) 328-9000

Institute on Black Chemical Abuse
2614 Nicollet Avenue
Minneapolis, MN 55408
(612) 871-7878

International Commission for the Prevention of Alcoholism and Drug Dependency
12501 Old Columbia Pike
Silver Springs, MD 20904
(301) 680-6719

"Just Say NO" International
2101 Webster Street, Suite 1300
Oakland Creek, CA 94612
(510) 451-6666

Narcotics Anonymous
P.O. Box 9999
Van Nuys, CA 91409
(818) 780-3951

National Association for Children of Alcoholics, Inc.
31582 Coast Highway, Suite B
South Laguna, CA 92677
(714) 499-3889

National Association for Native American Children of Alcoholics (NANACoA)
P.O. Box 18736
Seattle, WA 98114
(206) 322-5601

National Council on Alcoholism and Drug Dependence
12 West 21st Street
New York, NY 10010
(212) 206-6770
(800) NCA-CALL

National Institute on Drug Abuse
Parklawn Building, 5600 Fishers Lane
Rockville, MD 20857
(301) 443-6480

Reach Out—A Community Intervention
14950 44th Avenue SE
North Bend, WA 98054
(206) 888-3739

Smoker's Anonymous World Services
2118 Greenwich Street
San Francisco, CA 94123
(415) 922-8575

CHAPTER 16   DELIRIUM, DEMENTIA, AND AMNESTIC AND OTHER COGNITIVE DISORDERS

Alzheimer's Association (formerly the Alzheimer's Disease and Related Disorders Association)
360 North Michigan Avenue, Suite 1102
Chicago, Il 60601
(800) 621-0379 (toll free)
(800) 572-6037 (toll free in Illinois)

Alzheimer's Disease Education and Referral Center (A Division of the National Institute on Aging)
P.O. Box 8250
Silver Spring, MD 20907-8250
(800) 438-4380

Alzheimer's Disease International: The International Federation of Alzheimer's Disease and Related Disorders Society, Inc.
919 North Michigan Avenue, Suite 1000
Chicago Il 60611-1676
(312) 335-5777

Family Caregiver Alliance (formerly the Family Survival Project)
1736 Divisadero Street
San Francisco, CA 94115
(415) 434-3388

CHAPTER 17   DISORDERS OF CHILDHOOD AND ADOLESCENCE

Association for Children with Down Syndrome
2616 Martin Avenue
Bellmore, NY 11710
(516) 221-4700

Federation for Children with Special Needs
95 Berkeley Street, Suite 104
Boston, MA 02116
(617) 482-2915

National Association of Developmental Disabilities Council
1234 Massachusetts Avenue NW, Suite 103
Washington, DC 20005
(202) 347-1234

National Attention-Deficit Disorder Association
42 Way to the River
West Newbury, MA 01985
(508) 462-0495

CHAPTER 18   EATING DISORDERS

American Anorexia/Bulimia Association (AABA)
418 East 76th Street
New York, NY 10021
(212) 734-1114

Anorexia Bulimia Care, Inc.
545 Concord Avenue
Cambridge, MA 02138-1122
(617) 492-7670

Anorexia Nervosa and Related Eating Disorders
P.O. Box 5102
Eugene, OR 97405
(503) 344-1144

Eating Disorders Awareness and Prevention
255 Alhambra Circle #321
Coral Gables, FL 33134
(305) 444-3731

National Anorexic Aid Society
1925 East Dublin-Granville Road
Columbus, OH 43229
(614) 436-1112

National Association of Anorexia Nervosa and Associated Disorders
P.O. Box 7
Highland Park, IL 60035
(708) 831-3438

Overeaters Anonymous
P.O. Box 92870
Los Angeles, CA 90009
(310) 618-8835

CHAPTER 25   SURVIVORS OF VIOLENCE

Batterers Anonymous
8485 Tamarind, Suite D
Fontana, CA 92335
(714) 355-1100

International Society for Prevention of Child Abuse and Neglect
12-5 Oneida Street
Denver, CO 80220
(303) 321-3963

National Woman Abuse Prevention Project
1112 16th Street NW, Suite 920
Washington, DC 20036
(202) 857-0216

People Against Rape
P.O. Box 5318
River Forest, IL 60305
(708) 452-0737

Survivors of Incest Anonymous
P.O. Box 21817
Baltimore, MD 21222
(410) 433-2365

Women in Crisis
133 West 21st Street, 11th Floor
New York, NY 10011
(212) 242-4880

CHAPTER 28   PERSONS WITH AIDS

AIDS Action Council
729 Eight Street SE, Suite 200
Washington, DC 20003

AIDS Information Ministries
P.O. Box 136116
Ft. Worth, TX 76136
(817) 237-0230

AIDS Prevention League
291 Crosby Street
Akron, OH 44303
(216) 476-4384

World Hemophilia AIDS Center
10 Congress Street, Suite 340
Pasadena, CA 91105
(818) 577-4336

CHAPTER 30   PERSONS WITH CHRONIC MENTAL ILLNESS

International Committee Against Mental Illness
P.O. Box 1921, Grand Central Station
New York, NY 10163
(914) 359-7387

National Alliance for the Mentally Ill
2101 Wilson Boulevard, Suite 302
Arlington, VA 22201

CHAPTER 31   COMMUNITY MENTAL HEALTH AND HOME CARE

Association of Community Health Nursing Educators
315 Con/HSLC Building
Lexington, KY
(606) 233-6534

Center for Family Support
386 Park Avenue, South
New York, NY 10016
(212) 481-1082

Emotional Health Anonymous
P.O. Box 63236
Los Angeles, CA 90063-0236
(213) 268-7220

National Association of Psychiatric Survivors
P.O. Box 618
Sioux Falls, SD 57101
(605) 334-4067

GENERAL MENTAL HEALTH ORGANIZATIONS

American Mental Health Foundation
2 East 86th Street
New York, NY 10028
(212) 737-9027

American Public Health Association
1015 Fifteenth Street, NW
Washington, DC 20005
(202) 789-5600

National Association for Mental Health, Inc.
1800 North Kent Street
Rosslyn Station
Arlington, VA 22209

National Mental Health Association
1021 Prince Street
Alexandria, VA 22314

National Mental Health Consumers Association
P.O. Box 1166
Madison, WI 53701

People First International
P.O. Box 12642
Salem, OR 97309
(503) 362-0331

World Federation for Mental Health
1021 Prince Street
Alexandria, VA 22314
(703) 684-7722

APPENDIX D

Clinical Pathways

Alcohol Dependence
Bipolar Affective Disorder
Dementia
Major Depression

DRG#/DIAGNOSIS/DESCRIPTION: Alcohol Dependence-Requiring inpatient detox due to #1–(Alcohol withdrawal delirium ICD 291.0) #2–(Severe comorbid medical condition requiring hospitalization for safe withdrawal or treatment of comorbid condition DSM 303.90, ICD 303)

ALLOWABLE LENGTH OF STAY (LOS): _____

DAY OUTLIER: ☐ NO ☐ YES DATE: _____

COST OUTLIER: ☐ NO ☐ YES DATE: _____

PHYSICIAN: _____ ADMITTING: _____ SURGEON: _____

ADDRESSOGRAPH

* = OUTCOME

TIMING SEQUENCE	DAY 1	DAY 2	DAY 3	DAY 4 (DISCHARGE)
PREDICTED LOCATION	OPEN DETOX UNIT	OPEN DETOX UNIT	OPEN DETOX UNIT	OPEN DETOX UNIT
PROCEDURES (LABS, DIAGNOSTIC TESTS)	• Routine labs, ekg • Chest x-ray if indicated • Toxicology screens, alcohol blood level • Labs for comorbid conditions • Studies obtained if delirium with head injury (MRI) or GI bleed.	• Labs in chart • Neuro/GI tests complete if ordered • Additional labs/studies as indicated	• Anticonvulsant level if on med	
	☐ Yes ☐ No	☐ Yes ☐ No	☐ Yes ☐ No	☐ Yes ☐ No
PHYSIOLOGIC	• On I.V. • Seizure precautions • Nursing assessment, initial V.S. q 4 hours • P.E. by attending or consultant • I&O if indicated • Adjunctive medical tx. as needed (P.T., etc.)	• On I.V., seizure precautions • V.S. q 4 hours • I&O as needed • Adjunctive medical treatments as needed	• I.V. discontinued	• Specific medical treatments confirmed for aftercare (CPT, Resp. Therapy, etc.)
	☐ Yes ☐ No	☐ Yes ☐ No	☐ Yes ☐ No	☐ Yes ☐ No
PSYCHOSOCIAL	• S.W. assessment completed following contacts with significant others • Discharge options identified • S.W. and nursing assessment of supports	• S.W. assessment in chart • Specific discharge plan formulated • Socialization/safety assess q shift	• D/C living situation and medical aftercare confirmed with all parties • Discharge transportation confirmed	• Discharge to least restrictive environment (nursing home, residential program, home with day treatment, or visiting nurses)
	☐ Yes ☐ No	☐ Yes ☐ No	☐ Yes ☐ No	☐ Yes ☐ No
MEDICATIONS	• Liberal anxiolytic sedatives routine and prn's to titrate • Routine symptomatic prn's • Meds for comorbid conditions as needed • Anticonvulsants considered • Meds. parenteral or oral	• Sedative antidytics on qid schedule reflecting baseline requirement in 1st 24 hours	• Qid sedatives dropped 25% • Meds oral • Routine meds for comorbid conditions • Anticonvulsants stabilized if indicated	• Rx written for 1–2 days for close follow-up • Qid sedatives dropped to 50% of baseline • Specific aftercare plan formulated to complete detox in 2–10 days
	* ☐ Yes ☐ No	* ☐ Yes ☐ No	* ☐ Yes ☐ No	* ☐ Yes ☐ No
ACTIVITY	• Bed rest, OOB to bathroom only • Q 15 minute checks • Restraints if needed • Special precautions as needed (suicide, violence, escape, etc.)	• Per M.D. orders and nursing assessment • Restraints discontinued	• OOB but unit restricted • Continue 15 minute checks • Discontinue special precautions	• Special needs for discharge finalized (exercise restrictions, appliances, etc.)
	* ☐ Yes ☐ No	* ☐ Yes ☐ No	* ☐ Yes ☐ No	☐ Yes ☐ No
NUTRITION	• Assess appetite and GI tolerance • Check weight • Clear fluids, bland diet as indicated	• Dietary consult considered	• Special dietary instructions as needed and tolerated	• Routine aftercare diet achieved • Recheck weight • Patient sign-off on special instructions
	* ☐ Yes ☐ No	* ☐ Yes ☐ No	* ☐ Yes ☐ No	* ☐ Yes ☐ No

Continued

TIMING SEQUENCE	DAY 1	DAY 2	DAY 3	DAY 4 (DISCHARGE)
PREDICTED LOCATION	OPEN DETOX UNIT	OPEN DETOX UNIT	OPEN DETOX UNIT	OPEN DETOX UNIT
PATIENT/FAMILY EDUCATION	• Patient/family oriented to unit and MAP • Meds and patient rights reviewed • Aftercare plan devised with family • 12-Step/codependency materials introduced as needed. * ☐ Yes ☐ No	• Family session to address discharge contingencies, codependency factors (SW or nursing directed) * ☐ Yes ☐ No	• Family understands: 1) Aftercare plans and meds for patient 2) Supports and phone numbers • Family meeting to review finalized aftercare plans * ☐ Yes ☐ No	• Check off aftercare plans with patient and family * ☐ Yes ☐ No
M.D. CONSULTS	• Ordered as indicated by attending • Neuro consult begun if mentative changes with head injury • GI consult begun question GI bleed * ☐ Yes ☐ No	• Neuro/GI consults completed if ordered • Others ordered as appropriate * ☐ Yes ☐ No	• Plans/Appointments made for outpatient completion of incomplete consults * ☐ Yes ☐ No	• Follow-up appointments and consults confirmed with patient and family * ☐ Yes ☐ No
COMORBIDITY	• Medical conditions noted in M.D. admit note and nursing plans • Adjunctive medical therapies as needed (P.T., Resp therapy) * ☐ Yes ☐ No	• Other specialists follow patient every day as needed * ☐ Yes ☐ No	• Follow-up outpatient appointments scheduled with other specialists * ☐ Yes ☐ No	• Follow-up appointments confirmed with patient and family * ☐ Yes ☐ No
THERAPIES	• After mentation clear, staff confirms that patient has had basic orientation to 12-Step approach, aftercare program, and patient has 12-Step literature * ☐ Yes ☐ No	• Attending sees qd for ongoing assessment and D/C planning * ☐ Yes ☐ No	* ☐ Yes ☐ No	• Attending reviews discharge plan in detail with patient * ☐ Yes ☐ No
LEGAL	• Involuntary process considered, if necessary • Patient rights orientation * ☐ Yes ☐ No	• Guardianship process initiated if legally justified and likely necessary for aftercare compliance * ☐ Yes ☐ No	* ☐ Yes ☐ No	• Discharge voluntary or per guardian or court • Discharge order in chart • Discharge diagnosis in chart * ☐ Yes ☐ No

Notes: 1) Routine alcohol withdrawal defined as outpatient procedure (e.g., residential setting, day program, home health program, nursing home). 2) Open unit assumed, with detox capability defined as appropriate access to acute nursing. May be on an open mental health unit. 3) Involuntary patient due to delirium may be treated in restraints initially, on open unit. Developed by and reprinted with permission of Dr. Marshall Lewis, M.D., La Mesa, California

Barnes and Jewish Hospitals
Department of Nursing
Patient Clinical Management Path

Admission _____

D/C Date _____

Estimated LOS _____

Case Manager _____

Case Type & Number **(DRG – 430) Bipolar Affective Disorder**

	Day 1/Adm. Loc ( )	Var. n/d m u	Day 2 – 3 Loc ( )	Var. n/d m u	Day 4 – 6 Loc ( )	Var. n/d m u	Day 7 – 9 Loc ( )	Var. n/d m u
Date								
Procedure/Test	Organic Workup (MD), EEG (MD), CT (MD), MRI (MD), EKG (MD), CXR (MD), Electrolytes (MD), Lithium Level (MD), Drug Screen (MD), Thyroid Studies (MD), Routine Labs (MD), Other _____ (MD)		Lab Results (ID abnormals)		- - - - -> Psych Testing complete		Labs _____ Tests _____ Med. Blood Levels _____	
Consults	Medical (MD) Behavior Med. (MD) Psych Testing (MD) Other _____ (MD)		ID additional consults		- - - - ->		- - - - ->	
Meds/Tx	Meds ordered per MD including PRN to control behavior. ECT (MD) – permits (Nsg) – teaching (Nsg) – team notified (Nsg)		Monitor antidepressant, lithium, tegretol, valproic acid, PRN Meds. Other anti-psychotic meds; if mania DC antidepressant - - - - ->		- - - - -> - - - - ->		- - - - -> - - - - ->	
Activity	Voluntary/Involuntary SP/EP (MD, Nsg) Fall precautions (MS, Nsg)		Assess ADL's - - - - -> - - - - -> Integrate into milieu Participate in groups Individual therapy		- - - - -> Assess precautions - - - - -> - - - - -> - - - - ->		- - - - -> - - - - -> - - - - -> - - - - -> - - - - ->	
Nutrition	Assess appetite (MD, Nsg) Assess elimination patterns (MD, Nsg)		- - - - -> - - - - -> Teaching diet		- - - - -> - - - - -> - - - - ->		- - - - -> - - - - -> - - - - ->	
Discharge Planning	Legal Guardian ID (Nsg) Assess support system (Nsg, MD, SW, AT) Initial Plan (MD/Nsg)		SW Acknowl. note Placement issues MTP signed (MD/Nsg/SW)		Family Mtg		Plans discussed with patient (MD) - - - - -> Weekly Progress Note (MD, SW, Nsg, TR) Completes SW assess Referrals Resources MTP developed	
INTERVENTIONS: Assessment Functional Assessment	H+P & Psych orders (MD) Nsg Assessment and ADB SW notified – pt/family Proper envir. assessed Mini Mental (Nsg) Assess LOF (Nsg, SW, AT) Assess methods to control behavior (Nsg) Remove ext. stimuli (Nsg)		Ongoing assess & treatment (MD, Nsg, SW, TR) BM initial Assess. Assess for dystonia If ADL assess needed OT referral		- - - - -> Assess: – thought patterns – orientation – cog. skills – task completion		- - - - -> Assess task completion Encourage incr. LOF - - - - -> Assess lifestyle changes - - - - ->	
Patient Teaching	Orient pt/family to unit (Nsg) Bill of Rights Given (Nsg)		Ed. Pt/family to various therapies MED Educ. Primary Nurse (Nsg)		- - - - -> - - - - ->		- - - - -> - - - - ->	

Signature & Initials   Refer to Nurses Notes for documentation regarding variances.

_____ _____ _____

_____ _____ _____

_____ _____ _____

_____ _____

	Day 10 – 12 Loc ( )	Var. n/a m u	Day 13 – 14 Loc ( )	Var. n/a m u	Day 15 Loc ( )	Var. n/a m u	Discharge Expected Outcome
Date							
Procedure/Test	Labs _____ Tests _____ Med. Blood Levels _____		Labs _____ Tests _____ Chart copied if appropriate		DC Orders Written		
Consults	- - - - ->		F/u appts made		- - - - ->		
Meds/Tx	- - - - -> - - - - -> Begin ECT outpt. arrangements		- - - - -> - - - - -> - - - - ->		Perscriptions written		Pt will verbalize/ demonstrate imp. of medication +/or other therapies in maintaining optimal level of fcn after DC as evidenced by _____
Activity	- - - - -> - - - - -> - - - - -> - - - - -> - - - - ->		Do teaching r/t follow up therapy		Plans finalized r/t outpt therapy		
Nutrition	- - - - -> - - - - -> - - - - ->		DC teaching r/t nutrition		- - - - ->		
Discharge Planning			DC teaching w/family Weekly progress notes (MD, SW, TR, Nsg) DC teaching on utilization of skills learned while in hosp and how to integrate to home. Written information r/t resource given.		MTP closed or remains ongoing Final DC instructions given to pt/family F/U appt finalized		Pt will return to least restrictive/most supportive environment after DC with improved coping skills and identified resources as demonstrated by _____ _____.
INTERVENTIONS: Assessment	- - - - -> - - - - ->		- - - - -> - - - - ->		Final assessments & DC summary written.		
Functional Assessment	MMSE (Neg) - - - - -> - - - - -> - - - - -> - - - - ->		- - - - ->		- - - - ->		
Patient Teaching	- - - - -> - - - - ->		- - - - -> - - - - -> DC teaching		Final DC teaching to patient. Patient's responses to teaching documented		

*SW works M – F

Teaching (initial and date when complete)
1. Medication Education _____
2. Education on illness _____
3. Social Skills _____
4. Coping Skills _____
5. ADL's _____
6. Self-Esteem _____

7. Dealing with Anger _____
8. Communication Skills _____
9. Dealing with Sadness _____
10. Decision Making _____
11. Other _____
*Document patient response in progress notes

Addressograph:

DEMENTIA CRITICAL PATH
NORTON HOSPITAL
DRG 429 PATH # N0024

Patient label:

Admit date: _____
Expected LOS: 14
Treatment date: _____
Disch. date: _____
Actual LOS: _____

Suicide attempts #
Psychotic features
Patient falls #
Readmits within 31 days
Readmits within 1 year
Transfer to _____ /from _____
a medical/surgical unit
Treatment of concurrent medical problems/
Dx:

	DAY 1 (admit)	DAY 2	DAY 3	DAY 4	DAY 5	DAYS 6–10	DAYS 11–14
ASSESSMENTS/ EVALUATIONS	H&P, MMSE, nrsg assess, VS, lifestyle questionnaire, continent care evaluation, elimination pattern evaluation	SW contact with family, dietary evaluation	audiology appt scheduled, PT evaluation, continent care re-evaluation, elimination pattern re-evaluation	Reevaluate privilege level	SW evaluation, psych testing, OT evaluation, Tolerates Meds, Free from falls	SW contact with family, continent care re-evaluation, elimination pattern re-evaluation, Leisure Assessment	stabilization of meds, SW family conference, continent care re-evaluation
TESTS	EKG	routine labs, CRX	BDI	CT scan, EEG	PPD	BDI - day 9	BDI - day
CONSULTS		MD consults notified				MD consults complete	
DIET/FLUID BALANCE	calorie count, I&O, weigh (2x/wk - Tues. & Fri.)			nutrition/hydration assessment		nutrition/hydration stable	
ACTIVITY/ SAFETY	unit privilege, falls protocol	ambulation asst guidelines, AM exercise	sleep disturbance assessment, AM exercise	AM exercise, OT Group, Therapy Group	AM exercise, Restraints utilized -passive -posy vest -leather waist -wheelchair	Sleep pattern stable, AM exercise daily	AM exercise daily
EDUCATION				Tuesday Nite family Nite referral		'The 36-Hour Day' given, educational film shown, ADRDA referral, Family Nite	d/c instructions given

Each column header includes N | M | U check columns.

NOO24.XLS 2/6/92 ngv

1 of 2

Treatment date: ___/___/___

	DAY 1 (admit)	DAY 2	DAY 3	DAY 4	DAY 5	DAYS 6–10	DAYS 11–14
	N|M|U	N|M|U	N|M|U	N|M|U	N|M|U	N|M|U	N|M|U
TREATMENT TEAM PLANNING/ DISCHARGE PLANNING						multi-disciplinary team mtg D/C plans complete	multi-disciplinary team mtg O.P. f/u scheduled living arrangements finalized transfer form
VARIANCE ANALYSIS							
FACTS RE: VARIANCE							
STEPS TO CORRECT VARIANCE							

Developed by and reprinted with permission from Connie Anton and David A. Casey, M.D., Norton Psychiatric Clinic, Alliant Health System, Louisville, Kentucky

ST. JOSEPH HOSPITAL

DRG Number :
Primary Physician :
Physician(s) in Consult :
Anticipated Discharge Date :
Actual Discharge Date :
Financial :

MAJOR DEPRESSION CLINICAL PATHWAY©

CARE NEEDS	DAY OF ADMIT	LEVEL 1	LEVEL 2	LEVEL 3	LEVEL 4	LEVEL 5
CONSULTS/ASSESSMENTS:	MD. CM. SW. RN. OT. Consults? Medical? Other?	Psy eval? Fam mtg? Complete all assess.	Complete family mtg. Complete psy testing if ordered.	SW/CM process family mtg w/pt. Complete psy consult if ordered.	OT reassess? Transfer summaries.	Send results of assess to out-pt Tx.
HEALTH MAINTENANCE Sleep Disturbance. ADL's. Diet. Med Dx ___	Chem 19. CBC. UA. Tox? T3T2Tsh? Pg? TCA/Li/Other? Sleep? ADL? Medical (below)? Nutri? VS ___ Ortho? ------ >	Lab results? Nutri? Sleep? ADL? Review prot? Medical? VS ___ --------- >	Nutri? Sleep? ADL? Review prot? Medical? VS ___ --------- >	Nutri? Sleep? ADL? Review prot? Medical? VS ___ --------- >	Nutri? Sleep? ADL? Review prot? Medical? Med refer to med f/u. VS ___ --------- >	VS ___
PROGRAM: Target Sx ___ / Meds. Teaching needs. Stressors. Compliancy. Tx	Orientation Prot. Rest 24"? Sx? Groups? Med orders? Consent form? Teaching needs? Stressors? Tx compliancy?	Shift Assess Prot. Multidis Tx plan mtg. Assess need for alt pathway. Groups per prot. Comm mtg: ___ Meds/SE? Chart to target Sx. Tx compliancy?	Shift Assess Prot. Groups per prot. ___ Tx compliancy? Med/SE? Chart to target Sx. Prov med sheets.	Shift Assess Prot. Groups per prot. Med group. D/C planning Tx compliancy? Med/SE? Chart to target Sx. 1 unit resp.	Shift Assess Prot. Multidis Tx plan? Groups per prot. ___ Chart to target Sx. Med/SE? Tx compl?	Daily Assess Prot. D/C Prot.
SAFETY - Harm to self, others, and destruction of property. Elopment. Potential for falls. Sexually acting out.	Suicide Prot.? Safety Prot.? SFC? Verbal contract? Mental status? E?	Suicide Prot.? Mental status? Safety Prot.? SFC? E? OW Prot.?	Suicide Prot.? Mental status? Safety Prot.? SFC? E? OW Prot.?	Suicide Prot.? Mental status? Safety Prot.? SFC? E? OW Prot.?	Suicide Prot.? Mental status? Safety Prot.? SFC? E? SI review opt if ret. OW Prot.?	Review opt if SI reoccurs. Use of support systems.
DISCHARGE PLANNING: Compliancy. F/u. Teaching. MHC / Financial	CM/SW 1 data - family? placement? F/up? Release of info. LOS expectation. DSHS form? Insurance?	Housing? LOS. F/up resources? Support system? Contact fam. Assign fam. grp. Contact MHC/out-pt Tx.	Placement? MHC call liaison? Formulate f/up plan. Fam. attend sup/ed group. LOS.	Finalize f/up plan. LOS. Arrange for trans on day of D/C. Assess for therapeutic pass.	Liaison from MHC to see. Review Sx & cues to reoccurrence. Consider long-term care. Resources for meds. Coord D/C w/fam.	Check transportation & meds by 8 am for D/C by 11 am.

MAJORDEP.PIH 2/28/92

Axis I ___   Axis II ___   Axis III ___   Axis IV ___   Axis V ___

PERMANENT PART OF THE PATIENT RECORD

NOTE: This is not a Physician Order

Glossary

Abstinence Voluntary refraining from a behavior or the use of a substance that has caused problems in psychosocial, biologic, cognitive/perceptual, or spiritual/belief dimensions of life, especially with regard to food, alcohol, or drugs.

Abuse A maladaptive pattern of substance use leading to problems in psychosocial, biologic, cognitive/perceptual, or spiritual/belief dimensions of life.

Acculturation The process of adapting to another culture.

Acting-out The expression of internal affective states through external activities and behaviors, which are often destructive and/or maladaptive.

Activities of daily living (ADLs) Categories of personal care (for example, bathing, grooming, toileting, etc.).

Activity theory Supports that maintaining an active lifestyle and social roles offsets the negative effects of aging.

Acute grief The initial response to loss. While diminishing over time, acute grief may last for as long as several years, primarily depending on the meaning of the lost person/object for the survivor.

Adaptation A constant, ongoing process that occurs along the time continuum and includes the dimensions of health and illness, beginning with birth and ending with death. It involves both cognitive and physiologic neural-chemical-endocrine processes.

Adjunct therapy An action-oriented process with the primary intention of fostering adaptation and productivity for the purpose of minimizing pathology and promoting the maintenance of health.

Adjustment disorder A short-term disturbance in mood or behavior with nonpsychotic manifestations resulting from identifiable stressors. The severity of the reaction is not predictable by the severity of the stressor.

Adult developmental theory This theory suggests that although persons may complete developmental tasks of childhood, they continue to evolve as maturity progresses. Adulthood is divided into four age categories, and central themes of adult experience and development are articulated.

Adverse drug reaction An unintended effect of a medication resulting in severe, unwanted symptoms or consequences.

Affect Outward, bodily expression of emotions, ranging through joy, sorrow, anger, etc. **Blunted affect** Restricted expression of emotions. **Flat affect** Lack of outward expression of emotions. **Inappropriate affect** Affect that is not congruent with the emotion being felt (for example, laughing when sad). **Labile affect** Rapid changes in emotional expression.

Affective instability Rapidly fluctuating moods in which the individual is emotionally reactive to external events and lacks coping skills to manage feeling states.

Ageism Systematic stereotyping and discrimination against the elderly.

Agnosia The loss of comprehension of auditory, visual, or other sensations, although the senses are intact.

Agonist A chemical that results in stimulation of activity of the target receptor.

Agranulocytosis A drop in the production of leukocytes, specifically the neutrophil cell line, leaving the body defenseless against bacterial infection.

AIDS dementia complex (ADC) A progressive neurologic syndrome caused by a subacute chronic HIV encephalitis. Cognitive impairment indicative of damage to the central nervous system is evidenced in these clients.

AIDS wasting syndrome (AWS) During the later stages of AIDS, clients may experience a significant weight loss. A condition of an unexplained weight loss of 10%, along with chronic diarrhea, fatigue, or unexplained fever, and a loss of muscle mass, may occur during the later stages of AIDS.

Akathisia Literally, "not sitting." A syndrome caused by dopamine-blocking drugs characterized by both motor restlessness and a subjective feeling of inner restlessness.

Alcoholism A chronic, progressive, and potentially fatal biogenic and psychosocial disease characterized by impaired control over drinking, tolerance, and physical dependence that lead to loss of control, distorted thinking, and other social consequences.

Allopathic The health beliefs and practices that are derived from the scientific models of the present time and involve the use of technology and other modalities of present-day health care, such as immunization, proper nutrition, and resuscitation.

Alpha$_1$ blockade The process of inhibiting alpha$_1$ receptors that may result in orthostatic hypotension and reflex tachycardia.

Alter ego A function of the therapist to reflect back the client's attitudes and feelings without including the client's negative connotations.

Alzheimer's disease A neurodegenerative disease characterized by progressive, irreversible, and lethal structural damage to the brain due to the presence of β-amyloid proteins and leading to loss of cognitive functions and symptoms of progressive dementia.

Analysis Taking apart collected data to examine and interpret each piece and identify variations from typical behaviors or responses. Discovering patterns or relationships in the data that may be cues or clues that require further investigation.

Anhedonia The loss of pleasure and interest in activities previously enjoyed, or in life itself.

Anorexia nervosa An eating disorder classified in DSM-IV, characterized by self-starvation, weight loss below minimum normal weight, intense fear of being fat even when emaciated, distorted body image, and amenorrhea in females.

Antagonist A chemical that results in inhibition of activity of the target receptor.

Anticholinergic delirium Toxic effects of anticholinergic drugs characterized by confusion, perceptive disturbances, sleep disturbance, increased or decreased psychomotor activity, and change in level of consciousness. Also called atropine psychosis, this syndrome may present as a psychotic state.

Anticipatory grief Grief experienced before death or loss occurs, for example, when a loved one has a terminal illness.

Antiretroviral therapy The use of drugs, such as AZT, ddI, and ddC. These drugs, often administered to clients via drug trials, treat the major opportunistic diseases associated with AIDS. Treatment with antiretroviral therapy can significantly impact the progression of AIDS by preventing opportunistic infections.

Anxiety A vague, subjective, nonspecific feeling of uneasiness, tension, apprehension, and sometimes dread or pending doom. Occurs as a result of a threat to one's biologic, physiologic, or social integrity arising from external influences. A universal experience and an integral part of human existence.

Aphasia **Expressive aphasia** - The inability to speak or write (also known as Broca's aphasia). **Global aphasia** - The complete loss of all motor and sensory uses of oral and written speech; expression and comprehension are severely impaired. **Receptive aphasia** - The inability to comprehend what is being said or written (also known as Wernicke's aphasia).

Appraisal As related to crisis, the ongoing perceptual process by which a potentially harmful event is distinguished from a potentially beneficial or irrelevant event.

Apraxia The loss of the ability to carry out purposeful, complex movements and to use objects properly.

Art medium Material or technical means of artistic expression.

Art therapy The use of artistic activities, such as painting and clay modeling, in psychotherapy and rehabilitation.

Assimilation To become absorbed into another culture and to adopt its characteristics.

Attending Demonstrating to a client attention to what he is saying.

Atypical depression Depression with features that include hypersomnia, weight gain, mood reactivity, and sensitivity in interpersonal relationships.

Autism A pervasive developmental disorder characterized by marked impairment of social and cognitive abilities.

Autodiagnosis Self-examination of one's own thoughts, feelings, perceptions, and attitudes about a particular client.

Autonomy versus shame and doubt Erikson's term for the second developmental crisis. Parental encouragement toward self-sufficiency in basic tasks of toileting, dressing, and feeding foster autonomy. Thwarted efforts by over- or under-controlling parents result in the polar opposite, or shame and doubt. Shame is rage turned against the self. Doubt is an internal feeling of badness.

Battered wife Women who are abused physically or mentally by their male intimates or those with whom they have been intimate.

Behavioral reorganization A new way of viewing development emphasizing that new developmental capabilities are fit together and organized into previous capabilities in an orderly, patterned, and predictable fashion, and build in a cumulative manner from earlier capabilities in a direction of greater complexity.

Bereavement The state of grieving.

Binge eating disorder (BED) A pattern of binge eating without the purging characteristic of bulimia nervosa. BED is commonly known as compulsive overeating. It is included in DSM-IV as a proposed diagnosis for further study.

Bioavailability The amount, usually described as a percentage, of a drug administered that reaches the blood.

Bipolar disorder A mood disorder characterized by episodes of mania and depression.

Blackout Acute anterograde amnesia without recognition formation of long-term memory, e.g., a period of memory loss during which there is no recall for activities, resulting from the ingestion of alcohol and/or other drugs.

Body image disturbance A perceptual disturbance in the way individuals subjectively perceive and experience their body shape, size, weight, and proportions. Typically, persons with anorexia complain of feeling "fat" or see their stomach/hips/thighs as fat when they are clearly underweight.

Body knowledge An "embodied" knowledge that allows a person to recognize familiar and unfamiliar mental, emotional, and body mechanisms—a sense of balance/imbalance changes.

Boundary The definition and separation of the self from others through the clarification of the limits and extent of responsibilities and duties of one's self in relationship to others.

Boundary violations Going beyond the established therapeutic relationship standards.

Bulimarexia An obsession with thinness, dieting, and a compulsive cycle of bingeing and purging. This syndrome is now labeled Bulimia nervosa.

Bulimia nervosa An eating disorder classified in DSM-IV, characterized by recurrent episodes of binge eating subjectively experienced as out of control, followed by inappropriate compensatory behavior to prevent weight gain, such as self-induced vomiting; overuse of laxatives, diuretics, diet pills; fasting; or excessive exercise. Also present is excessive preoccupation with body shape and weight.

Case finding The methodical and deliberate identification of people of any age who are ill and in need of care or who are at risk for incurring illness and injury.

Catastrophic reaction A sudden or gradual negative change in the behavior of dementia clients caused by their inability to understand and cope with stimuli in the environment.

CD₄ count The CD_4 lymphocyte count (T_4 cell count) is the most commonly used marker to determine HIV progression. HIV attacks CD_4 cells that help fight infections.

Chemical restraint The use of psychotropic drugs and sedatives to reduce or eliminate psychiatric symptoms.

Childhood incest Any type of exploitative sexual experience between relatives or surrogate relatives before the victim reaches the age of 18.

Child neglect Harm or threatened harm to a child's health or welfare by a parent, legal guardian, or any other person responsible for the child's health or welfare through either 1) failure to provide adequate food, clothing, shelter, or medical care, or 2) placing the child at unreasonable risk to health or welfare.

Child physical abuse Inflicted injury to a child that can range from minor bruises and lacerations to severe neurologic trauma and death. Psychologic abuse is also included.

Child psychologic abuse Rejection, degradation/devaluation, terrorization, isolation, corruption, exploitation, denying essential stimulation to a child, and unreliable and inconsistent parenting.

Chronic mental illness A psychiatric disorder that persists over time with remissions and recurrence of severe, disabling symptoms.

Chronic sorrow Grief in response to an ongoing loss such as chronic illness in a loved one.

Chronically mentally ill Persons who have manifested the symptoms of chronic mental illness.

Clear and convincing evidence A burden of proof that requires more than the preponderance of evidence used in a civil proceeding and less than beyond a reasonable doubt used in a criminal proceeding.

Clinical pathway A standardized format used to provide and monitor client care and progress by way of the case management, interdisciplinary health care delivery system. (Also known as critical pathway, care path, or Care Map.)

Closure Also called sharing. The last stage in a psychodrama or movement/dance therapy experience in which the experience is processed (verbally and nonverbally), and insight and a sense of completion are promoted.

Codependency An emotional, psychologic, and behavioral pattern of coping that an individual develops as a result of prolonged exposure to a dysfunctional pattern of behavior within the family of origin. The individual experiences difficulty with identity development and setting functional boundaries, which lead to taking care of others rather than self.

Cognition Awareness and subjective meaning of an event.

Cognitive rigidity The inability to adequately identify problems and corresponding solutions.

Cognitive triad A pattern of thinking noted in depressed people and characterized by 1) a negative self-assessment, 2) a negative view of the present, and 3) a negative view of the future.

Cohort A group united due to one or more common factors.

Collegiality Working within a body of associates or colleagues, for example, a team of home care providers.

Commitment A court order certifying that an individual is to be confined to a mental health facility for treatment.

Communication A reciprocal process of sending and receiving messages between two or more people and their environment; the vehicle for establishing a therapeutic relationship.

Community-linked health care Care provided by public and/or private partnerships using grant and government funds.

Comorbidity The co-occurrence of two or more psychiatric or other disorders. The simultaneous appearance of the disorders may be due to a causal relationship between the two, an underlying predisposition to both, or the disorders may be completely unrelated. For example, depression is a common comorbid disorder in clients with eating disorders. There are different theories about the association between eating disorders and mood disorders. Also known as dual diagnosis.

Compensatory developmental task Developmental tasks that deal with replacing losses with some other mechanism (for example, developing new skills or hobbies after retirement).

Competency to stand trial The ability of the individual to understand the charges and the consequences, the nature and object of the legal proceedings, and to advise an attorney and assist in the defense.

Compulsion An unremitting, repetitive impulse to perform a behavior (for example, hand washing, ordering, checking) or mental acts (for example, praying, counting, or repeating words silently), the goal of which is to prevent or reduce anxiety or distress and not to provide pleasure or gratification. In most cases, the person feels driven to perform the compulsion to reduce the distress that accompanies an obsession or to prevent some dreaded event or situation.

Concentrated care Also called "intensive" care. Home care services delivered during a crisis, usually on a short-term basis, and designed to meet a specific, acute need.

Concrete operational period Piaget's term for the third stage of cognitive development whereby the child begins to think and reason in logical ways about the present and the past.

Confidentiality The right of the psychiatric client to keep information from people outside the health care team.

Congruence Consistency of agreement between verbal and nonverbal behavior.

Conscious suicidal intention A state of awareness characterized by a person's desire to accomplish death through self means.

Continuity theory Promotes the premise that people become "more like themselves" as they age, maintaining continuity of habits, beliefs, and values.

Conventional morality Kohlberg's second stage of morality whereby moral decisions consider the perspective of the victim and are first based on a desire for approval from others to avoid guilt, and later based on defined rights, assigned duty, rules of the community, and respect for authority.

Conversion reaction A repression of an emotional problem by replacing it with a physical symptom. Most often involves the sensory organs or voluntary nervous system.

Coping Various strategies used, consciously or unconsciously, to deal with stress and tensions arising from perceived threats to psychologic integrity. It is the process of attempting to solve life problems.

Countertransference The nurse's irrational and inappropriate responses to a client because of a personal problem.

Creativity The ability to apply original ideas to the solution of problems; the development of theories, techniques, or devices; or the production of novel forms of art, literature, philosophy, or science.

Crisis A turning point marked by sharp improvement or sharp deterioration. A decision or event of great psychologic significance for an individual.

Crisis intervention Therapeutic techniques for helping individuals experiencing a crisis.

Crisis theory A theory that examines conscious coping abilities and unconscious defense mechanisms and how they help or inhibit interaction with the individual. Crises are separated into three categories: maturational, situational, and adventitious.

Cross-tolerance A condition in which a tolerance to one drug often results in a tolerance to chemically similar drugs. Tolerance is originally produced by long-term administration of one drug, which is manifested toward a second drug that has not been administered previously (for example, tolerance to alcohol is accompanied by cross-tolerance to volatile anesthetics of barbiturates).

Decanoate Decanoic (10 carbon) acid ester which is linked to the antipsychotics fluphenazine and haloperidol to create the long-acting antipsychotics. Dissolved in sesame oil and injected intramuscularly or subcutaneously, the rate-limiting pharmacokinetic step is the cleavage of the decanoate bond to release the active drug.

Defense A means or method of protecting oneself; an unconscious mental activity or mental structure (for example, a defense mechanism) that protects the ego from anxiety.

Defense mechanism A structure of the psyche that protects the ego against unpleasant feelings or impulses. Defense mechanisms are unconscious and deny, falsify, or distort reality.

Deinstitutionalization The process of returning psychiatric clients to the community, which includes limited admission and commitment policies.

Delayed grief Grief that is not expressed or experienced until well after a loss, often as a result of circumstances such as being focused on survival (as among refugees).

Delirium A disturbance of consciousness and a change in cognition that develop over a short period of time and tend to fluctuate during the course of the day, characterized by disorientation to time and place; reduced ability to focus, sustain, or shift attention; incoherent speech; and continual aimless physical activity.

Delusions False beliefs that are fixed and resistant to reasoning.

Dementia A global impairment of intellectual (cognitive) functions (e.g., thinking, remembering, reasoning) that usually is progressive and of sufficient severity to interfere with a person's normal social and occupational functioning.

Denial A range of psychologic maneuvers designed to decrease awareness of the fact that substance use is the cause of an individual's problems rather than a solution to the problems.

Dependence, physical A physiologic state of adaptation to a drug or alcohol, usually characterized by the development of tolerance to drug effects and the emergence of a withdrawal syndrome during prolonged abstinence.

Dependence, psychologic The compulsive use of substances leading to a state of craving a drug or alcohol for its positive effect or to avoid negative effects associated with its absence, or the inability to exercise behavioral restraint.

Dependency ratio The number of individuals below the age of 18 and over the age of 64 who are dependent on those persons ages 18–64.

Depo-Lupron Leuprolide A synthetic analog of naturally occurring gonadotropin-releasing hormone. It inhibits gonadotropin secretion, thus suppressing testicular testosterone. **Depo-Lupron Medroxyprogesterone acetate** A medication used in the adjunctive treatment of sexual disorders; a sexual appetite suppressant; lowers testosterone level to a prepubescent level.

Derealization The feeling that the surrounding world is not real or is distorted.

Dereism A loss of connection with reality and logic that occurs just prior to autistic thinking. Thoughts become private and idiosyncratic. Dereism is seen in schizophrenia.

Detoxification A treatment that helps the individual withdraw from the physical effects of alcohol and/or other addictive substances and helps eliminate severe withdrawal symptoms that can occur with abrupt withdrawal. It can be provided in a hospital setting, day treatment, or outpatient setting.

Devaluation A method of coping whereby a person deals with emotional conflict or stressors by attributing exaggerated negative qualities to self or others.

Developmental contexts The necessary circumstances that must exist for development to occur; some circumstances are related to nature (genes, inheritance), and others are related to nurture (environment).

Dichotomous thinking A cognitive distortion common to people with eating disorders, in which an individual views a situation as all or nothing, black or white, all good or all bad. If a situation is less than perfect, it is perceived as a failure.

Disaffiliated A person who does not associate with family, friends, or service providers.

Disengagement theory The process of mutual withdrawal between the aging individual and society.

Dissociation Occurs when an overwhelming event or experience is separated from an individual's conscious awareness.

Distress A subjective response to internal or external stimuli that are threatening or perceived as threatening to the self.

Diurnal variation Feeling worse or more depressed in the morning and better in the evening.

Double The individual in psychodrama who operates as the "inner voice" of the protagonist, to express repressed thoughts, feelings, and conflicts.

Double-bind A situation in which contradictory messages are given to one person by another, demanding a response or choice between two opposing alternatives.

Dual diagnosis A term used when the individual has two identified primary psychiatric diagnoses, most commonly used when one diagnosis is drug- or alcohol-related. For example, the person may have both a psychoactive substance use disorder and a mood disorder.

Duty to warn The legal obligation of a mental health professional to warn an intended victim of potential harm from a client with mental illness.

Dysarthria Difficulty in articulating words: this is especially frustrating because the client knows what words to use but has trouble forming them (more commonly found in vascular dementias and strokes).

Dysfunctional grief Grief expressed to a significantly greater or lesser intensity over a significantly longer or shorter time than is culturally expected. It may manifest itself in serious physical and/or emotional disabilities.

Dysthymia A state of chronic, low-level depression lasting more than two years that may lead to more severe depression if untreated.

Dystonic Pertaining to unstable states or to some disorder.

Ego Freud's word for the self, whose major role is to find safe and appropriate ways for needs (instincts) to be met (gratified) in the external world. Lies mostly in the conscious.

Ego defenses Automatic psychologic processes that keep out the threat of internal and external stressors and dangers or deny awareness to protect the self. (Also known as defense mechanisms or mental mechanisms.)

Ego dissonance Inconsistency between attitudes and behaviors.

Ego dystonic pedophile A person who is cognitively aware that his or her behavior is inappropriate and is truly affected by this. This person might voluntarily seek treatment to deal with the disorder.

Ego state A coherent set of feelings developed by the child's organization of similar life experiences and accompanied by a related set of coherent and observable behavior patterns. There are three ego states defined in transactional analysis: parent, adult, and child.

Ego syntonic pedophile A person who is cognitively aware that his or her behavior is inappropriate; however, he or she is not troubled by this. This person will not voluntarily seek treatment because he or she sees no need to do so.

Elder abuse Includes psychologic or emotional neglect, psychologic or emotional abuse, violation of personal rights, financial abuse, physical neglect, direct physical abuse to persons over age 65.

Empathy Projecting sensitivity and understanding of another's feelings and communicating the understanding in a way the client understands.

Enactment The action portion in psychodrama in which a scene, or sequence of scenes, is portrayed.

Encopresis The repeated passage of feces into inappropriate places (for example, clothing or floor), whether involuntary or intentional.

Endogenous agonist/antagonist A substance that occurs naturally in a cell or tissue that stimulates or inhibits a receptor (for example, dopamine, GABA).

Enmeshed An individual's inability to differentiate or establish a personal identity. Enmeshed individuals have diffuse boundaries within the family and live solely for each other. Member roles are permeable with a tendency to cut off outside interactions.

Enmeshed families A pattern of family relationships in which children are pressured to conform to parental expectations rather than express their individuality. Overinvolvement among family members, discouragement of outside relationships, and blurring of boundaries occur (for example, a mother will "feel" her daughter's emotions).

Enuresis The repeated voiding of urine into bed or clothing, whether involuntary or intentional.

Epigenesis A developmental concept developed by Erikson that genetics and environmental experiences, which begin with conception and continue throughout life, determine the person's personality and the mentally healthy or destructive responses to the world.

Equilibrium A state of emotional balance.

Estradiol Endocrine testing for the female that determines the level of estradiol in the bloodstream. Estradiol levels may reflect level of sexual desire.

Ethnicity A cultural group's sense of identification associated with the group's common social and cultural heritage.

Ethnocentrism The tendency of members of one cultural group to view the members of other cultural groups in terms of the standards of behavior, attitudes, and values of their own group. Belief in the superiority of one's own group.

Ethnomethodology The study of people in context, through inductive, qualitative methods.

Eustress A nonspecific stress response associated with desirable events such as marriage, birth of a child, job promotion, etc., from the Greek word *eu* or "good."

Euthymia A mood that is normal and level.

Expert witness Someone with education and experience on a specialized subject who is qualified as an expert and allowed to testify in order to assist the jury in understanding technical information.

External vacuum pump A cylindrical vacuum pump applied to the penis. When operated it brings blood into the penis and traps it there, thus improving erection.

Extrapyramidal symptoms (EPS) The collective term used to describe the motor side effect of dopamine-blocking medications. EPS includes acute dystonia, akathisia, parkinsonism, and tardive dyskinesia.

Faulty information processing Fixed and rigid patterns of thinking that block the contextual aspects of a situation and are characteristic of depressed people.

Feedback The measure by which the effectiveness of the message is gauged.

Feminist theory Includes four major dimensions of wife abuse: 1) the explanatory utility of the constructs of gender and power, 2) the analysis of the family as a historically situated institution, 3) the crucial importance of understanding and validating women's experiences, and 4) the employment of scholarship for women.

Figure-background formation The concept that an organism's foremost need or specific interest will define the reality of the moment.

First-pass effect Refers to the process of orally administered drugs, when absorbed, first passing through the liver where substantial percentages of the administered dose may be metabolized before the drug is distributed to the tissues.

Flight of ideas The rapid shifting from one idea to another without completion of the preceding idea, commonly manifested in mania.

Forensic psychiatry A branch of psychiatry that studies individuals who commit crimes and enter the court system, some of whom are incarcerated.

Formal operations period Piaget's term for the fourth stage of cognitive development whereby the child learns to think in abstract and hypothetical ways about future events and learns to develop strategies for solving complex problems.

Generativity In Erikson's personality theory, the positive outcome of one of the stages of adult personality development; the ability to do creative work or to contribute to the raising of one's children. The opposite of stagnation.

Generic approach A method that focuses on the characteristic course of the particular kind of crisis rather than on the psychodynamics of each individual in crisis.

Genuineness A quality of an effective nurse that encompasses openness, honesty, and sincerity.

Gerontology The scientific study of the aging process involving multiple disciplines and settings.

Grief The dynamic natural psychologic and physiologic responses to loss. Grief affects physical, cognitive, behavioral, emotional, social, and spiritual aspects of the individual.

Grief work   The intense psychologic effort to 1) fully express the feelings associated with grief, 2) understand the relationship with the deceased, and paradoxically, 3) carry on with essential activities of daily living.

Half-life   The time required for the serum concentration of a drug to decrease by 50%. Drugs dosed at intervals less than their half-life will accumulate in the body, often to toxic levels.

Hallucination   A subjective disorder of perception in which one of the five senses is involved in the absence of external stimuli.

Hardiness   A sense of mastery or self-confidence needed to appropriately appraise and interpret health stressors.

Heritage consistency   The observance of the beliefs and practices of one's traditional cultural belief system.

Holism   A term with various interpretations and meanings. Holism in the broadest sense refers to a belief system in which persons are unified, complex, interdependent systems with interrelated physical, mental, emotional, spiritual, and social dimensions.

Homeopathic   Health beliefs and practices derived from traditional cultural knowledge to maintain health, prevent changes in health status, and restore health.

Humanistic nursing   A view of nursing as an interactive process that occurs between two people, one needing help and one willing to give help. Developed by Josephine Patterson and Loretta Zderad and based on existential theory and the phenomenological method.

Hypochondriasis   A long-standing dependency. A preoccupation with the "sick role." A fear or belief that one has a serious illness, in spite of medical reassurances to the contrary.

Hypomania   The mood of elation with higher-than-usual activity and social interaction; not as expansive as full mania.

Id   The basic level of the personality that lies in the unconscious and consists of primitive drives and instincts aimed at self-preservation.

Ideas of influence   Delusional beliefs that one's thought processes are being influenced by an external source, such as radar, space aliens, or another person.

Ideas of reference   Incorrect interpretations of incidents and external events as having a particular or special meaning specific to the person.

Identified client   In family therapy, the member of the family (or group) whose behavior is seen as causing the problem for the family (or group).

Identity versus role confusion   Erikson's term for the fifth developmental crisis. Self-assurance of the previous stage leads to the adolescent's gaining a self-identity and the development of an ability to determine where the adolescent fits in society. Failure to develop a self-identity leads to role confusion, poor self-confidence, and alienation.

Imminence   The likelihood that an event will occur within a specific time period.

Incidence   The frequency of occurrences of a specific disorder within a designated time period; number of new cases.

Independent activities of daily living (IADLs)   Activities an individual requires in order to function in the community (for example, shopping, preparing meals, and transportation).

Indifference   The manner in which the nurse interacts with the client that manifests disconnectedness and unconcern.

Individual approach   The individual approach differs from the generic approach in its emphasis on assessment, by a professional, of the interpersonal and intrapsychic processes of the person in crisis.

Industry versus inferiority   Erikson's term for the fourth developmental crisis. From the initiative achieved in the previous stage, the child develops an ability to master learning and develop peer relationships that lead to self-assurance or industry. Failure to master academic and social pursuits leads to inferiority and hinders attempts to try new things.

Inference   The interpretation of behavior, assumption of motive, and formation of a conclusion without having all the information.

Initiative versus guilt   Erikson's term for the third developmental crisis. Self-sufficiency allows the child to undertake and plan tasks and join with others in cooperative efforts resulting in increased initiative. If the child's desire to show initiative causes excessive conflict in the family, guilt results.

Insight   The ability to perceive oneself realistically and understand oneself.

Institutionalization   The act of placing or confining persons with mental disorders in state-run facilities, such as residential treatment programs designed to treat such disorders.

Interactive context of behaviors   Behavior is shaped and reinforced by interaction with one's social system while the social system is being shaped and reinforced by the same interaction.

Intermediate care   Short-term home care services designed to assist the client and family to achieve a planned, higher level of functioning.

Interoceptive deficits   The inability to correctly identify and respond to bodily sensations. Individuals with eating disorders are often out of touch with their bodies and either fail to recognize or mistrust physical sensations such as hunger, satiety, fatigue, or pain, as well as emotional states.

Interpersonal communication   Communication between two or more persons containing both verbal and nonverbal messages.

Intracorporal injections   Injections of various medications into the right and left corpus cavernosum to improve erection.

Intrapersonal communication   Communication occurring within oneself that can be functional or dysfunctional.

Intrapsychic   Pertaining to the mind or mental process.

Intuition   Insight into a situation without the benefit of critical analysis. (Also known as intuitive reasoning.)

Isolation   A feeling of aloneness with perceived social rejection or lack of support from others during a crisis.

Kindling   The creation of electrophysiologic sensitivity in the brain from stress that results in alteration of neural functioning.

Learned helplessness   The perception that events are uncontrollable, leading to apathy, helplessness, powerlessness, and depression.

Least restrictive alternative   Providing the least restrictive treatment in the least restrictive setting for a mental health client.

Legal duty   Something that an individual is required to do by law.

Lethality   The potential for causing death related to the level of danger associated with the suicidal plan; along a continuum from low to high probability, for example, aspirin overdose versus a gunshot wound to the head. (A) **High** involves a precise suicide plan for the next 24–72 hours, with a lethal method, available means, intent to die, poor impulse control, and no rescue plan. (B) **Moderate** involves a less immediate or less lethal method and plan. (C) **Low** involves

plans that are vague, imprecise, and sometimes include plans for rescue.

Libido The energy of the instincts held in the id.

Life span The maximum length of survival genetically fixed for each species.

Locus of control An aspect of personality that deals with the degree of control an individual perceives over one's own destiny. **Internal locus of control** refers to the ability to actively control one's own destiny. **External locus of control** refers to the inability to control one's own destiny.

Loosening of associations Thought disturbance in which the speaker rapidly shifts expression of ideas from one subject to another in an unrelated manner.

Loss A process characterized by a series of overlapping stages that include common psychologic and behavioral manifestations of recognition, adjustment, and resolution.

Lovemap A term coined by John Money that refers to an idiosyncratic image in the mind-brain that depicts the idealized lover and lovemaking activities.

Machismo Compulsive masculinity characterized by a male's excessive need to control and dominate his wife at all costs.

Maintenance care Home care services provided when the client has reached a stable, higher level of functioning, such as surveillance, client and family education, and emotional support. Concentrated and intermediate care is performed by skilled providers, and maintenance by less skilled providers.

Mandatory outpatient treatment The legal requirement that an individual undergo mental health treatment in an outpatient setting. The individual usually has been noncompliant and allegedly has a propensity for dangerous acts.

Mania An elevated, expansive, or irritable mood accompanied by hyperactivity, grandiosity, and loss of reality.

Melancholic depression Severe depression characterized by anhedonia, feeling worse in the morning, weight loss, psychomotor retardation.

Message The information (feelings or ideas) being sent and received.

Metabolism The biotransformation of a drug molecule into a new molecule.

Metabolite The result of biotransformation of a drug. Although most metabolites tend to be pharmacologically inactive and less toxic, there are important exceptions (for example, fluoxetine is metabolized into the active metabolite nor-fluoxetine; ethanol is metabolized into the more toxic acetaldehyde).

Metamemory One's self-perceptions of memory changes.

Metaneeds As the physiologic and safety needs are met, the need for belonging and love emerges.

Milieu therapy Re-creates a community atmosphere on an inpatient hospital unit, a partial hospitalization unit, and a day treatment setting, in order to facilitate interaction between client peers to identify and problem-solve issues that occur while relating to others.

Mirroring A technique in psychodrama and movement/dance therapy in which one individual imitates the behavior patterns of another in order to show the person how other people perceive and react to him or her.

Mood A feeling state reported by the client that can vary with external and internal changes.

Mourning Feeling or expressing grief or sorrow.

Movement Kinesthetic behavior in which individuals communicate by the use of body motions rather than formal language.

Movement/dance therapy The use of movement to promote increased awareness of the body and changes in feeling states, cognition, and behavior.

Music The science or art of assembling or performing intelligible combinations of tones in an organized, structured form.

Music therapy The use of music to provide a variety of listening and participatory experiences adapted to the needs of the individual clients, such as an opportunity for nonverbal communication, shared experience, emotional expression, relaxation, and nonthreatening enjoyment.

Negative symptoms A syndrome that includes flat affect, poverty of speech, poor grooming, withdrawal, and disturbance in volition.

Neuritic plaques The maltese-cross-appearing clumps composed of amyloid fibers found in the brains of Alzheimer's victims.

Neurofibrillary tangle The accumulation of twisted filaments inside brain cells, which is one of the characteristic structural abnormalities found on autopsy that confirms the diagnosis of Alzheimer's disease.

Neuroleptic Literally, "to clasp the neuron"; the term used to describe what are now called the typical antipsychotic medications (for example, chlorpromazine/Thorazine, haloperidol/Haldol).

Neuroleptic malignant syndrome A rare but potentially lethal toxic reaction to dopamine-blocking drugs that presents with a constellation of symptoms, including fever, automatic instability, increased muscular rigidity, and altered mental status.

Neurotransmission The process by which electrochemical signals are sent throughout the brain.

Neutrality The manner in which the nurse interacts with the client that shows respect and acceptance regardless of the client's appearance or behavior.

Nihilism Belief that existence is meaningless and useless.

Nocturnal penile tumescence A test that uses a strain gauge around the penis to depict the pattern of arousal while the client sleeps.

Nonadrenergic A neuronal system or neuron that manufactures and/or responds to norepinephrine.

Nonverbal communication The nonverbal behaviors displayed by individuals during the process of an interaction.

Norms The group's standards for behavior, attitudes and, at times, perceptions of their members and, as such, represent the shared expectations of appropriateness in behavior.

Nuclear family A family made up of the parental dyad and the individual's siblings.

Object constancy The ability to maintain a relationship regardless of frustration and changes in the relationship.

Object relations The stability and depth of an individual's relations with significant others as manifested by warmth, dedication, concern, and tactfulness.

Objectivity The state of remaining free from bias, prejudice, and personal identification in an interaction with another person.

Obsession The persistent ideas, thoughts, impulses, or images about death, sexual matters, or religious matters that lead to efforts to resist them, are associated with marked distress or interference, and result in marked anxiety or distress.

Occupation The goal-directed use of time, energy, interest, and attention to foster adaption and productivity, to minimize pathology, and to promote the maintenance of health.

Occupational therapy The application of goal-directed, purposeful activity in the assessment and treatment of individuals with psychologic, physical, or developmental disabilities.

Opportunistic diseases Diseases that commonly appear with AIDS clients, especially when their T-cells drop; these diseases include cytomegalovirus and mycobacterium.

Organismic self-regulation The concept that once the need is satisfied, it will recede and allow the emergence of the next need.

Overselect A behavior commonly noted in children with psychiatric disorders. The child tends to be so specific about the stimuli that he or she selects to respond to, it appears as if there is no response at all.

Paradigm A side-by-side example to show a clear pattern.

Paraphilia A category of sexual deviations/disorders presenting with inappropriate sexual fantasies involving deviant sexual acts, inappropriate sexual urges, and acting-out of these fantasies and urges.

Parasitic One's total dependence on someone else for one's every need.

Parasuicidal behavior Suicidal gestures and attempts that are unsuccessful and of low lethality. For example, superficial cutting of the wrists.

Penile-brachial index (PBI) A test that determines the difference between the penile and brachial blood pressure that assesses vascularization to the penis.

Penile plethysmograph A diagnostic test that determines a person's arousal pattern and level of arousal. This test may reveal the source of the client's arousal and the degree of its significance.

Performance inadequacy The fear beginning nurses may feel that they will not know what to say to help clients resolve their problems.

Perseveration A disturbance in thought association in which there is a persistent repetition of the same idea in response to different questions.

Personality traits Enduring patterns of perceiving, relating to, and thinking about the environment and oneself that are exhibited in a wide range of social and personal contexts.

Perturbation A determination of an individual's level of distress, developed by Shneidman, and rated on a scale of 1–9. Refers to how upset, disturbed, or perturbed the individual is.

Pervasive developmental disorder A collection of disorders in which the child experiences deficits in a broad range of developmental areas.

Phobias A group of disorders primarily characterized by avoidance of a specific situation or escape, if that situation is unexpectedly encountered.

Pleasure principle The goal of experiencing pleasure while avoiding pain. This principle represents the id's goal in the personality to satisfy a person's innate needs and instincts.

Positive affirmation A self-supporting message that reinforces confidence and enhances performance.

Positive cognitive set The belief that success is possible and that one can achieve what one believes.

Positive regard Acceptance of and respect for a client.

Positive symptoms A syndrome that includes hallucinations, increased speech production with loose associations, and bizarre behavior.

Postconventional morality Kohlberg's third stage of morality in which moral decisions reflect underlying ethical principles that consider societal needs and are first based on a sense of community respect and disrespect and later based on principles of justice, the reciprocity and quality of human rights, and respect for the dignity of human beings as individuals.

Postvention Grief therapy after a death occurs, but before pathology develops.

Poverty of thought A psychopathologic thought disturbance in schizophrenia. The client's inability to think logically and sequentially is reflected in **Poverty of Content Speech,** which is vague, repetitious, and disconnected.

Preconventional morality Kohlberg's first stage of morality whereby moral decisions are self-centered, and the child's behavior is first based on avoidance of punishment and later based on a desire to gain rewards or benefits.

Premorbid The period just preceding the onset of a mental illness. Characteristics of the personality may indicate the type of disorder that may occur.

Preoperational period Piaget's term for the second stage of cognitive development whereby the child remains egocentric, is oriented in the present, and only guesses about cause and effect.

Pressured speech Rapid speech with an urgent quality.

Prevalence The number of cases of a specific disorder in a normal population at a given point in time; the number of existing cases.

Primary prevention Prevention efforts that focus on reduction of the incidence of mental disorders within the community. It is directed toward occurrence of mental health problems with emphasis on health promotion and prevention of disorders.

Primary process thinking Prelogical thought that aims for wish fulfillment. It is associated with the pleasure principle characteristic of the id portion of the personality.

Privileged communication Communication between a professional and a client that is confidential and protected from forced disclosure in court, unless authorized by the client. The privilege is delegated by statutes in the various states.

Problem solving The process involved in discovering the correct sequence of alternatives leading to a goal or to an ideational solution.

Prodromal symptoms Early symptoms, such as a deterioration in functioning, that may mark the onset of a mental illness.

Projection The process whereby a person deals with his or her emotional conflicts or stressors, both internal and external, by unconsciously and falsely attributing to another person his or her own unacceptable feelings, impulses, or thoughts.

Projective identification The process whereby a person projects his or her emotional conflicts and stressors to another; however, this individual does not fully disavow what is projected. The individual remains aware of his or her own affects or impulses but misattributes them as justifiable reactions to the other person.

Protagonist The individual, in psychodrama, who presents and acts out his or her emotional problems and interpersonal relationships.

Protein binding The holding of a drug in the blood by circulating protein molecules. The percentage of a drug that is protein-bound varies widely. The percentage of a drug that is protein-bound is not pharmacologically active until released.

Psyche The mind as the center of thought processes, emotions, and behavior.

Psychodrama A form of psychotherapy in which an individual reenacts life situations in order to examine subjective experiences, promote insight, and alter specific behavior patterns.

Psychoeducation A type of therapy that educates the client with a paraphilic disorder to identify situations/objects that may trigger inappropriate sexual activity, develop awareness of relapse prevention strategies, and acknowledge the importance of treatment compliance.

Psychological morbidity The prevalence of psychologic impairment in a specific population. With respect to AIDS, psychologic morbidity refers to the prevalence of emotional distress and syndromic conditions in persons with AIDS (PWAs).

Psychomotor agitation Agitated motor activity.

Psychomotor retardation The slowing of physiologic processes resulting in slow movement, speech, and reaction time.

Psychosis Having impaired ability to recognize reality, and thus being unable to deal with life's demands.

Psychosocial stages Theory by Erikson. A series of eight stages, distinct periods in a person's social development; each stage is marked by a particular type of crisis resulting from the ego's attempt to meet the demands of social reality.

Psychosomatic illness Pertaining to a physical disorder that is notably influenced or caused by emotional or mental factors, involving the mind and the body.

Psychotropic Literally, "mind nutrition." The term used to describe drugs that affect the central nervous system.

Purging The use of self-induced vomiting and/or the abuse of laxatives, diuretics, syrup of ipecac, diet pills, or enemas to avoid weight gain following a binge. One or more of these behaviors as well as periods of fasting and excessive exercise during an episode of bulimia nervosa may be used.

Reality principle The goal of postponing immediate gratification until a suitable object for this satisfaction is found. The ego is ruled by this principle.

Receiver The individual who both receives and interprets the message.

Receptors Protein molecules located in the cell walls of tissues that receive chemical stimulation resulting in stimulation or inhibition of activity of the target cell.

Recreation To create again by some form of play, amusement, or relaxation.

Recreational therapy The use of recreational activities as an integral part of the rehabilitation or therapeutic process. The purpose is to increase enjoyment of life, stimulate activity and self-expression, enhance socialization, and counterbalance self-concern.

Reframing A technique of changing the viewpoint of a situation and replacing it with another viewpoint that fits the facts equally well but changes the entire meaning.

Regressive developmental task Developmental tasks that focus on adjustments to physical, psychologic, and functional changes due to aging.

Relapse/relapse prevention The resumption of a pattern of substance use or dependency after a period of sobriety, and/or the process in which indicators or warning signs appear prior to the individual's actual resumption of the substance. Relapse prevention is a means of helping the chemically dependent individual maintain behavioral changes over a prolonged period of time.

Repression The involuntary exclusion of a painful, threatening experience. Begins in infancy and continues throughout life. Underlies all other defense mechanisms but also operates as its own defense mechanism.

Residual symptoms Minor disturbances that may remain after an episode of schizophrenia but do not include delusions, hallucinations, incoherence, or gross disorganization.

Resistance The inability, whether conscious or unconscious, to accept change; the denial of new problems.

Restrictive admission policies A component of the deinstitutionalization process that limits the length of stay until symptoms are under control.

Restrictive commitment policies A component of the deinstitutionalization process that limits commitment to a psychiatric facility to threat to harm self and/or others.

Restrictive environment An environment that restricts the client's activity in order to help him or her regain control of his or her behavior. The individuals may be placed in open-door or closed-door seclusion during periods of extreme agitation, suicidal ideations, or threats of violence to self or others.

Rites of passage Rituals associated with life transitions that facilitate maturational development, such as puberty, marriage, birth, and death. These rites are commonly composed of three stages: separation, transition, and incorporation.

Roles The socially expected behavior patterns usually determined by an individual's status in a particular group. Peplau identified four roles for the psychiatric nurse: 1) resource person, 2) counselor, 3) surrogate, and 4) technical expert.

Safeguards Relapse prevention strategies employed to assist the individual in developing control over inappropriate sexual acting-out (reoffending) behaviors.

Safety The sense of security developed within the therapeutic relationship when the responsibilities and expectations of each party are clearly defined. Safety develops from knowing the boundaries of a relationship and acting within them.

Schemata The cognitive set of the self and world through which situations are perceived, coded, and interpreted.

Seasonal affective disorder (SAD) A mood disorder that occurs at a regular time each year.

Secondary gain Any benefit, such as personal attention, sympathy from others, or escape from unwanted responsibilities, as a result of illness. May be experienced when family or friends pay a great deal of attention to the client's eating behavior, for example, preparing special meals or making special arrangements in an attempt to encourage him or her to eat.

Secondary prevention Prevention efforts directed toward reduction in the prevalence of mental disorders through early identification of problems and early treatment of those problems. This stage occurs after the problem arises and aims at shortening the course or duration of the episode.

Selective attention The ability to discriminate and focus on relevant information.

Self-actualization A concept developed by Maslow as an ongoing actualization of potentials, capacities, and talents as fulfillment of a mission, and as a greater knowledge and acceptance of one's own intrinsic nature.

Self-system Sullivan's term for the system that infants develop to cope with anxiety associated with the interpersonal process of need satisfaction and security. The individual develops self-appraisal as a result of significant others' responses to actions from the individual. Actions that cause anxiety result in "bad-me" self-appraisals. Actions that cause no anxiety result in "good-me" self-appraisals. Actions of disapproval cause severe anxiety, emotional withdrawal, and "not-me" self-appraisals.

Sender The individual who initiates the transmission of information.

Sensate focus A learned exercise developed by Masters and Johnson that involves concentrating on the sensations produced by touching.

Sensorimotor period Piaget's term for the first stage of cognitive development in which children use their senses and motor skills to manipulate the environment and develop the ability to differentiate self from objects.

Sero status The presence or absence of HIV antibodies in the bloodstream. HIV status is determined through laboratory tests and is either seropositive or seronegative.

Seroconversion The term used to signify that HIV antibodies are discernible in the individual's laboratory blood tests. A person who was previously exposed to the HIV virus and showed no presence of the virus but subsequently tests positive for the virus has experienced seroconversion.

Serum level monitoring The process of obtaining blood samples to determine drug concentration.

Sick role A set of social expectations that an ill person meets such as 1) being exempt from usual social role responsibilities, 2) not morally responsible for being ill, 3) obligation to "want to get well," and 4) obligation to seek competent help.

Side effect An undesired nontherapeutic and often predictable consequence of medication. Frequently diminished with time. Contrast with adverse drug reaction.

Sleep reversal A state in which normal sleeping patterns are reversed; the individual sleeps during the day and is active during the night.

Sobriety The state of complete abstinence from alcohol and/or other drugs of abuse in conjunction with a satisfactory quality of life.

Social learning The process by which children acquire the behaviors they need to survive and function in society, that result from repeated interactions in their environments.

Social learning theory Bandura's theory that aggression is not instinctual but a learned behavior.

Social support The presence of other individuals who are able to give understanding, encouragement, and other assistance in life, especially during difficult times.

Socialization The process of being raised within a culture and acquiring the characteristics of the given group.

Somatization The conversion of mental states or experiences into bodily symptoms, associated with anxiety.

Splitting The process by which a person keeps the positive and negative aspects of self or others separate from each other. An individual who utilizes the unconscious defense mechanism of splitting cannot tolerate ambiguity; therefore, people, events, or ideas are either good or bad, right or wrong, black or white, but not gray.

State disorders The diagnoses made on Axis I are considered state diagnoses. They constitute behavior patterns that are not as pervasive or long-lasting as trait disorders.

Stereotype To form an oversimplified, standardized opinion of a person or group of people that is often determined without adequate information.

Stress 1) A term that refers to both a stimulus and response. It can denote a nonspecific response of the body to any demand placed on it, whether the causal event is negative (a painful experience) or positive (a happy occasion). 2) A state produced by a change in the environment that is perceived as challenging, threatening, or damaging to the person's dynamic equilibrium. 3) The wear and tear on the body over time. 4) Psychologic stress has been defined as all processes, whether originating in the external environment or within the person, that demand a mental appraisal of the event prior to the involvement or activation of any other system.

Subjectivity Emphasizing one's own moods, attitudes, and opinions in an interaction with another person.

Suicide The act of taking one's own life.

Suicide ideators Those persons who experience suicidal thinking on a consistent basis.

Suicidology The scientific and humane study of human self-destruction.

Sundowner's syndrome The confusion and irritation common in dementia clients at the end of the day, probably due to general tiredness and an inability to process anymore information after a long day of struggling to interpret their environment correctly.

Superego The portion of the mind, differentiated from the ego that contains the traditional values and taboos of society as interpreted by the child's parents, that becomes part of the self. Lies in the preconscious.

Sustained release Medications designed to provide slow, controlled dissolution, which allows longer dosing intervals.

Synthesis Combining several parts of relevant data into a single piece of information. Comparing behavioral patterns to learned theories or typical patterns of behavior in order to identify strengths and seek explanations for symptoms.

Syntonic Pertaining to a state of stability.

Tardive dyskinesia A syndrome of abnormal, involuntary movements occurring after months or years of treatment with drugs that block dopamine type 2 receptors. These movements, often described as oral, buccal, lingual, or masticatory, can occur throughout the body.

Taxonomy A classification of known phenomena under a hierarchial structure.

Teratogen A substance that causes developmental malformations in the fetus.

Tertiary prevention Prevention efforts that have the dual focus of reduction of residual effects of the disorder and rehabilitation of the individual who experienced the mental disorder.

Themes The recurring patterns of interactions the client experiences in relationships with self and/or others.

Therapeutic communication The interaction that takes place between the nurse and client. The content has meaning and focuses on the client's concerns.

Therapeutic milieu An environment designed to promote emotional health and, based on the assumption that the client is an active participant in his or her own life, the client therefore needs to be involved in the management of his or her behavior and environment.

Therapeutic play Age-appropriate play activities used purposefully by the nurse for assessment, intervention, and promotion of normal growth and development in children.

Therapeutic relationship A personal relationship convened to help one of the participants deal more effectively and maturely with some difficulty in life. It is a goal-directed, client-centered, and objective relationship.

Theme development The part of movement/dance therapy in which a specific issue or feeling is actively being explored.

Thought blocking The abrupt interruption in the flow of thoughts or ideas due to a disturbance in the speed of associations.

Tic A sudden, rapid, recurrent, nonrhythmic, stereotyped movement or vocalization that is considered irresistible but is often suppressible for short periods of time.

Tolerance Physiologic adaptation to the effect of drugs in order to diminish effects with constant dosages or to maintain the intensity and duration of effects through increased dosage.

Trait disorders Trait disorders are used to describe Axis II diagnoses. Axis II is used exclusively for the description of personality disorders and mental retardation, which are considered trait diagnoses. The symptoms of a personality disorder or mental retardation are not time-limited, nor do they occur only in a time of crisis.

Transference The unconscious response whereby clients associate the nurse with someone significant in their lives.

Transgenerational violence When violence within the family is an accepted everyday occurrence, a natural, normal component of family living.

Transindividual perspective Looking beyond individuals to the family or community as the unit of care.

Transinstitutionalization A process in which clients are transferred from one institution to another, such as from a psychiatric hospital to a nursing home.

Transitional objects Objects that remind one of a significant person. For example, the boss keeps a picture of his wife on his desk, which reminds him of her during work hours.

Triggers Stimuli that heighten unacceptable sexual cravings.

Trust The reliance on the truthfulness or accuracy of the therapeutic relationship developed through a congruency between the therapist's words and actions.

Trust versus mistrust Erikson's term for the first developmental crisis that the child tries to resolve. Consistent, predictable, and continuous care results in developing a sense of trust in oneself, others, and the world. Inconsistent, unpredictable, or discontinuous care results in the polar opposite, or mistrust of oneself, others, and the world.

Unconditional positive regard The stance of therapist modeling the unconditional acceptance of the client and based on the belief that the client is competent to direct himself or herself in his or her natural tendency to move forward toward integration.

Unconscious suicidal intention A state outside of awareness during which persons engage in risk-taking behaviors that have a high likelihood of causing their deaths.

Underselect The inability of children with psychiatric disorders to select which stimuli are most important; manifested by inappropriate responses to routine events.

Unipolar A depressive disorder characterized by episodes of depression with no mania.

Vaginal dilators A graduated series of cylindrical dilators introduced into the vagina to decrease involuntary spasm.

Vaginal plethysmography A test that uses a vaginal probe to assess blood flow to the female vagina. Blood flow is an indicator of arousal.

Verbal communication Spoken or written words that compose the symbols of language.

Vicarious learning Learning through imagining the experiences of others as if they are one's own.

Victimizer Another term used to define a sex offender. This term may be used when discussing familial transmission of the paraphilia.

Vigilance The ability to sustain attention over longer periods of time.

Warm up A stage of psychodrama and movement/dance therapy that focuses on introducing group members, increasing the comfort level, and determining the theme or issue to be addressed.

Xenophobia A morbid fear of strangers and those who are not of one's own ethnic group.

Yohimbine An alpha adrenoreceptor blocker that may facilitate blood flow to the genitalia and therefore improve sexual arousal.

Index

GENERIC: amitriptyline (a-mee-trip'ti-leen)
TRADE: Elavil

CLASSIFICATION Tricyclic antidepressant

INDICATIONS & USES Major depression, anxiety, panic, eating disorders, chronic pain.

USUAL ADULT DOSAGE RANGE 50-300 mg/day. In major depression: 150-300 mg/day. Initial dosing is 50-75 mg/day in divided doses.

AVAILABE FORMS Tabs 10, 25, 50, 75, 100, 150 mg; inj IM 10 mg/mL.

PHARMACOKINETICS/DYNAMICS Half-life varies from 10-46 hr in adults to 17-46 hr in the elderly. Partially metabolized to nortriptyline. Plasma therapeutic range: (amitriptyline + nortriptyline) 120-250 ng/mL. Full therapeutic effects may not be apparent for 2-4 wk. Initial multiple daily dosing can often be consolidated to once or twice a day, once tolerant to side effects.

SIDE EFFECTS Sedation, dizziness, blurred vision, dry mouth, constipation, urinary retention, nausea, vomiting, tachycardia, orthostatic hypotension, tremor, cardiac conduction abnormalities, decreased libido, weight gain, allergic dermatitis, skin photosensitivity, reduced seizure threshold.

ADVERSE REACTIONS Exacerbation of untreated narrow-angle glaucoma, induction of mania, reduced seizure threshold, **potentially fatal in overdose.**

INTERACTIONS Increased levels—cimetidine, fluoxetine, antipsychotics, methylphenidate, propoxyphene. Decreased levels—barbiturates, phenytoin, chronic carbamazepine. Increased effects of epinephrine, norepinephrine, CNS depressants. **Severe hypertension with MAOIs.** Antacids reduce absorption.

CONTRAINDICATIONS Caution in clients with cardiovascular disease, arrhythmias, strokes, and acute myocardial infarction and thyroid disease medications. May exacerbate signs and symptoms of glaucoma, benign prostatic hypertrophy, diabetes. Avoid in pregnant and lactating women.

NURSING CONSIDERATIONS Monitor level of sedation and vital signs carefully during dose titration. Suicide risk may be increased during initial improvement, particularly as psychomotor depression abates.

CLIENT TEACHING Therapeutic effects may take several weeks. Caution about initial sedation and dizziness. Instruct to change positions slowly. Use hats and sunscreens to reduce risk with sun exposure.

AVAILABLE IN CANADA Apo-Amitriptyline, Levate, Meravil, Novotriptyn, Rolavil, Elavil

bold—Life-threatening reactions

GENERIC: alprazolam (al-pray'zoe-lam)
TRADE: Xanax

CLASSIFICATION Antianxiety—benzodiazepine

INDICATIONS & USES Anxiety, anxiety associated with depression, panic disorder.

USUAL ADULT DOSAGE RANGE 0.5-4 mg/day in anxiety; up to 10 mg/day in panic disorder in divided doses. Initial dosing is 0.25-0.5 mg bid to tid. Lower doses for geriatric clients.

AVAILABLE FORMS Tab 0.25, 0.5, 1 mg

PHARMACOKINETICS/DYNAMICS Rapidly absorbed. Average half-life is 12-15 hr. In some individuals, antianxiety effects may last <12 hr. Antianxiety effects may be rapidly apparent. Antipanic effects may be apparent in 1-2 wk.

SIDE EFFECTS Drowsiness, dizziness, ataxia. Rarely—nausea, vomiting, GI upset, blurred vision.

ADVERSE REACTIONS Rarely increased aggression/irritability. **Oversedation and respiratory depression with other CNS depressants,** seizures on withdrawal.

INTERACTIONS Serum levels increased by cimetidine, oral contraceptives, disulfiram, nefazodone, erythromycin.

CONTRAINDICATIONS Coma, shock, alcohol intoxication, pregnancy. Use with caution in history of drug abuse/addiction. Use with caution in clients with liver or kidney disease.

NURSING CONSIDERATIONS Schedule IV controlled substance. Risk of respiratory depression when used with other CNS depressants. Abrupt discontinuation associated with anxiety, rebound insomnia, and seizures. Discontinuation titration may need to be as slow as 0.25 mg/day every week in some clients. Rapid absorption causing a "buzz" may reinforce drug-seeking behavior or may be perceived dysphoricly in non-drug abuse population.

CLIENT TEACHING Avoid hazardous activities during initiation; avoid alcohol; caution against sudden discontinuation.

AVAILABLE IN CANADA Apo-Alpraz, Novo-Alpazol, Nu-Alpraz, Xanax

bold—Life-threatening reactions

GENERIC: bupropion (byoo-proe'pee-on)
TRADE: Wellbutrin

CLASSIFICATION Aminoketone antidepressant

INDICATIONS & USES Major depression. Often used in clients who have failed to respond to or cannot tolerate other antidepressant drugs. Seldom used as a first-choice drug.

USUAL ADULT DOSAGE RANGE 200-450 mg/day. Initial dosing is 100 mg bid. Maximum dose is 150 mg tid. Never administer more than 150 mg at one time to minimize risk of seizure.

AVAILABLE FORMS Tabs 75, 100 mg

PHARMACOKINETICS/DYNAMICS Half-life varies from 10-21 hr in adults. Full therapeutic effects may not be apparent for 2-4 wk.

SIDE EFFECTS Agitation, insomnia, headache, dizziness, slight weight loss, slight increases in blood pressure. Occasional mild, dry mouth, blurred vision, constipation, nausea, and tremor.

ADVERSE REACTIONS Dose-related increased incidence of seizures, induction of mania, rare depersonalization and psychotic symptoms.

INTERACTIONS MAOIs increase side effects; L-dopa may increase side effects. Other drugs that reduce seizure threshold may increase seizure activity.

CONTRAINDICATIONS Preexisting seizure disorder, anorexia nervosa, bulimia. (Clients with eating disorders may be at increased risk for seizures.)

NURSING CONSIDERATIONS Suicide risk may be increased during initial improvement, particularly as psychomotor depression abates. Low risk of fatality in overdose.

CLIENT TEACHING Therapeutic effects may take several weeks.

AVAILABLE IN CANADA not available

bold—Life-threatening reactions

GENERIC: carbamazepine (kar-ba-maz'e-peen)
TRADE: Tegretol

CLASSIFICATION Anticonvulsant

INDICATIONS & USES Generalized tonic-clonic and complex partial seizures, mixed seizure patterns, trigeminal neuralgia. Other uses: mood stabilizer in depression and bipolar disorder with and without lithium; aggression, rage, and impulse control disorders; adjunct in benzodiazepine withdrawal.

USUAL ADULT DOSAGE RANGE 200-1800 mg/day. Initial dosing is 200 mg bid.

AVAILABLE FORMS Tabs, chewable 100 mg; tabs 200 mg; oral susp 100 mg/5 mL

PHARMACOKINETICS/DYNAMICS Initial half-life averages 36 hr in adults. Carbamazepine induces its own metabolism. After 4-6 wk the average half-life is 24 hr. Once adequate serum levels are obtained, efficacy may be rapid in seizure disorders while taking 1-3 wk in mood disorders. Plasma therapeutic range is 4-12 μg/mL. Persistent side effects can be serum level-related and increase substantially in some clients at levels > 7 μg/mL.

SIDE EFFECTS Blurred or double vision, drowsiness, hypotension, hypertension, urinary retention, rash, pruritus, nystagmus, paraesthesia, nausea, vomiting, visual hallucinations, ataxia, photosensitivity, chills, confusion, leucocytosis, dizziness.

ADVERSE REACTIONS **Aplastic anemia, agranulocytosis, thrombocytopenia, Stevens-Johnson syndrome,** eosinophilia, antidiuretic effects leading to water intoxication, seizures upon abrupt withdrawal.

INTERACTIONS Increases carbamazepine levels—erythromycin, fluoxetine, verapamil, propoxyphene, valproate, cimetidine, TCAs, diltiazem, INH, terfenadine. Decreases carbamazepine levels—phenobarbital, phenytoin, primidone. Carbamazepine decreases levels and potentially the efficacy of oral contraceptives, warfarin, cyclic antidepressants, phenothiazines, haloperidol, clonazepam, thyroid hormone, theophylline, doxycycline.

CONTRAINDICATIONS Bone marrow suppression, hypersensitivity to TCAs or carbamazepine. Use with caution in severe liver, renal, or cardiac disease and with increased intraocular pressure.

NURSING CONSIDERATIONS Monitor for decrease in WBC. Monitor for neurotoxicity in clients receiving lithium. Shake oral suspension well. Notify prescriber if symptoms of fever, sore throat, mouth ulcers, bleeding, or easy bruising occur. Take with food to minimize GI upset.

CLIENT TEACHING Risks of initial sedation, potential for failure of oral contraceptive. Teach client to notify if signs and symptoms of infection occur.

AVAILABLE IN CANADA Apo-Carbamazepine, Mazepine, Novo Carbamaz, Tegretol

bold—Life-threatening reactions

GENERIC: benztropine (benz'troe-peen)
TRADE: Cogentin

CLASSIFICATION Antiparkinsonian, anticholinergic

INDICATIONS & USES Parkinsonism, treatment and prevention of extrapyramidal symptoms caused by antipsychotic medications (excluding tardive dyskinesia).

USUAL ADULT DOSAGE RANGE 1-6 mg/day; Typical starting dose is 0.5-1 mg bid. Most clients have significant side effects at doses ≥ 6 mg/day.

AVAILABLE FORMS Tabs 0.5, 1, 2 mg; inj IM, IV 1 mg/mL.

PHARMACOKINETICS/DYNAMICS Rapidly absorbed PO with effects in 1-2 hr. Very rapidly absorbed IM with effects in 10-30 min. The pharmacokinetics are not well-characterized. Usually given bid, elimination is slow enough in some clients to allow qd dosing.

SIDE EFFECTS Dry mouth, blurred vision, tachycardia, urinary retention, constipation, nervousness, confusion.

ADVERSE REACTIONS **Paralytic ileus.** Anticholinergic delirium (also called anticholinergic intoxication and atropine psychosis)—confusion, disorientation, stupor, Flushing, hyperthermia, extreme agitation, hallucinations, hypotension, supraventricular tachycardia, markedly diminished or absent bowel sounds.

INTERACTIONS Additive anticholinergic effects with other medications, esp. antipsychotics, tricyclic antidepressants.

MAOIs, digoxin, furosemide (Lasix). Additive effects with CNS depressants.

CONTRAINDICATIONS Severe cardiac or GI disorders, benign prostatic hypertrophy, angle-closure glaucoma, neuroleptic malignant syndrome.

NURSING CONSIDERATIONS Increased risk of heat stroke. Evaluate for adequate hydration and constipation. May aggravate the movements of tardive dyskinesia. Elderly at increased risk for confusion and anticholinergic delirium.

AVAILABLE IN CANADA Apo-benztropin, Bensylate

bold—Life-threatening reactions

GENERIC: chloral hydrate (klor-al hye'drate)
TRADE: Noctec

CLASSIFICATION Hypnotic

INDICATIONS & USES Short-term treatment of insomnia.

USUAL ADULT DOSAGE RANGE 500-2000 mg at bedtime.

AVAILABLE FORMS caps 250, 500 mg; syr 250, 500 mg/5mL; supp 325, 500 650 mg

PHARMACOKINETICS/DYNAMICS Rapidly absorbed and metabolized in minutes. The active metabolite, trichloroethanol, has a half-life of 8-11 hr. Sleep is usually attained in 30-60 min and is effective for 4-8 hr.

SIDE EFFECTS GI irritant causing nausea, vomiting, diarrhea. Next-day sedation and impaired motor coordination are common. Drowsiness, dizziness.

ADVERSE REACTIONS Continued use is associated with gastritis, skin ulceration, and renal damage; **5000-10,000 mg can be fatal in overdose.**

INTERACTIONS Additive effects with CNS depressants including alcohol. Furosemide can cause flushing, diaphoresis, and unsteady blood pressure.

CONTRAINDICATIONS Severe hepatic cardiac or renal disease, porphyria, ulcer, pregnancy.

NURSING CONSIDERATIONS Schedule IV controlled substance. Risk of respiratory depression when used with other CNS depressants. Monitor for next-morning sedation,

reduced cognitive functioning, incoordination. Administer with plenty of water to minimize GI upset.

CLIENT TEACHING Avoid hazardous activities; avoid alcohol; caution against sudden discontinuation after long-term use.

AVAILABLE IN CANADA Novochlorhydrate, Noctec

bold—Life-threatening reactions

GENERIC: amantadine (a-man'ta-deen)
TRADE: Symmetrel

CLASSIFICATION Antiparkinsonian/antiviral

INDICATIONS & USES Parkinsonism, prophylaxis and treatment of extrapyramidal symptoms, prophylaxis and treatment of influenza A.

USUAL ADULT DOSAGE RANGE For adults with normal renal function: 100 mg bid. Dosage must be reduced with decreasing renal function.

AVAILABLE FORMS Caps 100 mg; syr 50 mg/5 mL.

PHARMACOKINETICS/DYNAMICS Average half-life is 24 hr with normal renal function. Renal elimination. Full effects may be seen in 4-5 days. Amantadine may facilitate the release of dopamine in CNS neurons.

SIDE EFFECTS Dizziness, insomnia, impaired concentration, hypotension, irritability, depression, anxiety, ataxia, nausea, anorexia, livedo reticularis (blotchy spots on the skin) with chronic use.

ADVERSE REACTIONS Hallucinations and psychotic reactions, particularly in clients not on antipsychotics or if doses are not reduced for impaired renal function. May exacerbate eczema.

INTERACTIONS May cause hypertension with MAOIs. May cause insomnia, irritability, seizures, and irregular heartbeat

with stimulants. May increase side effects of anticholinergic medications.

CONTRAINDICATIONS Uncontrolled psychosis, eczema, seizures.

NURSING CONSIDERATIONS Generally used for EPS when anticholinergics are contraindicated or ineffective. Monitor vital signs and for level of consciousness initially. Monitor for continued efficacy; may lose effectiveness over time. Abrupt discontinuation may result in acute worsening of symptoms.

AVAILABLE IN CANADA Symmetrel

bold—Life-threatening reactions

GENERIC: buspirone (byoo-spear'own)
TRADE: Buspar

CLASSIFICATION Antianxiety/azaspirone

INDICATIONS & USES Anxiety disorders, adjunct in treatment of anxiety and aggression in developmentally disabled, adjunct treatment of behavioral problems in brain-injured and elderly clients, adjunct treatment in partial responders to SSRIs (e.g., fluoxetine) of depression and obsessive-compulsive disorder.

USUAL ADULT DOSAGE RANGE 15-60 mg/day; Typical starting dose 5 mg tid. Due to the short half-life, tid dosing is usually required.

AVAILABLE FORMS Tabs 5, 10 mg

PHARMACOKINETICS/DYNAMICS Average half-life is 2-4 hr. Buspirone is a 5-HT1 (serotonin) partial agonist. Efficacy in anxiety may not appear until the second week of therapy. Full therapeutic effects may not be apparent for 2-4 wk.

SIDE EFFECTS Nausea, dizziness, headache, excitement, lightheadedness. Rare insomnia, drowsiness.

ADVERSE REACTIONS Rare reports of increased liver enzymes when used with trazodone.

INTERACTIONS Do not use with MAOIs. May increase haloperidol serum levels.

CONTRAINDICATIONS Severe hepatic or renal disease, pregnancy.

NURSING CONSIDERATIONS Many clients being treated for anxiety are accustomed to rapid antianxiety and sedative effects of benzodiazepines.

CLIENT TEACHING Educate clients to potential side effects and delayed antianxiety effects of buspirone.

AVAILABLE IN CANADA Buspar

bold—Life-threatening reactions

GENERIC: clonazepam (kloe-na'zi-pam)
TRADE: Klonopin

CLASSIFICATION Anticonvulsant—benzodiazepine

INDICATIONS & USES Lennox-Gastaut syndrome (petit mal variant epilepsy), antianxiety; adjunctive treatment of bipolar disorder.

USUAL ADULT DOSAGE RANGE 0.5-10 mg/day in divided doses, bid or tid. Typical starting dose 0.5 mg bid or tid.

AVAILABLE FORMS Tabs 0.5, 1, 2 mg

PHARMACOKINETICS/DYNAMICS Rapidly absorbed. Half-life ranges from 20-40 hr.

SIDE EFFECTS Drowsiness, ataxia, hypotonia, hypersalivation. Rarely—nausea, vomiting, GI upset, blurred vision.

ADVERSE REACTIONS Rarely—euphoria followed by dysphoria; increased aggression/irritability. Oversedation and **respiratory depression with other CNS depressants,** seizures on withdrawal

INTERACTIONS CNS depressants, may increase levels of phenytoin, digoxin. Effects reduced by smoking, rifampin. Serum levels increased by cimetidine, valproate, disulfiram, oral contraceptives.

CONTRAINDICATIONS Coma, shock, alcohol intoxication, pregnancy, narrow-angle glaucoma. Use with caution in history of drug abuse/addiction.

NURSING CONSIDERATIONS Schedule IV controlled substance. Risk of respiratory depression when used with other CNS depressants. Abrupt discontinuation associated with anxiety, rebound insomnia, and seizures. Discontinuation titration may need to be as slow as 1 mg/day each week in some clients. Increased risk of ataxia and falls in the elderly.

CLIENT TEACHING Avoid hazardous activities during initiation; avoid alcohol; caution against sudden discontinuation.

AVAILABLE IN CANADA Rivotril, Klonopin

bold—Life-threatening reactions

GENERIC: diphenhydramine (dye-fen-hye'dra-meen)
TRADE: Benadryl, Benalyn, various OTC products

CLASSIFICATION Antihistamine (H₁ blocker)

INDICATIONS & USES Acute and chronic treatment of drug-induced extrapyramidal reactions; hypnotic; sedation; allergy and cold symptoms; nausea, vomiting, vertigo, motion sickness.

USUAL ADULT DOSAGE RANGE 25-50 mg tid to qid. Acute dystonic reactions: 25-50 mg IM.

AVAILABLE FORMS Caps 25, 50 mg; tabs 25, 50 mg; elix 12.5 mg/5 mL; syr 12.5 mg/5 mL; inj IM, IV 10, 50 mg/mL.

PHARMACOKINETICS/DYNAMICS Rapidly absorbed. 50% bioavailable. Half-life varies considerably between 3-9 hr in adults. IM effects begin in 15-30 min. Sedative effects after oral dosing are maximal at 1-3 hr. Nonspecific sedative effects are the result of histamine blockade. Substantial anticholinergic effects.

CONTRAINDICATIONS Severe cardiac or GI disorders, benign prostatic hypertrophy, angle-closure glaucoma, stenosing peptic ulcer, asthma, nursing mother, infants.

NURSING CONSIDERATIONS Increased risk of heat stroke. Evaluate for adequate hydration and constipation. May aggravate the movements of tardive dyskinesia. Elderly at increased risk for confusion and anticholinergic delirium. Injections should be deep IM as superficial injections can be locally irritating.

AVAILABLE IN CANADA Alledryl, Insomnal, Benadryl, Benalyn

bold—Life-threatening reactions

GENERIC: chlorpromazine (klor-proe'ma-zeen)
TRADE: Thorazine

CLASSIFICATION Typical antipsychotic

INDICATIONS & USES Symptomatic management of psychotic disorders, initial management of psychotic manic states, intractable hiccoughs.

USUAL ADULT DOSAGE RANGE 60-2000 mg/day. Initial dosing is 20-75 mg every day in divided doses. Doses greater than 1000 mg/day are seldom required. Typical IM dose is 25-50 mg.

AVAILABLE FORMS Tabs 10, 25, 50, 100, 200 mg; time-rel caps 30, 75, 150, 200, 300 mg; syr 10 mg/5mL; conc 30, 100 mg/mL; supp 25, 100 mg; inj IM, IV 25 mg/mL

PHARMACOKINETICS/DYNAMICS Rapidly absorbed; half-life averages 10-20 hr. Onset of action: 30-60 min. Full therapeutic effects may not be apparent for 6-12 wk. Initial multiple daily dosing can often be consolidated to once or twice a day, once tolerant to side effects.

SIDE EFFECTS Sedation, dizziness, blurred vision, dry mouth, constipation, urinary retention, nausea, vomiting, tachycardia, orthostatic hypotension, acute dystonic reaction, stiffness, cogwheel rigidity, bradykinesia, akathisia, gynecomastia, galactorrhea, amenorrhea, decreased libido, retrograde ejaculation, weight gain, allergic dermatitis, skin photosensitivity, reduced seizure threshold.

ADVERSE REACTIONS Risk of tardive dyskinesia, **neuroleptic malignant syndrome.** Rarely—jaundice.

INTERACTIONS Additive effects with CNS depressants and anticholinergic drugs. Potentiates hypotensive effects of clonidine. Serum levels are increased by antidepressants and propranolol, reduced by carbamazepine and phenytoin. Epinephrine may result in reverse (hypotensive) effects. Antacids reduce absorption. Do NOT mix liquid concentrate with apple juice, cranberry juice, grape juice, or Tang.

CONTRAINDICATIONS Contraindicated in coma, severe hypotension, acute subcortical brain damage. Relatively contraindicated in liver disease, renal insufficiency, blood dyscrasias, Parkinson's disease. May exacerbate signs and symptoms of glaucoma, benign prostatic hypertrophy, diabetes. Avoid in pregnant and lactating women.

NURSING CONSIDERATIONS Monitor level of sedation and vital signs carefully during dose titration. Topical contact with drug can lead to dermatitis. IM injections cause a burning pain. Rapid dose increases, IM injections, dehydration, and agitation are associated with increased incidence of neuroleptic malignant syndrome.

CLIENT TEACHING Rise from bed and change positions slowly to avoid dizziness; sugarless gum and candy for dry mouth; use hats and sunscreens to reduce risk with sun exposure.

AVAILABLE IN CANADA Chlorpromanyl, Largatil, Novo-Chlorpromazine, Thorazine.

bold—Life-threatening reactions

GENERIC: desipramine (diss-ip'ra-meen)
TRADE: Norpramin

CLASSIFICATION Tricyclic antidepressant

INDICATIONS & USES Major depression, anxiety, panic, eating disorders, chronic pain.

USUAL ADULT DOSAGE RANGE 50-300 mg/day. In major depression: 150-300 mg/day. Initial dosing is 50-75 mg/day in divided doses.

AVAILABLE FORMS Tabs 10, 25, 50, 75, 100, 150 mg; caps 25, 50 mg

PHARMACOKINETICS/DYNAMICS Half-life varies from 11-46 hr in adults. Plasma therapeutic range: 115-300 mg/mL. Full therapeutic effects may not be apparent for 2-4 wk. Initial multiple daily dosing can often be consolidated to once or twice a day, once tolerant to side effects.

SIDE EFFECTS Sedation, dizziness, blurred vision, dry mouth, constipation, urinary retention, nausea, vomiting, tachycardia, orthostatic hypotension, tremor, cardiac conduction abnormalities, decreased libido, weight gain, allergic dermatitis, skin photosensitivity, reduced seizure threshold.

ADVERSE REACTIONS Exacerbation of untreated narrow-angle glaucoma, induction of mania, reduced seizure threshold, **potentially fatal in overdose. Unexplained cardiac events resulting in sudden death have been reported in four children in the United States.**

INTERACTIONS Increased levels—cimetidine, fluoxetine, antipsychotics, methylphenidate, propoxyphene, quinidine.

Decreased levels—barbiturates, phenytoin, chronic carbamazepine, chronic ethanol. Increased effects of epinephrine, norepinephrine, CNS depressants. **Severe hypertension with MAOIs.** Antacids reduce absorption.

CONTRAINDICATIONS Caution in clients with cardiovascular disease, arrhythmias, strokes, and acute myocardial infarction and thyroid disease/medications. May exacerbate signs and symptoms of glaucoma, benign prostatic hypertrophy, diabetes. Avoid in pregnant and lactating women.

NURSING CONSIDERATIONS Monitor level of sedation and vital signs carefully during dose titration. Suicide risk may be increased during initial improvement, particularly as psychomotor depression abates.

CLIENT TEACHING Therapeutic effects may take several weeks. Caution about initial sedation and dizziness. Instruct to change positions slowly. Use hats and sunscreens to reduce risk with sun exposure.

AVAILABLE IN CANDADA Norpramin

bold—Life-threatening reactions

GENERIC: clozapine (kloz-a'pin)
TRADE: Clozaril

CLASSIFICATION Atypical antipsychotic

INDICATIONS & USES Treatment refractory (failed to respond to typical antipsychotic medication) schizophrenia, and schizoaffective disorders. Also used in treatment refractory bipolar disorder, tardive dyskinesia, and emergent psychosis in the treatment of Parkinson's disease.

USUAL ADULT DOSAGE RANGE 300-600 mg/day. Initial dosing is 12.5 mg once or twice a day.Total daily dose should not exceed 900 mg.

PHARMACOKINETICS/DYNAMICS Rapidly absorbed; half-life averages 10-20 hr. PO onset of action:30-60 min. Full therapeutic effects may not be apparent for 2-4 mo. Initial multiple daily dosing can often be consolidated to once or twice a day, once tolerant to side effects.

SIDE EFFECTS Sedation, fatigue, dizziness, blurred vision, dry mouth, constipation, diarrhea, urinary retention, nausea, vomiting, tachycardia, orthostatic hypotension, hypertension, weight gain, allergic dermatitis, skin photosensitivity, increased salivation, gastrointestinal discomfort, diaphoresis, fever, neutropenia, eosinophilia.

ADVERSE REACTIONS **Agranulocytosis, seizures, possible neuroleptic malignant syndrome.**

INTERACTIONS Additive effects with CNS depressants (esp. benzodiazepines). Epinephrine may result in reverse

(hypotensive) effects. Serum levels are increased by antidepressants, cimetidine and propranolol; reduced by carbamazepine and phenytoin. Antacids reduce absorption.

CONTRAINDICATIONS Contraindicated in coma, severe hypotension, acute subcortical brain damage, and emergent dyscrasias. Relatively contraindicated in liver disease, renal insufficiency. May exacerbate signs and symptoms of glaucoma, benign prostatic hypertrophy, diabetes. Avoid in pregnancy and lactating women.

NURSING CONSIDERATIONS Monitor level of sedation and vital signs carefully during dose titration.

CLIENT TEACHING Use hats and sunscreens to reduce risk with sun exposure. Clients should report lethargy, weakness, fever, sore throat, or other signs and symptoms of infection without delay. Weekly WBC monitoring required. Do not start or give if WBC <3500/mm³.

AVAILABLE IN CANADA Clozaril

bold—Life-threatening reactions

GENERIC: fluoxetine (floo-ox'e-teen)
TRADE: Prozac

CLASSIFICATION Antidepressant—serotonin selective reuptake inhibitor

INDICATIONS & USES Major depression, obsessive-compulsive disorder

USUAL ADULT DOSAGE RANGE 10-80 mg/day. Initial dosing is 20 mg qam. Maximum dose is 80 mg/day.

AVAILABLE FORMS Pulvules 20 mg; cap 10 mg; liquid 20 mg/5mL

PHARMACOKINETICS/DYNAMICS In adults, half-life is 2-6 days for fluoxetine and 4-16 days norfluoxetine (active metabolite).Thus steady state may not be achieved for a month or more after dosage changes. Full therapeutic effects may not be apparent for 2-4 wk.

SIDE EFFECTS Agitation, irritability, insomnia, headache, dizziness, gastrointestinal upset, drowsiness, fatigue, diarrhea, tremor, sexual dysfunction, slight weight loss, akathisia, nervousness, sweating, occasionally extrapyramidal symptoms, rarely bradycardia.

ADVERSE REACTIONS Induction of mania, rash.

INTERACTIONS **Potentially fatal hypertensive crisis when MAOIs (including selegiline) are used within 5 wk of discontinuation.** Increased levels of haloperidol, tricyclic antidepressants, propranolol, benzodiazepines. Loss of therapeutic efficacy with cyproheptadine.

CONTRAINDICATIONS MAOI use within 5 wk. Avoid in pregnant and nursing mothers. May accumulate substantially in hepatic and renal disease and in the debilitated.

NURSING CONSIDERATIONS Suicide risk may be increased during initial improvement, particularly as psychomotor depression abates. Low risk of fatality in overdose. Sexual dysfunction (loss of libido, delayed ejaculation, anorgasmia) may persist and interfere with compliance.

CLIENT TEACHING Therapeutic effects may take several weeks.

AVAILABLE IN CANADA Prozac

bold—Life-threatening reactions

GENERIC: clomipramine (klom-ip'ra-meen)
TRADE: Anafranil

CLASSIFICATION Tricyclic antidepressant

INDICATIONS & USES Obsessive-compulsive disorder, major depression, phobias, panic, chronic pain.

USUAL ADULT DOSAGE RANGE 100-250 mg/day. Initial dosing is 25 mg/day at bedtime. Initial daytime doses should be given with meal to minimize GI upset.

AVAILABLE FORMS Caps 25, 50, 75 mg.

PHARMACOKINETICS/DYNAMICS In adults, half-life varies from 19-37 (mean, 32) hr for clomipramine and 54-77 (mean, 69) hr for desmethyl-clomipramine (active metabolite).Thus steady state may not be achieved for nearly 2 wk after dosage changes. Full therapeutic effects may not be apparent for several weeks. Initial multiple daily dosing can often be consolidated to once or twice a day, once tolerant to side effects.

SIDE EFFECTS Sedation, dizziness, blurred vision, dry mouth, constipation, urinary retention, nausea, vomiting, tachycardia, orthostatic hypotension, tremor, cardiac conduction abnormalities, decreased libido, weight gain, allergic dermatitis, skin photosensitivity, reduced seizure threshold, appetite disturbance, myoclonus, sweating.

ADVERSE REACTIONS Exacerbation of untreated narrow-angle glaucoma, induction of mania, reduced seizure threshold, **potentially fatal in overdose.**

INTERACTIONS Increased levels—cimetidine, fluoxetine, antipsychotics, methylphenidate, propoxyphene. Decreased levels—barbiturates, phenytoin, chronic carbamazepine. Increased effects of epinephrine, norepinephrine, CNS depressants. **Severe hypertension with MAOs.** Antacids reduce absorption.

CONTRAINDICATIONS Caution in clients with cardiovascular disease, arrhythmias, strokes, and acute myocardial infarction and thyroid disease/medications. May exacerbate signs and symptoms of glaucoma, benign prostatic hypertrophy, diabetes. Avoid in pregnant and lactating women.

NURSING CONSIDERATIONS Monitor level of sedation and vital signs carefully during dose titration. Suicide risk may be increased during initial improvement, particularly as psychomotor depression abates.

CLIENT TEACHING Therapeutic effects may take several weeks. Caution about initial sedation and dizziness. Instruct to change positions slowly. Use hats and sunscreens to reduce risk with sun exposure.

AVAILABLE IN CANADA Anafranil

bold—Life-threatening reactions

GENERIC: diazepam (dye-az'e-pam)
TRADE: Valium

CLASSIFICATION Antianxiety, anticonvulsant—benzodiazepine

INDICATIONS & USES Anxiety disorders, acute alcohol withdrawal, status epilepticus, adjunctive therapy in seizure disorders, skeletal muscle relaxant.

USUAL ADULT DOSAGE RANGE 2-40 mg/day.

AVAILABLE FORMS Tabs 2, 5, 10 mg; caps ext rel 15 mg. IM/IV inj.

PHARMACOKINETIC/DYNAMICS Average half-life including active metabolites 100 hr. Very rapid PO absorption. IM absorption is erratic and unpredictable. Use in status epilepticus is IV.

SIDE EFFECTS Drowsiness, dizziness, ataxia. Rarely—nausea, vomiting, GI upset, blurred vision.

ADVERSE REACTIONS Anterograde amnesia. Rarely increased aggression/irritability. Oversedation and **respiratory depression with other CNS depressants.**

INTERACTIONS CNS depressants, may increase levels of phenytoin, digoxin. Effects reduced by smoking, rifampin. Serum levels increased by cimetidine, valproate, oral contraceptives, disulfiram.

CONTRAINDICATIONS Coma, shock, alcohol intoxication, pregnancy. Use with caution in history of drug abuse/addiction.

NURSING CONSIDERATIONS Schedule IV controlled substance. Active metabolites with long half-life may result in accumulating effects over time. Risk of respiratory depression when used with other CNS depressants. Abrupt discontinuation associated with anxiety, rebound insomnia, and seizures. Rapid absorption causing a "buzz" may reinforce drug-seeking behavior or may be perceived dysphorically in non-drug abuse population.

CLIENT TEACHING Avoid hazardous activities during initiation; avoid alcohol; caution against sudden discontinuation.

AVAILABLE IN CANADA D-Tran, E-Pam, Meval, Novodipam, Stress-Pam, Vivol, Valium

bold—Life-threatening reactions

GENERIC: fluphenazine (floo-fen'a-zeen)
TRADE: Prolixin, Permitil

CLASSIFICATION Typical antipsychotic

INDICATIONS & USES Symptomatic management of psychotic disorders, initial management of psychotic manic states.

USUAL ADULT DOSAGE RANGE 1-20 mg/day. Initial dosing is 2.5-10 mg/day every day in divided doses. Fluphenazine decanoate 12.5-25 mg IM every 1-3 wk.

AVAILABLE FORMS HCl tabs 1, 2.5, 5, 10 mg; elix 2.5 mg/5 mL; conc 5 mg/mL; inj IM 10 mg/mL, enanthate, decanoate, inj sc, IM 25 mg/mL

PHARMACOKINETICS/DYNAMICS Rapidly absorbed; half-life averages 10-20 hr. Onset of action: 30-60 min. Full therapeutic effects may not be apparent for 6-12 wk. Initial multiple daily dosing can often be consolidated to once or twice a day, once tolerant to side effects. The half-life of fluphenazine decanoate is approximately 14 days.

SIDE EFFECTS Sedation, nausea, vomiting, acute dystonic reaction, stiffness, cogwheel rigidity, bradykinesia, akathisia, gynecomastia, galactorrhea, amenorrhea, decreased libido, weight gain, allergic dermatitis, skin photosensitivity, reduced seizure threshold.

ADVERSE REACTIONS Risk of tardive dyskinesia, **neuroleptic malignant syndrome, seizures.**

INTERACTIONS Additive effects with CNS depressants. Serum levels are increased by antidepressants and propranolol, reduced by carbamazepine and phenytoin. Antacids reduce absorption. Do NOT mix liquid concentrate with coffee, tea, cola, or apple juice.

CONTRAINDICATIONS Contraindicated in coma, severe hypotension, acute subcortical brain damage. Relatively contraindicated in liver disease, renal insufficiency, blood dyscrasias, Parkinson's disease. May exacerbate signs and symptoms of glaucoma, benign prostatic hypertrophy, diabetes. Avoid in pregnant and lactating women.

NURSING CONSIDERATIONS Monitor level of sedation and vital signs carefully during dose titration. Rapid dose increases, dehydration, IM injections, and agitation are associated with increased incidence of neuroleptic malignant syndrome.

CLIENT TEACHING Use hats and sunscreen to reduce risk with sun exposure. Clients should immediately report fever and increasing stiffness.

AVAILABLE IN CANADA Prolixin, Permitil, Modecate Decanoate, Moditen Enanthate

bold—Life-threatening reactions

GENERIC: haloperidol (ha-loe-per'idole)
TRADE: Haldol

CLASSIFICATION Typical antipsychotic

INDICATIONS & USES Symptomatic management of psychotic disorders, initial management of psychotic manic states.

USUAL ADULT DOSAGE RANGE 6-20 mg/day. Initial dosing is 0.5-10 mg/day every day in divided doses. Total daily doses as high as 100 mg/day may be required. Typical IM dose is 2-5 mg. Haldol decanoate, 25-100 mg IM q 4 wk.

AVAILABLE FORMS Tabs 0.5, 1, 2, 5, 10, 20 mg; conc 2 mg/mL; inj IM 5 mg/mL

PHARMACOKINETICS/DYNAMICS Rapidly absorbed; half-life averages 10-20 hr. Onset of action: 30-60 min. Full therapeutic effects may not be apparent for 6-12 wk. Initial multiple daily dosing can often be consolidated to once or twice a day, once tolerant to side effects. The half-life of haloperidol decanoate is approximately 21 days.

SIDE EFFECTS Sedation, nausea, vomiting, acute dystonic reaction, stiffness, cogwheel rigidity, bradykinesia, akathisia, gynecomastia, galactorrhea, amenorrhea, decreased libido, weight gain, allergic dermatitis, skin photosensitivity, reduced seizure threshold.

ADVERSE REACTIONS Risk of tardive dyskinesia, **neuroleptic malignant syndrome, seizures.**

INTERACTIONS Additive effects with CNS depressants. Serum levels are increased by antidepressants and propranolol, reduced by carbamazepine and phenytoin. Antacids reduce absorption. Do NOT mix liquid concentrate with milk, coffee, tea, grape or grapefruit juice.

CONTRAINDICATIONS Contraindicated in coma, severe hypotension, acute subcortical brain damage. Relatively contraindicated in liver disease, renal insufficiency, blood dyscrasias, Parkinson's disease. May exacerbate signs and symptoms of glaucoma, benign prostatic hypertrophy, diabetes. Avoid in pregnant and lactating women.

NURSING CONSIDERATIONS Monitor level of sedation and vital signs carefully during dose titration. Rapid dose increases, dehydration, IM injections, and agitation are associated with increased incidence of neuroleptic malignant syndrome.

CLIENT TEACHING Use hats and sunscreens to reduce risk with sun exposure. Clients should immediately report fever and increasing stiffness.

AVAILABLE IN CANADA Apo-Haloperidol, Haldol LA, Novoperidol, Peridol, Haldol

bold—Life-threatening reactions

GENERIC: lithium (li'thee-um)
TRADE: Eskalith, Eskalith CR, Lithane, Lithobid, Cibalith-S syrup

CLASSIFICATION Antimanic

INDICATIONS & USES Bipolar disorder, adjunctive therapy in depression, adjunctive therapy in schizophrenia, adjunctive treatment in aggression.

USUAL ADULT DOSAGE RANGE 300-1800 mg/day in divided doses. Typical initial dosing—300 mg tid. Subsequent dosing is determined by serum level monitoring.

AVAILABLE FORMS Caps 150, 300, 600 mg; tabs 300 mg; tabs cont rel 300, 450 mg; syrup 300 mg/5 mL

PHARMACOKINETICS/DYNAMICS Average half-life in healthy adults is 18-27 hr. Half-life varies widely and is dependent on renal function. Maintenance therapeutic range in adults is 0.8-1.2 mEq/L.

SIDE EFFECTS Fine tremor, mild GI upset, diarrhea, polyuria, polydipsia, muscle weakness, lethargy, leucocytosis, hypothyroidism, exacerbation of psoriasis, acne, alopecia, weight gain.

ADVERSE REACTIONS (including symptoms that may predict serious lithium toxicity)—coarsening of tremor, confusion, excessive sedation, ataxia, dysarthria, mental status deterioration, seizure, coma, **cardiovascular collapse.** Severe polyuria, polydipsia, and GI upset, goiter formation.

INTERACTIONS Increases lithium levels— hydrochlorothiazide, nonsteroidal antiinflammatory drugs (e.g., ibuprofen, indomethacin), angiotensin converting enzyme inhibitors (e.g., captopril, enalapril). Decreases lithium levels—sodium bicarbonate, sodium chloride, theophylline, caffeine, urea. Potential for neurotoxicity when used with carbamazepine, calcium channel blockers. **Risk factor for neuroleptic malignant syndrome when used with typical antipsychotics.** Reductions in dietary sodium or excessive sweating result in increased or toxic lithium levels.

CONTRAINDICATIONS Severe renal disease, cardiovascular disease, organic brain syndrome, dehydration. Use in pregnancy may increase risk of Ebstein's anomaly (cardiac valve formation).

NURSING CONSIDERATIONS Draw blood 12 hr after previous dose. Monitor for peripheral edema or sudden weight gain. May give with meals to reduce GI disturbance. GI disturbance common on initiation, but subsides. A return of GI symptoms may indicate lithium toxicity. Report excessive thirst or water consumption.

CLIENT TEACHING Report GI upset, sedation, ataxia, or increasing tremor immediately. It is important to maintain stable salt intake in diet.

AVAILABLE IN CANADA Carbolith, Lithizine, Eskalith, Eskalith CR, Lithane, Lithobid, Cibalith-S syrup

bold—Life-threatening reactions

GENERIC: loxapine (lox'apeen)
TRADE: Loxitane

CLASSIFICATION Typical antipsychotic

INDICATIONS & USES Symptomatic management of psychotic disorders, initial management of psychotic manic states.

USUAL ADULT DOSAGE RANGE 60-100 mg/day. Initial dosing is 10 mg bid. Total daily doses as high as 200 mg/day may be required. Typical IM dose is 12.5-50 mg.

AVAILABLE FORMS Caps 5, 10, 25, 50 mg; conc 25 mg/mL; inj IM 50 mg/mL.

PHARMACOKINETICS/DYNAMICS Rapidly absorbed; half-life averages 4-12 hr. PO onset of action: 30-60 min. Full therapeutic effects may not be apparent for 6-12 wk. Initial multiple daily dosing can often be consolidated to once or twice a day, once tolerant to side effects.

SIDE EFFECTS Sedation, dizziness, blurred vision, dry mouth, constipation, urinary retention, nausea, vomiting, tachycardia, orthostatic hypotension, acute dystonic reaction, stiffness, cogwheel rigidity, bradykinesia, akathisia, gynecomastia, galactorrhea, amenorrhea, decreased libido, retrograde ejaculation, weight gain, allergic dermatitis, skin photosensitivity, reduced seizure threshold.

ADVERSE REACTIONS Risk of tardive dyskinesia, **neuroleptic malignant syndrome, seizures.**

INTERACTIONS Additive effects with CNS depressants. Serum levels are increased by antidepressants and propranolol, reduced by carbamazepine and phenytoin. Antacids reduce absorption.

CONTRAINDICATIONS Contraindicated in coma, severe hypotension, acute subcortical brain damage. Relatively contraindicated in liver disease, renal insufficiency, blood dyscrasias, Parkinson's disease. May exacerbate signs and symptoms of glaucoma, benign prostatic hypertrophy, diabetes. Avoid in pregnant and lactating women.

NURSING CONSIDERATIONS Monitor level of sedation and vital signs carefully during dose titration. Rapid dose increases, dehydration, IM injections, and agitation are associated with increased incidence of neuroleptic malignant syndrome.

CLIENT TEACHING Use hats and sunscreens to reduce risk with sun exposure. Clients should immediately report fever and increasing stiffness.

AVAILABLE IN CANADA Loxapac, Loxitane

bold—Life-threatening reactions

GENERIC: imipramine (im-ip'ra-meen)
TRADE: Tofranil

CLASSIFICATION Tricyclic antidepressant

INDICATIONS & USES Major depression, anxiety, panic, eating disorders, chronic pain, childhood enuresis.

USUAL ADULT DOSAGE RANGE 50-300 mg/day. In major depression: 150-300 mg/day. Initial dosing is 50-75 mg/day in divided doses.

AVAILABLE FORMS Tabs 10, 25, 50 mg; inj IM 25 mg/2 mL

PHARMACOKINETICS/DYNAMICS Half-life varies from 6-28 hr in adults to 21-35 hr in the elderly. Partially metabolized to desipramine. Plasma therapeutic range: (imipramine + desipramine) 200-300 mg/mL. Full therapeutic effects may not be apparent for 2-4 wk. Initial multiple daily dosing can often be consolidated to once or twice a day, once tolerant to side effects.

SIDE EFFECTS Sedation, dizziness, blurred vision, dry mouth, constipation, urinary retention, nausea, vomiting, tachycardia, orthostatic hypotension, tremor, cardiac conduction abnormalities, decreased libido, weight gain, allergic dermatitis, skin photosensitivity, reduced seizure threshold.

ADVERSE REACTIONS Exacerbation of untreated narrow-angle glaucoma, induction of mania, reduced seizure threshold, **potentially fatal in overdose.**

INTERACTIONS Increased levels—cimetidine, fluoxetine, antipsychotics, methylphenidate, propoxyphene. Decreased levels—barbiturates, phenytoin, chronic carbamazepine.

Increased effects of epinephrine, norepinephrine, CNS depressants. **Severe hypertension with MAOIs.** Antacids reduce absorption.

CONTRAINDICATION Caution in clients with cardiovascular disease, arrhythmias, strokes, and acute myocardial infarction and thyroid disease/medications. May exacerbate signs and symptoms of glaucoma, benign prostatic hypertrophy, diabetes. Avoid in pregnant and lactating women.

NURSING CONSIDERATIONS Monitor level of sedation and vital signs carefully during dose titration. Suicide risk may be increased during initial improvement, particularly as psychomotor depression abates.

CLIENT TEACHING Therapeutic effects may take several weeks. Caution about initial sedation and dizziness. Instruct to change positions slowly. Use hats and sunscreens to reduce risk with sun exposure.

AVAILABLE IN CANADA Apo-imipramine, Impril, Tofranil

bold—Life-threatening reactions

GENERIC: nefazodone (ne-faz'o-doan)
TRADE: Serzone

CLASSIFICATION Triazolopyridine antidepressant.

INDICATIONS & USES Major depression.

USUAL ADULT DOSAGE RANGE 300-600 mg/day. Initial dosing is 100 mg bid (50 mg bid in the elderly) for 1 wk then increased 150 mg bid. Maximum dose is 600 mg/day in divided doses.

AVAILABLE FORMS Tabs 100, 150, 200, 250 mg

PHARMACOKINETICS/DYNAMICS In adults, half-life is approximately 2-4 hr. Full therapeutic effects may not be apparent for 2-4 wk.

SIDE EFFECTS Weakness, dry mouth, nausea, constipation, somnolence, dizziness, lightheadedness, confusion, blurred vision, abnormal vision (visual flashes). The abnormal vision that may occur with initiation and/or dose increase is of short duration and not clinically significant.

ADVERSE REACTIONS Induction of mania.

INTERACTIONS **Potentially fatal cardiac arrhythmias with astemizole and terfenadine. Potentially fatal hypertensive crisis when MAOIs (including selegiline) are used within 2 wk of discontinuation.** May increase triazolam serum levels by 75% and alprazolam levels by 50%.

CONTRAINDICATIONS Never use with astemizole and terfenadine. Avoid in pregnant and nursing mothers.

NURSING CONSIDERATIONS Suicide risk may be increased during initial improvement, particularly as psychomotor depression abates.

CLIENT TEACHING Therapeutic effects may take several weeks. Warn of excessive sedation during initiation. Watch for orthostatic hypotension.

AVAILABLE IN CANADA Serzone

bold—Life-threatening reactions

GENERIC: fluvoxamine (floo-vox'a-meen)
TRADE: Luvox

CLASSIFICATION Antiobsessional—serotonin selective reuptake inhibitor

INDICATIONS & USES Obsessive-compulsive disorder, major depression

USUAL ADULT DOSAGE RANGE 100-300 mg/day. Initial dosing is 50 mg hs. Maximum dose is 300 mg/day; bid dosing is recommended for doses > 100 mg/day. In unequal doses, larger dose should be at bedtime.

AVAILABLE FORMS Tabs 50, 100 mg

PHARMACOKINETICS/DYNAMICS In adults, half-life is approximately 16 hr. Full therapeutic effects may not be apparent for 2-4 wk.

SIDE EFFECTS Somnolence, insomnia, nervousness, nausea, constipation, sweating, tremor, dyspepsia, anorexia, vomiting, sexual dysfunction, weakness, dry mouth, dizziness.

ADVERSE REACTIONS Induction of mania, rash, seizures.

INTERACTIONS **Potentially fatal hypertensive crisis when MAOIs (including selegiline) are used within 2 wk of discontinuation.** Diazepam should not be used. Alprazolam and triazolam doses should be halved. Increased astemizole and terfenadine levels may lead to cardiac arrhythmias. Theophylline dose should be decreased and serum levels monitored closely. Warfarin may be increased by nearly 100%; monitor prothrombin times closely.

CONTRAINDICATIONS MAOI use within 2 weeks. Avoid in pregnant and nursing mothers; May accumulate substantially in hepatic and renal disease and in the debilitated. **Do not use with astemizole or terfenadine.**

NURSING CONSIDERATIONS Suicide risk may be increased during initial improvement, particularly as psychomotor depression abates. Low risk of fatality in overdose. Sexual dysfunction (loss of libido, delayed ejaculation, anorgasmia) may persist and interfere with compliance.

CLIENT TEACHING Therapeutic effects may take several weeks.

AVAILABLE IN CANADA Luvox

bold—Life-threatening reactions

GENERIC: lorazepam (lor-a'ze-pam)
TRADE: Ativan

CLASSIFICATION Antianxiety agent—benzodiazepine

INDICATIONS & USES Anxiety; adjunct in agitation and irritability in other psychiatric disorders, sometimes used for insomnia.

USUAL ADULT DOSAGE RANGE 2-6 mg/day in divided doses (bid or tid). Acute use: 1-2 mg IM q 4-6 hr.

AVAILABLE FORMS Tabs 0.5, 1, 2 mg; IM/IV inj 2, 4 mg/mL

PHARMACOKINETICS/DYNAMICS Average half-life is 10-20 hr. Absorption is considerably more rapid with PO concentrate and IM administration. Initial therapeutic effects may be observed within 15 min. Some clients require tid dosing to avoid breakthrough symptoms. No active metabolites.

SIDE EFFECTS Drowsiness, dizziness, ataxia. Rarely—nausea, vomiting, GI upset, blurred vision.

ADVERSE REACTIONS Anterograde amnesia, rarely increased aggression/irritability. Oversedation and respiratory depression with other CNS depressants.

INTERACTIONS CNS depressants, may increase levels of phenytoin, digoxin. Effects reduced by smoking, oral contraceptives.

CONTRAINDICATIONS Coma, shock, alcohol intoxication, pregnancy. Use with caution in history of drug abuse/addiction.

NURSING CONSIDERATIONS Schedule IV controlled substance. Risk of respiratory depression when used with other CNS depressants. Abrupt discontinuation associated with anxiety, rebound insomnia, and seizures.

CLIENT TEACHING Avoid hazardous activities during initiation; avoid alcohol; caution against sudden discontinuation.

AVAILABLE IN CANADA Apo-Lorazepam, Novolorazem

bold—Life-threatening reactions

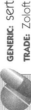

GENERIC: phenelzine (fen'el-zeen)
TRADE: Nardil

CLASSIFICATION Antidepressant, monoamine oxidase inhibitor

INDICATIONS & USES Atypical depression, treatment refractory depression, panic disorder.

USUAL ADULT DOSAGE RANGE 45-90 mg/day. Can be given in divided doses. Thereafter may be increased 15 mg/day each week. Maximum dose is 90 mg/day.

AVAILABLE FORMS Tabs 15 mg

PHARMACOKINETICS/DYNAMICS Well-absorbed. Irreversibly inhibits monoamine oxidase (MAO). Maximal inhibition at a particular enzyme site is complete in 5-10 days. After discontinuation, 2 weeks are required for resynthesis of MAO. Full therapeutic effects may not be apparent for 2-6 wk.

SIDE EFFECTS Orthostatic hypotension, dizziness, weight gain, edema, sexual dysfunction, insomnia, paresthesia, sweating, flushing.

ADVERSE REACTIONS **Hypertensive crisis secondary to tyramine-rich foods, stimulant drugs (e.g., nasal decongestants). Serotonin syndrome (autonomic instability, hyperthermia, rigidity, myoclonus, altered mental status—confusion, delirium, coma) with SSRIs.**

INTERACTIONS **Tyramine-rich foods, sympathomimetic drugs (e.g., phenylpropanolamine, ephedrine),** dextromethorphan, antihypertensives

(reserpine, guanethidine), L-dopa, narcotics, antiasthmatics (epinephrine, isoproterenol), diuretics, general anesthetics.

CONTRAINDICATIONS Relatively contraindicated in renal disease, cardiovascular disease, hyperthyroidism, Parkinson's disease, asthma. May alter glucose treatment requirements in diabetes.

NURSING CONSIDERATIONS Monitor blood pressure closely. Assess for symptoms of hypertensive crisis reaction.

CLIENT TEACHING Dietary restrictions, symptoms of hypertensive crisis reaction (pounding headache, neck stiffness, nausea, sweating), drug interactions. Advise not to take cough, cold preparation, or weight loss pills without professional counsel.

AVAILABLE IN CANADA Nardil

bold—Life-threatening reactions

GENERIC: paroxetine (par-oh'xe-teen)
TRADE: Paxil

CLASSIFICATION Antidepressant—serotonin selective reuptake inhibitor

INDICATIONS & USES Major depression, obsessive-compulsive disorder.

USUAL ADULT DOSAGE RANGE 10-50 mg/day. Initial dosing is 20 mg/day (10 mg/day in the elderly or debilitated). Maximum dose is 50 mg/day.

AVAILABLE FORMS Tabs 20, 30 mg

PHARMACOKINETICS/DYNAMICS In adults, half-life is approximately 21 hr. Full therapeutic effects may not be apparent for 2-4 wk.

SIDE EFFECTS Agitation, irritability, insomnia, headache, dizziness, gastrointestinal upset, dry mouth, constipation, sedation, sexual dysfunction, slight weight loss, tremor, akathisia, sweating, somnolence, nervousness, occasionally extrapyramidal symptoms.

ADVERSE REACTIONS Induction of mania, rash.

INTERACTIONS **Potentially fatal hypertensive crisis when MAOIs (including selegiline) are used within 2 wk of discontinuation.** Loss of therapeutic efficacy with cyproheptadine.

CONTRAINDICATIONS MAOI use within 2 wk. Avoid in pregnant and nursing mothers.

NURSING CONSIDERATIONS Suicide risk may be increased during initial improvement, particularly as psychomotor depression abates. Low risk of fatality in overdose. Sexual dysfunction (loss of libido, delayed ejaculation, anorgasmia) may persist and interfere with compliance.

CLIENT TEACHING Therapeutic effects may take several weeks.

AVAILABLE IN CANADA Paxil

bold—Life-threatening reactions

GENERIC: thioridazine (thye-or-rid'a-zeen)
TRADE: Mellaril

CLASSIFICATION Typical antipsychotic

INDICATIONS & USES Symptomatic management of psychotic disorders; initial management of psychotic manic states; short-term management of depression, anxiety, and agitation.

USUAL ADULT DOSAGE RANGE 50-800 mg/day. Initial dosing is 50-100 mg bid or tid. Absolute maximum dose is 800 mg/day.

AVAILABLE FORMS Tabs 10, 15, 25, 50, 100, 150, 200, 300 mg. conc 30, 100 mg/mL; susp 25, 100 mg/5 mL; syrup 10 mg/15 mL.

PHARMACOKINETICS/DYNAMICS Rapidly absorbed; half-life averages 10-20 hr. Onset of action: 30-60 min. Full therapeutic effects may not be apparent for 6-12 wk. Initial multiple daily dosing can often be consolidated to once or twice a day, once tolerant to side effects.

SIDE EFFECTS Sedation, dizziness, blurred vision, dry mouth, constipation, urinary retention, nausea, vomiting, tachycardia, orthostatic hypotension, acute dystonic reaction, stiffness, cogwheel rigidity, bradykinesia, akathisia, gynecomastia, galactorrhea, amenorrhea, decreased libido, retrograde ejaculation, weight gain, allergic dermatitis, skin photosensitivity, reduced seizure threshold.

ADVERSE REACTION Risk of tardive dyskinesia. Doses >800 mg/day **neuroleptic malignant syndrome.** Doses >800 mg/day

have been associated with pigmentary retinopathy and blindness.

INTERACTIONS Additive effects with CNS depressants and anticholinergic drugs. Serum levels are increased by antidepressants and propranolol, reduced by carbamazepine and phenytoin. Epinephrine may result in reverse (hypotensive) effects. Antacids reduce absorption.

CONTRAINDICATIONS Contraindicated in coma, severe hypotension, acute subcortical brain damage. Relatively contraindicated in liver disease, renal insufficiency, blood dyscrasias, Parkinson's disease. May exacerbate signs and symptoms of glaucoma, benign prostatic hypertrophy, diabetes. Avoid in pregnant and lactating women.

NURSING CONSIDERATIONS Monitor level of sedation and vital signs carefully during dose titration. Rapid dose increases, dehydration, and agitation are associated with increased incidence of neuroleptic malignant syndrome. Do NOT mix liquid concentrate with mild coffee, tea, cola; apple, grape, pineapple, prune, or tomato juice; or Tang.

CLIENT TEACHING Rise from bed and change positions slowly to avoid dizziness; sugarless gum and candy for dry mouth; use hats and sunscreens to reduce risk with sun exposure.

AVAILABLE IN CANADA Novoridazine, Mellaril

bold—Life-threatening reactions

GENERIC: risperidone (riss-pair'-i-doan)
TRADE: Risperdal

CLASSIFICATION Atypical antipsychotic

INDICATIONS & USES Symptomatic management of psychotic disorders.

USUAL ADULT DOSAGE RANGE 4-8 mg/day. Initial dosing is 1 mg bid. Total daily doses as high as 16 mg/day may be required.

AVAILABLE FORMS Tab 1, 2, 3, 4 mg

PHARMACOKINETICS/DYNAMICS Rapidly absorbed; half-life averages 10-20 hr. PO onset of action: 30-60 min. Full therapeutic effects may not be apparent for 6-12 wk.

SIDE EFFECTS Mild sedation, dizziness, nausea, vomiting, tachycardia, orthostatic hypotension, acute dystonic reaction, stiffness, cogwheel rigidity, bradykinesia, akathisia, gynecomastia, galactorrhea, amenorrhea, decreased libido, retrograde ejaculation, weight gain, allergic dermatitis, skin photosensitivity, reduced seizure threshold, anxiety, constipation, rhinitis, rash. Extrapyramidal symptoms are minimal at doses ≤6 mg/day, but increase with increasing dose.

ADVERSE REACTIONS Risk of tardive dyskinesia, **neuroleptic malignant syndrome.**

INTERACTIONS Additive effects with CNS depressants. Serum levels are increased by antidepressants and propranolol, reduced by carbamazepine and phenytoin. Antacids reduce absorption.

CONTRAINDICATIONS Contraindicated in coma, severe hypotension, acute subcortical brain damage. Relatively contraindicated in liver disease, renal insufficiency; blood dyscrasias, Parkinson's disease. May exacerbate signs and symptoms of glaucoma, benign prostatic hypertrophy, diabetes. Avoid in pregnant and lactating women.

NURSING CONSIDERATIONS Monitor level of sedation and vital signs carefully during dose titration.

CLIENT TEACHING Use hats and sunscreens to reduce risk with sun exposure. Clients should immediately report fever and increasing stiffness.

AVAILABLE IN CANADA Risperdal

bold—Life-threatening reactions

thiothixene (thye-oh-thix'een)

GENERIC: thiothixene (thye-oh-thix'een)
TRADE: Navane

CLASSIFICATION Typical antipsychotic

INDICATIONS & USES Symptomatic management of psychotic disorders, initial management of psychotic manic states, acute agitation.

USUAL ADULT DOSAGE RANGE 6-30 mg/day. Initial dosing is 2-5 mg/day every day. Total daily doses as high as 60 mg/day may be required. Typical IM dose is 2-4 mg.

AVAILABLE FORMS Caps 1, 2, 5, 10, 20 mg; conc 5 mg/mL; inj IM 2 mg/mL; powder for inj 5 mg/mL.

PHARMACOKINETICS/DYNAMICS Rapidly absorbed; half-life averages 10-20 hr. PO onset of action: 1-2 hr. Full therapeutic effects may not be apparent for 6-12 wk. Initial multiple daily dosing can often be consolidated to once or twice a day, once tolerant to side effects.

SIDE EFFECTS Sedation, blurred vision, dry mouth, constipation, urinary retention, nausea, vomiting, tachycardia, orthostatic hypotension, acute dystonic reaction, stiffness, cogwheel rigidity, bradykinesia, akathisia, gynecomastia, galactorrhea, amenorrhea, decreased libido, retrograde ejaculation, weight gain, allergic dermatitis, skin photosensitivity, reduced seizure threshold.

ADVERSE REACTIONS Risk of tardive dyskinesia, **neuroleptic malignant syndrome, seizures.**

INTERACTIONS Additive effects with CNS depressants. Serum levels are increased by antidepressants and propranolol, reduced by carbamazepine and phenytoin. Antacids reduce absorption. Do NOT mix liquid concentrate with coffee, tea, apple juice, or cola.

CONTRAINDICATIONS Contraindicated in coma, severe hypotension, acute subcortical brain damage. Relatively contraindicated in liver disease, renal insufficiency, blood dyscrasias, Parkinson's disease. May exacerbate signs and symptoms of glaucoma, benign prostatic hypertrophy, diabetes. Avoid in pregnant and lactating women.

NURSING CONSIDERATIONS Monitor level of sedation and vital signs carefully during dose titration. Rapid dose increases, dehydration, IM injections, and agitation are associated with increased incidence of neuroleptic malignant syndrome.

CLIENT TEACHING Use hats and sunscreens to reduce risk with sun exposure. Clients should immediately report fever and increasing stiffness.

AVAILABLE IN CANADA Navane

bold—Life-threatening reactions

---

triazolam (trye-ay'zoe-lam)

GENERIC: triazolam (trye-ay'zoe-lam)
TRADE: Halcion

CLASSIFICATION Hypnotic—benzodiazepine

INDICATIONS & USES Short-term (7-10 days) treatment of insomnia.

USUAL ADULT DOSAGE RANGE 0.25 mg starting dose in adults; 0.125 mg in elderly or debilitated; 0.5 mg should be reserved for exceptional cases and should not be exceeded.

AVAILABLE FORMS Tabs 0.125, 0.25, 0.5 mg

PHARMACOKINETICS/DYNAMICS Rapidly absorbed. Half-life averages 2 hr. Rapid onset of sleep.

SIDE EFFECTS Sedation, fatigue, drowsiness, dizziness, ataxia.

ADVERSE REACTIONS Anterograde amnesia. Rare—agitation, excitability, psychotic symptoms.

INTERACTIONS Addition of nefazodone, erythromycin may notably increase and prolong effects; CNS depressants; may increase levels of phenytoin, digoxin. Effects reduced by smoking, rifampin. Serum levels increased by cimetidine, valproate, oral contraceptives, disulfiram.

CONTRAINDICATIONS Coma, shock, alcohol intoxication, pregnancy. Use with caution in history of drug abuse/addiction.

NURSING CONSIDERATIONS Schedule IV controlled substance. Risk of respiratory depression when used with other CNS depressants. Monitor for next-morning sedation and reduced cognitive functioning. Abrupt discontinuation associated with anxiety, rebound insomnia.

CLIENT TEACHING Avoid hazardous activities during initiation; avoid alcohol; caution against sudden discontinuation.

AVAILABLE IN CANADA Apo-Triazo, Novotriolam, Nu-Triazol

bold—Life-threatening reactions

---

valproic acid, valproate sodium, divalproex sodium (val-proe'ate)

GENERIC: valproic acid, valproate sodium, divalproex sodium (val-proe'ate)
TRADE: Depakene, Depakene Syrup, Depakote, Depakote Sprinkle

CLASSIFICATION Anticonvulsant, antimanic

INDICATIONS & USES Simple and complex absence seizures, tonoclonic seizures, mixed seizures, bipolar disorder, episodic dyscontrol disorder.

USUAL ADULT DOSAGE RANGE Initially 15 mg/kg/day to a maximum of 60 mg/kg/day. Starting doses typically used vary from 250-500 mg bid. Some clinicians treat acute mania with starting doses of 500 mg tid.

AVAILABLE FORMS Caps 250 mg; tabs 125, 250, 500 mg; syr 250 mg/5 mL; 125 mg sprinkle capsules

PHARMACOKINETICS/DYNAMICS Average half-life is 8-20 hr in adults. Efficacy in seizures may occur over several days after achieving therapeutic levels. Efficacy in mania may occur over 1-2 wk, but as quickly as 3 days with aggressive dosing (e.g., starting at 500 mg tid). Therapeutic range for seizures is 50-120 µg/mL. Efficacy equivalent to lithium has been found when dosed to serum levels of 150 µg/mL. Therapeutic efficacy is seldom seen at levels <50 µg/mL.

SIDE EFFECTS Drowsiness, nausea, vomiting, diarrhea, tremor, weight gain, transient hair loss, elevated serum ammonia, mild thrombocytopenia, pruritus.

ADVERSE REACTIONS Excess sedation, pancreatitis, liver enzymes >3 times normal. Rare—**liver failure.**
Teratogenic—associated with neural tube defects, most commonly spina bifida.

INTERACTIONS Decreases valproate levels—carbamazepine, phenobarbital, primidone, phenytoin. Increased valproate effect—salicylates, erythromycin.

CONTRAINDICATIONS Severe hepatic dysfunction, coma, pregnancy.

NURSING CONSIDERATIONS Monitor liver function tests.

CLIENT TEACHING Initial sedation. May take with food to reduce GI upset. Do not crush the coated (enteric) product Depakote.

AVAILABLE IN CANADA Epival, Depakene, Depakene Syrup, Depakote, Depakote Sprinkle

bold—Life-threatening reactions

---

zolpidem (zole-pi'-dem)

GENERIC: zolpidem (zole-pi'-dem)
TRADE: Ambien

CLASSIFICATION Hypnotic—imidazopyridine

INDICATIONS & USES Short-term treatment of insomnia.

USUAL ADULT DOSAGE RANGE 5-10 mg at bedtime. Usual adult dose is 10 mg; use 5 mg in the elderly and physically debilitated. Dose should not exceed 10 mg.

AVAILABLE FORMS Tabs 5 mg & 10 mg (in the United States)

PHARMACOKINETICS/DYNAMICS Rapid onset of action; sleep is generally attained in 20-30 min after administration. Average half-life is 2.5 hr. Zolpidem is a nonbenzodiazepine hypnotic. Does NOT appear to alter normal sleep architecture.

SIDE EFFECTS Ataxia, dizziness, confusion, euphoria, insomnia, vertigo, diplopia, diarrhea.

ADVERSE REACTIONS Rarely: doses >10 mg have been associated with psychotic reactions; anterograde amnesia.

INTERACTIONS Additive effects with CNS depressants including alcohol.

CONTRAINDICATIONS None known.

NURSING CONSIDERATIONS Schedule IV controlled substance. Dizziness commonly associated with increased doses. Abrupt discontinuation has NOT been associated with rebound insomnia.

CLIENT TEACHING Avoid hazardous activities during initiation; avoid alcohol. Medication works quickly. Take right before going to bed.

AVAILABLE IN CANADA Not available.

bold—Life-threatening reactions

Psychiatric-Mental Health Nursing
Drug Cards

GENERIC: trihexyphenidyl (trye-hex-ee-fen'i-dill)
TRADE: Artane

CLASSIFICATION Antiparkinsonian, anticholinergic

INDICATIONS & USES Parkinsonism, treatment and prevention of extrapyramidal symptoms caused by antipsychotic medications (excluding tardive dyskinesia).

USUAL ADULT DOSAGE RANGE 1–5 mg bid to qid. Typical starting dose 5 mg bid.

AVAILABLE FORMS Tabs 2.5 mg; caps sus-rel 5 mg; elix 2 mg/5 mL.

PHARMACOKINETICS/DYNAMICS Rapidly absorbed. Peak effects in 1–2 hr. The pharmacokinetics are not well-characterized. Usually given in divided doses. Duration of efficacy varies from 6–12 hr.

SIDE EFFECTS Dry mouth, blurred vision, tachycardia, urinary retention, constipation, nervousness, confusion, excitation, euphoria.

ADVERSE REACTIONS Paralytic ileus. Anticholinergic delirium (also called anticholinergic intoxication and atropine psychosis)—confusion, disorientation, stupor, flushing, hyperthermia, extreme agitation, hallucinations, hypotension, supraventricular tachycardia, markedly diminished or absent bowel sounds.

INTERACTIONS Additive anticholinergic effects with other medications, esp. Antipsychotics, tricyclic antidepressants, MAOIs, digoxin, furosemide (Lasix).

CONTRAINDICATIONS Severe cardiac or GI disorders, benign prostatic hypertrophy, angle-closure glaucoma, neuroleptic malignant syndrome.

NURSING CONSIDERATIONS Increased risk of heat stroke. Evaluate for adequate hydration and constipation. May aggravate the movements of tardive dyskinesia. Elderly at increased risk for confusion and anticholinergic delirium. More stimulating than benztropine. Euphoric side effect can result in drug-seeking behaviors by substance abusers.

AVAILABLE IN CANADA Novohexidyl

bold—Life-threatening reactions

GENERIC: trazodone (tray'zoe-done)
TRADE: Desyrel

CLASSIFICATION Triazolopyridine antidepressant

INDICATIONS & USES Major depression, sleep disturbance, anxiety.

USUAL ADULT DOSAGE RANGE 50–600 mg/day. Initial dosing is 50–150 mg/day; Maximum dose is 600 mg/day in divided doses.

AVAILABLE FORMS Tabs 50, 100, 150, 300 mg

PHARMACOKINETICS/DYNAMICS In adults, half-life is approximately 6–11 hr. Full therapeutic effects may not be apparent for 2–4 wk.

SIDE EFFECTS Very sedating, dry mouth, blurred vision, constipation, urinary retention, somnolence, dizziness, orthostatic hypotension. Rare priapism in males.

ADVERSE REACTIONS Induction of mania, rare priapism.

INTERACTIONS Increased effects with CNS depressants, alcohol. Addition of fluoxetine may dramatically increase trazodone levels.

CONTRAINDICATIONS Avoid in pregnant and nursing mothers.

NURSING CONSIDERATIONS Suicide risk may be increased during initial improvement, particularly as psychomotor depression abates.

CLIENT TEACHING Therapeutic effects may take several weeks. Warn of excessive sedation during initiation. Priapism is a medical emergency.

AVAILABLE IN CANADA Desyral

bold—Life-threatening reactions

---

alprazolam (Xanax)
amantadine (Symmetrel)
amitriptyline (Elavil)
benztropine (Cogentin)
bupropion (Wellbutrin)
buspirone (Buspar)
carbamazepine (Tegretol)
chloral hydrate (Noctec)
chlorpromazine (Thorazine)
clomipramine (Anafranil)
clonazepam (Klonopin)
clozapine (Clozaril)
desipramine (Norpramin)
diazepam (Valium)
diphenhydramine (Benadryl, Benalyn)
fluoxetine (Prozac)
fluphenazine (Prolixin, Permitil)
fluvoxamine (Luvox)
haloperidol (Haldol)
imipramine (Tofranil)
lithium (Eskalith, Eskalith CR, Lithane, Lithobid, Cibalith, Cibalith-S
Syrup)
lorazepam (Ativan)
loxapine (Loxitane)
nefazodone (Serzone)
nortriptyline (Pamelor, Aventyl)
paroxetine (Paxil)

perphenazine (Trilafon)
phenelzine (Nardil)
propranolol (Inderal)
risperidone (Risperdal)
sertraline (Zoloft)
thioridazine (Mellaril)
thiothixene (Navane)
trazodone (Desyrel)
triazolam (Halcion)
trihexyphenidyl (Artane)
valproic acid, valproate sodium, divalproex sodium
   (Depakene, Depakene Syrup, Depakote, Depakote Sprinkle)
venlafaxine (Effexor)
zolpidem (Ambien)

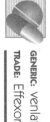

GENERIC: venlafaxine (ven-lah-fax'een)
TRADE: Effexor

CLASSIFICATION Phenethylamine antidepressant. Norepinephrine and serotonin reuptake inhibitor.

INDICATIONS & USES Major depression.

USUAL ADULT DOSAGE RANGE 150–350 mg/day. Initial dose is 75 mg/day as 25 mg tid or 37.5 mg bid. Maximum dose is 375 mg/day in divided doses. Dose increases should be made at no less than 4-day intervals.

AVAILABLE FORMS Tab 25, 37.5, 50, 75, 100 mg

PHARMACOKINETICS/DYNAMICS In adults, venlafaxine's half-life is approximately 3–7 hr, and the active metabolite O-desmethyl-venlafaxine's half-life is approximately 9–13 hr. Doses should be reduced in clients with severe hepatic or renal disease and in the elderly. Full therapeutic effects may not be apparent for 2–4 wk.

SIDE EFFECTS Asthenia, sweating, nausea, vomiting, constipation, anorexia, somnolence, dry mouth, dizziness, nervousness, anxiety, tremor, blurred vision, sexual dysfunction, insomnia

ADVERSE REACTIONS Induction of mania, hypertension.

INTERACTIONS Potentially fatal hypertensive crisis when MAOIs (including selegiline) are used within 2 wk of discontinuation.

CONTRAINDICATIONS Avoid in pregnant and nursing mothers.

NURSING CONSIDERATIONS Suicide risk may be increased during initial improvement, particularly as psychomotor depression abates.

CLIENT TEACHING Therapeutic effects may take several weeks. Warn of excessive sedation during initiation. Should not be discontinued suddenly.

AVAILABLE IN CANADA Effexor

bold—Life-threatening reactions

LIST OF KEY FEATURES